Oculoplastic, Lacrimal and Orbital Surgery

Francesco M. Quaranta Leoni
David H. Verity • Dion Paridaens
Editors

Oculoplastic, Lacrimal and Orbital Surgery

The ESOPRS Textbook: Volume 2

Springer

Editors
Francesco M. Quaranta Leoni
Oftalmoplastica Roma
Roma, Italy

David H. Verity
Moorfields Eye Hospital
London, UK

Dion Paridaens
Rotterdam Eye Hospital
Rotterdam, The Netherlands

ISBN 978-3-031-39637-3 ISBN 978-3-031-39638-0 (eBook)
https://doi.org/10.1007/978-3-031-39638-0

This Springer imprint is published by the registered company Springer Nature Switzerland AG
The registered company address is: Gewerbestrasse 11, 6330 Cham, Switzerland

Paper in this product is recyclable.

Foreword

The year 2020 will remain in people's memories for a very long time: the year of the COVID pandemic that effectively closed down the world for travel, created a lasting and devastating effect on world economies, prevented most normal social interactions, and led to many tragic personal losses. However, many good things arose in the face of adversity and necessity. Valuable advances were made at the global level—such as the rapid emergence of internet-based technologies for virtual meetings, or advances in the development and design of vaccines—and also at the personal level, with many people working more closely at home than at previous times.

Francesco M. Quaranta-Leoni—at that difficult time as President of the European Society of Oculo-Plastic and Reconstructive Surgeons—seized the opportunity to draw together a team to edit a multi-authored textbook of oculoplastic surgery. Drawn from the core administration of ESOPRS, Dion Paridaens and David Verity agreed to join him in undertaking this daunting task. And what a task it proved to be! This triumvirate of editors had to not only choose a broad spectrum of authors drawn largely from continental Europe, but also organise this diverse assembly of writers into an effective working group.

The result of this gargantuan effort is immediately evident in the 90 chapters of the two volumes of this book that cover all aspects of oculoplastic diseases and surgery. Despite the potential for overlap between chapters, within the book there is relatively little duplication, and the large number of authors from many backgrounds provides an attractive spectrum of views—some of which may ride contrary to one's own knowledge and experience. The book certainly achieves its objective, to provide a comprehensive textbook of current oculoplastic diagnosis and therapy.

The chief editors are to be thoroughly congratulated on seeing this work to completion, with more than three years of constant work. Our thanks must also be extended to the many colleagues who reviewed and edited the individual chapters. The huge effort can only be fully appreciated when one has undertaken such an editorship: this effort, together with the sacrifice of personal time, has at last made this magnificent work a reality.

London, UK — Geoffrey E. Rose
London, UK — J. Richard O. Collin

Preface

This first edition of the *ESOPRS Textbook on Oculoplastic, Lacrimal and Orbital Surgery* is written for all clinicians who wish to be informed about the state of the art and recent insights in all the subfields of ophthalmic plastic, lacrimal, and orbital surgery.

In 2018 the first steps were made towards a European Board of Ophthalmology—European Society of Ophthalmic Plastic and Reconstructive Surgery (EBO-ESOPRS) examination.

During the pandemic of 2020, the Executive Council of ESOPRS (Francesco M. Quaranta Leoni, David Verity, and Dion Paridaens), with FQL in a leading role, felt that a textbook, written by members of our Society, could serve as an educational instrument for young colleagues, including those preparing for the EBO-ESOPRS exam, and colleagues of other subspecialties with an interest in oculoplastic, lacrimal, and orbital surgery. The EBO-ESOPRS—a reality thanks to the input and determination of Michèle Beaconsfield, Brigita Drnovšek-Olup, and Andrea Papp—is aimed at those who have already completed an oculoplastic, lacrimal, orbital, and aesthetic fellowship, and are beginning or already practicing independently; the Diploma awarded to successful candidates will indicate a certified advanced knowledge in our subspecialty.

This book is comprised of both functional and cosmetic periocular surgery and is divided into two volumes: the first volume includes chapters on functional eyelid disorders, rejuvenation of periorbital region, and lacrimal disorders, the second volume focuses on socket surgery, orbital diseases, and on thyroid-associated orbitopathy. Each chapter is written by authors with an indisputable expertise on the specific topic, being evidence and experience based.

We hope that this book will become an important asset to the European oculoplastic community and a useful tool for fellows and residents, especially for those colleagues who wish to sit the subspecialty exam.

The planning, writing, and editing of this book lead to a frequent exchange of ideas and opinions, deepening our mutual respect, understanding, and sincere friendship. It has been an immense task spanning more than 3 years, entailing countless virtual meetings and communications with our excellent illustrators and artists Jessica Leenen, Frank Stoute, and Linda Zoon, and with our publishers. We are also indebted to ESOPRS for the Society's financial support of the book's beautiful illustrations.

We are sincerely indebted to our authors who gave their time and expertise in writing this text—we cannot thank you all enough! A special acknowledgement goes to Carole Jones, Geoffrey Rose, and Kaveh Vahdani, who reviewed many chapters, together with Dan Georgescu, Naresh Joshi, Ilse Mombaerts, Marco Sales Sanz, and Vladimir Thaller.

We offer a note of dedication to our colleague and friend Bruno Fayet, co-author of two lacrimal chapters, who sadly passed away in August 2022.

Particular thanks are offered to all who have been instrumental in mentoring our community: we are so grateful for your tireless dedication to our specialty.

Rome, Italy — Francesco M. Quaranta Leoni
London, UK — David H. Verity
Rotterdam, The Netherlands — Dion Paridaens

March 2024

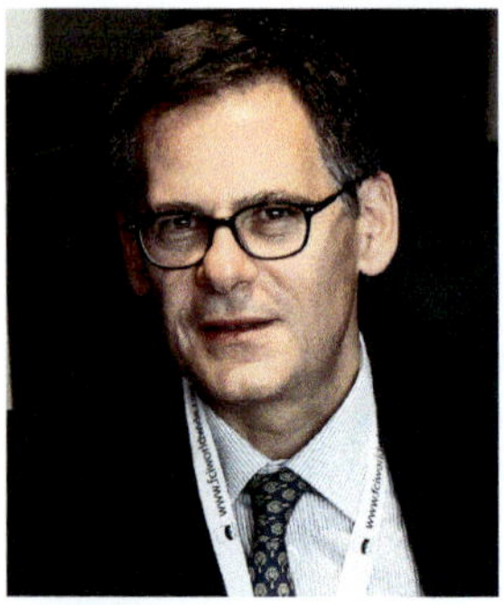

Francesco M. Quaranta Leoni

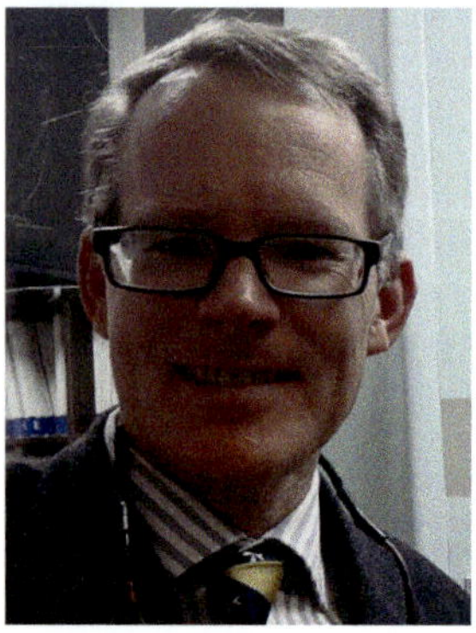

David Harding Verity

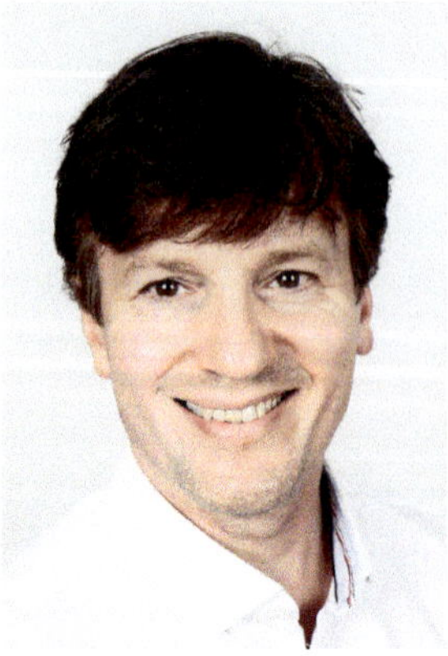

Dion Paridaens

Acknowledgements

To my teachers and mentors: Richard Collin, Geoffrey Rose, Michèle Beaconsfield, and the late John Wright, outstanding characters, true friends, and instrumental in shaping my personality: your greatness was attained by hard work, and the will to do one's best.

And to Antonella, Flavia, and Claudia, who have always been loving and supportive.

Francesco M. Quaranta Leoni

This work is dedicated to our mentors who have freely imparted their knowledge, and to our dear families for their patience. A reflective note of thanks to the late Tony Tyers, and to Richard Collin and Geoffrey Rose; you have taught us values beyond knowledge, and your wisdom and kindness have been a guiding light.

David H. Verity

To my teacher and friend Willem van den Bosch. To my teachers Maarten Mourits, Jack Rootman, the late John Hungerford, and the late Alison McCartney. To my sister Désirée and my late parents, and—last but not least—to my wife Femke and children Maartje, Niek, and Mark for their loving support and understanding.

Dion Paridaens

Contents

Part II Orbital Disease

Contributors

Segun Awotesu Ophthalmology Department, Leicester Royal Infirmary, Leicester, UK

Shirin Hamed Azzam Baruch Padeh Medical Center, Poriya, Israel

Lelio Baldeschi Department of Ophthalmology, Catholic University of Louvain, Academic Hospital Saint Luc, Brussels, Belgium

Ronald L. A. W. Bleys Department of Anatomy, University Medical Center Utrecht, Utrecht, The Netherlands

Elin Bohman Oculoplastic and Orbital Services, St. Erik Eye Hospital, Stockholm, Sweden

Paola Bonavolontà Maxillofacial Unit, University of Naples Federico II, Naples, Italy

Davide Johan Bottini Department of Plastic and Reconstructive Surgery, Università degli Studi di Roma Tor Vergata, Rome, Italy

Cornelia Caron Orbital Center, Department of Maxillofacial Surgery, Erasmus MC, Rotterdam, The Netherlands

Valerio Cervelli Department of Plastic and Reconstructive Surgery, Università degli Studi di Roma Tor Vergata, Rome, Italy

George C. Charonis Athens Vision Eye Institute, Athens, Greece

Eva Dafgård Kopp Department of Oculoplastic, Lacrimal and Orbital Surgery, St. Erik Eye Hospital, Karolinska Institutet, Stockholm, Sweden

Ronald O. B. de Keizer Department of Orbital Surgery, The Rotterdam Eye Hospital, Rotterdam, The Netherlands

Alain Ducasse Department of Ophthalmology, Reims CHR, Reims, France

Suzanne K. Freitag Ophthalmic Plastic Surgery Service, Department of Ophthalmology, Massachusetts Eye and Ear, Harvard Medical School, Boston, MA, USA

Renske Gahrmann Department of Radiology and Nuclear Medicine, Erasmus Medical Center, Rotterdam, The Netherlands

Mayke Gardeniers Department of Radiology and Nuclear Medicine, Erasmus Medical Center, Rotterdam, The Netherlands

Sri Gore Clinical and Academic Department of Ophthalmology, Great Ormond Street Hospital for Children, London, UK

Dyonne T. Hartong Orbital Center, Department of Ophthalmology, Amsterdam University Medical Center, University of Amsterdam, Amsterdam, The Netherlands

Ludwig M. Heindl Department of Ophthalmology, University of Cologne, Cologne, Germany

Christoph Hintschich Department of Ophthalmology, Ludwig-Maximilians-University, Munich, Germany

Leonard Holbach Department of Ophthalmology, Friedrich-Alexander University Erlangen-Nürnberg, Erlangen, Germany

Simon Holmes Department of Oral and Maxillofacial Surgery, Barts Health NHS Trust, London, UK

Gijsbert J. Hötte Department of Oculoplastic, Orbital and Lacrimal Surgery, The Rotterdam Eye Hospital, Rotterdam, The Netherlands

Adriana Iuliano Orbital Unit, University of Naples Federico II, Naples, Italy

Aaron Jamison Department of Ophthalmology, NHS Greater Glasgow and Clyde, Glasgow, Scotland, UK

Lama Jurdy Orbital Center—Amsterdam University Medical Center, Amsterdam, The Netherlands

Rachel Kalmann Department of Ophthalmology, University Medical Center Utrecht, Utrecht, The Netherlands

Mikhail Kataev Oculoplastic Department, S. Fyodorov Eye Microsurgery Federal Institute, Moscow, Russia

William Rocamora Katowitz Division of Ophthalmology, The Children's Hospital of Philadelphia, Philadelphia, PA, USA

Michelle Khan Department of Ophthalmology and Vision Sciences, Univeristy of Toronto, Toronto, ON, Canada

Arthur Klett Eye Clinic, East-Tallinn Central Hospital, Tallinn, Estonia

Onur Konuk Department Ophthalmology, Oculoplastic and Orbital Unit, Gazi University Medical School, Ankara, Turkey

Maarten Koudstaal Orbital Center, Department of Maxillofacial Surgery, Erasmus MC, Rotterdam, The Netherlands

Vladimir Kratky Oculoplastic and Orbital Surgery Unit, 1st Medical Faculty, Charles University, Prague, Czech Republic - Queen's University , Kingston, ON, Canada

Raman Malhotra Corneoplastic Unit, Queen Victoria Hospital, East Grinstead, UK

Stijn van der Meeren Department of Ophthalmology, Leiden University Medical Center, Leiden, The Netherlands

Alessandra Modugno Ocularistica Italiana, Rome, Italy

Ilse Mombaerts Department of Ophthalmology, University Hospitals Leuven, Leuven, Belgium

Maarten P. Mourits Orbital Center, Department of Ophthalmology, Amsterdam University Medical Centers, Amsterdam, The Netherlands

Rachna Murthy Face Restoration, Harley St, London, UK

Ioannis Ntountas Athens Ophthalmic Plastic Center, Athens, Greece

Santiago Ortiz-Pérez Department of Ophthalmology, Hospital Universitario Virgen de las Nieves, Granada, Spain

Department of Surgery, University of Granada - Instituto de Investigación Biosanitaria ibs.GRANADA, Granada, Spain

Andrea Papp Department of Ophthalmology and Optometry, Medical University of Vienna, Vienna, Austria

Dion Paridaens Department of Oculoplastic, Orbital and Lacrimal Surgery, The Rotterdam Eye Hospital and Erasmus Medical Center, Rotterdam, The Netherlands

Francesco M. Quaranta Leoni Oftalmoplastica Roma, Rome, Italy

Marie Louise Roed Rasmussen External and Adnexal Service, Department of Ophthalmology, Rigshospitalet, Copenhagen, Denmark

Department of Clinical Medicine, University of Copenhagen, Copenhagen, Denmark

Eyvind Rødahl Department of Ophthalmology, Haukeland University Hospital, Bergen, Norway

Department of Clinical Medicine, University of Bergen, Bergen, Norway

Jonathan C. P. Roos Face Restoration, Harley St, London, UK

Geoffrey E. Rose Adnexal Service, Moorfields Eye Hospital, London, UK

Peerooz Saeed Orbital Centre, Department of Ophthalmology, Amsterdam University Medical Center, Amsterdam, The Netherlands

Sven Sahlin Department of Clinical Neuroscience, Karolinska Institutet, Stockholm, Sweden

Marco Sales-Sanz Oculoplastic Surgery Unit, Ophthalmology Department, Hospital Universitario Ramón y Cajal, Madrid, Spain

Oculoplastic Surgery Unit, IMO Madrid, Grupo Miranza, Madrid, Spain

Raghavan Sampath Department of Ophthalmology, University Hospitals of Leicester NHS Trust, Leicester Royal Infirmary, Leicester, UK

Gustavo Savino Department of Ophthalmology, Fondazione Policlinico Universitario A. Gemelli IRCCS, Rome, Italy

Michael Schittkowski Section for Strabismus and Neuroophthalmology, Department of Ophthalmology, University Medicine Goettingen, Goettingen, Germany

Pari N. Shams Adnexal Service, Moorfields Eye Hospital, London, UK

Haraldur Sigurdsson Department of Ophthalmology, Landspitali University Hospital, Reykjavik, Iceland

Diego Strianese Orbital Unit, University of Naples Federico II, Naples, Italy

Dario Surace LaVista Eye Center, Venice, Italy

Theodora Tsirouki Athens Ophthalmic Plastic Center, Athens, Greece

Jimmy M. Uddin Adnexal Service, Moorfields Eye Hospital, London, UK

Kaveh Vahdani Adnexal Service, Moorfields Eye Hospital, London, UK

Robert M. Verdijk Department of Pathology, Section Ophthalmic Pathology, Erasmus MC & the Rotterdam Eye Hospital, Rotterdam, The Netherlands

Department of Pathology, Leiden University Medical Center, Leiden, The Netherlands

David H. Verity Adnexal Service, Moorfields Eye Hospital, London, UK

St John Eye Hospital Group, London, UK

Eppo Wolvius Orbital Center, Department of Maxillofacial Surgery, Erasmus MC, Rotterdam, The Netherlands

Part I

Socket Surgery

Enucleation

Ioannis Ntountas, Theodora Tsirouki, Arthur Klett, Haraldur Sigurdsson, and Dion Paridaens

Key Messages

- Enucleation is indicated in case of intraocular malignancy, which is not treated by non-surgical modalities, or when optimal histopathological examination of a (painful) blind eye is desired.
- For patients with a blind and painful and or cosmetically disturbing eye, evisceration yields better results than enucleation.
- An important step prior to enucleation is to ensure repeatedly that the correct eye is (prepared to be) removed.
- Wrapped, non-porous implants show similar outcomes and lower complication rates compared to porous implants.
- Pegging of porous implants has a high complication rate and should be avoided.
- Enucleation with placement of an orbital implant and conformer/artificial eye aims to achieve aesthetic results by maintaining normal eyelid shape and function, and preserving adequate fornix volume.

I. Ntountas (✉) · T. Tsirouki
Athens Ophthalmic Plastic Center, Athens, Greece
e-mail: Yanni-nt@otenet.gr

A. Klett
Eye Clinic, East-Tallinn Central Hospital, Tallinn, Estonia

H. Sigurdsson
Department of Ophthalmology, Landspitali University Hospital, Reykjavik, Iceland

D. Paridaens
Department of Oculoplastic, Orbital and Lacrimal Surgery, The Rotterdam Eye Hospital and Erasmus Medical Center, Rotterdam, The Netherlands

1 Introduction

Enucleation is a surgical procedure in which the globe and the anterior portion of the optic nerve are removed from the orbit. The eyeball is separated from the extraocular muscles and the surrounding tissues and removed along with the anterior portion of the optic nerve. The procedure aims to eradicate any (intra)ocular malignancy whilst achieving aesthetic results and prosthetic motility.

2 Indications and Contraindications for Enucleation

2.1 Indications for Enucleation

Enucleation is the procedure of choice in cases of intraocular malignancy that cannot be managed medically because the eyeball and its contents should be removed intact (choroidal melanoma, retinoblastoma) (Fig. 1). The segment of the optic nerve removed with the globe, is studied histopath-

F. M. Quaranta Leoni et al. (eds.), *Oculoplastic, Lacrimal and Orbital Surgery*,
https://doi.org/10.1007/978-3-031-39638-0_1

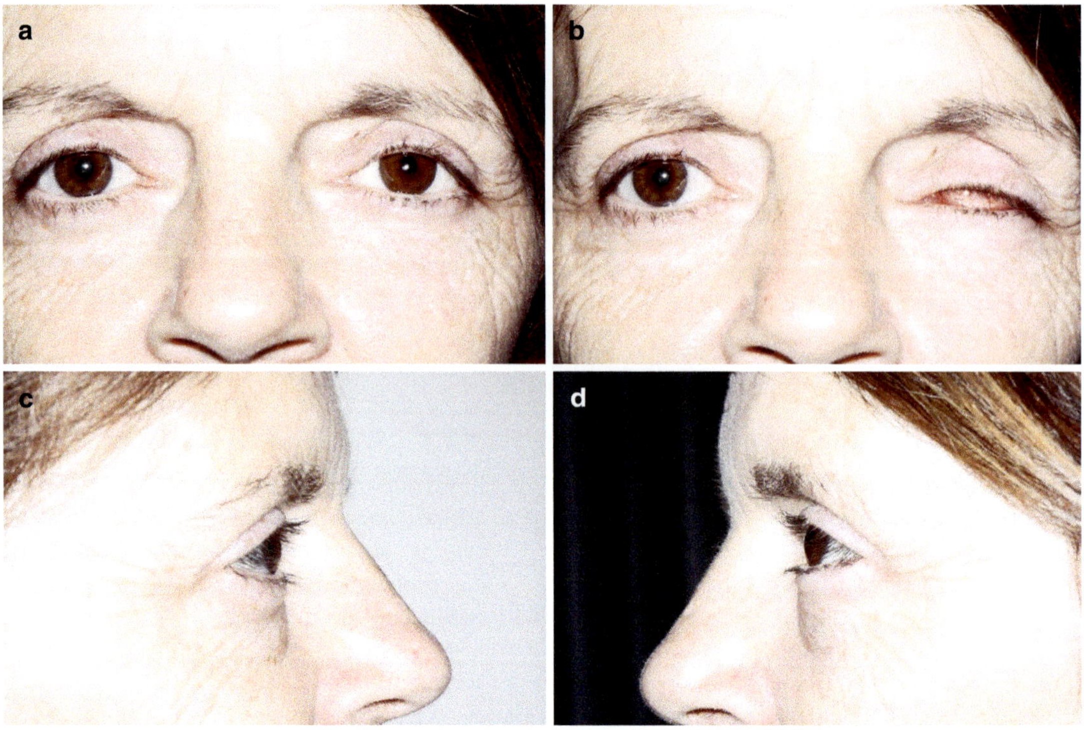

Fig. 1 (**a–d**) A 57-year old woman with a left artificial eye (glass) in situ, following enucleation with placement of a 22 mm acrylic spherical implant, wrapped in donor sclera, 1 year earlier. The indication for surgery was a large intraocular malignant melanoma. (**a**) Note the symmetry of eyelids and globe/artificial eye position. (**b**) Patient without the artificial eye in place. (**c**) Lateral right view. (**d**) Lateral left view showing the prosthesis

ologically for tumor extension, which is especially important in case of retinoblastoma. In addition, it may be considered for painful, blind eyes for which optimal histopathological examination is needed. Evisceration is a sclera-preserving eye-removal procedure. It is contraindicated in cases of suspected intraocular malignancy but is the treatment of choice in case of painful, blind eyes and cosmetically disturbing, blind eyes, often secondary to intractable glaucoma or trauma. Evisceration provides better post-surgical esthetic rehabilitation, better prosthesis motility, and less orbital trauma [1–5], both in adults and in children.

When, in the case of a painful, blind eye, fundoscopy is not possible, MRI scan and/or ultrasound of the globe must be performed to rule out an intraocular tumour. If that is not possible, enucleation is the procedure of choice [6, 7].

Enucleation is preferred to evisceration when the remaining sclera is not normal or adequate for scleral modification, as in advanced phthisis bulbi [6] following scleral buckling procedures, severe trauma, buphthalmos, scleromalacia, or staphyloma.

In cases of trauma with rupture of the globe and diffuse uveal exposure, the development of sympathetic ophthalmia (SO) in the contralateral eye represents a serious potential complication. In that case, the surgical goal is to complete removal the eye and the uvea, and enucleation is therefore the surgery of choice. However, SO is unlikely to develop, with a 1-year incidence of 0.03 per 100,000 people [8]; it is a granulomatous panuveitis that can be observed months to years after scleral rupture, and attacks both eyes—the injured and the healthy eye. It is an acquired immune reaction to the previously unexposed ocular antigens. Uveal self-antigens are mainly considered to cause SO [9]; however antigens of the lens, retina, and RPE have also been implicated [10, 11]. During evisceration, it is not possible to completely remove all uveal tissue, as microscopic quantities of uveal pigment are always left in the scleral channels at the points where the vortex veins exit the globe. Consequently, it is considered that the risk of sympathetic ophthalmia, however minimal, is greater with evisceration than with enucleation [12] (see chapter "Evisceration").

2.2 Contraindications for Enucleation

Enucleation is contraindicated in cases of intraocular malignancy with orbital invasion. In these cases, orbital exenteration is mandatory [6, 13].

3 Significant Notes Before Surgery

- Enucleation is indicated for eradication of an (intra)ocular malignancy.
- Enucleation without implant leads to a reduced volume of orbital contents and alterations of their anatomic location. Thus, the procedure is followed by the replacement of the evacuated orbital tissues by an orbital implant of adequate size.
- Enucleation with placement of an orbital implant aims to achieve a satisfactory aesthetic result by maintaining normal eyelid shape and function, and preserving adequate fornices and orbital volume.
- The post-enucleation socket syndrome (PESS) is observed in cases where the socket is not filled with an appropriately sized orbital implant, or where -after years- a gradual loss of orbital fat tissues developed. It is characterized by enophthalmos, a deep superior sulcus, blepharoptosis, lower eyelid laxity and posterior tilt of the prosthesis [6].
- The extraocular muscles must be adequately fixated to the anterior aspect of the orbital implant to ensure that the prosthesis has adequate motility. Many techniques are currently used, with the purpose to accomplish satisfactory implant motility and achieve transfer of the movement of the implant to the prosthesis.
- Haemostasis is crucial after globe removal. Haemorrhage from the ophthalmic artery may be difficult to control and may lead to an orbital hematoma. This situation leads to deposition of blood and haemosiderin and may result in reactive fibrosis of the orbital tissues, increasing the danger of extrusion of the orbital implant.
- Meticulous closure of Tenon's capsule and conjunctiva reduces the risk of implant extrusion.
- The surgeon should be aware that traction of the extraocular muscles and the optic nerve during surgery may lead to bradycardia due to the 'oculocardiac reflex'.

4 Pre-operative Evaluation

4.1 Examination and Patient History

The examination and history of the patient who will undergo an enucleation needs to be thorough. The surgeon should examine the patient, identify the causes that lead to the necessity of this operation, and evaluate any imaging studies of the eye and possible extent of the malignancy. With other indications for enucleation, such as a blind eye with sclero-malacia, or when whole eye histopathology is required, the surgeon should detect any possible intraocular tumour prior to enucleation. Systemic conditions and treatment define the type of anaesthesia and provide information for possible post-operative complications. For example, impaired blood supply, diabetes, previous radiation therapy to the orbital area, and immunosuppression affect wound closure and are associated with implant extrusion. Nonsteroidal anti-inflammatory agents, aspirin, or other anticoagulants must be temporarily discontinued, in agreement with the prescribing physician.

4.2 Patient Preparation

Enucleation is a psychologically traumatic event for each patient. Good pre- and post-operative care by the surgeon and the nursing team is mandatory. The permanent loss of the eye and its personal and social consequences must be thoroughly explained to the patient and his/her family. The surgeon and supporting staff should analyse the patient's expectations, show pictures of patients with and without the prosthesis, and explain its expected motility. The patient should not leave the surgeon's office with unrealistic expectations about his/her future appearance. A prosthesis should be shown to the patient. Additionally, the details of the procedure must be explained to the patient, as well as post-surgical anticipations, such as the post-surgical risk of pain for several days, and the temporary placement of the conformer/temporary prosthesis before the definite prosthesis fitting, that can usually be scheduled 6–8 weeks following surgery. Finally, the possible complications must be clarified, such as reduced prosthesis motility, asymmetric appearance, infection, and exposure or extrusion of the orbital implant. During the counselling of the patient, the surgeon should always explain that this procedure has a major impact on the patient's quality of life [14].

5 Surgical Technique

5.1 Equipment

The equipment that are required for the surgery of enucleation are:

- Eye speculum
- Wescott scissors
- Straight and curved tenotomy scissors (Stevens)
- Needle holder and St Martin's forceps
- Haemostatic forceps
- Squint hook
- Enucleation scissors (Metzenbaum) and/or enucleation snare
- Retractors
- Carter sphere introducer (if desired)
- Conformer/temporary prosthesis
- Bipolar cautery set
- Suture material and wrapping material (e.g. whole donor sclera)
- Orbital spherical implant (silicone, acrylic, porous polyethylene, hydroxyapatite)

5.2 Surgical Preparation

The patient must be offered adequate time to discuss any concerns.

An important step prior to enucleation is to ensure repeatedly that the correct eye is prepared for removal [6]. Even though this possibility seems distant, correct-side surgery needs to be confirmed by the surgeon and the supporting staff in the operating room through the usual peri-operative 'time-out' protocols. Pre-operatively, the eye to be removed is marked on the forehead by the surgeon. Immediately before the surgery, the surgeon must check the clinical chart of the patient, the informed consent, and ensure s/he is correct, taking the opinion of the anesthesiologist and the surgical nurse [14]. In addition, following dilation of the pupil with mydriatic drops—in case of a malignancy—pre-operative fundoscopy is performed (if possible) to confirm the presence of the intraocular tumour.

5.3 Anaesthesia

Although the surgery can be performed under local retrobulbar anaesthesia, general anaesthesia is usually preferred. General anaesthesia is accompanied by a retrobulbar injection of a mixture of about 4–5 mL of xylocaine, epinephrine and bupivacaine, which reduces intra and post-operative pain. Some centres use ropivacaine only, which provides prolonged reduction of post-operative pain and reduction of the patient's discomfort (Fig. 2).

5.4 Peritomy

A sterile field is in position and an eyelid speculum is applied. A Westcott scissors is used for the 360° conjunctival peritomy adjacent to the corneal limbus. Tenon's capsule is gently separated from the underlying sclera to the level of the equator using a Stevens tenotomy scissors, taking care to avoid damage to the rectus muscle insertions. 5-0 Vicryl® sutures are placed in the four quadrants of Tenon's capsule and conjunctiva (at 2, 4, 8, and 10 clock hours), and the ends of the sutures are clamped to the surrounding drape with a haemostat.

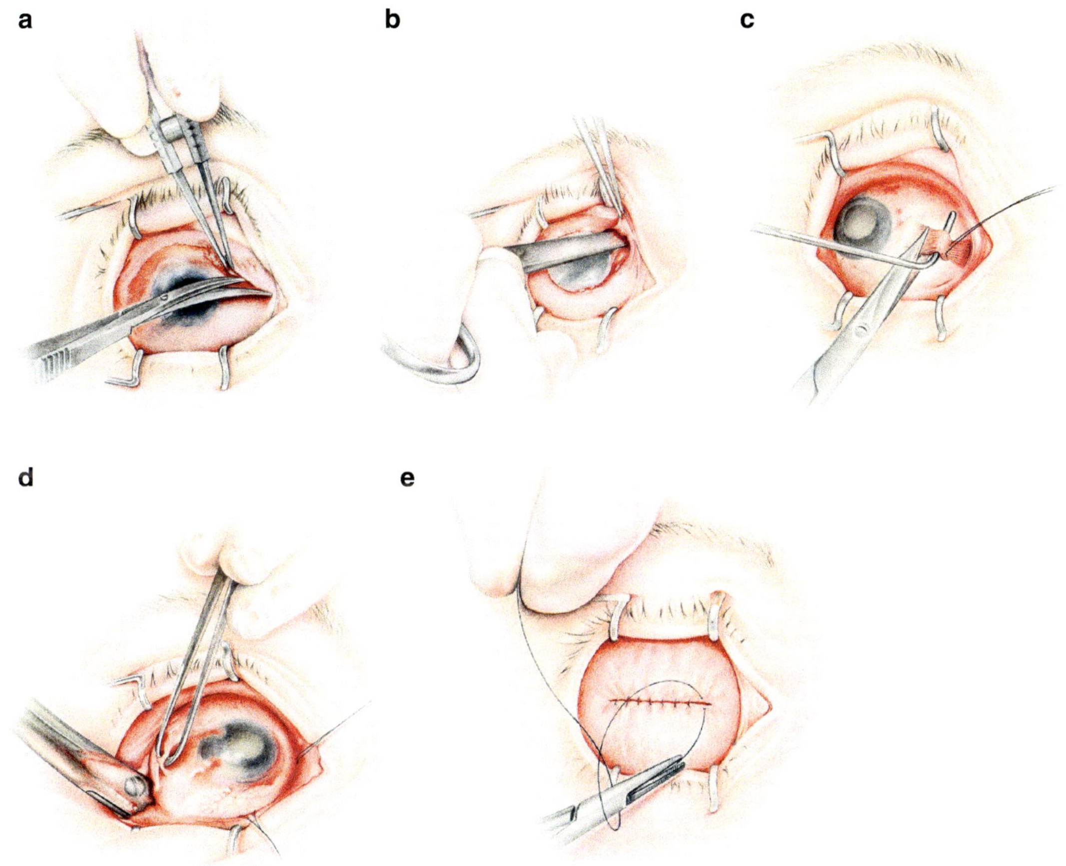

Fig. 2 (**a–e**) Illustration of the technique of enucleation with placement of a wrapped implant without an inserter, (**a**) 360° conjunctival peritomy, (**b**) Tenon's capsule is gently separated from the underlying sclera to the level of the equator, taking care to avoid damage to the rectus muscle insertions, (**c**) A muscle insertion is identified, and isolated by a squint hook. A locking suture is passed in the muscle tendon near the insertion. The muscle is disinserted, (**d**) A curved enucleation scissors is passed behind the globe, the nerve is transected and the globe is removed. (**e**) Following the positioning of an adequate size wrapped implant, a meticulous closure of Tenon's capsule and conjunctiva is performed

5.5 Detaching the Extraocular Muscles from the Globe

The following procedure is repeated for the four recti muscles, and the inferior oblique: muscle insertions are identified, and isolated by a squint hook. A locking suture of double-armed 4-0 or 5-0 Vicryl® (spatula) is passed in the muscle tendon near the insertion. At the medial and lateral rectus tendon, the surgeon should leave a 1- to 2-mm stump, so as to facilitate the future traction of the globe. Consequently, each muscle is disinserted, with care so as not to damage it, and is isolated, with the ends of the sutures also clamped to the surgical drape. Some surgeons prefer to attach the inferior oblique muscle to the inferior border of the lateral rectus close to its insertion, providing a "Hammock" to support the implant. This might reduce any post-operative implant migration towards the lower temporal quadrant. The superior oblique muscle is identified with a muscle hook, detached from the globe, and usually left to glide back.

5.6 Removing the Globe

Stevens scissors are used for the detachment of the remaining adherent tissues from the globe, as far posterior as possible. The medial or lateral horizontal rectus muscle stump on the globe is grasped with a haemostat and the globe is rotated laterally so that the optic nerve becomes more accessible. Alternatively, 4-0 silk sutures are placed on the medial and lateral muscle stumps, which are gently elevated, elevating the globe, and detaching it from the posterior portion of the muscle cone. The globe is now only attached to the optic nerve.

Some surgeons prefer to clamp the optic nerve with a large curved haemostat, preferably passing at the medial or lateral quadrant, as far posteriorly as possible. The haemostat is passed behind the globe with closed tips to identify the optic nerve, and separate it from the adherent tissues. The haemostat is then placed around the optic nerve as far posteriorly as possible. This placement of the haemostat helps to increase the space behind the globe. The nerve is clamped for about 5 min to obtain satisfactory haemostasis. A curved enucleation scissors (Metzenbaum) is passed behind the globe, usually with the haemostat in place, the nerve is transected – with special care not to damage the rectus muscles – and the globe is removed. In case of intraocular tumour, at least 7–10 mm of the optic nerve should be resected. The less the orbital fat is manipulated, the less the risk of atrophy and volume loss.

If Metzenbaum scissors are not available, the optic nerve can be transected with the enucleation snare, using the 18-gauge wire loop. The globe is gently pulled upwards, the loop is placed medially, and the wire is slowly tightened as the snare is placed posteriorly.

5.7 After Globe Removal

The globe is removed and carefully checked for evidence of extrascleral extension of the tumour, or involvement of the transected part of the optic nerve. In the latter case, removal of an additional part of the optic nerve is necessary. The globe is photographed, and sent for histopathologic examination (Fig. 3). Some surgeons prefer to place reference sutures in one or more extraocular muscle stump(s) for exact localization of the intraocular tumour by the pathologist.

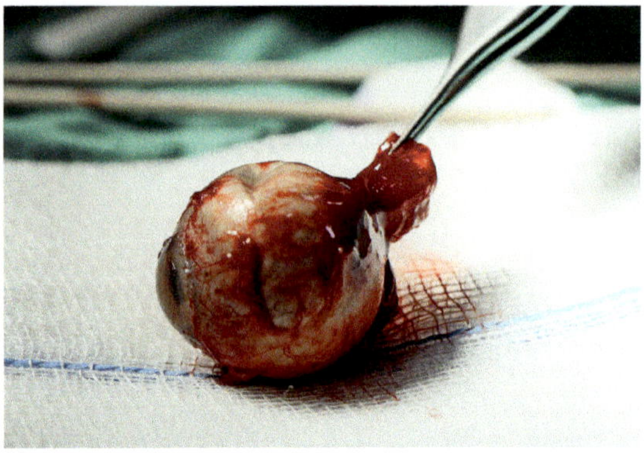

Fig. 3 The enucleated globe, with a part of the anterior optic nerve

5.8 Haemostasis

After globe removal, the remaining segment of the optic nerve and the ophthalmic artery are cauterised with bipolar cautery. The haemostat is then removed, and gauze pads are pressed in the socket for several minutes. When no haemostat is used, the gauze pads should be pressed in the socket for at least 5 min. The gauzes are removed, and any residual bleeding vessel is cauterised. Haemostasis is crucial at this point, because an orbital haematoma carries an increased risk of extrusion of the orbital implant.

5.9 Implant Insertion to the Socket

The size of the implant is typically chosen at surgery, and depends on the size of the eye that is removed, the volume of the bony orbit and the quality and quantity of the ocular and eyelid lining (conjunctiva). In case of a normally sized eye and intact conjunctiva, most Caucasian patients can be fitted with a 20 or 22 mm diameter spherical implant. Several centres have developed a preference towards 22 mm implants for better long-term results regarding orbital filling and prevention of a deep upper eyelid sulcus.

The implant should be soaked in antibiotics before introduction to the anophthalmic socket to minimise infection of the implant. Currently, most surgeons prefer placing the implant in a large 40–60 mL syringe with a solution of gentamicin. The exit port is closed by the plug, and the implant is compressed with the antibiotic solution for about 1 min, until it is adequately saturated [15]. Alternatively, surgeons may prefer to soak the implant (and wrapping material) in a container with gentamicin solution.

Where a wrapping material is used, e.g. donor-sclera, the alloplastic spheric implant is placed in the donor sclera cavity which is then closed with one or two Vicryl® 5.0 sutures. The closed side of the donor sclera with optic nerve stump should be faced posteriorly.

The implant should be placed as far posteriorly into the anophthalmic cavity as possible to avoid its exposure. In some cases, it is necessary to enlarge the space where the implant will be placed, with retractors, or a smooth glide, to avoid the *cactus syndrome*. The *cactus syndrome* is provoked when the implant is forced into the anophthalmic socket, drawing superficial tissues into the deeper orbit. With tissue restitution, they return to their initial position, drawing the implant anteriorly, resulting in thinning of the tissues overlying the implant and extrusion of the implant (see Chapter "Secondary Orbital Implants, Dermis-Fat Graft, and Socket Volume Enhancement Techniques"). A specialised tool such as a smooth glide (a single use enucleation implant introducer) prevents dragging of superficial tissues by the implant, which can thus be placed into the socket without tension [16]. Deep insertion of the ball can also be assisted with the use of specialised equipment, such as "Carter sphere introducer and holder" (Fig. 4) or with orbital spatulas. Smooth surfaced alloplastic implants, such as silicone spherical implants, are less likely to cause tissue drag.

5.10 Muscle Suturing for the Achievement of Optimal Prosthetic Motility

A great variety of surgical techniques have been tried for muscle suturing on the implant in an attempt to minimise implant migration and maximise prosthesis motility. Prosthesis motility depends on the transmission of movement from the implant to the prosthesis (Fig. 5). While the implant is separated from the prosthesis by Tenon's capsule and the conjunctiva, the most important factor limiting prosthesis motility is the forniceal space, especially medially and laterally [17] (Fig. 6).

In case of non-porous implants, the rectus muscles are sutured on the anterior surface of the implant, offering adequate motility. However, the imbrication of the muscles over the non-porous implant, due to their possible future contraction, may lead to implant migration. Use of wrapping in these cases is helpful for the attachment of the muscles on the wrapping material (Fig. 7).

In case of porous implants, the muscles are attached directly onto the implant, or on pre-drilled holes and tunnels. The location of attachment of the muscles to the wrapping or to the implant is paracentral, corners to each other, or are central over each other.

The myoconjunctival technique is an alternative to the usual suturing of the muscles on the implant. This technique is based on the theory that prosthesis motility is not only a result of the implant motility but also provided by contraction of the fornices. It is performed as follows: after the implant insertion, the rectus muscles (with the inferior oblique sutured on the inferior rectus muscle) are identified with their sutures clamped to the surrounding drape. The posterior layer of the Tenon's capsule is sutured with 4-0

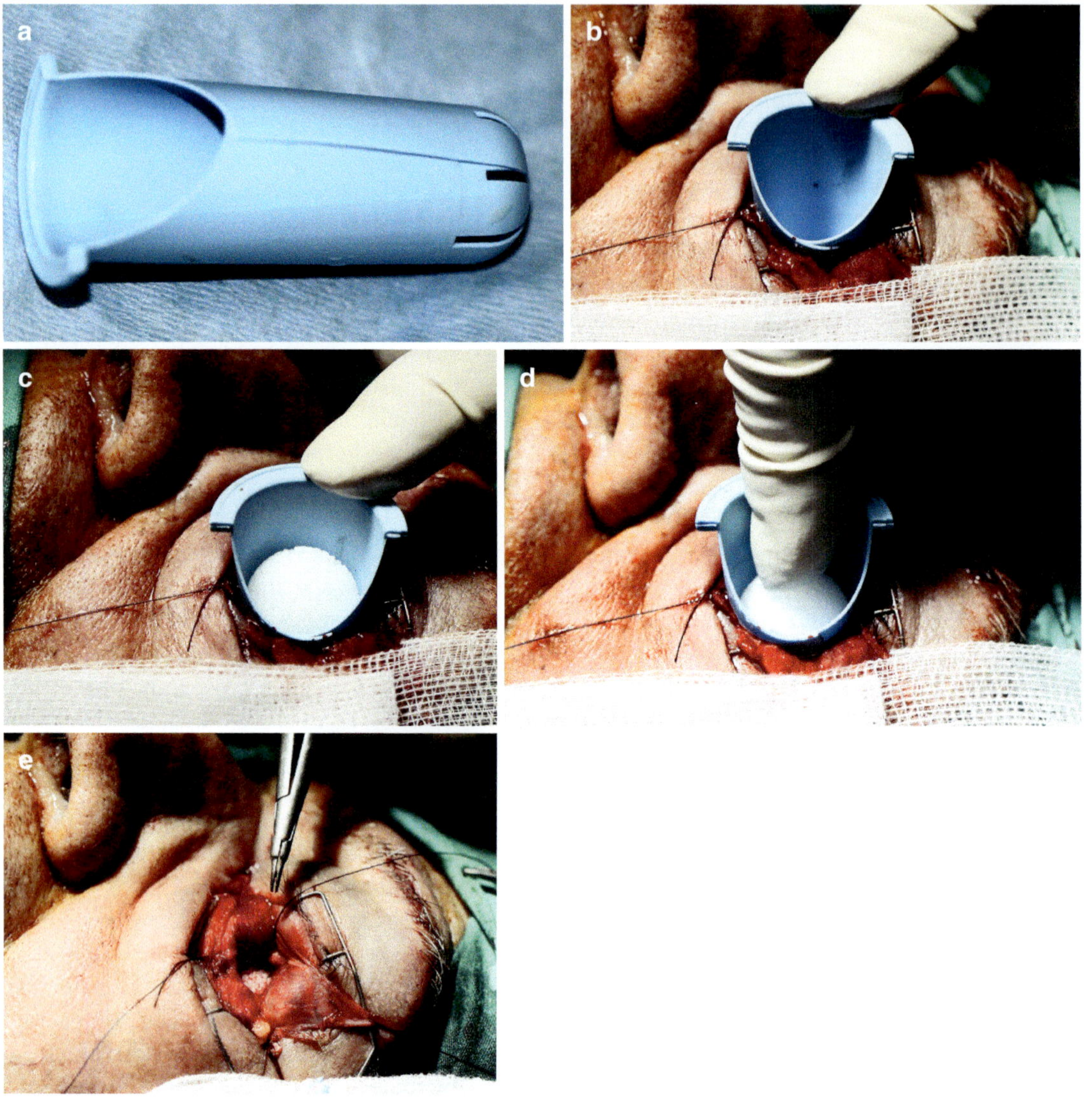

Fig. 4 The implant should be placed as far posteriorly into the anophthalmic cavity as possible. In some cases, it is necessary to enlarge the space where the implant will be placed with retractors. Deep insertion of porous implants with a rough surface can be assisted with the use of specialised equipment such as the "single use enucleation implant introducer" (**a**). This may prevent tissue drag into the orbit (**b**, **c**, **d**)

Vicryl® interrupted sutures, from opposite oblique quadrants, i.e. superotemporal to inferonasal and superonasal to inferotemporal. The muscles are drawn anteriorly and sutured with their double-armed sutures secured to their ends, through the anterior layer of the Tenon's capsule and the conjunctiva, into their corresponding fornices. The superior and inferior rectus are sutured each in their respective fornix, 10–12 mm from the horizontal edges of the conjunctival wound. The medial and lateral recti are also attached to their respective fornix, about 25 mm apart from each other. The anterior layer of the Tenon's capsule and the conjunctiva receive no tension this way. Tenon's capsule is sutured with 5-0 Vicryl® interrupted sutures and conjunctiva with a continuous 6-0 Vicryl® suture.

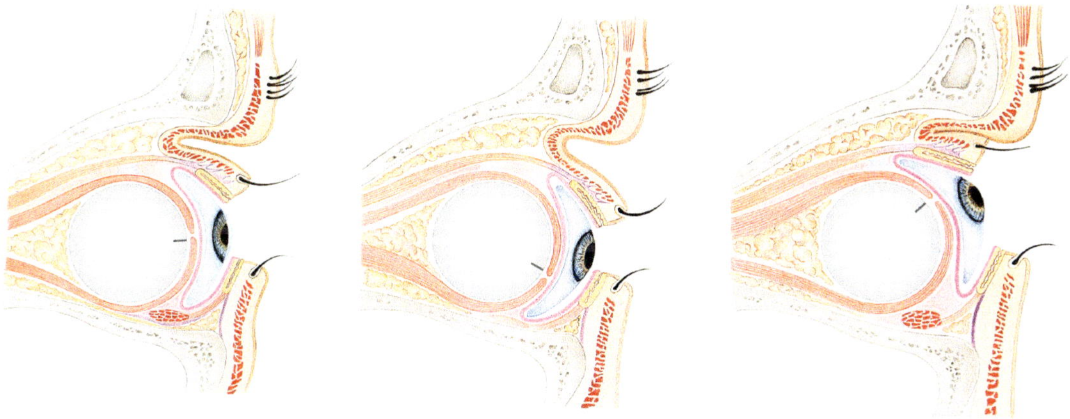

Fig. 5 Implant and prosthesis motility following enucleation (*left*). Due to the limited depth of the fornices and the lack of direct mechanical coupling of prosthesis to orbital implant, there is limitation of prosthesis' motility in downgaze (*middle*) and upgaze (*right*)

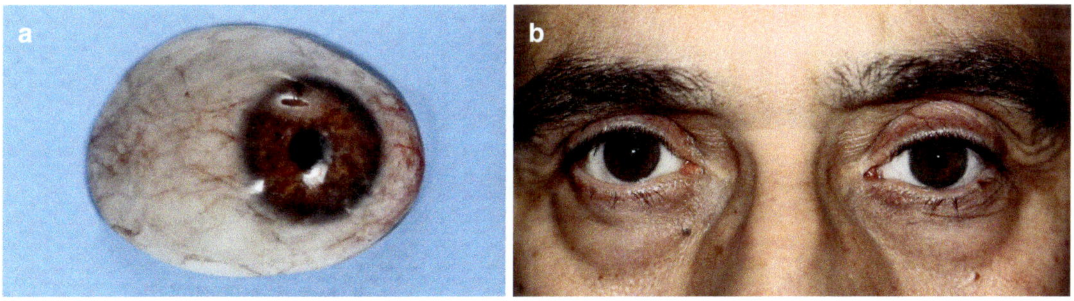

Fig. 6 Prosthesis motility following enucleation. The *left* eye was enucleated, and a prosthesis was placed. (**a**) In this patient, the prosthesis has minimal motility (**b**, **c**, **d**, **e**), but in some—especially vertical motility—may be much better. Note the limited prosthesis motility in extremes of gaze due to restricted fornix motility and elasticity

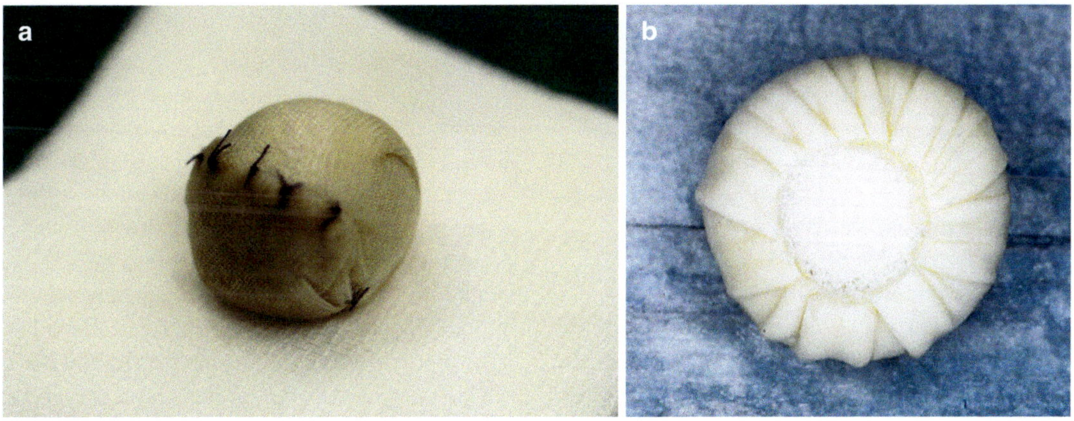

Fig. 7 Wrapping of the implant with donor-sclera. (**a**) In case of use of porous implants small openings in the donor-sclera may assist in fibrovascular ingrowth for better integration. (**b**) In case of silicone, acrylic or porous implants the donor-sclera wrap can be wrapped around the implant with the opening posteriorly. The donor optic nerve points anteriorly and is only slightly trimmed after insertion into the socket and fixation of the extraocular muscles to the donor-sclera. During the insertion of such a wrapped implant, the donor optic nerve can be used as a joy-stick to check if the implant is well situated without evidence of tissue drag

5.11 Closure of Tenon's Capsule and Conjunctiva

Meticulous closure of Tenon's capsule and conjunctiva decreases the danger of implant extrusion. However, tension between the sutured segments should be avoided, and eyelid fornices should be preserved and provide enough space for placement of the prosthesis.

Tenon's capsule, as mentioned, may be sutured either behind, or in front of the sutured rectus muscles, with 5-0 or 6.0 Vicryl® interrupted sutures. The conjunctiva is closed with a continuous 6-0 Vicryl® (spatula) suture. Alternatively, a two layer closure with several interrupted fast-absorbing Vicryl® 6.0 sutures has been shown to be equally effective as closure in two separate layers [18].

Topical antibiotic ointment is applied to the fornices and eyelids. Finally, a temporary conformer or artificial eye is inserted. Placement of a suitable conformer is extremely important, because it maintains the fornices, until the definitive prosthesis is fitted, after several (e.g. 6–12) weeks.

Retro-orbital injection with liposomal bupivacaine or ropivacaine gives good post-operative pain control. A temporary tarsorrhaphy suture is frequently inserted between the lateral, upper, and lower eyelids with a 5-0 prolene suture to reduce chemosis and prevent the conformer from falling out. These sutures are removed 7–12 days after surgery. The orbit is covered with a pressure bandage for 1 up to 5 days to reduce post-operative oedema.

6 Post-operative Care

6.1 After Surgery

The patient is usually discharged the next day after surgery, and a course of post-operative oral antibiosis is prescribed. Analgesics are essential for the first days after the surgery, usually during the first 48 h. The pressure bandages are removed up to 7 days post-operatively, and antibiotic ointment is put for 2–3 weeks afterwards.

6.2 Patient Instructions

When the pressure bandages are removed, the surgeon must assure that the eyelids retain the conformer/artificial eye. At this point the patient is confronted with the appearance of the conformer or temporary prosthesis and swollen eyelids: a temporary artificial eye gives the patient a more natural appearance. The surgeon should discuss with the patient any possible short- and long-term concerns that might arise [19]. It should be explained that the conformer (or artificial eye) is left until the definite prosthesis is ready. During the first few weeks, patients who could previously see with the eye in question will need to adapt to monocular vision, including loss of stereopsis and reduction of horizontal visual field. During this critical period the patient has to be careful not to injure the healthy eye, and should protect it with protective glasses. In case of a temporary cosmetically disturbing appearance the use of a covering shield can help in the social interaction of the patient.

6.3 Prosthesis Fitting

The conformer or temporary artificial eye is left until the definite prosthesis is ready: it maintains the fornices, it prevents socket contraction and—in case of an artificial eye—helps to improve the patient's appearance, adding to the quality of life. A definite prosthesis can be fitted after 6–8 weeks, when the oedema has largely subsided and the wound has healed. Prosthesis size depends on the implant size. A small implant creates enophthalmos, that requires a larger prosthesis. The material of the prosthesis is either glass, or acrylic. During prosthesis fitting, the ocularist usually explains to the patient the details on how to insert, remove and clean it.

7 Orbital Implant Selection

Orbital implants have been used in enucleation surgery for more than 135 years. The first descriptions of orbital implant placement are in 1885, in which a glass sphere was placed within an eviscerated socket [20, 21]. Various orbital implants and methods for their placement have been described since then, and are currently in use. In 2015, Mourits et al. published a survey that investigated the enucleation technique for retinoblastoma, chosen by 58 oculoplastic surgeons across the world. Almost no one followed the same surgical technique, implant material, or wrapping or pegging choice. The article underlines that there is no consensus among oculoplastic surgeons for the "correct" method, especially because they are offered various alternatives [22].

Common reasons that determine the technique and the implant materials are implant cost, availability, surgical experience, recurrence and complications risk, and final cosmetic outcome. The most common complications that surgeons try to avoid are socket infection, implant exposure or extrusion and socket contraction, post enucleation socket syndrome (PESS), cyst formation, pyogenic granuloma, and minor prosthetic motility.

Thus, the choices that concern every oculoplastic surgeon on implant selection are implant volume, implant material selection, implant wrapping, pegging, choice of implant technique, and suturing of the muscles on (or in front of) the implant.

7.1 Implant Volume

The volume deficit of the anophthalmic socket is corrected by an orbital implant of proper size during surgery and by the ocular prosthesis. Subsequent in spite of the danger of extrusion, the largest implant that fits into the socket should be inserted into the anophthalmic cavity. Decreased size of the orbital implant (combined with the orbital fat atrophy that usually follows enucleation), can lead to PESS, with a deep superior sulcus, ptosis or eyelid retraction, enophthalmos, and displacement of the prosthesis [6]. On the other hand, larger implants leave minimal space to the ocularist, resulting in difficult fitting of the appropriate prosthesis.

The diameter of the implants for enucleation surgery ranges between 12–24 mm. A 20 or 22 mm diameter implant is used for the majority of adult cases. The adult globe has an average volume of 7.0 mL. The volume of a 20-mm diameter implant is 4.19 mL, and that of a 22-mm diameter implant is 5.58 mL, whilst the average size of the artificial prosthesis is 1.5–2.0 mL. A larger prosthesis is heavy, and leads to ptosis of the upper and lower eyelids [7, 23].

Each surgeon prefers to estimate the implant of choice with different means. There are surgeons that decide based on their experience, depending on the size of the socket during surgery. Others use "sizers". Sizers are metallic spheres, of various diameters, placed temporarily in the position of the future implant. Testing each sizer in the specific socket, leads to the proper implant dimension. Another method is by calculating the volume of the removed globe, based on the A-scan of the contralateral eye [24].

7.2 Implant Material

Various implant materials have been used since 1885, such as fat, aluminium, cork, bone, ivory, cartilage, rubber, gold, and silver. Since then, a variety of implants have been tested, aiming to reduce the risk of extrusion. These implants are categorised based on their shape (spherical, oval, or conical), their material (autoplastic, integrated, or non-integrated) and their surface smoothness (porous or nonporous) [1, 25]. Primary dermis fat graft is the most common autoplastic implant and is still used by some oculoplastic surgeons [22].

At the beginning of the twentieth century, orbital implants were non-porous, made initially of glass, and later rubber, silicone, steel, gold, and silver [7]. Currently, the favoured non-porous implants are silicone and polymethylmethacrylate (PMMA). Non-porous implants do not have attachments for the extraocular muscles and do not allow ingrowth of vessels and fibrous tissue into their substance. However, compared to no implant, these devices provide volume replacement. The Universal, the Iowa, and the Allen have been popular orbital implants over the last 50 years, all made of PMMA [26, 27].

Porous implants were introduced in 1985, changing the scenery of enucleation surgery [28]. The hydroxyapatite (HA) orbital implant is manufactured out of natural hydroxyapatite, an extremely porous material which comprises calcium carbonate, a component of skeletal bones. Due to its composition, vascular and fibrovascular tissues grow into its stroma, providing immune cells within the implant. Therefore, it becomes 'integrated', preventing future migration. Additionally, HA implant is nontoxic, non allergenic, and biocompatible [28, 29]. However, following the introduction of HA, numerous studies reported prolonged orbital inflammation to the implant, with increased exposure rates compared to silicone implants [30–34].

During the following years, a variety of other porous implants were manufactured, such as synthetic HA, porous polyethylene (PP), bioceramics and others. The new porous implants are structurally strong, non-dissolving, nontoxic, bioinert, and non allergenic, presenting low rates of inflammation and exposure. They are less expensive than the HA implant and ecologically acceptable (in contrast to HA that causes environmental damage). PP is softer compared to HA, providing the potential of direct suturing of the rectus muscles to the implant [26, 28].

In general, definitive conclusions cannot be made about the extrusion rate between porous and non-porous implants, which seems to be mainly determined by surgical technique [35].

The choice of material (silicone, acrylic, hydroxyapatite, porous polyethylene, etc.) depends on the preference of the surgeon and the size of the implant. The alleged advantage of (partially wrapped) porous implants with regard to motility has not been demonstrated [17]. Some surgeons have a preference for porous polyethylene implants. These have predrilled tunnels for muscle fixation and a smooth anterior surface that enables insertion without wrapping, and with low extrusion and migration rates. However, when porous implants, especially those with a rough anterior surface without a wrap, do erode through the conjunctiva, they are difficult to remove and replace without marked disruption of orbital tissues.

7.3 Implant Wrapping

The necessity of wrapping implants is not accepted by all surgeons. Wrapping is mostly indicated in case of non-porous implants or porous implants with a rough anterior surface. In the latter, several small windows can be cut in the posterior half of the wrapping material to enhance fibrovascular ingrowth.

Surgeons that advocate wrapping the implant do so to provide a barrier between the surface of the implant and the overlying soft tissue, providing protection from implant exposure. Wraps also facilitate entry of the implant into the orbit and allow reattachment of extraocular muscles onto the implant, providing motility and reduced implant migration [31, 36] (Fig. 7).

In case of porous implants, wrapping has also been used, but is probably unnecessary because unwrapped implants are considered to have better potential for fibrovascular ingrowth. In case of porous polyethylene implants, studies demonstrate no significant difference in the exposure rate between wrapped and unwrapped implants [37, 38].

Wrapping materials are either organic (autologous and heterologous) or artificial. Organic materials include donor sclera, autologous dermis, autologous or preserved human fascia lata, rectus abdominis sheath, temporalis fascia, posterior auricular muscle complex graft, and processed bovine pericardium. Synthetic wraps include Vicryl® mesh (Polyglactin 910), Gore-Tex (PTFE), Dexon mesh (polyglycolic acid), polyester-urethane, polytetrafluoroethylene, and others [7].

Organic wraps are widely used with good results, but are not always available, requiring a separate surgery to obtain the wraps. Vicryl® mesh avoids creating a second surgical site for reception of autogenous wraps, reducing operating time and risks. Vicryl® mesh comprises a multi-porous structure, which permits fibrovascular ingrowth over the surface of the implant. It is less expensive than most wraps, and readily available. It is easy to use, bioinert, nontoxic, absorbable, and nonantigenic. However, cases of implant exposure have been reported with Vicryl® mesh wrapped implants [39, 40].

7.4 Pegged Implants

Transmitting movement from the implant to the prosthesis leads to prosthetic motility, and depends on surface tension of the conjunctival-prosthetic interface and movement of the fornices. This can be achieved through *pegging*, enabling an external coupling mechanism. Pegging is the insertion of a motility peg into the implant, through the conjunctiva and the Tenon's capsule, on which the prosthesis is attached. A second surgery needs to be performed after the enucleation for the insertion of the peg. A drill hole of 5–9 mm depth and 3 mm diameter is performed through the conjunctiva into the anterior portion of the implant. The peg is inserted, and the conjunctiva is allowed to epithelialize. The prosthesis is fashioned with a central posterior concavity which holds the peg.

Pegging offers improved prosthesis motility, but is associated with significant disadvantages, such as infections and an audible click when the peg is disinserted from the prosthesis at extremes of gaze. Additionally, peg decentration leads to a worse aesthetic result compared to no pegging at all. Currently, pegging is rarely performed, due to increased complication rates, and the fact that most surgeons feel that pegging is not necessary for an adequate cosmetic result [25, 32, 41].

8 Conclusions

Enucleation is a very stressful but possibly life-saving procedure for the patient. Mostly, it provides a satisfactory aesthetic outcome.

References

1. Kord Valeshabad A, Naseripour M, Asghari R, et al. Enucleation and evisceration: indications, complications and clinicopathological correlations. Int J Ophthalmol. 2014;7:677–80.
2. Idowu OO, Ashraf DC, Kalin-Hajdu E, Ryan MC, Kersten RC, Vagefi MR. Efficacy of care for blind painful eyes. Ophthalmic Plast Reconstr Surg. 2019;35:182–6.
3. Lundin AM, Azari AA, Kanavi MR, Potter HD, Lucarelli MJ, Burkat CN, Albert DM. Ocular trauma resulting in enucleation: a 12-year experience from a large regional institution. WMJ. 2014;113:99–101.
4. Bauza AM, Emami P, Son JH, Langer P, Zarbin M, Bhagat N. Work-related open-globe injuries: demographics and clinical characteristics. Eur J Ophthalmol. 2013;23:242–8.
5. Al-Dahmash SA, Bakry SS, Almadhi NH, et al. Indications for enucleation and evisceration in a tertiary eye hospital in Riyadh over a 10-year period. Ann Saudi Med. 2017;37:313–6.
6. Fu L, Patel BC. Enucleation. In: StatPearls [Internet]. Treasure Island: StatPearls; 2021, Jan 2021–Feb 25.
7. Moshfeghi DM, Moshfeghi AA, Finger PT. Enucleation. Surv Ophthalmol. 2000;44:277–301.
8. Savar A, Andreoli MT, Kloek CE, et al. Enucleation for open globe injury. Am J Ophthalmol. 2009;147:595–600.e1.
9. Holmes CJ, McLaughlin A, Farooq T, et al. Outcomes of ocular evisceration and enucleation in the British Armed Forces from Iraq and Afghanistan. Eye (Lond). 2019;33:1748–55.
10. Rofail M, Lee GA, O'Rourke P. Prognostic indicators for open globe injury. Clin Experiment Ophthalmol. 2006;34:783–6.
11. Campbell M, Humphries P. The blood-retina barrier: tight junctions and barrier modulation. Adv Exp Med Biol. 2012;763:70–84.
12. Payal AR, Foster CS. Long-term drug-free remission and visual outcomes in sympathetic ophthalmia. Ocul Immunol Inflamm. 2017;25:190–5.

13. Gündüz AK, Mirzayev I, Temel E, et al. A 20-year audit of retinoblastoma treatment outcomes. Eye (Lond). 2020;34:1916–24.
14. Wester ST. Enucleation and techniques of orbital implant placement. In: Johnson TE, editor. Anophthalmia, the expert's guide to medical and surgical management. Cham: Springer Nature; 2020. p. 60.
15. Badilla J, Dolman PJ. Methods of antibiotic instillation in porous orbital implants. Ophthalmic Plast Reconstr Surg. 2008;24:287–9.
16. Sagoo MS, Rose GE. Mechanisms and treatment of extruding intraconal implants: socket aging and tissue restitution (the "Cactus Syndrome"). Arch Ophthalmol. 2007;125:1616–20.
17. Colen TP, Paridaens DA, Lemij HG, Mourits MP, van Den Bosch WA. Comparison of artificial eye amplitudes with acrylic and hydroxyapatite spherical enucleation implants. Ophthalmology. 2000;107:1889–94.
18. Verhoekx JSN, Rengifo Coolman A, Tse WHW, Paridaens D. A single- versus double-layered closure technique in anophthalmic surgery. ophthalmic. Plast Reconstr Surg. 2017;33:329–33.
19. Verhoekx JSN, Tse WHW, Rengifo Coolman A, van Kinderen YB, Wubbels RJ, Paridaens D. Complications following enucleations and subsequent oculoplastic surgeries. Ophthalmic Plast Reconstr Surg. 2018;34:320–3.
20. Luce CM. A short history of enucleation. Int Ophthalmol Clin. 1970;10:681–7.
21. Mules PH. Evisceration of the globe with artificial vitreous. 1884–1895. Adv Ophthalmic Plast Reconstr Surg. 1990;8:69–72.
22. Mourits DL, Hartong DT, Bosscha MI, et al. Worldwide enucleation techniques and materials for treatment of retinoblastoma: an international study. PLoS One. 2015;10:e0121292.
23. Custer PL, Trinkaus KM. Volumetric determination of enucleation implant size. Am J Ophthalmol. 1999;128:489–94.
24. Wester ST. Enucleation and techniques of orbital implant placement. In: Johnson TE, editor. Anophthalmia, the expert's guide to medical and surgical management. Cham: Springer Nature; 2020. p. 66–7.
25. Goiato MC, Haddad MF, dos Santos DM, et al. Orbital implants insertion to improve ocular prostheses motility. J Craniofac Surg. 2010 May;21:870–5.
26. Su GW, Yen MT. Current trends in managing the anophthalmic socket after primary enucleation and evisceration. Ophthalmic Plast Reconstr Surg. 2004;20:274–80.
27. Wells TS, Harris GJ. Direct fixation of extraocular muscles to a silicone sphere: a cost-sensitive, low-risk enucleation procedure. Ophthalmic Plast Reconstr Surg. 2011;27:364–7.
28. Custer PL, Trinkaus KM. Porous implant exposure: incidence, management, and morbidity. Ophthalmic Plast Reconstr Surg. 2007;23:1–7.
29. Chuo JY, Dolman PJ, Ng TL, Buffam FV, White VA. Clinical and histopathologic review of 18 explanted porous polyethylene orbital implants. Ophthalmology. 2009;116:349–54.
30. Karsloglu S, Serin D, Simsek I, Ziylan S. Implant infection in porous orbital implants. Ophthalmic Plast Reconstr Surg. 2006;22:461–6.
31. Wang JK, Liao SL, Lai PC, et al. Prevention of exposure of porous orbital implants following enucleation. Am J Ophthalmol. 2007;143:61–7.
32. Yoon JS, Lew H, Kim SJ, Lee SY. Exposure rate of hydroxyapatite orbital implants a 15-year experience of 802 cases. Ophthalmology. 2008;115:566–72.e2.
33. Lin CW, Liao SL. Long-term complications of different porous orbital implants: a 21-year review. Br J Ophthalmol. 2017;101:681–5.
34. Hui JI. Outcomes of orbital implants after evisceration and enucleation in patients with endophthalmitis. Curr Opin Ophthalmol. 2010;21:375–9.
35. Wladis EJ, Aakalu VK, Sobel RK, et al. Orbital implants in enucleation surgery: a report by the American Academy of Ophthalmology. Ophthalmology. 2018;125:311–7.
36. Perry J, Tam RC. Safety of unwrapped spherical orbital implants. Ophthalmic Plast Reconstr Surg. 2004;20:281–4.
37. Trichopoulos N, Augsburger JJ. Enucleation with unwrapped porous and nonporous implants: a 15-year experience. Ophthalmic Plast Reconstr Surg. 2005;21:331–6.
38. Li T, Shen J, Duffy MT. Exposure rates of wrapped and unwrapped orbital implants following enucleation. Ophthalmic Plast Reconstr Surg. 2001;17:431–5.
39. Heimann H, Bechrakis NE, Zepeda L, et al. Exposure of orbital implants wrapping with polyester-urethane after enucleation for advanced retinoblastoma. Ophthalmic Plast Reconstr Surg. 2005;21:123–8.
40. Jordan DR, Klapper S, Gilberg S. The use of Vicryl mesh in 200 porous orbital implants: a technique with few exposures. Ophthalmic Plast Reconstr Surg. 2003;19:53–61.
41. Jordan DR, Klapper SR. A new titanium peg system for hydroxyapatite orbital implants. Ophthalmic Plast Reconstr Surg. 2000;16:380–7.

Evisceration

Gijsbert J. Hötte, Marco Sales-Sanz,
and Dion Paridaens

Key Messages

- Intraocular malignancy should be ruled out pre-operatively, and if it cannot be reliably excluded with fundus examination, B-scan ultrasonography should be performed.
- For patients with a blind and painful and or cosmetically disturbing eye, evisceration yields better results than enucleation.
- The risk of sympathetic ophthalmia is extremely low, but specific informed consent is mandatory
- Scleral modification techniques allow placement of larger implants with improved cosmesis.
- Non-porous implants show similar outcomes and lower complication rates compared to porous implants.
- Pegging of porous implants has a high complication rate.

1 Introduction

Evisceration, first described in 1817, is a procedure in which all intraocular structures (lens, uvea, vitreous, retina, and cornea) are removed while preserving the conjunctiva, sclera and extraocular muscles. Historically, enucleation has been preferred for eye removal due to the theoretical increased risk of sympathetic ophthalmia after evisceration, but in recent years, evisceration has gained popularity for a number of indications and has become the first-choice procedure for many surgeons [1].

2 Contra-indications and Indications

2.1 Contra-indications for Evisceration

When considering eye removal for treatment of a suspected intraocular malignancy, evisceration must be avoided, and enucleation should be performed instead. Enucleation may also be preferable for establishing histological diagnosis in certain benign conditions, such as a painful blind eye caused by scleritis of uncertain cause, or where there is insufficient sclera to cover the implant (for example, following inflammation, trauma, or scleromalacia).

G. J. Hötte (✉) · D. Paridaens
Department of Oculoplastic, Orbital and Lacrimal Surgery, The Rotterdam Eye Hospital and Erasmus Medical Center, Rotterdam, The Netherlands
e-mail: g.hotte@oogziekenhuis.nl

M. Sales-Sanz
Oculoplastic Surgery Unit, Ophthalmology Department, Hospital Universitario Ramón y Cajal, Madrid, Spain

Oculoplastic Surgery Unit, IMO Madrid, Grupo Miranza, Madrid, Spain

F. M. Quaranta Leoni et al. (eds.), *Oculoplastic, Lacrimal and Orbital Surgery*,
https://doi.org/10.1007/978-3-031-39638-0_2

2.2 Indications for Evisceration

2.2.1 Painful and Blind Eye

The most common indications for evisceration are a blind and painful eye, and a cosmetically disturbing eye [2]. These are often associated with phthisis bulbi as a result of previous trauma, congenital abnormalities, or multiple surgeries. Other indications include neovascular glaucoma and a fulminant corneal ulcer.

2.2.2 Endophthalmitis

Evisceration in the setting of post-operative refractory endophthalmitis or panophthalmitis is debatable. Some favour evisceration over enucleation in these cases as the remaining scleral shell may act as a barrier, reducing the risk of meningitis, though the extent of this protection is questionable. With the advent of modern scleral modification techniques, transecting the sclera may also facilitate abscess drainage [3]. On the other hand, it has been argued that necrotic sclera may not provide an effective protective cover for the implant and will likely become a source of persistent infection, particularly in cases involving virulent organisms such as Pseudomonas [3]. Overall, evisceration is considered a safe option in the context of endophthalmitis.

2.2.3 Trauma

Eviscerating a non-salvageable traumatised eye is controversial due to the theoretical risk of sympathetic ophthalmia, but studies have shown that it is safe [4, 5]. Despite the poor visual prognosis of penetrating ocular trauma, every effort should be made to restore globe integrity, and evisceration should be postponed to a later stage, only if needed, and when the patient is more prepared to accept it. Moreover, patients and surgeons should be aware that prosthetic motility is usually better when the prosthesis is fitted on a phthisical eye than on an eviscerated eye.

3 Less Invasive Alternatives to Evisceration

3.1 Treatment Options for Discomfort in Phthisis Bulbi

Discomfort in (pre-)phthisical eyes is a common problem. Lubricants and or topical steroids may help to relieve symptoms in some cases. Covering the cornea with a conjunctival flap is another option for reducing corneal discomfort [6]. However, if evisceration or enucleation is needed at a later stage, conjunctival shortage may be an issue since the previous conjunctival flap will be removed together with the cornea. Conjunctival deficiency may also limit the insertion of a sufficiently large implant, resulting in shallow fornices and consequent difficulties with wearing a prosthesis.

3.2 Cosmetic Contact Lenses and Shells

A cosmetic contact lens or shell worn over the damaged eye can be considered if the eye is cosmetically unappealing but not painful. If the eye is not enophthalmic, a contact lens or thin shell (Fig. 1) should be used; otherwise, a thicker cosmetic shell (similar to what is worn after eye removal surgery) may be considered. Although the contact lens or shell can be worn over the

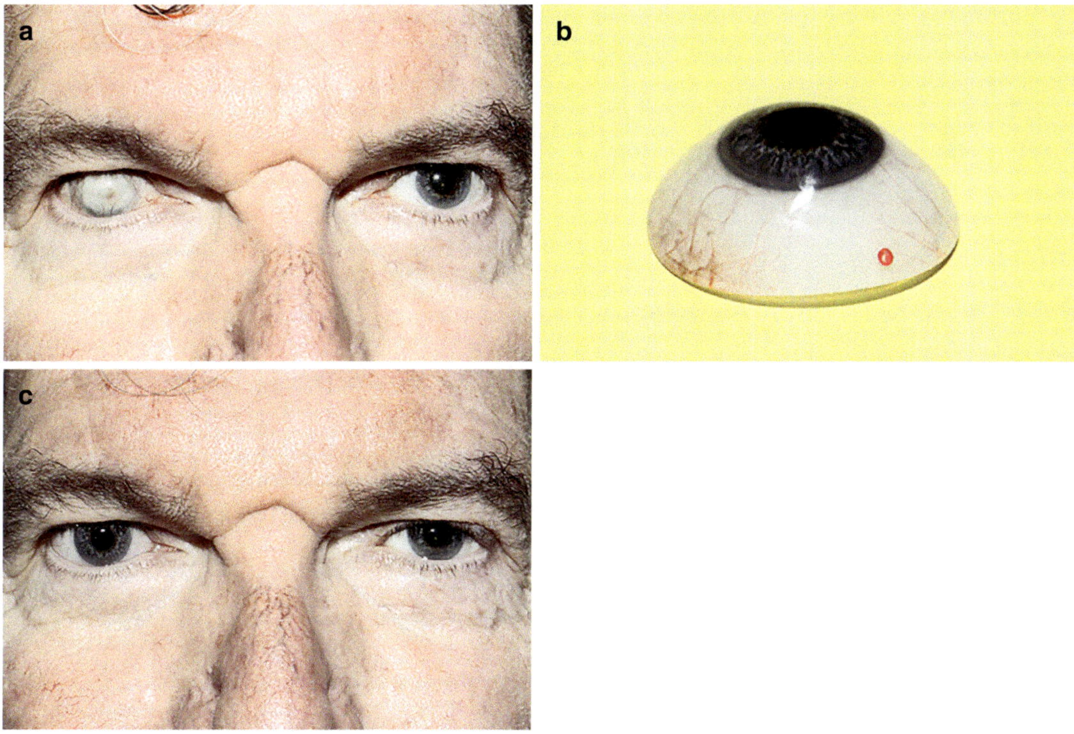

Fig. 1 Cosmetic shell. (**a**) A cosmetically disturbing but painless right eye. Corneal sensitivity was absent, therefore no conjunctival flap was required to cover the cornea. (**b**) View of the thin scleral shell. (**c**) The shell provides a good cosmetic result without the need for surgery

naked eye, corneal sensitivity may be an issue. If this occurs, covering the cornea with a conjunctival flap may allow the lens or shell to be worn [6]; however, as aforementioned, this may result in conjunctival shortage, with implications for future evisceration and implant size.

4 Advantages and Disadvantages of Evisceration Over Enucleation

4.1 Advantages

4.1.1 Preservation of Tissue

The orbital tissues, particularly the pulley system, are better preserved in eviscerated eyes than in enucleated eyes, which may lead to better implant motility. Moreover, tissue disruption during enucleation may result in fat atrophy and enophthalmos [7].

4.1.2 Improved Cosmesis

Although no studies have been conducted to compare the overall aesthetic results of eviscerated and enucleated eyes, evisceration does result in less enophthalmos and better sulcus contour [7], and an ocularist survey indicated that its overall cosmesis was superior to enucleation [8].

4.1.3 Improved Motility

Implant motility is better in eviscerated eyes than in enucleated eyes, which is attributed in part to less disturbance of the pulley system and extraocular muscles [2]. However, from an aesthetic standpoint, mobility of the overlying prosthesis is more important to the patient. There are no comparative studies of prosthetic motility after enucleation versus evisceration, though an ocularist survey concluded that evisceration resulted in better motility [8].

4.1.4 Less Risk of Implant Exposure

Evisceration has been associated with a lower risk of implant exposure compared to enucleation [7].

4.1.5 No Need for Donor Material

The use of donor sclera in enucleation carries the risk of prion transmission, which can lead to Creutzfeldt-Jakob disease, whereas standard evisceration techniques do not require donor material [9].

4.1.6 Possibility of Local Anaesthesia

Evisceration can be performed under local (peribulbar or retrobulbar) anaesthesia, with or without sedation, when a patient is unfit for general anaesthesia.

4.1.7 Easier, Faster, Cheaper

Technically, evisceration is easier to learn than enucleation, making it accessible to more surgeons. In addition, fewer surgical consumables, such as donor sclera and other implant wrapping material and sutures, are required, reducing operation costs. The surgical time and duration of general anaesthesia are also considerably reduced since there is no need to disinsert and reinsert the extraocular muscles [10].

4.2 Disadvantages

4.2.1 Risk of Sympathetic Ophthalmia

Sympathetic ophthalmia was first described after evisceration in 1887 by Frost and it has since become one of the most feared complications of this procedure. It is associated with intraocular surgery or penetrating trauma, and is characterised by a devastating non-necrotising granulomatous panuveitis of the fellow eye that is thought to be induced by ocular antigen exposure to the conjunctival lymphatic system in the injured eye [11]. Nevertheless, the extremely low incidence of sympathetic ophthalmia in the literature has contributed to the rising popularity of evisceration over enucleation in recent years [12].

4.2.2 Risk of Undetected Malignancy

As previously emphasised, evisceration is contraindicated in cases of intraocular malignancy. There have been reports of inadvertent evisceration in the presence of an undiagnosed intraocular tumour [13]; therefore, if intraocular malignancy cannot be reliably ruled out with fundus examination, B-scan ultrasonography should be performed.

5 Pre-operative Evaluation

5.1 Patient History

A detailed ophthalmic history is important for establishing the cause of painful blind eye, as well as disclosing previous interventions that could complicate evisceration, such as scleral buckles and glaucoma implants. Past medical history should also be reviewed to identify any complicating factors, such as anticoagulant therapy and conditions that may influence post-operative wound healing (for example, diabetes or previous radiotherapy in the orbital area).

5.2 Examination

Several factors are considered in the pre-operative examination. Most importantly, intraocular malignancy should be ruled out, and B-scan ultrasonography should be performed if media opacities preclude adequate evaluation of the fundus. Risk factors for post-operative complications or unfavourable outcomes must be identified, including scleral abnormalities (for example, scleromalacia), which may predispose to implant exposure, or conjunctival shortage, which may cause problems with prosthesis fitting. Evaluating ductions may help in estimating post-operative implant motility. Finally, corneal sensitivity and exophthalmometry should be assessed, if an alternative to evisceration is considered.

5.3 Risks and Expectations

The expectations and risks of evisceration, as well as any alternative treatment options, should be thoroughly discussed with the patient, taking into account the history and clinical findings. It is also advisable to show the patient a prosthesis prior to surgery and instruct them on how to use it, this aiding psychological preparation for the post-operative appearance.

6 Surgical Technique

The surgical technique is described in more detail in Fig. 2.

6.1 Anaesthesia

It is imperative to confirm with the patient and the entire team which eye will be eviscerated, just before anaesthesia. Most surgeons and patients prefer general anaesthesia, and additional retrobulbar block with a mixture of short-acting and long-acting anaesthetics can significantly reduce post-operative pain. If the patient is not fit for general anaesthesia, the procedure can be performed under retrobulbar anaesthesia alone, with or without sedation. In cases of severe inflammation (for example, endophthalmitis), hyaluronidase can be added to boost the effectiveness of the retrobulbar block.

6.2 Peritomy

Before placing the eyelid speculum, the eye to be eviscerated is again confirmed by the surgeon and the rest of the team. The conjunctiva is opened by making a small radial cut at the level of the lateral limbus with Wescott scissors. The scissors are then used to enter the sub-Tenon's space and conjunctiva and Tenon's capsule are bluntly dissected off the scleral surface for approximately 10 mm while performing a 360° peritomy. It is important not to dissect too far posteriorly to avoid injuring the extraocular muscle insertions. A further radial incision is made at the medial limbus. When there is conjunctival scarring as a result of previous surgery or trauma, care is taken to preserve as much conjunctiva as possible. Depending on the scleral modification technique (see discussion below), adhesions between Tenon's capsule and sclera in the four quadrants between the recti muscles are bluntly dissected using straight Stevens scissors.

6.3 Removing the Cornea

Using a scalpel (nr. 11 or nr. 15), a temporal limbal incision is made, entering the anterior chamber in a plane parallel to the iris. The cornea can then be removed by completing the incision for 360° with the scalpel or scissors. A small strip of conjunctiva is normally attached to the limbus, and if left behind, this could result in the formation of inclusion cysts; thus, the limbal incision should be placed just posterior to this tissue, so that it is removed together with the cornea. Pay special attention to areas where scarring has not allowed to completely dissect the conjunctiva. Alternatively, residual conjunctival tissue may be removed with scissors or cauterised after the cornea has been removed.

6.4 Removing the Intraocular Contents

The scleral shell is grasped with toothed forceps and an evisceration spoon (or a freer periosteal elevator) is used to enter the space between uvea (choroid) and sclera. The spoon is moved around for the entire 360° to separate the choroid from the inner surface of the sclera, and the intraocular contents are removed *en bloc* from the scleral shell. A long-standing phthisis bulbi may occasionally undergo extensive calcification and ossification resulting in a scleral cavity cast (Fig. 3). Although intraocular malignancy should have been ruled out before surgery, some cases of malignancy have been inadvertently eviscerated [13], hence all eviscerated tissues should be sent for histological examination. Residual choroidal

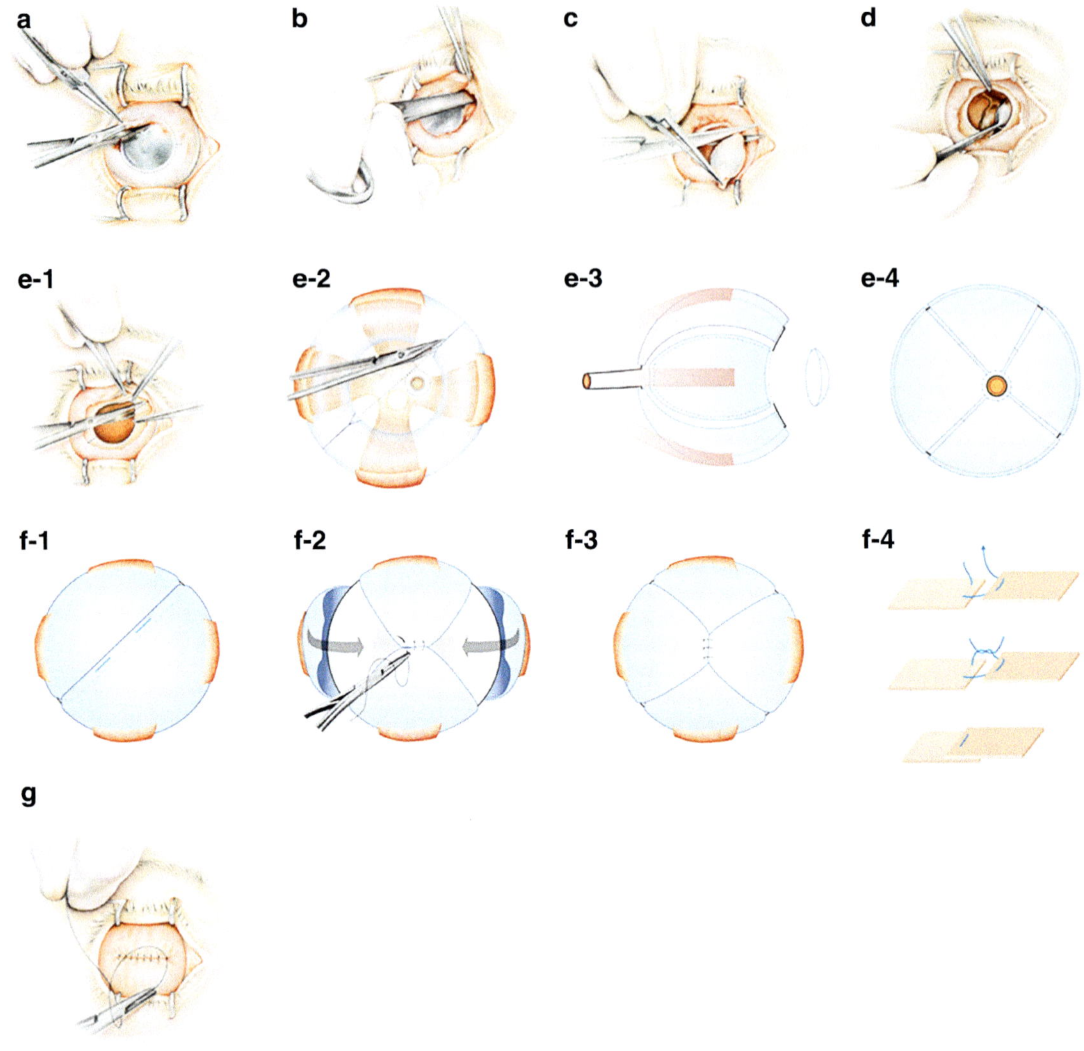

Fig. 2 Surgical technique for evisceration with two-flap or four-flap scleral modification and optic nerve disinsertion. (**a**) *Peritomy*: 360° peritomy is made with two radial cuts at the lateral and medial aspects. Care is taken to make the peritomy close to the limbus. The conjunctiva and Tenon's capsule are dissected off the sclera for approximately 10 mm. (**b**) *Dissection in four quadrants*: straight Stevens scissors are used to bluntly dissect posteriorly in between the four recti muscles. (**c**) *Removing the cornea*: the temporal limbus is incised with a scalpel, and the cornea is removed by completing the incision for 360° with the scalpel or scissors. Care is taken not to leave residual conjunctival tissue attached to the limbus. (**d**) *Removing the intraocular contents*: the scleral shell is grasped with toothed forceps and an evisceration spoon is used to enter the space between choroid and sclera. The spoon is then moved circumferentially, and the intraocular contents are removed *en bloc* from the scleral shell. (**e**) *Scleral modification*: (**e-1**) when using a two-flap technique, sclerotomies are made in two opposing quadrants, while in the four-flap technique sclerotomies are made in all four quadrants. Note that the sclera is put on stretch to facilitate cutting it, while the conjunctiva and Tenon's capsule are kept away from the scissors. The sclerotomies are extended posteriorly and the optic nerve is released. (**e-2**) In the two-flap technique each flap is attached to two recti muscles. (**e-3**, **e-4**) In the four-flap technique each flap is attached to one rectus muscle. (**f**) *Closing the sclera*: (**f-1**) if two scleral flaps are used, they are advanced over the implant so that there is sufficient overlap between the flaps and then closed with one or two 5-0 polyglactin horizontal mattress sutures. (**f-2**, **f-3**) If four flaps are used, first the vertical flaps are closed over the implant with 5-0 polyglactin interrupted or horizontal mattress sutures and then the horizontal flaps are similarly closed over the vertical ones. (**f-4**) Note that if mattress sutures are used, it is advisable to place the knot in between the flaps to prevent disruption of the overlying Tenon's and conjunctiva. (**g**) *Closure of Tenon's capsule and conjunctiva*: Tenon's capsule and conjunctiva are closed separately or in one layer with 6-0 polyglactin

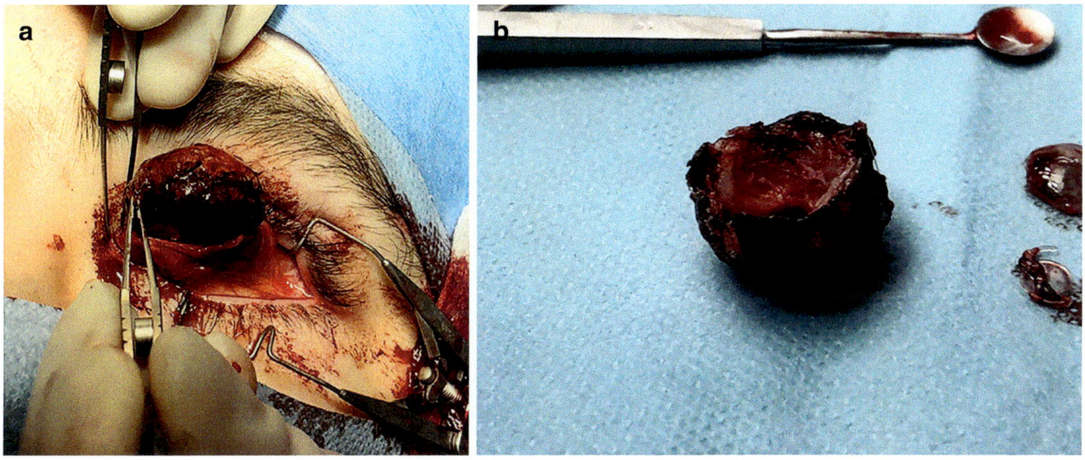

Fig. 3 Intraocular contents in phthisis bulbi. (**a**) Removing the intraocular content in a long-standing phthisical eye. (**b**) Solidified intraocular contents (scleral cavity cast) after removal

tissue is pared off the sclera with the evisceration spoon. Some surgeons irrigate the scleral cavity with alcohol to denature residual choroidal tissue which in theory might reduce the risk of sympathetic ophthalmia, however there is no evidence to support this. Furthermore, alcohol can cause an inflammatory response which may impair wound healing, increasing the risk of implant extrusion. Therefore, if alcohol is used it should be rinsed copiously with saline or sterile water. Haemostasis is achieved with bipolar cautery, particularly in the area of the optic nerve insertion and the entry points of the vortex veins and ciliary arteries.

6.5 Removing Epibulbar Remains of Previous Surgery

Following removal of the intraocular contents, any material from previous interventions (such as glaucoma drainage devices or scleral buckles) is more easily accessible and should be removed as it may cause persistent post-operative discomfort and pain. Removal is facilitated by identifying the extraocular muscles with a squint hook. The capsule around a glaucoma drainage device can be quite large and difficult to separate from the surrounding tissues (Fig. 4), and care should be taken not to damage the conjunctiva, sclera, or extraocular muscles.

6.6 Scleral Modification

One of the main goals of evisceration is to restore orbital volume with an adequately sized implant. Historically, the scleral shell was not modified, which allowed for the placement of implants with a maximum diameter of 13–16 mm [14]. Several techniques have been described for modifying the scleral shell to allow for the insertion of a larger implant, thereby improving enophthalmos, superior sulcus deformity, and cosmetic appearance. Scleral modification also minimises the wound tension, reducing the risk of implant exposure [15].

Quadrisection is a scleral modification technique that involves four scleral incisions between the recti muscles from the limbus down to the optic nerve [16]. The optic nerve can also be released circumferentially from the sclera, resulting in four separate scleral flaps (also known as petals), each attached to a single rectus muscle [14, 17]. Some surgeons prefer a two-flap technique with optic nerve disinsertion by sclerotomies in two opposing quadrants, with each flap containing two recti muscles [18]. In both tech-

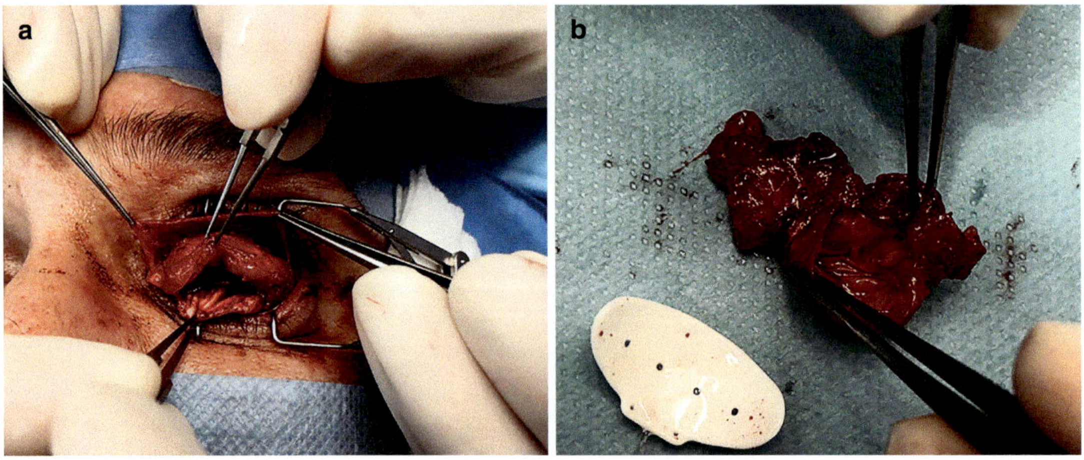

Fig. 4 Removal of glaucoma drainage devices. (**a**) Glaucoma drainage devices can be extensively encapsulated and difficult to separate from the conjunctiva, extraocular muscles and sclera. Note that the eye has already been eviscerated, which facilitates removal of the device. (**b**) The device and its capsule after complete removal

niques, damage to the conjunctiva is avoided by stretching the sclera to allow Stevens scissors to cut it down to the optic nerve while the assistant keeps the conjunctiva and Tenon's capsule away from the scissors. During optic nerve disinsertion, care must also be taken not to injure the recti muscles which may cause brisk bleeding and problems with post-operative implant motility. Although these flap techniques with optic nerve disinsertion leave the posterior aspect of the implant uncovered, implant migration is not a problem for both porous and non-porous implants [14]. Moreover, scleral modification does not appear to impair implant motility [19].

6.7 Implant Placement

The implant of choice (see discussion below) is inserted into the modified scleral cavity. An implant injector can be used if desired, however it is generally not necessary if the sclera is modified. In flap techniques with optic nerve disinsertion, the sclera is readily advanced anteriorly over the implant, with the flaps overlapping one another. If four flaps are used, first the vertical flaps are closed over the implant with 5-0 polyglactin sutures and then the horizontal flaps are similarly closed over the vertical ones [17]. If two flaps are used, they are advanced over the implant so that there is sufficient overlap between the flaps which can be closed with 5-0 polyglactin horizontal mattress sutures [18, 20].

6.8 Closure of Tenon's Capsule and Conjunctiva

Tenon's capsule and conjunctiva should be closed meticulously. The goal is to reduce tension on the wound and to maintain adequate conjunctival fornices, which are important for proper prosthetic wear. Most surgeons close Tenon's capsule and conjunctiva separately with 6-0 polyglactin as it is believed to create a stronger closure with less tension on the wound, reducing the risk of implant exposure and epithelial inclusion cysts. However, a one-layered closure of Tenon's capsule and conjunctiva with interrupted 6-0 polyglactin sutures is as effective and safe, with similar exposure rates and cyst formation, and a shorter operating time [20]. Following wound closure, an adequately sized conformer or temporary prosthesis is placed (to prevent conjunctival contraction), along with antibiotic ointment. We prefer a temporary prosthesis that matches the contralateral eye, which significantly improves the immediate post-operative appearance and helps the patient's acceptance. A temporary tarsorrhaphy may be placed to keep the conformer or shell in place, although this is not required in most cases. Finally, a pressure dressing is applied over the socket for up to one week.

7 Post-operative Care

7.1 After Surgery

Systemic antibiotics are not routinely given [21]. Patients are usually admitted for one night, and the following day the pressure bandage can be removed for inspection. At this point, it is advisable to show patients what it looks like in a mirror so that they can ask questions should they have them. A new pressure dressing can then be applied for approximately 5–7 days, particularly if there is significant post-operative swelling or if the patient is on anticoagulants. After removal of the bandage, topical antibiotics and steroids are used for 10–14 days and follow-up consultation is planned after 3–6 weeks.

7.2 Patient Instructions

Patients are warned that the temporary prosthesis or conformer may fall out due to residual swelling, and they are advised to avoid pressure on the wound for the first two weeks following surgery, as this may increase the risk of wound dehiscence. If visual function was still present in the period before the evisceration, patients should be counselled about the loss of stereopsis and or visual field. Low vision clinics can help patients to regain self-confidence and self-reliance after loss of an eye. Patients must also be advised to wear protective glasses, to protect their only eye.

7.3 Prosthesis Fitting

Patients are advised to make an appointment with an ocularist approximately 2–6 weeks after surgery for fitting a temporary prosthesis, after the swelling has subsided (Fig. 5). Patients can decide

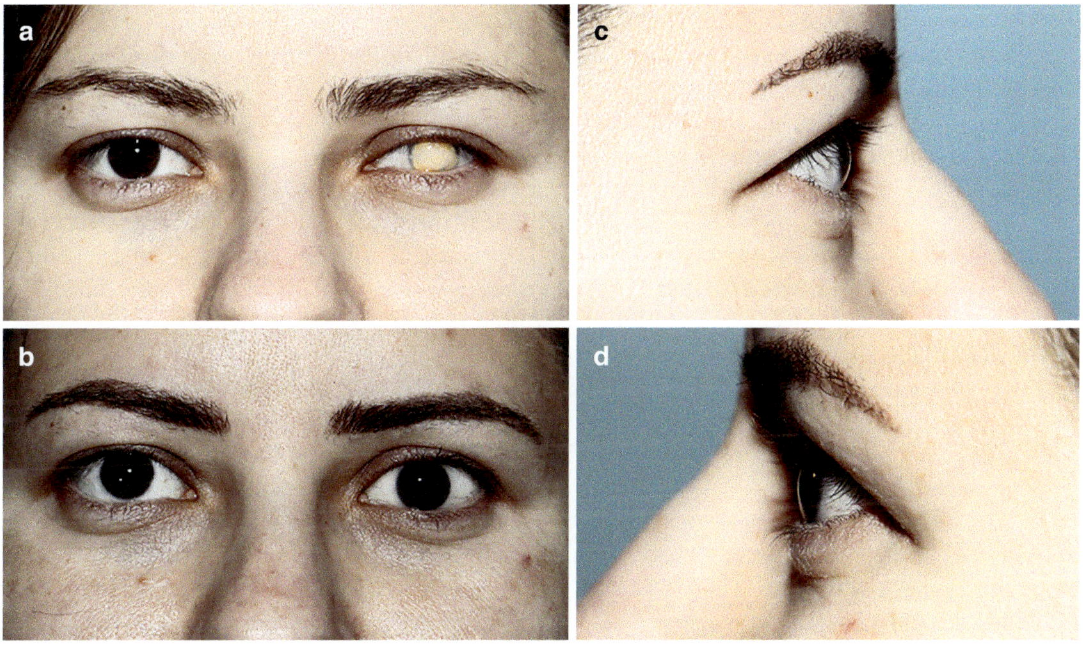

Fig. 5 Results of evisceration. (**a**) Pre-operative appearance of a 35-year-old woman with a blind, painful and cosmetically disturbing left eye. (**b–d**) Post-operative appearance after evisceration and a 20 mm silicone sphere implant

whether they prefer a glass or acrylic prosthesis. Glass prostheses are moulded from heated glass, however, unlike acrylic prostheses, their shape cannot be altered afterwards. Glass prostheses are also quite fragile and break easily; nonetheless, most patients find that they appear more natural, shinier, and more comfortable than acrylic. Recent evidence suggests that patients wearing cryolite glass artificial eyes are more comfortable than those wearing polymethyl methacrylate prostheses [22]. Enophthalmos due to small implant may be compensated to some extent by a thicker prosthesis, although a thicker and heavier prosthesis may lead to lower eyelid laxity.

7.4 Handling the Prosthesis

The ocularist or a trained nurse will instruct patients how to insert, remove, and clean their prosthesis. Frequent or vigorous manipulation of the artificial eye should be avoided as it may cause conjunctival irritation or abrasion. Excessive manipulation of the prosthesis may also be responsible for microbial imbalance of the conjunctival flora, which has a negative impact on prosthetic comfort [23]. The frequency of maintenance varies per patient, but it is not necessary to remove and clean the prosthesis on a daily basis.

8 Implants in Evisceration

When choosing an implant, the size and material should be considered.

8.1 Size

The main goal of an implant is to restore volume, and if the lost volume is not adequately replaced, enophthalmos and superior sulcus deformity may ensue. Historically, the scleral shell was not modified, allowing to place only relatively small implants, with insufficient final socket volume in most cases [14]. With the advent of scleral modification techniques, the size of the implant is no longer limited by the scleral shell, which is particularly useful in phthisical eyes, although conjunctival shortage may cause limitations in some cases. The volume that is lost with an evisceration is approximately 4–5 mL which can be replaced by an implant of 20 mm in diameter [14]. According to a survey of United Kingdom surgeons, most surgeons prefer to use an implant of 18–20 mm, while a 22 mm implant may be preferable to compensate for the additional volume loss caused by fat atrophy [1]. In cases of conjunctival shortage due to previous surgery or scarring, the implant size should be smaller (18–20 mm), permitting tension-free closure of the Tenon's layer and conjunctiva and preservation of deep fornices. Alternatively, using implants with a diameter 3 mm less than the axial length of the contralateral healthy eye have been proposed [24]. Hence, with orbital implants, one size does not fit all, and the surgeon should consider the volume of the contralateral eye, orbital size, and availability of sufficient conjunctival lining.

8.2 Material

The first implant that was used by Mules in 1885 consisted of a hollow glass sphere [11]. Since then, a variety of materials and shapes have been used to improve cosmesis.

8.2.1 Porous vs. Non-porous

Implants can be categorised as porous and non-porous implants. Porous implants, such as hydroxyapatite, polyethylene, or bioceramic, have holes or channels that allow fibrovascular ingrowth; theoretically, this reduces the risk of implant migration and extrusion, and small areas of exposure may heal spontaneously (see Chapter "Enucleation") [25, 26]. Hydroxyapatite is a popular porous material composed of calcium phosphate minerals. Despite the theoretical benefit of porous implants, hydroxyapatite implants have been associated with high rates of exposure and extrusion (due to abrasive effects on the conjunctiva), though the incidence of these complications has declined over time [7, 26, 27]. Polyethylene (Medpor) is a less expensive synthetic porous material that, due to its rough surface, also tends to erode the Tenon's capsule and conjunctiva [28]. Although alterations of the material have given the implant a smoother surface [28], studies have shown higher exposure rates for Medpor compared to hydroxyapatite and bioceramic [29]. Bioceramic (aluminium oxide) is a porous inert material that is used as an alternative to Hydroxyapatite and Medpor. Porous implants are notoriously difficult to remove or exchange due to fibrovascular ingrowth.

Non-porous implants, such as acrylic (PMMA) and silicone, are solid and do not allow for fibrovascular ingrowth. They are less expensive and, due to their smooth surface, have a low risk of extrusion and other complications [27, 30], though this smooth surface may predispose to implant migration [14]. Implant motility, is similar in non-porous and unpegged porous implants (see below) [31, 32].

8.2.2 Integrated vs. Non-integrated Implants

Implants can be also categorised as integrated and non-integrated. Furthermore, the integrated implants can be coupled to the prosthesis by a peg that protrudes from the implant through a small opening in the conjunctiva. Pegging aims to enhance prosthetic motility and can be done in any porous implant (mostly with Hydroxyapatite), but it is now seldom used due to the high complication rate (up to 45%) [32]. If pegging is needed, a titanium peg and sleeve system is favoured [30]. Semi-integrated implants (such as Allen Implant) lack a protruding peg through the conjunctiva, but have an irregular surface allowing for some indirect coupling between the implant and the modified overlying prosthesis [33].

8.2.3 Choosing Your Material

The choice of material depends mostly on the surgeon's preference, with most using porous implants [1, 30]. However, the Authors prefer silicone spheres for the following reasons:

- Silicone implants have low complications rates such as exposure and extrusion. Rates of implant migration are acceptable.
- Silicone implant motility is similar to non-pegged porous implants. Pegging can give superior motility, but it has a very high complication rate and is rarely performed.
- Silicone implants are easy to remove or exchange; porous implants are very difficult to remove without damaging the overlying conjunctiva.
- Silicone implants are cheap.

8.3 Implants in Cases with Endophthalmitis

The use of an implant in the setting of endophthalmitis is controversial, with many surgeons preferring secondary implants or none given the risk of implant exposure or extrusion [1], although primary implant complication rates in infected and non-infected cases are similar [3]. If a primary implant is planned, a nonporous silicone implant is preferable due to lower risk of infection [3]. Other risk factors for infection and poor wound healing, such as diabetes and microorganism virulence, must also be taken into account when considering an implant in the context of endophthalmitis [3].

References

1. Viswanathan P, Sagoo MS, Olver JM. UK national survey of enucleation, evisceration and orbital implant trends. Br J Ophthalmol. 2007;91:616–9.
2. Roelofs KA, Aghazadeh H, Cheema M, Weis E, Badilla J. Enucleation and evisceration: an analysis of indications, histopathological findings, and surgi-

cal trends over 23 years at a tertiary care hospital in western Canada. Can J Ophthalmol. 2019;54:106–10.
3. Tripathy D, Rath S. Evisceration with primary orbital implant in fulminant endophthalmitis/panophthalmitis. Orbit. 2015;34:279–83.
4. Reed D, Papp A, Brundridge W, Mehta A, Santamaria J, Valentin F, et al. Evisceration versus enucleation following ocular trauma, A retrospective analysis at a level one trauma center. Mil Med. 2020;185:409–12.
5. Zheng C, Wu AY. Enucleation versus evisceration in ocular trauma: a retrospective review and study of current literature. Orbit. 2013;32:356–61.
6. Ding J, Chen T, Hou Z, Qin Y, Hao L, Li D. Cosmetic shell fitting over a sensitive cornea in mild phthisis bulbi using total conjunctival flap. Aesthet Plast Surg. 2013;37:398–401.
7. Nakra T, Simon GJ, Douglas RS, Schwarcz RM, McCann JD, Goldberg RA. Comparing outcomes of enucleation and evisceration. Ophthalmology. 2006;113:2270–5.
8. Timothy NH, Freilich DE, Linberg JV. Evisceration versus enucleation from the ocularist's perspective. Ophthalmic Plast Reconstr Surg. 2003;19:417–20; discussion 20
9. Mehta JS, Franks WA. The sclera, the prion, and the ophthalmologist. Br J Ophthalmol. 2002;86:587–92.
10. Yousuf SJ, Jones LS, Kidwell ED Jr. Enucleation and evisceration: 20 years of experience. Orbit. 2012;31:211–5.
11. Migliori ME. Enucleation versus evisceration. Curr Opin Ophthalmol. 2002;13:298–302.
12. Levine MR, Pou CR, Lash RH. The 1998 Wendell Hughes Lecture. Evisceration: is sympathetic ophthalmia a concern in the new millennium? Ophthalmic Plast Reconstr Surg. 1999;15:4–8.
13. Eagle RC Jr, Grossniklaus HE, Syed N, Hogan RN, Lloyd WC 3rd, Folberg R. Inadvertent evisceration of eyes containing uveal melanoma. Arch Ophthalmol. 2009;127:141–5.
14. Dave TV, Ezeanosike E, Basu S, Ali MJ, Kaliki S, Naik MN. Effect of optic nerve disinsertion during evisceration on nonporous implant migration: a comparative case series and a review of literature. Ophthalmic Plast Reconstr Surg. 2018;34:336–41.
15. Vijlbrief JW, Hafezi F, Paridaens D. [Anterior surface breakdown following evisceration: "Classic", "scleral modification", and "scleral patch techniques"] Anteriorer Durchbruch nach Eviszeration: "Klassisch", "Skleramodifikation" und "Sklera-Patch-Technik". Ophthalmologe. 2010;107:246–50.
16. Yang JG, Khwarg SI, Wee WR, Kim DM, Lee JH. Hydroxyapatite implantation with scleral quadrisection after evisceration. Ophthalmic Surg Lasers. 1997;28:915–9.
17. Sales-Sanz M, Sanz-Lopez A. Four-petal evisceration: a new technique. Ophthalmic Plast Reconstr Surg. 2007;23:389–92.
18. Massry GG, Holds JB. Evisceration with scleral modification. Ophthalmic Plast Reconstr Surg. 2001;17:42–7.
19. Masdottir S, Sahlin S. Patient satisfaction and results after evisceration with a split-sclera technique. Orbit. 2007;26:241–7.
20. Verhoekx JSN, Rengifo Coolman A, Tse WHW, Paridaens D. A single- versus double-layered closure technique in anophthalmic surgery. Ophthalmic Plast Reconstr Surg. 2017;33:329–33.
21. Pariseau B, Fox B, Dutton JJ. Prophylactic antibiotics for enucleation and evisceration: a retrospective study and systematic literature review. Ophthalmic Plast Reconstr Surg. 2018;34:49–54.
22. Rokohl AC, Koch KR, Adler W, Trester M, Trester W, Pine NS, et al. Concerns of anophthalmic patients-a comparison between cryolite glass and polymethyl methacrylate prosthetic eye wearers. Graefes Arch Clin Exp Ophthalmol. 2018;256:1203–8.
23. Toribio A, Marrodan T, Fernandez-Natal I, Martinez-Blanco H, Rodriguez-Aparicio L, Ferrero MA. Study of conjunctival flora in anophthalmic patients: influence on the comfort of the socket. Graefes Arch Clin Exp Ophthalmol. 2017;255:1669–79.
24. Kaltreider SA, Lucarelli MJ. A simple algorithm for selection of implant size for enucleation and evisceration: a prospective study. Ophthalmic Plast Reconstr Surg. 2002;18:336–41.
25. Tari AS, Malihi M, Kasaee A, Tabatabaie SZ, Hamzedust K, Musavi MF, et al. Enucleation with hydroxyapatite implantation versus evisceration plus scleral quadrisection and alloplastic implantation. Ophthalmic Plast Reconstr Surg. 2009;25:130–3.
26. Yoon JS, Lew H, Kim SJ, Lee SY. Exposure rate of hydroxyapatite orbital implants a 15-year experience of 802 cases. Ophthalmology. 2008;115:e2.
27. Nunery WR, Heinz GW, Bonnin JM, Martin RT, Cepela MA. Exposure rate of hydroxyapatite spheres in the anophthalmic socket: histopathologic correlation and comparison with silicone sphere implants. Ophthalmic Plast Reconstr Surg. 1993;9:96–104.
28. Jung SK, Cho WK, Paik JS, Yang SW. Long-term surgical outcomes of porous polyethylene orbital implants: a review of 314 cases. Br J Ophthalmol. 2012;96:494–8.
29. Lin CW, Liao SL. Long-term complications of different porous orbital implants: a 21-year review. Br J Ophthalmol. 2017;101:681–5.
30. Shoamanesh A, Pang NK, Oestreicher JH. Complications of orbital implants: a review of 542 patients who have undergone orbital implantation and 275 subsequent PEG placements. Orbit. 2007;26:173–82.
31. Colen TP, Paridaens DA, Lemij HG, Mourits MP, van Den Bosch WA. Comparison of artificial eye amplitudes with acrylic and hydroxyapatite spherical enucleation implants. Ophthalmology. 2000;107:1889–94.

32. Gonzalez-Candial M, Umana MA, Galvez C, Medel R, Ayala E. Comparison between motility of bio-integratable and silicone orbital implants. Am J Ophthalmol. 2007;143:711–2.

33. Fan JT, Robertson DM. Long-term follow-up of the Allen implant. 1967 to 1991. Ophthalmology. 1995, 102:510–6.

Management of the Anophthalmic Socket

Ludwig M. Heindl, Alessandra Modugno, Leonard Holbach, and Dyonne T. Hartong

Key Messages

- Integrated care provided by a multidisciplinary team including ocularists and ophthalmologists is beneficial.
- Clinical socket evaluation should focus on dry anophthalmic socket syndrome (DASS), chronic socket infection, socket cysts, socket granulomas, and socket melanosis.
- For contracted sockets, a non-surgical compressor treatment can be applied to form stable fornices and allow adequate prosthesis fitting.

L. M. Heindl (✉)
Department of Ophthalmology, University of Cologne, Cologne, Germany
e-mail: ludwig.heindl@uk-koeln.de

A. Modugno
Ocularistica Italiana, Rome, Italy

L. Holbach
Department of Ophthalmology, Friedrich-Alexander University Erlangen-Nürnberg, Erlangen, Germany

D. T. Hartong
Orbital Centre, Department of Ophthalmology, Amsterdam University Medical Center, Amsterdam, The Netherlands

1 Rehabilitation with Prosthetic Eyes

The first known ocularists, constructing artificial eyes from glass during the golden age of Italian glassmaking, came from Venice in the sixteenth century. In 1868, Ludwig Müller-Uri (1811–88), a maker of doll's eyes, and his nephew Friedrich Müller-Uri developed a new form of glass called cryolite. In 1880, Herman Snellen, a Dutch eye surgeon, produced a light-weight hollow prosthetic eye made from cryolite glass. The advantages of cryolite glass included a better aesthetic appearance, better tolerability, easier processing, and longer durability than previous glass eyes. Throughout the nineteenth century, teams of German ocularists would dispense artificial eyes while visiting towns and cities in Europe and America. When German cryolite glass eyes became unavailable at the start of the second world war, outside the German-speaking area, particularly in the USA, polymethyl methacrylate (PMMA) became a substitute material for prosthetic eyes. Although PMMA is currently the most commonly used material for the production of ocular prostheses worldwide, over 90% of ocularists in Germany, Austria, and Switzerland still manufacture customised prostheses using cryolite glass from Thuringia (Fig. 1). Cryolite prostheses are also still produced in Italy, but they represent less than 10% of the national production. The learning curve for producing a cryolite prosthesis

F. M. Quaranta Leoni et al. (eds.), *Oculoplastic, Lacrimal and Orbital Surgery*,
https://doi.org/10.1007/978-3-031-39638-0_3

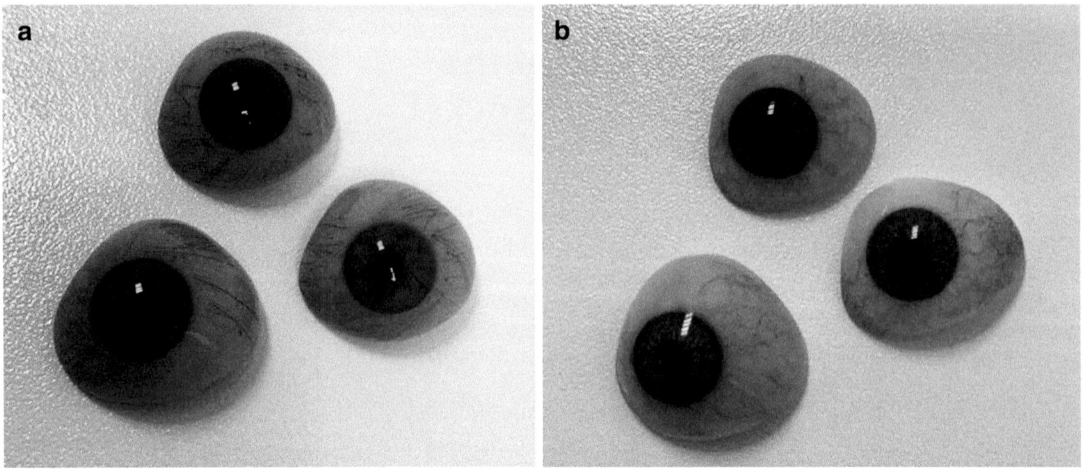

Fig. 1 Rehabilitation with prosthetic eyes. These can be made from cryolite glass (**a**) or polymethyl methacrylate (PMMA, **b**)

is much longer than for a PMMA prosthesis; moreover, PMMA is unbreakable [1, 2]. These are probably the two main reasons why more PMMA prostheses are produced worldwide. The advantage of PMMA is the ability to use the same mould technique as for dental prostheses, obtaining excellent conformation to the contour of the socket or the atrophic eye. Despite the long history of both materials being used in the manufacture of prostheses, there are few comparative studies regarding the concerns of cryolite glass and PMMA prosthetic eye wearers [3].

An ocular prosthesis allows patients to recover their aesthetic appearance. After enucleation/evisceration a conformer is inserted into the socket. As soon as the socket is well healed, the aesthetic prosthesis can be fitted. Patients often experience depression after eye removal surgery, especially in cases of eye tumours (e.g., uveal melanoma) or trauma. In paediatric cases, malformations or tumours (retinoblastoma) generate significant emotional stress not only for the children, but also for their parents. The early aesthetic rehabilitation of the patient is of great importance from a psychological point of view, both for the patient and for the whole family. The modern and innovative surgical techniques described in this book allow for excellent prosthetic mobility. The earlier the prosthesis is fitted, the better the emotional response of the patient. The main concern of patients who wear an ocular prosthesis is the health of the fellow eye and the aesthetic outcome they can achieve with their prosthesis. They may also be hesitant to discuss the issue with people close to them in their emotional and social lives. In order to reassure patients, they are advised to undergo an examination of the fellow eye at least once a year, and if there are signs of depression, the patient should be encouraged to participate in a psychological support course [4].

The use of ocular prostheses is not only intended for patients undergoing eye removal surgery; they are also very useful in cases of painless blind atrophic eye due to medical or traumatic reasons. In such cases, shell prostheses are used, which are very thin prostheses moulded directly on the phythisis eye and provide the same motility as the fellow eye with a very good aesthetic result. They are also used at an early stage in congenital eye malformations, particularly in microphthalmos, when there is no possibility of visual recovery. The positive psychological impact in this case is immediately noticed by the patient and family [4].

The ocular prosthesis should be kept in the socket all day and only be removed for cleaning, which must be carried out at least once a month, or more often according to the clinical case. Even if the patient has an atrophic eye, the prosthesis can be worn all day after a period of progressive adaptation, first during the day and then at night. Cleaning should be done with neutral liquid soap to remove any deposits that may form on the anterior surface of the prosthesis and rinsed before fitting in the socket [5–8].

2 Clinical Evaluation of the Anophthalmic Socket

For standard maintenance, it is advised to have the prosthesis polished (only acrylic prosthesis) or renewed (both glass and acrylic prosthesis) on a regular basis. Polishing should be done every 6–12 months where protein deposits and superficial scratches will be removed and the surface is smoothened [9].

2.1 Medical History

A complete medical history, including a general medical history and the reason for enucleation/evisceration is required for the evaluation of a patient with an anophthalmic socket or with phthisis bulbi. Any socket or cosmetic eyelid surgery or intervention including radiotherapy and medication use should be investigated, and the type of prosthesis (glass, acrylic) noted, with dates of last renewal and polishing. Wearing and cleaning habits should be considered: does the patient sleep with or without the prosthesis? How often is the prosthesis cleaned?

2.2 Maintenance of the Prosthesis

Frequency of renewal depends on type of prosthesis, age, and changes experienced by the patient. With growth in children, long-term prosthetic wear, and involutional or post-operative changes, the socket will change over time, resulting in fitting issues. These include prosthesis instability, and changes in prosthetic eye appearance (size, contour and position, and colour of the prosthesis). Children will need more frequent renewal because of orbital growth, this being faster in the first 3–5 years of life; earlier renewal is often required in all age groups in the first year due to volume changes in the post-operative period. Acrylic prosthesis can be adapted by grinding and polishing, and renewal is often performed between 2 and 5 years. Glass prostheses cannot be polished or adapted and will have to be renewed more frequently. Some medical issues require regular monitoring of the socket patient, for example following malignant tumour excision, while others may come for check-up of the fellow eye, or only present to the ophthalmologist when problems arise. We recommend a combined clinic with ocularist and ophthalmologist at least once a year for at least a subset of patients for the following reasons: (1) complex problems need accurate workup and planning, like the fabrication of custom-made conformers to use during surgery, and (2) interventions often have an impact on the fit of the prostheses; likewise changes on the prosthesis can influence surgical options. Direct communication will improve patient care.

2.3 Clinical Socket Evaluation

The general appearance should look natural, with dynamic and static symmetries being equally important, especially for the prosthesis and eyelid. Asymmetric appearance may be from deviations in the prosthesis (size, iris colour and position) or due to abnormalities in eyelid position, such as ptosis, en- or ectropion, retraction, and lagophthalmos. Furthermore, deficient periocular volume might occur, often presenting as enophthalmos, deep superior sulcus, and increased pre-tarsal show. In cases with pain or irritation, the periocular region should be checked for redness, swelling, crusts, and spontaneous discharge. While removing the prosthesis, eye care clinicians should check the amount of discharge, bleeding, and pain. The prosthesis should be inspected for accumulation of debris, sharp edges or cracks (acrylic), and excessive size and weight. It is also critical to check the socket for any implant exposure, remaining sutures, conjunctival redness, melanosis, swelling, papillae, granulomas, hairs, cysts, and discharge or pus. Palpation might be helpful to note the presence and position of a solid ocular implant or dermis-fat-graft. The fornix should also be evaluated for general cicatrisation, localised symblephara, or excessively large superior fornix. A computed tomography (CT) or magnetic resonance imaging (MRI) scan is performed if orbital inflammation, infection, tumours, or cysts are suspected, or if further information is required for pre-operative planning (e.g., implant replacement, potential bony reconstruction). When indicated, the lacrimal drainage system is evaluated, and the orbital rims and trochlear region are palpated for masses, irregularities, or pain.

3 Dry Anophthalmic Socket Syndrome (DASS)

The dry anophthalmic socket syndrome (DASS) is a disease of the socket surface characterised by a loss of tear film homeostasis accompanied by socket discomfort, in which tear film instability, conjunctival inflammation, and damage as well as eyelid and neurosensory abnormalities play aetiological roles [10].

The following clinical criteria should remind eye care practitioners of DASS—at least one of the four following clinical abnormalities:

1. Significant conjunctival inflammation resulting in conjunctival staining
2. Reduced tear meniscus height
3. Anterior blepharitis
4. Posterior blepharitis in combination with the presence of subjective symptoms in the anophthalmic socket evaluated with standardised measurements of dry eye questionnaires: Ocular Surface Disease Index (OSDI) with values $\geq$13, or 5-Item Dry Eye Questionnaire (DEQ-5) with values $\geq$6, or Symptom Assessment iN Dry Eye (SANDE) with values $\geq$13.

A detailed evaluation of external and systemic factors potentially causing dry anophthalmic socket and dry eye complaints, such as SANDE and DEQ-5 scores, should be undertaken in patients with increased bilateral scores. Due to a positive correlation between OSDI, SANDE, and DEQ-5, only one of these questionnaires is necessary for a fast and easy evaluation of patients' complaints regarding a dry anophthalmic socket. Furthermore, one of these established dry eye questionnaires should be used separately for the anophthalmic socket and the healthy fellow eye by eye care clinicians when examining the anophthalmic socket routinely.

In patients with significantly higher scores for the anophthalmic socket compared to the healthy fellow eye, the treatment principles of dry eye syndrome, including artificial tears, are recommended [10, 11].

4 Medical Diseases of the Socket

4.1 Chronic Socket Infection/Discharge

Mild chronic mucoid discharge is normal, and often exacerbated by the common cold, but symptoms may change to chronic mucopurulent discharge and discomfort (Fig. 2a) due to multiple factors that are yet not completely understood. Patient questionnaires have shown chronic discharge to be one of the highest concerns in anophthalmic patients [5, 12].

One factor that contributes to chronic discharge is the anatomic alteration after enucleation or evisceration where the bulbar conjunctiva is now behind the prosthesis and no longer in direct contact with the wiping effect of the eyelids. The mucus and tears produced by the conjunctiva can accumulate behind the prosthesis, creating an environment where micro-organisms can easily grow. This is supported by the fact that more pathogenic micro-organisms are found in the socket compared to a healthy eye, especially when a large dead space exists between the prosthesis and the conjunctiva (i.e., giant fornix syndrome, absence of ocular implant) or when lacrimal obstruction is present. Other associated findings are lagophthalmos, and decreased tear production compared to the healthy eye. In addition, patients with severe complaints frequently remove their prosthesis for cleaning, which may cause conjunctival irritation. Also, the surface of the prosthesis is likely to play a role in the mucosal reaction, where it is postulated that at least some mucoid deposition after intermediate wear serves as a protective biofilm, and high mucus deposi-

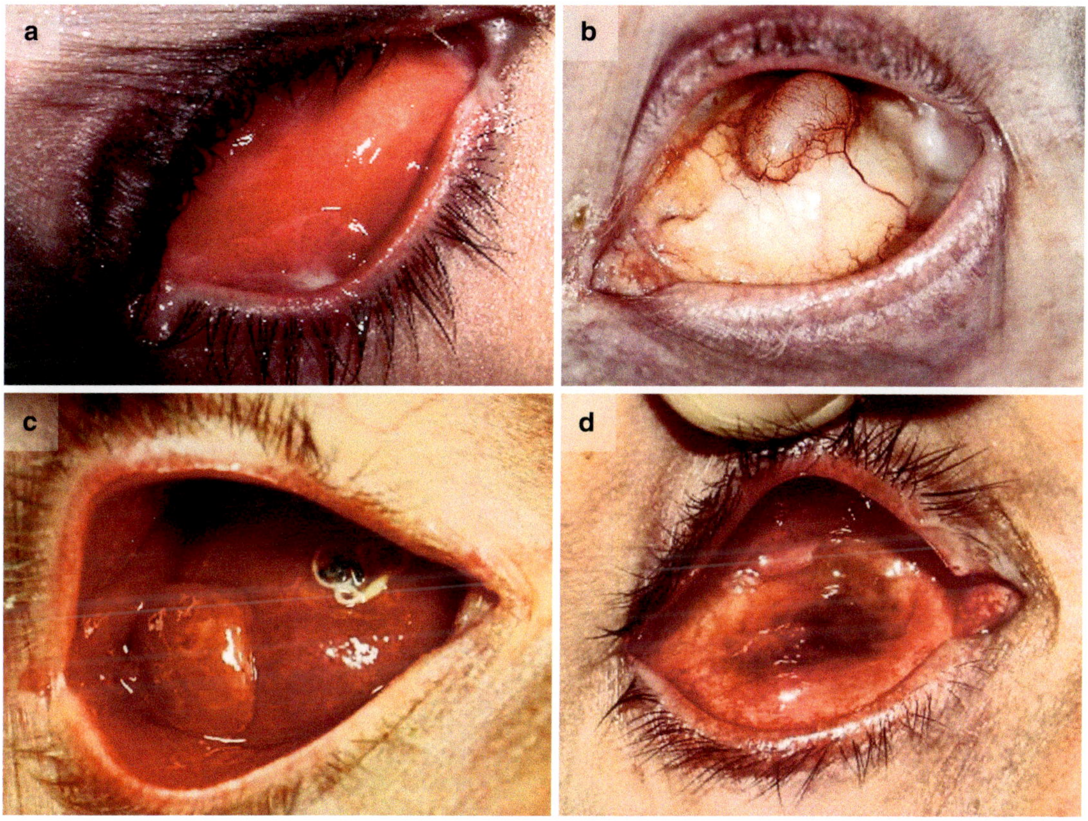

Fig. 2 Medical diseases of the socket. (**a**) Chronic socket infection. (**b**) Socket cyst. (**c**) Socket granuloma. (**d**) Socket melanosis

tion, debris and scratches from long-term wear will have a negative effect. Furthermore, irregularities of the conjunctiva (granuloma, cyst, giant papillae, exposed implant, stitches) and mechanical pressure from the prosthesis will also influence the mucosal reaction [13]. Symptoms include increased mucopurulent discharge, decreased comfort, pain, crusts, and rarely bleeding. Signs include mucopurulent discharge, periocular redness and crusts, conjunctival hyperaemia and swelling. There are no established protocols for treatment, but management should first be aimed at identifiable causes, and non-invasive methods are preferred whenever possible. The socket should be treated for acquired irregularities or inflammation (conjunctival cyst, exposed implant, granuloma, allergic conjunctivitis). Scratched or irregular prostheses should be polished or renewed, and the model of the prosthesis can be adapted if a poor fit is suspected (i.e., large empty space, pressure points). Lubricants can improve comfort, vitamin A ointment is often advised for night time use in case of lagophthalmos, and low dose (maintenance) steroids help to reduce the mucosal reaction. Patients are often advised to lower the frequency of prosthetic cleaning, to achieve a better equilibrium in prosthetic surface deposits and minimise potential harm from the prosthetic handling. A hole in the inferior border of the prosthesis may improve the mucosal flow. Antibiotic eyedrops should be used with caution. They will relieve short-term symptoms, but they can also increase the antibiotic resistance (including the resistance in the healthy eye). Antibiotics should only be used in acute infections and for the full course, to eradicate the pathogenic microorganisms. The suggested preferred antibiotics are quinolones (ofloxacin) and macrolides (azithromycin). Surgical procedures to decrease dead space include conjunctivoplasty-Müllerectomy for giant superior fornix, and implant insertion (dermis-fat graft or solid) in case of sockets without (or small) implant. Lacrimal drainage surgery is advised for concurrent tearing or chronic dacryocystitis [14, 15].

4.2 Cysts

Conjunctival cysts (Fig. 2b) are a rare complication after socket surgery; they can be superficial (often at the level of conjunctival closure) or deep. Deep cysts are more frequently reported after secondary implants. The cysts are thought to result from surgical epithelial entrapment within the socket. Symptoms are discomfort, prosthetic protrusion or fitting problems, and sometimes increased discharge due to an irregular surface. Signs include a visible translucent cystic structure, with or without conjunctival redness. Deeper cysts cause implant protrusion or displacement with or without a palpable mass, with shallow or absent fornices. Diagnosis is made with ultrasound, MRI or CT scan, that show extent of the cyst. Treatment consists in total excision of the cyst, with direct epithelial closure, but care should be taken to preserve sufficient conjunctival lining. Oral mucosa or dermis-fat-grafts can be used to restore the socket lining if necessary. Excision of deeper cysts may require replacement of the implant. Sclerosing agents are an alternative to surgery, and different concentrations of trichloroacetic acid can be used to successfully treat socket cysts [16–20].

4.3 Granulomas

Socket granuloma (Fig. 2c) is an acquired benign capillary lesion occurring during an inflammatory event (e.g., after surgery such as dermis-fat-graft, exposed implant or peg, or irritation from wrong-fitted prosthesis). Symptoms include spontaneous bleeding from the socket, irritation, discharge or visible mass, and it is usually painless. Signs are a pedunculated or lobulated vascular or fleshy mass in the socket with or without surrounding hyperaemia. Management includes observation for spontaneous resolution or topical steroids. Recalcitrant cases can be easily excised. Recent reports have shown a good response to topical timolol [21–23].

4.4 Melanosis

Pigmentation in the socket (Fig. 2d) may result from trauma, chemical irritation, and chronic inflammation, or represent racial melanosis, naevus, primary acquired melanosis (PAM), primary or recurrent melanoma. Although usually asymptomatic, the patient may notice the pigmentary changes after prosthesis removal. In the case of a growing melanoma, fitting changes and intermittent bleeding can be noticed. Signs of racial melanosis are usually bilateral and occur in dark-skinned individuals. Pigmentary changes from previous trauma, chemical irritation, or inflammation have a specific history, and are generally stable. A naevus is commonly present from childhood, involves deeper layers, and often has cysts. PAM may be difficult to detect in a pink-coloured socket, but is suspected when acquired and unilateral, with flat intraepithelial, patchy or multifocal pigmentation of variable size. The surrounding skin may show lentigo maligna. Melanoma presents as a raised pigmented (or non-pigmented) lesion with feeder vessel and often surrounding melanosis. Treatment of PAM and melanoma should be discussed with an experienced ophthalmic oncologist, and may include excisional biopsy, adjuvant topical chemotherapy (mitomycin C), topical immunotherapy, radiotherapy or cryotherapy. Differential diagnosis should also include the rare case of melanoma recurrence in an anophthalmic orbit (Fig. 3) [24, 25].

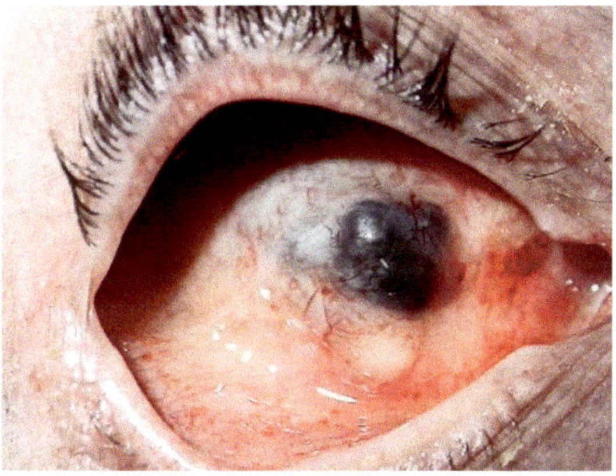

Fig. 3 Recurrence of a malignant melanoma in an anophthalmic orbit

5 Non-surgical Treatment of the Contracted Socket

The aim is to describe a simple non-surgical method for reshaping shallow fornices in a contracted socket that cannot be fitted with a prosthesis. This procedure is highly beneficial for patients who are not medically fit for surgery [26–32].

5.1 Procedure for the Contracted Socket

The socket is fitted with a customised conformer. A mark is made on the conformer at the centre of the eyelid opening. The conformer is removed from the socket and a cylindrically shaped piece is glued onto the previously marked area to form the so-called *compressor*. The compressor is then inserted into the socket (Fig. 4a, b). To keep the compressor in the socket while applying pressure, two patches are positioned to form a cross. The patient is asked to wear this device all day for the first seven days; the compressor can be removed as necessary for daily cleaning. After one week, the device can be alternated with a customised conformer for a few hours a day, increasing the hours without the compressor according to each individual clinical case (customised strategy). The patient is instructed to continue wearing the compressor at night for at least one month, gradually decreasing the time step by step. After the use of the compressor both fornices will appear to be deeper. When the patient wears the conformer properly and can use the compressor only overnight, a customised prosthesis is fitted to start cosmetic rehabilitation. The patient is asked to continue using the compressor every other day, then every 2–3 days, and then once a week, until the fornices are fully stabilised and the prosthesis is properly fitted into the socket (Fig. 4c, d).

5.2 Procedure for Mild Contraction

If the patient can wear the prosthesis but this comes out easily from the socket (mainly due to a shallow lower fornix) a compressor is made and used only overnight. As with a contracted socket, the compressor is made from a customised conformer and applied following the same procedure. After the use of the compressor, the prosthesis will fit better into the socket and will not come out again. The patient will continue to use the compressor alternately, as described above, until the prosthesis stays firmly into the socket.

5.3 Use After Surgery

This device can also be used after graft surgery to minimise graft contraction and to stabilise the fornices. When a contracted socket is operated on for fornices or socket reconstruction with a graft, and a temporary tarsorrhaphy is applied, as soon as the tarsorrhaphy is opened, the compressor can be fitted to prevent graft contraction, and used as described above. The aim is remove

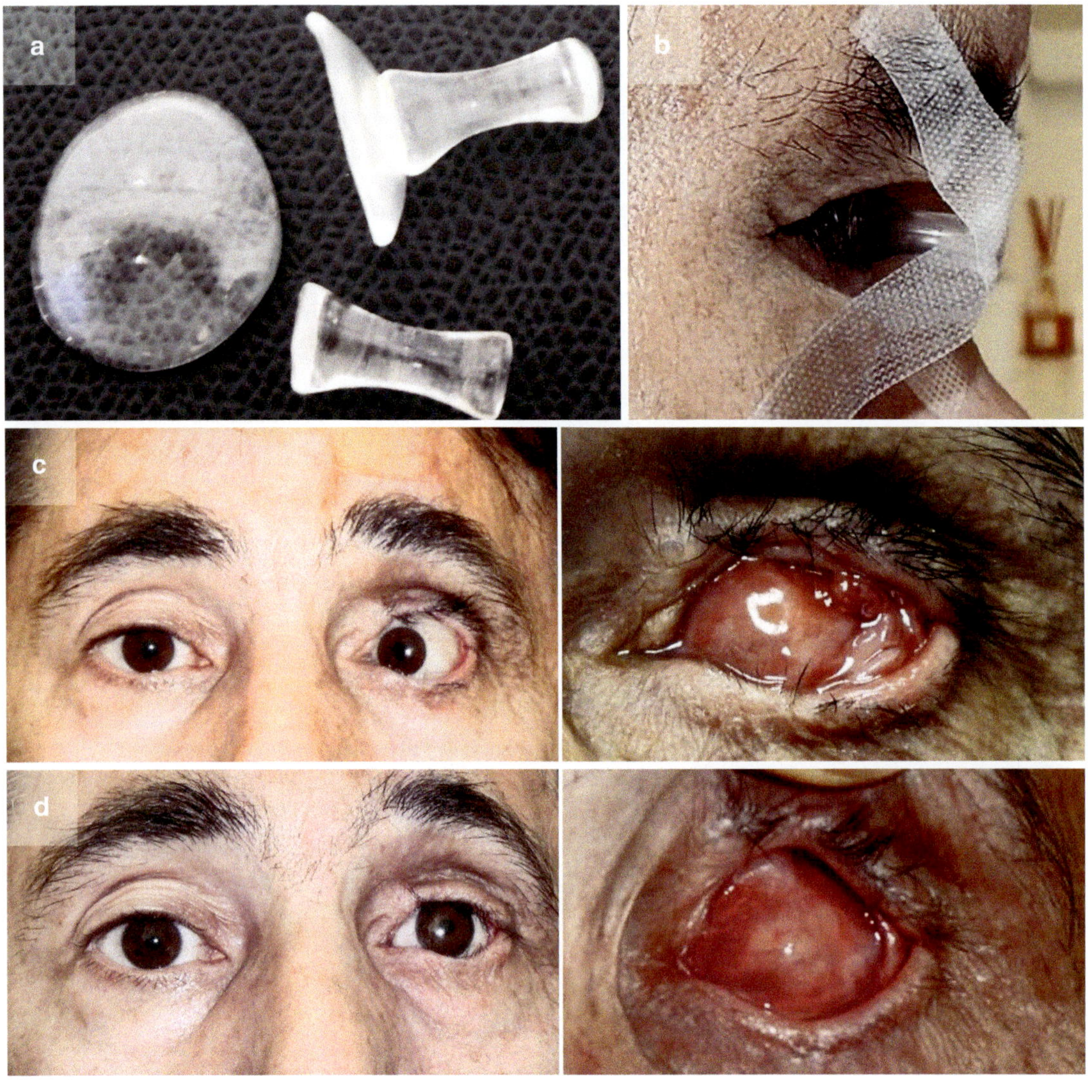

Fig. 4 Compressor treatment for a contracted socket. (**a**) A cylindrical shaped piece is glued to the customised conformer to form the so-called *compressor*. (**b**) The compressor is inserted, and two patches are positioned to form a cross to apply adequate pressure. (**c**) Contracted socket prior to compressor treatment. (**d**) Stable fornices and properly fitted prosthesis following treatment with the compressor

the tarsorrhaphy earlier, avoiding excessive stretching of the eyelids. As soon as the graft has properly healed, a customised prosthesis can be easily fitted.

References

1. Rokohl AC, Adler W, Koch KR, et al. Cryolite glass prosthetic eyes-the response of the anophthalmic socket. Graefes Arch Clin Exp Ophthalmol. 2019;257:2015–23.
2. Rokohl AC, Trester M, Mor JM, Loreck N, Heindl LM. Customizing a cryolite glass prosthetic eye. J Vis Exp. 2019;152
3. Heindl LM, Rokohl AC. Orbital implants: material matters. Br J Ophthalmol. 2021;105:1337.
4. Heindl LM, Trester M, Guo Y, et al. Anxiety and depression in patients wearing prosthetic eyes. Graefes Arch Clin Exp Ophthalmol. 2021;259:495–503.
5. Shapira Y, Worrell E, Litwin AS, Malhotra R. The UK National Artificial Eye Questionnaire study: predictors of artificial eye wearers' experience Part 1—comfort and satisfaction. Eye (Lond). 2021;35:2233–40.

6. Korani H, Pine KR, Sood M, Vyas A. Concerns regarding Indian prosthetic eye wearers. Clin Exp Optom. 2021;104:85–9.
7. Rokohl AC, Koch KR, Adler W, et al. Concerns of anophthalmic patients—a comparison between cryolite glass and polymethyl methacrylate prosthetic eye wearers. Graefes Arch Clin Exp Ophthalmol. 2018;256:1203–8.
8. Rokohl AC, Koch KR, Trester M, Trester W, Pine KR, Heindl LM. Concerns of anophthalmic patients wearing cryolite glass prosthetic eyes. Ophthalmic Plast Reconstr Surg. 2018;34:369–74.
9. Rokohl AC, Trester M, Pine KR, Heindl LM. Prevention of socket complications in anophthalmic patients. Curr Eye Res. 2020;45:1625–6.
10. Rokohl AC, Marc T, Yongwei G, et al. Dry anophthalmic socket syndrome—standardized clinical evaluation of symptoms and signs. Ocul Surf. 2020;18:453–9.
11. Rokohl AC, Trester M, Naderi P, et al. Dry anophthalmic socket syndrome—morphological alterations in meibomian glands. Eye (Lond). 2021;35:3358–66.
12. Pine K, Sloan JRJ. Deposit buildup on prosthetic eyes and implications for conjunctival inflammation and mucoid discharge. Clin Ophthalmol. 2012;6: 1755–62.
13. Pine NS, Terte ID, Pine KR. An investigation into discharge, visual perception, and appearance concerns of prosthetic eye wearers. Orbit. 2017;36:1–6.
14. Mourits DL, Hartong DT, Budding AE, Bosscha MI, Tan HS, Moll AC. Discharge and infection in retinoblastoma post-enucleation sockets. Clin Ophthalmol. 2017;11:465–72.
15. Toribio A, Marrodán T, Fernández-Natal I, Martínez-Blanco H, Rodríguez-Aparicio L, Ferrero M. Conjunctival flora in anophthalmic patients: microbiological spectrum and antibiotic sensitivity. Int J Ophthalmol. 2019;12:765–73.
16. Owji N, Aslani A. Conjunctival cysts of the orbit after enucleation: the use of trichloroacetic acid. Ophthal Plast Reconstr Surg. 2005;21:264–6.
17. Smit TJ, Koornneef L, Zonneveld FW. Conjunctival cysts in anophthalmic orbits. Br J Ophthalmol. 1991;75:342–3.
18. Sánchez EM, Formento NA, Pérez-López M, Jiménez AA. Role of trichloroacetic acid in treating posterior conjunctival cyst in an anopthalmic socket. Orbit. 2009;28:101–3.
19. Bagheri A, Shahraki K, Yazdani S. Trichloroacetic acid 10% injection for treatment of conjunctival inclusion cysts. Orbit. 2020;39:107–11.
20. McCarthy RW, Beyer CK, Dallow RL, Burke JF, Lessell S. Conjunctival cysts of the orbit following enucleation. Ophthalmology. 1981;88:30–5.
21. Demaria LN, Silverman NK, Shinder R. Ophthalmic pyogenic granulomas treated with topical timolol—clinical features of 17 cases. Ophthal Plast Reconstr Surg. 2018;34:1.
22. Nair AG, George RJ, Natarajan S, Jain V. Topical timolol for the treatment of conjunctival pyogenic granulomas: Outcomes and effect on intraocular pressure. Indian J Ophthalmol. 2020;68:2170–4.
23. Oke I, Alkharashi M, Petersen RA, Ashenberg A, Shah AS. Treatment of ocular pyogenic granuloma with topical timolol. JAMA Ophthalmol. 2017;135:383–5.
24. Shields C, L., Shields, Jerry, A. Conjunctival primary acquired melanosis and melanoma: tales, fairy tales, and facts. Ophthalmic. Plast Reconstr Surg. 2009;25:167–72.
25. Shields JA, Shields CL, Mashayekhi A, Marr BP, Eagle RC. Primary acquired melanosis of the conjunctiva: risks for progression to melanoma in 311 eyes. The 2006 Lorenz E. Zimmerman lecture. Ophthalmology. 2008;115:511–19.e2.
26. Toribio A, Marrodán T, Fernández-Natal I, Martínez-Blanco H, Ferrero M. Study of conjunctival flora in anophthalmic patients: influence on the comfort of the socket. Graefes Arch Clin Exp Ophthalmol. 2017;255:1669–79.
27. Rose GE. The giant fornix syndrome: an unrecognized cause of chronic, relapsing, grossly purulent conjunctivitis. Ophthalmology. 2004;111:1539–45.
28. Jones DF, Lyle CE, Fleming JC. Superior conjunctivoplasty-mullerectomy for correction of chronic discharge and concurrent ptosis in the anophthalmic socket with enlarged superior fornix. Ophthalmic Plast Reconstr Surg. 2010;26:172–5.
29. Kashkouli MB, et al. Tear film, lacrimal drainage system, and eyelid findings in subjects with anophthalmic socket discharge. Am J Ophthalmol. 2016;165:33–8.
30. Pine KR, Sloan BH, Jacobs RJ. A proposed model of the response of the anophthalmic socket to prosthetic eye wear and its application to the management of mucoid discharge. Med Hypotheses. 2013;81:300–5.
31. Tyers AG, Collin JR. Baseball orbital implants: a review of 39 patients. Br J Ophthalmol. 1985;69:438–42.
32. Rokohl AC, Trester M, Pine KR, Heindl LM. Risk of breakage of cryolite glass prosthetic eyes. Graefes Arch Clin Exp Ophthalmol. 2019;257:437–8.

Orbital Exenteration

Raghavan Sampath, Kaveh Vahdani,
and Geoffrey E. Rose

Key Messages

- Orbital exenteration is a mutilating, but potentially life-saving, treatment.
- Pre-operative counselling is necessary to manage psychosocial issues.
- The biological behaviour, extent of lesion, and presence of perineural spread should guide the extent of resection.
- The least-disfiguring approach to exenteration should be used, whilst ensuring complete oncological clearance.
- Skin-muscle sparing exenteration allows for rapid rehabilitation and maximises psychological adjustment, particularly in the terminally-ill patient with limited life-expectancy.

1 Introduction

Mainly performed for management of advanced adnexal malignancies, orbital exenteration is a radical surgery that involves complete removal of the eyeball, retrobulbar soft tissues, and most, or all, of the eyelids. It was first described by Bartisch in 1583, with Golovine publishing the first report of orbital exenteration in the early twentieth century [1].

The aim of exenteration is to achieve total local control of disease whilst, whenever possible, preserving normal tissues to optimise surgical rehabilitation [2]. It requires careful pre-operative counselling and surgical planning in order to achieve an acceptable cosmetic outcome and minimise the psycho-social impact for the patient.

2 Indications for Exenteration

Orbital exenteration is generally reserved for certain pervasive malignant or benign orbital diseases [3–5] (Table 1) and the typical patient will have already undergone various treatments, such as surgery, radiotherapy and chemotherapy.

Exenteration is mostly performed in the following contexts:

1. As part of resection for tumours extending into the orbit from the eyelids, conjunctiva, paranasal sinuses or intracranial space.
2. Primary malignant tumours of the orbit.
3. Major extrascleral extension of intraocular tumours (e.g. choroidal melanoma).
4. Fulminant infections (e.g. orbital mucormycosis, especially in the immune-compromised patient).

R. Sampath
Department of Ophthalmology, University Hospitals of Leicester NHS Trust, Leicester Royal Infirmary, Leicester, UK

K. Vahdani (✉) · G. E. Rose
Adnexal Service, Moorfields Eye Hospital, London, UK
e-mail: kaveh.vahdani@nhs.net

F. M. Quaranta Leoni et al. (eds.), *Oculoplastic, Lacrimal and Orbital Surgery*,
https://doi.org/10.1007/978-3-031-39638-0_4

Table 1 Indications for orbital exenteration

Malignant disease	Carcinomas (basal cell, squamous, or sebaceous)
	Invasive melanomas (eyelid, conjunctival or major extrascleral extension of choroidal melanoma)
	Sarcomas and malignant mesenchymal tumours
	Solitary metastases
Benign disease	Uncontrolled inflammatory disease
	Pervasive benign disease with malignant potential (recurrent pleomorphic adenoma, aggressive solitary fibrous tumour)
	Severe trauma defying effective reconstruction
	Severe developmental and vascular anomalies
	Severe ischaemic necrotising infections (e.g. mucormycosis)

Invasive eyelid tumours are the commonest indication for orbital exenteration, basal cell carcinoma being (historically) the most frequent entity [6], followed by squamous cell carcinoma, sebaceous gland carcinoma, and Merkel cell carcinoma. Primary orbital malignancies are the second most frequent indication for exenteration, although in the recent decades there has been a shift towards globe-sparing treatment modalities for certain orbital tumours such as lacrimal gland carcinomas. Invasive surface melanoma or squamous carcinoma are the most common conjunctival tumours requiring exenteration [2], often as a palliative measure [7].

Sinonasal or intracranial tumours that extend into the orbit may also necessitate exenteration as part of cranio-facial resection, particularly if they involve the extraocular muscles, globe or orbital apex.

3 Investigations and Pre-operative Preparation

Most orbital exenterations are performed under general anaesthesia and patients with significant medical comorbidities may benefit from loco-regional nerve blocks combined with intravenous sedation [8]. Pre-operative investigations should generally include full blood count, renal and liver function tests, clotting profile, and electrocardiography. Anaemic patients should also be cross-matched for possible blood transfusion. Systemic hypertension and glycaemia must be adequately controlled and, if possible, all antiplatelet agents and anticoagulants should be stopped before surgery.

Pre-operative computerised X-ray tomography is required to assess orbital bone involvement, and magnetic resonance imaging with contrast may also help to define the extent of soft tissue involvement, as well as detecting dural or perineural invasion [9].

A multidisciplinary approach is essential in planning the management of cases with sino-nasal or intracranial tumours invading the orbit and this may require involvement of head and neck surgeons, neurosurgeons, otorhinolaryngologists, plastic surgeons and medical or radiation oncologists.

4 How to Avoid Exenteration?

Orbital invasion by periocular cutaneous malignancies is the commonest indication for performing exenteration [10, 11], and so early detection, referral to secondary care, and adequate and timely treatment (surgery and/or adjunctive treatments) are critical for reducing the risk of future exenteration. Targeted therapies, such as BRAF inhibitors (e.g. vemurafenib, dabrafenib) for advanced conjunctival melanoma and sonic hedgehog signalling pathway inhibitors (e.g. vismodegib) for locally advanced basal cell carcinoma, may also be beneficial in selected cases (see Chapters "Management of Locally Invasive and Metastatic Eyelid Tumours" and "Secondary Orbital Tumours and Orbital Metastases") [12].

5 Types of Orbital Exenteration

In planning the type of exenteration, it is important to consider the extent and biologic behaviour of the orbital condition, the presence of local or distant spread, the reconstructive options, and the patient's preference.

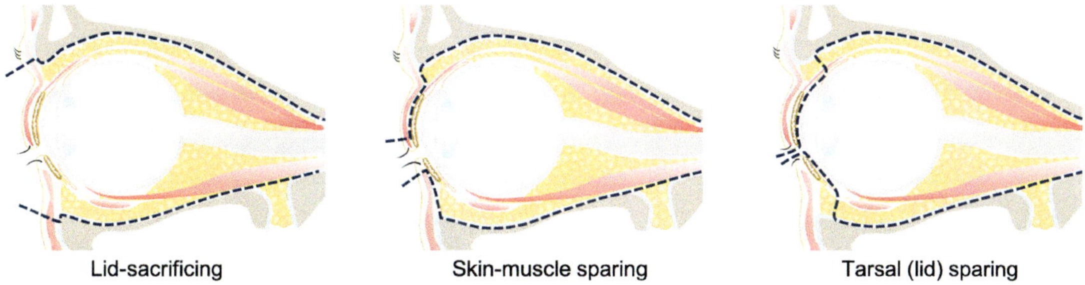

Fig. 1 Types of orbital exenteration

Methods of orbital exenteration (Fig. 1) can be considered as:

1. Lid-sacrificing, where all orbital soft tissues and eyelids are removed, with or without the eyebrow. This is usually required for extensive eyelid malignancies involving the orbit.
2. Skin-muscle sparing, where some of the skin and muscle from one or both eyelids is preserved, with primary closure of the skin-muscle flaps over the cavity. This method enables a very rapid rehabilitation [13] and is particularly useful for benign disease, post-septal intraorbital malignancy and for the palliation of fungating terminal malignancy.
3. Tarsal (eyelid sparing), where the tarsal plates and conjunctiva are spared, and may be applicable for posterior orbital malignancies. Preservation of tarso-conjunctiva allows formation of a rudimentary socket and use of an ocular prosthesis.

The extent of an orbital exenteration can be either "anterior partial" or "deep", the latter leaving a 5–8 mm soft tissue plug at the apex of the orbit. If safe to do so, the supraorbital nerve may also be spared.

Extended exenteration (combined exenteration; "superexenteration") involves removal of all soft tissues together with adjacent structures, such as bony walls and the neighbouring sinuses, and is usually performed for locally-advanced malignancies or sino-nasal tumours invading the orbit [14].

Orbital exenteration defects can also be classified into "Type I defects" limited to the orbit, "Type II defects" characterised by loss of one or more walls, "Type III defects" affecting the skull base, or "Type IV defects" with oro-orbital communication and usually seen after resection of extensive maxillary malignancies [15].

6 Surgical Technique

General anaesthesia with controlled hypotension is preferable, although the periorbital tissues can be infiltrated with either 2% lidocaine with 1:200,000 epinephrine, or 0.5% bupivacaine with 1:100,000 epinephrine (Fig. 2a). Intravenous tranexamic acid also helps to reduce intra-operative blood loss and the need for transfusion [16]. To minimise the local venous pressure, the head-end of the operating table should be elevated during surgery.

The eyelids are closed with a 2/0 silk traction suture (Fig. 2b). After marking a margin of at least 5 mm around the tumour, an incision is made either near the orbital rim (if dealing with extensive eyelid malignancy invading the orbit), or in the eyelid if a skin-muscle sparing exenteration is planned; if skin-muscle sparing, the sub-orbicularis (preseptal) plane is dissected widely out to the orbital rim (Fig. 2c), to create 1 or 2 intact skin-muscle flaps that can be slung aside with additional traction sutures during the procedure (Fig. 2d). Using monopolar in cutting mode aids in haemostasis and makes this dissection easier.

The periosteum is incised circumferentially (Fig. 3a) just outside the orbital rim, and reflected intact over the rim using a periosteal elevator (Rollet's rougine or Freer) (Fig. 3b). Most of the periosteum is loosely adherent to the bone, with resistance encountered at the arcus marginalis,

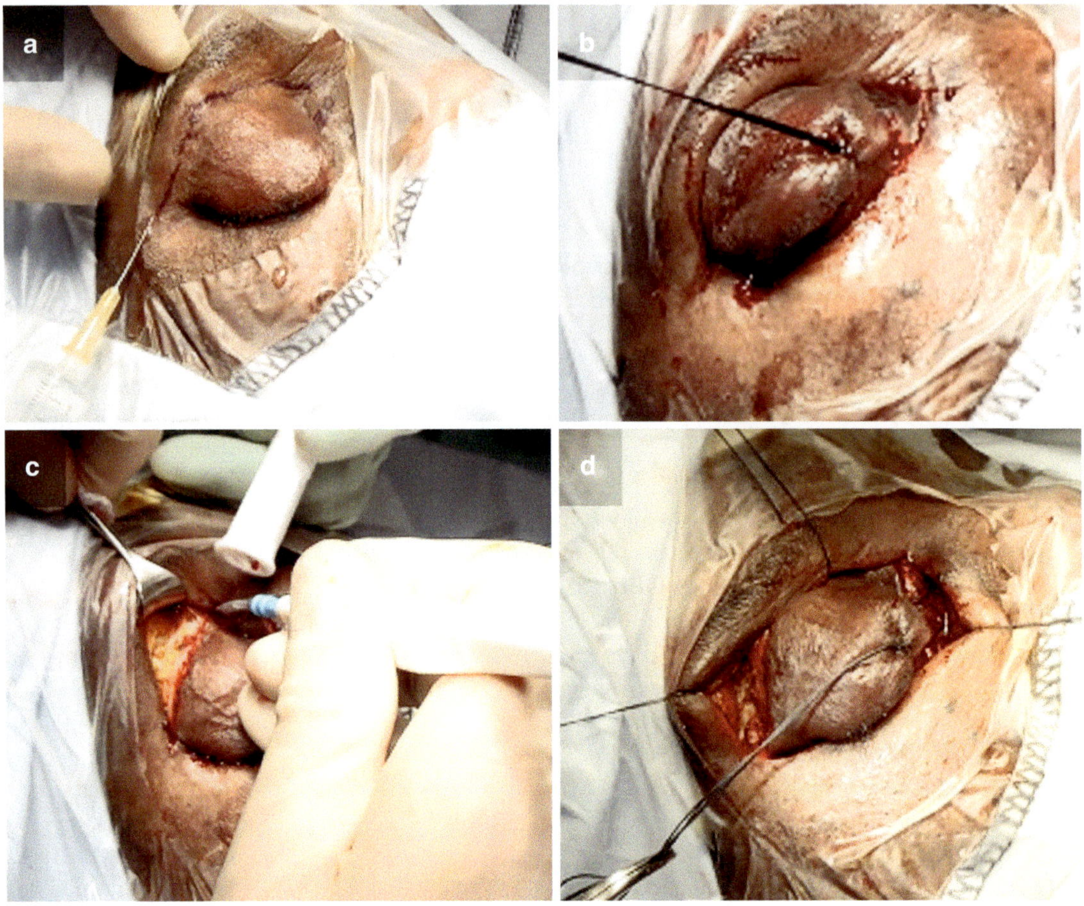

Fig. 2 Skin-muscle sparing exenteration—exposure of the orbital rim (**a**) infiltration of periorbital tissues with local anaesthesia. (**b**) Closure of the eyelid with 2/0 silk traction suture. (**c**) Dissection in the sub-orbicularis plane to expose the orbital rim. (**d**) Skin-muscle flaps are slung aside with additional traction sutures

the trochlear fossa, the interosseous suture lines and the lacrimal crests. Along the upper rim, the supraorbital and supratrochlear neurovascular bundles are identified and cauterised, the angular vessels are cauterised at the medial canthus, and the medial canthal tendon is divided and reflected laterally.

The periosteum is then raised from the orbital walls, aided by a wide malleable retractor (Fig. 3c), with particular care along the medial wall (Fig. 3d) to avoid fracturing the lacrimal bone and lamina papyracea that may lead to a chronic sino-orbital fistula. The anterior and posterior ethmoidal arteries, zygomatico-facial and zygomatico-temporal vessels, as well as the inferior and superior orbital fissures, are cauterised and divided, and the upper nasolacrimal duct freed.

Once the orbital contents have been mobilised within the periosteum, the posterior tissues are transected about 5–10 mm from the orbital apex using a monopolar diathermy in a blended cutting and coagulation mode (Fig. 3e, f); a snare or curved enucleation scissors can be used to divide the apical tissues, although this often leads to profuse haemorrhage. Meticulous haemostasis should be obtained with bipolar diathermy and bone wax applied to any bleeding perforating vessels.

With skin-muscle sparing exenteration, the orbicularis oculi on the upper and lower myocutaneous flaps is closed with multiple buried 5/0 soluble sutures to produce an airtight union, and the skin closed with a running 6/0 nylon suture. Drain placement in the socket should be avoided, as the goal is to create an air-tight closure of the

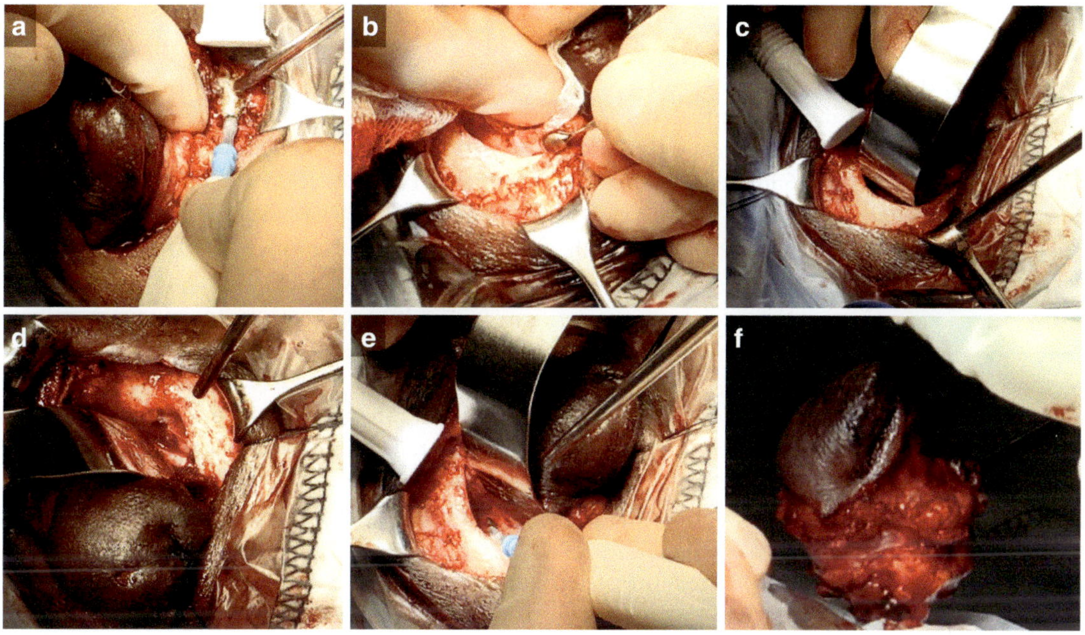

Fig. 3 Skin-muscle sparing exenteration—isolating and removal of the orbital contents. (**a**) Periosteum is incised just outside the orbital rim, and (**b**) raised 360° from the rim and the orbital walls (**c**, **d**). (**e**) Transection of the posterior orbital tissues using a monopolar diathermy. (**f**) Exenterated specimen

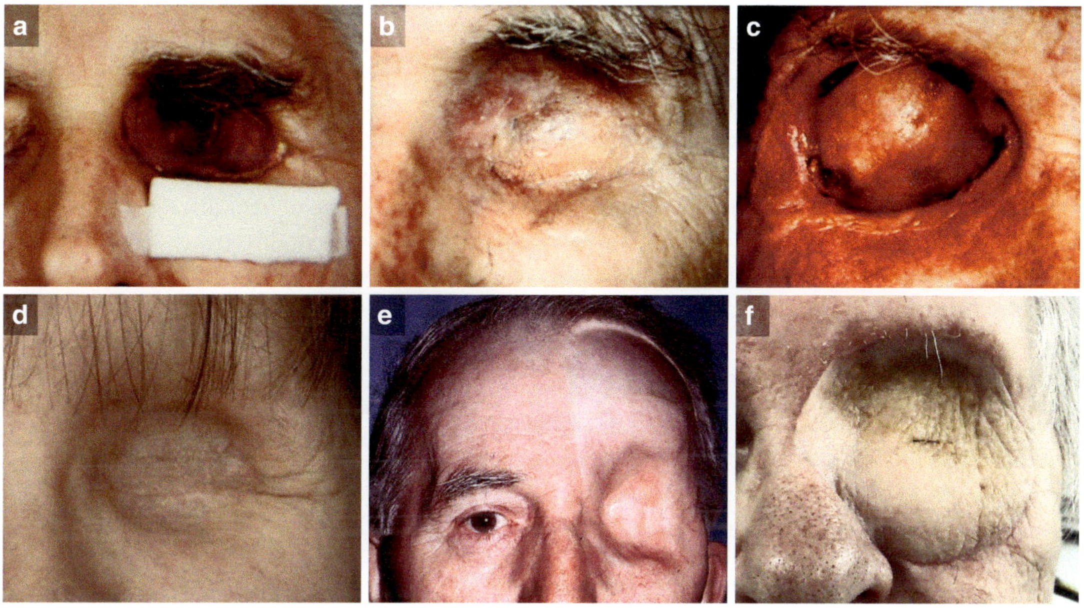

Fig. 4 Healed sockets after various repair methods. (**a**) Early granulation and (**b**) subsequent epithelialisation with deep socket formation following laissez-faire. (**c**) Split skin graft. (**d**) Skin muscle closure. (**e**) Rotation forehead flap. (**f**) Antero-lateral thigh free flap

closed cavity. If a lid-sacrificing (complete) exenteration has been performed, the socket can either be left to granulate or covered with split-thickness skin grafts (Fig. 4). A moderately firm dressing is applied for 1 week, and the patient discharged on a systemic oral antibiotic, with clear instruction to avoid nose-blowing for 2 weeks after surgery.

If the socket is left to granulate (laissez-faire), dressings are applied daily after the first week until granulation and epithelialization is complete, which usually takes 6 months, or longer in previously irradiated sockets. Small gauzes should be avoided as they can disappear into the granulation tissue.

7 Restoration of the Exenteration Cavity

The choice of reconstruction (Table 2) depends on the exenteration type and extent, on the proposed adjuvant treatment, and on the ability for the patient to tolerate multiple reconstructive procedures.

1. **Complete laissez-faire** involves removal of orbital contents and allowing spontaneous granulation to occur over a period of 14 weeks to 6 months [17] (Fig. 4a, b). Advantages of laissez faire include reduced surgical intervention, especially in elderly or frail patients, and the ability to monitor recurrences. Disadvantages include the prolonged healing, the need for frequent monitoring and dressings, and a high rate of sino-orbital fistula formation [18]. It also leaves a deep socket when healed, often with a large and "moist" air-space behind the epithesis.

Table 2 Reconstruction options for various types of orbital exenteration

Eyelid-sacrificing	Complete laissez-faire Partial laissez-faire Split skin grafting Local myocutaneous flap (e.g. rotational forehead flap) Temporalis transposition into the cavity and overlying skin-graft Larger free flaps (e.g. free myocutaneous graft)
Skin-muscle sparing	Direct closure Enhanced closure (glabellar flap, or cheek advancement flap)
Tarsal-sparing (True eyelid-sparing)	Direct conjunctival closure Secondary intention healing

2. **Partial laissez-faire,** where the residual skin is flapped backwards into the cavity and packed, to allow the skin to adhere to the underlying bone and any residual bare areas left to heal by granulation.
3. **Partial thickness skin grafting to the orbital cavity**. A split thickness skin is harvested, usually from the thigh, and secured into the orbital cavity. This technique is associated with a deep socket (Fig. 4c) and more difficult socket hygiene due to skin secretions.
4. **Skin-muscle closure:** where the eyelids are closed directly across the cavity, allowing rapid rehabilitation with the initial fitting of a prosthetic a few weeks after surgery and permitting early adjunctive orbital radiotherapy if required [13]. It also avoids the risk of donor-site morbidity associated with other reconstructive techniques, although additional local skin-muscle flaps may occasionally be necessary to allow complete cover of the cavity.
5. **Temporalis muscle transposition** into the cavity with or without overlying skin-graft. Advantages include covering orbital bones and reducing the risk of fistula formation, less socket care than the laissez-faire approach, and is particularly beneficial in patients due for early post-operative radiotherapy [19]. It adds volume to the orbit, but does result in deformity in the temporal fossa and possible difficulties with mastication [20].
6. **Loco-regional flaps**
   (a) Paramedian forehead flap, based on the supra-trochlear artery, is recommended for repair of nasal defects and especially for sinonasal fistulae near the nasal walls [21]. A limitation of this approach is that it must be performed as a two-stage procedure.
   (b) Cheek- advancement flap, a modification of the cervico-facial flap, permits a one-stage procedure allowing osseo-integration at the time of repair or at a later date [22]. It may be used in conjunction with a forehead advancement flap to cover any residual upper orbital defect [23].
   (c) Pericranial flap. The pericranium refers to the periosteum and subgaleal loose connective tissue which can be raised as a

thin, pliable and well-vascularized flap [21]. Direct coverage of the socket can be achieved with a galeal fascia flap, pedicled on the contralateral supraorbital vessel, this allowing faster epithelialization than spontaneous granulation [24]

(d) Pedicle flaps involve distant tissues being transferred to the recipient orbit bed and still perfused by the original arterial supply [17]. The frontal island flap is an example of pedicled flap based off the frontal branch of the superficial temporal artery [21].

7. **Microvascular free flaps** are useful for reconstructing large defects from extended exenteration, and involve harvesting autologous tissue from remote anatomical sites along with their vasculature and re-establishing blood supply by anastomosis with the recipient superficial temporal artery and vein [25]. Free flaps offer adequate tissue volume to cover the exenteration cavity and are beneficial in the setting of prior irradiation; however, they are difficult to perform and time consuming, with the risk of flap failure and donor site morbidity [2]. Commonly used free flaps include rectus abdominis [26], latissimus dorsi [27], radial forearm [25, 28] and antero-lateral thigh flap—the latter being described as a "workhorse" for repairing complex cranio-orbital defects [29].
8. **Other techniques**
   (a) Dermis-fat graft harvested from the abdomen may be used to reconstruct the orbit after subtotal exenteration in conjunction with a myocutaneous flap to provide the anterior vascular supply [30]. A meshed acellular dermal allograft or a synthetic bilayer matrix wound dressing can also be used as an alternative lining to split-thickness skin grafts [31, 32].

8 Complications Following Orbital Exenteration

Complications of exenteration are summarised in Table 3.

Table 3 Complications of orbital exenteration

Intra-operative	Breach of lamina papyracea
	Haemorrhage
	Exposure of dura mater
	Cerebrospinal fluid leak
Post-operative	Haemorrhage
	Infection
	"Blow-hole" fistula formation from sinus (sino-orbital fistula)
	Spontaneous necrosis of skin flaps and grafts, particularly if previously irradiated (orbito-cutaneous fistula))
	Delayed or incomplete socket granulation
	Osteonecrosis (especially with previously irradiated bone)
	Meningitis

8.1 Intra-operative Complications

Cerebrospinal fluid (CSF) leak during surgery has a reported incidence of 0.6% [33], mostly occurring in the context of extended exenteration with resection of orbital walls. Treatment may involve conservative measures, such as bed rest, or may require surgical closure [34]. Persistent haemorrhage, exposure of dura mater, and intracranial arterial avulsion of the temporal branch of the middle cerebral have also been reported [2, 35, 36].

8.2 Post-operative Complications

Infections should be treated with topical and broad-spectrum oral antibiotics, and sloughing of the graft or flap can be managed with cleaning and antibiotics, and/or debridement of devitalised tissue. Obliterating the orbit using local or free flaps is occasionally required to reduce the risk of serious intracranial infection [37].

Flap or graft necrosis (Fig. 5a) are usually encountered in the context of prior radiotherapy, multiple previous reconstructive procedures, diabetes and smoking. A localised break-down of the skin flaps may lead to formation of dry sinus to the exenteration cavity (Fig. 5b). Delayed socket granulation may also occur with laissez-faire or split-skin graft repair techniques, particularly in previously irradiated sockets.

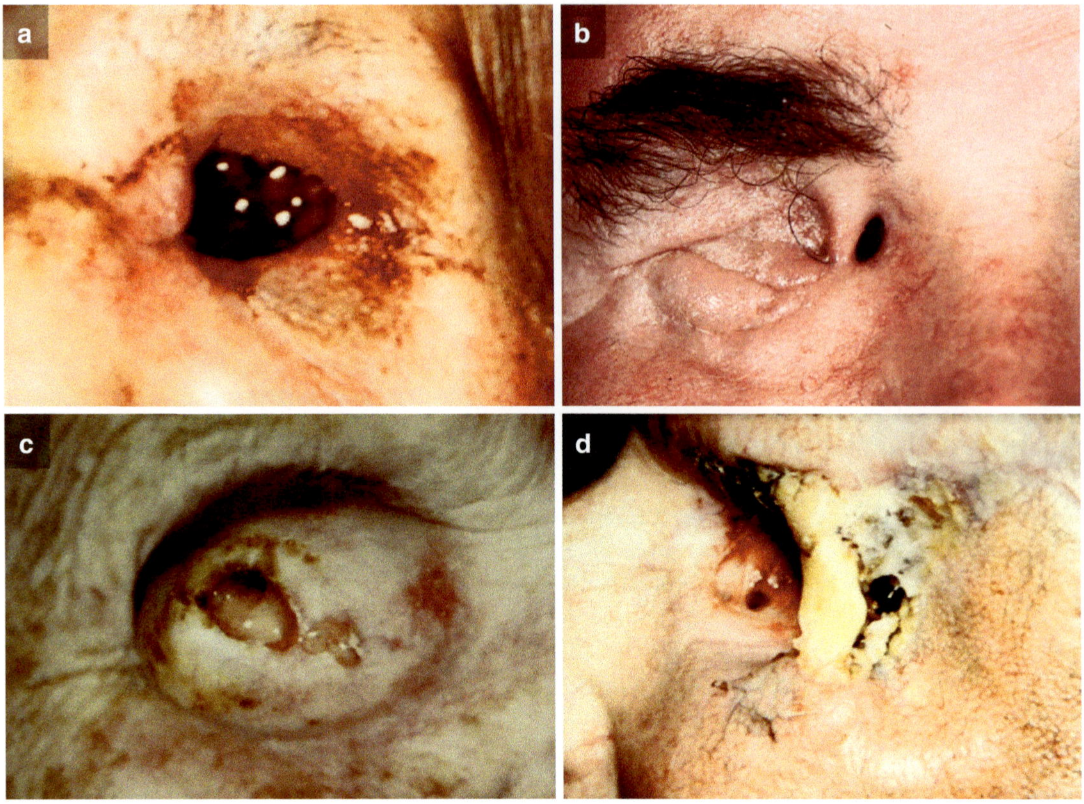

Fig. 5 Complications of exenteration. (**a**) Spontaneous necrosis of the skin flaps. (**b**) Formation of dry sinus to exenteration cavity. (**c**) Sinus blow-hole (sino-orbital fistula). (**d**) Ischaemic necrosis of the lateral orbital wall

A sino-orbital fistula, or "blow-hole", results from breakdown of the lamina papyracea, leading to communication between the ethmoid sinuses and the exenteration cavity, and a mucus-secreting surface in the socket (Fig. 5c). Non-healing fistulae can cause foul-smelling discharge, crusting, breakdown of skin, infection, and difficulty in wearing an epithesis. They are most commonly observed with spontaneous healing or skin grafting, but other risk factors including radiation, sinus disease, or immunocompromise [38]. Small fistulae may be managed conservatively, but larger ones may require ethmoidectomy and/or cover with flaps [2].

Osteoradionecrosis occurs where exposed previously-irradiated and devitalised bone fails to heal over 3 months (Fig. 5d), and management is difficult although debridement is indicated in severe cases. It is important to distinguish this from tumour recurrence, metastases or infection [39].

Cluster headache has been well documented following exenteration and may require targeted pain relief [40–42]. Chronic phantom eye pain and vision have also been reported in patients that have undergone exenteration and may require psychological input [43, 44].

9 Rehabilitation of the Exenterated Socket

Rehabilitation is accelerated to within weeks after surgery when the cavity is closed at the time of exenteration and skin-muscle flaps raised from as little as half an eyelid enable such direct closure. Larger defects may necessitate local flaps or free grafts, with associated donor-site morbidity and a higher complication rate. Rehabilitation of the exenterated patient and various types of exenteration prosthesis are described in Chapter "Rehabilitation of the Exenterated Socket".

References

1. Bartisch G, Stöckel M, Lessing J. Rosenwald. Ophthalmodoulei; das ist, Augendienst. Newer vnd wolgegründter Bericht von Vrsachen vnd Erkentnüs aller Gebrechen, Schäden vnd Mängel der Augen vnd des Gesichtes, wie man solchen anfenglich mit gebürlichen Mitteln begegenen, vorkommen vnd wehren, auch wie man alle solche Gebresten künstlich durch Artzney, I nstrument vnd Handgrieffe curiren, wircken vnd vertreiben sol. Colophon: Gedruckt zu Dressden durch Matthes Stöckel; 1583, 28 p.l., 274 numb. l., 15 pp.
2. Sagili S, Malhotra R. Orbital exenteration: indications, techniques and complications. Expert Rev Ophthalmol. 2016;11:201–13.
3. Vartanian JG, Toledo RN, Bueno T, Kowalski LP. Orbital exenteration for sinonasal malignancies: indications, rehabilitation and oncologic outcomes. Curr Opin Otolaryngol Head Neck Surg. 2018;26:122–6.
4. Ali MJ, Pujari A, Dave TV, Kaliki S, Naik MN. Clinicopathological profile of orbital exenteration: 14 years of experience from a tertiary eye care center in South India. Int Ophthalmol. 2016;36:253–8.
5. Rose GE, Wright JE. Exenteration for benign orbital disease. Br J Ophthalmol. 1994;78:14–8.
6. Tyers AG. Orbital exenteration for invasive skin tumours. Eye (Lond). 2006;20:1165–70.
7. Paridaens AD, McCartney AC, Minassian DC, Hungerford JL. Orbital exenteration in 95 cases of primary conjunctival malignant melanoma. Br J Ophthalmol. 1994;78:520–8.
8. Bhat MT, Hegde HV, Santhosh MC, Rao RP. Orbital exenteration under trigeminal block: An innovative method of regional anesthesia. Saudi J Anaesth. 2013;7:470–3.
9. Traylor JI, Christiano LD, Esmaeli B, Hanasono MM, Yu P, Suki D, Zhang W, Raza SM, Hanna EY, DeMonte F. Outcomes of orbital exenteration for craniofacial lesions. Cancer. 2021;127:2465–75.
10. Goldberg RA, Kim JW, Shorr N. Orbital exenteration: results of an individualized approach. Ophthalmic Plast Reconstr Surg. 2003;19:229–36.
11. Ben Simon GJ, Schwarcz RM, Douglas R, Fiaschetti D, McCann JD, Goldberg RA. Orbital exenteration: one size does not fit all. Am J Ophthalmol. 2005;139:11–7.
12. Sagiv O, Ding S, Ferrarotto R, Glisson B, Altan M, Johnson F, Elamin Y, Thakar SD, Nagarajan P, Esmaeli B. Impact of food and drug administration approval of vismodegib on prevalence of orbital exenteration as a necessary surgical treatment for locally advanced periocular basal cell carcinoma. Ophthalmic Plast Reconstr Surg. 2019;35:350–3.
13. Jayaprakasam A, Vahdani K, Rose GE, Saleh GM, Hussain B, Verity DH, Collin JRO. Rapid rehabilitation with skin-muscle sparing orbital exenteration: a single-center series. Ophthalmic Plast Reconstr Surg. 2021;37:51–4.
14. Sugawara T, Aoyagi M, Ogishima T, Kawano Y, Tamaki M, Yano T, Tsunoda A, Ohno K, Maehara T, Kishimoto S. Extended orbital exenteration for sinonasal malignancy with orbital apex extension: surgical technique and clinical analysis. J Neurosurg. 2015;123:52–8.
15. Kesting MR, Koerdt S, Rommel N, Mücke T, Wolff KD, Nobis CP, Ringel F, Frohwitter G. Classification of orbital exenteration and reconstruction. J Craniomaxillofac Surg. 2017;45:467–73.
16. Martin JP, Wang JS, Hanna KR, Stovall MM, Lin KY. Use of tranexamic acid in craniosynostosis surgery. Plast Surg (Oakv). 2015;23:247–51.
17. Levin PS, Ellis DS, Stewart WB, Toth BA, Orbital exenteration. The reconstructive ladder. Ophthalmic. Plast Reconstr Surg. 1991;7:84–92.
18. Mohr C, Esser J. Orbital exenteration: surgical and reconstructive strategies. Graefes Arch Clin Exp Ophthalmol. 1997;235:288–95.
19. Wirth-Welle RB, Chaloupka K. Early surgical rehabilitation due to modified exenteration technique. Klin Monbl Augenheilkd. 2013;230:380–4.
20. Levin PS, Dutton JJ. A 20-year series of orbital exenteration. Am J Ophthalmol. 1991;112:496–501.
21. Jategaonkar AA, Vernon D, Byrne PJ. Regional reconstruction of orbital exenteration defects. Semin Plast Surg. 2019;33:120–4.
22. Sira M, Malhotra R. Reconstruction of orbital exenteration defects by primary closure using cheek advancement. Br J Ophthalmol. 2013;97:201–5.
23. Bilge AD, Yazici B, Efe AC. Reconstruction of orbital exenteration defect with cheek or combined cheek and forehead advancement flaps. Ophthalmic Plast Reconstr Surg. 2021;37:346–51.
24. Zwahlen RA, Grätz KW, Obwegeser JA. The galea fascia flap in orbital reconstruction: innovative harvest technique. Eur J Surg Oncol. 2006;32:804–7.
25. López F, Suárez C, Carnero S, Martín C, Camporro D, Llorente JL. Free flaps in orbital exenteration: a safe and effective method for reconstruction. Eur Arch Otorhinolaryngol. 2013;270:1947–52.
26. Pryor SG, Moore EJ, Kasperbauer JL. Orbital exenteration reconstruction with rectus abdominis microvascular free flap. Laryngoscope. 2005;115:1912–6.
27. Donahue PJ, Liston SL, Falconer DP, Manlove JC. Reconstruction of orbital exenteration cavities. The use of the latissimus dorsi myocutaneous free flap. Arch Ophthalmol. 1989;107:1681–3.
28. Tahara S, Susuki T. Eye socket reconstruction with free radial forearm flap. Ann Plast Surg. 1989;23:112–6.

29. Parkes WJ, Krein H, Heffelfinger R, Curry J. Use of the anterolateral thigh in cranio-orbitofacial reconstruction. Plast Surg Int. 2011;2011:941742.
30. Shore JW, Burks R, Leone CR, McCord CD. Dermis-fat graft for orbital reconstruction after subtotal exenteration. Am J Ophthalmol. 1986;102:228–36.
31. Young SM, Park JW, Kim YD, Woo KI. Use of meshed acellular dermal allograft as a lining material after orbital exenteration. Ophthalmic Plast Reconstr Surg. 2020;36:349–54.
32. Rafailov L, Turbin RE, Langer PD. Use of bilayer matrix wound dressing in the exenterated socket. Orbit. 2017;36:397–400.
33. Limawararut V, Valenzuela AA, Sullivan TJ, McNab AA, Malhotra R, Davis G, Jones N, Selva D. Cerebrospinal fluid leaks in orbital and lacrimal surgery. Surv Ophthalmol. 2008;53:274–84.
34. Massoud VA, Fay A, Yoon MK. Cerebrospinal fluid leak as a complication of oculoplastic surgery. Semin Ophthalmol. 2014;29:440–9.
35. de Conciliis C, Bonavolontà G. Incidence and treatment of dural exposure and CSF leak during orbital exenteration. Ophthalmic Plast Reconstr Surg. 1987;3:61–4.
36. Gonzalez LF, Bilyk JR. Intracranial arterial avulsion during orbital exenteration. Orbit. 2012;31:190–3.
37. Spiegel JH, Varvares MA. Prevention of postexenteration complications by obliteration of the orbital cavity. Skull Base. 2007;17:197–203.
38. Limawararut V, Leibovitch I, Davis G, Rees G, Goldberg RA, Selva D. Sino-orbital fistula: a complication of exenteration. Ophthalmology. 2007;114:355–61.
39. Peter NM, Laitt R, Leatherbarrow B. Osteoradionecrosis of the exenterated orbit. Orbit. 2014;33:220–2.
40. Bond JB, Wesley RE. Cluster headache after orbital exenteration. Ann Ophthalmol. 1987;19:438.
41. McKinney AS. Cluster headache developing following ipsilateral orbital exenteration. Headache. 1983;23:305–6.
42. Evers S, Sörös P, Brilla R, Gerding H, Husstedt IW. Cluster headache after orbital exenteration. Cephalalgia. 1997;17:680–2.
43. Rasmussen ML, Prause JU, Toft PB. Phantom pain after eye amputation. Acta Ophthalmol. 2011;89:10–6.
44. Maloof AJ. Phantom vision: a graphic description. Ophthalmic Plast Reconstr Surg. 2004;20:80–1.

Rehabilitation of the Exenterated Socket

Valerio Cervelli and Davide Johan Bottini

Key Messages

- Epitheses are the preferred rehabilitative option for exenterated orbits due to their ease of use, bio-tolerability and low cost.
- Osseointegrated prostheses are particularly beneficial in extended exenterations and severe orbito-cranio-facial trauma.
- Titanium implants can be positioned in a one-step procedure under local anaesthesia with mild sedation.
- Osseointegrated implantation is an effective alternative to autologous reconstructive flaps and grafts for complex orbital defects, where traditional reconstructive methods have failed or are contraindicated.

1 Introduction

Orbital exenteration is a radical procedure that causes significant functional and psychosocial morbidity, and rehabilitation following exenteration is crucial for minimising its negative impact on patients' quality of life.

Cosmetic and social rehabilitation can be challenging in patients with large or complex orbital defects, and it may be unattractive because of the need for additional interventions and cost. The extent of the defect and the type of reconstruction have a major impact on rehabilitation, with a satisfactory aesthetic appearance feasible in the presence of an intact bony orbit and adequate soft tissue cover. Cosmesis is best achieved with an orbital prosthesis, although some patients may prefer to conceal the defect with an eye patch. Types of exenteration prosthesis include stick-on (adhesive) prosthesis with or without glasses, glasses-borne prosthesis, obturator prosthesis (when some eyelid is preserved), and osseointegrated mountings.

With advances in anaplastology, epitheses have become the preferred rehabilitative option, owing to their ease of use, bio-tolerability, and low cost, albeit a stable fixation to the orbit is difficult to establish, particularly with glass-borne and adhesive prostheses. To overcome this limitation, prostheses retained by bone-anchored implants have been designed, based on the concept of implant osseointegration first described by Brånemark et al. in 1969 [1]. Since then, several protocols have been developed according to the material type, biocompatibility, and the osseointegration process [2–5], with modern anaplastology allowing the fabrication of high-quality prostheses that replicate the contralateral orbit and eye [4, 5]. Osseointegrated prostheses are particularly beneficial in the context of extended exenterations, malformations, and severe orbito-cranio-facial trauma. This chapter describes the use of bone-anchored prostheses in

V. Cervelli · D. J. Bottini (✉)
Department of Plastic and Reconstructive Surgery, Università degli Studi di Roma Tor Vergata, Rome, Italy
e-mail: d.bottini@me.com

F. M. Quaranta Leoni et al. (eds.), *Oculoplastic, Lacrimal and Orbital Surgery*,
https://doi.org/10.1007/978-3-031-39638-0_5

craniofacial reconstructive surgery, focusing on the rehabilitation of the exenterated orbit.

2 Surgical Technique

2.1 Stage One: Placement of the Implants

Osseointegrated titanium implants, specifically designed for extraoral use, are placed in a one-step procedure under local anaesthesia with mild sedation. The site and orientation of the implants are determined by the anatomy and quality of the bone, as well as the stability requirements of the epithesis. A pre-operative computed tomography scan (CT) is necessary for assessing the bone thickness and density, and optimising implant placement.

The orbital rim is exposed by raising a subperiosteal flap of soft tissues and retention holes are created with a low speed and high torque drill, using specifically designed drill cutters. Progressive widening of the holes enables primary and stable retention of the implants (Fig. 1). Fixtures with a diameter of 3 or 4 mm and a length of 5 mm provide adequate stability, and once the implants are positioned and secured, the healing abutment is placed on the fixture and the flap is repositioned to fit the protruding abutment.

Prophylactic antibiotics are used during and after surgery, and post-operative analgesia with paracetamol is sufficient for most patients; persistent post-operative pain is unusual in the absence of post-operative complications. The surgical wound usually heals in 7–10 days, following which the sutures are removed. Once the skin has healed completely, the print transfer and manufacture of the epithesis are carried out.

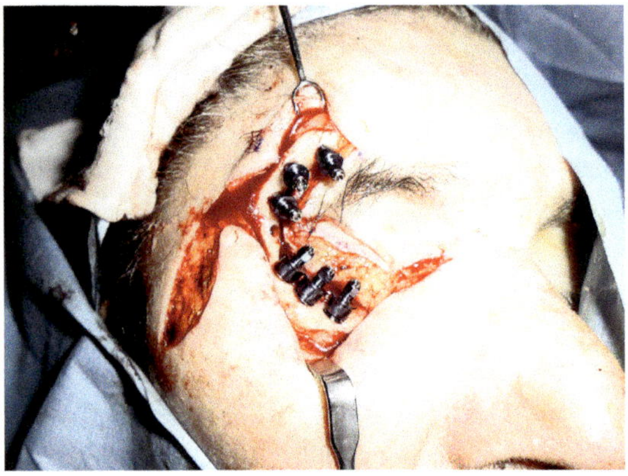

Fig. 1 Intra-operative view of the implants fixed to the bony orbital rim

The implants may cause a foreign body inflammatory reaction, albeit this is minimal with titanium implants, which have a low risk of long-term rejection. Proteoglycans and sparse inflammatory cells form a thin, non-reactive layer around the implant. Osseous integration occurs as a result of interactions between implants and recipient tissues, leading to formation of a layer of titanium oxide 20–50 Å thick, which promotes the development of chemical bonds in the tissue and prevents titanium decay over time. This one-step procedure and the early reconstruction allows a fast rehabilitation of the exenterated socket.

2.2 Stage Two: Prosthesis Manufacturing and Anchoring

Following the healing of the soft tissues, the second step begins with the manufacture of the prosthesis by specialised anaplastologists. The epithesis is created using a wax model, and consists of two parts: an acrylic plate that holds the clips (to be anchored) and a soft silicon part modelled on the contralateral orbit with a similar chromatic shade (Fig. 2a, c). A plaster model is utilised as a reference, with the abutment position reproduced, to create the structure that will allow the abutments to be positioned.

There are several retaining systems, and the most commonly used is a gold-platinum-iridium bar (Fig. 2b) soldered to white gold rings and positioned to correspond with the transcutaneous titanium cylinders. Resin and silicon, the components that comprise the epithesis, degrade over time and must be replaced every 2 years. For the summer months, a differently coloured prosthesis can be made to better blend in with the patient's

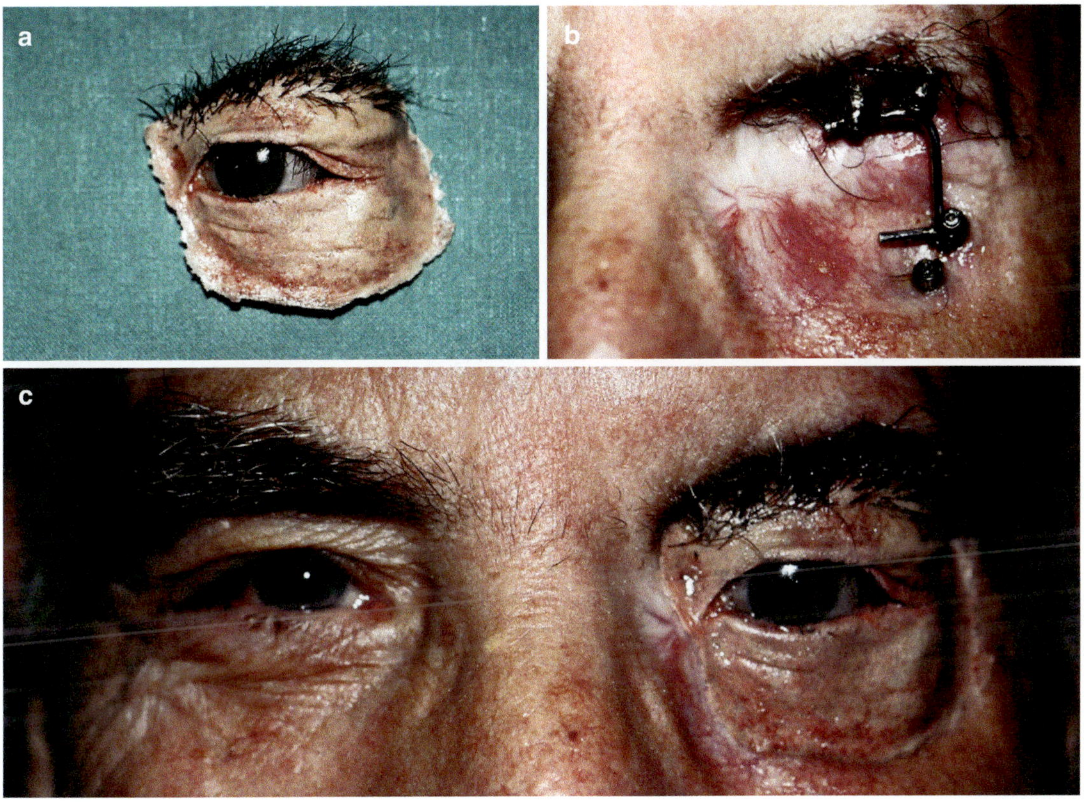

Fig. 2 (**a**) Ocular and orbital prosthesis. (**b**) Anchorage bar over-structure for attachment of the prosthesis. (**c**) Appearance of the mounted prosthesis

skin tone. Cleaning of the prosthesis should include the holding structures, abutments, and surrounding skin.

In most patients only the orbit and periorbital soft tissues are reconstructed, while other cases require complex repair of both the orbit and the maxilla.

Patient selection and a careful pre-operative evaluation of anatomical abnormalities caused by trauma (Fig. 3) or tumour ablative surgery are essential, as well as photographic documentation in three standard projections. All patients require a 2D and 3D CT to rule out local tumour recurrence and to plan the position of bone fixtures and the manufacture of the epithesis.

Fixtures may be applied immediately after orbital exenteration or after a recovery period, depending on the probability of disease recurrence. They can be implanted 9–12 months following radiotherapy.

During surgery, bone-anchored implants are placed on the orbital rim to provide support for the epithesis. Post-operatively, incisions, scars, and implants are checked for stability and infection. Single-photon emission computerised tomography (S.P.E.C.T.) or bone scintigraphy can be used to assess the metabolism of the tissues surrounding the implant, which is helpful in monitoring the functional dynamics of the bone-anchoring and detecting fixture failure caused by bone resorption.

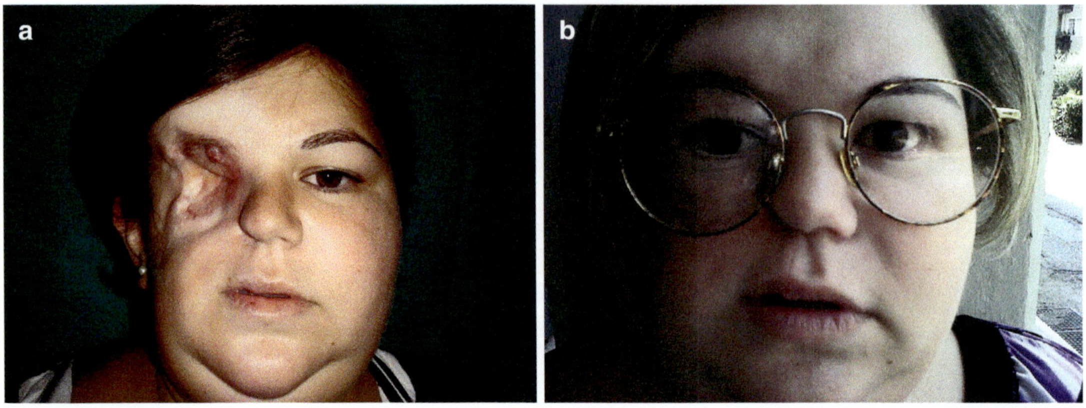

Fig. 3 (**a**) Cranio-orbito-facial trauma in a 14-year-old female. This patient sustained craniofacial trauma to the right fronto-temporal-orbital region, resulting in loss of the right eye and periorbital tissues, and was referred for rehabilitation following neurosurgical intervention with fracture repair. Due to scarred skin and inadequate local soft tissues, a bone-anchored prosthesis was chosen. Surgery was performed under local anaesthesia with sedation, and five fixtures were placed on the lateral and superolateral orbital rim. The patient was discharged the following day, the sutures were removed 8 days later, and the print transfer procedure started, with a manufactured prosthesis covering the deformity 20 days after surgery. (**b**) Appearance with bone-anchored prosthesis. During a 5-year follow-up period, there were no complications or implant failure

3 Alternative Techniques for Orbital Reconstruction

Orbital reconstructive procedures aim to create a bowl-shaped cavity for future prosthesis placement. The skeletal component can be restored using autologous rib, calvarial bone [6], iliac crest grafts, or free fibula flaps [7], while the soft tissues can be repaired with direct skin-muscle closure (where possible) [8], various loco-regional flaps such as sliding pedicled flaps of the temporal muscle and fascia [9], or distant microvascular flaps, as indicated in Chapter 4 "Orbital Exenteration". Combined flaps using temporalis muscle fascia and facial-cervical-perioral fascia are also described for reconstruction of extensive soft tissue defects [10]. The condition of periorbital tissues is crucial in reconstructions using local flaps or grafts, with previous irradiation or scarring potentially compromising the local vascular supply, resulting in unfavourable outcomes.

Ocular prostheses can be used after reconstructive procedures to improve cosmetic rehabilitation. Direct skin-muscle closure over an exenteration cavity provides a shallow cavity ideal for fitting an episthesis [8]. Skin-grafting or secondary intention healing, on the other hand, forms an extremely deep cavity, which promotes skin maceration in the humid environment behind an epithesis. Tarsal plates and conjunctival preservation allow for the formation of a rudimentary socket and the use of an ocular prosthesis (see chapter "Orbital Exenteration").

4 Complications of Osseointegrated Implants

Most of the extraoral bone-anchored prosthesis complications are due to failure of the osseointegration, with implant loss occurring at any point after surgery. Early post-operative causes of failure include surgical wound dehiscence or infection. Late bone exposure, peri-implantitis, and implant loss are usually the result of inadequate bone/implant margin care and may be avoided with proper wound hygiene and disinfection. Although relatively uncommon, peri-implantitis can result in loss of the implants within 6 months. Additional fixtures can be placed to maintain the bone anchoring stability for epithesis when an implant is lost.

Implant malposition is another complication, leading to fixation loss of the prosthesis. We have encountered three such cases, referred from other centres requiring implant exchange; in one case, a fixture had penetrated the anterior skull base, causing epileptic seizures. The bone-retaining system can occasionally break due to trauma, and if the fixture is not damaged, the over-structure can be replaced. We have observed one such case, which was managed by replacing the broken abutment and bar.

In summary, osseointegrated implantation is an effective alternative to autologous reconstructive flaps and grafts, when traditional reconstructive methods have failed or are inapplicable; it can also be a primary reconstructive option for complex defects. It is relatively simple to perform and has good cosmesis and biotolerability. Materials such as titanium offer durability, mechanical resistance, and, most importantly, bio-integration into the bone. The quality of the reconstruction is influenced by pre-procedure planning, precise implant positioning, and the expertise of the anaplastologists; hence, close collaboration between the surgeon and the anaplastologist is essential for achieving best outcomes [4]. Daily cleaning of the skin around the implants and the supporting structures is also important for optimal long-term outcomes, which requires education of patients and caregivers.

References

1. Brånemark PI, Breine U, Adell R, Hansson BO, Lindström J, Ohlsson A. Intra-osseous anchorage of dental prostheses: I. Experimental studies. Scand J Plast Reconstr Surg. 1969;3:81–100.
2. Gentile P, Bottini DJ, Colicchia GM, Trimarco A, Cervelli V. Burns: Bone-anchored, Extra-oral implantology. J Burn Care Res. 2008 Jul;29:627–31.
3. Brånemark PI, Albrektsson T. Titanium implants permanently penetrating human skin. Scand J Plast Reconstr Surg Hand Surg. 1982;16:17–21.
4. Cervelli V, Bottini DJ, Arpino A, Colicchia M, Mugnaini F, Trimarco A, et al. Orbital reconstruction: bone-anchored implants. J Craniofac Surg. 2006;17:848–53.
5. DeSerres JJ, Budden CR, Wolfaardt JF, Wilkes GH. Long-term follow-up of osseointegrated orbital prosthetic reconstruction. J Craniofac Surg. 2017;28:1901–5.
6. Artico M, Ferrante L, Pastore FS, Ramundo EO, Cantarelli D, Scopelliti D, et al. Bone autografting of the calvaria and craniofacial skeleton: Historical background, surgical results in a series of 15 patients, and review of the literature. Surg Neurol. 2003;60:71–9.
7. Chang DW, Langstein HN. Use of the free fibula flap for restoration of orbital support and midfacial projection following maxillectomy. J Reconstr Microsurg. 2003;19:147–52.
8. Jayaprakasam A, Vahdani K, Rose GE, Saleh GM, Hussain B, Verity DH, Collin JRO. Rapid rehabilitation with skin-muscle sparing orbital exenteration: a single-center series. Ophthalmic Plast Reconstr Surg. 2021;37:51–4.
9. Cordeiro PG. Reverse temporalis muscle flap for the reconstruction of orbital exenteration defects: Invited discussion. Ann Plast Surg. 2002;48:526–7.
10. Cuesta-Gil M, Concejo C, Acero J, Navarro-Vila C, Ochandiano S. Repair of large orbito-cutaneous defects by combining two classical flaps. J Craniomaxillofac Surg. 2004;32:21–7.

Post Enucleation Socket Syndrome

Christoph Hintschich and Mikhail Kataev

Key Messages

- Post-enucleation socket syndrome (PESS) is characterised by enophthalmos of the artificial eye, deep upper eyelid sulcus, and eyelid malposition as a result of socket volume deficiency and soft tissue redistribution after eye removal.
- The loss of the eyeball and absence of primary implant account for most of the volume deficit, with other factors such as chronic inflammation, orbital infection, trauma, and radiation also playing a role.
- PESS can be associated with various degrees of socket contraction.
- Primary insertion of an adequate orbital implant is the most effective way to prevent the development of PESS.
- Surgical management of PESS aims to correct orbital volume deficit, eyelid malpositions (such as eyelid laxity, entropion, ptosis, or retraction), and any associated socket contraction.
- Orbital volume deficiency should be addressed prior to any eyelid surgery.

1 Clinical Features of Post-enucleation Socket Syndrome

Removal of an eye causes orbital volume deficiency and soft tissue architectural changes leading to the clinical features of the post-enucleation socket syndrome (PESS), a term originally coined by Tyers and Collin [1]. PESS can occur after both enucleation and evisceration and is characterised by:

- enophthalmos of the artificial eye
- deep upper eyelid sulcus
- lower eyelid laxity
- upper eyelid malposition, such as eyelid retraction or ptosis
- tilting of the prosthesis, associated with an anterior-to-posterior and superior-to-inferior rotation of orbital tissues [2]

Patients with PESS often have an undesirable appearance due to enophthalmos, hollow upper eyelid sulcus, or eyelid malposition (Figs. 1a, 2a, and 3a); however, a prosthesis can usually be fitted and retained unless there is concurrent high degree of socket contraction (see chapter "Management of Contracted Socket").

Mild socket contraction results in lagophthalmos, entropion, lower eyelid retraction, and forniceal shortening due to the contraction of the conjunctiva and underlying orbital soft tissues; however, an artificial eye can usually be retained.

C. Hintschich (✉)
Department of Ophthalmology, Ludwig-Maximilians-University, Munich, Germany
e-mail: christoph.hintschich@med.uni-muenchen.de

M. Kataev
Oculoplastic Department, S. Fyodorov Eye Microsurgery Federal Institute, Moscow, Russia

F. M. Quaranta Leoni et al. (eds.), *Oculoplastic, Lacrimal and Orbital Surgery*,
https://doi.org/10.1007/978-3-031-39638-0_6

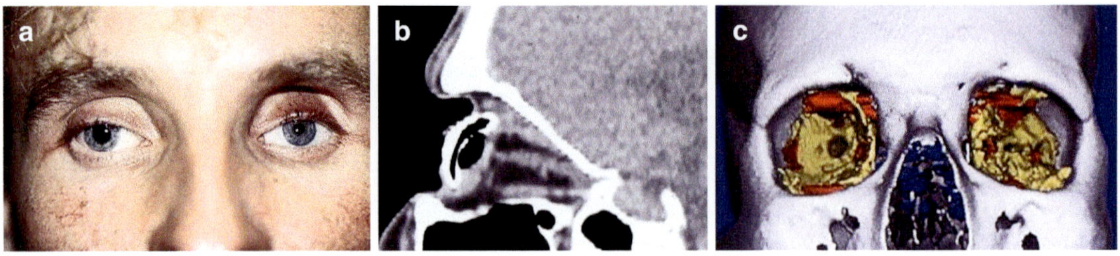

Fig. 1 (**a**) Clinical photography of a young male patient with left acquired anophthalmos showing typical signs of a post-enucleation socket syndrome (PESS) with deep upper sulcus and enophthalmos of the artificial eye. (**b**) CT-scan (sagittal plane) of the same patient showing the typical radiological findings of PESS with enophthalmos and tilting of the artificial eye, deep superior sulcus and anterior shift of the inferior fat pad. (**c**) CT-based volumetric reconstruction of the bony orbit, extraocular muscles and orbital fat compartment shows a displacement of orbital fat tissue, but no orbital fat atrophy (Orbital fat volume Orb enuc [L]: 9.0 mL, Δ: +15.5%)

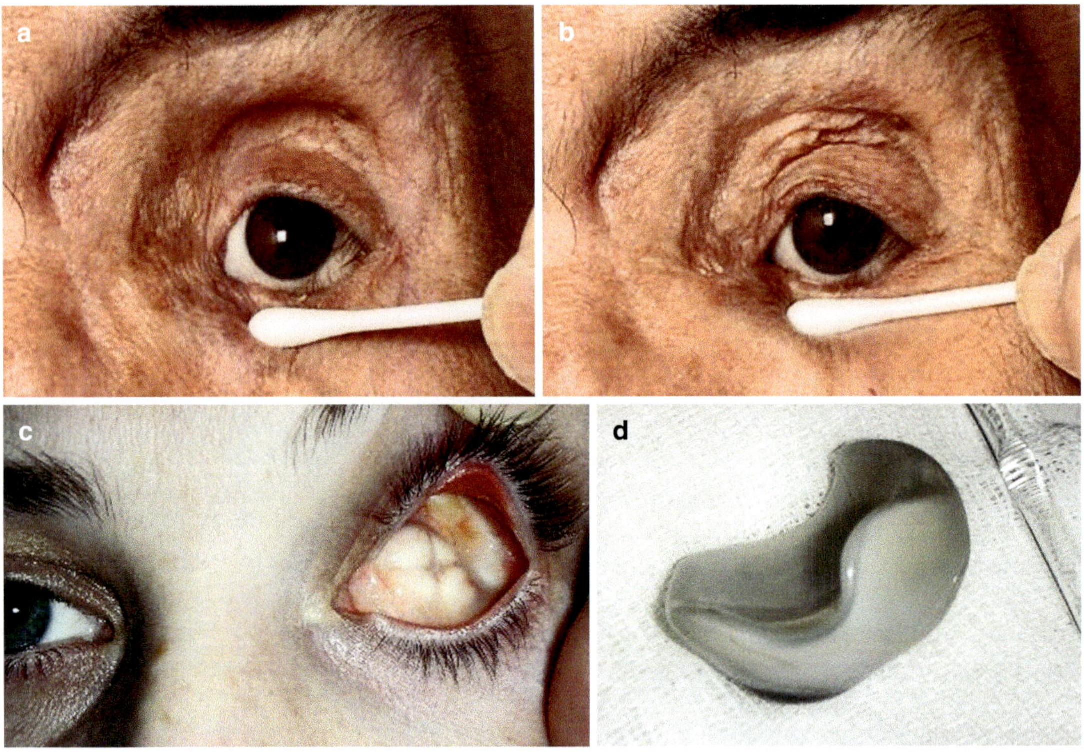

Fig. 2 (**a**) Clinical picture of left PESS showing signs of volume deficit with a deep upper sulcus. A cotton swab is gently apposed without pressure on the lower eyelid. (**b**) Same patient, now with the cotton swab gently pressing on the inferior orbital septum, resulting in filling of the upper sulcus and demonstrating mobile orbital fat compartments, a good indication for secondary orbital implantaction with a favorable prognosis. (**c**) Socket appearance after evisceration without orbital implant showing volume deficiency and a deep supero-temporal fornix. (**d**) Artificial eye of the same patient. A large prosthesis had to be fitted in the socket to fill the volume deficit. The asymmetric unbalanced shape is associated with further gradual shifting of orbital soft tissue downwards and anteriorly

More advanced forniceal contraction causes spontaneous loss of the prosthesis, whilst severe socket contraction with total loss of the conjunctival lining or ankyloblepharon precludes the use of an artificial eye. Often, there is associated secretion and chronic discharge. Features of both conditions (PESS and contracted socket) may co-occur in any combination.

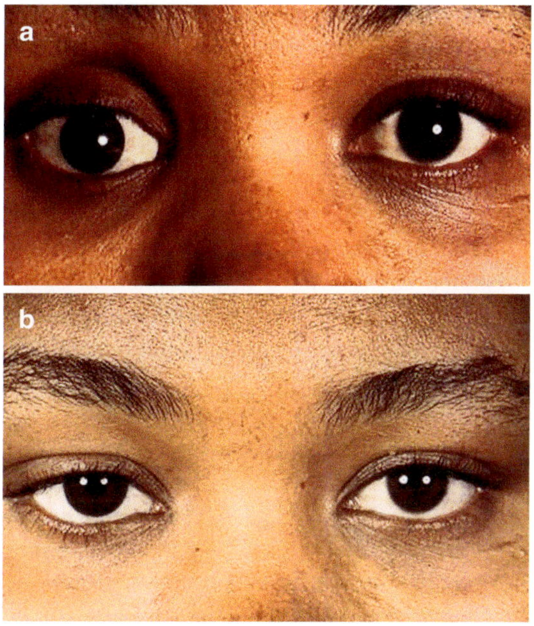

Fig. 3 (**a**) A young female patient with right PESS. (**b**) Same patient six months after right secondary orbital implant (Mersilene-mesh covered silicone sphere)

2 Pathophysiology

The anophthalmic socket is a complex system that includes orbital soft tissues such as extraocular muscles, orbital fat, and fibrous connective tissue with its vessels and nerves, as well as the orbital implant and prosthetic eye, if present (Fig. 1b, c).

Numerous pathophysiologic mechanisms are implicated in the development of PESS, including volume deficiency, structural changes and disorganisation of the remaining orbital contents, fat atrophy, retraction or stretching of extraocular muscles, loss of support for the levator system, and displacement of the Tenon's capsule [1, 3–13].

The loss of the eyeball accounts for most of the volume deficit, which can be variable due to significant inter-individual variations; the mean eyeball volume is 7.3 mL (5.7–11.1 mL). Extraocular muscle volumes are also reduced by up to 16%, but due to their relatively small volume (4.5 mL), this has a limited impact on overall volume changes [14]. Orbital fat atrophy is not always present in PESS (Fig. 1c), however persistent inflammation, trauma, orbital abscess, socket radiation, and secondary orbital implantation can cause fat atrophy and contribute to the development of PESS [14]. On the other hand, long-standing acquired anophthalmos, both in children and adults, is associated with a reduction in bony orbital volume. However, the bony orbital changes are smaller than generally assumed and tend not to cause obvious facial asymmetry [15].

The pathophysiology of PESS and its clinical features differ slightly in cases of enucleation and evisceration. Following evisceration, the internal fascial network of the orbit remains intact, resulting in less displacement of the orbital content.

To summarise, PESS is caused by an inadequate orbital volume replacement and possibly volume redistribution, as well as changes in eyelid supporting structures and ligaments. This condition can be prevented by primary positioning of an adequate orbital implant.

3 Pre-operative Assessment

Before considering any surgical correction, the patient's concerns and clinical features must be thoroughly evaluated. History taking should determine the most troublesome symptom(s), its duration, any associated pain or discomfort, cosmetic issues, spontaneous loss of the artificial eye, incomplete eyelid closure or eyelid malposition. Previous surgeries, type of orbital implant (if present), prior radiotherapy and difficulties in fitting the prosthesis should all be explored.

Clinical evaluation should include the overall appearance, symmetry, position, and stability of the artificial eye, spontaneous loss or inability to wear a prosthesis, the presence of enophthalmos, and the shape and depth of the upper eyelid sulcus (Fig. 2a–d). Palpation of the socket aids in the detection of an alloplastic orbital implant, whilst slit lamp examination is useful in examining the fornices, the lining (conjunctiva, mucous membrane, skin), and the presence of conjunctival or subconjunctival scars or symblepharon [16]. Volume deficit and signs of possible implant erosion or extrusion must be investigated. In patients with a history of chronic discharge or significant secretion, it is essential to meticulously search for conjunctival dehiscence or erosion, and a moist cotton bud is usually helpful. Finally, the prosthetic eye should be assessed in terms of size, shape, surface deposits, and roughness of edges.

3.1 Orbital Imaging.

Imaging is very useful in assessing the altered anatomy of bone and orbital soft tissues. MRI and CT scans both show the position of the extraocular muscles (EOM), their relationship to each other and to adjacent structures, and the displacement of fat compartments within the bony orbit (Fig. 1b). CT can also reveal previous undiagnosed orbital fractures with consequent displaced orbital contents.

Imaging allows to analyse:

- *Orbital implant*
  The presence, size, shape and position of an orbital implant should be evaluated by inspecting the coronal, the axial and the sagittal planes.
- *Extraocular muscles*
  The recti muscles still form the muscle cone, but occupy less space. The superior rectus and levator muscles, in particular, sag downward from their original position, whereas the inferior oblique muscle shifts anteriorly, determining shallowing of the inferior fornix.
- *Orbital fascial network*
  Gravity appears to be the main mechanism of soft tissue dystopia, which is normally counteracted by the orbital connective tissue network. Enucleation disrupts the attachments of this network's fibres to the globe, leading to sequential disintegration of the peri- and retrobulbar suspension meshwork, which is particularly notable in elderly patients. [17, 18]
- *Orbital fat pad*
  Extra- and intraconal portions of the orbital fat are interconnected by fibres. Therefore, displacement of one compartment causes displacement of the adjacent one. The descent of the central fat pad induces sagging of the superior rectus/levator muscle complex, drawing the retro-septal upper fat pad backward, resulting in significant deepening of the upper eyelid sulcus. Fat depletion exacerbates the signs of PESS in cases of severe trauma or malignancy.
- *Conjunctival space*
  The spatial configuration of the socket in PESS is characterised by an expanded volume of the cavity with a nearly spherical shape, and deepening of the supero-lateral fornix due to the lack of an adequate orbital implant.

3.2 Prosthesis Fitting

To adequately fit an empty socket, the prosthesis will typically have a thicker upper part and a thinner bottom part for the superior and inferior fornices, respectively (Fig. 2d). Such imbalance of the artificial eye is rather harmful to the socket because it will inevitably lead to further deformity over time. Every successive ocularist adjustment exacerbates this uneven shape, with long-term use of progressively unbalanced prostheses causing inferior fornix shallowing and eyelid malposition.

In a "balanced" shaped socket, the depth of the superior and inferior fornices corresponds to the normal proportions of the conjunctival *cul-de-sacs*. Such sockets have an even crescent-like profile that allows adequate prosthesis fitting, although a slight antero-inferior displacement of the orbital soft tissues is acceptable.

4 Principles of Socket Surgery

If PESS persists despite adequate prosthesis fit, several surgical procedures can be performed to improve prosthetic wear, comfort, and cosmesis, while taking individual requirements and expectations into account. Orbital volume deficiency, eyelid malpositions (such as eyelid laxity, entropion, ptosis, or retraction), and socket contraction can be addressed. Often more than one procedure will be necessary to improve the aesthetic appearance. Sequential surgery is recommended, and any orbital volume deficit should be addressed before performing eyelid surgery.

4.1 Volume Deficit

Surgical rehabilitation in cases of severe volume deficiency or socket contraction can be very challenging for both the patient and the surgeon, due to a variable degree of orbital soft tissue volume loss and structural deformities in the socket. A contracted socket, particularly when combined with volume deficiency, makes fitting and wearing an artificial eye extremely difficult or even impossible.

Socket surgery comprises a variety of procedures aimed at enhancing orbital volume and conjunctival lining. Volume replacement can be achieved with secondary orbital implants (Fig. 3a, b), taking care not to damage the orbital fat, which may induce fat atrophy or tissue restitution—also known as 'cactus-syndrome' [14, 19]. Dermis fat graft is useful for correction of combined PESS and socket contraction. Fat grafts and dermal fillers have also been used successfully (see chapter "Secondary Orbital Implants, Dermis-Fat Graft, and Volume Enhancement Techniques").

In severely contracted sockets, fornix reconstruction with mucous membrane grafting will reconstitute socket architecture and enhance prosthetic fitting. In patients with shallow inferior fornix—due to disinsertion of subconjunctival structures—but sufficient lining, a fornix-deepening procedure, often combined with horizontal eyelid tightening, can suffice. The amount of existing conjunctiva can be easily assessed by gently pushing a wet cotton swab into the fornix (Fig. 4a, b).

Finally, eyelid malpositions such as upper and lower entropion, lower eyelid laxity, or acquired ptosis can be corrected with standard eyelid procedures such as horizontal eyelid shortening, retractor plication, or ptosis repair, while a contralateral upper blepharoplasty may help conceal residual asymmetry. Close collaboration with the ocularist is mandatory for optimal aesthetic and functional outcomes.

4.2 Correction of Shallow Lower Fornix

Fornix repositioning or deepening techniques are described in chapter "Management of Contracted Socket". If lower eyelid laxity is present, fornix repositioning or deepening is usually combined with an eyelid shortening procedure such as lateral tarsal strip (Fig. 5a–g). The fornix deepening sutures are placed before tying the lateral canthal tightening sutures, followed by the insertion of an adequately sized conformer.

Lower fornix reconstruction can be achieved by fixing the conjunctiva close to the Lockwood's ligament, creating a more posteriorly oriented vector. The fornix is reformed by blunt dissection and scar tissue is excised as necessary. In the upper fornix, care is taken not to transect the levator complex, which could result in post-operative ptosis. In severe contractions, both the

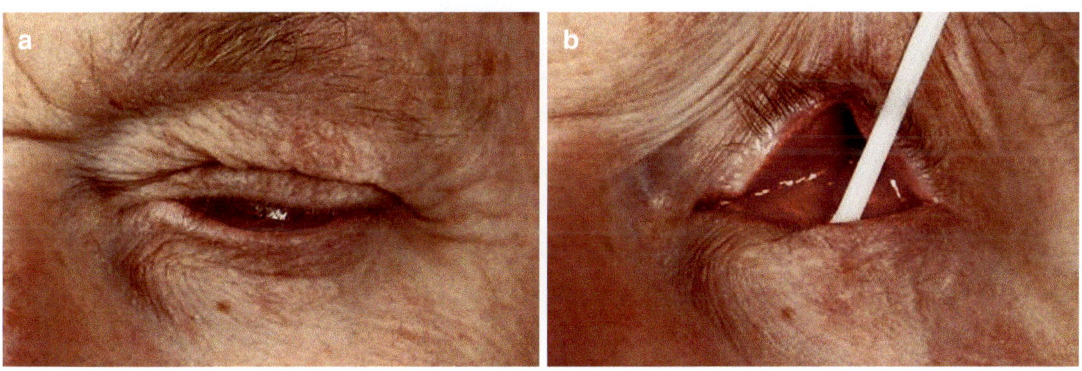

Fig. 4 (**a**) Left anophthalmic socket with presumed lower fornix deficiency and lower eyelid laxity. (**b**) Moist cotton swab gently pushed into the lower fornix showing sufficient conjunctival lining without conjunctival or subconjunctival scarring

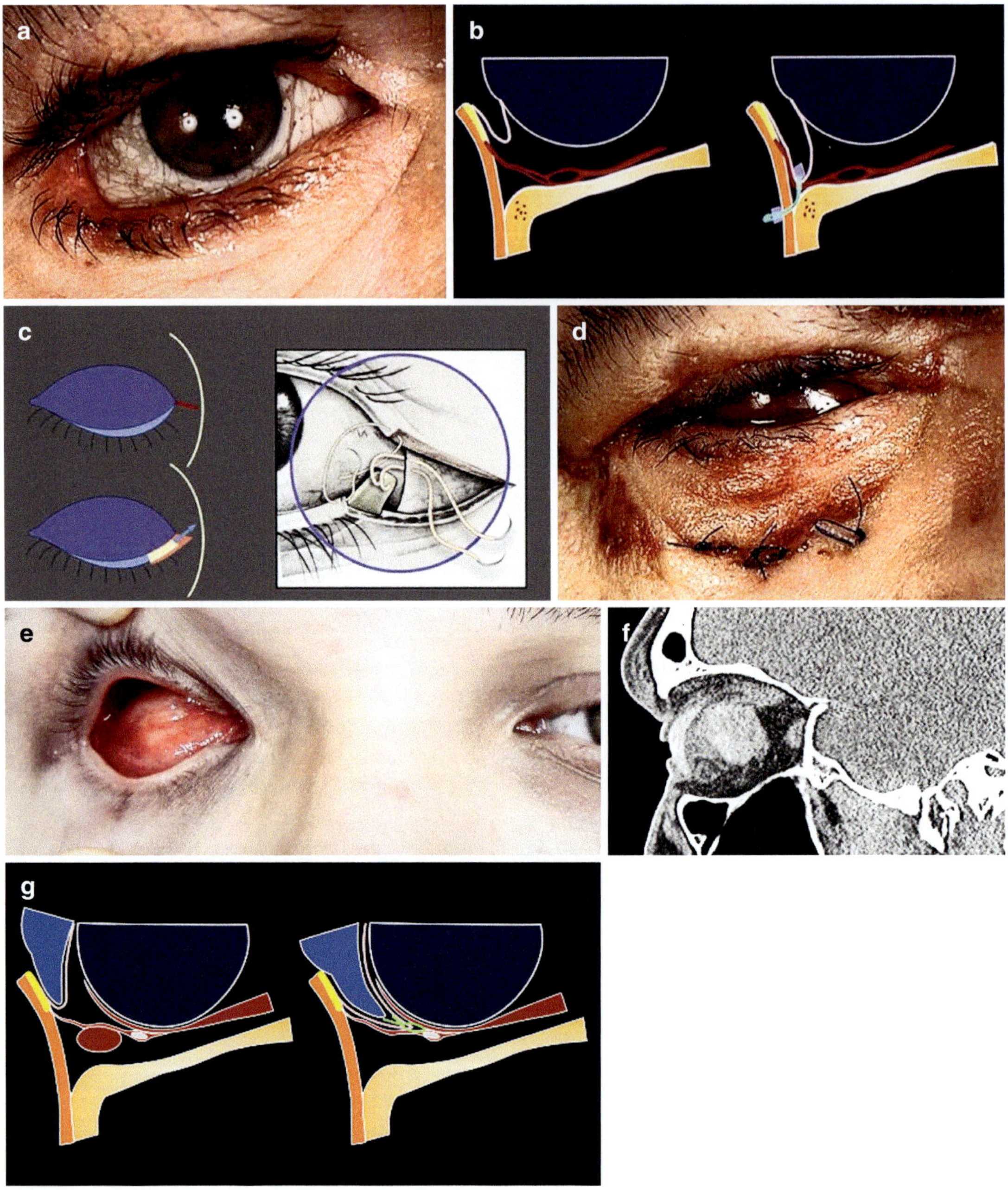

Fig. 5 (**a**) Right lower eyelid laxity in a patient with inadequate artificial eye fitting and recurrent spontaneous loss of the unstable prosthesis. (**b**) Schematic illustration (sagittal view) of lower fornix deepening procedure using a gutter and silicone bolsters. (**c**) Schematic illustration of lower eyelid lateral canthal sling procedure. (**d**) Clinical picture of right socket after fornix deepening procedure and lower eyelid tightening. (**e**) Clinical picture of right shallow inferior fornix (fornix prolapse). (**f**) CT-scan (sagittal plane) of the same patient showing typical radiological findings of shallow inferior fornix (fornix prolapse) with tilting of the artificial eye and relative superior-anterior shift of the inferior oblique, that can be seen distinctly as a rounded body between the fornix and orbital implant. (**g**) Schematic picture (sagittal view) of a lower fornix deepening procedure using fixation sutures tied close to Lockwood ligament

upper and lower fornices are dissected, and the extended defect is then covered with a single large mucous membrane graft. A paper template is used to estimate the size of the defect and required graft. This is inserted into the defect and tested by placing a conformer shell on top of it. If the conformer still does not fit, the dissection can be continued or the template can be adjusted.

Fixing the inferior fornix to the orbital rim periosteum may tend to immobilise the eyelid and to produce a non physiological vertically-oriented fornix. The normal lower fornix vector is oriented towards Lockwood's ligament and retractors, and fornix deepening by suturing conjunctiva close to Lockwood's ligament produces a more natural profile; the correct identification of the inferior oblique facilitates this procedure.

4.3 Eyelid Surgery

Eyelid surgery can improve cosmesis in anophthalmic patients by correcting any residual upper eyelid ptosis or retraction, entropion, and ectropion, following volume enhancement procedures. It can be performed ipsilaterally, bilaterally, or just in the contralateral eyelid to camouflage unilateral sulcus deformity.

4.3.1 Lower Eyelid Laxity Correction

Lower eyelid laxity is a common feature in PESS. Lateral canthal repositioning and lower eyelid tightening are easy procedures that will improve the position of the artificial eye and the overall aesthetic appearance. In case of moderate laxity, a lateral canthoplasty will suffice [20]. The anchoring sutures must be placed posterior to the bony orbital rim and within the anterior orbit (Fig. 5c, d). The Authors prefer absorbable sutures, such as 5-0 polyglycolic acid sutures. Although orbital volume should be augmented before any eyelid surgery, in cases with mild volume deficit and good conjunctival lining, a lateral canthal tendon tightening procedure may help to improve prosthesis retention (Fig. 5c).

4.3.2 Entropion Correction

Upper and lower eyelid entropion are often indicative of a mild form of contracted socket syndrome. If the malposition is mainly due to eyelid laxity, lateral canthal tightening will solve the problem; however, if there is conjunctival scarring but sufficient forniceal depth, retractor plication will improve the eyelid margin position [21]. Upper eyelid entropion can be successfully corrected by anterior lamella repositioning [22].

4.3.3 Upper Blepharoplasty

If there is only a mild upper sulcus deepening due to moderate volume deficiency, a contralateral upper blepharoplasty with skin excision and remodelling of the preaponeurotic fat pad can help to camouflage any residual asymmetry (Fig. 6a, b).

4.3.4 Ptosis Correction

Upper eyelid ptosis in anophthalmic patients is mainly due to involutional changes, with the typical pattern of good levator function and high skin crease. Surgery is recommended if ptosis persists despite increasing the volume of the prosthesis (Fig. 6c, d) (See chapters "Involutional Ptosis" and "Ptosis repair in Aesthetic Surgery"). In cases of post-traumatic ptosis with no residual levator function, a unilateral brow suspension procedure can be performed, albeit the outcome may be unsatisfactory, since active brow function is dependent on visual stimulation. Alternatively, an internal sling can be used, but with both procedures impaired eyelid closure may promote formation of deposits on the surface of the prosthesis.

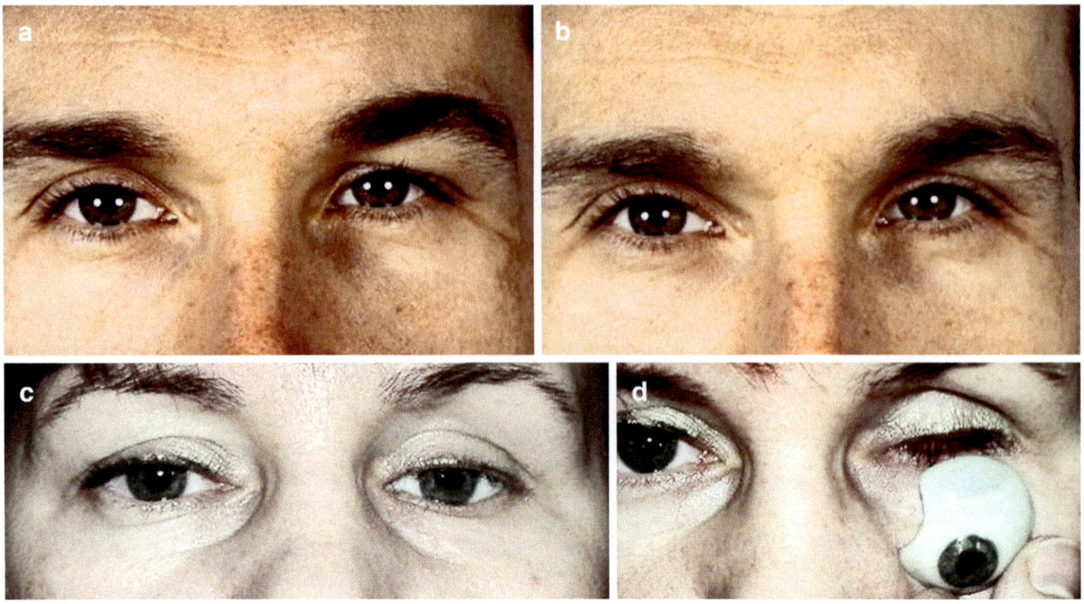

Fig. 6 (**a**) Clinical appearance of mild right PESS with signs of upper sulcus volume deficiency and mild left dermatochalasis. (**b**) Same patient after left upper blepharoplasty improving symmetry. (**c**) Clinical picture of left upper eyelid ptosis caused by long-standing wear of an extremely unbalanced prosthesis. (**d**) Same patient—the upper part of the prosthesis had been increased in size in an attempt to compensate the deep sulcus and raise the upper eyelid. However, ptosis worsened with time due to permanent pressure on the levator complex

References

1. Tyers AG, Collin JRO. Orbital implants and post enucleation socket syndrome. Trans Ophthalmol Soc U K (1962). 1982;102:90–2.
2. Smit AJGM. The postenucleation socket syndrome. University of Amsterdam; 1991.
3. Baylis H, Shorr N. Corrections of problems of the anophthalmic socket. In: McCord CDJ, editor. Oculoplastic surgery. New York: Raven Press; 1981. p. 327–47.
4. Culler AM. Enucleation and cosmetic rehabilitation. Arch Ophthalmol. 1951;45:445–57.
5. DeVoe AG. Experiences with the surgery of the anophthalmic orbit. Am J Ophthalmol. 1945;28:1346–51.
6. Sherman AE. The retracted socket. Am J Ophthalmol. 1952;35:89–101.
7. Silverstone PJ, Beyer-Machule CK, Schaefer DP, et al. Treatment of anophthalmos and socket reconstruction. In: Smith BC, Della Rocca RC, Nesi FA, et al., editors. Ophthalmic plastic and reconstructive surgery. St. Louis: CV Mosby; 1987. p. 1329–59.
8. Soll DB. The anophthalmic socket. Ophthalmology. 1982;89:407–23.
9. Stone WJ, editor. Complications of evisceration and enucleation. 2nd ed. Philadelphia: WB Saunders; 1965. p. 388–425.
10. Vistnes LM. Pathomechanism of the anophthalmic orbit syndrome. In: Surgical reconstruction in the anophthalmic orbit. Birmingham: Aesculapius; 1987. p. 36–51.
11. Vistnes LM, Iverson RE, Laub DR. The anophthalmic orbit: surgical correction of lower eyelid ptosis. Plast Reconstr Surg. 1973;52:346–51.
12. Hatt M. Orbitaplastiken bei Prothesenträgern. Klin Mbl Augenkeilkd. 1992;200:424–7.
13. Clodius L, Martin O. Problems of the anophthalmic orbit. In: Aston SJ, Hornblass A, Meltzer MA, et al., editors. Third international symposium of plastic and reconstructive surgery of the eye and adnexa. Baltimore: Williams & Wilkins; 1982. p. 244–7.
14. Hintschich C, Zonneveld F, L. K. Normal orbital volumes and its pathology in orbital socket surgery. Oper Tech Oculoplastic Orb Reconstr Surg. 2001;4:03–14.
15. Hintschich C, Zonneveld F, Baldeschi L, et al. Bony orbital development after early enucleation in humans. Br J Ophthalmol. 2001;85:205–8.
16. Hintschich C. Anopthalmic socket. In: Medel R, Vásquez LM, editors. Orbital surgery ESASO Course Series. Basel: Karger; 2014. p. 92–112.
17. Koornneef L. The architecture of the musculo-fibrous apparatus in the human orbit. Acta Morphol Neerl Scand. 1977;15:35–64.
18. Koornneef L. Details of the orbital connective tissue in the adult. Acta Morph Neerl-Scand. 1977;15:1–34.

19. Sagoo M, Rose G. Mechanisms and treatment of extruding intraconal implants: socket aging and tissue restitution (the "Cactus Syndrome"). Arch Ophthalmol. 2007;125:1616–20.
20. Anderson RL, Gordy DD. The tarsal strip procedure. Arch Ophthalmol. 1979;97:2192–6.
21. Jones LT, Reeh MJ, Wobig JL. Senile entropium: a new concept for correction. Am J Ophthalmol. 1982;100:1313–8.
22. Hintschich CR. "Anterior lamellar reposition" for the correction of upper eye lid entropion. Ophthalmologe. 1997;94:436–40.

Secondary Orbital Implants, Dermis-Fat Graft, and Socket Volume Enhancement Techniques

Francesco M. Quaranta Leoni, Christoph Hintschich, and George C. Charonis

Key Messages

- Secondary orbital ball implantation can restore adequate orbital volume and improve the motility of the prosthesis if no implant had been positioned at the time of primary surgery.
- Dermis-fat graft eliminates the possibility of implant extrusion, but it involves an additional surgical site, and the possibility of atrophy or hypertrophy at a later stage should be borne in mind.
- Large implant exposures should be managed by simultaneous explantation and dermis-fat graft to address the volume deficit and reduce the risk of a contracted socket by increasing the conjunctival lining.
- Repair of an orbital floor fracture should be addressed before any socket surgery. Subperiosteal implants are useful to correct residual enophthalmos and superior sulcus deformity persisting after implantation, but do not improve the mobility of the orbital contents and of the eyelids.
- Volume augmentation with dermal fillers is a useful minimally invasive alternative for orbital volume enhancement, and it can be combined with various surgical techniques.

F. M. Quaranta Leoni (✉)
Oftalmoplastica Roma, Rome, Italy
e-mail: fquarantaleoni@gmail.com

C. Hintschich
Department of Ophthalmology, Ludwig-Maximilians-University, Munich, Germany

G. C. Charonis
Athens Vision Eye Institute, Athens, Greece

1 Indications and Goals of Surgery

The aim of socket surgery is to minimise any disfigurement, either related to volume or lining deficiency in the socket, or to eyelid malpositions. In consideration of the significant psychological strain of patients with an unsatisfactory appearance due to the anophthalmic socket syndrome, primary surgery for eyeball removal plays a crucial role. Choosing the optimal surgical procedure helps to avoid long hours of unsuccessful prosthesis fitting.

If there is no implant, or a small implant is present, and the patient has problems getting fitted with an adequate eye prosthesis or is impaired by obvious disfigurement, surgical correction is required. Before that, it is necessary to carefully analyse patients' complaints, symptoms and expectations, and to evaluate possible conservative options. Modification of the prosthesis should always be considered and collaboration with the ocularist is mandatory.

F. M. Quaranta Leoni et al. (eds.), *Oculoplastic, Lacrimal and Orbital Surgery*,
https://doi.org/10.1007/978-3-031-39638-0_7

2 General Principles: Patient Evaluation

A complete medical and surgical history should be obtained to be aware of previous surgeries and/or previous radiotherapy.

The examination of patients with socket volume deficiency begins by looking at the whole face, at the periorbital areas and at the relative position of the prosthesis inside the orbit. The amount of superior sulcus deformity is estimated, the palpebral fissure length and height is measured, and the motility of the globe (in case of patients with phthisis bulbi), of the prosthesis and of the orbital implant is documented. The degree of enophthalmos or pseudo-enophthalmos (when a prosthesis is worn) can be measured with exophthalmometry, and clinical photographs should be obtained. Shallowing of the fornices should be inspected, and the socket should be palpated to investigate the presence and location of an orbital implant. Imaging is useful to verify the type, the size and location of the implant and possible bony asymmetry due to previous trauma (see chapter "Post Enucleation Socket Syndrome").

Different surgical and non-surgical procedures are available for socket volume enhancement. These include the insertion of a secondary orbital implant, an autologous dermis-fat graft (DFG), subperiosteal implants, fat transfer, dermal fillers [1, 2].

Volume augmentation with secondary ball implantation should be considered if the soft tissue components in the socket are reasonably soft and malleable, with no significant fibrosis. This can be assessed by pushing the orbital content backwards into the socket by gentle pressure on the lower eyelid: if the upper sulcus is filled by existing orbital fat and bulges anteriorly, secondary ball implantation can be suggested [3].

Alternatively, a DFG can be considered: this combines excellent compatibility with simultaneous increase of volume and lining, and usually provides satisfactory aesthetic and functional results.

Any residual volume deficit might then be corrected with an orbital floor implant, if necessary combined with fornix deepening procedures; finally, a DFG can be placed in the superior sulcus, or fillers can be suggested [1].

Follow up imaging studies are useful to determine the exact position of the secondary ball implant, of the subperiosteal implant, or the amount of filler placement.

3 Secondary Ball Implant

Indications for secondary orbital ball implantation are:

- Restore adequate orbital volume and improve the motility of the prosthesis when no implant had been positioned at the time of primary evisceration or enucleation
- Volume deficit following implant extrusion
- Implant exchange due to inadequate volume of primary implant [1–4]

Before surgery, the motility of the socket without an artificial eye is checked at slit lamp examination.

Surgery is generally performed under general anaesthesia. Polyglactin mesh-wrapped bioceramic implants or Mersilene mesh-wrapped acrylic implants are suitable for this procedure. All the implants should be soaked in antibiotic solution for 5 min at the time of implantation.

- Standard 2-0 traction sutures are positioned on upper and lower eyelids; a delicate speculum can be used alternatively.
- The virtual sagittal axis is marked on the conjunctival surface. Then, the conjunctiva is opened horizontally at this mark. Conjunctiva and Tenon's capsule flaps are maintained open by four 4-0 traction sutures.
- In previously enucleated patients, deep tissues are opened with a single central cut with sharp-pointed scissors, and the intraconal space is explored, verifying by palpation the position of the inferior rectus and medial rectus muscles. An implant between 18 and 22 mm in size is positioned deep in the intraconal space, carefully avoiding dragging of

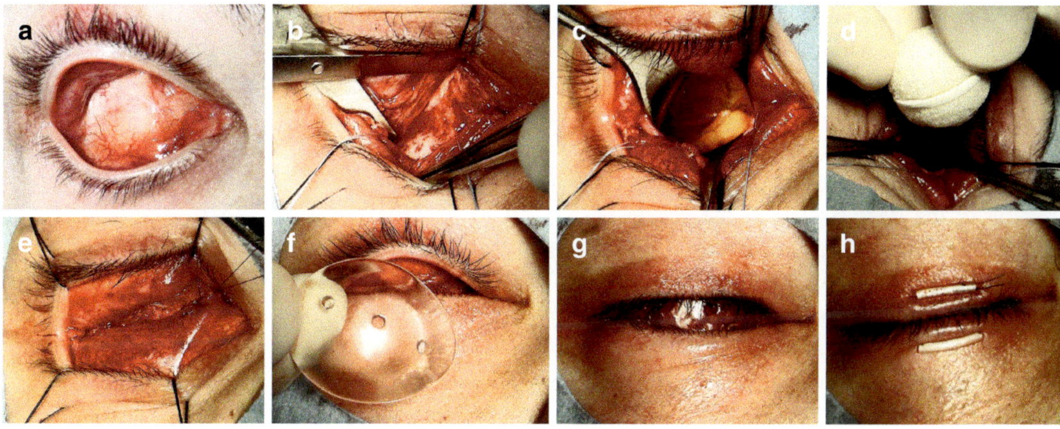

Fig. 1 Secondary ball implantation. (**a**) Empty socket following primary enucleation with no implant. (**b**) Opening of the socket with a central cut with sharp-pointed scissors. (**c**) The intraconal space is explored. (**d**) Positioning of an intraconal wrapped implant. (**e**) Socket closure is made in three separate layers. (**f**, **g**) A right size conformer is positioned to maintain adequate fornices. (**h**) A temporary tarsorrhaphy is applied (Courtesy of F. Quaranta Leoni)

orbital tissues. Deep tissues are then sutured together with a 5-0 polyglactin suture.

- In previously eviscerated patients the implant is positioned intraconal behind the remnant scleral tissues, and sutured together on top with multiple interrupted 5-0 polyglactin sutures. In all patients, Tenon's capsule and then conjunctiva are separately tied and closed in two layers with a polyglactin 6-0 suture.
- An adequate-sized polymethyl methacrylate conformer is positioned within the conjunctival fornices, a central temporary tarsorrhaphy can be applied, and a firm dressing is left in place for up to 5 days (Fig. 1) [5].
- Patients are treated with topical antibiotic and steroid drops for 14 days following removal of the eye pad.
- Slit lamp examination should be performed at each follow-up examination to evaluate signs of infection and the morphology of the socket.

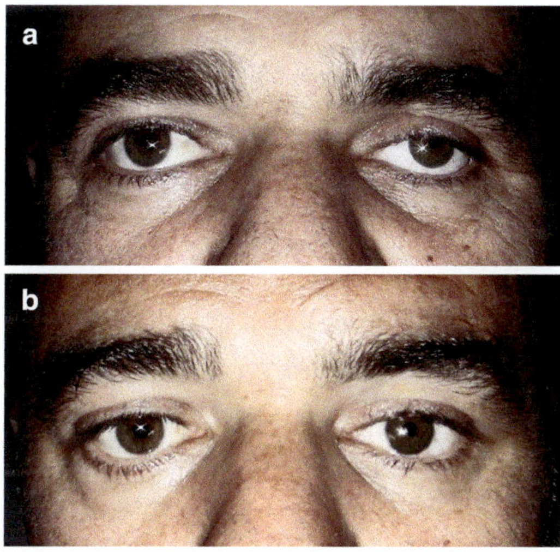

Fig. 2 (**a**) Left orbital volume deficiency post left enucleation with no primary implant. (**b**) Adequate orbital volume following left secondary ball implantation (From: Anophthalmic Socket Syndrome: Prevalence, Impact and Management Strategies. Quaranta-Leoni F et al. Clinical Ophthalmology 2021:153267–3281)

Stable secondary ball implantation can be achieved long term [4, 6, 7] (Fig. 2) and in our experience extrusion rate is lower in patients with previous evisceration than in patients with previous enucleation, although not significantly. In patients who had wrapped secondary porous implants following evisceration, sclera and polyglactin mesh appear to act as duplicate barriers between anterior surface of implants and overlying tissues [4].

Some authors advise to identify the extraocular muscles at surgery, and have found a reduced rate of extrusion or exposure after secondary implantation in patients in whom the muscles were identified and reattached to the implant, in comparison with patients whose extraocular muscles had not been individually identified [8].

Localization of the extraocular muscles may not be necessary, provided that the implant is placed deep in the orbit, above the inferior rectus and lateral to the medial rectus, following careful opening of the deep tissues of the socket [1, 4]. According to our experience, extensive dissection may induce orbital fat atrophy at a later stage [9].

Other surgeons described high complication rates following secondary orbital ball implantation and observed that further surgery was needed in an elevate number of cases, suggesting a shift towards dermis-fat graft (DFG) as preferred technique for secondary implantation [10].

An incorrect surgical procedure might be the main cause for high exposure rate, and this may be related to a superficial positioning of the implant that drags orbital fat deep down the socket and causes late tissue restitution, determining the so-called *cactus syndrome* (Fig. 3). This can be avoided at surgery by gently positioning the implant deep into the orbit through a polythene glide [7], or carefully exposing the intraconal space and avoiding rough contact of the surface of the implant or the mesh with the orbital tissues while positioning the implant in the intraconal space [4].

Orbital volume deficit should be corrected before performing any eyelid surgery (see chapter "Post Enucleation Socket Syndrome") [1, 2].

4 Dermis-Fat Graft

DFG eliminates the possibility of extrusion and foreign body reactions, and is less expensive than alloplastic implants.

Indications for DFG are:

- primary or secondary orbital implantation after trauma
- volume replacement when extra lining is needed (contracted socket)
- replacement of an extruded implant
- implant exchange in chronic socket pain
- primary implant in children with congenital anophthalmia, or implant exchange in children with congenital anophthalmia and previous implantation of orbital expanders (see chapter "Congenital Anophthalmia and Microphthalmia")
- primary implant in children with microphthalmos and cyst, if cyst and/or the microphthal-

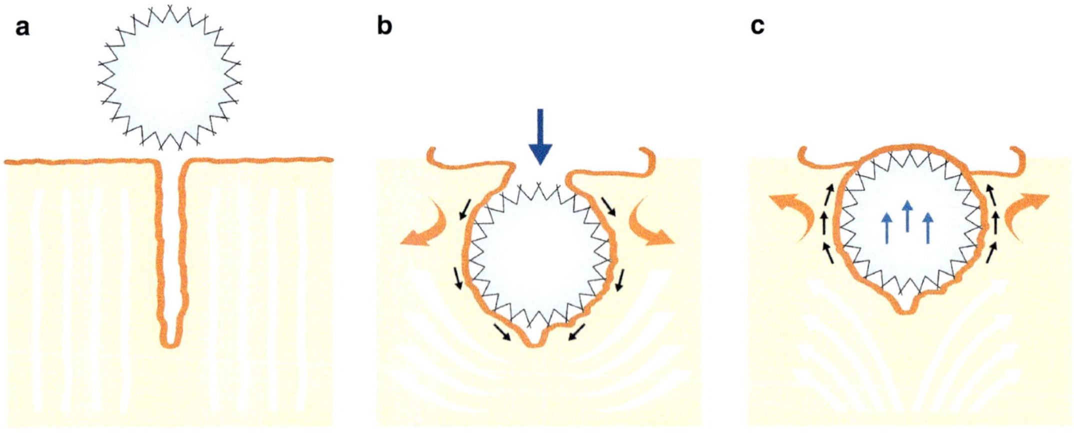

Fig. 3 Cactus syndrome. (**a**) Pre-implantation of rough-surfaced implant. (**b**) Forced implantation may drag superficial tissues down the orbit. (**c**) Tissue restitution during the healing process pushes the implant anteriorly with increased risk of exposure or extrusion (Modified from Sagoo MS, Rose GE. Mechanisms and treatment of extruding intraconal implants: socket ageing and tissue restitution (the "Cactus Syndrome"). Arch Ophthalmol. 2007 Dec;125(12):1616–20)

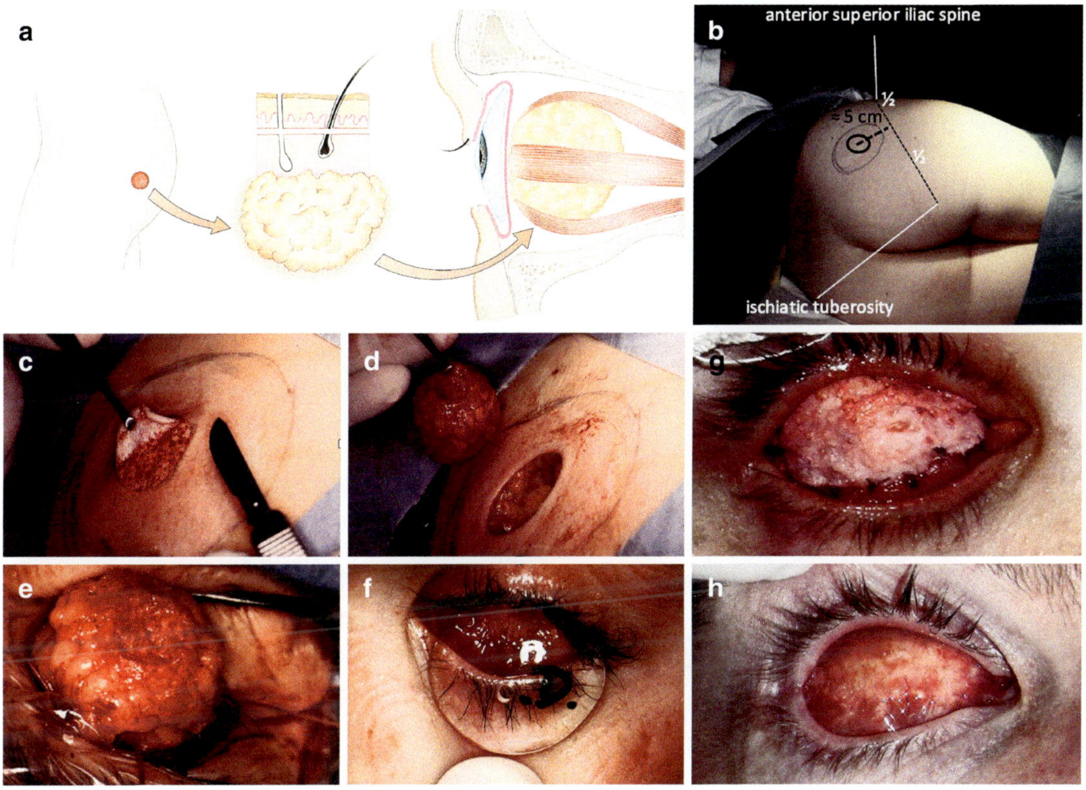

Fig. 4 Dermis-fat grafting (DFG). (**a**) DFG (schematic). De-epithelialized skin with adjacent subcutaneous fatty tissue is transplanted from the gluteal region into the socket. (**b**) DFG—Donor site. DFG is harvested from an area 5 cm superior to the centre point of a line connecting the anterior iliac crest and the sciatic tuberosity. Incision: circle of 25 mm diameter. (**c**) DFG—Harvesting the transplant (surgical site). Removal of epidermis with a no. 20 blade. Note: The blade is rather large and parallel to the surface, no islands of epidermal cells should be left behind. (**d**) En-bloc harvesting of the dermis-fat graft from the donor site. (**e**) Implantation of the DFG into the anophthalmic socket. (**f**) Insertion of a clear conformer shell size D fitting without tension at the end of the procedure. (**g**) Appearance of the socket at day five. (**h**) Dermis-fat graft well healed and fully conjunctivalised after 5 months (Courtesy of C Hintschich and F. Quaranta Leoni)

mic eye need removal (see chapter "Congenital Anophthalmia and Microphthalmia")

- deep upper sulcus correction persisting after secondary ball implant and/or subperiosteal implant.

The surgical procedure involves two steps: harvesting the transplant, and preparation of the recipient site and implantation of the graft (Fig. 4a) [1, 2, 11–18].

4.1 Harvesting the Transplant

The procedure is usually performed under general anaesthesia. The first step is harvesting of the DFG. The favourite donor site is the upper outer quadrant of the gluteal region, as this is not a weight-bearing area and there is no risk of damaging the sciatic nerve (Fig. 4b). Furthermore, the dermis itself in this area is thicker, and this is advantageous for graft stability. Harvesting from the left side of the abdomen (not to confuse the scar with a previous appendicectomy), or from the periumbilical area is a possible alternative, but cannot be considered in thin patients.

To harvest the graft from the gluteal region it is necessary to place the patient in a sideways position on his contralateral hip. Any damage to one of the extremities or the neck must be avoided by meticulous bedding, which is usually performed with the help of the anaesthesiologist.

- After an accurate disinfection of the surgical region with 10% povidone-iodine solution the dermis-fat graft is harvested from an area five centimetres below the centre point of a line joining the anterior iliac crest and the sciatic tuberosity.
- A circle with a maximal diameter of 25 mm, or alternatively a banana-shaped ellipse with the centre allowing a 25 mm graft removal, is marked on the skin before it is incised superficially with a D-15 blade, the incision not exceeding into the dermis. Intradermal injection of saline solution into the demarcated area facilitates the de-epithelialization of the skin.
- Using a D-20 blade, positioned nearly parallel to the skin surface and moved in a rotational manner, facilitates removal of the epidermis (Fig. 4c).
- A deep incision is then made along the incision line perpendicular to the surface, through the dermis and into the subcutaneous fat.
- The graft is severed from the donor site, paying attention not to damage the muscle fascia (Fig. 4d).
- The graft is preserved in isotonic saline solution, while the donor site is closed with multiple interrupted 2-0 or 3-0 absorbable sutures placed through the fatty tissue and subcutaneous tissue.
- Skin closure is performed with 2/0 or 3/0 nonabsorbable horizontal mattress sutures. Steri-Strips are placed across the wound; a pressure dressing with eudermic elastic plaster is applied.

4.2 Implanting the Transplant

After repositioning the patient into a supine position, the socket is prepared to receive the graft. The procedure varies depending on the socket. In the case of an exposed or extruding orbital implant, the conjunctiva is incised in a circular fashion around the extruding part of the implant. It is mandatory not to leave any conjunctival tissue in the depth of the orbital tissue, to avoid the development of conjunctival cysts. The orbital implant is then mobilised and finally explanted.

If no implant is present, the space for the DFG is accomplished by a careful blunt dissection. Preparation and dissection in the orbital soft tissues should be as atraumatic as possible and any attempt to expose remnants of the extraocular muscles should be avoided. Usually, bleeding can be controlled by applying some pressure. Four double-armed absorbable 5-0 Vicryl® sutures are placed superiorly, inferiorly, medially and laterally, in any firm tissue available in the socket, strong enough to keep the sutures.

In case of contracted socket, traction sutures into the upper and lower eyelid are usually necessary, as retractors cannot be inserted due to shallow fornices. The conjunctival incision is performed horizontally from the caruncle through the centre to the lateral canthus. A few millimetres of the conjunctiva are then mobilised along the incision line by subconjunctival dissection, and a space to accommodate the graft is created by blunt dissection; bands of scar tissue need to be divided. If there is adequate space to accommodate the graft, sutures are placed as described above. The DFG is then inserted into the socket, applying only slight pressure (Fig. 4e). If there is a discrepancy between the available space and the size of the graft, any undue pressure should be avoided. The space in the socket can be enlarged, or alternatively the graft can be trimmed, custom shaped, and gently positioned into the socket. Sutures are then passed from underneath through the dermis about 2 mm apart from its margin at the 12-o'clock position, the remaining sutures at 3-, 6- and 9-o'clock positions are placed sequentially as in primary grafting. In a contracted socket, the conjunctiva is sutured just to the margin of the dermis: conjunctival fornices are preserved and the dermis is left bare to granulate to increase the socket lining (Fig. 4e).

At the end of the procedure it is mandatory to insert a conformer with a rather shallow curvature of an appropriate size (Fig. 4f). This stabilises the graft and helps to maintain the fornices. A pressure dressing is applied. Post-operatively, antibiotic eye drops are applied for one week following removal of the dressing. Integration of the graft and conjunctival epithelialisation across the dermis surface usually takes 4–6 weeks. The sutures in the gluteal region are removed after 10–12 days.

Dermis acts as a scaffold for conjunctival spontaneous epithelialisation, and helps to provide vascularization and to reduce the risk of fat atrophy [13, 14]. Results may vary: a recent study showed better motility following secondary DFG with respect to primary DFG implantation [14]. Other studies reported better motility after a primary DFG than after secondary implantation [13, 17].

Post-operative fat atrophy should always be considered, and for this reason DFG is usually oversized by 10–20% to obtain an adequate orbital volume [1]. Excessive grafts may lead to excessive compression of the surrounding tissues, can compromise vascularization and cause central necrosis and insufficient conjunctival lining; on the other hand, small grafts may not completely restore an acceptable orbital volume for the possibility of fat atrophy [1, 14]. Some studies documented a greater fat atrophy after secondary procedures, maybe related to insufficient socket vascularization [13]. DFG can be combined with a mucous membrane graft (MMG) if conjunctiva does not allow to create adequate fornices [1, 13].

The most significant drawbacks are that DFG is a time-consuming procedure, there is higher morbidity due to an additional surgical site, and the possibility of atrophy or hypertrophy at a later stage [1, 2, 14].

Graft necrosis may occur in 2.9% of patients after primary procedures and in 4.5% of patients after secondary implantation [13]; cyst formation is caused by persistence of epithelial islands and occurs in up to 11% of patients [13, 18]. Late shallowing of the fornices and superior sulcus deformity are also possible.

Other complications can be granulomas formation, infection, atrophy, keratinization of the socket, hair growth, fat prolapse, seroma and posterior haemorrhage [1, 12, 13].

Patients can usually wear a temporary prosthesis 3–6 weeks after the operation, but a definitive custom made prosthesis should be made approximately 3 months after surgery, when healing of the socket is usually completed.

In our experience DFG is useful in paediatric patients both as primary or secondary implant. It is a suitable option in children affected by clinical congenital anophthalmia (CCA), following adequate eyelid and socket expansion, as it exerts adequate orbital pressure and continues to expand the eyelids and the soft tissues of the socket [15, 16]. The implant may grow at puberty, and in our experience patients with CCA submitted to early dermis-fat graft may need local fat debulking and transposition of the conjunctivalized derma to reconstruct a shallow lateral fornix years following primary surgery [1].

5 Management of Implant Exposure and Migration

Ideal orbital implants should restore the orbital volume, be biocompatible, be cost effective, and ensure satisfactory motility of the prosthesis [1, 2].

Modern implants offer peculiar features, but there are still uncertainties about the outcomes of integrated implants (hydroxyapatite (HA), porous polyethylene (PP), bioceramic composites and non-integrated (polymethylmethacrylate—PMMA/acrylic and silicone) orbital implants (see chapter "Enucleation") [1, 19].

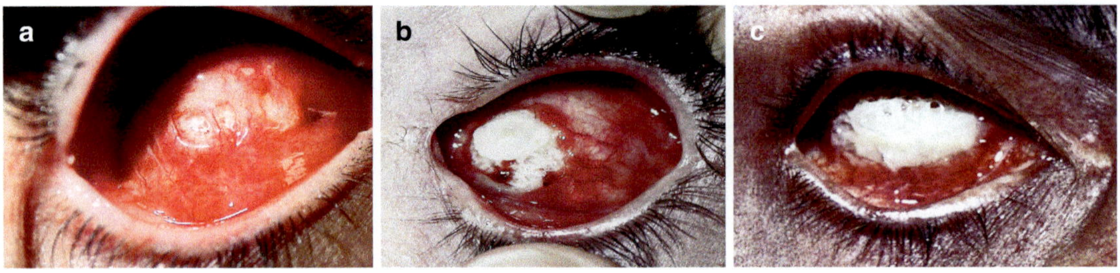

Fig. 5 (**a**, **b**) Different degrees of implant exposure, (**c**) large exposure is managed by explantation and DFG (Courtesy of F Quaranta-Leoni)

PMMA implants are economical, easy to place and to remove, provide overall satisfactory clinical outcomes, and reports suggesting there are few advantages to the use of porous implants compared to nonporous implants when these implants are properly placed in the orbit [20–22]. Acrylic implants are particularly useful in paediatric patients for ease of removal, as there is the possible need for implant exchange with time [23].

Careful selection of implant type, size and of surgical technique is mandatory. Placing an implant larger than 22 mm might be related to a higher exposure rate in the early post-operative period, as overlying tissues tend to be closed with greater tension [24]. Soaking porous implants in antibiotic solution at the time of implantation is recommended to promote fibrovascular ingrowth and reduce the risk of infection [24, 25].

Adequate wrapping may help to reduce the risk of exposure, and an increased rate of exposure can be related to different wrapping material rather than to the implant itself [26–28]. Finally, pegging [29] and history of smoking and immunomodulatory therapy appear associated with a higher rate of implant exposure [30].

Management of implant exposure is still controversial. Spontaneous healing takes place in a small percentage of cases, and vascularized flaps of conjunctiva may be effective for limited areas of exposures. The high failure rate after attempted repair of exposures with direct closure, scleral or mucous membrane patches could be related to the fact that the underlying cause, that is the anterior migration of the implant due to the *cactus syndrome*, remains untreated [24].

Large-area implant exposures can be managed by a thin dermis fat graft (DFG) [1] or by a myoperiosteal graft, as the thick composite nature of this graft provides a durable and vascularised coverage [31].

In cases of either recurrence of a large exposure or infection of the implant, explantation should be performed (Fig. 5). Adequate tissue ingrowth through the pores of the implant allows biointegration, reducing the risk of exposure and infection. Anterior exposure allows instead bacterial colonisation of the implant, and a subsequent heavy inflammatory infiltrate. Exposed porous implants show a reduction of fibrovascular ingrowth with associated inflammatory infiltrate tissue, that results in poor integration of the implant, and poor tissue ingrowth may limit the penetration of topical or systemic antibiotic therapy, leading to the necessity for explantation [24].

In our experience, simultaneous explantation and DFG is a suitable surgical option to address the volume deficit following removal of exposed implants and prevents the chance of a contracted socket by increasing the conjunctival lining.

Primary replacement of exposed implants, either porous and non-porous, is another possibility and it has shown a successful outcome even in cases with infection [32].

Implant migration is relatively uncommon following enucleation and evisceration; it may happen following secondary ball implantation and tends to be less frequent with porous implants. Treatment is necessary when it affects the correct placement of the prosthesis: imaging is mandatory, and options include implant exchange and DFG (Fig. 6) [1].

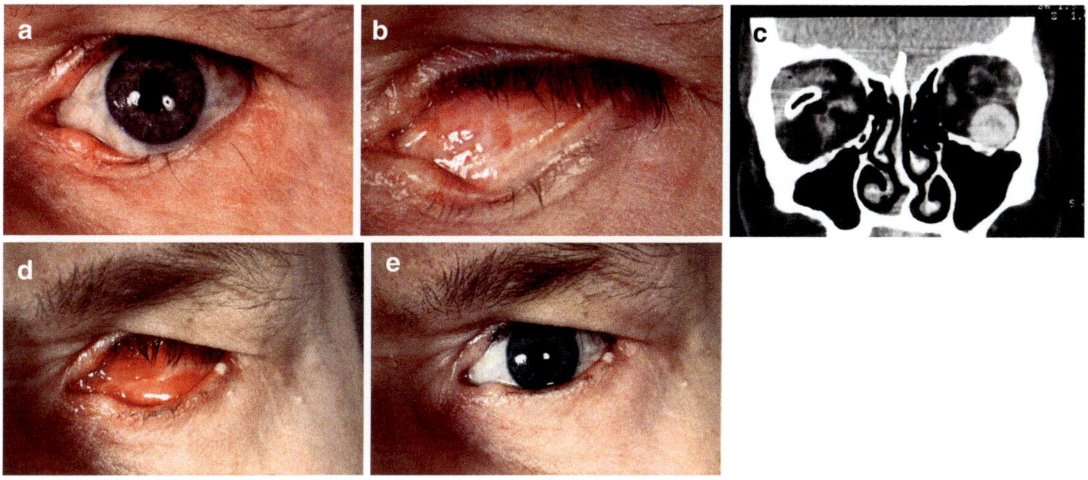

Fig. 6 Patient with bilateral acquired anophthalmos. (**a**) Left contracted socket and unstable prosthesis, after multiple surgical procedures. Note: artificial eye is riding on the lower eyelid margin, the lateral 2/3 of the prosthesis sits anterior to the eyelid. (**b**) Socket without artificial eye, severe shallowing of lower fornix. (**c**) Same patient, coronal CT. Left side: infero-lateral dislocation of the alloplastic orbital implant. (**d**) Socket without artificial eye, after implant removal and secondary DFG: adequate conjunctival lining and inferior fornix. (**e**) Satisfactory prosthesis fitting (Courtesy of C Hintschich)

6 Subperiosteal Implants

Indications for an orbital floor implant are:

- Repair of an orbital floor fracture. This is sometimes overlooked in anophthalmic patients: an orbital floor fracture may determine a dystopia that should not be addressed with other surgical procedures. For this reason, imaging is mandatory in post-traumatic sockets.
- Enophthalmos and/or superior sulcus deformity persisting after implantation. It may happen if the implant is small or if there is an excess of orbital fat reabsorption. A subperiosteal implant is indicated if an increase of the size of the prosthesis cannot compensate for volume deficiency [33].

Implants may be autogenous, such as bone or cartilage grafts, or non autogenous, such as silicon, porous polyethylene (Medpor®), synthetic porous composite of Teflon polymer and alumina (Proplast II) (1–2), and can be positioned via a subciliary incision or via transconjunctival approach [33–35]. The transconjunctival approach can be performed using a pre- or post-septal dissection, with infratarsal or fornix incision associated with lateral canthotomy and inferior cantholysis. Sparing the lateral canthus minimises lower eyelid dissection and offers sufficient exposure to allow insertion of large floor implants [36].

Infection, extrusion or anterior displacement are possible complications, and systemic antibiotics should be given peri- and post-operatively to reduce the risk of infection or extrusion of the implant. Sensory changes of the maxillary division of the fifth nerve may happen, but tend to recover with time. In our experience, a moderate shallowing of the lower fornix post-operatively is not uncommon, and care must be taken in choosing the correct size and a careful positioning of the implant. A skin-muscle approach should be preferred in case of shallow lower fornix, and the implant can be fixed to the orbital floor to prevent migration. However, the mobility of the orbital contents and of the upper eyelid is usually not improved by this procedure [37].

7 Fat Grafting - Fillers

Volume augmentation with fat grafting and dermal fillers can be combined with various surgical techniques [38]. Possible alternatives are:

- micro-fat grafting
- DFG to upper orbital sulcus
- injectable calcium hydroxyapatite
- hyaluronic acid fillers

The ideal filler should be safe, easy to administer, not expensive and have predictable outcomes, with acceptable longevity and a low migration ratio.

There are two main indications for minimally invasive orbital volume augmentation:

- *Phthisis bulbi:* This may develop after severe ocular trauma, or after serious ocular diseases or failed multiple intra-ocular surgeries. The aesthetic deformity might not be fully compensated by a prosthesis, and the gradual progression of this condition makes lipofilling and/or fillers a reasonable alternative in patients who do not wish further surgeries.
- *Post Enucleation Socket Syndrome (PESS):* Injectables can be combined with other surgical techniques and can be considered in patients reluctant to undergo extensive surgical reconstructions.

7.1 Patient Evaluation

Drug allergies or previous adverse events related to fillers must be investigated. For early phthisical eyes, documentation of visual function is mandatory. Although intraorbital filler injections have been performed for sighted enophthalmic eyes [39–41], the surgeon should be aware of the visual function in all cases; there is a potential risk for vision deterioration due to inadvertent intravascular injection or to a compartment syndrome. In cases of congenital microphthalmia, documentation of potential vision should be carried out with visual evoked potentials [42]. Intraorbital filler injections usually work better when the soft tissue contents of the orbit are soft and malleable.

7.2 Fat Grafting

Autologous fat has been used for many decades for soft tissue volumisation [42]. It has no immunogenicity and therefore has no risk for rejection. The variability in the amount of fat resorption makes autologous fat quite unpredictable in providing long term volumisation, and there is the need for adequate anaesthesia and a hospital setting. However, orbital fat grafting can result in a gain of orbital fat volume for up to 5 years, and micro-fat grafting usually produces minimal donor site morbidity [43, 44]. Reported complications include a lumpy appearance when fat is injected into the orbicularis oculi muscle and embolism in case of intravascular injections [43].

7.3 DFG to Superior Sulcus

A DFG positioned at the level of the superior orbital rim periosteum improves a superior deep sulcus still present after positioning of an adequate intraconal implant and a subperiosteal implant. The fat is placed to fill the preaponeurotic fat pad and the dermis is sutured to the periosteum of the superior orbital rim (Fig. 7). The levator muscle can be advanced at the same time to correct ptosis, if present [33]. Oversizing of 10% to prevent reabsorption is adequate, and outcomes are usually satisfactory and more stable than with fat transfer [1].

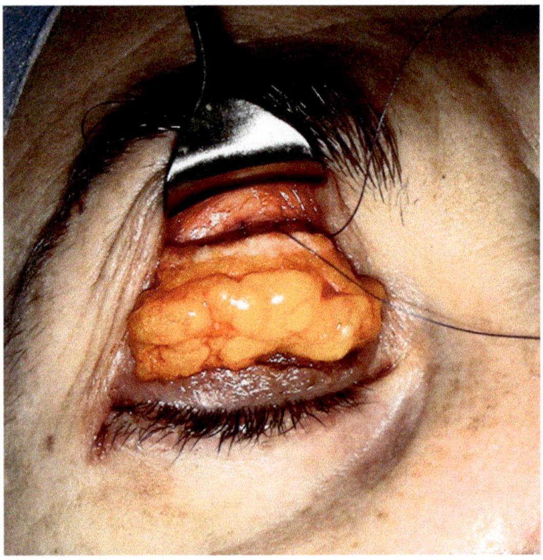

Fig. 7 DFG to upper sulcus. The dermis is sutured to the superior orbital rim periosteum (From: Anophthalmic Socket Syndrome: Prevalence, Impact and Management Strategies. Quaranta-Leoni F et al. Clinical Ophthalmology 2021:153267–3281)

7.4 Injectable Calcium Hydroxyapatite

Calcium hydroxyapatite gel (Radiesse) consists of CaOH microspheres (25–45 μ) in a gel carrier of sterile water, glycerin and carboxymethylcellulose [45]. Radiesse acts as a volumizing agent and has collagen stimulation properties. Compared to HA gels, it has shown an increased duration of effect, but there is no available material to dissolve the filler should it be required. The decrease of enophthalmos per mL of product injected is approximately slightly less than 1:2, and clinical improvement has been shown to persist for up to 1.5 years in most patients [46]. It is indicated in orbits that demonstrate significant fibrosis resulting from multiple surgeries, trauma, or radiation and it has shown relatively low complication rates [45, 46].

7.5 Hyaluronic Acid Fillers

Hyaluronic acid (HA) fillers are relatively easy to administer, and the low immunogenicity, the ease of administration, and the reversibility make HA a useful tool for socket volume enhancement. For orbital volume augmentation are required fillers that tend to keep their shape during deformation (i.e. fillers with a high elastic modulus-G').

HA fillers injections can improve the appearance of both deep upper sulcus due to soft tissue volume loss and enophthalmos related to trauma or phthisis bulbi (Fig. 8) [47]. Successful out-

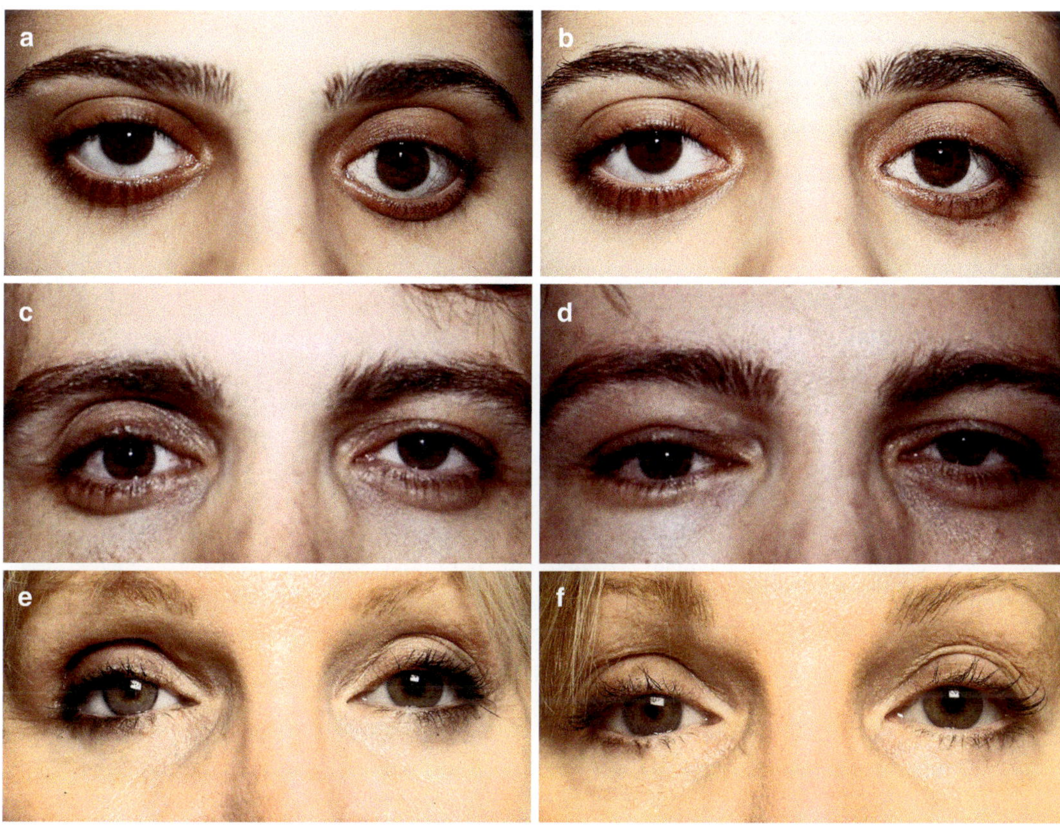

Fig. 8 Fillers in the anophthalmic socket. (**a**, **b**) Images before and after injection of 1 mL of HA gel to the left lower periorbital area. The patient wears a prosthesis on the left side. The filler was injected over the lateral part of the orbital rim to provide eyelid support. (**c**, **d**) Images before and after injection of 0.8 mL of HA gel to the right upper eyelid sulcus of a patient wearing a prosthesis on the right side. (**e**, **f**) Images before and after two sessions (1 mL in each session) of intraorbital injection of HA gel to address the volume deficit of the right orbit (Images **a**, **b**, **c**, **d** courtesy of G Charonis; images **e**, **f** courtesy of R.A Goldberg)

comes have been described with the use of both Restylane Sub-Q (Q-Med, Uppsala, Sweden) [40, 41, 48] and Juvederm Voluma (Allergan) [49]. The achieved effect follows an approximate 1:1 ratio (i.e. 1 mL of product achieves a 1 mm correction of enophthalmos) [40, 41].

Volume loss is usually corrected in most cases with a single injection. However, the reduction of enophthalmos tends to decrease over time and a significant loss of volume may occur by 6 months [40, 41]. Persistent oedema and ptosis requiring surgical treatment have been reported as possible complications [49].

7.6 Other Fillers

Polyacrylamide gel (Aquamid) is a permanent filler that is used for facial volumisation. It consists of a 2.5% polymer backbone of cross-linked polyacrylamide and 97.5% water. The theoretical advantage is indefinite longevity, with the drawback of no reversibility [50].

Hydrogel pellet expanders [51] have been proposed for treatment of orbital volume deficiency in congenital microphthalmia (see chapter "Congenital Anophthalmia and Microphthalmia"), although in our experience they might migrate [1].

7.7 Technique of Injection

1. *Estimation of injection volume*

   There are several ways to determine the required volume for an adequate volume restoration:

   (a) By orbital imaging

      The orbital volume can be calculated by means of graphic computation after drawing the orbital contour in each axial CT image and generating a 3D module of the orbit. The volume deficit is calculated by subtracting the volume of the deficient orbit from the normal contralateral orbit [50].

   (b) By injecting normal saline or local anaesthetic

      Some injectors prefer to inject normal saline or local anaesthetic prior to the filler to determine the volume required [50].

   (c) By direct observation during product injection

      Most injectors estimate the amount required while constantly observing the contralateral orbit during the injection process.

   (d) By using the data from published papers

      Some of the published studies provide information on the amount of enophthalmos reduction (in mm) per mL of product injected. This is often quite variable depending on the type of filler used. For instance, for one type of Hyaluronic acid gel, Restylane SQ, this ratio is approximately 1:1 (for up to 2 mm of enophthalmos reduction. No additional effect is observed for injected volumes greater than 2 mL). For CaOH (Radiesse), it was found to be slightly less than 1:2 (1.3 mL of product resulted in 2.4 mm reduction in enophthalmos) [45, 46].

2. *Anaesthesia*

   Most adult cases can be performed in an office setting with topical tetracaine drops and a mild pre-procedure sedation if needed. However, both surgeons and patients should be prepared for possible post-operative orbital pain and vasovagal responses. Most hyaluronic acid gels contain lidocaine and a prior local anaesthetic injection is usually not required. A slow, controlled injection lessens the discomfort significantly. Paediatric cases require general anaesthesia. Autologous fat transfer usually requires intravenous IV sedation or general anaesthesia.

3. *Antiseptic technique*

   Standard skin sterilisation regimens with povidone iodine or other type of appropriate skin disinfectants should be used to prevent infection. A head drape and surgical gloves are also necessary.
4. *Entry point*

   The injection can be performed via a transcutaneous or transconjunctival route. The choice depends on the injector's preference. The most common entry point is along the inferolateral orbit; a transcutaneous approach is required when the filler is placed on the upper eyelid preaponeurotic space to camouflage a deep superior sulcus; both retrobulbar and direct sulcus injection are safe and effective methods for the correction of a deep superior sulcus [47].
5. *Location of material placement/Injection pearls*

   The material can be placed in the intraconal or extraconal space. Basic principles include:
   - Start the injection when the needle or cannula is past the equator of the globe or implant.
   - Aspirate before injection.
   - Inject in either retrograde or anterograde fashion in small volumes and very slowly.
   - Placing a *lake* of material along the inferolateral extraconal orbit, an area with no critical neurovascular structures, is safe and effective.
   - If correction of significant axial enophthalmos is required, the injection can target the intraconal retrobulbar (or retro-implant) space. This space provides more efficient anterior projection of the globe or implant and the chance of anterior migration or shallowing of the fornices is lower. However, the possibility of a decreased implant motility and vasovagal response following the injection should be considered.
   - If the implant is displaced inferiorly in the orbit, filler injection on the orbital floor pushes the implant superiorly and helps to reduce superior sulcus deformity.
   - Care should be taken to avoid the superior orbital fissure with posterior injections.
   - Needles or cannulas can be used. Needles for hyaluronic acid gels, CaOH or polyacrylamide gel, measure between 18G and 27G, with length of 1–1.5 in [40, 41, 47, 49]. For autologous fat, larger needles or cannulas (14–16G) are helpful [43].
6. *Post-operative care: Complications*

   Patients should be observed for the risk of haemorrhage, or the possibility of a vasovagal response. This is due to an oculocardiac reflex and may occur after intraconal injections that stretch the muscle cone, resulting in bradycardia and hypotension. Cold compresses are applied before discharge and oral analgesics can be prescribed in case of pain [50].

   Other reported complications are: central nervous system morbidity due to inadvertent cavernous sinus thromboembolic sequelae; pressure sensation, or rarely severe orbital pain; headaches; chemosis; ecchymosis; infection; inflammatory granulomas; anterior migration with lower eyelid fullness and poor prosthesis fitting [40, 41, 43, 45, 50, 51]. Most complications are self-limited. However, rate of filler absorption in the orbit is faster than in the dermis, and this must be considered and included in patient counselling, as multiple injections are needed to maintain a satisfactory aesthetic appearance and repeated treatment could represent a potential source of inflammation [1].

A system for socket volume enhancement is proposed in Fig. 9.

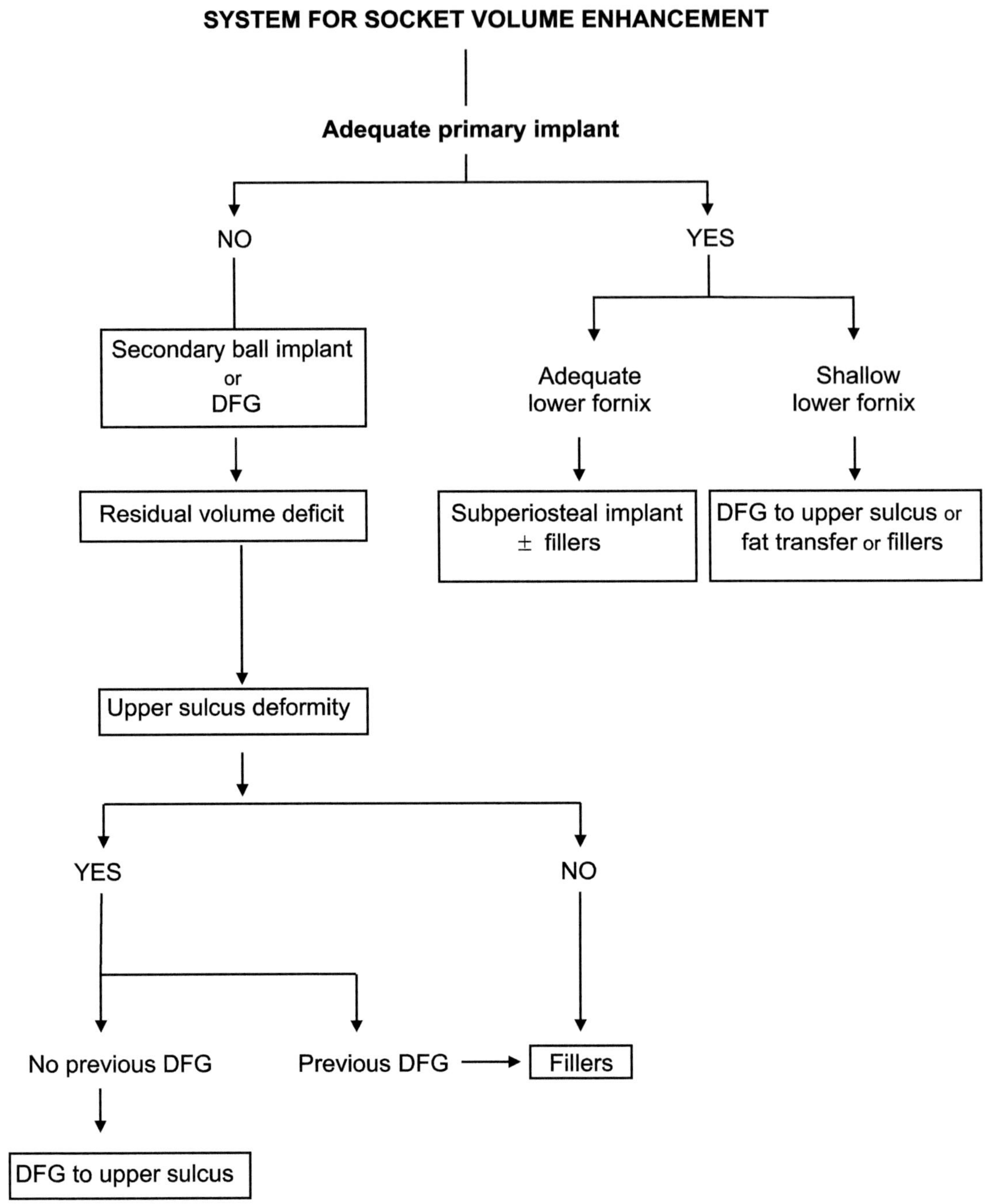

Fig. 9 System for socket volume enhancement (From: Anophthalmic Socket Syndrome: Prevalence, Impact and Management Strategies. Quaranta-Leoni F et al. Clinical Ophthalmology 2021:153267–3281)

References

1. Quaranta-Leoni FM, Fiorino MG, Quaranta-Leoni F, Di Marino M. Anophthalmic socket syndrome: prevalence, impact and management strategies. Clin Ophthalmol. 2021;15:3267–81.
2. Quaranta-Leoni FM. Treatment of the anophthalmic socket. Curr Opin Ophthalmol. 2008;19:422–7.
3. Hintschich C. Anophthalmic socket. In: Medel R, Vasquez LM, editors. Orbital surgery, ESASO course series, vol. 5. Basel: Karger; 2014. p. 92–112.
4. Quaranta-Leoni FM, Sposato S, Lorenzano D. Secondary orbital ball implants after enucleation and evisceration: surgical management, morbidity, and long-term outcome. Ophthalmic Plast Reconstr Surg. 2015;31:115–8.
5. McGrath LA, McNab AA. Temporary suture tarsorrhaphy at the time of orbital ball implantation. Graefes Arch Clin Exp Ophthalmol. 2018;256:2437–41.
6. Hintschich C, Zonnefeld FW, Baldeschi L, Koornneef L. Long-term outcome after secondary orbital implants. Ophthalmologe. 1999;96:34–9.
7. Sagoo MS, Rose GE. Mechanisms and treatment of extruding intraconal implants: socket aging and tissue restitution (the "Cactus Syndrome"). Arch Ophthalmol. 2007;125:1616–20.
8. Axmann S, Paridaens D. Anterior surface breakdown and implant extrusion following secondary alloplastic orbital implantation surgery. Acta Ophthalmol. 2018;96:310–3.
9. Hintschich C, Zonneveld F, Koornneef L. Normal orbital volumes and its pathology in orbital socket surgery. Oper Tech Oculoplastic Orbital Reconstr Surg. 2001;4:03–14.
10. Sundelin KC, Dafgård Kopp EM. Complications associated with secondary orbital implantations. Acta Ophthalmol. 2015;93:679–83.
11. Smith B, Petrelli R. Dermis-fat graft as a movable implant within the muscle cone. Am J Ophthalmol. 1978;85:62–6.
12. Hintschich C. Dermis-fat graft. Possibilities and limitations. Ophthalmologe. 2003;100:518–24.
13. Nentwich MM, Schebitz-Walter K, Hirneiss C, Hintschich C. Dermis fat grafts as primary and secondary orbital implants. Orbit. 2014;33:33–8.
14. Jovanovic N, Carniciu AL, Russell WW, Jarocki A, Kahana A. Reconstruction of the orbit and anophthalmic socket using the dermis fat graft: a major review. Ophthalmic Plast Reconstr Surg. 2020;36:529–39.
15. Tarantini A, Hintschich C. Primary dermis-fat grafting in children. Orbit. 2008;27:363–9.
16. Quaranta-Leoni FM, Sposato S, Raglione P, Mastromarino A. Dermis-fat graft in children as primary and secondary orbital implant. Ophthalmic Plast Reconstr Surg. 2016;32:214.
17. Shams PN, Bohman E, Baker MS, et al. Chronic anophthalmic socket pain treated by implant removal and dermis fat graft. Br J Ophthalmol. 2015;99:1692–6.
18. Baum SH, Schmeling C, Pförtner R, et al. Autologous dermis—fat grafts as primary and secondary orbital transplants before rehabilitation with artificial eyes. J Craniomaxillofac Surg. 2018;46:90–7.
19. Schellini S, Jorge E, Sousa R, Burroughs J, El-Dib R. Porous and nonporous orbital implants for treating the anophthalmic socket: A meta-analysis of case series studies. Orbit. 2016;35:78–86.
20. Custer PL, Kennedy RH, Woog JJ, Kaltreider SA, Meyer DR. Orbital implants in enucleation surgery: a report by the American Academy of Ophthalmology. Ophthalmology. 2003;110:2054–61.
21. Viswanathan P, Sagoo MS, Olver JM. UK national survey of enucleation, evisceration and orbital implants trends. Br J Ophthalmol. 2007;91:616–9.
22. Quaranta-Leoni FM. Reply re: "Management of porous orbital implants requiring explantation: a clinical and histopathological study". Ophthalmic Plast Reconstr Surg. 2014;30:528–9.
23. Piest KL, Welsh MG. Pediatric enucleation, evisceration, and exenteration techniques. In: Katowitz JA, editor. Pediatric oculoplastic surgery. New York: Springer; 2002. p. 617–27.
24. Quaranta-Leoni FM, Moretti C, Sposato S, Nardoni S, Lambiase A, Bonini S. Management of porous orbital implants requiring explantation: a clinical and histopathological study. Ophthalmic Plast Reconstr Surg. 2014;30:132–6.
25. Badilla J, Dolman PJ. Methods of antibiotic instillation in porous orbital implants. Ophthal Plast Reconstr Surg. 2008;24:287–9.
26. Jordan DR, Klapper SR, Gilberg SM. The use of vicryl mesh in 200 porous orbital implants: a technique with few exposures. Ophthal Plast Reconstr Surg. 2003;19:53–61.
27. Tabatabaee Z, Mazloumi M, Rajabi MT, et al. Comparison of the exposure rate of wrapped hydroxyapatite (Bio-Eye) versus unwrapped porous polyethylene (Medpor) orbital implants in enucleated patients. Ophthal Plast Reconstr Surg. 2011;27:114–8.
28. Sobti MM, Shams F, Jawaheer L, Cauchi P, Chadha V. Unwrapped hydroxyapatite orbital implants: our experience in 347 cases. Eye (Lond). 2020;34:675–82.
29. Lin CW, Liao SL. Long-term complications of different porous orbital implants: a 21-year review. Br J Ophthalmol. 2017;101:681–5.
30. Habib LA, North VS, Freitag SK, Yoon MK, Lefebvre DR, Grace LN. Medical comorbidities and orbital implant exposure. Acta Ophthalmol. 2022;100:e813–9.
31. Medel R, Cicinelli MV, Arboleda Hurtado JC, Sánchez España JC, Bahamondes AT, Vasquez LM. Retroauricular myoperiosteal autograft for orbital implant exposure: 11 years of experience. Orbit. 2020;39:342–9.
32. Curragh DS, Kamalarajah S, Lacey B, et al. Primary replacement for the management of exposed orbital implant. Orbit. 2019;38:461–7.
33. Collin JRO. Enucleation, evisceration and socket surgery. In: 3rd, editor. A manual of systematic eyelid

surgery. London: Elsevier-Butterworth-Heinemann; 2006. p. 203–28.
34. Choi BH, Lee SH, Chung WS. Correction of superior sulcus deformity and enophthalmos with porous high-density polyethylene sheet in anophthalmic patients. Korean J Ophthalmol. 2005;19:168–73.
35. Jordan DR. Microplate fixation of prefabricated subperiosteal orbital floor implants. Ophthalmic Surg. 1995;26:78–9.
36. Bernardini FP, Nerad J, Fay A, Zambelli A, Cruz AA. The revised direct transconjunctival approach to the orbital floor. Ophthalmic Plast Reconstr Surg. 2017;33:93–100.
37. Rose GE, Sigurdsson H, Collin R. The volume-deficient orbit: clinical characteristics, surgical management, and results after extraperiorbital implantation of Silastic block. Br J Ophthalmol. 1990;74:545–50.
38. Tan P, Kwong TQ, Malhotra R. Non-aesthetic indications for periocular hyaluronic acid filler treatment: a review. Br J Ophthalmol. 2018;102:725–35.
39. Tay E, Olver J. Intraorbital hyaluronic acid for enophthalmos. Ophthalmology. 2008;115:1101.
40. Malhotra R. Deep orbital Sub-Q restylane (nonanimal stabilized hyaluronic acid) for orbital volume enhancement in sighted and anophthalmic orbits. Arch Ophthalmol. 2007;125:1623–9.
41. Vagefi MR. Minimally invasive approaches to orbital volume augmentation. Int Ophthalmol Clin. 2013;53:67–86.
42. Neuber G. Fettrsnsplantation [Fat transplantation]. Bericht über die Verhandlungen der Deutschen Gesellschaft für Chirurgie Zbl Chir. 1893;22:66. [German]
43. Hardy TG, Joshi N, Kelly MH. Orbital volume augmentation with autologous micro-fat grafts. Ophthal Plast Reconstr Surg. 2007;23:445–9.
44. Fox DM. Orbital fat injection: technique and 5-year follow-up. Aesthetic Plast Surg. 2019;43:123–32.
45. Vagefi MR, McMullan TF, Burroughs JR, Georgescu D, McCann JD, Anderson RL. Orbital augmentation with injectable calcium hydroxyapatite for correction of postenucleation/evisceration socket syndrome. Ophthalmic Plast Reconstr Surg. 2011;27:90–4.
46. Aletaha M, Salour H, Yadegary S, Fekri Y, Tavakoli M. Orbital volume augmentation with calcium hydroxyapatite filler in anophthalmic enophthalmos. J Ophthalmic Vis Res. 2017;12:397–401.
47. Sung Y, Goldberg RA, Lew H. Periorbital injection of hyaluronic acid gel in patients with deep superior sulcus. J Craniofac Surg. 2020;31:271–3.
48. Zamani M, Thyagarajan S, Olver JM. Adjunctive use of hyaluronic acid gel (Restylane Sub-Q) in anophthalmic volume deficient sockets and phthisical eyes. Ophthal Plast Reconstr Surg. 2010;26:250–3.
49. Crochelet O, Maalouf T, Duron S, et al. Efficacité et tolérance des injections d'acide hyaluronique hautement réticulé dans la prise en charge des énophtalmies. J Fr Ophtalmol. 2012;35:1–7.
50. Da Silva AL, Bredemeier M, Gebrim ES, et al. Intraorbital polyacrylamide injection for the treatment of anophthalmic enophthalmos. Ophthal Plast Reconstr Surg. 2008;24:367–71.
51. Schittkowski MD, Guthoff RF. Injectable self-inflating hydrogel pellet expanders for the treatment of orbital volume deficiency in congenital microphthalmos: preliminary results with a new therapeutic approach. Br J Ophthalmol. 2006;90:1173–7.

Management of the Contracted Socket

Marco Sales-Sanz and Dyonne T. Hartong

Key Messages

- Socket contraction is characterised by the loss of the fornices, with or without orbital volume deficiency, resulting in the inability to wear an ocular prosthesis.
- Reconstruction of the contracted socket is usually challenging and must address the underlying pathophysiological mechanisms.
- Fornix contraction usually requires reconstruction with buccal mucosa grafts.
- Posterior lamella grafts are usually required when fornix contraction is associated with eyelid retraction.
- Placement of a large conformer and fixation of the fornix (fornix-deepening or quilting sutures) and eyelids are essential to prevent recurrence.
- Vascularised flaps, such as temporalis muscle flap or free microvascular flaps, may be required in severely contracted and ischemic sockets.

1 Definition

Socket contraction results from shrinkage and shortening of part or all of the soft tissues in the anophthalmic socket, leading to loss of fornices, with or without orbital volume loss, and inability to wear an ocular prosthesis.

2 Causes

Socket contraction can be caused by:

- Scar tissue and fibrosis secondary to the initial injury
- Poor surgical techniques with extensive traumatic dissection and cauterisation of the orbital tissues
- Multiple socket operations
- Cicatrising conjunctival diseases (ocular mucous membrane pemphigoid, Stevens-Johnson Syndrome, toxic epidermal necrolysis)
- Radiotherapy
- Alkali or acid burns
- Poor vascular supply
- Chronic inflammation
- Infection
- Not wearing a conformer or prosthesis, or wearing a poorly fitting prosthesis

M. Sales-Sanz (✉)
Oculoplastic Surgery Unit, Ophthalmology Department, Hospital Universitario Ramón y Cajal, Madrid, Spain

Oculoplastic Surgery Unit, IMO Madrid, Grupo Miranza, Madrid, Spain
e-mail: marco@sales-sanz.com

D. T. Hartong
Orbital Centre, Department of Ophthalmology, Amsterdam University Medical Center, Amsterdam, The Netherlands

F. M. Quaranta Leoni et al. (eds.), *Oculoplastic, Lacrimal and Orbital Surgery*,
https://doi.org/10.1007/978-3-031-39638-0_8

3 Pathophysiology of Socket Contraction

Tissue contracture occurs as a result of an inflammatory response induced by external or internal (auto-immune) factors, or during post-operative wound healing, where inadequate or prolonged activity of myofibroblasts is thought to play a role [1]. Contraction of orbital tissues can result in a variety of functional or cosmetic outcomes. Shortening or obliteration of the conjunctival fornices can cause discomfort, entropion, eyelid retraction, limited prosthesis motility, contour changes, or inability to retain the prosthesis. Contracture of the levator–superior rectus muscle complex can result in upper eyelid retraction and lagophthalmos, or loss of the normal eyelid crease, while involvement of deeper socket tissues may lead to enophthalmos.

4 Classification of Socket Contraction

Various classifications have been proposed, but many of them fail to address all the factors that contribute to the inability to retain an ocular prosthesis. One of the most widely accepted classifications divides socket contraction into four categories [2]:

- Grade 1: Minimal or no actual contraction. Patients usually complain of inability to retain the prosthesis for a long time. Horizontal lid laxity is common, with subsequent prolapse or retraction of the inferior fornix. Patients with an unusually large or anteriorly displaced implant also fall into this category.
- Grade 2: Mild contraction of the inferior and or the superior fornix. Patients either complain of inability to wear the prosthesis or a cosmetic disfigurement due to inward rolling of the upper and lower eyelid margins.
- Grade 3: More advanced scarring than grade 2, with cicatrisation involving the entire upper and lower fornices. Wearing the prosthesis is impossible.
- Grade 4: Severe phimosis of the palpebral fissure both vertically and horizontally. This category includes recurrent cases and irradiated sockets.

5 Principles of Management

The goal is to enable the patient to comfortably wear a prosthesis with acceptable cosmetic appearance. Reconstruction of the contracted socket should adequately address conjunctival deficiency, orbital volume and eyelid position. Where possible, a one-step procedure is preferred, although secondary procedures are often required.

6 Non-surgical Management

It is important to determine whether the prosthesis is the cause of the problem (for example, an inadequate fit or an old prosthesis with chronic irritation) and/or whether the prosthesis can be adjusted or renewed, which requires close collaboration with an ocularist.

Non-surgical fornix expansion can be offered to patients with mild contraction, when surgery is not an option, or in cases where socket expansion is desirable prior to socket surgery. This involves applying pressure to the socket using a custom-made conformer (a compressor) that gradually stretches the fornices. Pressure can be applied with patches or with a customised facial mask that allows continuous pressure to the socket [3], as described in chapter "Management of the Anophthalmic Patient".

7 Surgical Management

Treatment options are summarised in Table 1.

7.1 Grade 1

Lower eyelid laxity, which can result in fornix flattening or prolapse, is the main pathogenic mechanism for failure to retain the prosthesis in grade 1 contractions. This category is associated with a lack of orbital implant and the ocular prosthesis is often large and heavy. Mild fornix shortening and eyelid displacement or ectropion may be present. Prosthetic modifications to improve fit may exacerbate the eyelid laxity.

Table 1 Treatment options

Type of contraction	Cause/problem	Treatment options	Notes
Grade 1	Inferior fornix loss due to eyelid laxity	Prosthetic adjustment	Fitting a larger/heavier prosthesis may aggravate the problem
		Horizontal eyelid shortening	lateral tarsal strip, lateral en-bloc excision (Bick's procedure)
		Fornix repositioning	Open or closed procedure
	+ Conjunctival shortage/ contraction	Fornix repositioning + posterior lamella lengthening using oral mucosa	
Grade 2	Mild conjunctival contraction	Prosthetic adjustment	
		Non-surgical fornix expansion with compressor	
	Entropion + stable prosthetic fit	Standard eyelid everting procedures	Anterior lamella repositioning, transcutaneous retractor plication, tarsotomy
	Entropion + unstable prosthetic fit	Oral mucosal graft	
		Amniotic membrane graft	The presence of healthy conjunctival epithelial cells is required for re-epithelialisation to occur
Grade 3	Moderate/severe conjunctival contraction	Oral mucosal graft	
		Skin graft (if mucous membrane graft is contraindicated)	Risk for foul odour and increased socket discharge in moist sockets
	+ Lower eyelid retraction	Hard palate graft	Can be done in conjunction with oral mucosal graft
		Auricular cartilage graft	Only possible if sufficient healthy conjunctiva is left to allow for re-epithelialisation
		Nasal mucosal graft	Potentially good, but sparse literature Risk for septal perforation
		Tarso-conjunctival graft	Ideal tissue, but often insufficient in size
	+ Volume deficiency	Dermis-fat graft • Total socket filling, or • Local add-on in addition to retained implant	A sufficiently vascularised socket and healthy conjunctiva are required for survival and re-epithelialisation
		Autologous fat grafting or non-permanent fillers	May help to reduce scarring and slightly improve eyelid position
Grade 4	Severe contraction due to superficial vascular insufficiency (also recurrent contractions)	Large oral mucosal graft with long-term fixation	
	Total vascular insufficiency + volume loss	Pedicle flap: temporalis muscle transposition + oral/dermis-fat graft	
		Free flaps with or without skin	Radial forearm, groin, dorsalis pedis, scapular, deltopectoral, or lateral thigh flaps

Surgery in grade 1 may include the following procedures:

- Horizontal eyelid shortening
- Fornix repositioning
- Posterior lamella lengthening

Horizontal eyelid shortening. In the absence of conjunctival retraction, horizontal tightening procedures such as lateral tarsal strip may provide sufficient inferior fornix depth by improving lower eyelid position and support [4].

Fornix repositioning or deepening can be performed through a "closed" or "open" procedure. In the "closed" approach, several 3-0 non-braided double-armed sutures are passed from the fornix through the inferior orbital rim periosteum and lower eyelid skin and tied over a bolster for 3–6 weeks.

In the "open" method, the conjunctiva is incised transversally at least 10 mm below the lower eyelid margin, at the level of the intended fornix (note that a higher incision closer to the eyelid margin increases the risk of lower eyelid contraction and retraction). The lower eyelid retractors are incised, and dissection is continued inferiorly until reaching the orbital floor periosteum, 5–10 mm posterior to the inferior orbital rim. Three 6-0 polyglycolic horizontal mattress sutures are then placed, incorporating the posterior conjunctival edge, the periosteum of the orbital floor, and the anterior conjunctival edge. Inadvertent incorporation of tissues other than the anterior conjunctival edge, or closure with excessive tension, may result in entropion or eyelid retraction [5, 6].

Posterior lamella lengthening with spacer is indicated in relatively more advanced lower eyelid retraction with fornix contraction. Since the retraction is mild in grade 1 cases, it is usually sufficient to use "surface" grafts, like oral mucous membrane, rather than "support" grafts, such as hard palate, ear cartilage, or nasal septum. For technical description, see method described in Grade 2.

7.2 Grade 2

The inferior fornix is affected before the superior fornix, with lower eyelid contraction causing more significant aesthetic deformities than upper eyelid contraction. Reduced superior fornix depth may impair eyelid closure and prosthesis retention [7].

Eyelid everting procedures such as transverse tarsal incision (tarsotomy) with marginal rotation or anterior lamella repositioning may yield acceptable results in patients with mild upper or lower eyelid entropion but good prosthesis stability [8–10]. Fornix reconstruction is necessary when prosthetic fitting is difficult or impossible, or when standard entropion surgery fails. Oral mucous membrane is the most commonly used graft in grade 2 contracted sockets. Amniotic membrane can also be used in selected cases.

Oral mucous membrane grafting. The conjunctiva is incised horizontally over the recipient area and gently undermined along its margins. Scar tissue is excised while avoiding aggressive cauterisation, and dissection is continued until the eyelid is freely mobile and a large conformer can be inserted with complete approximation of the eyelid margins. A mucous membrane graft is harvested from the mouth, and it should be about 40–50% larger than the observed conjunctival defect (to compensate for subsequent graft contraction). The graft can be harvested from the lower lip (easier access) or from the cheek (larger grafts possible) with a D15 blade for the incision and blunt-tipped scissors for the dissection. In the cheek, care must be taken not to damage the salivary duct near the second molar. The donor site can be left to re-epithelialise spontaneously or closed with 5-0 absorbable sutures. Using blunt scissors, the graft is freed of submucosal tissue before being sutured to the conjunctival edges of the recipient area with a 6-0 absorbable running suture (Fig. 1). Grafts vascularise from the base rather than the edges, therefore apposition with the underlying vascularised socket tissue is crucial, and this can be achieved by:

- Placement of a large conformer with temporary tarsorrhaphy (4–5 weeks).
- Fornix-deepening sutures (see also Grade 1).
- Anchoring a silastic tube in the fornix, adjacent to the periosteum.

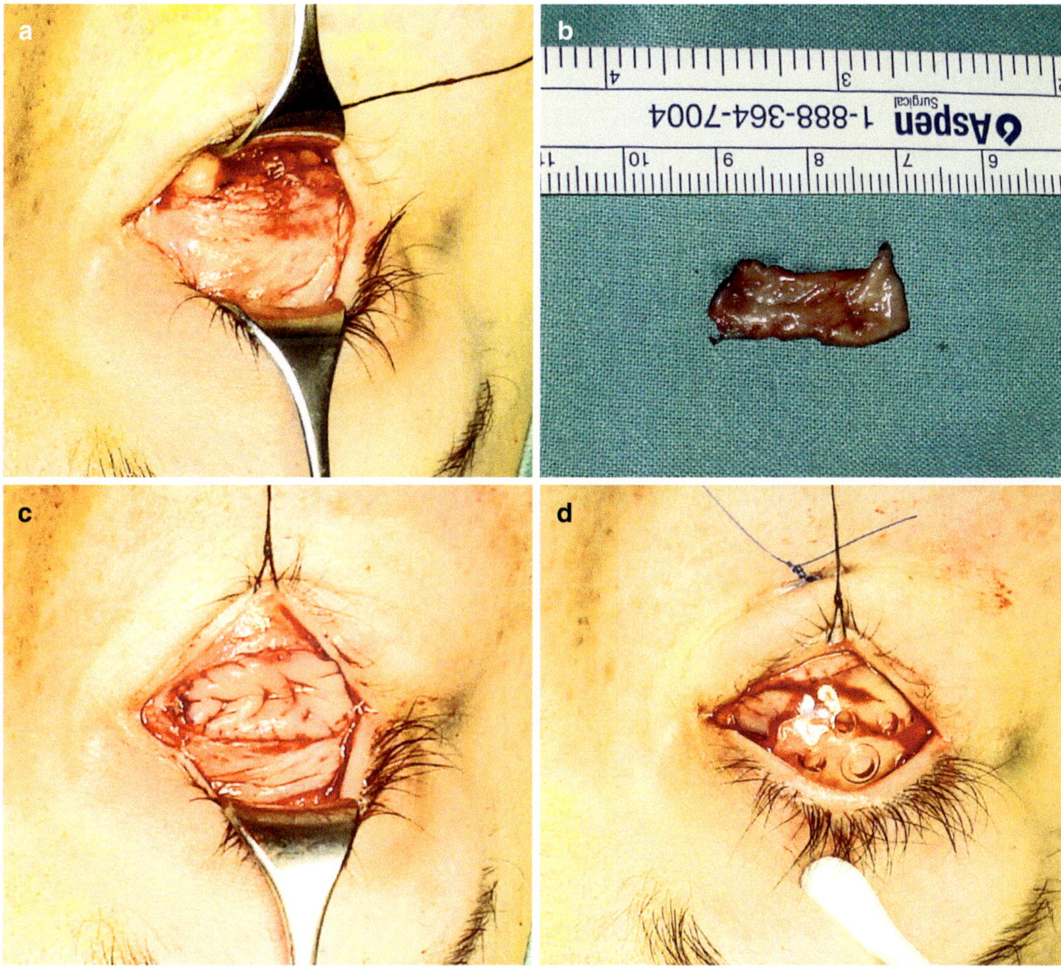

Fig. 1 Grade 2 contracted socket reconstruction with oral mucosa graft. (**a**) Incised conjunctiva and direction of a virtual plane to reconstruct the inferior fornix. (**b**) Harvested oral mucosal graft. (**c**) Graft sutured to the conjunctival defect. (**d**) Quilting (fornix-deepening) sutures and a large conformer are placed to maintain the inferior fornix

Amniotic membrane grafts act as "substrate grafts" in contrast to a mucous membrane graft that acts as "substitute graft". Amniotic membrane promotes normal conjunctival epithelial cell migration and differentiation over the graft by serving as a basement membrane and secreting growth factors [11]. It also reinforces basal epithelial adhesion and inhibits subconjunctival fibrosis by downregulation of transforming growth factor beta. However, it requires healthy conjunctival epithelial cells to grow over the graft, and can only be used in moderate socket contractions. The amount of normal conjunctiva needed has yet to be determined. The mucous membrane is regarded as a 'substitute graft' and does not need healthy epithelial cells as a prerequisite for implantation.

The advantages of amniotic membrane transplantation include its wide availability, lack of donor site morbidity, and proven antifibroblastic activity. While some studies have shown its superiority over mucous membrane grafts [11],others have found similar favourable outcomes in both groups [12], with one study reporting a 20% recurrence rate of forniceal contraction and loss of prosthetic hold [13].

Antifibrotic agents, such as topical mitomycin C 0.02% (intra-operatively) [14] or 5 fluorouracil (5FU) injections (post-operatively) [15], have also been proposed as adjunctive treatments to reduce recurrence rate, though their role in unhealthy sockets has yet to be established, and both substances should be used with caution due to their potential conjunctival toxicity.

7.3 Grade 3

Management of grade 3 contracted sockets aims to address:

- Moderate or severe eyelid conjunctival deficiency
- Moderate or severe eyelid retraction
- Orbital volume loss

7.3.1 Contracted Sockets with Mainly Conjunctival Deficiency

Oral mucosal grafts can be harvested and positioned as described in grade 2 contraction. Splitting the harvested graft allows using separate grafts for the lower and upper fornices. Alternatively, a large graft can be placed in the centre, with the remaining conjunctiva used for the palpebral parts of the socket. In these cases, it is important to adequately release the conjunctiva from its underlying tissue and use fornix-fixating sutures. It is also recommended to use a conformer with temporary tarsorrhaphy for at least 6 weeks.

Skin grafts are occasionally used when the size of the oral mucosal graft is deemed insufficient to cover the entire socket, though in our experience, it is always possible to obtain enough mucosa. Skin grafts can be used in dry sockets (if harvesting oral mucosa is contraindicated), but they should be avoided in moist sockets, where adding cutaneous components is generally associated with foul odour, keratinisation and discharge. Anterior lamella deficit can also be addressed with skin grafts.

7.3.2 Contracted Sockets with Moderate to Severe Lower Eyelid Retraction

Fornix contraction associated with moderate or severe eyelid retraction, requires a posterior lamella spacer that both lengthens the retracted conjunctiva and provides a strong vertical support, which the oral mucosa lacks. Reconstruction can be performed using various autologous, allogenic or synthetic materials. While synthetic materials are readily available, they carry risks of extrusion, exposure, and infection [16–19]. Autogenous grafts, such as hard palate, auricular cartilage, nasal chondro-mucosa, and tarsoconjunctiva, are generally preferred and more commonly used in the lower eyelid.

The *surgical technique* for suturing posterior lamella spacer grafts in the lower eyelid is similar in most cases. A conjunctival incision is made along the inferior tarsal border across the length of the lower eyelid. The lower eyelid retractors are dissected from the septum and orbicularis muscle, and any scar tissue is released. The inferior border of the graft is sutured to the recessed retractors and conjunctiva with a buried 6-0 polyglyconate or polyglactin absorbable suture. The superior border of the graft is sutured to the inferior border of the tarsus with a running 6-0 polyglactin, and both ends are externalised and secured over the skin. Fornix-deepening sutures and a temporary conformer are placed (see also grade 1 and 2) and the lower eyelid is held in position with a Frost suture for several days [20], or temporary tarsorrhaphy sutures.

Hard Palate Graft

Hard palate fibro-mucous grafts are more rigid and contract less than oral mucosa grafts. They are usually used to reconstruct the tarsal conjunctiva, particularly when lower eyelid elevation is desired [21], and may be combined with buccal mucosal graft [22]. The hard palate comprises the anterior two-thirds of the palate, while the soft palate (more red and softer) constitutes the posterior third. Under general anaesthesia, retractors are used to gain access to the mouth, and the desired hard palate graft is marked, staying lateral to the central raphe and medial to the alveolar ridge (bumpy part directly behind the teeth). The technique of harvesting the hard palate is thoroughly described in chapter "Management of Eyelid Retraction". The donor site is left open for spontaneous granulation, and comfort can be improved by applying a dental plate prepared by a dentist.

Auricular Cartilage Graft

The concha and scapha are the two main donor sites for auricular cartilage grafts, which can be harvested either anteriorly or posteriorly. The Authors prefer the posterior approach as it has less risk of visible scar, and the graft from the scaphoid fossa is generally favoured over the concha because of its flat surface, albeit it may not always be large enough to correct severe retractions. The graft is sized to match the horizontal length of the recipient site, and the height is determined by the degree of lower eyelid retraction (approximately 1–2 mm for every millimetre of eyelid retraction). Trimming of the cartilage may be necessary for an optimally shaped graft with no visible or palpable irregularities. The lack of mucosal lining limits the use of cartilage grafts to sockets with healthy epithelium that allows epithelisation of the graft or if there is enough conjunctiva to cover the implant [20, 23–26].

Nasal Mucosa Graft

Nasal septal composite chondro-mucosal grafts combine the advantages of the palatal graft (mucosal lining) with the auricular graft (the rigidity of the septal cartilage). A single graft with a mucosal "excess" much larger than the cartilaginous part can be utilised to reconstruct both the tarsal and bulbar conjunctiva. Care should be taken to avoid septal perforation.

Tarso-conjuntival Graft

The upper eyelid tarso-conjunctival unit provides an ideal tissue match, however the amount of the donor tissue is limited and may be insufficient to correct moderate or severe fornix contractions.

Dermis-fat Grafts

Dermis-fat grafts (DFG) can be used to treat lower eyelid retraction as well as volume deficit in the anophthalmic socket [27, 28].

DFG not only improves orbital volume but also increases conjunctival surface area by allowing the migration of conjunctival cells over its dermis surface. As with amniotic membrane grafts, some normal recipient conjunctiva is necessary for a successful outcome. It also requires a healthy vascularised socket as its viability depends on fibrovascular ingrowth; hence, it should be used with caution in cases of previous orbital radiotherapy, recurrent scarring, or poor orbital vascularity. As with mucous membrane grafts, a large conformer shell is mandatory (with temporary tarsorrhaphy) to prevent socket contraction. Advantages and drawbacks of DFG have been discussed in chapter "Secondary Orbital Implants, Dermis-Fat Graft and Volume Enhancement Techniques". Porous implants have been used in conjunction with mucus membrane grafting to minimise fat resorption [29], which requires sufficient vascular tissue to cover the implant and nourish the mucous membrane graft.

Autologous fat transfer is another option for enhancing the orbital or palpebral volume. Adipose tissue is harvested by gentle manual negative pressure aspiration from the abdomen or medial thighs, in multi-layered "feathered" passes. The processed fat can be injected into the intraconal space, subcutaneous or submuscular layer of the eyelids using a closed blunt cannula technique with multiple passes. The procedure is simple, minimally invasive and can be repeated (at several month intervals) until satisfactory cosmesis is achieved [30, 31] (Fig. 2). Non-permanent fillers can also be used for small touch-ups, with generally good results and durability in the periocular region (see chapter "Secondary Orbital Implants, Dermis-Fat Graft and Volume Enhancement Techniques").

7.4 Grade 4

Patients with severe or recurrent socket scarring tend to have poor vascularisation, and management is challenging as ischemia increases the risk

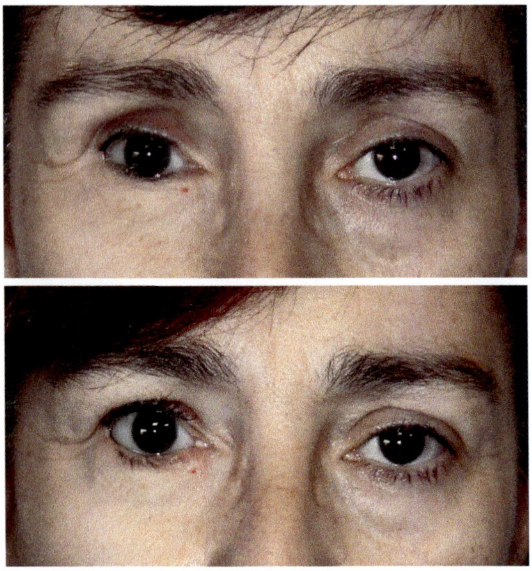

Fig. 2 *Top*: Contracted socket with enophthalmos and inferior fornix shortening with entropion. *Bottom*: Same patient after orbital lipofilling to correct the enophthalmos and oral mucosa graft to enlarge the inferior fornix

of graft failure, with further scarring and socket contraction. Surgery should be postponed for at least 9–12 months after any socket inflammation has subsided.

Grade 4 contraction can primarily affect the anterior part or the entire socket. The 'mainly anterior group' is characterised by extensive superficial scarring and vascular deficit, but relatively normal blood supply in the deeper socket, commonly after chemical injury or trauma with multiple surgeries. They can be treated with a large mucosal graft attached to the deeper vascular bed and long-term placement of an adequately sized conformer [32, 33]. The 'totally contracted sockets' have poor vascularisation of the entire socket, often with significant volume deficiency, and are typically associated with previous socket irradiation.

Vascularisation, volume, and epithelial lining should all be addressed, usually by staged surgery. Flaps provide a good vascular bed for mucosal or skin grafts, with options including local flaps (such as temporalis muscle flap) or free flaps (for example, radial forearm or dorsalis pedis flap). On-lay bone grafts or orbital osteotomies can be used to address bony orbit asymmetry, providing enough space for the prosthesis to be fitted [34–39].

It is essential to carefully discuss the cosmetic expectations, the prolonged treatment course, and the possibility of additional procedures, as well as alternative options (including no ocular prosthesis, or episthesis). Levator function and prosthesis movement are often poor, and any lash loss or malposition is unlikely to improve after surgery.

7.4.1 Socket Preparation

Surgery for severely contracted socket usually starts with placing 4-0 silk traction sutures through upper and lower eyelid margins. An incision is made along the existing mucosa, and the underlying scar tissue is removed. Dissection is continued until the orbital rim is reached, creating a virtual space in which a large conformer can be placed.

7.4.2 Large Oral Mucosal Graft with Long-term Conformer Fixation

The cheek generally allows for larger grafts than the lip. A large graft of freely mobile buccal mucosa, preferably sized around 3–5 cm is obtained (or less if considerable conjunctival lining is still present) while taking care not to interfere with the Stensen's duct. It is advisable to oversize the graft because of potential shrinkage; if necessary, both the lip and the cheek, or both cheeks, can be used. The graft should be freed of submucosal tissue, and further extension is achieved by multiple full-thickness releasing incisions. If there is no or little residual conjunctiva, the graft should be sized to completely wrap around the conformer.

Customised conformers created by an ocularist or an approved 3D printer (for example, from dental or maxillofacial practices), or commercially available conformers with preformed holes in different sizes can be used. We prefer to prepare customised conformers, 4 mm wider than the eyelid length (2 mm beyond the nasal and temporal fornices), with varying heights (16, 18, 20 or 22 mm) to fit the available space and mucosal size. A wing-shaped extension with fixation-holes at the lower third of the conformer helps long-term fixation of the eyelids (as a central tarsorrhaphy), while fixation-holes at the edges allow fornix-deepening sutures to pass. The conformer with the greatest height (while permitting eyelid closure without traction) is placed, and the buccal mucosal graft is sutured to the conjunctival margins with a running 6-0 polyglactin that is exteriorised and fixed over the skin. The nasal and temporal fornices are formed with double–armed 5-0 sutures, in the same manner. Fornix fixation sutures can be passed through the holes at the conformer edges. Central fixation sutures (temporary tarsorrhaphy) are placed either on bolsters or at the wing-shaped extension of the conformer. The fixation sutures and conformer should be left in situ for two months to counteract the contraction during the healing phase, with combined antibiotic-steroid drops and/or cyclosporine drops used during this period. Crust formation from wound debris is normal and can gently be cleaned. After removing the conformer, it can be replaced by a similarly-shaped ocular prosthesis. The cyclosporine drops are continued if the mucosa remains inflamed (Fig. 3).

7.4.3 Temporalis Muscle Transposition

The temporalis muscle flap is pedicled on the deep temporalis vessels and may be approached through a variety of skin incisions, including the coronal approach. The skin is incised and dissection is carried out until the superficial temporalis fascia is reached, maintaining the plane of the dissection between the deep and superficial temporalis fasciae, or through both layers of the deep temporalis fascia to avoid injuring the frontal branch of the facial nerve.

The posterior part of the temporalis muscle is dissected subperiosteally from the temporal fossa along its superior and posterior borders, taking care not to damage the underlying blood vessels, particularly the muscular branches of the middle temporal artery that run along its undersurface. The

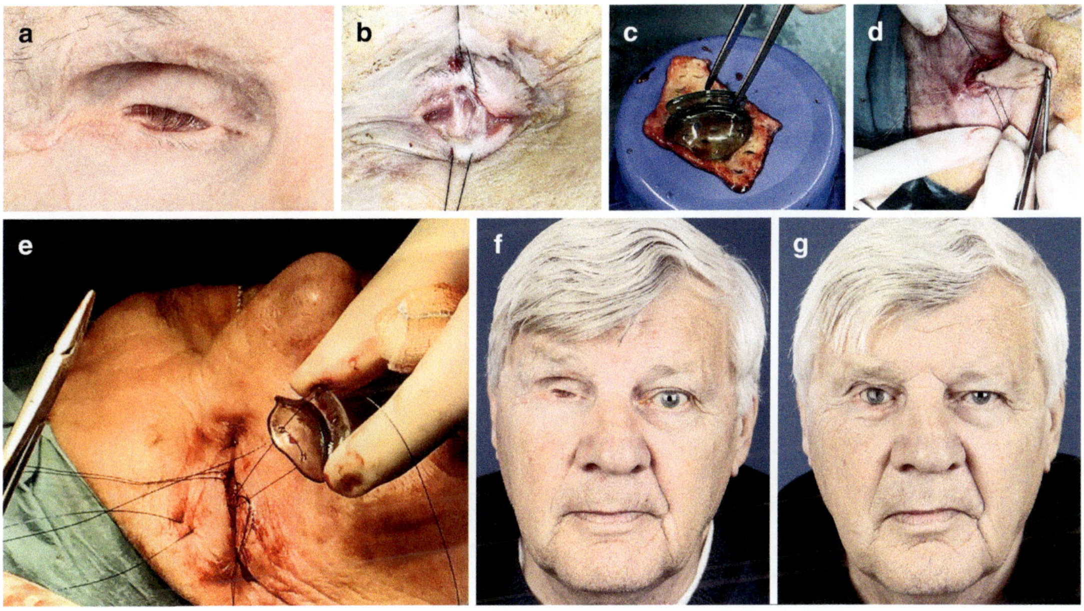

Fig. 3 Grade 4 recurrent contracted socket. (**a**, **b**) Pre- and intra-operative views of a contracted socket with inability to wear a prosthesis due to loss of fornices. (**c**) A large cheek (buccal) mucosal graft with perforation holes is assessed to ensure that it can fully cover the conformer. (**d**) The lateral (and medial) fornix fixation is performed before suturing the oral mucosal margins to the conjunctival remnants. (**e**) Double-armed sutures are passed through the conformer openings, superior and inferior fornices, and skin before being tied over a bolster. The conformer will glide into the pre-prepared socket and push the oral mucosa into the correct position, in contact with the deeper vascular bed. The eyelids can be sutured with a temporal tarsorrhaphy. (**f**) Pre-operative appearance and (**g**) post-operative result

flap is then dissected inferiorly to the coronoid process of the mandible, and depending on the defect size, it can be transferred totally or partially.

The periosteum of the lateral orbital wall is raised to create a bony window, with or without rim preservation; when the rim is preserved or repositioned, care must be taken to minimise compression on the flap's vascular pedicle. The temporalis muscle flap is transposed through the bone window into the socket and sutured to the surrounding subcutaneous or sub-orbicularis tissue using a 4-0 absorbable suture; in some cases, the flap can also be fixed to the orbital rim through drill holes.

Once the flap is positioned in the orbit, mucous membrane grafts or a dermis-fat graft is sutured over the temporalis flap to the epithelial margins of the socket. A conformer with temporary suture tarsorrhaphy is used for at least 4–6 weeks until the prosthesis is fitted.

The coronal incision is closed in two layers and a drain is placed into the temporalis muscle bed (usually for 48 h), along with a compressive bandage over the socket and temporalis region (Fig. 4). Over the following months, mild to moderate muscle flap atrophy and mucosal graft contraction are expected (Fig. 5).

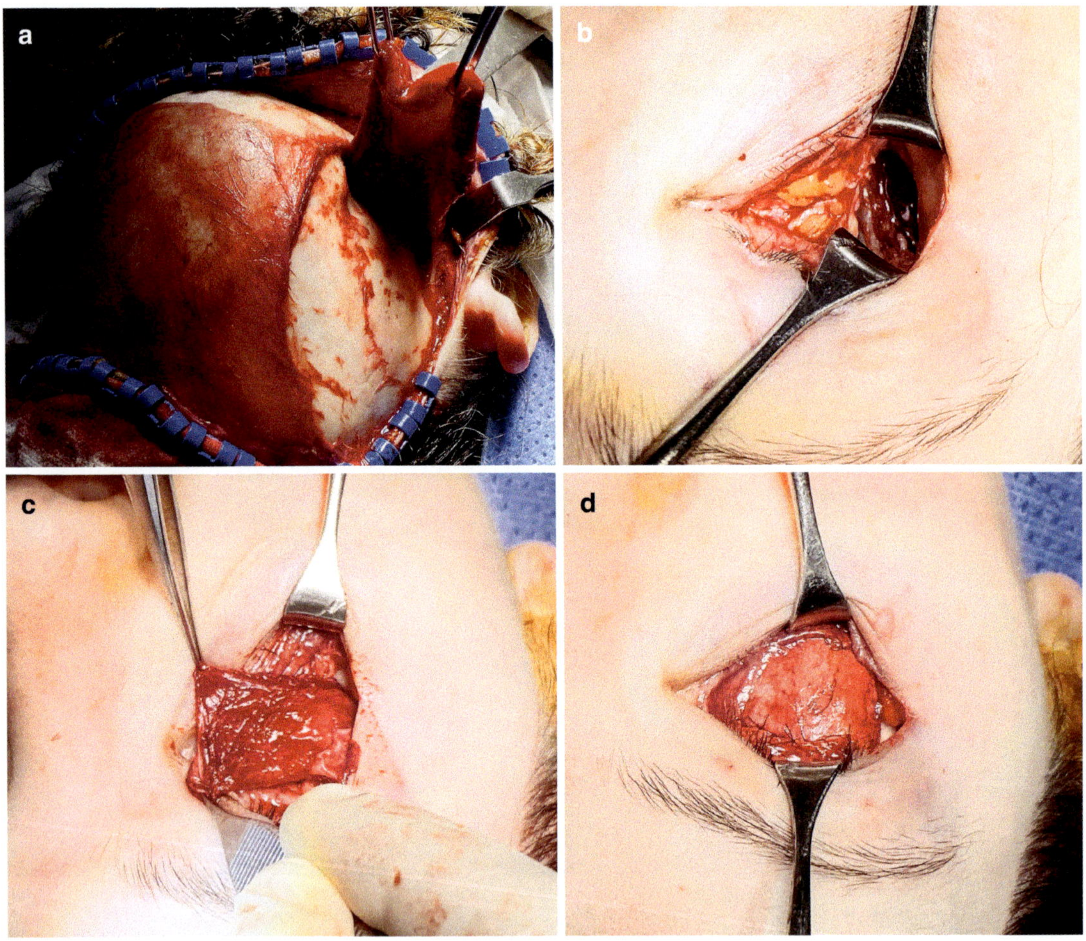

Fig. 4 Temporalis muscle flap for grade 4 contracted socket. (**a**) The muscle flap is dissected through a coronal approach. (**b**) The contracted cavity is dissected to enable placement of a large conformer and a bony window is created on the lateral orbital wall to allow for the transposition of the temporalis flap. (**c**) The flap is transposed into the orbit, and in severe cases, it should cover the entire anterior surface of the orbit. (**d**) The flap is sutured to the orbital rim and the edges of the socket dissection before being covered with oral mucosa grafts

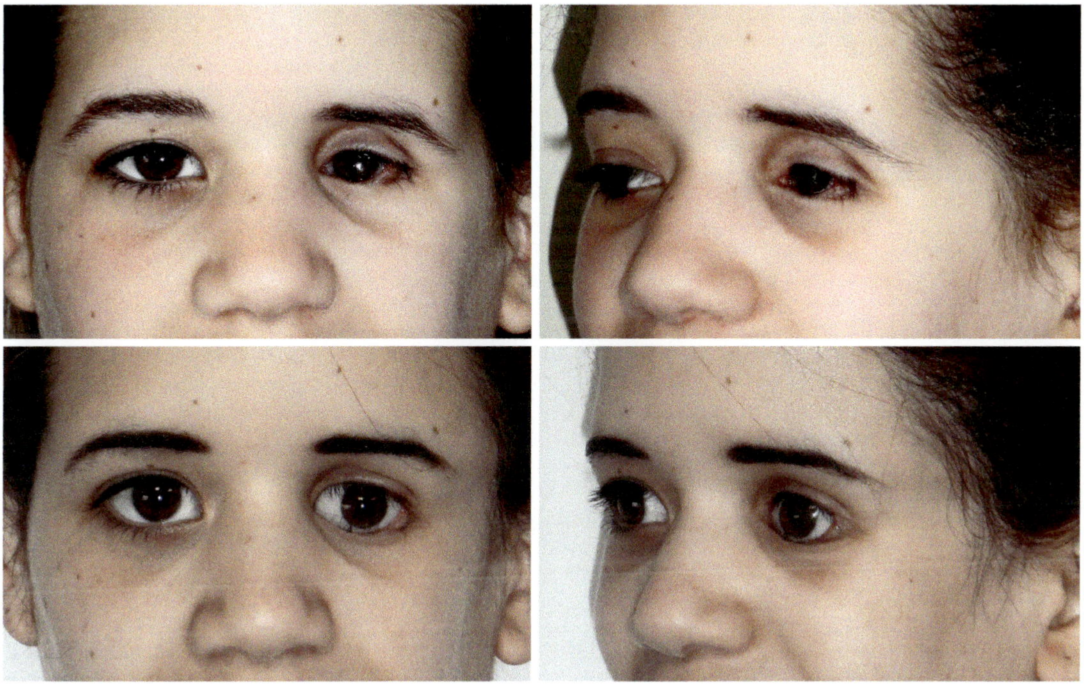

Fig. 5 *Top*: Pre-operative pictures of a grade 4 contracted socket. *Bottom*: Post-operative pictures after orbital reconstruction with a temporalis muscle flap and oral mucosa grafts. Note the improvement in orbital volume and the deeper fonices permitting placement of a considerably larger ocular prosthesis

7.4.4 Free Flap Transposition

Several flaps, including radial forearm, groin, dorsalis pedis, scapular, deltopectoral, and lateral thigh flaps, have been used for socket repair, with the choice of flap depending on the extent of the orbital depression and the presence of any conjunctival remnants. Thin flaps can be easily folded to match the contour of the socket, but they may not have sufficient volume. Free muscle flaps without a skin paddle can be used when there is enough residual conjunctiva; otherwise, a flap with a skin paddle can be folded to fill the whole socket. The donor vessels are anastomosed microsurgically to the superficial temporal or the facial vessels. Auricular cartilage or autologous fat grafts have also been used in combination with free flaps [23, 38, 40, 41].

References

1. Tawfik HA, Abdulhafez MH, Fouad YA, Rashed HO, Osman WM. Revisiting the role of the myofibroblast in socket surgery: an immunohistochemical study. Ophthalmic Plast Reconstr Surg. 2016;32:292–5.
2. Tawfik HA, Raslan AO, Talib N. Surgical management of acquired socket contracture. Curr Opin Ophthalmol. 2009;20:406–11.
3. Kuijten MMP, Remmers JS, Mourits DL, Moll AC, Hartong DT. Three-dimensionally printed facial mask to aid the treatment of contracted socket after radiation damage in retinoblastoma. Ophthalmic Plast Reconstr Surg. 2018;34:178–9.
4. Anderson RL. Tarsal strip procedure for correction of eyelid laxity and canthal malposition in the anophthalmic socket. Ophthalmology. 1981;88:895–903.
5. Ma'Luf RN. Correction of the inadequate lower fornix in the anophthalmic socket. Br J Ophthalmol. 1999;83:881–2.

6. Neuhaus RW, Hawes MJ. Inadequate inferior cul-de-sac in the anophthalmic socket. Ophthalmology. 1992;99:153–7.
7. Jordan DR, Klapper SR. Evaluation and management of the anophthalmic socket and socket reconstruction. In: Black EH, et al., editors. Smith and Nesi's ophthalmic plastic and reconstructive surgery. New York: Springer Science; 2012. p. 1131–73.
8. Quaranta-Leoni FM. Treatment of the anophthalmic socket. Curr Opin Ophthalmol. 2008;19:422–7.
9. Kersten RC, Kleiner FP, Kulwin DR. Tarsotomy for the treatment of cicatricial entropion with trichiasis. Arch Ophthalmol. 1992;110:714–7.
10. Wies FA. Surgical treatment of entropion. J Int Coll Surg. 1954;21:758–60.
11. Bajaj MS, Pushker N, Singh KK, Chandra M, Ghose S. Evaluation of amniotic membrane grafting in the reconstruction of contracted socket. Ophthal Plast Reconstr Surg. 2006;22:116–20.
12. Kumar S, Sugandhi P, Arora R, Pandey PK. Amniotic membrane transplantation versus mucous membrane grafting in anophthalmic contracted socket. Orbit. 2006;25:195–203.
13. Oonyathalang A, Preechawat P, Pomsathit J, Mahaisaviriya P. Reconstruction of contracted eye socket with amniotic membrane graft. Ophthalmic Plast Reconstr Surg. 2005;21:359–62.
14. Mandour SS, Elmazar HM, Marey HM, Rahman AKA, Sakr RA. mucous membrane grafting augmented with topical Mitomycin C application in contracted socket repair surgeries. J Ocul Pharmacol Ther. 2016;32:691–4.
15. Kamal S, Kumar S, Goel R, Bodh SA. Serial subconjunctival 5-Fluorouracil for early recurrent anophthalmic contracted socket. Graefes Arch Clin Exp Ophthalmol. 2013;251:2797–802.
16. Wong JF, Soparkar CN, Patrinely JR. Correction of lower eyelid retraction with high density porous polyethylene: The Medpor((R)) Lower Eyelid Spacer. Orbit. 2001;20:217–25.
17. Fenton S, Kemp EG. A review of the outcome of upper lid lowering for eyelid retraction and complications of spacers at a single unit over five years. Orbit. 2002;21:289–94.
18. Tan J, Olver J, Wright M, Maini R, Neoh C, Dickinson AJ. The use of porous polyethylene (Medpor) lower eyelid spacers in lid heightening and stabilisation. Br J Ophthalmol. 2004;88:1197–200.
19. Lee YJ, Khwarg SI. Polytetrafluoroethylene as a spacer graft for the correction of lower eyelid retraction. Korean J Ophthalmol. 2005;19:247–51.
20. Barrancos C, García-Cruz I, Ventas-Ayala B, Sales-Sanz M. The addition of a conjunctival flap to a posterior lamella auricular cartilage graft: A technique to avoid corneal complications. Eur J Ophthalmol. 2021;31:2165–70.
21. Mai C, Bertelmann E. Oral mucosal grafts: old technique in new light. Ophthalmic Res. 2013;50:91–8.
22. Lee AC, Fedorovich I, Heinz GW, Kikkawa DO. Socket reconstruction with combined mucous membrane and hard palate mucosal grafts. Ophthalmic Surg Lasers. 2002;33:463–8.
23. Hashikawa K, Terashi H, Tahara S. Therapeutic strategy for the triad of acquired anophthalmic orbit. Plast Reconstr Surg. 2007;119:2182–8.
24. Smith RJ, Malet T. Auricular cartilage grafting to correct lower conjunctival fornix retraction and eyelid malposition in anophthalmic patients. Ophthalmic Plast Reconstr Surg. 2008;24:13–8.
25. Zbylski JR, LaRossa DD, Rich JD. Correction of lower eyelid ptosis in the anophthalmic orbit with an autogenous ear cartilage graft. Plast Reconstr Surg. 1978;61:220–4.
26. Baylis HI, Rosen N, Neuhaus RW. Obtaining auricular cartilage for reconstructive surgery. Am J Ophthalmol. 1982;93:709–12.
27. Choi CJ, Tran AQ, Tse DT. Hard palate-dermis fat composite graft for reconstruction of contracted anophthalmic socket. Orbit. 2019;38:199–204.
28. Godfrey KJ, Tooley AA, Kazim M. Bipedicle dermis fat graft for orbital volume augmentation and repair of lower eyelid retraction in an anophthalmic socket with prior orbital implant placement. Ophthalmic Plast Reconstr Surg. 2019;35:e39–41.
29. Bhattacharjee K, Bhattacharjee H, Kuri G, Das JK, Dey D. Comparative analysis of use of porous orbital implant with mucus membrane graft and dermis fat graft as a primary procedure in reconstruction of severely contracted socket. Indian J Ophthalmol. 2014;62:145–53.
30. Hardy TG, Joshi N, Kelly MH. Orbital volume augmentation with autologous micro-fat grafts. Ophthalmic Plast Reconstr Surg. 2007;23:445–9.
31. Fox DM. Orbital fat injection: technique and 5-year follow-up. Aesthet Plast Surg. 2019;43:123–32.
32. Yang F, Li Z, Deng Y. A custom-made conformer wrapped in lower oral mucosa for the correction of severely contracted socket. Eur J Ophthalmol. 2021;31:3430–5.
33. Groot AL, Remmers JS, Kloos RJ, Saeed P, Hartong DT. Recurrent contracted sockets treated with personalized, three-dimensionally printed conformers and buccal grafts. Eur J Ophthalmol. 2022;32:717–24.
34. Tessier P, Krastinova D. La Transposition Du Muscle Temporal Dans L'orbite Anophtalme. Ann Chir Plast. 1982;27:213–20.
35. Bosniak S, Sachs M, Smith B. Temporalis muscle transfer: a vascular bed for autogenous dermis-fat orbital implantation. Ophthalmology. 1985;92:292–6.

36. Lee YH, Kim HC, Lee JS, Park WJ. Surgical reconstruction of the contracted orbit. Plast Reconstr Surg. 1999;103:1129–36.
37. Krastinova D, Kelly MB, Mihaylova M. Surgical management of the anophthalmic orbit, Part 1: congenital. Plast Reconstr Surg. 2001;108:817–26.
38. Zhang R. Reconstruction of the anophthalmic orbit by orbital osteotomy and free flap transfer. J Plast Reconstr Aesthet Surg. 2007;60:232–40.
39. Bonavolontà G. Temporalis muscle transfer in the treatment of the severely contracted socket. Adv Ophthalmic Plast Reconstr Surg. 1992;9:121–9.
40. Asato H, Harii K, Yamada A, Ueda K. Eye socket reconstruction with free-flap transfer. Plast Reconstr Surg. 1993;92:1061–7.
41. Tahara S, Susuki T. Eye socket reconstruction with free radial forearm flap. Ann Plast Surg. 1989;23:112–6.

Phantom Eye Syndrome

Marie Louise Roed Rasmussen and Elin Bohman

Key Messages

- Phantom eye syndrome is common in anophthalmic patients, and the diagnosis can be made when one or more of the following symptoms are present: phantom pain, phantom vision and phantom sensation.
- Phantom pain and phantom vision are reported by around a quarter and one-third of patients, respectively, while phantom sensation is rare (2%). Since phantom pain is a diagnosis of exclusion, phantom vision is in our opinion the most reliable parameter for diagnosing phantom eye syndrome
- A comprehensive history, clinical examination, and, if necessary, imaging are the first steps in assessing a patient with a painful or uncomfortable anophthalmic socket, and close collaboration with ocularists is helpful.

M. L. R. Rasmussen (✉)
External and Adnexal Service, Department of Ophthalmology, Rigshospitalet, Copenhagen, Denmark

Department of Clinical Medicine, University of Copenhagen, Copenhagen, Denmark
e-mail: marie.louise.roed.rasmussen@regionh.dk

E. Bohman
Oculoplastic and Orbital Services, St. Erik Eye Hospital, Stockholm, Sweden

Psychological aspects should be considered as they can modulate the perception of pain and discomfort and may need to be addressed. However, the presence of apparent psychiatric problems does not exclude the possibility of other non-psychogenic causes of pain.Phantom eye syndrome is defined as any sensation reported by a patient as originating in the eye after it has been amputated. Studies indicate that around 46–68% of patients present with phantom eye syndrome [1–4]. Its aetiology is surgical removal of the eye by either evisceration, enucleation or exenteration of the eye, affecting both sensory and motor nerves. Phantom eye syndrome includes phantom vision, phantom pain and phantom sensations. At least one of the symptoms must be present to get the diagnosis [3–6].

1 Phantom Pain

Phantom pain is a known sequela to amputations in all parts of the human body. Up to 80% of patients with limb amputation experience phantom pain [7], and as many as 70% are troubled even 25 years after amputation [8]. Phantom sensations and pain after amputation have been described in various organs: limbs [7–9], mammae [10], rectum [11], larynx [12], teeth [13], parts of the face [14], bladder [15], uterus and even the appendix [16].

F. M. Quaranta Leoni et al. (eds.), *Oculoplastic, Lacrimal and Orbital Surgery*,
https://doi.org/10.1007/978-3-031-39638-0_9

Table 1 Compilation of causes of orbital, periorbital pain or headache

Causes of orbital/periorbital pain or headache		Comments
Non-specific to the anophthalmic patient	Trochleitis/Trochleodynia	Tenderness over trochlear area [19]
	Intracranial lesions	Tumours or aneurysms may cause trigeminal pain through compression of the fifth cranial nerve
	Elevated intracranial pressure	Pain combined with other neurologic signs
	Idiopathic trigeminal neuropathic pain	Triggered chronic pain in one or more divisions of the trigeminal nerve. Usually electric shock-like or stabbing pain [20]
	Giant cell arteritis	Inflammatory disease classically affecting external carotid artery branches. May cause scalp tenderness, headache, jaw or tongue pain [21]
	Cluster headache	Recurrent episodes in clusters [22]
	Migraine	Often positive family history
	Herpes zoster ophthalmicus	Pain may precede the vesicles
	Dissection of internal carotid artery	Sudden onset of pain. Spontaneous for example in Marfan's syndrome Secondary to head or neck trauma
Specific to the anophthalmic patient	Implant exposure	
	Implant infection	Tenderness over the implant [23]
	Neuroma	Microneuromas may not be visible on imaging [24]
	Pyogenic granuloma	Recurrent granulomas may herald implant infection [25]
	Inclusion cysts	May be superficial or deep (uncommon [26–28])
	Psychological factors	
	Phantom eye pain	

The reported incidence of phantom eye pain ranges from 23% to 28% in various studies [3, 5, 6, 17, 18]. Most patients with phantom eye pain describe intermittent pain, with frequency ranging from many times a day to once every few months. The pain is often in the form of attacks that vary in duration from seconds to minutes. In one-third of the patients, the phantom eye pain is daily; this group also have the most intense pain [3, 6]. It has been suggested that younger women are more likely to report pain [4].

One of the most challenging issues that may arise in the anophthalmic socket is painful sensations that the patient refers to the amputated eye or persistent socket pain for which no cause can be found. However, it should be emphasised that phantom eye pain is a diagnosis of exclusion and several differential diagnoses should be considered.

Firstly, it is important to determine whether the patient is experiencing severe pain or a sensation of discomfort in the socket. Pain requires a more extensive work-up. Some of the causes of pain can occur in patients with intact eyes, while others are specific to the anophthalmic patient (Table 1). Intracranial or systemic causes of orbital and periorbital pain may be more difficult to identify in an anophthalmic patient as pupillary reaction, visual acuity and visual field cannot be tested, and ocular motility may be difficult to evaluate. Therefore, a detailed clinical history and meticulous examination is necessary.

1.1 Assessment of the Patient with Possible Phantom Pain

The history should reveal the speed of onset, progression, location, quality, and intensity of the pain, any triggers, and any associated symptoms such as increased discharge or bleeding from the anophthalmic socket. Furthermore, any neurological symptoms, such as numbness, weakness, imbalance, deafness/tinnitus, nausea or neck pain, which could indicate an extraorbital cause should be explored. General medical and surgical history are also important, especially if there was a history of previous malignancy, and the possibility of giant cell arteritis should be considered in patients over the age of 50.

The socket should be examined for signs of conjunctival irritation, implant exposure, pyogenic granulomas or inclusions cysts. The implant and the periorbital area are palpated for any localised tenderness, especially where the supraorbital nerve exits the orbit, the trochlear area and the temporal arteries. Facial sensation as well as orbicularis and facial muscle power are assessed, and the skin is inspected for changes such as herpetic vesicles. Imaging of the orbit, brain and sinuses is recommended if no obvious cause of pain is found, as some of the before mentioned causes, may be more difficult to diagnose in the anophthalmic patient.

Phantom eye pain may be considered if symptoms do not indicate a specific cause and examination of the anophthalmic socket is normal.

1.2 Pathophysiology

Phantom eye pain is caused by the interruption of sensory nerve impulses as a result of the sensory nerves being severed during eye removal surgery. The pathophysiological mechanisms contributing to phantom pain in general can broadly be categorised into supraspinal, spinal, and peripheral mechanisms. Supraspinal mechanisms, for example reorganisation of the somatosensory cortex, are thought to be the predominant cause of phantom eye pain [29]. In the spinal cord, the regulatory mechanisms for sensory input from the missing body part are affected, resulting in increased autonomous activity of the dorsal horn neurons [29]. This could most likely be similar to an amputated eye as the signal passes the same number of neurons, even though the trigeminal nerve enters the brain via the brain stem and not the spinal cord.

Peripherally, the severing of a nerve initiates inflammation and regenerative sprouting of the axons resulting in a neuroma [29, 30]. This may contribute to phantom pain but also to stump pain, that is pain localised to the remaining body part [29]. Five to ten percent of patients with a limb amputation experience persistent stump pain [31] although in studies of phantom eye pain, long-term persistent stump pain has not been found [6, 32]. Few amputation neuromas large enough to create an orbital mass have been described [33, 34]. Microneuromas have also been associated with persistent pain in anophthalmic sockets, with some patients reporting resolution of pain after neuroma excision [25, 36]. However, when treating phantom pain and stump pain in general the long-term outcomes of peripheral nerve surgery are varied [29, 31]. While there is no evidence to suggest that the type of surgery (enucleation or evisceration) or the aetiology of the underlying disease influence the development of phantom eye pain [6, 27], in our experience, patients who had their eye removed due to acanthamoeba keratitis and endophthalmitis are often among those who develop the most severe form of phantom eye pain. The nerve invasion appears to be central, which could argue for enucleation in these patients to diminish the risk of pain.

From studies on pain after limb amputation, it is known that the afferent fibres develop mechanical sensitivity and that ectopic discharge may be induced by emotional stress and temperature changes [29, 30]. This is consistent with the findings that cold and windy weather and psychological stress/fatigue were the most commonly reported triggers of phantom eye pain [4–6, 35]. There is a high correlation between ophthalmic pain before anophthalmic surgery and phantom pain afterward, which may be explained by sensitisation. A long duration of pre-amputation pain significantly increases the risk of developing phantom pain [31, 36]. A common indication for enucleation/evisceration is the presence of a painful blind eye, and one-third of these patients continue to have pain subsequently [3, 6, 17, 31]. The presence of an implant appears to be associated with phantom eye pain [6], albeit it is unknown whether this is due to the implant triggering pain or altering the psychological reaction of the patient.

1.3 Treatment and Prognosis

Phantom pain persisting more than 6 months after the inciting operation becomes very difficult to treat [8, 16]. Rest, sleep, heat, firm pressure, use of prosthesis, and distraction are patient-reported approaches to dealing with the pain [4–6, 35]. No effective pharmacological treatment of phantom eye pain can be found in the literature but the similarity with phantom pain in limbs suggests that medications used in these cases might also be useful in severe orbital cases. Conventional analgesics and opioids have been shown to be effective for phantom pain in limbs, and in severe cases, neuroleptics, anticonvulsants (carbamazepine), tricyclic antidepressants, beta- blockers, intravenous calcitonin, and N-methyl-D-aspartate receptor antagonist (ketamine) have been used [1].

Retrobulbar alcohol or chlorpromazine injections were historically used to treat anophthalmic socket pain with varying degrees of success in terms of duration or pain relief, but they are now seldom utilised due to a number of associated complications such as cellulitis, inflammation, facial paresis and ptosis [37–39].

The only surgical treatment for phantom eye pain with proven effectiveness is implant removal and replacement with a dermis-fat graft [40–42]. The association between presence of a firm non-autologous implant and phantom eye pain is well established, and it is believed to be due to the implant movement against or compressing the cut peripheral nerves (i.e. a peripheral mechanism for phantom pain). By extension, it seems reasonable that replacement with a soft dermis-fat graft would result in less pain; however, this is not effective in all patients. If the spinal or supraspinal mechanisms were the dominant cause of pain, implant removal would theoretically have no effect.

Anxiety and depression are found in up to 34% and 42% of patients with phantom pain, respectively [35, 43]. The incidences of anxiety and depression are lower in the subgroup of patients who develop phantom pain after eye removal for malignant melanomas [4]. This is in line with the findings that the quality-of-life in this selected group of patients are higher, due to the fact that participation in studies likes these always is conditional on survival [1] Patient education in phantom pain and psychological support is essential and recommended. No treatment eliminates the pain, and persistent long-term phantom pain may be resistant to any treatment, with fewer than 10% of patients reporting permanent pain relief [3, 6, 8, 16, 29–31, 44].

2 Phantom Vision

In many ways, phantom vision is the clearest form of phantom eye syndrome since it is more easily recognised and differentiated from other visual phenomena, as compared to phantom eye pain which is a diagnosis of exclusion.

Phantom vision is a visual hallucination [45]. A hallucination is a sensory experience, possessing the compelling sense of reality of a true perception, but occurring without external stimulation of the relevant sensory organ [46, 47]. The opposite is blindsight, where external stimulation can be transformed to retinal input, and used to respond to certain types of visual challenge but there is no visual awareness.

The cornerstones in phantom vision are that visual acuity in the remaining eye is within normal range (>6/24) and that the patient shows critical insight (i.e. awareness that their visual perception is not real). Unlike a dream, where all senses can come into play, the visual hallucination is not accompanied by sound, sensation, smell or taste.

Visual hallucinations can be divided into:

- Elementary visual hallucinations: These include all simple visual phenomena lacking meaning and form, such as simple geometric shapes, points of light, spots, and line elements [47, 48].
- Complex visual hallucinations: These include structured objects and scenes, sometimes related to past experiences [46, 47].
- Other visual hallucinations (in this setting): These include the sensation of seeing with two eyes, extreme sensitivity to light, difficulties focusing because of irritation from the non-existing eye, and other sensations which cannot be classified as elementary or complex visual hallucinations [32].

The elementary and complex hallucinations might be regarded as true hallucinations since there is no external perception in the course of it. In contrast, illusions and distortions occur when real visual input is modulated by endogenously generated activity, producing an alteration in the perception of the external world. Palinopsia, polyopsia, micropsia, macropsia and metamorphosis are examples of this (Table 2) [47].

Table 2 The differential diagnosis of visual hallucinations in phantom eye vision

	Elementary hallucinations	Complex hallucination	Duration	Age groups	Visual function	Awareness	Other comments
Phantom eye syndrome	Phosphenes constantly shining or moving (flash) Colours and kaleidoscopic features	Objects, scenes, faces. Often not filling the full visual field	Seconds to minutes Rare cases continuous	All	None in the removed eye. Normal in other seeing eye	All are aware that this is not real	
Charles Bonnet syndrome	Phosphenes and coloured and static elements	Landscapes, scenes, vehicles and small figures in hats Illusions and distortions (Micropsia/ Macropsia) (Palinopsia/ polyopsia)	Seconds to hours	All	Severe impairment, usually due to AMD	Majority are aware that the hallucination is unreal	Hallucinations tend to be sharper and more detailed than real objects
Migraine	Fortification spectra. Bright line elements orientated at angles to one another forming an arc	None	Minutes (5–60)	All	Normal, apart during the migraine Can be experienced as / followed by ictal blindness	When patients are diagnosed, they have full insight	
Visual snow	Perturbed perception of constant bilateral whole-visual field flickering or pixilation	None	Constantly described as a persistent dynamic visual noise. Can last for years	All (mostly young adults)	Normal	Patients know it is unreal	
Somatic delirium	None	Full-size people, animals and objects – even full tableaus	Constantly while diseased	All (mostly elderly)	Normal	Intense misinterpretation	

(continued)

Table 2 (Continued)

	Elementary hallucinations	Complex hallucination	Duration	Age groups	Visual function	Awareness	Other comments
Parkinson's disease	None	People, children, animals and objects		Mostly elderly	Normal	Approximately 50% are severely distressed by their experiences. The majority find it real	Visual hallucinations are associated with a more rapid cognitive decline and mortality
Epilepsy	Circular discs, phosphenes, coloured flicker, and motions	Figures and familiar faces Illusions and distortions (Micropsia/ Macropsia) (Palinopsia/ polyopsia)	Seconds	All	Normal – But can be experienced as / followed by ictal blindness	All are aware that this is not real	

Since most studies have been conducted in these types of hallucinations, and several parallels can be drawn, a brief description may be beneficial for differential diagnosis [47, 49–52]. However, a crucial question for differential diagnosis is if the visual disturbance originates in the seeing eye (if possible, to differentiate) and if they had any visual hallucinations before the eye was surgically removed

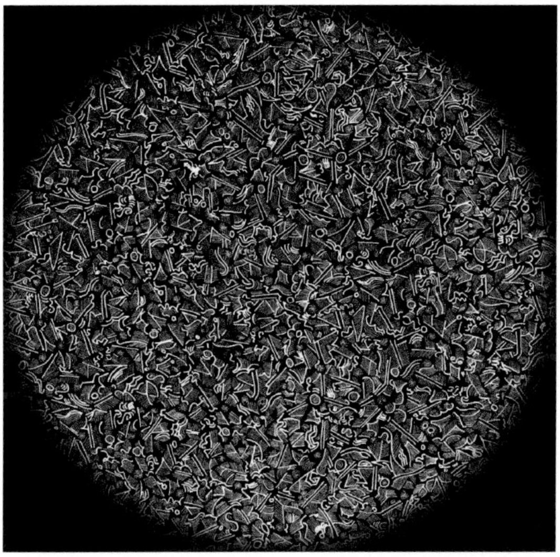

Fig. 1 Elementary visual hallucination. The picture is a drawing by a patient with phantom vision, described as multiple exploding and fading white line shapes. A single line lasts only 2 s, indicating that the hallucination is constantly moving. The most common description of a visual hallucination is a white light, like a desk lamp, shining directly in the patient's face every time she closes her eyes. This is neurologically termed a tessellopsia (geometric hallucination consisting of pellucid geometrical patterns featuring tiles, brickwork, triangles, hexagonal figures, grid like pattern, latticed patterns or network patterns)

2.1 Visual Hallucinations in Phantom Eye Syndrome

Visual hallucinations are reported by 30–42% of patients with phantom eye syndrome, mostly being elementary visual hallucinations (36–79%), and often described as white light dots constantly shining or moving (flash). Some experience the light in colours, while a minority have more kaleidoscopic features. Figure 1 is drawn by a patient with phantom vision and is an example of an elementary visual hallucination, specifically tessellopsia, which is a geometric hallucination consisting of repeated geometrical patterns featuring tiles, brickwork, triangles, hexagonal figures, grid like pattern, latticed pattern or network patterns [3, 4, 32, 35]. Figure 2 demonstrates this phenomenon in bright conditions with both eyes open.

Complex hallucinations are rare (1–6%) and are described as objects, scenes, landscapes or faces, often not filling the full visual field [4, 32] (see clinical vignette).

Other described visual hallucinations include photophobia and, more frequently, the visual sensation of seeing with both eyes. Almost all patients experience phantom vision in the dark or when they are tired, which might be explained by rod signal dominance in scotopic conditions. The cone-dependent stereopsis is missing in both the one-eyed and two-eyed patients; therefore, they use the same measurements for depth perception [1].

The frequency of phantom vision is for most patients weekly or less. However, 14–28% experience it every day. In a few extraordinary cases the experience is constant. An explanation for these cases could be ocular dominance. Some describe their phantom vision as difficulty in focusing, while others have it as a filter over the "real" visual stimulus from the remaining eye. Five percent of the patients have visual disturbances that interfere with their daily life. The emotional response towards phantom vision is for most patients pleasant or neutral. However, around 27% finds it disturbing and 13% have strong emotions towards it [1, 32].

The most common triggers are darkness, closing of the eyes, fatigue and psychological stress, although approximately half the patients have no known precipitating factor for their visual symptoms [3, 32, 53]. In a minority of patients (14%) the phantom vision disappears after 3–6 months, but in most cases it becomes chronic. Hallucinations can sometimes change over time, for example lose colours and become black and white [1, 32].

The aetiology of phantom vision is still unknown. One striking similarity with Charles

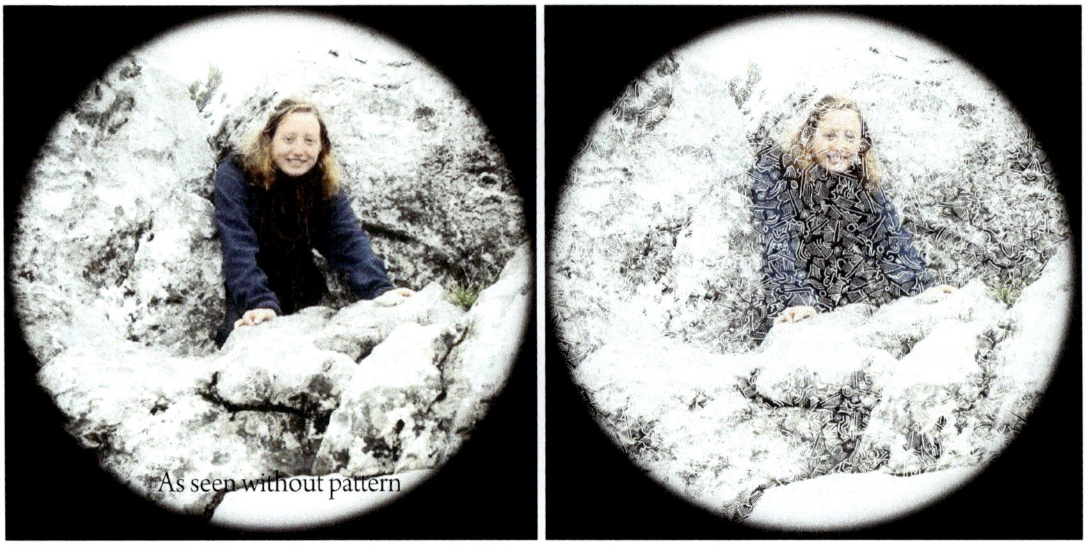

Fig. 2 Elementary visual hallucination, seen with the eyes open, by the same patient in Fig. 1. The hallucination is constantly present and adds a filter to the view of the external world. The patient is very disturbed by the hallucination, especially in dark and very bright conditions where she describes herself as functionally blind, causing an impact on her daily life

Bonnet syndrome is the reduction in visual input. However, the most common indication for eye removal is a painful blind eye where no visual input has been present for a while. In addition, studies have found no significant correlation between vision in the remaining eye and the risk of experiencing phantom vision. Similarly, there is no association with age, and none of the studies of phantom vision have included patients with dementia [1, 32].

Treatment for phantom vision is rarely needed. Most patients can be helped with information about the nature of their hallucinations and reassurance that their perceptions are not real. If required, pharmacological treatment is similar to that used for phantom pain.

3 Phantom Sensation

Phantom sensations are rare, occurring in 2% of the patients, mimicking itching around the eye and a feeling of non-existing eyelids. Patients with phantom sensations tend to have the full spectrum of phantom eye syndrome [1, 6, 32].

3.1 Psychological Aspects

Removal of an eye, regardless of its indication, has a significant psychological impact, with a significant proportion of anophthalmic patients experiencing depression, stress, or anxiety and have a lower health-related quality of life than the normal population [43, 54]. The psychological wellbeing is associated more with psychological than clinical factors [55]. Pain is highly subjective, and cognitive factors play a part in modulating the perception of pain. Depression is a significant predictive factor for severe pain after limb amputations [7, 30]. Emotional stress can exacerbate pain not only psychologically but also through increased amounts of circulating epinephrine that can trigger neuronal activity in neuromas [7, 30].

It is important that the clinician is aware of this aspect when evaluating a patient troubled by pain in the anophthalmic socket. When necessary, a multi-disciplinary approach is advisable; for example, referral for psychological interventions such as cognitive behavioural pain-management. It is recognised that limb amputees receiving adequate pre-counselling and support report less phantom-limb pain [65], thus the value of patient education should not be disregarded [56, 57]. With chronic pain syndromes, there is always a risk of the patient developing chemical dependency and this has been described with anophthalmic patients [1]. The physician needs to be cognisant of drug-seeking behaviour.

Patients with phantom vision may be concerned about mental health conditions or, in the older population, dementia as the cause of their experiences. Even when they have no personal doubt about the integrity of their mental state, they fear that family or medical professionals might judge them medically incompetent. Information and reassurance of mental status is critical for this group of patients [32, 47]. Written material for patients outlining that visual hallucination is common after eye removal is useful. Patient groups where they can discuss their concerns and perceptions might be of value. The surgeon should also keep an open mind and cultivate a positive connection with the patient, reassuring and acknowledging them, which is more valuable than any pharmacological treatment.

References

1. Rasmussen MLR. The eye amputated—consequences of eye amputation with emphasis on clinical aspects, phantom eye syndrome and quality of life. Acta Ophthalmol. 2010;88:1–26.
2. Andreotti AM, Goiato MC, Pellizzer EP, Pesqueira AA, Guiotti AM, Gennari-Filho H, et al. Phantom eye syndrome: a review of the literature. ScientificWorldJournal. 2014;2014:686493.
3. Sörös P, Vo O, Husstedt I-W, Evers S, Gerding H. Phantom eye syndrome: its prevalence, phenomenology, and putative mechanisms. Neurology. 2003;60:1542–3.
4. Hope-Stone L, Brown SL, Heimann H, Damato B, Salmon P. Phantom eye syndrome: patient experiences after enucleation for uveal melanoma. Ophthalmology. 2015;122:1585–90.
5. Nicolodi M, Frezzotti R, Diadori A, Nuti A, Sicuteri F. Phantom eye: features and prevalence. The predisposing role of headache. Cephalalgia. 1997;17:501–4.
6. Rasmussen MLR, Prause JU, Toft PB. Phantom pain after eye amputation. Acta Ophthalmol. 2011;89:10–6.
7. Flor H. Phantom-limb pain: characteristics, causes, and treatment. Lancet Neurol. 2002 Jul;1:182–9.
8. Sherman RA, Sherman CJ, Parker L. Chronic phantom and stump pain among American veterans: results of a survey. Pain. 1984;18:83–95.
9. Jensen TS, Krebs B, Nielsen J, Rasmussen P. Immediate and long-term phantom limb pain in amputees: incidence, clinical characteristics and relationship to pre-amputation limb pain. Pain. 1985;21:267–78.
10. Crone-Munzebrock A. Phantom sensation and phantom pain following amputation of the breast. Langenbecks Arch für Klin Chir. 1950;266:569–75.
11. Ovesen P, Krøner K, Ørnsholt J, Bach K. Phantom-related phenomena after rectal amputation: prevalence and clinical characteristics. Pain. 1991;44:289–91.
12. Mal RK, Baldwin DL. Phantom larynx: a clinical survey. Eur Arch Otorhinolaryngol. 2009;266:397–401.
13. Marbach JJ. Orofacial phantom pain: theory and phenomenology. J Am Dent Assoc. 1996;127:221–9.
14. Hoffman J. Facial phantom phenomenon. J Nerv Ment Dis. 1955;122:143–51.
15. Bors E. Phantom limbs of patients with spinal cord injury. AMA Arch Neurol Psychiatry. 1951;66:610–31.
16. Ramachandran VS, Hirstein W. The perception of phantom limbs. The D. O. Hebb lecture. Brain. 1998;121:1603–30.
17. Gerding H, Vo O, Husstedt IW, Evers S, Sörös P. Phantom pain after eye enucleation. Der Ophthalmol Zeitschrift der Dtsch Ophthalmol Gesellschaft. 2003;100:943–9.
18. Sörös P, Vo O, Gerding H, Husstedt IW, Evers S. Enucleation and development of cluster headache: a retrospective study. BMC Neurol. 2005;5:6.
19. Tran TM, McClelland CM, Lee MS. Diagnosis and Management of Trochleodynia, Trochleitis, and trochlear headache. Front Neurol. 2019;10:361.
20. Cruccu G, Di Stefano G, Truini A. Trigeminal neuralgia. N Engl J Med. 2020;383:754–62. Accessed 29 Jun 2021.
21. Lazarewicz K, Watson P. Giant cell arteritis [internet]. BMJ. 2019;365:1964. Accessed 29 Jun 2021.

22. Leroux E, Ducros A. Cluster headache. Orphanet J Rare Dis. 2008;3:20.
23. Custer PL, Trinkaus KM. Porous implant exposure: incidence, management, and morbidity. Ophthal Plast Reconstr Surg. 2007;23:1–7.
24. Abràmoff MD, Ramos LP, Jansen GH, Mourits MP. Patients with persistent pain after enucleation studied by MRI dynamic color mapping and histopathology. Invest Ophthalmol Vis Sci. 2001;42:2188–92.
25. Jordan DR, Brownstein S, Lee-Wing M, Ashenhurst M. Pyogenic granuloma following oculoplastic procedures: an imbalance in angiogenesis regulation? Can J Ophthalmol. 2001;36:260–8.
26. Tan CSH, Ang LPK, Choo C-T, Cheah EST, Chee S-P. Orbital cysts lined with both stratified squamous and columnar epithelia: a late complication of silicone implants. Ophthal Plast Reconstr Surg. 2006;22:398–400.
27. McCarthy RW, Beyer CK, Dallow RL, Burke JF, Lessell S. Conjunctival cysts of the orbit following enucleation. Ophthalmology. 1981;88:30–5.
28. Hanig CJ, Hornblass A. Treatment of postenucleation orbital cysts. Ann Ophthalmol. 1986;18:191–3.
29. Hsu E, Cohen SP. Postamputation pain: epidemiology, mechanisms, and treatment. J Pain Res. 2013;6:121–36.
30. Wolff A, Vanduynhoven E, van Kleef M, Huygen F, Pope JE, Mekhail N. 21. Phantom pain. Pain Pract. 2011;11:403–13.
31. Nikolajsen L. Postamputation pain: studies on mechanisms. Dan Med J. 2012;59:B4527.
32. Roed Rasmussen ML, Prause JU, Ocularist MJ, Toft PB. Phantom eye syndrome: Types of visual hallucinations and related phenomena. Ophthal Plast Reconstr Surg. 2009;25:390–3.
33. Messmer EP, Camara J, Boniuk M, Font RL. Amputation neuroma of the orbit. Report of two cases and review of the literature. Ophthalmology. 1984;91:1420–3.
34. Ng DT, Francis IC, Whitehouse SA, Kneale KL. Orbital amputation neuroma causing failure of prosthesis wear. Orbit. 2001;20:57–62.
35. Martel A, Baillif S, Thomas P, Almairac F, Galatoire O, Hamedani M, et al. Phantom eye pain: a multicentric study in 100 patients. Acta Ophthalmol. 2020;99:e753–60.
36. Nikolajsen L, Ilkjaer S, Krøner K, Christensen JH, Jensen TS. The influence of preamputation pain on postamputation stump and phantom pain. Pain. 1997;72:393–405.
37. Margo CE, Wilson T. Orbital cellulitis after retrobulbar injection of chlorpromazine. Arch Ophthalmol. 1993;111:1322.
38. Cotliar JM, Shields CL, Meyer DR. Chronic orbital inflammation and fibrosis after retrobulbar alcohol and chlorpromazine injections in a patient with choroidal melanoma. Ophthal Plast Reconstr Surg. 2008;24:410–1.
39. Giligson A, Dolman PJ, Buffam F. Comparison of retrobulbar analgesics for evisceration. Ophthal Plast Reconstr Surg. 2002;18:258–60.
40. Shams PN, Bohman E, Baker MS, Maltry AC, Kopp ED, Allen RC. Chronic anophthalmic socket pain treated by implant removal and dermis fat graft. Br J Ophthalmol. 2015;99:1692–6.
41. Christmas NJ, Gordon CD, Murray TG, Tse D, Johnson T, Garonzik S, et al. Intraorbital implants after enucleation and their complications: a 10-year review. Arch Ophthalmol. 1998;116:1199–203.
42. Hogeboom CSE, Mourits DL, Ket JCF, Tan HS, Hartong DT, Moll AC. Persistent socket pain postenucleation and post evisceration: a systematic review. Acta Ophthalmol. 2018;96:661–72.
43. Ahn JM, Lee SY, Yoon JS. Health-related quality of life and emotional status of anophthalmic patients in Korea. Am J Ophthalmol. 2010;149:1005–1011.e1.
44. Halbert J, Crotty M, Cameron ID. Evidence for the optimal management of acute and chronic phantom pain: a systematic review. Clin J Pain. 2002;18:84–92.
45. Cohn R. Phantom vision. Arch Neurol [Internet]. 1971;25:468–71.
46. Menon GJ, Rahman I, Menon SJ, Dutton GN. Complex visual hallucinations in the visually impaired: the Charles bonnet syndrome. Surv Ophthalmol. 2003;48:58–72.
47. Wilkinson F. Auras and other hallucinations: windows on the visual brain. Prog Brain Res. 2004;144:305–20.
48. Kölmel HW. Complex visual hallucinations in the hemianopic field. J Neurol Neurosurg Psychiatry. 1985;48:29–38.
49. O'Brien J, Taylor JP, Ballard C, Barker RA, Bradley C, Burns A, et al. Visual hallucinations in neurological and ophthalmological disease: pathophysiology and management. J Neurol Neurosurg Psychiatry. 2020;91:512–9.
50. Swann P, O'Brien JT. Management of visual hallucinations in dementia and Parkinson's disease. Int Psychogeriatr. 2019;31:815–36.
51. Gomperts SN. Lewy body dementias: dementia with Lewy bodies and Parkinson disease dementia. Continuum (Minneap Minn). 2016;22:435–63.
52. Santhouse AM, Howard RJ, Ffytche DH. Visual hallucinatory syndromes and the anatomy of the visual brain. Brain. 2000;123:2055–64.
53. Maloof AJ. Phantom vision: a graphic description. Ophthal Plast Reconstr Surg. 2004;20:80–1.

54. Rasmussen MLR, Ekholm O, Prause JU, Toft PB. Quality of life of eye amputated patients. Acta Ophthalmol. 2012;90:435–40.
55. McBain HB, Ezra DG, Rose GE, Newman SP. The psychosocial impact of living with an ocular prosthesis. Orbit. 2014;33:39–44.
56. Wilder-Smith CH, Schuler L. Postoperative analgesia: pain by choice? The influence of patient attitudes and patient education. Pain. 1992;50:257–62.
57. Mortimer CM, Steedman WM, McMillan IR, Martin DJ, Ravey J. Patient information on phantom limb pain: a focus group study of patient experiences, perceptions and opinions. Health Educ Res. 2002;17:291–304.

Congenital Anophthalmia and Microphthalmia

Alessandra Modugno, Michael Schittkowski, Dyonne T. Hartong, and Sri Gore

Key Messages

- Anophthalmia and microphthalmia are rare conditions with a prevalence of approximately 1–3 per 10,000 live births.
- Children should have a complete ophthalmological and paediatric screening to detect any other malformations.
- Imaging is required to visualise the orbital content and the presence of an associated cyst.
- Early expansion helps to achieve the best possible cosmetic outcomes.
- In anophthalmia and microphthalmia with cyst, the timing of cyst removal is important to avoid distortion of the periorbital tissues.

1 Introduction

Perturbation of early ocular embryogenesis, either due to genetic or environmental factors, can result in a lack of eye induction or abortion of development [1]. Anophthalmia and microphthalmia are severe ocular developmental anomalies characterised by the absence or reduced size of the globe compared to the population age-adjusted mean, respectively [2, 3].

True anophthalmia occurs when eye development is aborted at the stage of optic vesicle formation around 3–4 weeks of gestation, leading to the absence of the eye, optic nerve, and chiasm. These anomalies can be confirmed with MRI of the brain and orbit [4]. In microphthalmia, the eye has a smaller volume, with a reduced corneal diameter (microcornea, defined as a horizontal diameter <9 mm in neonates and <10 mm in children over 2 years) [5].

Anophthalmia and microphthalmia can be unilateral or bilateral. When there are no other associated congenital malformations, they are more commonly unilateral, whereas cases with chromosomal defects or other anomalies are often bilateral. However, in unilateral cases, the fellow eye may show abnormalities in 25–63% of cases, and therefore a thorough bilateral examination is warranted [6–8]. Co-existing extraocular abnormalities occur more frequently in severe cases, but can be present irrespective of the severity of the malformation [5, 7–10].

A. Modugno (✉)
Ocularistica Italiana, Rome, Italy
e-mail: modugno@ocularistica.it

M. Schittkowski
Section for Strabismus and Neuroophthalmology, Department of Ophthalmology, University Medicine Goettingen, Goettingen, Germany

D. T. Hartong
Orbital Centre, Department of Ophthalmology, Amsterdam University Medical Center, Amsterdam, The Netherlands

S. Gore
Clinic and Academic Department of Ophthalmology, Great Ormond Street Hospital for Children, London, UK

F. M. Quaranta Leoni et al. (eds.), *Oculoplastic, Lacrimal and Orbital Surgery*,
https://doi.org/10.1007/978-3-031-39638-0_10

2 Epidemiology, Aetiology and Genetics

2.1 Epidemiology

The reported prevalence of anophthalmia and microphthalmia, based mostly on national malformation registries, is around 1–3 per 10,000 live births [6–8, 11–16]. Additional anomalies of other organs or systems are present in 32–93% of cases [6, 7, 13, 16–18] and 20% of children with anophthalmia and microphthalmia, and/or coloboma have delayed psychomotor milestones [1, 15].

2.2 Aetiology

Aetiology is currently believed to be mainly genetic, at least for children with bilateral involvement and severe phenotype. No gene abnormalities are usually found for unilateral isolated cases. Exogenic and environmental factors have also been associated and include:

- Infections (cytomegalovirus, rubella, toxoplasmosis, Zika).
- Drugs (such as thalidomide), alcohol, smoking and maternal age during pregnancy [8, 19, 20].
- Bariatric surgery [21]. The deficit of fat-soluble vitamins caused by post-surgical malabsorption, particularly vitamin A (retinol) deficiency (VAD), seems to play a crucial role in embryogenesis. Within the embryonic tissues, retinol is metabolised to retinoic acid by a series of intracellular processes and is involved in the differentiation and development of ocular epithelia [21].

2.3 Genetics

Recent advances in the field of genetics, including high-throughput, next-generation sequencing technology, have enhanced our knowledge of the genetic basis of anophthalmia and microphthalmia [22–24].

In non-syndromic anophthalmia and microphthalmia, the incidence of chromosomal abnormalities identified by array comparative genomic hybridization (aCGH) is low [1, 25]. *SOX2* and *OTX2* are the two most frequently mutated genes known to cause monogenic anophthalmia and microphthalmia, accounting for 10% and 3% of cases of anophthalmia or severe microphthalmia, respectively [26]. Mutations in *VSX2* (*CHX10)*, *PAX6*, *RAX*, *FOXE3*, *BMP4*, and *GDF6* are less commonly detected [26].

Human eye development starts during the third week of gestation in the anterior neural plate. *OTX2* is required for forebrain specification, and allows the neural plate to become competent for eye development by coordinating expression of eye field initiators *SIX3*, *RAX* and PAX6 [27–30]. Approximately 100 additional genes have been associated with anophthalmia and microphthalmia [31], but only a minority of them have been reported more than once, and most will only account for a very small number of cases [1, 32].

The inheritance pattern can be autosomal dominant, recessive or X-linked. However, many mutations occur *de novo*, and the chance of finding a causative defect is much higher for bilateral severe anophthalmia and microphthalmia (70–80%) than unilateral cases (less than 10%) [1, 33, 34]. Increased genetic diagnosis will allow larger cohorts to be analysed for the genotype/phenotype relationships in anophthalmia and microphthalmia, including the identification of environmental factors or genetic modifiers which may result in the heterogeneity observed in affected patients [35].

3 Clinical Features

The severity of microphthalmia and anophthalmia varies depending on the stage at which the eye development was disrupted.

3.1 Anophthalmia

- Clinical observation shows the absence of an eye. Sometimes a small cystic remnant is

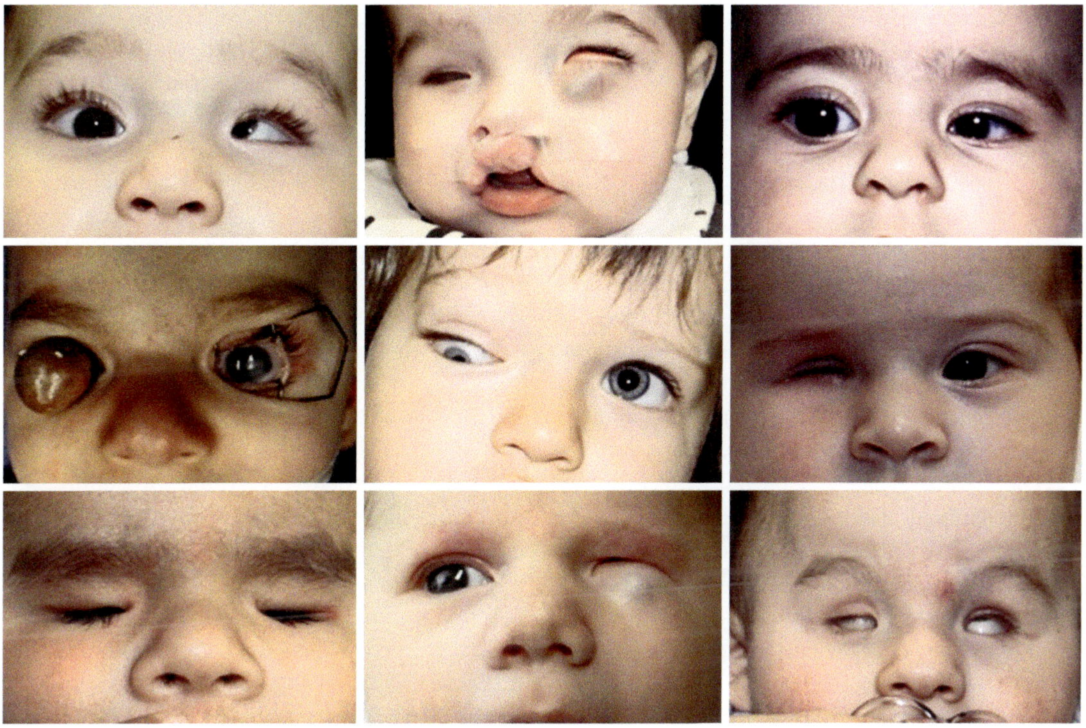

Fig. 1 Clinical features of congenital anophthalmia and microphthalmia. (Courtesy of Alessandra Modugno)

detectable in the socket, due to a degeneration of the optic vesicle [31]. The presence of a cyst of variable size in the socket can be identified.

- Orbital imaging may show eye remnants within the orbit, indicating a condition that is referred to as 'clinical congenital anophthalmia' (CCA) [36].
- In severe anophthalmia the eyelids are usually involved: the horizontal palpebral length (HPL) is rarely symmetric in bilateral cases and is reduced compared to the contralateral eyelid in unilateral cases [36]. Coloboma, microblepharon, incomplete development of the anterior or posterior lamellae are the most frequently associated malformations.
- The initial assessment in children with unilateral or bilateral anophthalmia can be made while the child is awake. In unilateral cases, the fellow eye should be carefully examined, and electro-functional tests should be performed. However, examination of both eyes and ultrasonography under general anaesthesia are recommended to detect non-clinically visible malformations (i.e. orbital cysts) that can be bilateral, although with different clinical features (Fig. 1).

3.2 Microphthalmia

- Microphthalmia spectrum ranges from rudimentary stumps to small eyes with axial lengths less than 2 standard deviations below normal [37]. The corneal diameter is often less than 10 mm at birth.
- In posterior microphthalmia, the axial length is reduced, but only the posterior part of the eye is affected, and both anterior segment and corneal diameter are within the normal range.
- Congenital cataract, glaucoma, persistent foetal vasculature, anterior or posterior segment dysgenesis are the most frequent associated features. The anterior chamber is often shallow or absent. Retinal dysplasia, chorioretinal atrophy, vascular abnormalities, and a hypoplastic or dysplastic optic disc may also be seen.
- Colobomas of the iris, ciliary body, choroid, retina and optic nerve may be present; involve-

ment can be unilateral or bilateral, symmetric or asymmetric [38].

4 Management of Anophthalmia

The management of congenital anophthalmia requires a coordinated approach, involving both oculoplastic surgeons and ocularists. An adequate prosthesis should be fitted shortly after birth, preferably within the first 2 months of life, as early socket expansion is necessary to achieve a satisfactory cosmetic appearance.

The expansion can be achieved with conservative or surgical methods, and due to the wide range of clinical features, each patient requires a customised treatment plan. Various approaches to congenital anophthalmic socket expansion have been developed over the past few decades, mainly through hydrophilic socket and orbital expanders, and cosmetic customised prosthesis (CCP).

4.1 Hydrophilic and Osmotic Expanders

Tissue expansion is a widely used technique in reconstructive surgery that was first introduced in the late 1950s, utilising rubber and then silicone balloons, which were initially filled with air, and later with saline solution [39].

4.1.1 Low Hydrophilic Expanders

The concept of using a soft hydrophilic contact lens polymer (HEMA) with an expansion capacity of only 20% was first reported in the early 1980s [40]. The minimal expansion properties of this material limited its use to cases of extremely contracted sockets where the insertion of a conformer was not possible; however, it paved the way for the conformer therapy [41–43].

4.1.2 Highly Hydrophilic Expanders

The use of polymers with up to 50-fold swelling capacities opened new possibilities for tissue expansion [44, 45]. The anhydrous expander is a solid body consisting of an interlaced, physiologically well-tolerated, hydraulic gel (copolymer based on methyl methacrylate and vinyl pyrrolidone—MMA-VP). The material can be used to manufacture expander devices of any shape and size. After implantation, it absorbs water from tears and intercellular fluid, and the volume automatically increases. These expanders were first used to manage clinical congenital anophthalmia in 1997 [46]. Since then, different sizes and shapes have been proposed, and several studies have shown their effectiveness [47–49].

4.1.3 Socket Osmotic Expansion

Socket expansion with an osmotically active expander is a relatively simple procedure, and no additional eyelid surgery is needed to fit a conformer. Although osmotic expanders are available in several sizes, their capacity to increase volume means that they seldom need to be exchanged with larger ones to attain the required volume. The hemispherical expander is left in the socket for about 2 months, and a temporary tarsorrhaphy is placed to prevent the child from manipulating the material, which is extremely soft [47]. If a shorter expansion time is required, cyanoacrylate glue can be used, obviating the need for sutures and general anaesthesia [50, 51].

A prosthesis or a conformer can be inserted immediately after the removal of the first expander, and consultations with the ocularist every 6–12 weeks are advisable to monitor the treatment plan and assess progress. A regular increase in the size of the prosthesis is necessary to adequately enlarge the palpebral fissure.

4.1.4 Orbital Osmotic Expansion

After socket expansion is completed, orbital volume expansion can be addressed. Previous socket expander therapy enlarges palpebral aperture and facilitates the subsequent step of expanding the orbit with a spherical expander or a dermis-fat graft (DFG). The spherical expander positioned in the orbit compensates for the volume deficit, helps to stabilise the prosthesis and may stimulate bony orbital growth [47–49].

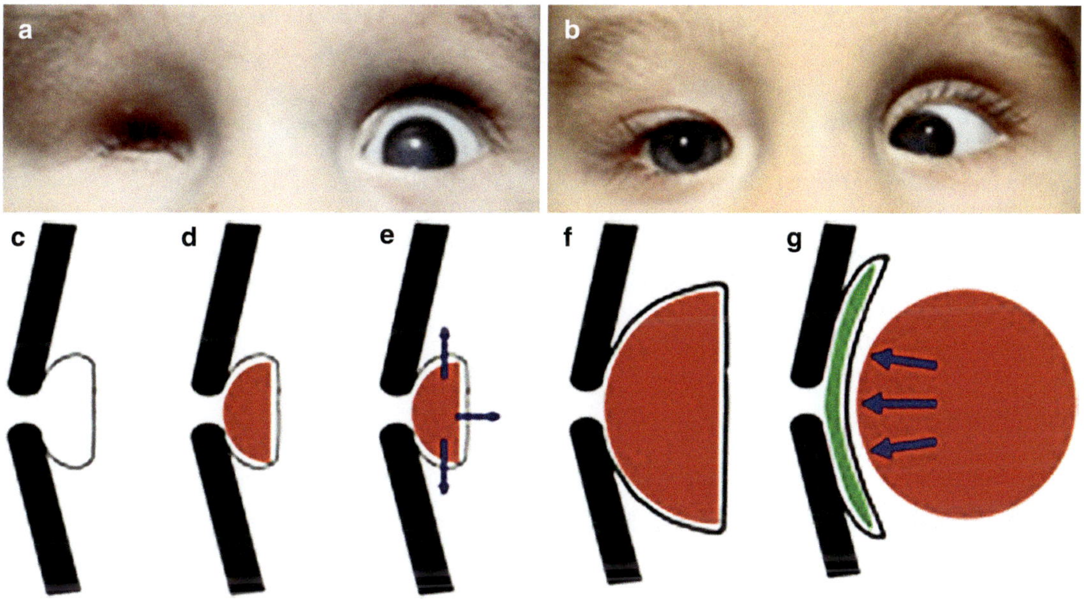

Fig. 2 Hydrogel expander treatment in a 4-month-old boy. (**a**) Clinical appearance at presentation. (**b**) 8 months later, after initial socket expansion for 2 months followed by orbital expansion and prosthetic management. (**c**) Schematic drawing: small empty socket. (**d**) Socket expander in place. (**e**) Generated expansion forces in all directions. (**f**) Expanded socket (surface enlarged). (**g**) Orbital expander and a first prosthesis are inserted. (Courtesy of Michael Schittkowski)

Since expander inflation does not occur continuously over time, the implant size can be increased in 1 mL increments, up to expanders of 4 and 5 mL (Fig. 2a–g). Alternatively, a DFG can be used [52].

Orbital hydrogel expanders can improve the orbital development in congenital anophthalmia. However, the enlargement is not as extensive as that observed in the normal orbit, and expanders associated with external conformers may not be sufficient to induce an adequate growth of eyelids and fornices [49].

Advantages

- The inflatable silicone expanders led to the development of an expanding copolymer without the potentially tissue-damaging effect of hyperosmolar solutions.
- The use of the hydrogel expanders allows the first prosthesis to be fitted in about 2 months, and thus within the first 6 months of life. This leads to a high compliance by the parents.

Disadvantages

- The expansion process may be more rapid than desired.
- Sometimes it is not possible to maintain the central position of the expander during the swelling process, which is a prerequisite for optimal prosthesis fitting.
- At present the expanders are not available in Europe.

4.2 Cosmetic Custom Made Prostheses (CCP)

CCP can be fitted at the time of the first clinical consultation without surgery, permitting a gradual and effective socket expansion. Progressively enlarging CCPs should be changed fortnightly for the first 2 months, then replaced every 3–4 weeks for the following 2–4 months. Afterwards, patients are followed up according to a customised plan every 2–6 months. A DFG can be then positioned to increase orbital volume and socket lining.

Replacement of enlarging CCPs can be performed without anaesthesia in an outpatient setting by means of a purpose-designed holder, with no need for tarsorrhaphy or cyanoacrylate glue. It is essential to have a specialised ophthalmologist-ocularist team capable of fitting and removing the prosthesis without anaesthesia; an accurate observation of the socket will allow the ocularist to manufacture custom made prostheses following the indications of the ophthalmologist.

CCPs are made of polymethylmethacrylate (PMMA) and reproduce the same colour of the sclera and the iris of the fellow eye, allowing an immediate cosmetic recovery, with no need for temporary transparent PMMA conformers (Fig. 3h).

Advantages

- No need for general anaesthesia.
- Immediate improvement of cosmesis.
- Family satisfaction and positive emotional impact.
- Highly beneficial for social integration of children.

Disadvantages

- A specialised team is needed to fit and remove CCPs without anaesthesia in an outpatient setting.
- A longer learning curve than with other techniques is required to achieve optimal results.

4.3 Dermis-Fat Graft

Congenital anophthalmia is characterised by a lack of conjunctival lining with shallow fornices and orbital volume deficit (Fig. 3a). DFG has been recognised in recent years as the state-of-

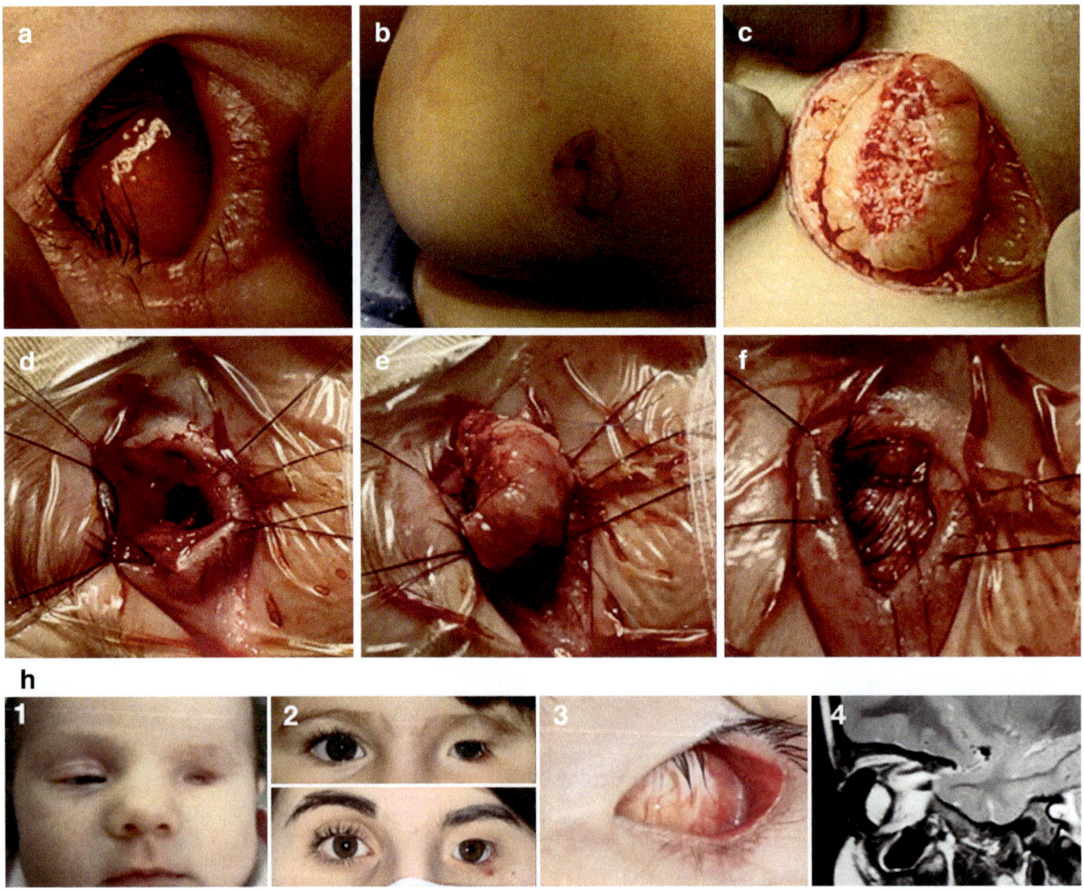

Fig. 3 (**a–f**) Surgical sequence for orbital volume enhancement with dermis-fat graft (DFG). (**h1**) Left congenital anophthalmia. (**h2**) Outcome after treatment with cosmetic customised prosthesis (CCP) (above), outcome after DFG (below). (**h3**) Homogeneously filled socket after DFG with adequate fornices. (**h4**) Imaging shows correct positioning of DFG. (Courtesy of Alessandra Modugno)

the-art implant for enhancing both volume and lining in sockets of children with congenital anophthalmia, helping to deepen shallow fornices after adequate socket expansion with either CCPs or hydrophilic expanders [52].

Magnetic resonance imaging is mandatory before performing a DFG for accurate evaluation of the socket shape and the exact position of the CCP, as well as detection of any cysts or eye remnants within the orbit. If a cyst is present, it is necessary to assess whether removal may be necessary before the DFG. After cyst removal, the orbital content tends to shift towards the socket centre, and it is not advisable to perform the DFG at the same time, as the graft may end up exactly in the place where the cyst was located. In our experience, this happens more frequently for the cysts in the lower orbital quadrants. Orbital volume replacement with DFG should therefore be considered as a secondary procedure approximately 6 months after the cyst is removed.

The surgical technique of DFG harvesting and positioning is described in Chapter "Secondary Orbital Implants, Dermis-Fat Graft and Volume Enhancement Techniques" (see Fig. 3a–h for surgical sequence).

Pre-operative MRI findings determine how to position the DFG inside the orbit. If no extraocular tissues are present, the DFG is placed centrally; if eye remnants or a small cyst are present and not removed at surgery, the DFG can be placed above or below the eye remnants or the cyst to fill up the socket homogeneously. The average size in children aged 1 to 2 years is an ellipse of 3 × 2.5 cm (Fig. 3c).

Following the DFG, the socket appears homogeneously filled and the fornices reshaped, facilitating the fitting and removal of the prosthesis by the children's parents. Increasingly sized prostheses will be fitted every sixth to twelve months to allow continued expansion of socket and eyelids until the best possible symmetry is achieved [36] (Fig. 3h).

4.4 Alternative Techniques for the Socket

4.4.1 Mucous Membrane and Dermal Grafts

An oral mucous membrane graft is useful for improving deficiencies in the conjunctival lining [51, 53], especially if there is extensive scarring from previous unsuccessful surgery or inflammation. A dermal graft is a viable alternative since it has a low rate of contraction after grafting, and will be covered by conjunctiva.

4.4.2 Amniotic Membrane

This can be an option for mild to moderate socket contraction in acquired anophthalmia; [54–56] its use in congenital anophthalmia should be limited to patients in whom conventional expansion has failed, or previous surgery has caused modest conjunctival scarring.

4.5 Alternative Techniques for the Orbit

4.5.1 Silicon Balloon Expanders

Classic balloon expanders require a complex surgical procedure, usually involving a coronal approach. Spherical expanders can be implanted intraconally, and C-shaped expanders subperiosteally [55]. The inflation tube is then passed through an osteotomy of the lateral orbital wall and connected to an injection port placed subcutaneously above the ear. Regular refilling of the depot with saline solution is necessary. Inflatable soft tissue expanders can be useful, but it is sometimes difficult to control the direction of expansion and maintain expansion pressure in every direction [57, 58].

These expanders can displace or lead to extrusion of the conformer, and the pressure exerted can cause atrophy of the surrounding tissue [59]. Moreover, the development of the fornices is not addressed. For this reason, this technique should be combined with conventional conformer therapy and/or mucosal grafting to help the adequate fitting of the prosthesis, which is essential for cosmesis.

4.5.2 Craniofacial Surgery

Craniofacial surgery is indicated in older children. These complex procedures are reserved for patients in whom adequate expansion or satisfactory facial symmetry has not been achieved despite previous aggressive conformer or expander therapy [53]. Surgery is usually performed after completion of cranial growth to avoid further interventions at a later stage [60]. However, additional eyelid and socket surgery are often necessary to enhance conjunctival lining and enable adequate prosthetic fitting.

5 Microphthalmia: Prosthetic Rehabilitation

Children with congenital microphthalmia should have a complete eye examination as soon as possible to evaluate the possibility of visual recovery. Visual impairment may be due to high myopia/hypermetropia or astigmatism or congenital optic nerve coloboma. Ultrasound, axial length measurement, visual evoked potential test (VEP) and electroretinogram (ERG) are useful for assessing eye residual function. MRI is preferable to computed tomography scan (CT) to avoid exposure to radiation.

Eyes with anterior segment dysgenesis or a shorter axial length can have a visual perception. In such cases, it is recommended to wait at least 6 months before considering fitting an ocular prosthesis, but not before reassessing the possibility of residual vision. If blindness of one or both eyes is established, the focus should be on restoring the child's aesthetic appearance.

Conjunctival fornices are usually adequate in congenital microphthalmia, allowing a cosmetic prosthesis to be readily fitted. The first prosthesis insertion is determined by the timing of diagnosing blindness; the earlier the diagnosis, the sooner the aesthetic rehabilitation may begin (Fig. 4).

In case of severe microphthalmia, the prosthesis will be replaced every fortnight during the first 2 months, then according to the socket/fornix expansion achieved. Prosthesis replacement is less frequent in mild cases, and the ophthalmologist should monitor the microphthalmic eye at every consultation and prescribe anti-inflammatory and lubricant drops to improve tolerance of the prosthesis and prevent ocular surface inflammation. The cornea should always be examined at the slit lamp.

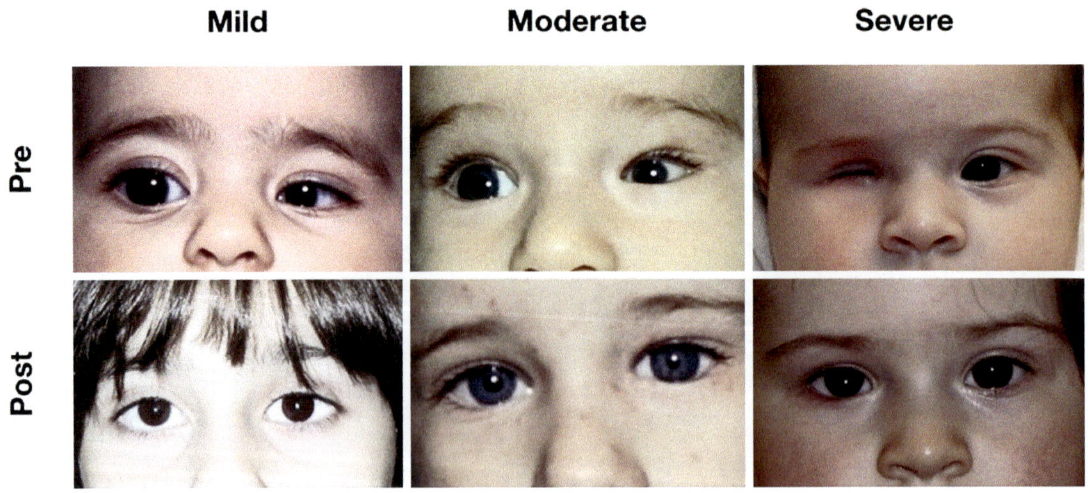

Fig. 4 Congenital microphthalmia: outcomes after customised cosmetic prosthesis treatment in mild, moderate, and severe cases. (Courtesy of Alessandra Modugno)

At approximately 4 years of age, the child will be able to cooperate, and a PMMA prosthesis can be fitted using the advanced impression technique with good cosmesis and tolerance. The prosthesis is manufactured with the same curvature of the eye and the socket, as reproduced by the impression mould. Self-inflating hydrogel pellet expanders [61] have been abandoned in favour of moulded prostheses for orbital volume enhancement in congenital microphthalmia.

Again, good collaboration between the ophthalmologist and ocularist is critical for optimal results.

6 Microphthalmia-Anophthalmia with Cyst

6.1 Anophthalmia-Associated Orbital Cysts

Orbital cysts (also known as 'colobomatous cysts' and 'congenital cystic eye') can be associated with the whole ocular malformation spectrum, affecting patients with posterior segment coloboma, anophthalmia and microphthalmia (Fig. 5). The full list of differential diagnoses for orbital cysts is not covered in this chapter, but meningoencephalocele and teratoma should be considered in differential diagnosis [62, 63]. Orbital cysts are uncommon; several studies have found a prevalence of approximately 12–16% in the anophthalmia microphthalmia population [64]. Natural history data is sparse, with very few large case series presenting longitudinal follow up data. In our experience, cysts may spontaneously regress or completely resolve but the time frame of this change is difficult to predict [64].

6.2 Classification and Histology

The classification of these cysts depends on the associated microphthalmia-anophthalmia condition:

- 'Congenital cystic eye' is associated with anophthalmia. There is no optic nerve remnant and no obvious eye remnant visible on MRI, and only the cyst is present within the socket. The cyst results from the failure of

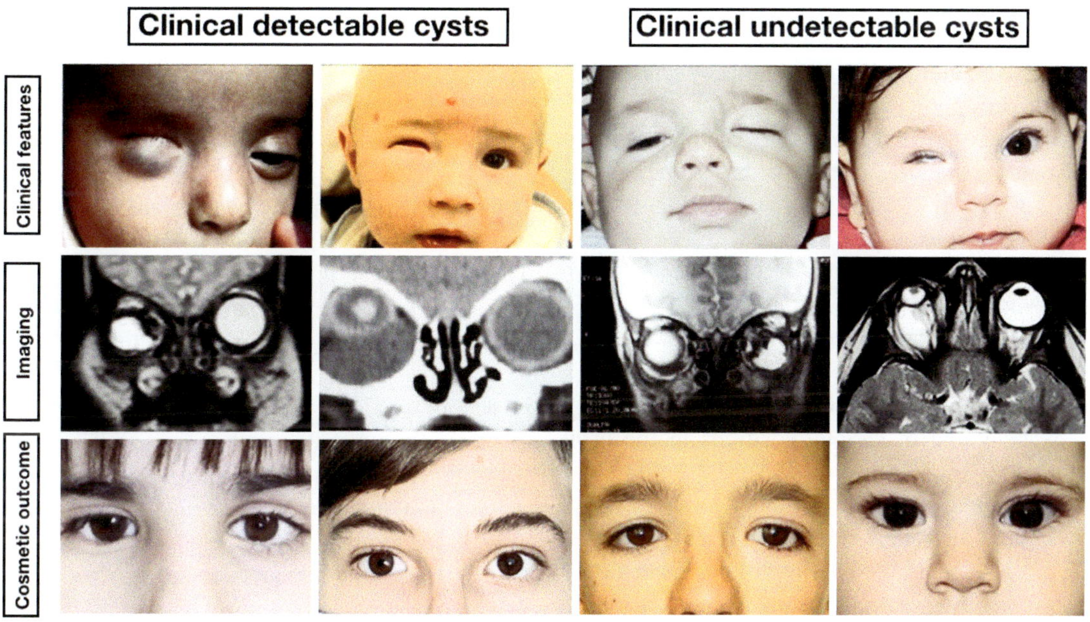

Fig. 5 Anophthalmia and microphthalmia with cyst: clinical features, imaging and cosmetic outcomes in detectable and undetectable cysts. (Courtesy of Alessandra Modugno)

optic vesicle invagination during the third week of gestation [31, 65].

- 'Microphthalmia with cyst' is associated with microphthalmia. There is usually a small eye with the optic nerve. The eye size may vary from remnants to well-formed but smaller structures. Microphthalmia with cyst would occur due to the failure of closure of the embryonic fissure at around the sixth week of gestation.

It is important to distinguish between these conditions to determine the risk of systemic abnormalities. Patients with anophthalmia (with or without cyst), had a disruption of normal development at around the third week of gestation when other organs such as the heart and kidneys develop [31]. Thus, the diagnosis has a significant impact on general management pathways in terms of genetic and medical screening and future family planning. MRI is mandatory for diagnosis and management planning.

Histology studies [66, 67] have demonstrated the following features in orbital cysts:

- A thin outer wall made of collagenous lining.
- An inner lining composed of neuroectodermal tissue with varying degrees of retinal cell differentiation.
- The cysts often contain fluid which is yellow or clear, and similar to vitreous or cerebrospinal fluid [66].
- True 'congenital cystic eyes' should have no ocular structures or tissues due to the disruption in molecular pathways prior to eye development.

6.3 Clinical Features

Orbital cysts can be unilateral or bilateral and may be found in various positions in the orbit [66–68]. Cysts can be:

- Clinically evident at birth or later in infancy as a translucent blue swelling of the lower lid.
- Clinically visible through the palpebral aperture.
- Present in the orbit and, although not visible, they may cause a deviation of the microphthalmic eye.
- May be discovered incidentally on screening imaging after birth, or with prenatal foetal MRI [69].

6.4 Radiological Features

Orbital cysts may be identified with ultrasound, but MRI is recommended to better identify the orbital contents and possible brain abnormalities. With B-scan ultrasound, the cyst appears as an echolucent lesion which may be in communication with the globe [70], and connections to the optic nerve sheath may be recognised. With MRI scan, it is possible to identify well-delineated cystic lesions with content that shows the same high signal as vitreous on T2-weighted images.

The cysts can be in any orbital quadrant—although more common inferiorly—and may vary in size, sometimes considerably larger than the microphthalmic eye. They can be multilobulated, and may extend intracranially or into the maxillary sinus. Colobomatous communications or connections to the microphthalmic eye [66] or the optic nerve can be recognised, although this may be difficult to delineate even on thin-slice MRI.

6.5 Management of Orbital Cysts

The management is related to the residual visual potential of the microphthalmic eye.

The main treatment strategies include:

- Maximise visual potential if any was recorded clinically, behaviourally or with ERG/VEP. Visual rehabilitation may be very intensive and it should be thoroughly discussed with the family.
- Leave the cyst untouched and proceed with prosthetic rehabilitation. The cyst may provide additional volume within the orbit to help

drive the bony growth, compensating for a reduced ocular volume. In our experience, cysts situated within the intraconal space or posteriorly may provide an optimal expansion. Traditional strategies recommend that cysts be retained until the age of 5 years when the orbital growth is thought to reach adult size. However, every clinical decision should be adapted to each patient [64, 71–74].

- Surgical treatment, prosthetic rehabilitation and orbital volume replacement if needed. The presence of the cyst may prevent the retention of a prosthesis, causing fornix contracture. Moreover, cysts may cause abnormal orbital bone expansion, shortage of fornices and lid maldevelopment [64, 73–75].

Treatment options for anophthalmia microphthalmia cysts include:

- Aspiration of fluid (with or without image guidance) [67, 75].
- Aspiration with various sclerosing agents [71, 76–78] such as ethanolamine oleate, or doxycycline and bleomycin.
- Surgical excision: although recurrence is possible, it appears to be lower after surgery than following aspiration. The microphthalmic eye may be preserved as it may provide useful orbital volume, but there are risks of inadvertent injury if the cyst has a colobomatous attachment to it or to the optic nerve [64].

6.5.1 Surgical Technique

1. The conjunctiva is incised at the horizontal midline of the socket.
2. The cyst capsule is separated from the surrounding conjunctiva and Tenon's capsule by blunt dissection.
3. Large cysts can be reduced in size by needle aspiration to facilitate removal. A traction suture positioned on the cyst wall acts as a marker and facilitates traction during removal.
4. Adequate cauterisation is used to prevent intra-operative bleeding, particularly if there is an extension to the orbital apex.
5. Gentle clamp and cautery can be applied to any connection between the microphthalmic eye and the cyst; the microphthalmic eye can be left in situ if the cyst can be easily separated.
6. After the removal of the cyst, the conjunctiva can be closed with interrupted 7/0 polyglactin sutures.
7. It is mandatory to insert a clear conformer of an adequate size into the socket.
8. The socket can be inspected 2–3 weeks after surgery, the conformer is removed, and a cosmetic prosthesis is fitted.

6.5.2 Orbital Volume Replacement Strategy Following Cyst Excision

Following fitting of the prosthesis, it is possible to assess whether there is volume deficit.

Orbital volume enhancement is not always necessary [64, 79], and we recommend this as a secondary procedure at least 6 months after cyst excision. Most children may have good cosmetic outcomes with simple prosthetic rehabilitation, even after excision of large orbital cysts. Moreover, orbital tissues should adequately settle before further surgery. If volume replacement is needed, DFG should be placed in the correct position to fill the socket homogeneously.

6.5.3 Key Points in the Management of Anophthalmia Microphthalmia-Associated Cysts

1. The diagnosis of anophthalmia or microphthalmia associated cyst is confirmed by thorough examination under general anaesthesia and imaging.
2. Visual potential is maximised if appropriate.
3. The following stages are dependent on whether a prosthesis could be adequately fitted and retained.
4. If a prosthesis is retained, the cyst does not need treatment, and prosthetic rehabilitation proceeds as with other patients with anophthalmia microphthalmia.
5. If the prosthesis cannot be retained, the cyst needs to be treated, but it is advisable to wait until the age of 6 months.

6. Following treatment, orbital volume replacement can be considered, but prosthetic rehabilitation should always be started and continued in the interim (Fig. 5).

References

1. Plaisancié J, Ceroni F, Holt R, Zazo Seco C, Calvas P, Chassaing N, Ragge NK. Genetics of anophthalmia and microphthalmia. Part 1: non-syndromic anophthalmia/microphthalmia. Hum Genet. 2019;138:799–830.
2. Chassaing N, Causse A, Vigouroux A, et al. Molecular findings and clinical data in a cohort of 150 patients with anophthalmia/microphthalmia. Clin Genet. 2014;86:326–34.
3. Slavotinek A. Genetics of anophthalmia and microphthalmia. Part 2: syndromes associated with anophthalmia-microphthalmia. Hum Genet. 2019;138:831–46.
4. Forrester MB, Merz RD. Descriptive epidemiology of anophthalmia and microphthalmia, Hawaii, 1986-2001. Birth Defects Res A Clin Mol Teratol. 2006;76:187–92.
5. Källén B, Robert E, Harris J. The descriptive epidemiology of anophthalmia and microphthalmia. Int J Epidemiol. 1996;25:1009–16.
6. Shah SP, Taylor AE, Sowden JC, Ragge N, Russell-Eggitt I, Rahi JS, Gilbert CE, Surveillance of Eye Anomalies Special Interest Group. Anophthalmos, microphthalmos, and Coloboma in the United Kingdom: clinical features, results of investigations, and early management. Ophthalmology. 2012;119:362–8.
7. Roos L, Jensen H, Grønskov K, Holst R, Tümer Z. Congenital microphthalmia, anophthalmia and coloboma among live births in Denmark. Ophthalmic Epidemiol. 2016;23:324–30.
8. Källén B, Tornqvist K. The epidemiology of anophthalmia and microphthalmia in Sweden. Eur J Epidemiol. 2005;20:345–50.
9. Schittkowski MP, Guthoff RF. Systemic and ophthalmological anomalies in congenital anophthalmic or microphthalmic patients. Br J Ophthalmol. 2010;94:487–93.
10. Groot ALW, Kuijten MMP, Remmers J, et al. Classification for treatment urgency for the microphthalmia/anophthalmia spectrum using clinical and biometrical characteristics. Acta Ophthalmol. 2020;98:514–20.
11. Bermejo E, Martínez-Frías ML. Congenital eye malformations: clinical-epidemiological analysis of 1,124,654 consecutive births in Spain. Am J Med Genet. 1998;75:497–504.
12. Busby A, Dolk H, Collin R, Jones RB, Winter R. Compiling a national register of babies born with anophthalmia/microphthalmia in England 1988-94. Arch Dis Child Fetal Neonatal Ed. 1998;79:F168–73.
13. Chambers TM, Agopian AJ, Lewis RA, Langlois PH, Danysh HE, Weber KA, Shaw GM, Mitchell LE, Lupo PJ. Epidemiology of anophthalmia and microphthalmia: prevalence and patterns in Texas, 1999-2009. Am J Med Genet A. 2018;176:1810–8.
14. Lowry RB, Kohut R, Sibbald B, Rouleau J. Anophthalmia and microphthalmia in the Alberta congenital anomalies surveillance system. Can J Ophthalmol. 2005;40:38–44.
15. Morrison D, FitzPatrick D, Hanson I, Williamson K, van Heyningen V, Fleck B, Jones I, Chalmers J, Campbell H. National study of microphthalmia, anophthalmia, and coloboma (MAC) in Scotland: investigation of genetic aetiology. J Med Genet. 2002;39:16–22.
16. Spagnolo A, Bianchi F, Calabro A, Calzolari E, Clementi M, Mastroiacovo P, Meli P, Petrelli G, Tenconi R. Anophthalmia and benomyl in Italy: a multicenter study based on 940,615 newborns. Reprod Toxicol. 1994;8:397–403.
17. Slavotinek AM. Eye development genes and known syndromes. Mol Genet Metab. 2011;104:448–56.
18. Tucker S, Jones B, Collin R. Systemic anomalies in 77 patients with congenital anophthalmos or microphthalmos. Eye (Lond). 1996;10:310–4.
19. Strömland K. Visual impairment and ocular abnormalities in children with fetal alcohol syndrome. Addict Biol. 2004;9:153–7; discussion 159–160.
20. Kava MP, Nagarajan L. Microphthalmia and microcornea: in congenital cytomegalovirus. Indian J Ophthalmol. 2009;57:323.
21. Gilchrist H, Taranath DA, Gole GA. Ocular malformation in a newborn secondary to maternal hypovitaminosis A. J AAPOS. 2010;14:274–6.
22. Hiler D, Chen X, Hazen J, et al. Quantification of retinogenesis in 3D cultures reveals epigenetic memory and higher efficiency in iPSCs derived from rod photoreceptors. Cell Stem Cell. 2015;17:101–15.
23. Balikova I, de Ravel T, Ayuso C, Thienpont B, Casteels I, Villaverde C, Devriendt K, Fryns J-P, Vermeesch JR. High frequency of submicroscopic chromosomal deletions in patients with idiopathic congenital eye malformations. Am J Ophthalmol. 2011;151:1087–1094.e45.
24. Delahaye A, Bitoun P, Drunat S, et al. Genomic imbalances detected by array-CGH in patients with syndromal ocular developmental anomalies. Eur J Hum Genet. 2012;20:527–33.
25. Raca G, Jackson CA, Kucinskas L, Warman B, Shieh JTC, Schneider A, Bardakjian TM, Schimmenti LA. Array comparative genomic hybridization analysis in patients with anophthalmia, microphthalmia, and coloboma. Genet Med. 2011;13:437–42.
26. Skalicky SE, White AJR, Grigg JR, Martin F, Smith J, Jones M, Donaldson C, Smith JEH, Flaherty M, Jamieson RV. Microphthalmia, anophthalmia, and coloboma and associated ocular and systemic features:

understanding the spectrum. JAMA Ophthalmol. 2013;131:1517–24.
27. Sinn R, Wittbrodt J. An eye on eye development. Mech Dev. 2013;130:347–58.
28. Chow RL, Lang RA. Early eye development in vertebrates. Annu Rev Cell Dev Biol. 2001;17:255–96.
29. Zagozewski JL, Zhang Q, Eisenstat DD. Genetic regulation of vertebrate eye development. Clin Genet. 2014;86:453–60.
30. Chuang JC, Raymond PA. Embryonic origin of the eyes in teleost fish. BioEssays. 2002;24:519–29.
31. Harding P, Moosajee M. The molecular basis of human anophthalmia and microphthalmia. J Dev Biol. 2019;7:E16.
32. Hever AM, Williamson KA, van Heyningen V. Developmental malformations of the eye: the role of PAX6, SOX2 and OTX2. Clin Genet. 2006;69:459–70.
33. Harding P, Brooks BP, FitzPatrick D, Moosajee M. Anophthalmia including next-generation sequencing-based approaches. Eur J Hum Genet. 2020;28:388–98.
34. Verma AS, Fitzpatrick DR. Anophthalmia and microphthalmia. Orphanet J Rare Dis. 2007;2:47.
35. Plaisancie J, Calvas P, Chassaing N. Genetic advances in microphthalmia. J Pediatr Genet. 2016;5:184–8.
36. Modugno AC, Resti AG, Mazzone G, Moretti C, Terreni MR, Albanese G, Savino G, Grimaldi G, Collin R. Long-term outcomes after cosmetic customized prostheses and dermis fat graft in congenital anophthalmia: a retrospective multicentre study. Eye. 2018;32:1803–10.
37. Bardakjian T, Weiss A, Schneider A. Microphthalmia/Anophthalmia/Coloboma Spectrum—retired chapter, for historical reference only. GeneReviews®; 1993.
38. Lingam G, Sen AC, Lingam V, Bhende M, Padhi TR, Xinyi S. Ocular coloboma—a comprehensive review for the clinician. Eye (Lond). 2021;35:2086–109.
39. Bennett RG, Hirt M. A history of tissue expansion. Concepts, controversies, and complications. J Dermatol Surg Oncol. 1993;19:1066–73.
40. Collin JR, Moriarty PA. Management of the contracted socket. Trans Ophthalmol Soc U K. 1982;102:93–7.
41. Downes R, Lavin M, Collin R. Hydrophilic expanders for the congenital anophthalmic socket. Adv Ophthalmic Plast Reconstr Surg. 1992;9:57–61.
42. Tucker SM, Sapp N, Collin R. Orbital expansion of the congenitally anophthalmic socket. Br J Ophthalmol. 1995;79:667–71.
43. Steinkogler FJ, Polzhofer K. Hema socket expander in primary conservative treatment of congenital anophthalmos. Klin Monatsbl Augenheilkd. 1987;191:240–2.
44. Wiese KG. Osmotically induced tissue expansion with hydrogels: a new dimension in tissue expansion? A preliminary report. J Craniomaxillofac Surg. 1993;21:309–13.
45. Wiese KG, Heinemann DE, Ostermeier D, Peters JH. Biomaterial properties and biocompatibility in cell culture of a novel self-inflating hydrogel tissue expander. J Biomed Mater Res. 2001;54:179–88.
46. Bacskulin A, Vogel M, Wiese KG, Gundlach K, Hingst V, Guthoff R. New osmotically active hydrogel expander for enlargement of the contracted anophthalmic socket. Graefes Arch Clin Exp Ophthalmol. 2000;238:24–7.
47. Schittkowski MP. Therapy options for blind microphthalmos and clinical anophthalmos. Ophthalmologe. 2012;109:1122–6.
48. Gundlach KK, Guthoff RF, Hingst VH, Schittkowski MP, Bier UC. Expansion of the socket and orbit for congenital clinical anophthalmia. Plast Reconstr Surg. 2005;116:1214–22.
49. Alanazi RR, Schellini SA, Alhussain H, Elkhamary S, Khandekar R, AlSheikh O. Outcomes of the use of orbital hydrogel expanders in the management of congenital anophthalmia: CT-based orbital parameter analysis. Orbit. 2021;28:1–9.
50. Trivedi D, McCalla M, Squires Z, Parulekar M. Use of cyanoacrylate glue for temporary tarsorrhaphy in children. Ophthalmic Plast Reconstr Surg. 2014;30:60–3.
51. Ragge NK, Subak-Sharpe ID, Collin JRO. A practical guide to the management of anophthalmia and microphthalmia. Eye (Lond). 2007;21:1290–300.
52. Quaranta-Leoni FM, Sposato S, Raglione P, Mastromarino A. Dermis-fat graft in children as primary and secondary orbital implant. Ophthalmic Plast Reconstr Surg. 2016;32:214–9.
53. Morax S, Hurbli T. Orbito-palpebral reconstruction in anophthalmos and severe congenital microphthalmos. Adv Ophthalmic Plast Reconstr Surg. 1992;9: 67–80.
54. Bajaj MS, Pushker N, Singh KK, Chandra M, Ghose S. Evaluation of amniotic membrane grafting in the reconstruction of contracted socket. Ophthalmic Plast Reconstr Surg. 2006;22:116–20.
55. Kumar S, Sugandhi P, Arora R, Pandey PK. Amniotic membrane transplantation versus mucous membrane grafting in anophthalmic contracted socket. Orbit. 2006;25:195–203.
56. Slentz DH, Joseph SS, Nelson CC. The use of umbilical amnion for conjunctival socket, fornix, and eyelid margin reconstruction. Ophthalmic Plast Reconstr Surg. 2020;36:365–71.
57. Lo AK, Colcleugh RG, Allen L, Van Wyck L, Bite U. The role of tissue expanders in an anophthalmic animal model. Plast Reconstr Surg. 1990;86:399–408; discussion 409–410.
58. Dunaway DJ, David DJ. Intraorbital tissue expansion in the management of congenital anophthalmos. Br J Plast Surg. 1996;49:529–35.
59. Tse DT, Abdulhafez M, Orozco MA, Tse JD, Azab AO, Pinchuk L. Evaluation of an integrated orbital tissue expander in congenital anophthalmos: report of preliminary clinical experience. Am J Ophthalmol. 2011;151:470–482.e1.

60. Marchac D, Cophignon J, Achard E, Dufourmentel C. Orbital expansion for anophthalmia and micro-orbitism. Plast Reconstr Surg. 1977;59:486–91.
61. Schittkowski MP, Guthoff RF. Injectable self inflating hydrogel pellet expanders for the treatment of orbital volume deficiency in congenital microphthalmos: preliminary results with a new therapeutic approach. Br J Ophthalmol. 2006;90:1173–7.
62. Tsitouridis I, Michaelides M, Tsantiridis C, Spyridi S, Arvanity M, Efstratiou I. Congenital cystic eye with multiple dermal appendages and intracranial congenital anomalies. Diagnostic and interventional radiology (Ankara, Turkey). 2009;16:116–21.
63. Guthoff R, Klein R, Lieb WE. Congenital cystic eye. Graefes Arch Clin Exp Ophthalmol. 2004;242:268–71.
64. Gore S, Grimaldi G, Mazzone G, Collin R, Savino G, Pagnoni M, Modugno A. Treatment strategies and long-term outcomes in patients with congenital microphthalmia-anophthamia with cyst. Br J Ophthalmol. 2022;107:750.
65. Pasquale LR. Congenital cystic eye with multiple ocular and intracranial anomalies. Arch Ophthalmol. 1991;109:985–7.
66. Decock CE, Breusegem CM, Van Aken EH, Leroy BP, Leroy BP, Van Den Broecke CM, Delanghe JR. High β-trace protein concentration in the fluid of an orbital cyst associated with bilateral colobomatous microphthalmos. Br J Ophthalmol. 2007;91:836–8.
67. Demirci H, Peksayar G, Demirci FYK, Buyukbabani N, Demiryont M. Bilateral Microphthalmos with Colobomatous orbital cyst. J Pediatr Ophthalmol Strabismus. 2002;39:110–3.
68. Timalsina BR, Shrestha GB, Thapa M. Congenital microphthalmia with intraorbital cyst: a rare case report. Case Reports in Ophthalmological Medicine. 2019;2019:e3640175.
69. Singer JR, Droste PJ, Hassan AS. Congenital cystic eye in utero: novel prenatal magnetic resonance imaging findings. JAMA Ophthalmol. 2013;131:1092–5.
70. Yagev R, Monos T, Shoham A, Lifshitz T. Microphthalmos and optic disc coloboma associated with a retrobulbar cyst. Journal of American Association for Pediatric Ophthalmology and Strabismus. 2000;4:381–2.
71. Cui Y, Li Y, Hou Z, Wang Y, Chang Q, Xian J, Li D. Management of congenital microphthalmos and anophthalmos with orbital cyst. Journal of American Association for Pediatric Ophthalmology and Strabismus. 2019;23:92.e1–6.
72. Lorenz B, Elflein HM, Hofstädter F. Ependymal tissue in microphthalmia with cyst. Ophthalmic Genet. 2006;27:165–8.
73. McLean CJ. The management of orbital cysts associated with congenital microphthalmos and anophthalmos. Br J Ophthalmol. 2003;87:860–3.
74. Chaudhry IA, Arat YO, Shamsi FA, Boniuk M. Congenital microphthalmos with orbital cysts: distinct diagnostic features and management. Ophthalmic Plast Reconstr Surg. 2004;20:452–7.
75. Kitthaweesin K. Orbital aspiration as treatment of microphthalmos with orbital cyst: a case report. J Med Assoc Thail. 2002;85:1024–7.
76. Cadet N, Dubois J, Codère F. Doxycycline injection in orbital cyst associated to microphthalmos. Can J Ophthalmol. 2017;52:e58–60.
77. Naik MN, Murthy RK, Raizada K, Honavar SG. Ethanolamine oleate sclerotherapy in the management of orbito-palpebral cyst associated with congenital microphthalmos. Am J Ophthalmol. 2005;139:939–41.
78. Naik MN, Honavar SG, Murthy RK, Raizada K, Thomas R. Ethanolamine oleate sclerotherapy versus simple cyst aspiration in the management of orbitopalpebral cyst associated with congenital microphthalmos. Ophthalmic Plast Reconstr Surg. 2007;23:307–11.
79. Wiwatwongwana D, Rootman J. Bilateral Microphthalmos with cyst: excision with orbital free fat graft. Ophthalmic Plast Reconstr Surg. 2009;25:241–3.

Part II

Orbital Disease

Embryonic Development of the Orbit

Ronald L. A. W. Bleys

Key Messages

- Bones of the skull base, including almost all orbital bones, form by endochondral ossification. The bones of the cranial vault and most facial bones form by intramembranous ossification.
- Cranial neural crest cells play a crucial role in orbital development. Only in the head neural crest cells form cartilage and bone. Moreover, neural crest cells form nerves, orbital fat, fibroblasts, and connective tissue elements, among others.
- Mesoderm is also involved in forming skull bones and orbital fat, and it forms the extraocular muscles.
- Interaction between neural crest cells and mesoderm seems to play a pivotal regulatory role in the complex development of the orbit.

1 Bone Formation

Bones in the human body develop from mesenchyme. Mesenchyme is a loosely woven tissue, typical for the embryo, which may differentiate into fibroblasts, chondroblasts and osteoblasts, the latter being the bone forming cells. The transition from mesenchyme to bone can take place in two different ways. One way is by the formation of a cartilaginous precursor. During this process of so-called endochondral ossification a cartilage model forms in the mesenchyme and is eventually replaced by bone. This is typical for most of the skeleton: spine, ribs, sternum, cranial base and the appendicular skeleton. The other way for bone to be formed is called intramembranous ossification, where bone forms directly from mesenchyme without prior formation of cartilage. This happens to the bones of the cranial vault and most of the bones of the face. Also part of the clavicle forms by intramembranous ossification.

Mesenchyme is derived from mesoderm, one of the three germ layers. The mesenchyme in the head is furthermore supplemented with cranial neural crest cells. As a consequence many bones in the head are derived not only from mesoderm but also from neural crest cells.

Thus, it can be concluded that the formation of the bones of the skull base including the orbit is characterised by endochondral ossification, hence the term chondrocranium, and the participation of neural crest cells. The neural crest forms during the process of neurulation: transformation of a dorsal part of the surface ectoderm into the neural plate and subsequently the neural tube (Fig. 1a–d). When the surface ectoderm covers the neural tube two groups of cells lie as neural crest cells between these two layers. These cells differentiate into mesenchyme and start migrating. This migration takes place along well defined pathways. Upon reaching their destinations throughout the body they form a wide range of cell types, such as sensory and autonomic gan-

Ronald L. A. W. Bleys (✉)
Department of Anatomy, University Medical Center Utrecht, Utrecht, The Netherlands
e-mail: r.l.a.w.bleys@umcutrecht.nl

F. M. Quaranta Leoni et al. (eds.), *Oculoplastic, Lacrimal and Orbital Surgery*,
https://doi.org/10.1007/978-3-031-39638-0_11

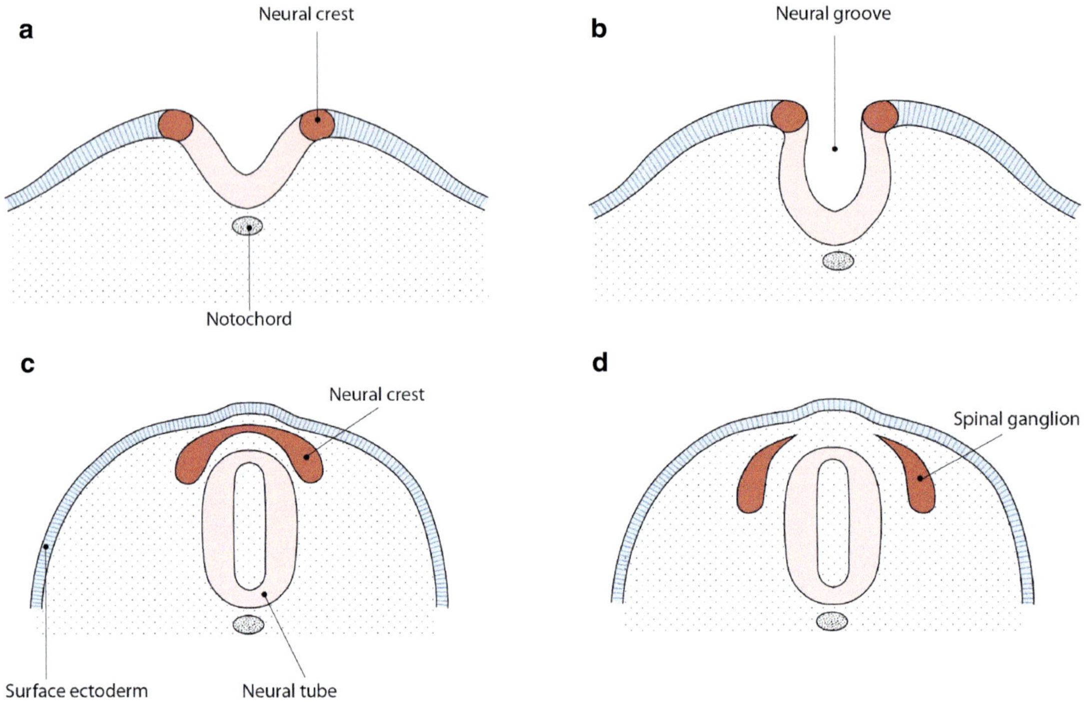

Fig. 1 Transverse sections through embryos showing the formation of the neural tube and neural crest. (**a**) A part of the dorsal surface ectoderm has thickened to become the neural plate, which shows a midline depression. The cells at the edges of the neural plate form the neural crests. (**b**) The midline depression has deepened and forms the neural groove. (**c**) The edges of the neural grooves fuse in the midline and as a result the neural tube is formed. The cells of the neural crests leave the ectoderm and undergo epithelium to mesenchymal transition. (**d**) Neural crest cells migrate and form a wide range of cell types, among others sensory ganglia

glia, Schwann cells, meninges, medulla of the adrenal gland, smooth muscle cells and in the head also cartilage and bones.

2 Formation of Skull Bones

Early in evolution the chondrocranium was formed to envelop and protect the brain, the olfactory organ, the eyes and the inner ears. Bones formed by intramembranous ossification are named dermal bones. These were overlying the chondrocranium and other dermal bones, derived from the first and second pharyngeal arches, formed the bones of the face, also known as the viscerocranium. Expansion of the brain in human development caused the chondrocranium to underlie the brain and the overlying dermal bones became the cranial vault. Cartilages derived from the first and second pharyngeal arches, respectively Meckel's cartilage and Reichert's cartilage, complete the skull bones by forming the auditory ossicles and a small part of the sphenoid bone (Fig. 2).

Tracing studies revealed the contribution from neural crest cells to the cranial bones more exactly. For the cranial vault it was found that in mouse embryos the frontal bones are derived from neural crest mesenchyme and parietal bones from mesodermal mesenchyme [1]. Neural crest cells are also present between the parietal bones. The fact that the coronal and sagittal sutures lie at the neural crest-mesoderm boundary is of interest with regard to mutations leading to craniosynostosis.

As for the skull base it was found that anterior to the sphenoid-occipital boundary the bones are neural crest derived. This includes the ethmoid and sphenoid bones. An exception, however, is the so-called hypochiasmatic cartilage which is derived from mesodermal mesenchyme. This cartilage contributes to part of the sphenoid bone (the lesser wing) and provides the attachment for the extraocular muscles [2].

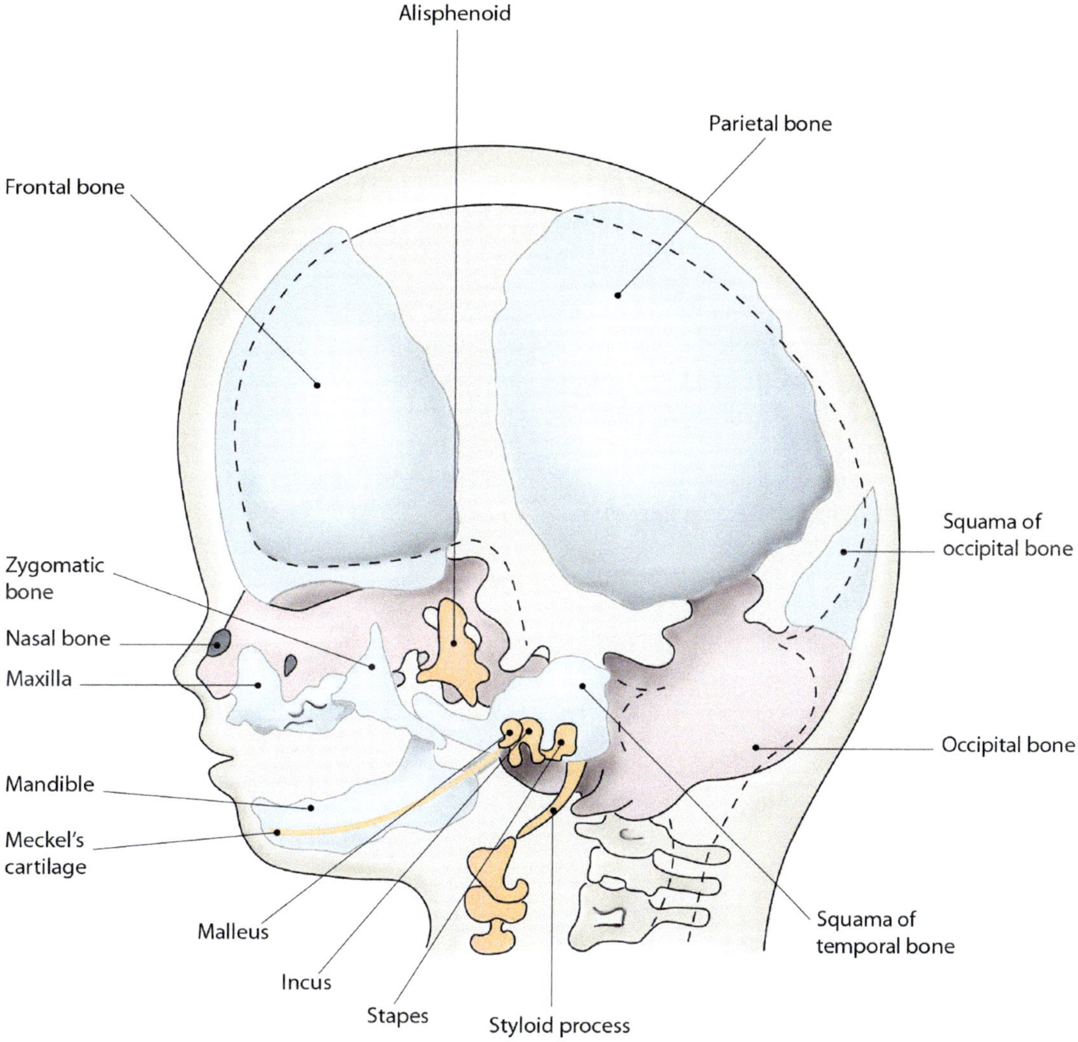

Fig. 2 Origin of the human skull bones. The chondocranium (purple) is formed by endochondral ossification and comprises the bones of skull base and the orbit. The dermal bones (blue) are formed by intramembranous ossification and form the bones of the cranial vault and the bones of the face. Bones derived from Meckel's and Reichert's cartilages are shown in orange

3 Orbit

The migration of cranial neural crest cells to the optic vesicle (see chapter "Embryology of Eyelid Development") is crucial for the development of the orbit [3]. These cells may form bone, cartilage, fibroblasts, smooth muscle cells, neurons and other cell types, and as a consequence many orbital structures are derived from neural crest cells. The optic vesicle itself plays an important role in guiding neural crest cell migration [4]. Disturbed development or migration of neural crest cells may result in diseases that manifest themselves as cranial defects, among others, such as Treacher Collins syndrome and DiGeorge syndrome [5].

A detailed and exhaustive narrative overview of the development of the orbit and its contents is presented by Tawfik et al. [6]. Remarkable highlights of development of orbital structures are the following.

By 8 weeks after fertilisation many major structures are present. These include the extraocular muscles which are derived from mesoderm that surrounds the developing eye, and the optic nerve, derived from the optic stalk as outgrowth of the forebrain. However, the structures do not have their definitive arrangement yet. Levator palpebrae superioris lies medial to superior rectus and both orbits still await a reorientation into a more medial position. Week 8 marks significant day-to-day changes. Ossification of the orbital bones starts, the optic nerve becomes filled with axons on their way to the diencephalon and the orbital floor is occupied by the orbital muscle of Müller (Fig. 3). This muscle is believed to cover the lateral orbital wall in animals that lack a complete bony lateral wall. In humans this muscle is replaced by connective tissue, gradually diminishes in size during development and the eventually remaining muscle fibres span the inferior orbital fissure and have an unclear function. Arterial supply and venous drainage is developing as well in this period. Also, the primordial lacrimal gland develops out of 5 to 6 epithelial buds which evaginate from the superior conjunctival fornix into the surrounding mesenchyme. After ingrowth of the lacrimal artery and the lacrimal nerve glandular acini develop [7].

In week 9 the lateral-to-frontal reorientation of the orbits proceeds much. As a result the intercanthal distance decreases in comparison to the width of the face. In week 10 Müller's orbital muscle is still very large since it covers the wide inferior orbital fissure and forms the greater part of the orbital floor which is far from completing the ossification process. In week 12 the orbits get closer together and levator palpebrae superioris moves above superior rectus.

Orbital fat has started to develop in week 13 as proliferations of primitive blood vessels and aggregations of mesenchymal cells, the preadipocytes (Fig. 3). There are strong indications that orbital fat has a dual origin in which both mesoderm and cranial neural crest cells contribute.

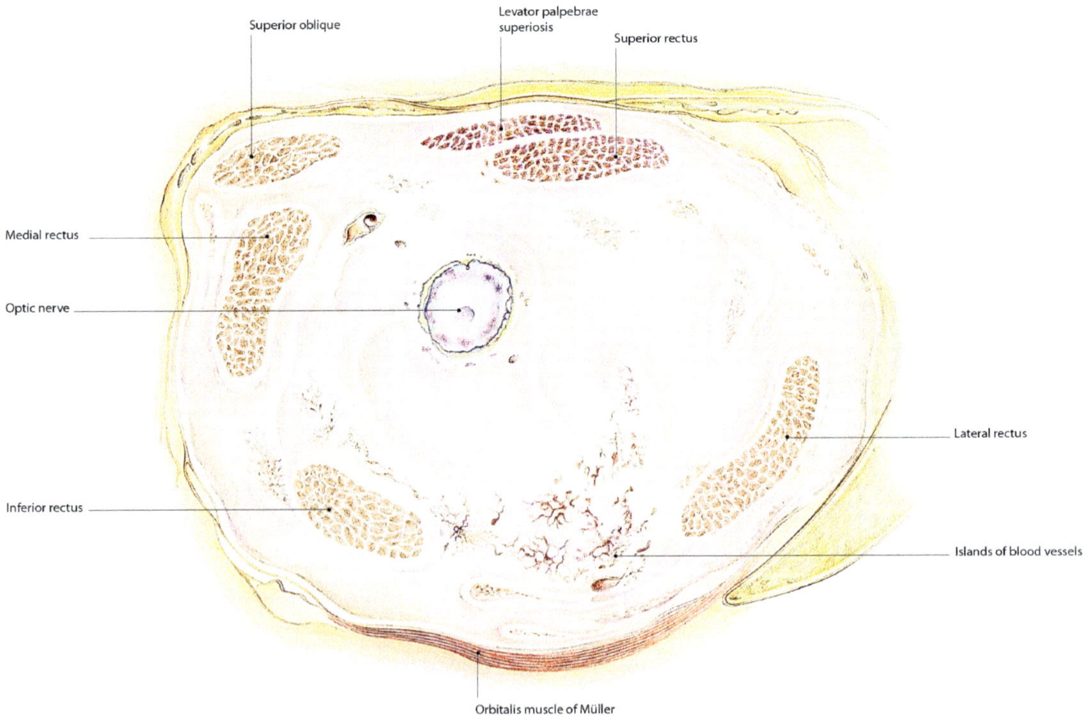

Fig. 3 Coronal cross-section of the orbit in week 14 showing the orbital muscle of Müller as part of the orbital floor. Levator palpebrae superioris is moving towards its position above the superior rectus. Islands of blood vessels are present as the precursor of orbital fat

Intraconal fat and the medial preaponeurotic fat pad originate from neural crest cells and the central preaponeurotic fat pad originates from mesoderm [8]. In week 16 adipose tissue can be seen throughout the orbit as fatty islands separated by connective tissue septa and in week 18 the amount of fat has increased considerably [6].

From week 17 the attachments of the extraocular muscles to the eyeball are visible but they have similar distances to the limbus. From week 22 the insertions start receding and obtain various distances to the limbus. In week 24 the cartilage at the apex of the orbit ossifies and the perichondrium becomes periosteum. A ring of dense periosteum forms the anulus of Zinn [9].

From week 26 there is an enormous increase of retrobulbar fat and in week 28 the number of axons in the optic nerve has reached the adult configuration. The last phase to term sees a substantial increase of the orbital dimensions and an increase of the fat/connective tissue ratio.

At full term the eye volume is 38% of the adult value, the orbital volume is 17.3% of the adult value and the distance of the insertion of the extraocular muscles to the limbus is 2 mm less than in adults [6].

References

1. Yoshida T, Vivatbusiri P, Morris-Kay G, Saga Y, Iseki S. Cell lineage in mammalian craniofacial mesenchyme. Mech Dev. 2008;125:797–808.
2. McBratney-Owen B, Iseki S, Bamforth SD, Olsen BR, Morris-Kay GM. Development and tissue origins of the mammalian cranial base. Dev Biol. 2008;322:121–32.
3. Cho RI, Kahana A. Embryology of the orbit. J Neurol Surg B Skull Base. 2021;82:2–6.
4. Langenberg T, Kahana A, Wszalek JA, Halloran MC. The eye organizes neural crest cell migration. Dev Dyn. 2008;237:1645–52.
5. Vega-Lopez GA, Cerrizuela S, Tribulom C, Aybar MJ. Neurocristopathies: new insights 150 years after the neural crest discovery. Dev Biol. 2018;444:S110–43.
6. Tawfik HA, Dutton JJ. Embryologic and fetal development of the human orbit. Ophthal Plast Reconstr Surg. 2018;34:405–21.
7. de la Cuadra-Blanco C, Peces-Peña MD, Mérida-Velasco JR. Morphogenesis of the human lacrimal gland. J Anat. 2003;203:531–6.
8. Korn BS, Kikkawa DO, Hicok KC. Identification and characterization of adult stem cells from human orbital adipose tissue. Ophthal Plast Reconstr Surg. 2009;25:27–32.
9. Sevel D. The origins and insertions of the extraocular muscles: development, histologic features, and clinical significance. Trans Am Ophthalmol Soc. 1986;84:488–526.

Orbital Surgical Anatomy

Alain Ducasse, Peerooz Saeed, and Vladimir Kratky

Key Messages

- Orbital anatomy is complex, with many structures that cross each other at different levels.
- The frequent variations demonstrate the difficulty in depicting a simple, standard and easy-to-learn view of this anatomy.
- Some aspects and variations are more common than others (for example, the association of an undercrossing ophthalmic artery-optic nerve with a meningolacrimal artery and a lateral muscular branch).
- A better knowledge of this anatomy, and future developments in orbital imaging, will lead to more precise localisation of orbital components, minimising the potential surgical difficulties.

A. Ducasse (✉)
Department of Ophthalmology, Reims CHR, Reims, France
e-mail: ducasse.alain24@orange.fr

P. Saeed
Orbital Center, Department of Ophthalmology, Amsterdam University Medical Center, Amsterdam, The Netherlands

V. Kratky
Oculoplastic and Orbital Surgery Unit, 1st Medical Faculty, Charles University, Prague, Czech Republic - Queen's University, Kingston, ON, Canada

1 Introduction

A solid knowledge of normal orbital anatomy and its most frequent variations is necessary to establish an accurate diagnosis of orbital disease and to perform meticulous orbital surgery, with the least amount of risk. While a great variability gives each orbit its unique characteristics, it is still possible to describe a general overview of the organization of the orbit, along with a description of the main variations.

The orbit contains the anterior part of the visual system—the eyeball and optic nerve—as well as the orbital muscles, the lacrimal gland, arteries, veins, other nerves and orbital fat. Usually, the orbit is described in two parts: the bony cavity and the soft tissue contents.

2 Location, Orientation and Dimensions

The orbits are located at the junction of the skull and the face, under the cerebral hemispheres and the frontal sinus, and above the maxillary sinus, on either side of the nasal cavities and the ethmoidal air cells. Orbit is also at the junction of the internal and external carotid systems, as well as the cranial and facial venous systems.

F. M. Quaranta Leoni et al. (eds.), *Oculoplastic, Lacrimal and Orbital Surgery*,
https://doi.org/10.1007/978-3-031-39638-0_12

Each orbit has the shape of a pyramid, lying on its side, with the tip (apex) placed posteriorly and the base (orbital opening) anteriorly. It has four walls which meet at four margins anteriorly, but only three of them reach the apex since the orbital floor ends at the sphenopalatine fossa.

This pyramidal cavity is angled forward and laterally, and its axis forms an angle of 23° with the visual axis in the anteroposterior direction, which determines the action of the ocular muscles. The medial walls are parallel to each other in the anteroposterior direction, whereas the lateral walls are oriented forward and laterally, together forming a 90° angle at the superior margin of the *sella turcica* (Fig. 1). The superior wall (roof) slopes downward and back towards the apex, whereas the inferior wall (floor) slopes upward and back.

The orbital depth in adults is usually between 42 to 50 mm, with an average of 45 mm. The distance between the two lateral margins is between 110 and 125 mm. The intercanthal distance varies from 27 to 33 mm, and the anterior orbital opening at the orbital rim measures on average 40 mm in width and 35 mm in height. The orbital volume plays an important role in surgery, measuring 24.9 mL (±3.03) in males and 23.09 mL (± 3.08) [1].

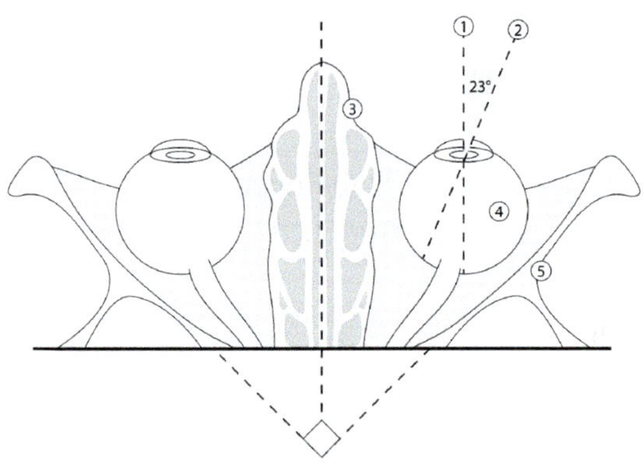

Fig. 1 Orbital orientation: (1) visual axis; (2) orbital axis; (3) medial wall of the orbit; (4) eyeball; (5) lateral wall of the orbit

3 The Bony Orbit

The bony orbit is comprised of seven bones: three skull bones (frontal, ethmoid and sphenoid) and four are facial bones (maxilla, zygomatic, lacrimal and palatine) (Fig. 2).

3.1 The Four Orbital Walls (Figs. 3 and 4)

3.1.1 The Orbital Roof

This wall is triangular in shape, with an anterior base. It is made up of the orbital nasal plate of the frontal bone anteriorly and the inferior plate of the lesser wing of the sphenoid bone posteriorly. The frontal bone forms the roof of the orbital cavity, with a concave shape in the anteroposterior and coronal cross section, a laterally placed lacrimal gland fossa, and a medially situated area of insertion of the trochlea, the trochlear spine. This wall is very thin and may have areas of spontaneous dehiscence, with a risk of perforation during orbital surgery. This roof is located under the anterior cranial fossa, with the frontal lobe of the cerebral hemisphere and the frontal sinus anteriorly.

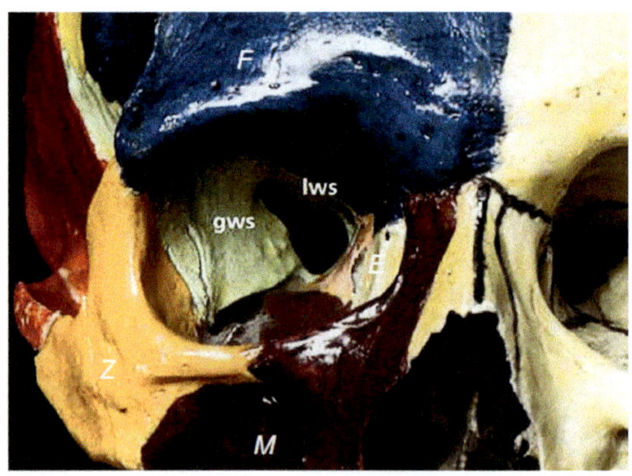

Fig. 2 Bones of the orbit: *F* frontal bone, *E* ethmoid, *M* maxilla, *Z* zygomatic bone, *lws* lesser wing of the sphenoid, *gws* greater wing of the sphenoid

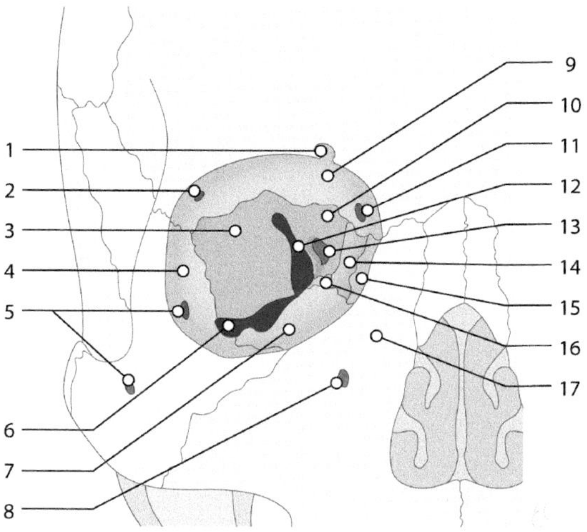

Fig. 3 Orbital foramina and fissures: (1) supraorbital foramen; (2) lacrimal gland fossa; (3) greater wing of the sphenoid; (4) zygomatic bone; (5) zygomatic foramen; (6) inferior orbital fissure; (7) maxilla; (8) infraorbital foramen; (9) frontal bone; (10) lesser wing of the sphenoid; (11) trochlear fossa; (12) superior orbital fissure; (13) optic canal; (14) ethmoid; (15) lacrimal bone; (16) palatine bone; (17) frontal process of the maxilla

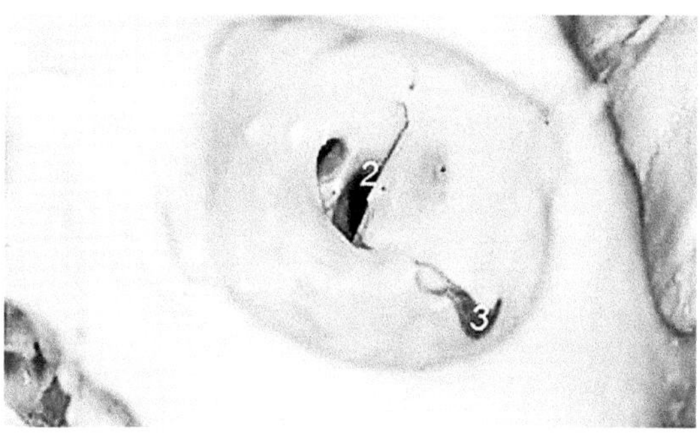

Fig. 4 Frontal view of the bony orbit: (1) optic canal; (2) superior orbital fissure; (3) inferior orbital fissure; (4) lacrimal sac fossa

3.1.2 The Lateral Wall

Directed forward and laterally, this wall is triangular in shape, with the apex being posterior. It is the strongest and thickest of the orbital walls and is formed by three bones: the frontal bone from above (its zygomatic process) with the zygomatic bone from below form the anterior part, while the greater wing of sphenoid completes this wall posteriorly. On the zygomatic bone, the zygomatico-orbital foramen is a Y-shaped channel containing the zygomatico-orbital nerve, branch of the zygomatic nerve and the zygomatico-orbital vessels. This foramen has three apertures, one on each of the three surfaces of the zygomatic bone. Laterally, is the temporal fossa with the temporalis muscle; posteriorly, this wall is in contact with the middle cranial fossa, enclosing the temporal lobe of the cerebral hemisphere.

3.1.3 The Orbital Floor

Unlike the other three walls, it forms only the anterior part of the orbit without reaching the orbital apex. It is also triangular in shape with an anterior base, very thin, and is directed backward, upward, and medially. Three bones participate in its formation: the orbital plate of the zygomatic bone anteriorly and laterally, the orbital face of the maxillary bone anteriorly and medially, and the orbital process of the palatine bone posteriorly. The infraorbital sulcus is located in the posterior part of the floor and is directed anteriorly and medially. This sulcus arises from the anterior part of the inferior orbital fissure and penetrates forward into the maxillary bone, forming the infraorbital canal which opens 5 to 6 mm under the infraorbital rim, as the infraorbital foramen. The sulcus, canal, and foramen contain the maxillary nerve, second terminal branch of the trigeminal nerve and the infraorbital artery, branch of the maxillary artery, and the infraorbital vein. The infraorbital nerve gives branches for the teeth, the upper lip and the cheek and can be damaged during orbital decompression and trauma. Inferior to the orbital floor is the maxillary sinus, and behind this bone are the infratemporal fossa laterally and the pterygopalatine fossa medially.

3.1.4 The Medial Wall

It is the most complex wall, consisting of four bones and measuring about 45 to 50 mm in length. From front to back, the four bones are: the lateral plate of the frontal process of the maxilla bearing the anterior lacrimal crest; the lateral plate of the lacrimal bone with the posterior lacrimal crest, and the lacrimal sac fossa between these two crests; the lateral plate of the lateral body of the ethmoid and the lateral plate of the sphenoid body, near the orbital apex. This wall is very thin, and trauma or surgery can easily create a bony dehiscence. The orbital septum attaches to the posterior lacrimal crest and represents the anterior limit of the true orbital cavity. The lacrimal sac is in fact extraorbital, as it is located in the lacrimal fossa, just in front of the orbit. Medially lies the lateral wall of the nasal cavity with the turbinates, and more posteriorly the ethmoid and sphenoid sinuses.

3.2 The Four Orbital Margins (Edges of the Orbital Pyramid)

1. *The superomedial margin* is situated between the superior and the medial walls, consisting of the fronto-maxillary, fronto-lacrimal, and fronto-ethmoidal sutures. It contains the anterior and posterior ethmoidal foramina, which correspond to the limit between the cranial fossa and the orbit (this is also the upper limit of an orbital decompression). The distance between the superomedial margin and the anterior cranial fossa is variable and may be less than 3 mm [2], with a risk of cerebrospinal fluid leakage during a dacryocystorhinostomy.
2. *The inferomedial margin* represents the junction between the medial and inferior walls, which is marked by the lacrimo-maxillary, ethmoido-maxillary and spheno-palatine sutures. Located anteriorly is the upper aperture of the nasolacrimal canal. This margin is very strong and often referred to as 'the strut' in surgery.
3. *The superolateral margin* is at the junction of the superior and lateral walls, bounded posteriorly by the superior orbital fissure, and is directed anteriorly, laterally and superiorly. Anteriorly, this margin runs along the frontal bone.
4. *The inferolateral margin* is between the inferior and lateral walls, mainly defined by the inferior orbital fissure directed anteriorly and laterally. It is limited by the posterior edge of the orbital plate of the maxilla and the inferior edge of the greater wing of the sphenoid, and laterally by the zygomatic bone. The fissure is covered by periosteum and separates the orbit from the pterygopalatine and infratemporal fossae. Anteriorly, the inferolateral margin continues onto the zygomatic bone.

3.3 The Orbital Apex (Fig. 5)

Located posteriorly at the junction of the orbital walls, it is a narrow space in the medial part of the superior orbital fissure, with the origin to the rectus muscles. Just above and medially is the optic canal which conducts the optic nerve and the ophthalmic artery [3]. These structures are crowded in this compact space and can be compressed, resulting in optic neuropathy, as is the case of enlarged extraocular muscles in thyroid-associated orbitopathy (TAO).

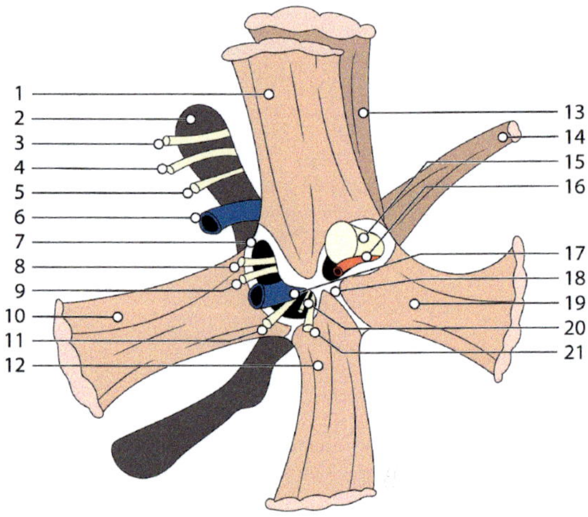

Fig. 5 Orbital apex: (1) superior rectus muscle; (2) superior orbital fissure; (3) lacrimal nerve; (4) frontal nerve; (5) trochlear nerve; (6) superior ophthalmic vein; (7) tendinous annulus; (8) abducens nerve; (9) oculomotor nerve: superior branch; (10) lateral rectus muscle; (11) oculomotor nerve: inferior branch; (12) inferior rectus muscle; (13) levator of the upper eyelid; (14) superior oblique muscle; (15) optic nerve; (16) ophthalmic artery; (17) medial ophthalmic vein; (18) Zinn's annulus; (19) medial rectus muscle; (20) sympathetic root of the ciliary ganglion; (21) nasociliary nerve

3.4 The Orbital Rim (Anterior Orbital Aperture)

The rim is quadrilateral in shape and opens medially as a key ring, made up of the posterior lacrimal crest on the lacrimal bone, the anterior margin of the frontal bone (with the supraorbital foramen or notch), the anterior margins of the zygomatic and maxillary bones, and finally by the anterior lacrimal crest on the maxillary bone. This rim is very thick and strong, protecting the eyeball in the event of facial trauma. The lateral rim is slightly recessed in comparison to the other three walls, and the globe may be more exposed to injury from this side.

3.5 The Foramina of the Bony Orbit

They are numerous, some can be absent, and their sizes vary.

3.5.1 The Optic Canal

Located between the two roots of the lesser wing and the body of the sphenoid bone, the optic canal courses obliquely forward, downward, and laterally. It measures 5 to 9 mm in length and 5 to 6 mm in diameter. It has a posterior intracranial orifice with a horizontal oval shape and an anterior orbital orifice with a vertical oval shape. It connects the orbit with the anterior cranial fossa. It contains the optic nerve with its sheaths and the ophthalmic artery, which usually crosses below the nerve into the canal and is found under and lateral to the nerve at the entrance to the orbit. The nerve and the artery then go through the superomedial part of the tendinous annulus. The medial wall of this canal is shared by the lateral wall of the sphenoid sinus, which is often very thin, sometimes even absent. It is therefore possible to reach the optic nerve by an endonasal surgical approach through this sinus.

3.5.2 The Superior Orbital Fissure

Directed upward, forward and laterally, the superior orbital fissure is usually comma- or pear-shaped, but it varies considerably in size and shape. It is between the inferior plate of the lesser wing of sphenoid and the upper edge of the orbital plate of the greater wing of sphenoid, and medially the lateral plate of the body of the sphenoid bone. It forms the anterior wall of the cavernous sinus and permits the transmission of several nerves and vessels between the middle cranial fossa and the orbit.

The tendon of Zinn is a ring of fibrous tissue on the sphenoid body and is the origin of the four recti muscles. It gives off two annuli, superomedial and superolateral, in front of the fissure. The superomedial part of the annulus conducts the optic nerve and the ophthalmic artery. The structures which go through the superolateral part of the annulus of Zinn, into the intraconal orbital space are the oculomotor nerve (IIIrd cranial nerve) which divides into two branches, superior and inferior; the abducens nerve (VIth cranial nerve); the nasociliary nerve, a branch of the ophthalmic nerve, which in turn is a branch of the trigeminal nerve (Vth cranial nerve), the sympathetic root of the ciliary ganglion and the inconsistent medial ophthalmic vein. Other structures that pass through the superior orbital fissure outside of the annulus into the extraconal orbital space include the trochlear nerve (IVth cranial nerve), the frontal and lacrimal nerves, branches of the ophthalmic nerve, and the superior ophthalmic vein.

3.5.3 The Inferior Orbital Fissure

This forms the inferolateral margin of the orbit, as described above. It is enclosed by periosteum, with only some small veins passing through it.

3.5.4 The Infraorbital Sulcus, Canal and Foramen

As described above, these structures transmit the maxillary nerve and the infraorbital vessels and open into the infraorbital foramen, on the anterior surface of the maxilla just under the inferior orbital rim. In a study of 133 cases [4], this foramen was found to be 6.33 ± 1.39 mm below the orbital rim and 25.69 ± 2.37 mm from the median line. Its caliber is on average 5.5 mm and multiple openings can be found in 21%.

3.5.5 The Nasolacrimal Canal

Directed downward, backward and medially, the canal opens under the inferior turbinate in the nose. Its upper aperture is located on the orbital floor anteriorly and medially, with the origin of the inferior oblique muscle just lateral to it. It contains the nasolacrimal duct.

3.5.6 The Supraorbital Foramen/Notch

Located on the superior orbital rim, it contains the supraorbital nerve (terminal branch of the frontal nerve), the supraorbital artery and vein. This foramen can be closed by a bony bridge or open, in which case it is called as supraorbital notch. In a study of 108 bony skulls [5], a bilateral closed foramen was found in 20.93% cases, and a unilateral closed foramen in 25%. Medial to the supraorbital foramen, a less consistent finding is that of a supratrochlear foramen, which conducts the supratrochlear nerve, a second terminal branch of the frontal nerve.

3.5.7 The Zygomatico-Orbital Foramen

This foramen has been described above.

3.5.8 The Ethmoidal Foramina

The anterior and posterior ethmoidal foramina are located at the superomedial margin of the orbit, at the level of the cribriform plate, and serve as an important landmark in orbital surgery, such as medial wall decompression, exenteration, or in case of nasal bleeding where a ligation of the anterior ethmoidal artery may be necessary.

- The anterior foramen contains the anterior ethmoidal artery and vein, and the anterior ethmoidal nerve, a terminal branch of the nasociliary nerve.
- The posterior foramen contains the posterior ethmoidal artery and vein, and the inconsistent posterior ethmoidal nerve, also a branch of the nasociliary nerve.

According to Kirchner et al. [6] the anterior foramen is located 14–18 mm behind the orbital rim. During dissections by Ducasse [7], it was found to be 9 to 34 mm behind the trochlea of the superior oblique muscle, usually between 18 to 22 mm with an average of 19.8 mm. The posterior foramen is classically located 10 mm behind the anterior, with a great variability. Studies by Cheng et al. [8] showed it on average to be 35.56 mm behind the anterior lacrimal crest and in our center [7], it was 15 mm behind the anterior foramen. The posterior foramen is 4–7 mm in front of the orbital opening of the optic canal.

Usually, there are two ethmoidal foramina, but accessory foramina have been described. Piagkou et al. [9] studied 240 orbits and reported only one foramen in 6% of the cases, two in 61%, three in 28.5%, and between three and six in 16.4%. These foramina contain accessory ethmoidal arteries.

3.5.9 The Orbito-Meningeal Foramina

These are inconsistent communicating foramina between the orbit and the cranium. Macchi et al. [10] found 54 of them in 100 patients, and up to five per orbit. Their diameter is less than 3 mm, on average 1.2 ± 0.3 mm, with those larger than 1 mm found only in 12% of the cases. They are channels for small arteries. One of the most frequent is the Hyrtl's canal on the lateral wall of the orbit, which conducts the meningolacrimal artery, arising from the middle meningeal artery.

3.6 The Orbital Periosteum

It is a thin fibrous membrane that lines the bony orbital cavity and surrounds the orbital contents, like a sac, perforated by the neurovascular structures. Except at the optic canal and the superior orbital fissure, where it is continuous with the dura mater of the optic nerve and the cavernous sinus, it is fairly easily separable from the underlying bone. It closes the inferior orbital fissure, along with a smooth muscle, also called the Muller's muscle. Anteriorly, at the orbital opening, it is continuous with the periosteum of the bones of the orbital rim.

4 The Orbital Contents

The orbital compartment is closed anteriorly 360° by the orbital septum, which extends from the edges of the tarsal plates to the orbital rim. Medially, it runs along the posterior lacrimal crest and laterally it is fixed on the lateral palpebral ligament. This septum defines the anterior limit of the orbital cavity and separates orbital fat and the orbicularis muscle. It is perforated superiorly by the levator palpebrae superioris muscle, which then leaves the orbit to reach the upper eyelid.

4.1 The Globe

Located at the anterior part of the orbit, the globe protrudes slightly beyond the orbital rim, especially laterally. With a diameter of 24 mm and a volume of about 7.5 cm^3, it is positioned closer to the lateral wall (6 mm) and the orbital roof (9 mm) than the inferior and medial walls (11 mm). Its arterial supply is provided by the ocular branches of the ophthalmic artery:

4.1.1 The Central Retinal Artery

Its presence is extremely constant, with mild variation in origin, arising directly from the ophthalmic artery in 49% of the cases, the medial ciliary artery in 37%, the inferior muscular artery in 8%, and the long lateral ciliary artery in 6% [11]. It is a small artery, usually with a diameter inferior to 0.5 mm, and range of 0.2 to 0.4 mm [12]. It quickly reaches the inferior part of the optic nerve and runs along it for 3 to 20 mm before penetrating the nerve 6 to 15 mm behind the eyeball and reaching to the optic nerve head, where it gives off its terminal branches.

4.1.2 The Posterior Ciliary Arteries

Usually there are two or three posterior ciliary arteries, which divide behind the globe into numerous smaller branches penetrating the sclera: the long and short posterior ciliary arteries. The long ciliary arteries run forward to supply the ciliary muscle, iris and anterior choroid, while the short ciliary arteries supply the optic nerve head and the rest of choroid.

The number of the long ciliary arteries varies according to different authors, most of them describing two or three arteries [13], and sometimes up to five arteries. There are between 15 and 20 short posterior ciliary arteries per orbit.

In fact, it seems logical to describe several posterior ciliary trunks, which give rise to the posterior long ciliary arteries, and many short posterior ciliary arteries. From our studies [13], there are usually two constant trunks, a medial and a lateral, which is always the largest. When a third trunk exists, it is often superior, and when a fourth trunk is present (very rare), it is lateral or inferior.

The lateral posterior ciliary trunk is more constant and arises from the ophthalmic artery in 92% of cases. Located at its origin on the lateral side of the optic nerve, it runs along this side to the eyeball, giving off numerous short ciliary arteries and one long lateral posterior ciliary artery, which penetrate into the sclera 4 mm away from the optic nerve head. The diameter of the trunk is between 0.3 and 1 mm, with an average of 0.56 mm.

The medial posterior ciliary trunk is more variable, arising from the ophthalmic artery in 82% of the cases, and from the inferior muscular artery in 17%. Its course depends of the location of its origin; when it starts inside the optic nerve, in 55% of cases, it goes along the medial side of the nerve to the sclera; when it starts outside the optic nerve, in 45% of cases, it crosses the nerve usually underneath (87%). It is usually smaller than the lateral trunk, with a diameter from 0.3 to 1 mm and an average of 0.51 mm [12].

According to Ducourneau [15], the short posterior ciliary arteries enter the sclera in two groups: one near the optic nerve—the paraoptic group (4 to 5 arteries)—and one at distance from the nerve head (5 to 10 arteries).

All these arteries, the central retinal artery, the long and short posterior ciliary arteries, and the long and short ciliary nerves form a great neurovascular bundle around the optic nerve, behind the optic nerve head.

4.2 The Optic Nerve

The second cranial nerve is a central nervous system expansion made up of retinal ganglion cell axons which exit the eyeball at the optic disc. It starts at the optic disc and can be divided into three parts as it passes through the sclera: prelaminar, laminar, and retrolaminar. The nerve runs posteriorly in the orbit to the optic canal, forming the axis of the muscle cone. Its orbital length is about 2.5 cm, with two S-shaped curves, the first one convex laterally and the second one convex medially. In its course it is crossed by the ophthalmic artery.

Along with the ophthalmic artery, the optic nerve then passes through the optic canal via the orbital optic foramen towards its cranial aperture. It is firmly fixed within the canal and may be susceptible to intracanalicular injury in cases of head trauma. After the nerve exits the optic canal inside the cranium, it joins the contralateral optic nerve to form the optic chiasm, which overlies the pituitary gland. It also crosses the anterior cerebral artery, making it vulnerable to compression by an aneurysm of this artery or a pituitary tumour in this region.

Within the canal, the nerve is surrounded by its sheaths, which are extensions of the cranial meninges: the pia, arachnoid and dura mater. At the cranial aperture of the canal, the dura mater leaves the nerve and continues with the dura mater of the skull. The intracranial portion of the nerve is covered only by the pia mater.

The arterial blood supply of the optic nerve also varies depending on the location. At the level of optic nerve head (lamina cribrosa), it is supplied by the peripapillary artery (also known as the circle of Zinn-Haller), which is derived from the short posterior ciliary arteries. The orbital portion is supplied by the central retinal artery, as it courses inside the nerve and beyond its point of penetration, by the arteries of the optic nerve, which are two or three very small branches of the ophthalmic artery. The intracanalicular part has a very poor vascularisation.

4.3 The Orbital Muscles

There are seven striated muscles found in each orbit: six oculomotors, directly fixed to the sclera and one elevator muscle of the upper eyelid. Four of the six oculomotors are recti muscles: superior, inferior, medial, and lateral. All of them insert on the eyeball in front of the equator. The other two are the superior and inferior oblique muscles, which insert on the eyeball behind the equator. Except for the inferior oblique muscle, all originate at the orbital apex. All the seven muscles are innervated by the three oculomotor nerves. The superior branch of the oculomotor nerve (III) supplies the levator and the superior rectus, while the inferior branch innervates the medial and inferior recti and the inferior oblique. The trochlear nerve (IV) supplies the superior oblique, and the abducens nerve (VI) innervates the lateral rectus muscle.

4.3.1 The Levator Muscle (Upper Eyelid Retractor)

The levator muscle originates at the orbital apex, directly on the periosteum, above and slightly medially to the optic canal. It is spindle-shaped and travels forward under the orbital roof, just above the superior rectus muscle. At the anterior part of the orbit, the levator muscle divides in two parts. The anterior part is the levator aponeurosis, which perforates the septum and inserts on to the anterior lower third of the tarsal plate, while sending fibers into the upper eyelid skin to form the lid crease. It is innervated by the upper branch of the oculomotor nerve and serves the function of elevating the upper eyelid. A few fibers reach the bony orbital rim laterally and medially, and are known as the horns of the levator muscle. The more important lateral horn, travels to the orbital tubercle and upwards to divide the lacrimal gland into orbital and palpebral lobes. The posterior part of the levator muscle forms the superior tarsal muscle or Muller's muscle, consisting of smooth muscular fibers, and has sympathetic innervation, which responds to epinephrine. At the level of the division of the anterior and posterior parts of the levator, there is a white band, the upper transverse ligament or Whitnall's ligament. Codère [16] also describes a white condensation just under this ligament, called the inferior ligament of Whitnall. The total length of the levator muscle is about 56 mm, with 15–20 mm for the aponeurotic part.

4.3.2 The Four Rectus Muscles

They extend from the orbital apex to the sclera with a length of about 40 mm. These four muscles with their connective fascias and their intermuscular septa define the muscle cone, around the optic nerve and the ophthalmic artery.

They arise from Zinn's tendon, originating from the lateral wall of the sphenoid body and which divides into four small bands of connective tissue. Each rectus muscle originates on two contiguous bands: the medial rectus from the superomedial and inferomedial bands, the superior rectus from the superomedial and superolateral bands, the lateral rectus from the superolateral and inferolateral bands, and the inferior rectus from the inferolateral and inferomedial bands.

Each muscle is spindle-shaped and travels forward following its orbital wall: the superior rectus follows the orbital roof, under the levator muscle, the medial rectus the medial wall, the lateral rectus the lateral wall, and the inferior rectus the orbital floor. While the medial rectus has an anteroposterior direction, along the visual axis, the other three muscles are directed forward and laterally, in relation to the orbital axis.

Anteriorly, the four recti muscles insert into the sclera in front of the equator, through a 10-mm-wide tendon. According to Porter [17], the distances between the muscular insertion and the corneal limbus are as follows: 5.5 mm for the medial rectus, 6.5 mm for the inferior rectus, 7 mm for the lateral rectus and 7.75 mm for the superior rectus, in the shape of an imaginary line called the spiral of Tillaux. De Gottrau [18] found some variability in the distances and gives a range for the medial rectus of 5.3 to 7.6 mm (average 6.2), the inferior rectus 5.8 to 8.1 mm (average 7), the lateral rectus 6.4 to 9 mm (average 7.7), and the superior rectus 7.3 to 9.9 mm (average 8.5).

Biomechanically, the horizontal recti muscles have only one action: abduction for the lateral rectus and adduction for the medial rectus. The vertical muscles each have three combined actions: elevation, adduction, and internal rotation (intorsion) for the superior rectus muscle, and depression, adduction and external rotation (extorsion) for the inferior rectus.

4.3.3 The Two Oblique Muscles

The Superior Oblique Muscle

The origin is at the periosteum of the orbital apex, above and medial to the optic canal, and consists of two parts: a muscular portion which travels anteroposteriorly along the medial wall of the orbit and a tendinous portion which goes backwards in an oblique, downward and lateral direction, crossing under the superior rectus and inserting directly into the sclera behind the equator of the globe. At the junction of these two sections is the trochlea, a fibrocartilaginous ring, located in the trochlear fossa of the frontal bone, at the anteromedial part of the orbital roof. The muscle goes through the trochlea, which acts as a fulcrum and changes its direction with an angle of 50 to 54° [17]. The total length of the muscle is about 50 mm, 30 for the muscular body and 20 for the tendon. Its action is depression, abduction, and internal rotation (intorsion).

The Inferior Oblique Muscle

It arises from the anteromedial part of the orbital floor, lateral to the superior opening of the nasolacrimal canal. It travels backward, laterally, and upward, crossing under the inferior rectus and attaching to the sclera behind the equator of the eyeball, near the macula. Its length is 30 to 35 mm and its action is elevation, abduction, and external rotation (extorsion).

4.3.4 The Arterial Blood Supply to the Muscles

The arterial muscular blood supply consists of numerous vessels, either large vascular trunks which supply several muscles, or smaller branches, arising directly from the ophthalmic artery or its branches and supply only one muscle.

The Muscular Trunks

One muscular trunk, the inferior muscular artery, is consistently present, whereas others are more variable. It is a fairly large trunk, with a diameter ranging from 0.8 to 1.2 mm. It usually arises from the inferior part of the ophthalmic artery, just after the crossing with the optic nerve. It dips toward the orbital floor, often crossing the medial side of the optic nerve and quickly divides into two or three terminal trunks: medial, lateral, and sometimes posterior. Each trunk has 6 to 25 collateral branches for the different muscles: the medial, lateral and inferior rectus. This artery usually terminates its course in the inferior oblique muscle at its posterior end.

A superior muscular artery is rare and only found in 9% of orbits [19]. When it exists, it supplies the superior rectus and the levator. A medial muscular artery, which is even rarer (found in 3% of orbits) and would supply the medial rectus. A lateral muscular artery is more frequent (23% of orbits) and it is usually encountered when the ophthalmic artery crosses under the optic nerve and a meningolacrimal artery supplies the lacrimal gland. It supplies the lateral rectus and sometimes the superior rectus.

The Small Muscular Branches

There are many small, terminal muscular branches which directly supply a single muscle, and originate from the ophthalmic artery or one of its branches.

The Muscular Blood Supply

Each muscle receives several arteries, organised in one or more bundles which nearly always enter its posterior and intraconal side.

The arteries that enter the rectus muscles travel forward, giving rise to one or two anterior ciliary arteries in the anterior part of each muscle. These arteries perforate the sclera in front of the muscular insertion and contribute to the blood supply of the major arterial circle of the iris.

The inferior oblique muscle normally receives two blood supplies: the inferior muscular artery, which terminates in the lateral third of its posterior edge (98% of the cases), and the infraorbital artery, a branch of the external carotid system, which sends a branch to the bony insertion of the muscle in 88% of the orbits. These two arteries were found together in 86% of our dissections, forming an anastomosis between the two carotid systems. In 12% of orbits, there was only one branch from the inferior muscular artery, while a single branch of the infraorbital artery was found in 2% of cases [19].

4.4 The Orbital Fascias (Connective Tissue)

The Tenon's capsule is a fibroelastic membrane that covers the sclera from the limbus to the optic nerve. It is perforated by the six oculomotor muscles before they insert into the sclera.

Each muscle has its own fascia, which in turn is interconnected with the other rectus muscles by an intermuscular fascia. These fascias permit the movements of the eyeball and create a cone-shaped space behind the eyeball with the tip at the orbital apex, known as the fasciomuscular or muscle cone. Many membranous expansions link the recti muscles with the other muscles. In particular, the fascias of the levator and superior rectus are connected to permit the elevation of the upper eyelid during the upgaze. Similarly, the fascias of the inferior rectus and inferior oblique are connected, forming a strong adherence, called Lockwood's ligament.

Each muscular fascia provides aponeurotic expansions to the conjunctiva, eyelids, and orbital walls. Two are very important: between the lateral rectus and the lateral wall, and between the medial rectus and the posterior lacrimal crest. Also, the fascia of the inferior rectus extends to the orbital floor and to the inferior edge of the tarsal plate.

Previously, Koornneef [20] described these fascias as "accessory locomotor system". According to him, these fascias consist of collagen fibers containing vessels, nerves, and smooth muscular fibers. They are mainly circumferential at the anterior part of the orbit and radiate out to the posterior orbit.

4.5 The Lacrimal Gland

Situated at the superolateral, anterior part of the orbit, the lacrimal gland sits in a depression of the frontal bone. It is a firm, yellowish pink structure with a lobular consistency and easily separable from the surrounding orbital fat, with an average length of 20 mm, a width of 15 mm, and depth of 5 mm.

4.5.1 Description

The gland has two parts: a larger orbital lobe and a smaller palpebral lobe, separated by the lateral horn of the levator muscle. The orbital part has two sides, a superolateral side in contact with the bone and an inferomedial side in contact with the anterior part of the lateral rectus, the lateral horn of the levator, and the lateral orbital expansion of the superior rectus. It also has two edges: an anterior in contact with the orbital septum and a posterior touching the orbital fat. The 3 to 5 excretory ducts of the gland open in the upper conjunctival fornix laterally.

4.5.2 The Arterial Supply to the Gland

There are two anatomic variants of the lacrimal artery:

The Classic Lacrimal Artery

In 83% of cases [21], it arises from the ophthalmic artery, usually at the point of crossing above the optic nerve, then travels forward and laterally, leaves the cone extending along the lateral wall to reach the lacrimal gland, at the superolateral orbital margin, above the superior border of the lateral rectus. In 54% of cases, an anastomosis, arising from the middle meningeal artery, the sphenoidal artery, joins the lacrimal artery just before it reaches the lateral wall.

The lacrimal nerve enters the orbit more laterally and crosses over the lacrimal artery. Together they arrive at the posterior part of the gland, where the artery gives off many branches. Past the gland, the artery gives branches to the skin of the temporal area, the two lateral palpebral arteries, and one or two zygomatic branches. During its course, it gives muscular branches for the lateral rectus (80%), superior rectus (69%) and levator (41%). It is a relatively large artery, measuring 0.3 to 1.8 mm in diameter, with an average of 0.99 [12].

The Meningolacrimal Artery

This arises from the external carotid system, most commonly from the middle meningeal artery, but rarely, it can also originate from the deep anterior temporal artery. It is found in 27% of the orbits [21]. It enters the orbit through a small opening in the lateral wall known as Hyrtl's canal, and is more anterior and lateral than the classic artery. It is smaller, 0.3 to 1.5 mm, with an average of 0.73 mm. It is usually separate from the lacrimal nerve and does not cross it. It has fewer muscular branches, with only 4 for the lateral rectus, 2 for the superior rectus and 8 for the levator in 27 orbits. These meningolacrimal arteries are more commonly found when the ophthalmic artery crosses under the optic nerve.

Thus, the vascular supply of the lacrimal gland can be divided into three types: type 1 with only one classic lacrimal artery (73%), type 2 with only one meningolacrimal artery (17%), and type 3 with both lacrimal arteries, one classic and one meningolacrimal (10%) [21].

4.5.3 Innervation of the Lacrimal Gland

The gland has two types of innervation:

The Lacrimal Sensory Nerve

This is the thinnest sensory orbital nerve, with a diameter of 0.5 to 0.8 mm. Located outside the cone, it travels along the superolateral orbital margin to join the lacrimal artery and together they reach the lacrimal gland. In 59.5% of the orbits, it divides into two branches before the gland [22]. After it passes through the gland, it provides sensory branches to the lateral third of the upper eyelid, the conjunctiva, and the temporal skin.

The Parasympathetic (Secretory) Innervation

The lacrimal gland is also supplied by parasympathetic fibers arising from the superior salivary nucleus in the pons. The preganglionic fibers follow the facial nerve to reach the pterygopalatine ganglion, where they synapse. The postganglionic fibers follow the maxillary nerve, then the zygomatic nerve, which perforates the lateral orbital wall and gives a branch, or two (15%), to reach the gland, at its inferior part in 92.5%. This branch is classically described as anastomosing with the lacrimal nerve, outside the gland, forming the lacrimal handle. However, this is rarely found, and innervation can be classified into three types [21]: type I with a lacrimal handle (7.5%), type II with two nerves reaching the gland separately and a macroscopically visible anastomosis in the gland (37.5%), and type III without any visible anastomosis (55%). According to Trauzettel and Jo [22], the secretory fibers reach the gland without joining the lacrimal nerve in 80.7% of cases.

4.6 The Orbital Fat

All the remaining space is filled with orbital fat, consisting of small lobules that are limited by a capsule and separated by different fascias. There is the central or intraconal fat around the optic nerve, and peripheral or extraconal fat, particularly abundant in the inferior orbit. Anteriorly, it is limited by the orbital septum and clinically discernible as separate fat pockets: three inferior and two superior.

5 Orbital Vascular Supply

5.1 The Arterial System

The arterial blood supply of the orbit depends mainly on the internal carotid system via the ophthalmic artery and partially on the external carotid system, with multiple anastomoses between the two. One characteristic of the orbital arterial tree is its great variability, with anatomic variations of the origin, diameter, location, actual pathway, and distribution of the arterial branches. Certain branches can even be absent. Therefore, a systematic description of standard orbital arterial supply is very difficult.

5.1.1 The Ophthalmic Artery (Fig. 6)

Its complex embryology, well described by Padget [23], accounts for the main variations of the orbital vascular supply. Originating from the internal carotid artery in the anterior cranial fossa, the ophthalmic artery reaches the orbit via the optic canal and provides numerous branches for the eyeball, orbital contents, and nasal cavity. It terminates its course at the anterosuperomedial angle of the orbit.

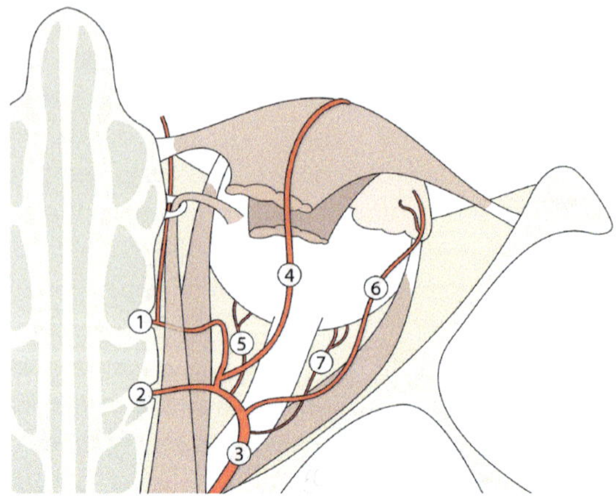

Fig. 6 Ophthalmic artery: intraorbital course: (1) anterior ethmoidal artery; (2) posterior ethmoidal artery; (3) ophthalmic artery; (4) supraorbital artery; (5) medial long ciliary trunk; (6) lacrimal artery; (7) lateral long ciliary trunk

The most common origin of the artery is a single collateral branch of the internal carotid artery, as it leaves the cavernous sinus and before giving rise to its four terminal cerebral branches. The ophthalmic artery starts on the anteromedial side of the internal carotid, under the anterior clinoid process. Numerous variations of this origin have been described, including origin from the internal carotid within the cavernous sinus, origin as two branches, or even from the middle meningeal artery. In a study of 170 orbits, Hayreh [24] found the origin of the ophthalmic artery on the internal carotid artery in 164 cases, and the middle meningeal artery in only 6 cases. In our experience with over 100 orbital dissections, the origin was always on the internal carotid artery. The initial diameter is between 0.7 to 1.4 mm [24], with a gender difference of 1.54 ± 0.4 mm for men and 1.31 ± 0.5 for women [12].

The course of the artery can be divided into three parts:

1. The intracranial part is located in the subdural space of the anterior cranial fossa and measures from 4.8 to 15.1 mm (average of 9 mm) according to Hayreh [25]. The artery reaches the optic canal with the optic nerve located above it. This part can occasionally be absent, with the artery starting right at the cranial aperture of the canal.

2. The intracanalicular part of the artery runs through the optic canal, from its cranial to its orbital apertures. In the canal it is usually under the optic nerve and crosses it from the inside to the outside. This part, like the optic canal measures 7 to 14 mm. At the orbital opening of the canal the artery is below and lateral to the nerve.
3. The intraorbital part measures up to 32.6 mm in length and can also be divided into three sections:
   (a) The 'latero-optic' part: the artery courses obliquely forward and upward, until it lies lateral to the optic nerve and enters the muscle cone with it, where it lies under the superior ophthalmic vein and is crossed by the nasociliary nerve.
   (b) The 'optic' part: the artery crosses the optic nerve from the outside to inside, usually superior to the nerve (Fig. 7) and between 13 and 29 mm behind the globe [11]. The incidence of crossing below the nerve ranges from 5.4 to 28%, with the lower rates found in Japanese studies [27–31], and higher in a study by Desantis et al. [31]. In our center, we found a rate of 23% out of 100 orbits [11] (Fig. 8a and b).

      At this level, the artery is found below the course of the nasociliary nerve, with the superior ophthalmic vein above it. The ciliary ganglion is located just anterior to this, on the lateral side of the optic nerve.
   (c) The 'medio-optic' section: after crossing the optic nerve, the ophthalmic artery travels to the medial wall of the orbit, while coursing over the nasociliary nerve several times. Then, in 76% of cases [33, the artery exits the muscle cone, passing between the medial rectus and the superior oblique muscles at an average of 16.5 mm behind the trochlea. In these cases, as the artery reaches the anterior ethmoidal foramen, it gives off the anterior ethmoidal artery and then continues forward along the medial orbital wall, terminating its course at the superomedial angle of the orbit. However, in some cases (24% in our study) [33], the artery remains inside the cone, outside the medial rectus and superior oblique muscles. The nasociliary nerve travels with the artery in this section and gives off its two terminal branches: the anterior ethmoidal nerve, which enters the anterior ethmoidal foramen and the infratrochlear nerve, which runs along the terminal part of the artery.

5.1.2 The Terminal Branches of the Ophthalmic Artery

The artery perforates the orbital septum, 14 mm above the medial palpebral ligament and gives off its terminal branches. There are one or two frontal branches which supply the forehead and the upper eyelid. There is one angular artery which usually anastomoses with the nasal artery, which is a terminal branch of the facial artery, part of the external carotid system. The artery has a terminal diameter of 0.5 to 1.5 mm.

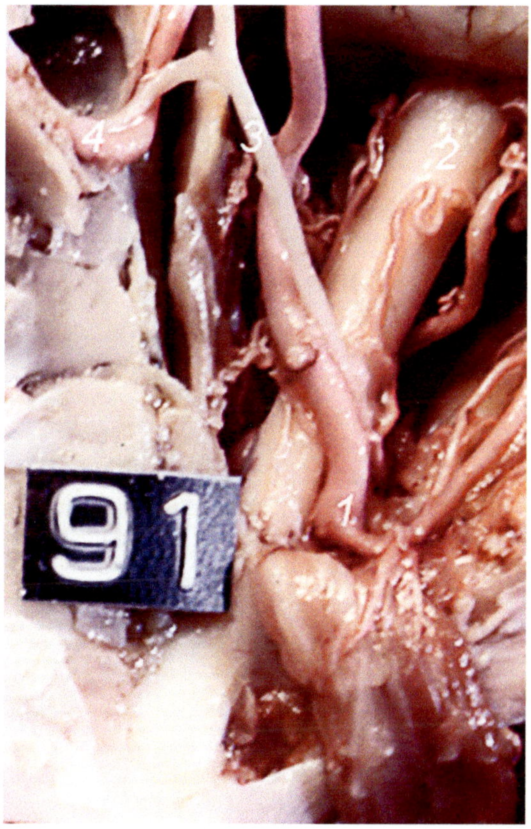

Fig. 7 Ophthalmic artery overcrossing: (1) ophthalmic artery; (2) optic nerve; (3) nasociliary nerve; (4) anterior ethmoidal artery and nerve

a

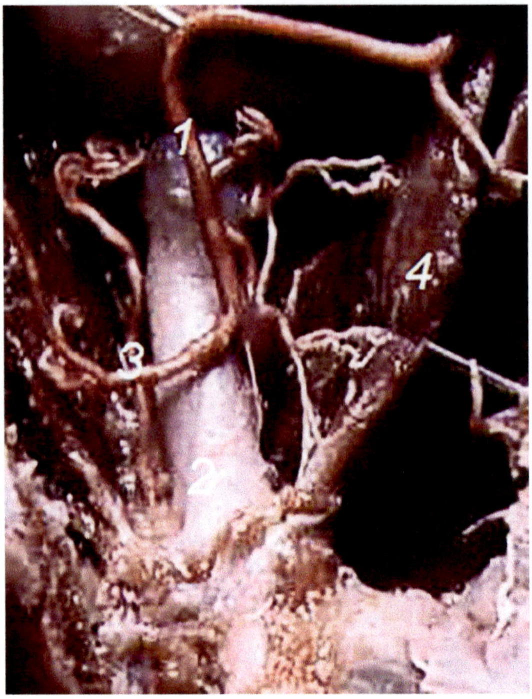

b

AUTHORS	YEAR	NUMBER OF ORBITS	UNDERCROSSINGS (%)
ZUCKERKANDL (26)	1876	20	15
TAGUCHI (27)	1898	56	5.4
ADACHI (28)	1928	108	6.5
SUDAKEVITCH(29)	1947	103	13.6
HAYREH-DASS(30)	1962	161	17.4
DESANTIS(31)	1981	243	28
LANG(12)	1990	71	18.6
JIMENEZ-CASTELLANOS(32)	1995	30	20
DUCASSE(11)	1985	100	23

Fig. 8 (**a**) Ophthalmic artery undercrossing: (1) ophthalmic artery; (2) optic nerve; (3) lateral muscular artery; (4) medial rectus muscle. (**b**) Frequency of under-crossings of the optic nerve by the ophthalmic artery

5.1.3 The Collateral Branches of the Ophthalmic Artery

There are numerous collateral branches of the artery (10 to 19 per orbit) which arise mainly from the intraorbital part, especially from the 'optic' and 'medio-optic' parts. Variations are common and depend mainly on the type of crossing, either over or under the optic nerve. The first collateral is usually the central retinal artery or one posterior ciliary artery.

These collateral branches can be divided in two groups: those for the visual structures, which are the central retinal artery, arteries of the optic nerve, and the ciliary trunks, already described above; and branches for the support or adnexal structures, the lacrimal and muscular arteries already described, as well as the supraorbital, ethmoidal and palpebral arteries discussed below.

The Supraorbital Artery

This artery most often arises from the ophthalmic artery in its 'medio-optic' part. It is absent in 12% of the orbits [11]. Its diameter varies from 0.2 to 1.2 mm (average of 0.57 mm) [24] and has a gender difference of 0.71 mm for men and 0.55 for women [12].

It starts within the muscle cone, courses up and forward, passing between the superior oblique and the levator muscles, before emerging outside of the cone. It then runs at the superior surface of the levator muscle under the orbital roof, and medial to the frontal nerve. Along with the external branch of the frontal nerve (the supraorbital nerve), it finally exits from the supraorbital foramen. It gives off branches to the skin of the forehead and some muscular branches to the levator muscle (80%), the superior oblique muscle (30%), and rarely to the superior rectus.

The Ethmoidal Arteries (Fig. 9)

These run a very short intraorbital course to reach the nose, where they provide an important blood supply.

The Anterior Ethmoidal Artery

The anterior ethmoidal artery is fairly consistent and large in volume. According to Hayreh, it is absent in 9% of orbits where the ophthalmic artery crosses over the optic nerve and absent in 20% of orbits where the artery crosses under the nerve [13]. In our centre [7], it was absent in only 2% of cases. Its diameter ranges from 0.2 to 1.5 mm, with an average of 0.76 mm.

This artery always arises from the medio-optic part of the ophthalmic artery. There are two configurations according to the course of the ophthalmic artery. When the ophthalmic artery exits the cone, the anterior ethmoidal artery starts outside the cone, often directly at the anterior ethmoidal foramen, with almost no intraorbital course (76% of cases [7]). When the ophthalmic artery remains inside the cone, the anterior ethmoidal artery reaches this foramen by a short intraorbital path, passing under the superior oblique muscle.

Along with the anterior ethmoidal nerve, it goes through the anterior ethmoidal foramen to reach the nasal cavity and supplies the anterior part of the nasal fossa. It also gives off the anterior meningeal artery at the level of the crista gali. In the orbit it may give off muscular branches in 49% of patients, mainly to the superior oblique muscle, and less often to the medial or superior rectus or the levator muscles.

The Posterior Ethmoidal Artery

Smaller than the anterior artery, with an average of 0.4 mm, it is also more frequently absent, in about 23% of orbits [7]. It originates usually from the 'medio-optic' part of the ophthalmic artery (75%), and sometimes from the supraorbital artery (17%), or the anterior ethmoidal artery (7%). Originating in the cone, it goes upwards and medially to come out of the cone, between the superior oblique and the levator muscles. Then it reaches the posterior ethmoidal foramen, with the inconsistent posterior ethmoidal nerve, crossing over the superior oblique muscle in 94% of the cases. At this level, it also goes under the trochlear nerve. The artery and the nerve leave the orbit through the posterior ethmoidal foramen to reach the posterior part of the nasal cavity. It gives branches to the superior oblique (59%), levator (37%), and less frequently, superior and medial rectus muscles.

The Medial Palpebral Arteries

The superior and inferior medial palpebral arteries are the last collateral branches of the ophthalmic

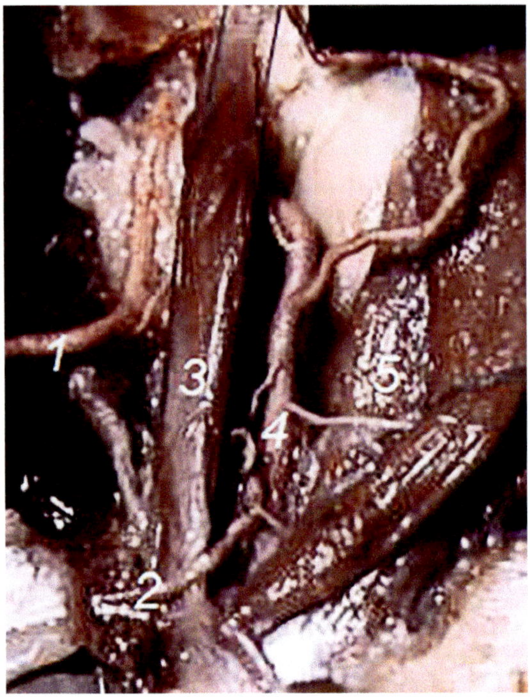

Fig. 9 Ethmoidal arteries: (1) anterior ethmoidal artery; (2) posterior ethmoidal artery; (3) superior oblique muscle; (4) ophthalmic artery; (5) superior rectus muscle

artery, and can be separate at their origin or have a common trunk. The diameter is small: 0.1 to 0.5 mm, the inferior being more often larger than the superior one. The superior is short, perforates the orbital septum, and gives two branches for the upper eyelid. The inferior artery passes behind the medial palpebral ligament and gives two branches to the lower eyelid. Along with the branches of the lateral palpebral arteries, originating from the lacrimal artery, these branches constitute the four palpebral arcades, two in each eyelid.

The Other Collateral Branches

These are solitary muscular branches, direct short ciliary arteries, or branches for the ethmoidal cells.

5.1.4 Anastomoses Between the Internal and External Carotid Systems

Two arteries originating in this system can participate to the collateral arterial blood supply of the orbit:

The Infraorbital Artery

This is a branch of the maxillary artery, itself a terminal branch of the external carotid artery, originating in the pterygopalatine fossa and entering the orbit along the inferior orbital fissure. It travels with the maxillary nerve through the infraorbital canal to the infraorbital foramen. It gives branches on the orbital floor, the superior aperture of the nasolacrimal duct, and in 88% of the cases a branch to the insertion of the inferior oblique muscle.

The Middle Meningeal Artery

This is a collateral branch of the maxillary artery of the external carotid system, and can give off a meningolacrimal artery, already described.

These two arteries participate in an intraorbital anastomosis between the two carotid systems [34]: in the inferior oblique muscle (86%), in the lacrimal gland (64%), directly between the lacrimal and meningolacrimal arteries (10%), and in over 54% of the cases with the sphenoidal artery.

There are additional anastomoses outside the orbit between these two systems, in the nose and on the cranial dura mater between the two ethmoidal arteries and the branches of the sphenopalatine artery, which is a branch of the maxillary artery. Also, in the periorbital area, there are multiple anastomoses between the angular, palpebral, supraorbital, and lacrimal arteries, as well as the branches of the facial and superficial temporal arteries.

5.2 The Orbital Venous Drainage

The venous drainage of the orbit mainly occurs via the superior ophthalmic vein and to a lesser extent by two smaller veins, the medial and the inferior ophthalmic veins. All these veins carry blood toward the cavernous sinus. The venous organisation is different from the arterial one. The veins are mainly dependent on the fascias, which form a "hammock" to support the venous network. The venous blood comes from all the orbital structures, including the eyeball through the central retinal vein and the four vortex veins; the lacrimal gland and the muscles have their own venous outflow.

5.2.1 The Superior Ophthalmic Vein

This large vein is consistently found in the superior orbit. It originates from two roots is in the superomedial angle of the anterior orbit: a superior one arising from the frontal veins and an inferior one arising from the angular vein. This is located under the trochlea and about 5 to 6 mm behind it. It then travels backward and laterally to reach the cavernous sinus at the superior orbital fissure, consisting of three parts: an initial extraconal part, followed by an intraconal part under the superior rectus, and finally an extraconal part towards the superior orbital fissure.

5.2.2 The Inferior Ophthalmic Vein

This vein is located at the inferior part of the orbit, it is variable, and consists of veins arising from the superior oblique and the lateral rectus muscles. It reaches the cavernous sinus after having joined the superior ophthalmic vein or sometime as a separate vessel.

5.2.3 The Medial Ophthalmic Vein

Also known as the middle ophthalmic vein, it is found in 40% of orbits. It arises from the medial, inferior, and lateral rectus muscles. It has an intraconal course above the optic nerve and reaches the cavernous sinus through the annulus of Zinn at the superior orbital fissure.

5.2.4 Organization of the Orbital Venous Drainage

The three ophthalmic veins carry blood toward the cavernous sinus and then to the internal jugular system. There is also a collateral venous drainage into the facial system by the angular vein, which receives the orbito-lacrimo-facial vein. The angular vein also receives blood from the eyelids, conjunctiva and the lacrimal sac. Thus, the orbital venous drainage, similar to the arterial system, has several areas of anastomosis between the cranial drainage via the cavernous sinus and the facial drainage.

5.3 The Orbital Lymphatics

While the lymphatics of the eyelids, conjunctiva and the lacrimal system are well known, the presence of lymphatics in the orbit has yet to be established. Classically, there are no lymphatics in the orbit, but recent studies [35, 36] have found lymphatic structures in the lacrimal gland, orbital muscles, and at the orbital apex in monkeys.

6 Orbital Innervation

6.1 Motor Innervation

The seven striated orbital muscles are innervated by three oculomotor nerves. The oculomotor nerve (IIIrd cranial nerve) innervates five muscles: the superior, medial, and inferior rectus, the inferior oblique and the levator muscles. It also carries parasympathetic fibers to the ciliary muscle and the sphincter of the iris. The trochlear nerve (IVth cranial nerve) innervates the superior oblique, while the abducens nerve (VIth cranial nerve) supplies the lateral rectus muscle.

Each cranial nerve has a nuclear origin in the brainstem of the central nervous system, an intracranial course, and an intraorbital course.

6.1.1 The Oculomotor Nerve

The oculomotor nuclear complex is found in the midbrain, at the level of the superior colliculus. The nucleus is divided into subnuclei for each muscle that is innervated. It emerges from the anterior face of the midbrain, near the posterior perforated substance (the interpeduncular fossa). During its intracranial course, it perforates the roof of the cavernous sinus, travels forward along the lateral wall of the sinus, and divides into two branches, superior and inferior. It then enters the orbit via the superior orbital fissure, passing through the annulus of Zinn. The superior branch is very short and quickly reaches the superior rectus and the levator muscles. The inferior branch, which is longer and larger, gives off one branch to the inferior rectus, one branch to the medial rectus, and reaches the posterior border of the inferior oblique muscle, along with the terminal part of the inferior muscular artery. The nerve and the artery terminate together in the muscle. Before reaching the inferior oblique muscle, the inferior branch also gives off a motor branch to the ciliary ganglion, which contains the preganglionic parasympathetic fibers of the third cranial nerve.

6.1.2 The Trochlear Nerve

This nerve's nucleus is also located in the midbrain, but below and in front of the inferior colliculus. In its intracranial course, it runs around the midbrain to reach the lateral wall of the cavernous sinus. It enters the orbit via the superior orbital fissure, outside of the annulus of Zinn. In the posterior part of the orbit, it remains extraconal, crosses the levator muscle, and quickly ends in the superior margin of the superior oblique muscle, at its posterior third. Usually, it also crosses the posterior ethmoidal artery.

6.1.3 The Abducens Nerve

The abducens nerve has its nucleus in the pons, in front of the fourth ventricle. Its intracranial origin is at the anterior side of the pons. In its course, it penetrates into the cavernous sinus, crossing the lateral side of the internal carotid artery. It reaches the orbit via the superior orbital fissure, passing through the annulus of Zinn, followed by a very short intraconal course before terminating at the posterior third of the medial side of the lateral rectus muscle.

6.2 The Sensory Innervation

Sensory innervation of the orbit and, in fact, the whole face is provided by branches of the trigeminal nerve, the Vth cranial nerve.

The trigeminal nerve has a complex nucleus, with three parts (the mesencephalic, chief sensory, and spinal trigeminal nucleus) extending through three parts of the cerebral trunk (midbrain, pons, and medulla). It has two intracranial roots, one motor and the other sensory, on the anterior face of the pons. At the trigeminal ganglion, on the petrous temporal bone, this nerve divides into three divisions: the ophthalmic nerve to the orbit, the maxillary nerve to the cheek, and the mandibular to the masticator muscles and the inferior third of the face. The ophthalmic division reaches the lateral wall of the cavernous sinus where it divides into three terminal branches: the frontal, the lacrimal, and the nasociliary nerves.

Except for the abducens, all orbital nerves are found in the lateral wall of the cavernous sinus (Fig. 10). At the anterior part of the lateral sinus wall, these nerves are arranged in the following order, from top to bottom: trochlear, lacrimal, frontal, the superior branch of the oculomotor, nasociliary and the inferior branch of the oculomotor. The three branches of the ophthalmic division pass through the superior orbital fissure and enter the orbit. The frontal and the lacrimal nerves travel outside the annulus Zinn, while the nasociliary passes through it.

The large flat frontal nerve, runs along the superior part of the levator, under the orbital roof where it is joined by the supraorbital artery. At about 5 mm behind the orbital rim, it divides in its two terminal branches: the supraorbital nerve, which exits via the supraorbital foramen, and the supratrochlear nerve which passes through the supratrochlear foramen more medially. These two nerves supply the sensory innervation of the forehead, frontal sinus, and medial two-thirds of the upper eyelid, along with its conjunctiva.

The lacrimal nerve has already been described above.

The nasociliary nerve is the only intraconal branch of the ophthalmic division. It runs forward and medially, crossing over the optic nerve and the ophthalmic artery. After crossing the artery several times anteriorly, it gives off two terminal branches: the anterior ethmoidal nerve and the infratrochlear nerve. The anterior ethmoidal nerve travels toward to the anterior ethmoidal foramen, crossing under the superior oblique muscle and reaching the nasal cavity with the anterior ethmoidal artery. The infratrochlear nerve, which runs along the medial wall with the terminal part of the ophthalmic artery, innervates the medial palpebral area, lacrimal sac, canaliculus, and caruncle. Along its course, the nasociliary nerve gives off several other branches: the posterior ethmoidal nerve, which is inconsistent, the two long ciliary nerves, medial and lateral, and the sensory root of the ciliary ganglion.

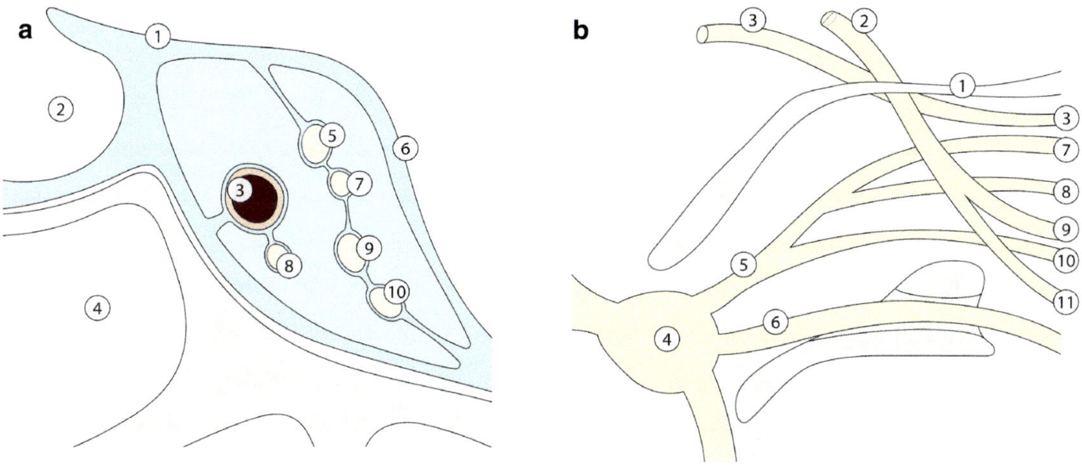

Fig. 10 Cavernous sinus: (**a**) posterior section: (1) superior wall; (2) pituitary gland; (3) internal carotid; (4) sphenoidal sinus; (5) oculomotor nerve; (6) lateral wall divided in two sheets; (7) trochlear nerve; (8) abducens nerve; (9) ophthalmic nerve; (10) maxillary nerve. (**b**) projection of the nerves: (1) superior wall; (2) oculomotor nerve; (3) trochlear nerve; (4) trigeminal ganglion; (5) ophthalmic nerve; (6) maxillary nerve; (7) lacrimal nerve; (8) frontal nerve; (9) superior branch of the oculomotor nerve; (10) nasociliary nerve; (11) inferior branch of the oculomotor nerve

6.3 The Ciliary Ganglion

The ganglion is located in the posterior part of the orbit, lateral to the optic nerve, and just after the crossing of the ophthalmic artery. It is about 1 cm in front of the optic canal, medial to the lateral rectus and measures 2.5 mm in length. This ganglion receives three roots: a motor (short) root, a sensory (long) root, and the sympathetic root. The motor root, arising from the inferior division of the oculomotor nerve, carries preganglionic parasympathetic fibers, which originate in the Edinger-Westphal nucleus of the IIIrd nerve. These fibers synapse in the ganglion with the postganglionic fibers. The sensory (or long) root is a collateral branch of the nasociliary nerve, containing sensory fibers, which pass through the ganglion without synapse. The third root is the sympathetic root, containing postganglionic sympathetic fibers. The preganglionic sympathetic fibers come from the thoracic medulla (C7 to T2) and synapse in the superior cervical sympathetic plexus. The postganglionic fibers then follow the internal carotid and the ophthalmic arteries and pass through the ciliary ganglion without synapse. About 9 to 14 short ciliary nerves emerge from the anterior part of the ciliary ganglion and penetrate the sclera around the optic nerve, along with the short ciliary arteries and the long ciliary arteries and nerves. The short ciliary nerves contain postganglionic sympathetic, parasympathetic, and sensory fibers that innervate the iris sphincter and dilator muscles, as well as to the ciliary muscle and cornea. Sympathetic innervation is also received by the two smooth muscles of the orbit, the orbital and palpebral Muller's muscles.

Acknowledgments All the pictures of dissections were created in the laboratory of Anatomy of Reims France, Pr JB Flament, Pr JF Delattre).

References

1. Andrades P, Cuevas P, Hernàndez R, Danilla S, Villalobos R. Characterization of the orbital volume in normal population. J Craniomaxillofac Surg. 2018;46:594–9.
2. Kurihashi K, Yamashita A. Anatomical consideration for dacryocysto-rhinostomy. Ophthalmologica. 1991;203:1–7.
3. Engin Ö, Adriaensen GFJPM, Hoefnagels FWA, Saeed P. A systematic review of the surgical anatomy of the orbital apex. Surg Radiol Anat. 2021;43:169–78.
4. Aggarwal A, Kaur H, Gupta T, Tubs RS, Sahni D, Batra YK, et al. Anatomical study of the infraorbital foramen: a basis for successful infraorbital nerve block. Clin Anat. 2015;28:753–60.

5. Webster RC, Gaunt JM, Hamdan US. Supraorbital and supratrochlear notches and foramina: anatomical variations and surgical relevance. Laryngoscope. 1986;96:311–5.
6. Kirchner JA, Yanagisawa E, Crelin S. Surgical anatomy of the ethmoidal arteries. A laboratory study of 150 orbits. Arch Otolaryngol. 1961;74:82–6.
7. Ducasse A, Segal A, Flament JB. Les artères ethmoïdales. Situation, variations. Ophtalmologie. 1993;7:361–3.
8. Cheng AC, Lucas PW, Yuen HK, Lam DS, So KF. Surgical anatomy of the Chinese orbit. Ophthalmic Plast Reconstr Surg. 2008;24:136–41.
9. Piagkou M, Skotsimara G, Dalaka A, Kanioura E, Korentzelou V, Skotsimara A, al. Bony landmarks of the medial orbital wall: an anatomical study of ethmoidal foramina. Clin Anat. 2014;27:570–7.
10. Macchi V, Regoli M, Bracco S, Nicoletti C, Morra A, Porzionato A, al. Clinical anatomy of the orbitomeningeal foramina: variational anatomy of the canals connecting the orbit with the cranial cavity. Surg Radiol Anat. 2016;38:165–77.
11. Ducasse A, Segal A, Delattre JF. Le contenu orbitaire. Etude anatomique des différents compartiments et de leur contenu. Ophtalmologie. 1992;6:180–5.
12. Lang J, Kageyama I. The ophthalmic artery and its branches: measurements and clinical importance. Surg Radiol Anat. 1990;12:83–90.
13. Hayreh SS. The ophthalmic artery: branches. Br J Ophthalmol. 1962;46:212–47.
14. Ducasse A, Segal A, Delattre JF. Aspects macroscopiques des artères ciliaires longues postérieures. Bull Fr Soc Ophtalmol. 1986;86:845–8.
15. Ducourneau D. La systématisation vasculaire de la choroïde. J Fr Ophtalmol. 1980;3:5–16.
16. Codère F, Tucker NA, Renaldi B. The anatomy of Whitnall ligament. Ophthalmology. 1995;102:2016–9.
17. Porter JD, Baker RS, Ragusa RJ, Brueckner JK. Extraocular muscles: basic and clinical aspects of structure and function. Surv Ophthalmol. 1995;39:451–84.
18. De Gottrau P. La chirurgie oculomotrice. Paris: Masson; 1995.
19. Ducasse A, Flament JB, Segal A. Etude anatomique de la vascularisation et de l'innervation des muscles obliques de l'œil. Ophtalmologie. 1991;5:5–8.
20. Koornneef L. Orbital septa: anatomy and function. Ophthalmology. 1979;86:876–80.
21. Ducasse A, Segal A, El Ladki S. Vascularisation artérielle et innervation de la glande lacrymale. A propos de 100 dissections. Ophtalmologie. 1990;4:129–33.
22. Trauzettel H, Jo A. Die topographie der nerven in der orbita. Verh Anat Ges. 1971;66:633–45.
23. Padget DH. The development of the cranial arteries in the human embryo. Carnegie Inst Washington Contrib Embryol. 1948;32:205–61.
24. Hayreh SS. Arteries of the orbit in the human being. Br J Surg. 1963;50:938–53.
25. Hayreh SS, Dass R. The ophthalmic artery: origin and intracranial and intracanalicular course. Br J Ophthalmol. 1962;46:65–98.
26. Zuckerkland E, Meyer F. Zur anatomie der orbitalarterien. Morph Jahrb. 1876;12:343–50.
27. Taguchi K. Uber das foramen clinoideo-ophthalmicum mit berücksich-tigung der arteria ophthalmica beim menschen. Tokyo Igakkwai Zassji. 1898;12:33–55.
28. Adachi B. Das arteriensystem der Japaner. Kyoto: Verlag der Kaiserlich-Japanischen Universität; 1928. p. 103–11.
29. Sudakevitch T. The variations in system of trunks of the posterior ciliary arteries. Br J Ophthalmol. 1947;31:738–60.
30. Hayreh SS, Dass R. The ophthalmic artery: intraorbital course. Br J Ophthalmol. 1962;46:165–85.
31. Desantis M, Anderson KJ, King DW. Variability in relationships of arteries and nerves in the human orbit. Anat Anz. 1984;75:227–31.
32. Jimenez-Castellanos J, Carmona A, Castellanos I. Microsurgical anatomy of the human ophthalmic artery: a mesoscopic study of its origin, course and collateral branches. Surg Radiol Anat. 1995;17:139–43.
33. Ducasse A, Delattre JF, Segal A, Desphieux JL, Flament JB. Anatomical basis of the surgical approach to the medial wall of the orbit. Anat Clin. 1985;7:15–21.
34. Ducasse A, Segal A, Delattre JF, Burette A, Flament JB. La participation de l'artère carotide externe à la vascularisation orbitaire. J Fr Ophtalmol. 1985;8:333–9.
35. Sherman DD, Gonnering RS, Wallon IH. Identification of orbital lymphatics: enzyme histochemical light microscopic and electron microscopic studies. Ophthal Plast Reconstr Surg. 1999;9:153–69.
36. Dickinson AJ, Gausas RE. Orbital lymphatics: do they exist? Eye. 2006;20:1145–8.

Further Reading

Ducasse A. Surgical orbital anatomy. In: Guthoff RF, Katovitz JA, editors. Essentials in ophthalmology. Oculoplastics and orbit. Berlin: Springer; 2007. p. 73–97.

Dutton JD. Clinical and surgical anatomy of the orbit. Philadelphia: WB Saunders; 1994.

Hayreh SS. Orbital vascular anatomy. Eye. 2006;20:1130–44.

Rothon A, Natori Y. The orbit and sellar region. Microsurgical anatomy and operative approaches. New York: Thieme; 1996.

Orbital Imaging

Renske Gahrmann and Mayke Gardeniers

Key Messages

- Computed tomography (CT) is often the first imaging method of choice in suspected orbital pathology due to its wide availability.
- Pre- and post-contrast T1-weighted (T1w) and T2-weighted (T2w) images with and without fat suppression are the main structural magnetic resonance imaging (MRI) sequences used in orbital imaging.
- Functional methods include diffusion-weighted-imaging (DWI) and perfusion imaging techniques with or without intravenous contrast-administration
- Restricted diffusion is commonly found in ischemia and in highly cellular lesions such as lymphoma and meningioma.
- Positron emission tomography (PET) can be used for evaluating systemic disease, such as malignancy, sarcoidosis or IgG4-related disease.
- Lymphoma can often be distinguished from inflammatory disease based on DWI-derived ADC values.

R. Gahrmann (✉) · M. Gardeniers
Department of Radiology and Nuclear Medicine, Erasmus Medical Center, Rotterdam, The Netherlands
e-mail: r.gahrmann@erasmusmc.nl

1 Introduction

Orbital Computed Tomography (CT) and Magnetic Resonance Imaging (MRI) can provide crucial information in various pathologies that are not easily visualised or diagnosed clinically. In this chapter, we discuss the basics of both CT and MRI and their use in commonly encountered traumatic, vascular, infectious, inflammatory, and neoplastic orbital disease.

2 Imaging Techniques

2.1 CT

In CT, cross-sectional images are constructed using a rotating x-ray tube emitting a spectrum of roentgen photons through the body. Tissue density and thickness determines x-ray absorption, which in turn determines the spectrum of photons measured by the detector. Tissue density is measured using the attenuation coefficient in Hounsfield Units (HU). Water is calibrated at a HU-value of zero. CT resolution and scanning speed have increased significantly with the introduction of multislice scanners and other new technologies and post-processing methods.

Since 2006, spectral CT scanners, including dual-source, single-source with rapid keV switching, and twin-beam source have been introduced and more recently advanced layered

F. M. Quaranta Leoni et al. (eds.), *Oculoplastic, Lacrimal and Orbital Surgery*,
https://doi.org/10.1007/978-3-031-39638-0_13

and photon-counting detectors have been developed. Using the different energy spectra created by these tubes, virtual monochromatic images (VMIs) can be created from 40 keV to 140 keV and after the administration of intravenous contrast, virtual non-contrast (VNC) and pure iodine maps can also be calculated [1]. Considering iodine density is dependent on keV, an iodine attenuation curve can be constructed for a specific region-of-interest. Different tissue types each show their own attenuation curve with a specific slope enabling tissue-characterization. With the latest spectral CT technique, photon-counting CT, a significant noise-reduction is achieved thus increasing the signal-to-noise ratio within images. This in turn makes it possible to significantly lower both the radiation exposure and required contrast-agent dosage [2]. Artefact reduction methods have improved as well with iterative reconstructions and (non-linear) blending of different energies generated with spectral CT.

Considering the availability of CT, it often is the first imaging method of choice in suspected orbital pathology. Pre- and postcontrast images are generally reconstructed in all 3 planes preferably using a soft-tissue window with 2–3 mm slice thickness. Additional bone-windows with thin 1 mm slice thickness should be reconstructed as well. CT remains superior to MRI for evaluating bony structures.

2.2 MRI

2.2.1 Sequences

In MRI, the patient is placed in a tube with a strong magnetic field consisting of a large superconducting magnet (usually with a field strength of 1.5 or 3 Tesla) and smaller adjustable gradient magnets. Frequency-encoded radio waves are transmitted through the body and detected returning signals are reconstructed into an image. Adjusting the radio-echo time (TE) and repetition time (TR), as well as a number of other parameters, different contrasts between tissues are created. In orbital imaging, either a head-coil or a smaller surface coil is used to transmit and/or detect the radiofrequency-signal.

T1-weighted (T1w), proton-density (PD) and T2-weighted (T2w) images are the main structural sequences in MRI. Intravenous paramagnetic gadolinium-contrast can be administered, which is mainly visible on T1-weighted images due to its magnetic properties. Water- or fat suppression techniques can be used in individual sequences or they can be reconstructed from chemical shift imaging (also known as the Dixon-technique). Another commonly used structural sequence often used in the cerebellopontine angle and orbit region is the steady-state high-resolution T2w sequence (CISS, FIESTA or DRIVE depending on the vendor) rendering a limited field of view to visualise the cranial nerves and cavernous sinus [3].

Functional methods include diffusion-weighted-imaging (DWI) and perfusion imaging techniques with or without intravenous contrast-administration. DWI is based on the Brownian motion (diffusivity) of water molecules within a voxel and is measured in at least 3 different directions. In the orbit, single-shot or multi-shot echo-planar imaging (EPI) and non-EPI sequences have been found more effective than 'normal' EPI-sequences [4, 5] because of artifact-reduction and higher resolution. On the down-side, these sequences have a lower signal-to-noise ratio and longer scan time [6]. Degree of diffusion is measured on an Apparent Diffusion Coefficient (ADC) map, which is usually automatically generated by the scanner. On this map a region-of-interest can be placed within a lesion to measure local diffusivity. Restricted diffusion is commonly found in ischemia and in highly cellular lesions such as lymphoma and meningioma.

In the dynamic contrast enhanced (DCE) sequence a preselected series of slices is repeatedly scanned before, during and after intravenous gadolinium administration. This allows the generation of a time-dependent intensity curve and measurement of different quantitative parameters such as blood flow, and different volumes including the extracellular-extravascular space (EES) volume (V_e), volume from EES back into blood plasma (k_{ep}) and the volume transfer constant K^{trans}, which can help characterise neoplasms and vascular malformations [7]. Perfusion techniques without an external contrast-agent include

Arterial Spin Labelling (ASL), time-of-flight (TOF) and time resolved imaging of contrast kinetics (TRICKS). Reconstruction of arterial, venous and dynamic series using intravascular flow as endogenous contrast make these techniques useful tools for evaluating vascular malformations and arteriovenous fistula. The field-of-view can be much larger compared to DCE and artefacts are limited.

2.2.2 Artefacts

Artefacts that should be considered in orbital MR-imaging include incomplete fat suppression, movement artefacts and susceptibility artefacts. Incomplete fat suppression is caused by distortions in the magnetic field at the air-tissue interface, appearing when the bandwidth used for fat suppression is too narrow. Movement artefacts include not only head and eye movement, but pulsation artefacts from nearby arterial structures as well. Susceptibility artefacts are caused by signal loss due to local distortions in the magnetic field, which occurs in the presence of iron, cobalt, nickel, and other heavy-metal substances. These substances can also be found in mascara and tattoos.

2.2.3 Scanning Protocol

A basic orbital scanning protocol should include axial 2D T1w and 2D T2w fast-spin echo (FSE) sequences parallel to the optic nerve, a coronal 2D T2w fat suppressed image perpendicular to the optic nerve and a DWI sequence, all with a preferred slice thickness of 3 mm (and 3 mm gap). T1w post-contrast images should be acquired in both the axial and coronal planes with fat suppression. Depending on the clinical question, additional structural sequences and dynamic techniques can be added to the protocol.

2.3 Molecular and Nuclear Imaging

The role of positron emission tomography (PET) and single-photon emission computed tomography (SPECT) for specific orbital pathologies is limited. Generally, these techniques are used in systemic disease, such as malignancy, sarcoidosis or IgG4-related disease. In PET, most commonly (^{18}F)-Fluorodeoxyglucose (FDG) is used as a tracer as the amount of uptake is directly related to increased glucose consumption seen in tumours and inflammatory/infectious disease. In suspected neuroendocrine tumour metastases or meningioma specific tracers such as ^{68}Gallium-labelled somatostatin analogues can be used. Further evaluation of orbital involvement tends to require additional diagnostic CT or MRI.

2.4 Imaging in Specific Pathologies

Depending on clinical information and history, the imaging method of choice is often either CT or MRI. Generally, in trauma cases, suspected bone abnormalities and in thyroid-associated orbitopathy, a non-contrast CT will suffice. When evaluating possible tumours, infection, and vascular structures post-contrast CT or MRI is required.

Regular T1w sequences are very useful for evaluating anatomical detail, considering orbital fat (T1w hyperintense) contrasts nicely with the extraocular muscles. Other entities showing hyperintense signals on T1 are normal bone marrow and pathological substrates such as a]subacute blood and melanin. T2w sequences are useful for determining the presence of oedema, especially when adding a fat-suppression technique. T1w post-contrast sequences, also generally performed with fat-suppression, will show enhancement patterns of vascular anomalies, space-occupying lesions, inflammation and possible perineural tumour growth. Diffusion weighted imaging (DWI) is added in (suspected) neoplasms to aid in the differentiation between benign and malignant lesions using ADC-values.

When assessing a scan, there are some universal lesion characteristics to consider. Benign lesions are more often sharply demarcated and tend to cause bony remodelling. Benign lesions also tend to be more homogeneous on different MRI sequences and will show high ADC-values. By contrast, malignant neoplasms grow more invasively into surrounding soft tissue, are more heterogeneous on different sequences and can cause bony erosions. In inflammatory and infectious disease diffuse changes are seen with fatty infiltration, enlargement of extraocular muscles and lacrimal gland with oedema and enhancement. Post-inflammatory changes include fibrosis (low signal on T2w and late enhancement) and volume loss due to atrophy.

Obviously not all lesions can be differentiated based on imaging and often a biopsy is needed, especially in atypical mass-lesions or inflammatory conditions. In these cases, the differential diagnosis can be directed somewhat, for instance by ADC values, which tend to be higher in benign lesions [8–10], or by iodine concentration derived from spectral CT, which tends to be higher in malignant lesions [11]. Dynamic perfusion derived time-intensity curves will give direction as well: persistent enhancement in a straight or curved line (type 1) is considered a benign pattern, while 'wash-out' of contrast after an initial peak (type 3) is often seen in malignant lesions. An increasing slope followed by a plateau of at least 90% peak intensity (type 2) can be seen in both [7, 12].

3 Injury

In suspected orbital fractures and associated soft-tissue damage, a non-contrast high-resolution CT is the imaging method of choice. It has completely replaced conventional imaging as it allows for much better visualisation of fractures and is nowadays readily available. An alternative in a non-emergency setting is cone-beam CT (CBCT) which is cheaper and can produce sharp images and 3D reconstructions with relatively low radiation exposure [13].

Most commonly, orbital injuries are caused by (motorised) vehicle accidents, assault or a fall from height. The extent of orbital and ocular injury in trauma does not seem directly related to the cause of the trauma, with the exception of gunshot wounds in which the severity of ocular injuries is considered significantly higher [14]. Aside from fracture assessment, evaluation of possible severe ocular injury, damage to the extraocular muscles and the presence of intra-orbital hematomas, posttraumatic connections to sinuses and to the intracranial space can have serious late consequences and should be taken into account during CT evaluation.

3.1 Fractures

Orbital fractures can be isolated, multiple or part of more extensive naso-orbito-ethmoidal (NOE), zygomatico-maxillary complex (ZMC), and LeFort II and III facial fractures. In >95% of cases, the orbital floor is involved and about 50% of patients have more than one fracture. In orbital floor fractures, herniation of orbital fat and the inferior rectus muscle can lead to entrapment when the orbital floor snaps back into

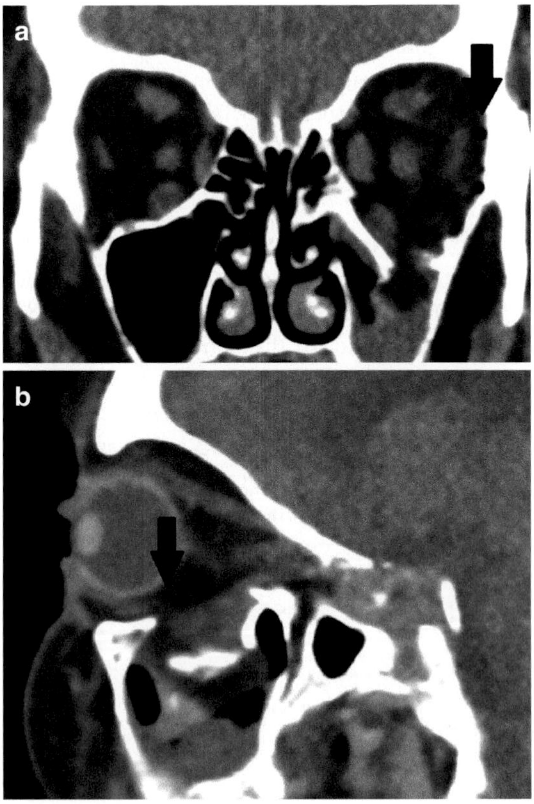

Fig. 1 Isolated orbital floor fracture with herniation of orbital fat and the inferior rectus in coronal (**a**) and sagittal (**b**) directions on unenhanced CT. There is a suspected partial rupture of the inferior rectus anteriorly (***arrow***)

place due to the classic ‘trap-door’ effect. An example of an isolated orbital floor fracture is shown in Fig. 1. Combined fractures of the orbital floor, medial wall and lateral wall are often blowout fractures, with outward displacement. Medial wall blow-out fractures are associated with herniation of fat and the medial rectus muscle into the defect and if the fracture is comminuted or anteriorly located it can cause rupture of the medial canthal tendon. An iatrogenic cause of medial wall fracture is shown in Fig. 2. Fractures of the orbital roof are commonly caused by direct impact and if displaced often turn inward (i.e. blow-in fracture) reducing orbital volume and causing hypoglobus and exophthalmos. Orbital apex fractures involving the optic canal and superior orbital fissure are associated with traumatic neuropathy [15, 16].

3.2 Ocular Injury

Risk of severe ocular injury increases when there are multiple or complex fractures and when patients are symptomatic with blurred vision, pain during eye movements, decreased visual acuity and/or restricted motility. About 25% of these patients have severe ocular injury including globe rupture, retinal tears or detachments, retrobulbar haemorrhage, hyphaema, neuropathy, and extraocular muscle damage [14, 17–19]. An example of severe ocular injury can be seen in Fig. 3. CT findings suggestive of globe rupture include ocular wall thickening, loss of contour (‘flat tire’ sign), intraocular air or haemorrhage, and lens extrusion. Absence of these findings does not exclude a rupture. Chorioretinal detachments can be invisible on unenhanced CT if the

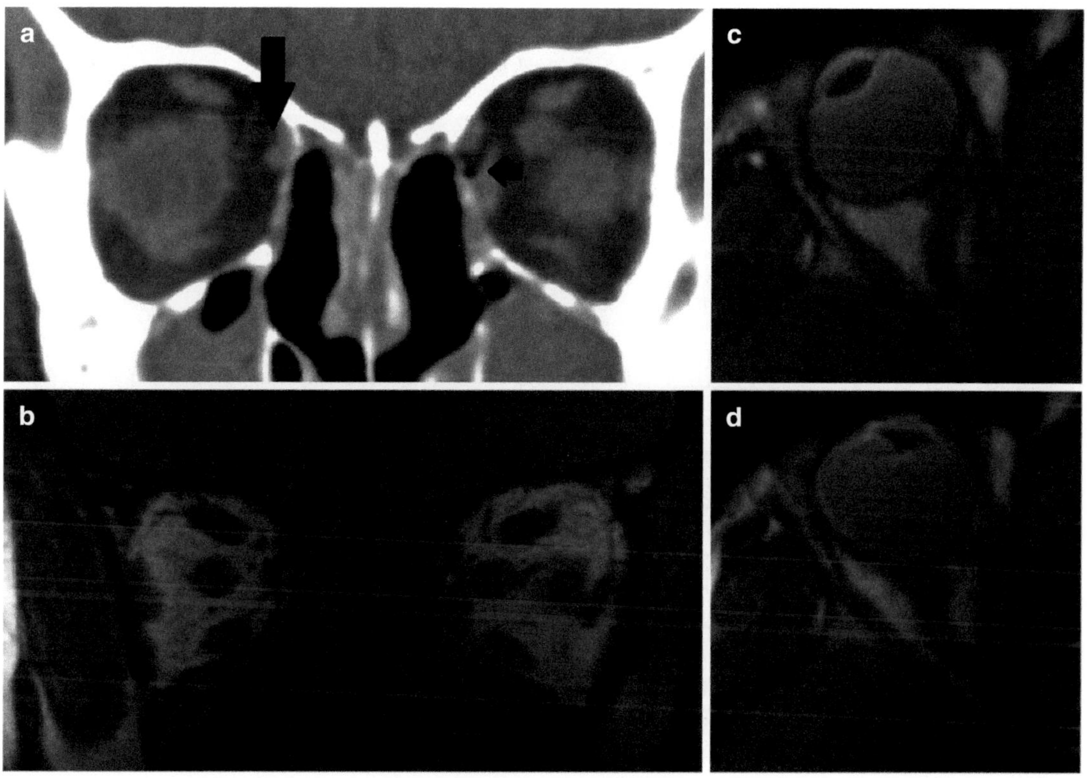

Fig. 2 Limited adduction on the right after functional endoscopic sinus surgery (FESS). Coronal unenhanced CT (**a**) and coronal PDw MRI (**b**) showing displacement and abnormal shape of the right medial rectus (***large arrow***). On CT a small air bubble in the left orbit (***small arrow***) is seen as well indicating bilateral perforation of the medial wall. Additional dynamic PDw MRI in abduction (**c**) and adduction (**d**) of the right eye shows limited adduction just reaching the midline. Findings were consistent with partial rupture of the right medial rectus

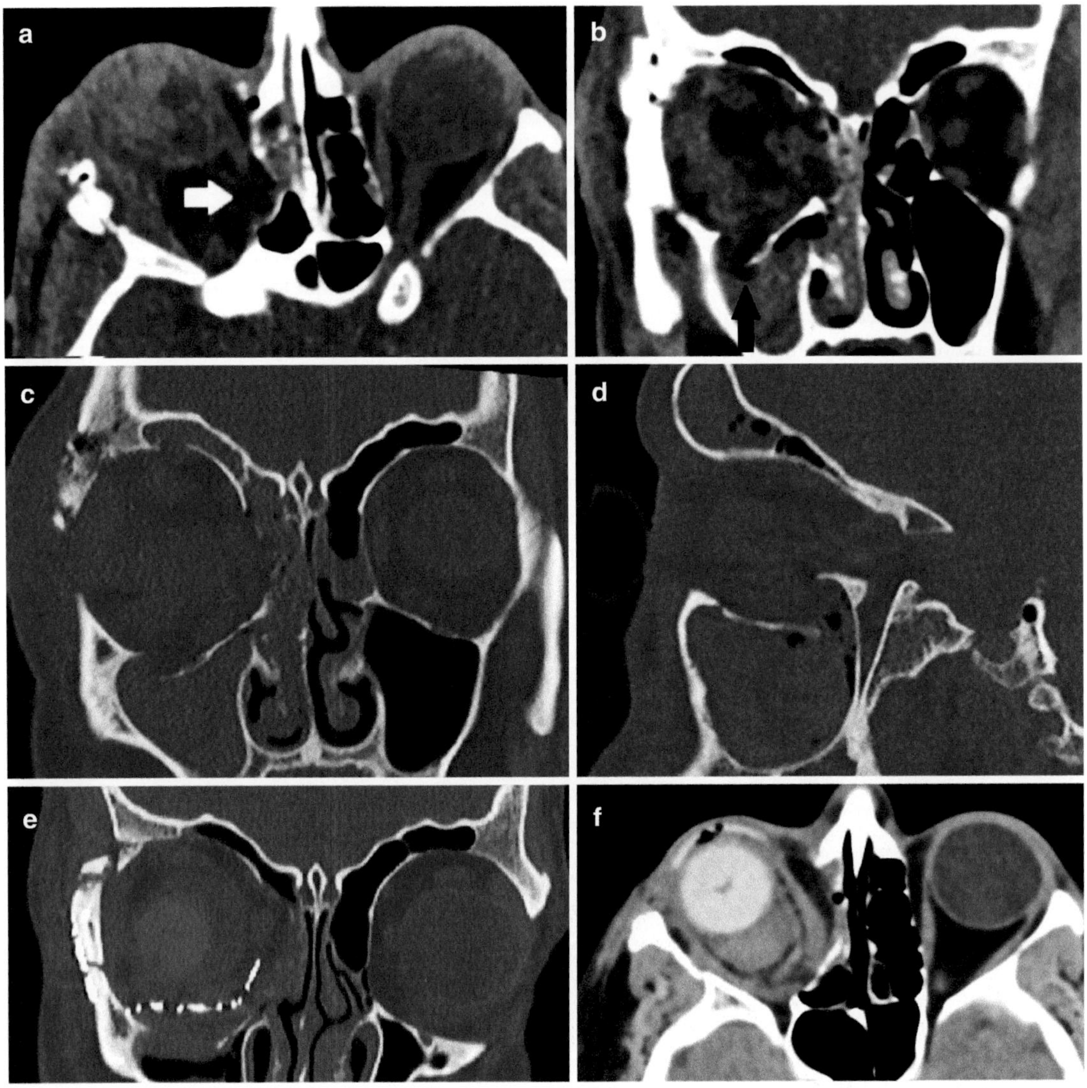

Fig. 3 Penetrating trauma of the right orbit on unenhanced CT. Soft tissue window (**a** and **b**) showing globe rupture, extensive intra-orbital fat stranding consistent with haematoma, medial rectus rupture (**a**; ***arrow***) and herniation of fatty tissue through the orbital floor (**b**; ***arrow***). Bone window (**c** and **d**) shows orbital blow-out fractures of the medial and lateral wall, orbital floor and roof. Post-operative CT (**e** and **f**) shows reconstruction of the orbital floor and prosthetic placement

haemorrhage is relatively hypodense. If clinically relevant, a post-contrast CT or MRI should be considered in these cases. Hyphema can be recognized as layered hyperdense fluid anterior to the lens. Traumatic optic neuropathy (TON) can be seen on MRI, with a hyperintense signal due to oedema on T2w fat-suppressed and diffusion restriction on DWI sequences [20].

Intraocular foreign bodies (IOFBs) can be encountered in penetrating trauma. Most IOFBs are of metallic origin and are seen in metalworkers or after ballistic damage. They can be visualised with either plain x-rays or CT, although CT has a higher sensitivity (almost 100% versus 87% for plain X-rays). MRI is generally contraindicated with metallic IOFBs. Non-metallic IOFBs, such as wood, plastic and glass, can be difficult to visualise with X-ray, CT and/or MRI depending on the location, configuration, and size. In suspected IOFB, imaging with either

X-ray or CT is a good start and if negative, ultrasound or MRI should be considered [21].

4 Vascular

Vascular malformations and tumours can be found throughout the body. Within the orbit, venous malformations (VMs) are by far the most common, followed by lymphatic malformations (LMs) [22]. A precise classification of vascular anomalies has been described by the International Society for the Study of Vascular Anomalies [23].

4.1 Venous Malformations

VMs can be categorised as cavernous malformations (most commonly encountered in the orbit), orbital varix or diffusely infiltrating VMs with or without lymphatic components [22]. Cavernous hemangioma is considered a misnomer as strictly speaking the term hemangioma is reserved for vascular tumours with endothelial proliferation. Instead, the term cavernous venous malformation should be used as the lesion consists of a cavernous space with non-dilated veins and some arterial vessels with low blood flow surrounded by a complete fibrous tissue capsule [24, 25]. They are generally located in the intraconal space and are quite common with an incidence of about 5–9%. The malformation can cause symptoms, but is often found incidentally on head CT or MRI performed for a different reason. The lesion is well-delineated on imaging with an oval, round or lobulated shape, and can have some mass effect with globe indentation or bony remodelling if adjacent. On MRI the lesion is T1-iso/hyperintense and T2-hyperintense with often early peripheral nodular enhancement and late gradual enhancement on dynamic-contrast series (type 1 curve). This distinguishes it from schwannoma and neurofibroma which both markedly enhance in the arterial/early phase. DWI-derived ADC values are relatively high, distinguishing it from rhabdomyosarcoma and lymphoma. There can be areas of T2-hypointensity due to thrombosis or haemorrhage. Typically, the lesion does not increase in size after Valsalva [22, 26, 27]. An example of a cavernous malformation can be seen in Fig. 4.

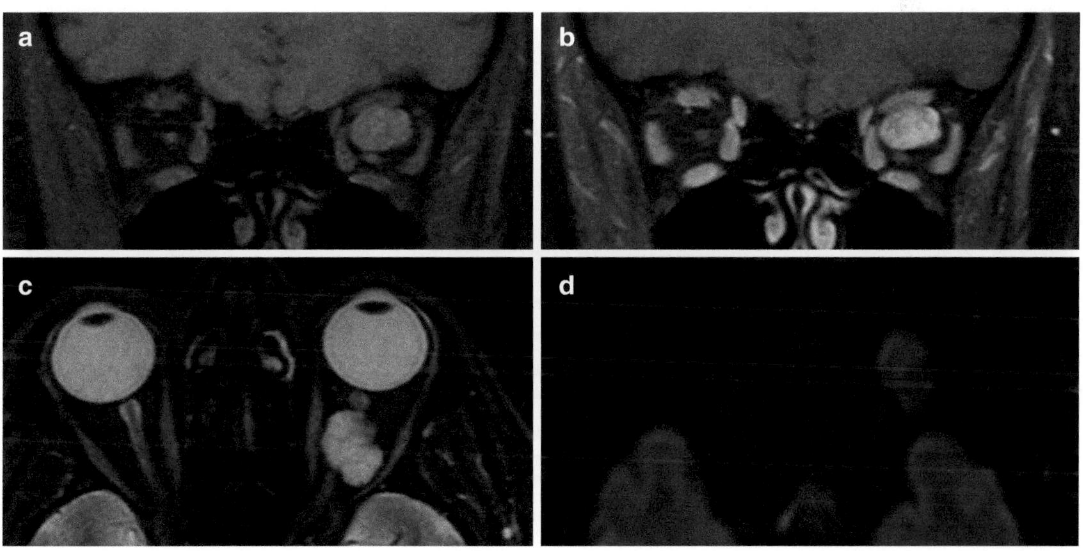

Fig. 4 Asymptomatic lobulated cavernous malformation in the left intraconal space on coronal pre- and postcontrast fat suppressed images (**a** and **b**) showing slight T1-hyperintensity and patchy enhancement in this late post-contrast phase. Also note the displacement of the optic nerve. The lesion is hyperintense on T2w imaging (**c**) and has relatively high ADC-values on DWI (**d**; $B = 1000$) measuring 1.166×10^{-3} mm^2/s

Orbital varices communicate with the venous network causing enlargement during Valsalva manoeuvre. If only a small communication with the venous network exists, thrombosis or haemorrhage can occur instead of distention. Often drainage to the cavernous sinus is present, but more elaborate connections to facial and cortical veins have been described as well. The distended venous structure can easily be identified on post-contrast CT or MRI. Imaging should be performed with and without Valsalva manoeuvre [28]. Using MRI, since it is not easy to employ Valsalva manoeuvre during complete cycles of image acquisition, the patient can alternatively be placed in a prone position. An example of an orbital varix with aberrant drainage can be seen in Fig. 5.

Diffusely infiltrating VMs are slow-flow malformations that can have lymphatic components. The presence of small calcifications, or phleboliths, that are formed after focal thrombophlebitis are considered pathognomonic. They are best seen on CT, but if they are sufficiently large and mineralized they are visible on MRI as well. If there are doubts regarding the drainage route, conventional angiography/venography can be performed to aid in treatment planning. Unlike LMs, VMs do not invade local structures. They often contain a central distensible component which has mass-effect when 'inflated' [22, 29, 30].

4.2 Lymphatic Malformations

Orbital and periorbital LMs are diffusely infiltrating lesions with microcystic and/or macrocystic lymphatic components. Lymphatic macrocysts are generally considered if they are >2 cm or >1 cm^3, but in orbital regions, considering the confined space, any cyst that can be penetrated by a needle should be considered a macrocyst [30]. If local connections between the lymphatic and venous systems are present, the lesion is considered a venolymphatic malformation (VLM) [22, 31]. MRI is the preferred imaging modality of choice. LMs follow a liquid-signal with T1-hypointensity and T2-hyperintensity. The lesion-rim and septae can enhance after contrast administration. If the cysts are so small that they are barely distinguishable on MRI, the enhancing septations can make the lesion appear mass-like.

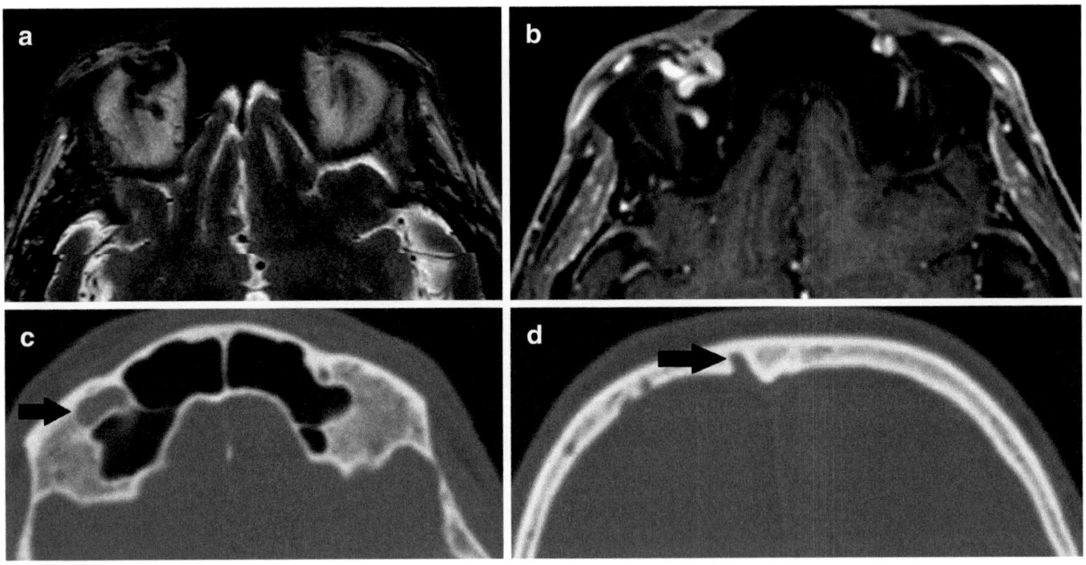

Fig. 5 Orbital varix on the right in a patient presenting with ptosis, diplopia and limited mobility. T2w and Tw1 post-contrast images (**a** and **b**) show enlargement of the right superior ophthalmic vein and also a slightly enlarged vein on the left. Additional CT-images (**c** and **d**) show an aberrant course (***arrows***) through the orbital roof and frontal bone draining into the anterior superior sagittal sinus

Larger cysts can be separate or interconnected and can contain fluid-fluid levels due to debris after infection or haemorrhage.

Percutaneous sclerotherapy of large cysts is often performed using a mix of bleomycin and doxycycline. This sclerosant-mix causes endothelial inflammation and damage, leading to obliteration of the lumen with limited secondary inflammation [30–33]. Complete response after sclerotherapy varies between 39% and 79% [34].

4.3 Arteriovenous Malformations

Orbital AVMs are rare. They are considered high-flow vascular malformations consisting of tangled arteries and veins connected by a capillary bed. Dynamic perfusion series and conventional angiography are required to evaluate the exact location, extent, feeding arteries, and venous drainage of the malformation. Most common feeding arteries include the ophthalmic artery, the superficial temporal artery, the terminal branch of the internal maxillary artery and the middle meningeal artery. Outflow veins include the ophthalmic vein, scalp veins and facial vein. Non-contrast structural MRI sequences can show flow-voids due to high arterial flow velocity [30, 35]. Other arterial malformations, such as carotid-cavernous fistulas or carotid aneurysms require a similar imaging work-up.

5 Infectious Disease

Orbital cellulitis (OC) has an incidence in children and adults of respectively 1.6 and 0.1 in 100,000 [36]. Sinusitis is by far the most common cause of OC [37]. Imaging is advised in case of proptosis, ophthalmoplegia, decreased vision and pain with eye-movements, and if it remains unclear whether OC is present in patients with periorbital cellulitis, as can be the case in children. Initial evaluation should be performed with post-contrast CT, as advised by the American College of Radiology 2018 Appropriateness Criteria (ACR) for orbital imaging [38]. Post contrast CT is very useful for evaluating the extent of disease, including abscess presence and bony destruction, and for surgical planning [39]. CT is readily available, has a high spatial resolution and is performed in seconds, making sedation in children unnecessary. As MRI is much more sensitive for detecting inflammation-related findings such as oedema and limited enhancement on fat-suppressed T2w and T1w post-contrast images, MRI can be helpful in cases with high clinical suspicion and negative CT. MRI is also indicated when intracranial complications are suspected [40]. When a repeat scan is performed, note that imaging findings may lag behind clinical improvement.

On both CT and MRI orbital cellulitis appears as diffuse heterogeneous soft tissue and fatty infiltration with diffuse enhancement, often combined with swelling. As stated, on MRI more subtle changes can be seen on fat suppressed T2w and T1w post-contrast images. On post-contrast CT and MRI, rim enhancement surrounding a fluid-like substance indicates an abscess. Note that abscess formation is a process and in the early stages rim enhancement may not yet be present. Abscess formation may be intraorbital or subperiosteal, the latter being more difficult to detect due to adjacent, often swollen, eye muscles. Considering sinusitis is the most common cause of OC, opacification of the paranasal sinuses and bony destruction should be evaluated as well. Presence of a fluid-level in a paranasal sinus is indicative of active sinusitis. Mucosal thickening and fluid in sinusitis tends to be T2-hyperintense, although variable signal is possible. The exceptions are fungal infections, which tend to be T2-hypointense.

Cavernous sinus thrombosis assessment requires a venous phase CT or MRI. In case of thrombosis there will be filling defects. Thrombosis of the superior ophthalmic vein is commonly seen in these cases as well. Secondary findings of cavernous sinus thrombosis such as bulging lateral walls and abnormal dural enhancement along the sinus lateral wall and orbital apex can be indicative if presence of a filling defect is questionable. An example of extensive thrombosis can be seen in Fig. 6.

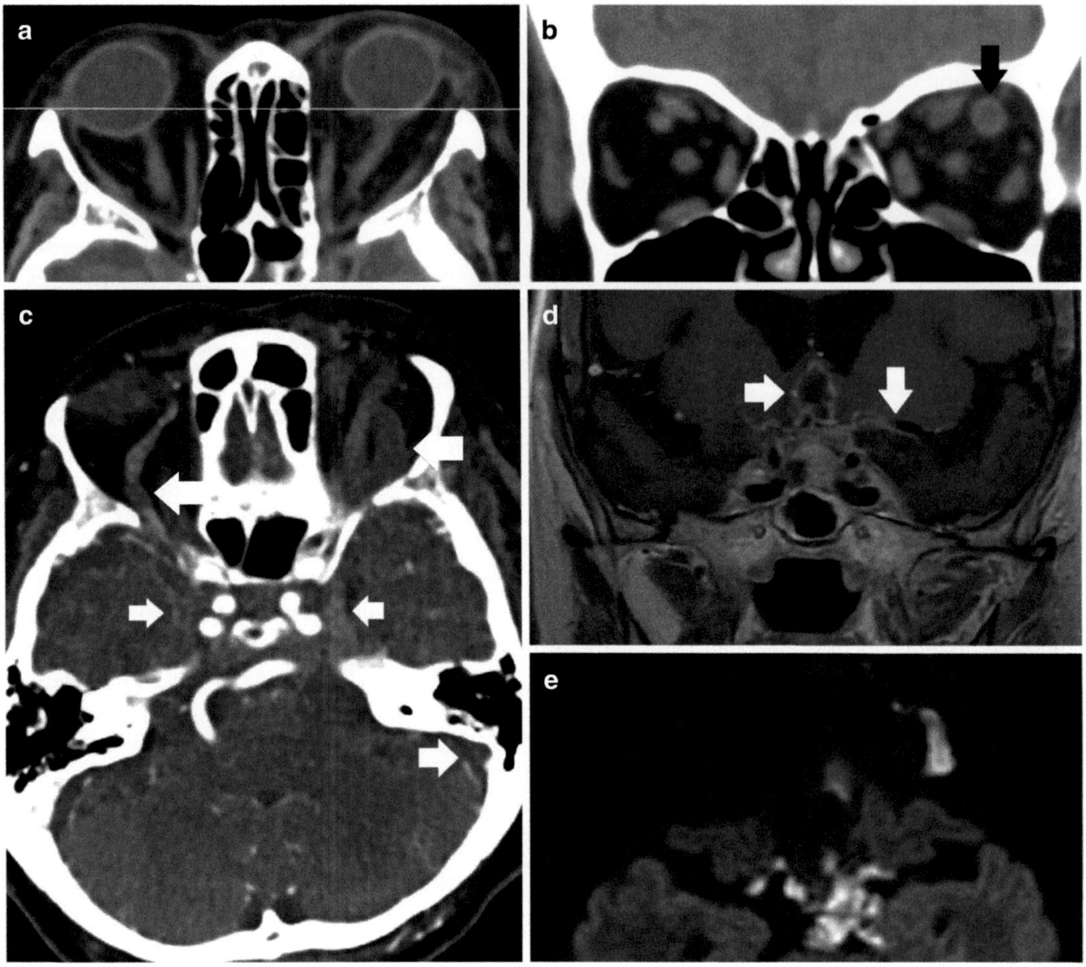

Fig. 6 Unenhanced axial (**a**) and coronal (**b**) CT showing infiltration of periorbital and orbital fat consistent with cellulitis. Additionally there is enlargement of the superior ophthalmic vein of the left (**b**; ***arrow***). Venous phase CT (**c**) shows (partial) thrombosis of both superior ophthalmic veins (**c**; ***black arrows***) and additional filling defects in both cavernous sinuses and the left sigmoid sinus (**c**; ***white arrows***). Post-contrast T1w image (**d**) shows additional leptomeningeal and perivascular enhancement (***arrows***) consistent with meningitis (and possible vasculitis). DWI (**e**) shows diffusion restriction within the basal cisterns which can be seen in purulent meningitis. Also note the restricted diffusion due to thrombosis of the left superior ophthalmic vein

A CT-based classification, suggested by Chandler et al., [41] can be used to describe the extent of disease. Chandler type I (periorbital cellulitis) and type II (orbital cellulitis) are considered uncomplicated OC, while Chandler type III (subperiosteal abscess), type IV (orbital abscess) and type V (cavernous sinus thrombosis) are considered complications that require more extensive treatment, possibly including surgical intervention. Intracranial complications include meningitis, empyema or abscess in the epidural or subdural space, intracerebral abscess, Pott's puffy tumour, cavernous sinus thrombosis and ischemic infarction. An example of OC with subperiosteal abscess can be seen in Fig. 7.

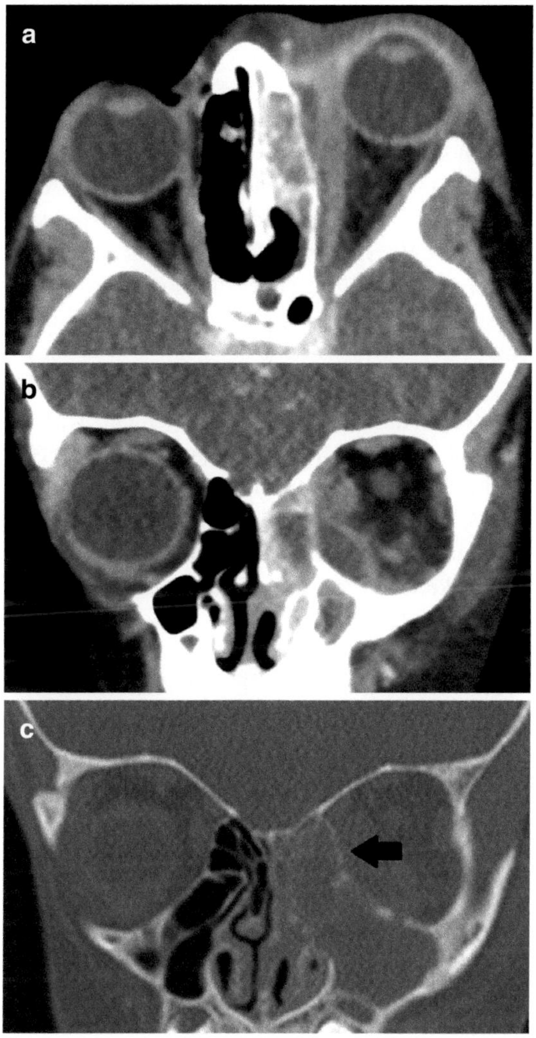

Fig. 7 Extensive left-sided periorbital and orbital cellulitis with clear proptosis and diffuse fatty infiltration as seen on axial post-contrast CT (**a**). An inferomedial subperiosteal abscess can be seen in the coronal reconstruction (**b**). Additionally, there is opacification of the ethmoid and maxillary sinuses on the left with bulging and irregularity of the medial orbital wall (**c**; ***arrow***)

6 Inflammatory and Lymphoproliferative Disease

The spectrum of orbital lymphoproliferative disease (OLPD) ranges from benign lesions such as idiopathic orbital inflammatory disease (IOID), lymphoid hyperplasia and IgG4-related disease, to malignant lymphoma. There is a significant overlap in imaging (and clinical) characteristics between different OLPDs and other inflammatory diseases often necessitating a biopsy. The exception is thyroid-associated orbitopathy which generally has a typical symmetrical appearance distinguishing it from other inflammatory diseases.

Disease location can give an indication of underlying pathology. For example, bilateral lacrimal gland involvement is most often seen in sarcoidosis, Sjögren syndrome and lymphoma. Also, preseptal involvement is more often seen in lymphoma as compared to IOID, infiltration of the infra-orbital nerve is often seen IgG4-ROD, and combined optic nerve and optic nerve sheath involvement could indicate sarcoidosis.

Independent of location, lymphoma can often be distinguished from inflammatory disease based on DWI-derived ADC values with a proposed threshold of $<0.775 \times 10^{-3}$ mm^{-2}/s. Vice versa inflammatory diseases tend to show higher ADC values compared to lymphoma with a proposed threshold of $>0.92 \times 10^{-3}$ mm^{-2}/s. Note that in between lies a range of indeterminate values [42]. In DCE-perfusion MRI, lymphoma tends to show a type 3 wash-out curve, although 'benign' curves have been described in lymphoma as well [7]. Combining information of location, DWI-derived ADC, DCE-perfusion and other characteristics such as age, medical history and presence of systemic disease will give the most likely diagnosis [43].

6.1 Thyroid-Associated Orbitopathy

Thyroid-associated orbitopathy (TAO), also known as thyroid eye disease (TED) or Graves orbitopathy, has a distinct pattern on imaging with relatively symmetrical inflammatory thickening of extraocular muscles described in the anagram I'M SLOw. The anagram describes the most commonly encountered order of affected muscles: inferior rectus, medial rectus, superior rectus, lateral rectus, and oblique muscles. In about 5–15% of cases there may be unilateral disease activity. TAO shows typical sparing of the tendinous insertion leading to a specific muscle shape in the axial plane which has been referred to as the 'Coca-Cola bottle' sign. Mid-muscle thickness of >5 mm is considered pathological, but considering the natural variety of extraocular muscle thickness, any increase in size is suspicious even if measures are <5 mm [44].

The inflamed muscles tend to enhance more vividly on post-contrast images compared to normal extraocular muscle tissue, and may show oedema. The signal intensity on T2w fat-suppressed images increases proportionally with disease activity as measured by the clinical activity score (CAS) and can be used for treatment monitoring [45–48]. An example of TAO is depicted in Fig. 8.

Aside from extraocular muscle enlargement, lacrimal gland enlargement, orbital fat hypertrophy, eyelid oedema, stretching of the optic nerve, and tenting of the posterior globe can be present. In the acute phase there will be signs of active inflammation with fatty infiltration, oedema and enhancement, while in the chronic phase muscles will atrophy with fatty replacement.

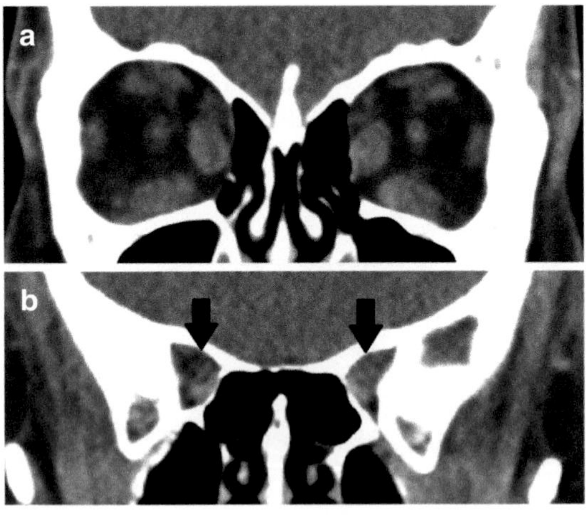

Fig. 8 Coronal unenhanced CT at the mid-muscle level (**a**) and orbital apex (**b**) in a patient with thyroid-associated orbitopathy. Almost symmetrical thickening of the inferior and medial rectus is seen and there is diffuse fuzzy infiltration of the orbital fat consistent with active inflammation. At the level of orbital apex, there is visible fatty tissue surrounding the right optic nerve, but on the left there is possible apical crowding (***arrows***)

6.2 Sarcoidosis

Sarcoidosis is a noncaseating granulomatous inflammatory disease that often shows ophthalmic and/or orbital involvement. Most commonly, patients present with (anterior) uveitis. On MRI, uveitis can be seen as nodular or diffuse thickening and enhancement of uveoscleral structures, although imaging is generally not performed in these patients as the diagnosis can be made clinically [49].

Within the orbit, sarcoidosis can cause diffuse (bilateral) lacrimal gland enlargement with or without infiltration of adjacent fat tissue. Infiltration of the optic nerve and/or optic nerve sheath can extend to (or from) the intracranial compartment and can appear as an enhancing mass-like lesion on imaging. Isolated optic nerve sheath involvement can easily mimic other pathologies such as meningioma, perineuritis, leptomeningeal metastases, and lymphoma. Combined disease of both optic nerve and optic nerve sheath however make sarcoidosis a likely diagnosis. Rare manifestations of orbital sarcoidosis include asymmetrical extraocular muscle infiltration and a retrobulbar focal or infiltrating mass [3, 49–51]. Cranial neuropathy may be present in case of granulomatous meningitis [52, 53].

6.3 Granulomatosis with Polyangiitis

Orbital involvement in granulomatosis with polyangiitis (GPA), previously known as Wegener's granulomatosis, is common with an incidence of 58–87%. About 8–16% of patients present with orbital symptoms at diagnosis. In early stages clinical features may be nonspecific making it difficult to differentiate GPA from other inflammatory diseases. As a small vessel vasculitis, GPA may cause conjunctivitis, (epi)scleritis, uveitis, retinitis and optic neuritis which tend to be detected clinically rather than radiologically. Orbital disease most often presents as diffuse infiltrative inflammation (sometimes extending from adjacent sinuses) and orbital pseudotumor. Extension of disease into the cavernous sinus can

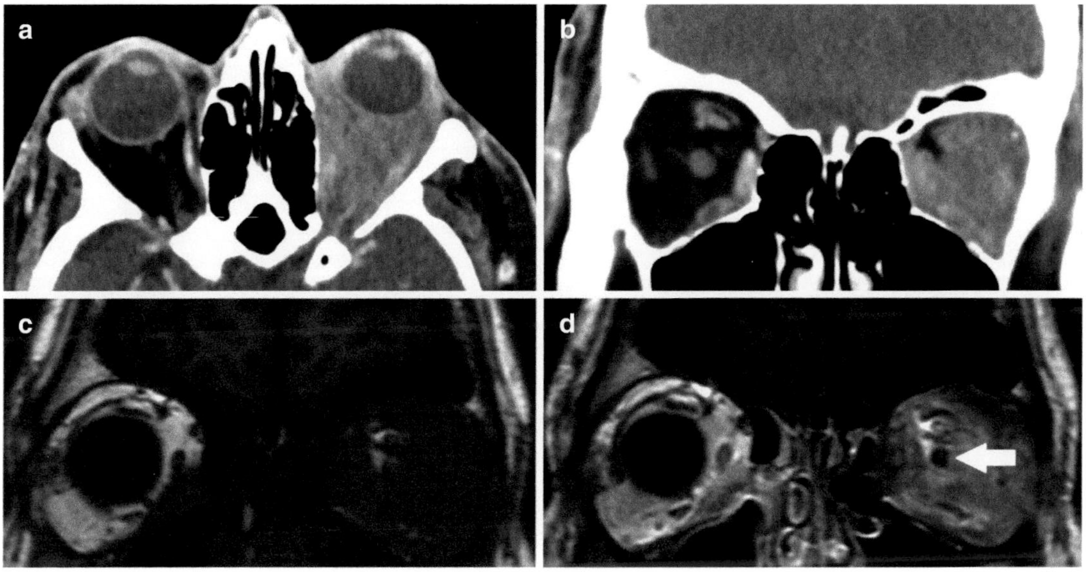

Fig. 9 Post-contrast CT (**a** and **b**) and T1w pre- (**c**) and post-contrast (**d**) images in GPA showing extensive infiltration of the left orbit with preseptal and postseptal (intra- and extraconal) disease with engulfment of orbital structures and exophthalmos. Note the sparing of the optic nerve visible on post-contrast MRI (**d**; ***arrow***) and the presence of limited infiltration of the right inferomedial orbit. There was no evidence of sinonasal disease in this patient

cause Tolosa-Hunt syndrome. An example of diffuse orbital infiltration in GPA can be seen in Fig. 9. Less common manifestations of the disease include extraocular muscle disease and lacrimal gland involvement. Optic neuropathy is generally caused by external compression. Presence of sinonasal and systemic disease aids in the diagnosis as well as elevated serum ANCA-titers, although serum titers may be negative in case of isolated orbital disease [53, 54].

GPA lesions tend to be hypointense on T1w images and will show enhancement after contrast administration. There is no diffusion restriction. At a late stage, fibrosis will give a characteristic low signal on both T1w and T2w images [55].

6.4 Idiopathic Orbital Inflammatory Disease

Idiopathic orbital inflammatory disease (IOID), also known as nonspecific orbital inflammation (NSOI), orbital pseudotumor, idiopathic orbital inflammation (IOI) and orbital inflammatory syndrome/disease, is a common cause of orbital pain in adults. IOID can show both unilateral and (asymmetrical) bilateral involvement of orbital fat, extraocular muscles, lacrimal gland, optic nerve sheath complex and uveoscleral structures. In case of extraocular muscle involvement, the medial rectus tends to be affected first. Both muscle belly and tendon are affected, as opposed to TAO in which the tendon is typically spared. IOID can present with diffuse orbital involvement or a focal mass-lesion. Mass-lesions tend to be T2-hypointense with contrast-enhancement and without diffusion restriction [55–57]. Examples of different IOID presentations can be seen in Figs. 10 and 11.

Extension of IOID through the orbital fissure into the cavernous sinus causes Tolosa-Hunt syndrome. Considering IOID shares many imaging (and clinical) characteristics with malignancies and other orbital inflammatory diseases, it is considered a diagnosis of exclusion.

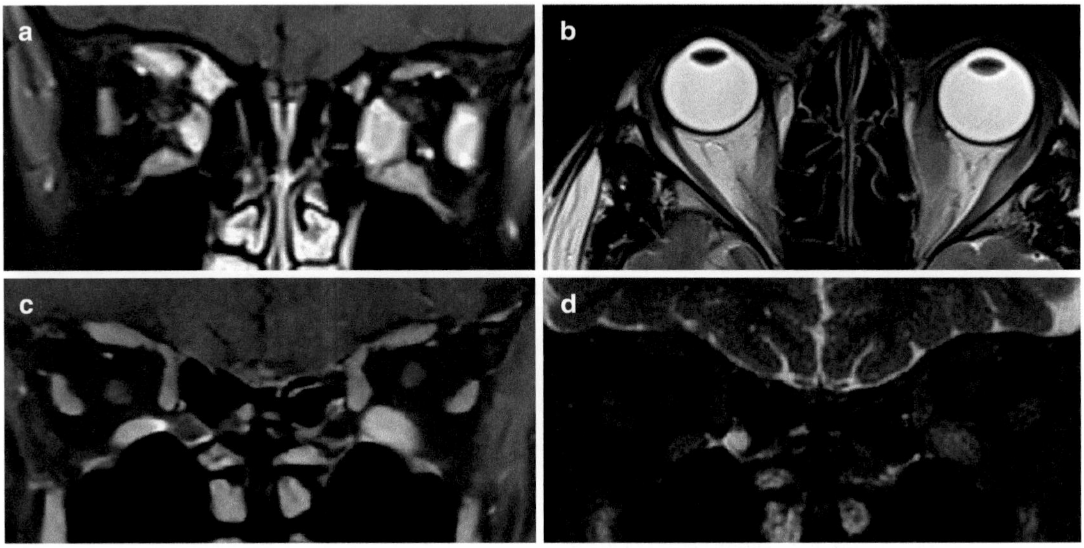

Fig. 10 Examples of IOID myositis in two different patients. Post-contrast T1w fat suppressed (**a**) and T2w image (**b**) in patient1 showing asymmetrical thickened, enhancing and T2-hyperintense extra-ocular muscles. There is also bilateral infiltration of the intraconal fat. Post-contrast T1w (**c**) and T2w fat suppressed (**d**) images in patient2 showing similar features limited to the left inferior rectus with limited perimuscular fatty infiltration

6.5 IgG4-Related Orbital Disease

The orbit is frequently involved in IgG4-related disease (IgG4-ROD). Other structures in the head- and neck area that are often affected are the salivary glands and lymph nodes, but IgG4-ROD has been described in almost all organs. Intracranial IgG4-ROD can present as hypertrophic meningitis which can spread along the optic nerve. In the orbit, symmetrical bilateral involvement of the lacrimal gland is the most frequent finding, followed by extraocular muscle, orbital fat and cranial nerve involvement. Increased awareness of the disease has led to an increase of diagnoses over the years [58].

Differentiating IgG4-ROD from other inflammatory diseases on imaging proves difficult and often a biopsy is needed for the final diagnosis. Infiltration of the infra-orbital nerve has been reported in up to 50% of patients, but this sign has a low sensitivity [59–61]. As lymphoplasmacytic infiltrates with (mainly) IgG4-positive plasma cells can cause both inflammation and fibrosis, imaging characteristics depend on disease stage and activity. Active disease imaging characteristics are similar to other inflammatory processes with T2-hyperintensity due to oedema, vivid enhancement and fatty infiltration. Fibrosis is commonly seen as diffusely infiltrating T2- and T1-hypointensity and may cause enophthalmos. An example of extensive IgG4-ROD with lacrimal gland, extraocular muscle, and nerve involvement is shown in Fig. 12.

6.6 Lymphoma

At the malignant end of the OPLD spectrum are lymphoma, the most common orbital malignancy in adults over 60 years of age. Most orbital lymphomas are primary low-grade B-cell non-Hodgkin lymphomas [44, 62]. Both B-cell and T-cell orbital lymphomas most commonly occur in the extraconal space and lacrimal gland. Other locations include the retrobulbar area, intraconal space and extraocular muscles. Overall roughly 80–90% of lymphoma are unilateral. Although specific subtypes such as the rare orbital mantle cell lymphoma can occur bilaterally in up to 43% of cases and is also more likely to reside in the conjunctiva and eyelids [56].

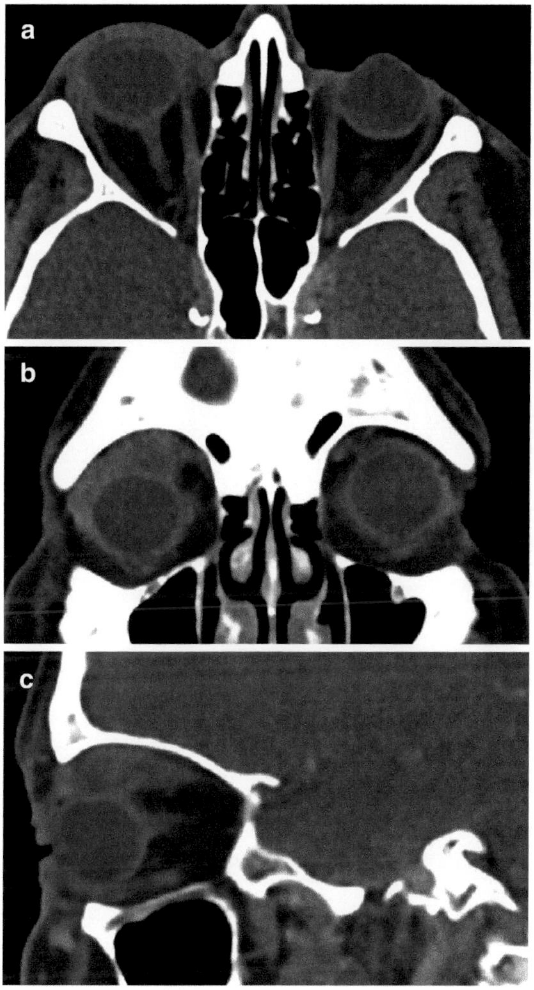

Fig. 11 Axial (**a**), coronal (**b**) and sagittal (**c**) unenhanced CT in a patient with biopsy proven IOID. There is a mass in and around the right superior rectus with exophthalmos and hypoglobus. Also note the reactive fat infiltration in the upper eyelid

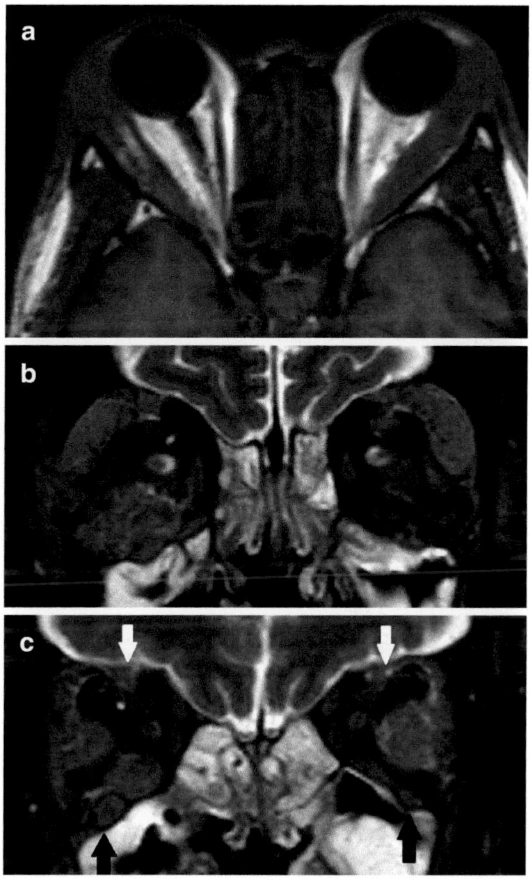

Fig. 12 Biopsy-proven IgG4-ROD in a patient with bilateral, almost symmetrical diffuse involvement of orbital structures. Unenhanced T1w image (**a**) shows bilateral enlargement of the lacrimal gland and lateral rectus. The lesions are hypointense on T2w fat suppressed (**b** and **c**) images on which diffuse asymmetrical muscle thickening. Also note the bilateral infiltration of the infraorbital (***black arrows***) and supraorbital nerves (***white arrows***)

On structural imaging, lymphoma tends to be relatively hyperdense on unenhanced CT with homogeneous enhancement after contrast on both CT and MRI. Most lesions are well-demarcated with T2-iso- or hypointense signals, the latter being quite specific if present. Flow voids can be present due to high vascularity. In case of malignant lacrimal gland disease (lymphoma or other), extraconal extension of mass towards the orbital apex creating a wedge or triangular appearance can be present. The wedge-sign can help substantiate the diagnosis of lymphoma as it is much less common in inflammatory disease [63].

Mean DWI-derived ADC values vary between studies from 0.47 to 1.25×10^{-3} mm^{-2}/s with higher values overlapping with inflammatory and other neoplastic lesions. A threshold value of <0.775×10^{-3} mm^{-2}/s has therefore been proposed to avoid false-positive results. There are no significant differences in ADC between different types and grades of lymphoma. Low ADC values at baseline tend to predict better treatment response and increasing ADC values during treatment may preclude

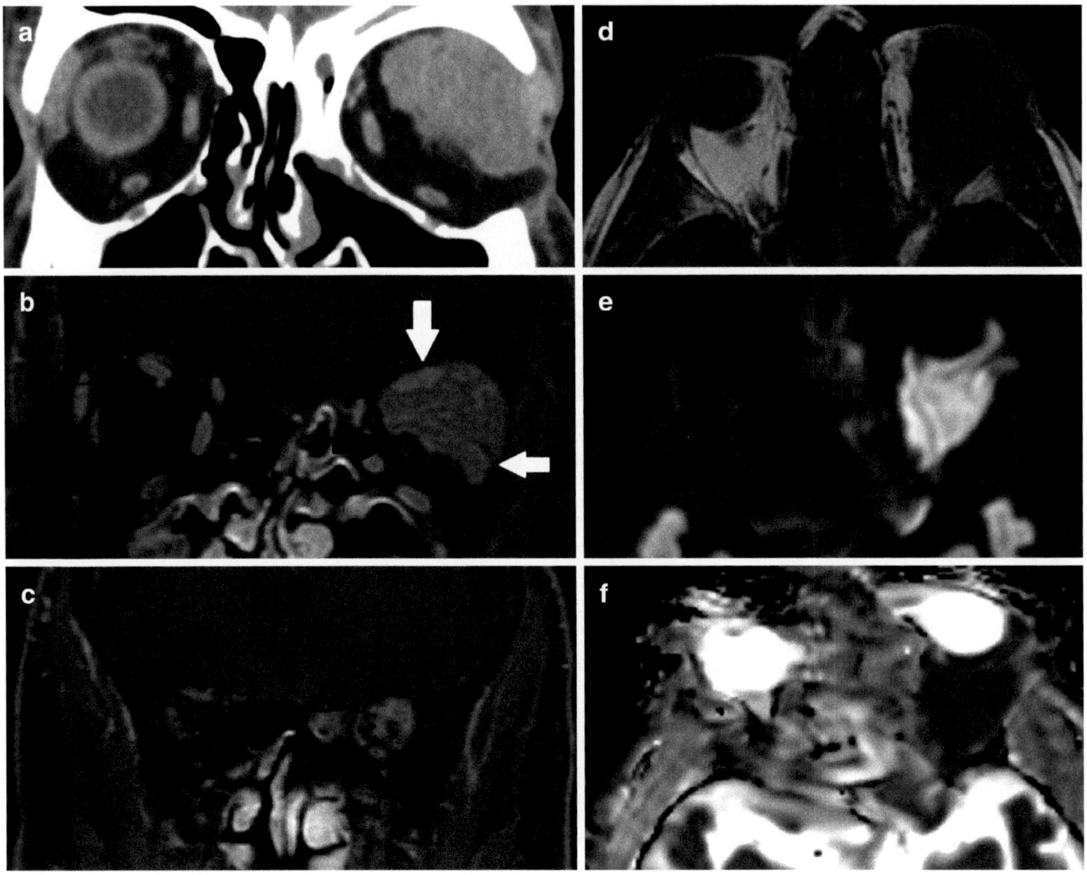

Fig. 13 Low-grade non-Hodgkin marginal zone lymphoma on the left. Unenhanced CT (**a**) shows a relatively hyperdense mass which seems to arise from the lacrimal gland. There is homogeneous enhancement on T1w-post-contrast images (**b** and **c**), engulfment of the lateral and superior rectus muscles (**b**; ***white arrows***) and the optic nerve (**b**; ***black arrow***) and extension into the orbital apex. On axial pre-contrast T1w (**d**) there is exophthalmos and possible infiltration of the bulb. On DWI (**e**) and the ADC-map (**f**) there are distortions but diffusion restriction is evident (ADC 0.567×10^{-3} mm^2/s)

tumour volume decrease [42, 64]. If ADC-values are $>0.775 \times 10^{-3}$ mm^{-2}/s, additional DCE-perfusion-derived parameters can further help to differentiate lymphoma from inflammatory disease if needed as lymphoma will often show a malignant type 3 curve with wash-out [7, 65, 66]. Examples of orbital lymphoma can be seen in Figs. 13 and 14.

CT is useful for evaluating possible bone destruction, which can be present in up to 7% of orbital lymphoma [67]. If MRI is contraindicated, spectral CT can help with tissue characterization as non-lacrimal gland lymphomas are found to have significantly higher iodine density and a steeper iodine attenuation slope compared to IOID and IgG4-ROD [68].

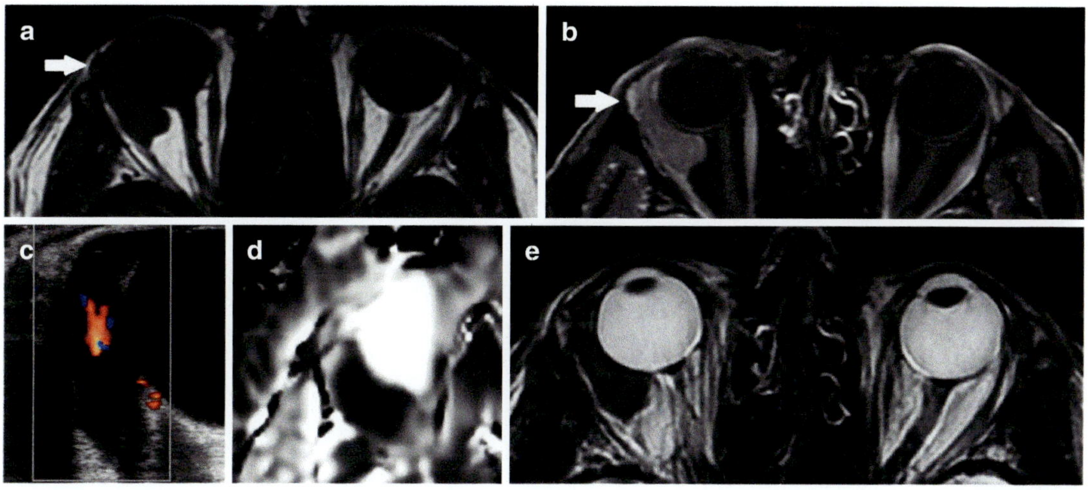

Fig. 14 Homogeneous subconjunctival mass in a patient with grade I MALT-lymphoma in the superolateral quadrant of the orbit on T1w pre-contrast (**a**) and post-contrast (**b**) images. Note the atrophied lacrimal gland (***white arrows***) anterior to the mass. Ultrasound with color Doppler (**c**) shows high vascularity. The DWI-derived ADC-map (**d**) shows diffusion restriction (ADC 0.450×10^{-3} mm^2/s) and the axial T2w image (**e**) shows a homogeneous hypointense signal, both consistent with high cellularity

7 Neoplasms

Many orbital tumours have specific imaging characteristics. Meningiomas, gliomas, peripheral nerve sheath tumours, dermoid and epidermoid cysts are relatively easy to recognize on CT and/or MRI. Lacrimal gland tumours with the exception of lymphoma and metastases can be more difficult to differentiate from inflammatory disease. Commonly encountered orbital tumours are discussed in this subchapter.

The value of DWI in distinguishing benign from malignant tumours is limited. While in lymphomas there is often clear diffusion restriction with low ADC values, non-lymphomatous malignant masses (including rhabdomyosarcoma and metastases) tend to have limited diffusion restriction with ADC values ranging between 0.84 and 0.99×10^{-3} mm^2/s. This means ADC-values in non-lymphomatous malignant masses are still relatively low compared to inflammatory lesions (with a proposed ADC cut-off>0.92×10^{-3} mm^{-2}/s), but the significant overlap means DWI is of limited value when evaluating many orbital tumours other than lymphoma [42].

7.1 Lacrimal Gland Tumours

Most tumours arising from the lacrimal gland are lymphomas (58%), which are discussed in an earlier subchapter. Tumours of epithelial origin are second most common and include the benign pleomorphic adenoma and several malignant lesions including adenoid cystic carcinoma (ACC), primary adenocarcinoma, carcinoma ex-pleomorphic adenoma, mucoepidermoid carcinoma, squamous cell carcinoma, and sebaceous carcinoma [69–71].

To differentiate between malignant and benign lacrimal gland lesions of epithelial origin some general imaging characteristics can be considered. Posterior orbital extension occurs in about 55% of all malignant epithelial tumours and can be seen as a 'wedge'-sign on imaging. Pleomorphic adenoma (either primary or recurrent) do not show this sign. Other malignant signs are bony erosions, local invasion of soft-tissue structures and perineural spread. Recurrent pleomorphic adenoma can mimic a malignant lesion however, as both are likely ill-defined and T1-heterogeneous [71, 72].

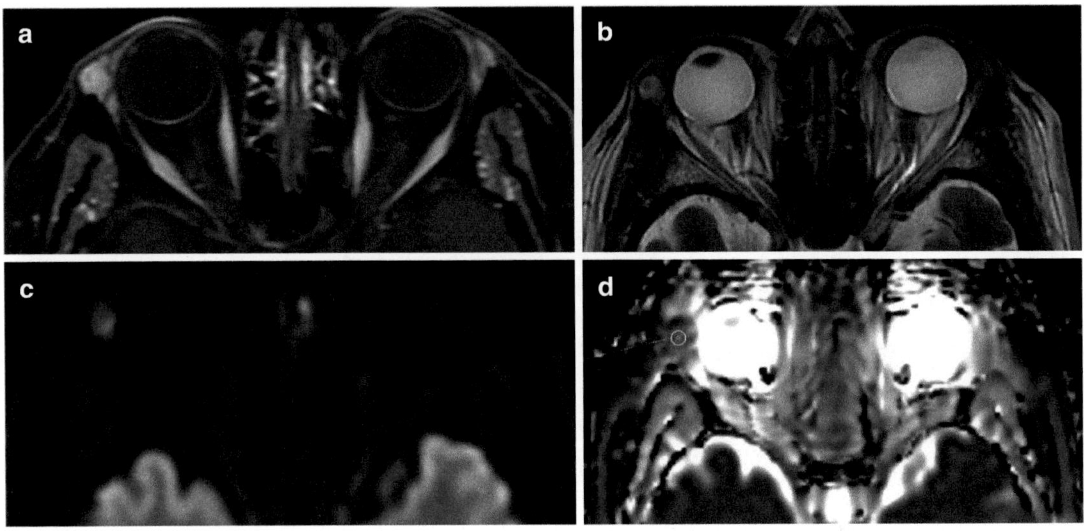

Fig. 15 Axial post-contrast T1w (**a**) image shows a solitary enhancing, well-demarcated lesion which is slightly inhomogeneous on T2w (**b**). DWI (**c**) and ADC-map (**d**) show increased diffusion with an ADC of 1.337×10^{-3} mm^2/s. These features are consistent with a benign lesion most likely pleomorphic adenoma, which was later histologically confirmed

Homogeneous enhancement and sharp demarcations indicate primary pleomorphic adenoma, but is only seen in a small percentage of these benign tumours. Cystic changes, calcifications, T2-inhomogeneity and vivid and/or inhomogeneous enhancement can occur in both benign and malignant lesions and do not aid in the diagnosis [71]. An example of a pleomorphic adenoma is shown in Fig. 15.

7.2 Dermoid and Epidermoid Cysts

Both dermoid and epidermoid cysts are congenital inclusion ectodermal cysts that grow in time due to the accumulation of debris. During folding near developing sutures there may be incomplete separation of ectoderm causing these cysts to form.

Dermoid inclusion cysts are lined by pluripotent ectodermal epithelium. In the orbit, superficial dermoid cysts can be found along the zygomaticofrontal and frontoethmoidal sutures with 80% occurring in the lacrimal fossa. They seldom appear in the intraconal space. Superficial dermoids tend to become apparent at an early age. Deeper lesions at the orbital apex are more often an incidental finding. An example of a dermoid at the orbital apex can be seen in Fig. 16. Dermoid cysts tend to be round or lobulated with well-defined margins. They contain fat tissue due to oily secretions of sebaceous glands, dense keratin debris and possible calcifications. This heterogeneous composition makes for its characteristic fat-fluid level, which is often seen. There might be some rim enhancement, although dermoid cysts typically do not enhance. There is often bony remodelling. Presence of perilesional oedema and enhancement suggests rupture with inflammation [44, 73].

Epidermoid inclusion cysts have a similar origin although they likely develop later during embryonic life when ectodermal cells are no longer pluripotent. Epidermoid cysts are lined by squamous epithelium only. The cyst is filled with white dry keratin material. Epidermoid cysts are also well-circumscribed but as they only contain keratin material the contents are T2-hyperintense with marked diffusion restriction. There can be slight rim enhancement [73]. Most epidermoid cysts are found in the periorbital region, differentiating them from dermoid cysts, but they can also occur in the orbit.

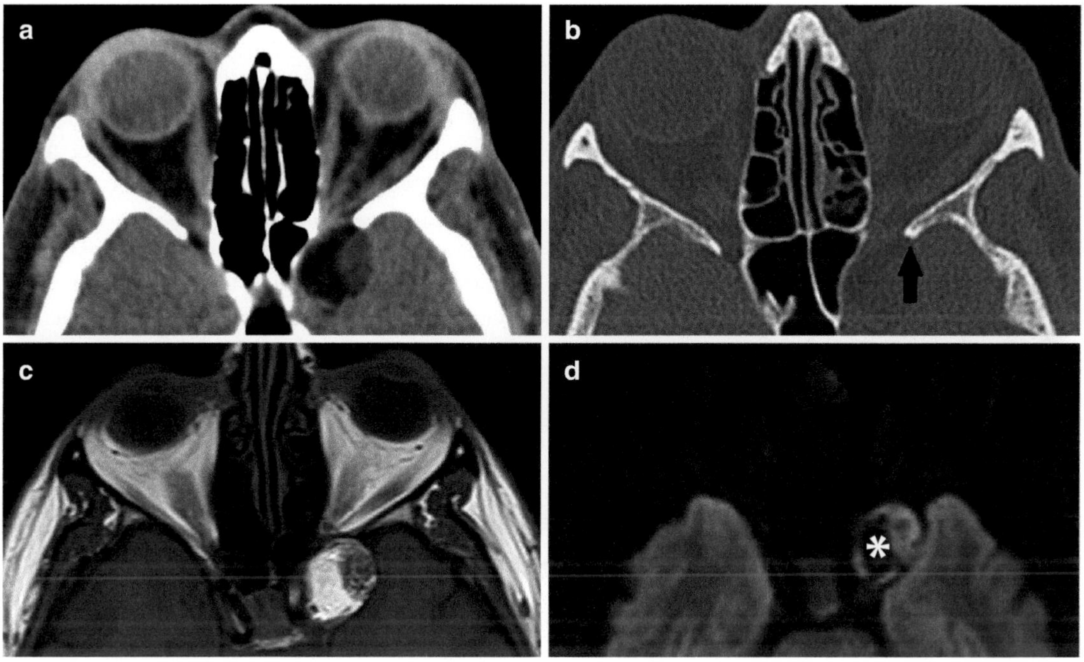

Fig. 16 Dermoid cyst at the orbital apex in a patient with periorbital pain and double vision. Unenhanced CT (**a** and **b**) shows a sharply demarcated fat-containing mass with adjacent bone remodeling (**b**; ***arrow***). Unenhanced T1w image (**c**) shows the lesion is located in the cavernous sinus. On DWI (**d**) fat is suppressed (*) and both the rim and central nodule show a slight hyperintense signal due to high cellularity

7.3 Peripheral Nerve Sheath Tumours

Schwannoma and neurofibroma are benign peripheral nerve sheath tumours (BPNSTs) in the orbit. Schwannomas commonly arise from trigeminal branches and can cause bony remodelling due to slow non-invasive growth. Schwannomas are encapsulated masses that are T1-iso and/or hypointense compared to grey matter. Generally, they are T2-hyperintense, except in the presence of calcifications or extensive collagen deposits. Enhancement may be variable, ranging from heterogeneous or rim-enhancement to homogeneous enhancement. The mass can be completely cystic (i.e. cystic schwannoma) or may contain smaller cysts. Arterial enhancement differentiates schwannoma from cavernous malformations. In clinical practice however, often only a static (late) post-contrast sequence is obtained, which can make differentiation difficult. Most schwannoma are cone-shaped modelling to the shape of the orbit or dumbbell shaped when extending through the superior orbital fissure. In smaller rounds of ovoid tumours eccentric perineural growth (as opposed to the concentric growth pattern of neurofibroma) might be seen [74].

Orbital neurofibromas are typically associated with neurofibromatosis type 1 (NF1) and tend to arise from trigeminal branches, similar to schwannomas. There is no capsule and the mass tends to be more heterogeneous on T1w and T2w sequences as compared to schwannoma. Enhancement can be heterogeneous as well. Neurofibromas can present as a focal mass or can be large and plexiform following the nerves path. When intersected on T2w images the mass can show a target sign with central T2-hypointensity surrounded by a T2-hyperintense rim, although it should be noted that this sign can be also present in schwannoma [44]. An example of an extensive plexiform neurofibroma can be seen in Fig. 17.

Malignant peripheral nerve sheath tumours (MPNSTs) should be suspected in case of fast growth, large tumour diameter, presence of peri-

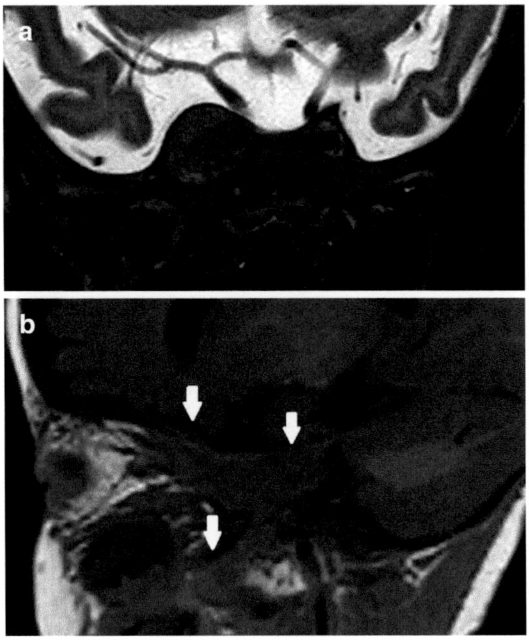

Fig. 17 Patient with NF1 suffering from vision loss and facial asymmetry. Coronal T2w image (**a**) shows a mass in the right cavernous sinus and sagittal unenhanced T1w image (**b**) shows an extensive plexiform neurofibroma extending from Meckel's cave, along N.V1 into the orbit (***upper arrows***) and along N.V2 (***lower arrow***) with foraminal widening

tumoral oedema, and ill-defined/infiltrative margins. ADC values also tend to be lower in MPNST and early arterial enhancement is more common, although large overlap with BPNST exists [75].

7.4 Meningioma

Meningiomas are generally benign (WHO grade I in 94.5%), although growth can cause considerable morbidity. Women are more often affected than men [76]. Orbital meningiomas can be divided into optic nerve sheath meningiomas and sphenoid-wing meningiomas.

Optic nerve sheath meningiomas (ONSM) comprise about 1–2% of all meningiomas. There is a female predilection similar to intracranial meningiomas. Paediatric ONSMs are rare and tend to be associated with neurofibromatosis type2. ONSM can arise from within or extend into the orbit, i.e. primary or secondary ONSM [77, 78]. The mass surrounds the optic nerve which may atrophy due to long-term compression. This is especially the case for small meningiomas located at the level of the optic canal (thus being a primary ONSM), which are frequently overlooked because of their size and location, allowing them ample time to cause considerable nerve damage. Meningiomas are generally hyperdense on CT and T1-hypointense with variable T2-signal (often hypointense) on MRI. There is vivid enhancement. Calcifications are common and best seen on CT. Diffusion is often somewhat restricted because of high cellularity with values ranging from 0.90 to 1.04×10^{-3} mm^{-2}/s. Because the tumour surrounds the optic nerve, typical tram-track (axial) and donut/target signs (coronal) can be seen in about 25% of patients, but this is not specific. There might be hyperostosis of adjacent bone. Subtle involvement of adjacent bone sometimes occurs without visible morphologic changes, but can be detected as signal changes in bone marrow on MRI. The mass can be tubular, globular, fusiform or focal. The differential diagnosis includes perineuritis (most common misdiagnosis), sarcoidosis, lymphoma, metastasis, peripheral nerve sheath tumour and solitary fibrous tumour [3, 42, 44, 77, 78]. In case of doubt somatostatin receptor PET-imaging can be considered, an example of which is shown in Fig. 18.

Sphenoid-wing or spheno-orbital meningiomas are generally meningiomas en plaque with extensive hyperostosis and sometimes invasion of the adjacent bone. Imaging characteristics are similar to other meningiomas, with T1-hypointensity, variable T2-signal and vivid enhancement [79]. Cavernous sinus and superior orbital fissure involvement are a frequent finding. Extensive intraosseous components with a surrounding mass instead of en plaque dural thickening could indicate a primary intraosseous location. An example of which can be seen in Fig. 19.

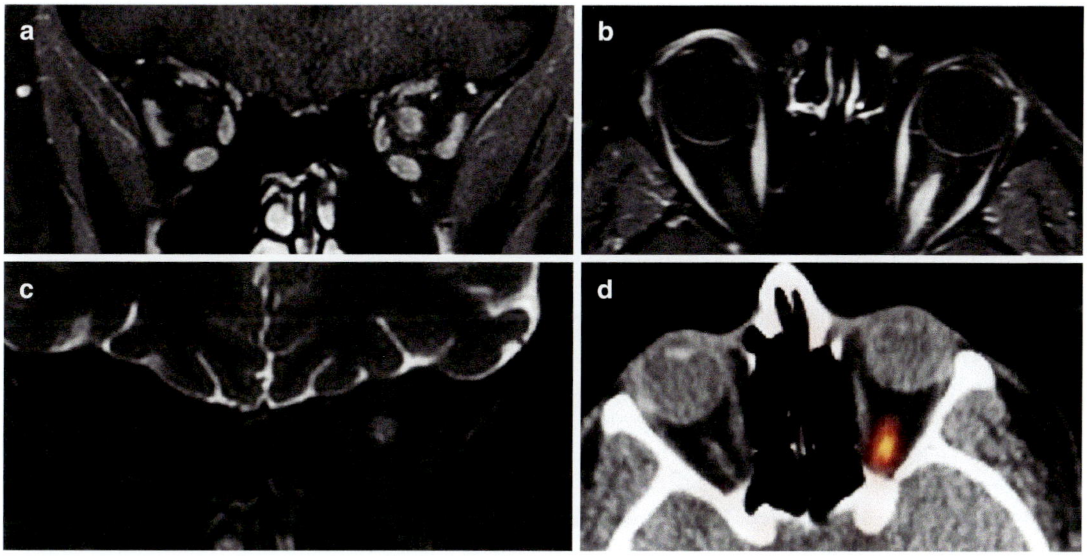

Fig. 18 Example of an ONSM on the left with almost homogeneous enhancement of the posterior orbital optic nerve on T1w post-contrast imaging (**a** and **b**) and hyperintense signal on T2w (**c**). A vague tram-track sign is seen on axial imaging (**b**). To rule out other diagnosis, a 68Ga-Dotatate PET-CT (**d**) was made showing clear uptake consistent with meningioma

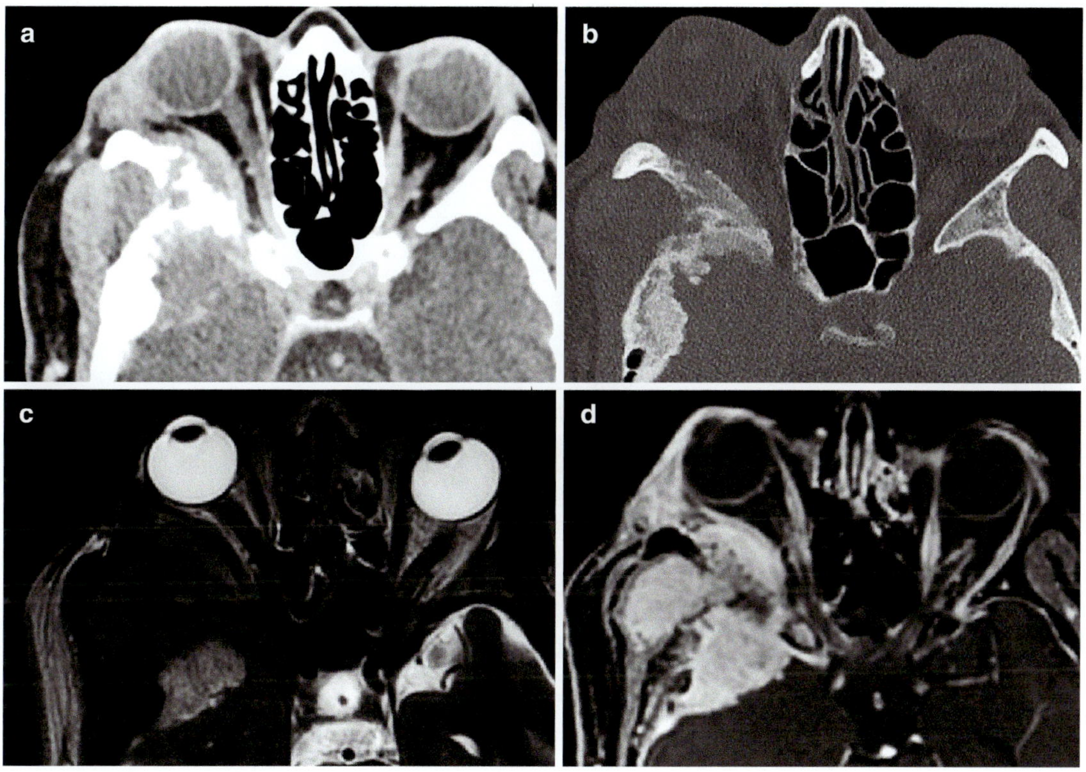

Fig. 19 Example of an sphenoid-wing meningioma on post-contrast CT (**a** and **b**) showing a large mass surrounding the sphenoid and temporal bone with hyperostosis and an intraosseous component. On T2w (**c**) and T1w post-contrast (**d**) MRI there is abnormal signal intensity of the bone with vivid enhancement also indicating a large intraosseous component. The mass has a large intra-orbital component causing exophthalmos. Considering the location and shape of the tumor it may be of primary osseous origin

7.5 Solitary Fibrous Tumour

Solitary fibrous tumour (SFT) of the orbit is a relatively rare entity arising from mesenchymal fibroblast-like cells similar to SFTs found elsewhere. Considering the overlap with entities such as hemangiopericytoma, giant cell angiofibroma, and fibrous histiocytoma of the orbit, it has been postulated that these all represent the same tumour that should be termed SFT [80]. Central nervous system SFT and hemangiopericytoma have already been merged into a single entity and a 3-tiered grading scheme has been suggested in the World Health Organization classification of CNS tumours [81].

SFT tends to be a solitary, well-circumscribed mass occurring in different orbital subsites both intra- and extraconal and preseptal. SFTs show relatively homogeneous signals on T1w-images and variable T2-signal intensity depending on the amount of mature fibrous tissue and presence of myxoid or cystic degeneration. As the tumours are highly vascular they markedly enhance. There can be linear or rounded non-enhancing areas due to the presence of hypovascular collagenous stroma [82]. On dynamic perfusion imaging the lesions show rapid early enhancement with washout (type 3 curve) [83]. Bony remodelling can be present in large slow-growing tumours, but bone destruction is rare and only occurs in a subset of locally aggressive or malignant cases. Note that more rapid growth can occur during pregnancy. Examples of SFTs can be seen in Fig. 20.

Imaging findings are very similar to peripheral nerve sheath tumours and meningioma and the mass can therefore easily be misdiagnosed. There

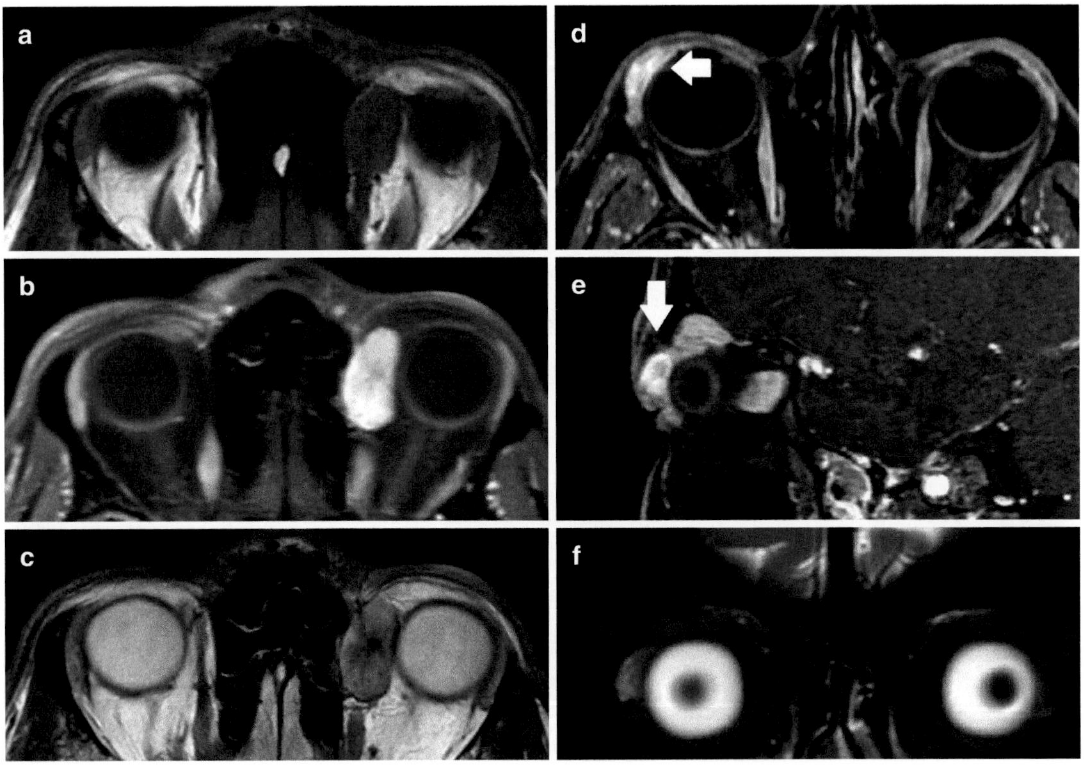

Fig. 20 Examples of SFT in two different patients. A well-demarcated SFT in the superomedial quadrant is seen in patient1 on unenhanced T1w (**a**), post-contrast T1w (**b**) and T2w (**c**) images with relatively homogeneous appearance and a central scar (likely due to presence of collagenous stroma). In patient 2 there is a homogeneously enhancing SFT on T1w post-contrast (**d** and **e**) images with also homogenous T2-hyperintensity (**f**). The lesions could not be completely delineated from the lacrimal gland, consistent with infiltrative growth, which was histopathologically confirmed

is a low risk of metastases from orbital SFT with an incidence of about 2.1%. Local recurrence occurs in up to 26% due to incomplete resection. As both recurrences and metastases can occur many years after resection, long-term follow-up is indicated [82, 84].

7.6 Optic Nerve Glioma

Optic nerve or pathway gliomas can occur isolated, but are much more common in patients with neurofibromatosis. In case of bilateral disease it is almost pathognomonic. CT is of limited value and can depict optic canal widening and possible tumour calcifications. MRI is necessary to evaluate both intra-orbital and intracranial extent of disease. There is fusiform enlargement and kinking or tortuosity of the optic nerve as well as possible dural ectasia. The tumour appears T1-hypointense and T2-iso/hyperintense with variable enhancement depending on tumour grade [3, 44]. Most tumours, in both children and adults are pilocytic astrocytoma. High-grade gliomas are very uncommon in this region [85].

7.7 Rhabdomyosarcoma

Rhabdomyosarcoma is the most common primary orbital malignancy in children. It arises from primitive mesenchymal cells rather than from the extraocular muscles and may be located next to or attached to an extraocular muscle. There is a correlation between location and histology with the embryonal subtype more frequently occurring in the superior orbit and the alveolar subtype more commonly occurring in the interior orbit. If small, the mass can appear well-circumscribed, but larger lesions tend to infiltrate and/or encase adjacent structures. Generally, rhabdomyosarcoma appears isodense and T1-isointense to muscle on respectively CT and MRI. T2-signal can be hyperintense or heterogeneous. Calcifications and haemorrhage are rare in orbital rhabdomyosarcoma. There is vivid enhancement after contrast administration, although non-enhancing central necrosis may be present in large tumours. Rhabdomyosarcoma has a high growth rate and can cause severe destruction of both bony and orbital structures. Intracranial extension and (pulmonary) metastases can occur as well [3, 44, 86].

7.8 Orbital Metastases

Orbital metastases most commonly originate from breast carcinoma, followed by lung carcinoma, melanoma, neuroendocrine tumours and renal cell carcinoma. Less frequent primaries include skin tumours and hepatocellular carcinoma. Prostate cancers often metastasize to the bone including the orbital bony structures [87]. In a subset of patients, orbital metastases can be the first presentation of cancer with metastases at other locations generally found during work-up. Orbital metastases tend to occur at more than one subsite, such as the retina, orbital adnexa and uveal tract and can extend beyond the orbit. They can present as an orbital mass (with typical mass effect symptoms), as a diffusely infiltrating lesion or as a sclerosing lesion, the last causing enophthalmos [88, 89]. Signal characteristics depend on the primary tumour, but generally metastases are T1-hypointense and T2-hyperintense. Similar to other malignant lesions there is contrast-enhancement and possible central necrosis. Margins are often irregular, although within extrinsic eye muscles they can appear quite smooth. Bony erosions may be present, while calcifications and cysts are rare [87]. Examples of orbital metastases are shown in Figs. 21 and 22.

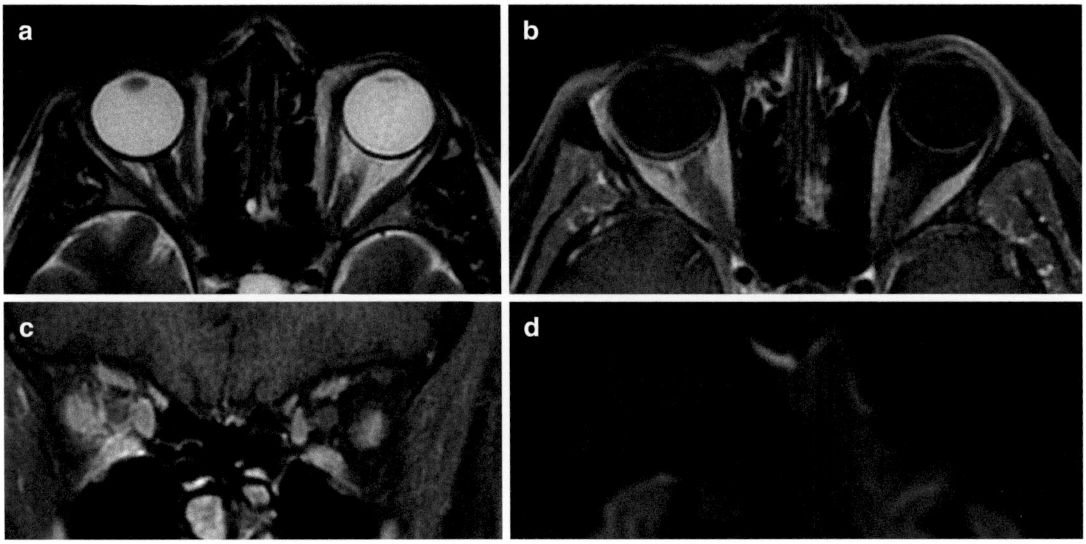

Fig. 21 Biopsy proven sclerosing breast cancer metastasis in the right orbit. Axial T2w image (**a**) showing enophthalmos and decreased orbital fat-volume. Axial T1w post-contrast image (**b**) showing marked enhancement of the intraconal fat as compared to the contralateral orbit. Similar infiltrating enhancement of intraconal and extraconal fat is seen on coronal T1w post-contrast image (**c**). There is no diffusion restriction on DWI (**d**)

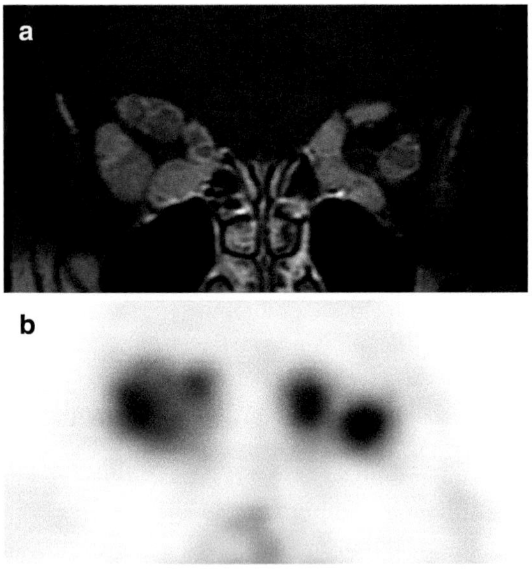

Fig. 22 Bilateral thickening of the extraocular muscles on coronal T1w post contrast (**a**) in a patient with a known neuroendocrine tumor. Axial ^{68}Ga-DOTATATE PET (**b**) shows specific tracer uptake consistent with neuroendocrine tumor extraocular muscle metastases

References

1. Forghani R, Mukherji SK. Advanced dual-energy CT applications for the evaluation of the soft tissues of the neck. Clin Radiol. 2018;73:70–80.
2. Higashigaito K, Mergen V, Eberhard M, Jungblut L, Hebeisen M, Rätzer S, et al. CT angiography of the aorta using photon-counting detector CT with reduced contrast media volume. Radiol Cardiothorac Imaging. 2023;5:e220140.
3. Becker M, Masterson K, Delavelle J, Viallon M, Vargas MI, Becker CD. Imaging of the optic nerve. Eur J Radiol. 2010;74:299–313.
4. Tanenbaum RE, Lobo R, Kahana A, Wester ST. Advances in magnetic resonance imaging of orbital disease. Can J Ophthalmol. 2022;57:217–27.
5. Bae YJ, Choi BS, Jeong HK, Sunwoo L, Jung C, Kim JH. Diffusion-weighted imaging of the head and neck: influence of fat-suppression technique and multishot 2D navigated interleaved acquisitions. Am J Neuroradiol. 2018;39:145–50.
6. Dudau C, Draper A, Gkagkanasiou M, Charles-Edwards G, Pai I, Connor S. Cholesteatoma: multishot echo-planar *vs* non echo-planar diffusion-weighted MRI for the prediction of middle ear and mastoid cholesteatoma. BJR Open. 2019;1:20180015.

7. Ang T, Juniat V, Patel S, Selva D. Evaluation of orbital lesions with DCE-MRI: a literature review. Orbit. 2022;1–9.
8. Ahmed Sultan A, HanyAl-backry M, Mohamed Alhefney E, Ezzat Mosa A, Elmetwally Abdallah Farahat H. Role of MR spectroscopy and diffusion-weighted imaging in diagnosis of orbital masses. Egypt J Radiol Nucl Med. 2018;49:45–53.
9. Kralik SF, Haider KM, Lobo RR, Supakul N, Calloni SF, Soares BP. Orbital infantile hemangioma and rhabdomyosarcoma in children: differentiation using diffusion-weighted magnetic resonance imaging. J Am Assoc Pediatr Ophthalmol Strabismus. 2018;22:27–31.
10. Pradeep T, Ravipati A, Melachuri S, Rajaii F, Campbell AA, Hodgson N, et al. Utility of diffusion-weighted imaging to differentiate benign and malignant solid orbital tumours. Can J Ophthalmol. 2022.
11. Luo S, Sha Y, Wu J, Lin N, Pan Y, Zhang F, et al. Differentiation of malignant from benign orbital tumours using dual-energy CT. Clin Radiol. 2022;77:307–13.
12. Yuan Y, Kuai XP, Chen XS, Tao XF. Assessment of dynamic contrast-enhanced magnetic resonance imaging in the differentiation of malignant from benign orbital masses. Eur J Radiol. 2013;82:1506–11.
13. Scarfe WC, Farman AG. What is cone-beam CT and how does it work? Dent Clin N Am. 2008;52:707–30.
14. Etheridge T, Brintz BJ, Jensen MS, Peralta E, Ayesha A, Jebaraj A, et al. Incidence and severity of asymptomatic ocular injury in adult and pediatric orbital fractures. Orbit. 2022;1–6.
15. Delpachitra SN, Rahmel BB. Orbital fractures in the emergency department: a review of early assessment and management. Emerg Med J. 2016;33:727–31.
16. Winegar BA, Gutierrez JE. Imaging of orbital trauma and emergent non-traumatic conditions. Neuroimaging Clin N Am. 2015;25:439–56.
17. Ho TQ, Jupiter D, Tsai JH, Czerwinski M. The incidence of ocular injuries in isolated orbital fractures. Ann Plast Surg. 2017;78:59–61.
18. Catherine Z, Courvoisier DS, Scolozzi P. Is the pure and impure distinction of orbital fractures clinically relevant with respect to ocular and periocular injuries? A retrospective study of 473 patients. J Craniomaxillofac Surg. 2019;47:1935–42.
19. Richani K, Do TH, Merritt HA, Pfeiffer ML, Chuang AZ, Phillips ME. Screening criteria for detecting severe ocular injuries in the setting of orbital fractures. Ophthal Plast Reconstr Surg. 2019;35:609–14.
20. Balakrishnan S, Harsini S, Reddy S, Tofighi S, Gholamrezanezhad A. Imaging review of ocular and optic nerve trauma. Emerg Radiol. 2020;27:75–85.
21. Rong AJ, Fan KC, Golshani B, Bobinski M, McGahan JP, Eliott D, et al. Multimodal imaging features of intraocular foreign bodies. Semin Ophthalmol. 2019;34:518–32.
22. Colletti G, Biglioli F, Poli T, Dessy M, Cucurullo M, Petrillo M, et al. Vascular malformations of the orbit (lymphatic, venous, arteriovenous): diagnosis, management and results. J Craniomaxillofac Surg. 2019;47:726–40.
23. ISSVA Classification of Vascular Anomalies ©2018 International Society for the Study of Vascular Anomalies. "issva.org/classification". Accessed Dec 2022.
24. Friedrich RE, Grzyska U, Kohlrusch FK, Von Kroge S, Vollkommer T, Luebke AM. Symptomatic intraosseous vascular malformation of infraorbital rim: a case report with literature survey. Anticancer Res. 2020;40:3333–43.
25. Zhang L, Li X, Tang F, Gan L, Wei X. Diagnostic imaging methods and comparative analysis of orbital cavernous hemangioma. Front Oncol. 2020;10:577452.
26. Jayaram A, Cohen LM, Lissner GS, Karagianis AG. A retrospective review of cases preoperatively diagnosed by radiologic imaging as cavernous venous malformations. Orbit. 2017;36:128–34.
27. Sullivan T. Vascular anomalies of the orbit—a reappraisal. Asia-Pac J Ophthalmol. 2018;7:356–63.
28. Ulus OS, Kararaslan E. Orbital varix: CT and MRI findings. Eur J Radiol Extra. 2010;75:e51–3.
29. Roelofs KA, Duckwiler G, Gundlach B, Yoo B, Diniz SB, Cohen LM, et al. Orbital vascular malformations: determining outflow with Valsalva maneuver-augmented computed tomography angiography. Ophthalmology. 2022;129:590–2.
30. Rootman DB, Diniz SB, Cohen LM. Clinical assessment and lesion-specific management of orbital vascular malformations. J Neurol Surg Part B Skull Base. 2021;82:116–28.
31. Kulungowski AM, Patel M. Lymphatic malformations. Semin Pediatr Surg. 2020;29:150971.
32. Dubois J, Thomas-Chaussé F, Soulez G. Common (cystic) lymphatic malformations: current knowledge and management. Tech Vasc Interv Radiol. 2019;22:100631.
33. Shergill A, John P, Amaral JG. Doxycycline sclerotherapy in children with lymphatic malformations: outcomes, complications and clinical efficacy. Pediatr Radiol. 2012;42:1080–8.
34. Horbach SER, Lokhorst MM, Saeed P, de Goüyon Matignon de Pontouraude CMF, Rothová A, van der Horst CMAM. Sclerotherapy for low-flow vascular malformations of the head and neck: a systematic review of sclerosing agents. J Plast Reconstr Aesthet Surg. 2016;69:295–304.
35. Yang P, Ren J, Yu JX, Zhai XD, Hu P, Hong T, et al. Comprehensive treatment and vascular architecture characteristic of high-flow vascular malformations in periorbital regions. J Craniofac Surg. 2021;32:187–92.
36. Murphy C, Livingstone I, Foot B, Murgatroyd H, MacEwen CJ. Orbital cellulitis in Scotland: current incidence, aetiology, management and outcomes: table 1. Br J Ophthalmol. 2014;98:1575–8.
37. Tsirouki T, Dastiridou AI, Ibánez Flores N, Cerpa JC, Moschos MM, Brazitikos P, et al. Orbital cellulitis. Surv Ophthalmol. 2018;63:534–53.
38. Kennedy TA, Corey AS, Policeni B, Agarwal V, Burns J, Harvey HB, et al. ACR appropriateness crite-

ria® orbits vision and visual loss. J Am Coll Radiol. 2018;15:S116–31.
39. Burek AG, Melamed S, Liljestrom T, Qi J, Kelly TG, Suelzer E, et al. Evaluation and medical management of the pediatric patient with orbital cellulitis/abscess: a systematic review. J Hosp Med. 2021;16:680–7.
40. Basily A, Mansukhani S, Anzeljc A, Gutierrez P. Orbital cellulitis—when computed tomography imaging is falsely reassuring. Pediatr Emerg Care. 2021;37:e48–50.
41. Chandler JR, Langenbrunner DJ, Stevens ER. The pathogenesis of orbital complications in acute sinusitis. Laryngoscope. 1970;80:1414–28.
42. Cameron CA, Tong JY, Juniat V, Patel S, Selva D. Diagnostic utility of diffusion-weighted imaging and apparent diffusion coefficient for common orbital lesions: a review. Ophthal Plast Reconstr Surg. 2022;38:515–21.
43. Hunt S, Pereni I, Ford R, Garrott H. Lymphoma and inflammatory disorders presenting in the orbit—a comparison of characteristics from a 10-year series in a tertiary hospital. Orbit. 2022;41:315–20.
44. Nagesh C, Rao R, Hiremath S, Honavar S. Magnetic resonance imaging of the orbit, part 2: characterization of orbital pathologies. Indian J Ophthalmol. 2021;69:2585–616.
45. Mayer E, Herdman G, Burnett C, Kabala J, Goddard P, Potts MJ. Serial STIR magnetic resonance imaging correlates with clinical score of activity in thyroid eye disease. Eye. 2001;15:313–8.
46. Mayer EJ, Fox DL, Herdman G, Hsuan J, Kabala J, Goddard P, et al. Signal intensity, clinical activity and cross-sectional areas on MRI scans in thyroid eye disease. Eur J Radiol. 2005;56:20–4.
47. Tortora F, Cirillo M, Ferrara M, Belfiore MP, Carella C, Caranci F, et al. Disease activity in graves' Ophthalmopathy: diagnosis with orbital MR imaging and correlation with clinical score. Neuroradiol J. 2013;26:555–64.
48. Higashiyama T, Iwasa M, Ohji M. Quantitative analysis of inflammation in orbital fat of thyroid-associated Ophthalmopathy using MRI signal intensity. Sci Rep. 2017;7:16874.
49. Chapman MN, Fujita A, Sung EK, Siegel C, Nadgir RN, Saito N, et al. Sarcoidosis in the head and neck: an illustrative review of clinical presentations and imaging findings. Am J Roentgenol. 2017;208:66–75.
50. Pollock JM, Greiner FG, Crowder JB, Crowder JW, Quindlen E. Neurosarcoidosis mimicking a malignant optic glioma. J Neuroophthalmol. 2008;28:214–6.
51. Prabhakaran VC. Orbital and Adnexal Sarcoidosis. Arch Ophthalmol. 2007;125:1657.
52. Lacomis D. Neurosarcoidosis. Curr Neuropharmacol. 2011;9:429–36.
53. Pakalniskis MG, Berg AD, Policeni BA, Gentry LR, Sato Y, Moritani T, et al. The many faces of granulomatosis with Polyangiitis: a review of the head and neck imaging manifestations. Am J Roentgenol. 2015;205:W619–29.
54. Tee QX, Wong A, Nambiar M, Lau KK. Granulomatosis with polyangiitis: common and uncommon presentations. J Med Imaging Radiat Oncol. 2022;66:1089–96.
55. Ferreira TA, Saraiva P, Genders SW, Buchem MV, Luyten GPM, Beenakker JW. CT and MR imaging of orbital inflammation. Neuroradiology. 2018;60:1253–66.
56. Olsen TG, Heegaard S. Orbital lymphoma. Surv Ophthalmol. 2019;64:45–66.
57. Yeşiltaş Y, Gündüz A. Idiopathic orbital inflammation: review of literature and new advances. Middle East Afr J Ophthalmol. 2018;25:71.
58. McNab AA, McKelvie P. IgG4-related ophthalmic disease. Part I: background and pathology. Ophthal Plast Reconstr Surg. 2015;31:83–8.
59. Soussan JB, Deschamps R, Sadik JC, Savatovsky J, Deschamps L, Puttermann M, et al. Infraorbital nerve involvement on magnetic resonance imaging in European patients with IgG4-related ophthalmic disease: a specific sign. Eur Radiol. 2017;27:1335–43.
60. Ohshima KI, Sogabe Y, Sato Y. The usefulness of infraorbital nerve enlargement on MRI imaging in clinical diagnosis of IgG4-related orbital disease. Jpn J Ophthalmol. 2012;56:380–2.
61. Lecler A, Zmuda M, Deschamps R. Infraorbital nerve involvement on magnetic resonance imaging in Igg4-related ophthalmic disease: a highly suggestive sign. Ophthalmology. 2018;125:577.
62. Demirci H, Shields CL, Shields JA, Honavar SG, Mercado GJ, Tovilla JC. Orbital tumors in the older adult population. Ophthalmology. 2002;109:243–8.
63. Lorenzano D, Rose GE. The "wedge sign": an imaging sign for aggressive lacrimal gland disease. Ophthalmology. 2017;124:1081–3.
64. Politi LS, Forghani R, Godi C, Resti AG, Ponzoni M, Bianchi S, et al. Ocular adnexal lymphoma: diffusion-weighted MR imaging for differential diagnosis and therapeutic monitoring. Radiology. 2010;256:565–74.
65. Eissa L, Abdel Razek AAK, Helmy E. Arterial spin labeling and diffusion-weighted MR imaging: utility in differentiating idiopathic orbital inflammatory pseudotumor from orbital lymphoma. Clin Imaging. 2021;71:63–8.
66. Sun B, Song L, Wang X, Li J, Xian J, Wang F, et al. Lymphoma and inflammation in the orbit: diagnostic performance with diffusion-weighted imaging and dynamic contrast-enhanced MRI. J Magn Reson Imaging. 2017;45:1438–45.
67. Juniat V, Cameron CA, Roelofs K, Bajic N, Patel S, Slattery J, et al. Radiological analysis of orbital lymphoma histological subtypes. Orbit. 2023;42:59–67.
68. Tunlayadechanont P, Panyaping T, Kaewkerd B. Role of quantitative spectral CT analysis for differentiation of orbital lymphoma and other orbital lymphoproliferative disease. Eur J Radiol. 2020;133:109372.
69. Andreoli MT, Aakalu V, Setabutr P. Epidemiological trends in malignant lacrimal gland tumors. Otolaryngol Neck Surg. 2015;152:279–83.

70. Shields CL, Shields JA, Eagle RC, Rathmell JP. Clinicopathologic review of 142 cases of lacrimal gland lesions. Ophthalmology. 1989;96:431–5.
71. Young SM, Kim YD, Shin HJ, Imagawa Y, Lang SS, Woo KI. Lacrimal gland pleomorphic adenoma and malignant epithelial tumours: clinical and imaging differences. Br J Ophthalmol. 2019;103:264–8.
72. See TRO, Stålhammar G, Tang T, Manusow JS, Jordan DR, Nerad JA, et al. Primary ductal adenocarcinoma of the lacrimal gland: a review and report of five cases. Surv Ophthalmol. 2020;65:371–80.
73. Chung EM, Smirniotopoulos JG, Specht CS, Schroeder JW, Cube R. Pediatric orbit tumors and Tumorlike lesions: nonosseous lesions of the extraocular orbit. Radiographics. 2007;27:1777–99.
74. Wang Y, Xiao LH. Orbital schwannomas: findings from magnetic resonance imaging in 62 cases. Eye. 2008;22:1034–9.
75. Demehri S, Belzberg A, Blakeley J, Fayad LM. Conventional and functional MR imaging of peripheral nerve sheath tumors: initial experience. Am J Neuroradiol. 2014;35:1615–20.
76. Lin D, Lin J, Deng X, Li W, Li D, Yin B, et al. Trends in intracranial meningioma incidence in the United States, 2004-2015. Cancer Med. 2019;8:6458–67.
77. Douglas VP, Douglas KAA, Cestari DM. Optic nerve sheath meningioma. Curr Opin Ophthalmol. 2020;31:455–61.
78. Solli E, Turbin RE. Primary and secondary optic nerve sheath meningioma. J Neurol Surg Part B Skull Base. 2021;82:027–71.
79. Watts J, Box G, Galvin A, Brotchie P, Trost N, Sutherland T. Magnetic resonance imaging of meningiomas: a pictorial review. Insights Imaging. 2014;5:113–22.
80. Furusato E, Valenzuela IA, Fanburg-Smith JC, Auerbach A, Furusato B, Cameron JD, et al. Orbital solitary fibrous tumor: encompassing terminology for hemangiopericytoma, giant cell angiofibroma, and fibrous histiocytoma of the orbit: reappraisal of 41 cases. Hum Pathol. 2011;42:120–8.
81. Louis DN, Perry A, Wesseling P, Brat DJ, Cree IA, Figarella-Branger D, et al. The 2021 WHO classification of tumors of the central nervous system: a summary. Neuro Oncol. 2021;23:1231–51.
82. Badawy M, Nada A, Crim J, Kabeel K, Layfield L, Shaaban A, et al. Solitary fibrous tumors: clinical and imaging features from head to toe. Eur J Radiol. 2022;146:110053.
83. Kim HJ, Kim HJ, Kim YD, Yim YJ, Kim ST, Jeon P, et al. Solitary fibrous tumor of the orbit: CT and MR imaging findings. Am J Neuroradiol. 2008;29:857–62.
84. René C, Scollo P, O'Donovan D. A review of solitary fibrous tumours of the orbit and ocular adnexa. Eye. 2023;37:858.
85. Park YW, Kim D, Eom J, Ahn SS, Moon JH, Kim EH, et al. A diagnostic tree for differentiation of adult pilocytic astrocytomas from high-grade gliomas. Eur J Radiol. 2021;143:109946.
86. Karcioglu ZA, Hadjistilianou D, Rozans M, DeFrancesco S. Orbital rhabdomyosarcoma. Cancer Control. 2004;11:328–33.
87. Wladis EJ, Lee KW, Nazeer T. Metastases of systemic malignancies to the orbit: a major review. Orbit. 2021;40:93–7.
88. Grajales-Alvarez R, Gutierrez-Mata A. Orbital metastases from breast cancer: a retrospective analysis of 28 cases. Cancer Treat Res Commun. 2020;24:100184.
89. Chaugule SS, Honavar SG, Finger PT, editors. Surgical ophthalmic oncology: a collaborative open access reference. Cham: Springer International; 2019. Accessed 15 Feb 2023.

Congenital Orbital Disorders

William Rocamora Katowitz and David H. Verity

Key Messages

- Apert and Crouzon syndromes are two of the most common syndromic craniosynostoses and are caused by mutations in the FGFR2 gene. They are characterised by craniosynostosis and midface hypoplasia
- Dermoid cysts should always be removed during infancy due to the risk for rupture, infection and fistulization. Consider an ultrasound if the lesion is in an atypical location, and MRI/CT to exclude intracranial, intra-orbital, and intra-nasal extension.
- Peribulbar dermolipomas can be observed unless visible hairs or keratinization are present. Excision and reconstruction present challenges to maintain cosmesis.
- A small or missing eye will result in a small bony orbit. To prevent facial asymmetry, orbital expansion should be considered at the time of diagnosis in infancy.
- MR imaging is the modality of choice when diagnosing vascular and soft tissue tumours of the orbit.
- MR Diffusion weighted imaging (DWI) is critical in diagnosing suspected malignancies.

W. R. Katowitz (✉)
Division of Ophthalmology, The Children's Hospital of Philadelphia, Philadelphia, PA, USA
e-mail: katowitzw@chop.edu

D. H. Verity
Adnexal Service, Moorfields Eye Hospital, London, UK

St John of Jerusalem Eye Hospital Group, London, UK

1 Malformations of the Bony Orbit

The development of the bony orbit is covered in great detail in Chapter "Embryonic Development of the Orbit". The most common orbital malformation is orbital hypoplasia. Hypoplasia (from ancient Greek ὑπο- hypo- 'under', and πλάσις - plasis - 'formation'; adjective form hypoplastic) is underdevelopment or incomplete development of a tissue or organ. Below is a list of the common deformities seen in congenital orbital bony malformations [1].

- Sphenoid wing dysplasia
- Craniosynostosis: Syndromic and Non-Syndromic
- Clefting syndromes
- Encephalocoele
- Orbital choristomas

1.1 Sphenoid Wing Dysplasia

Sphenoid wing dysplasia describes a complete absence or hypoplasia of the greater sphenoid wing, and is part of the diagnostic criteria of neurofibromatosis type 1 (Fig. 1). NF-1 is associated

F. M. Quaranta Leoni et al. (eds.), *Oculoplastic, Lacrimal and Orbital Surgery*,
https://doi.org/10.1007/978-3-031-39638-0_14

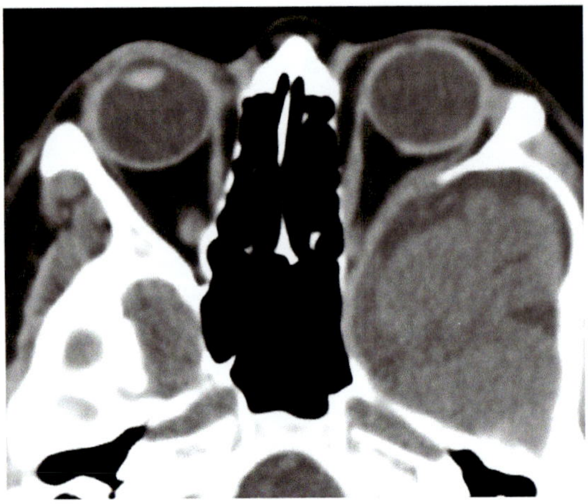

Fig. 1 Hypoplasia of the greater sphenoid wing in neurofibromatosis type 1

with a chromosomal anomaly on chromosome 17. Patients can present with exophthalmos and pulsatile proptosis; depending on the severity of symptoms, orbital reconstruction combined with craniofacial reconstruction can be considered.

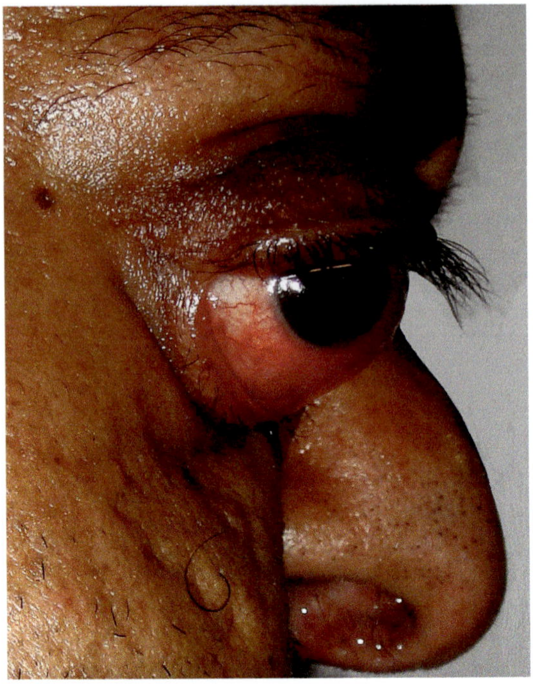

Fig. 2 Crouzon syndrome showing exophthalmos due to early fusion of the developing orbital bones, and psittichorhina (beak-like nose)

1.2 Craniosynostosis

Craniosynostosis (Table 1) describes the early closure of a cranial vault or base suture. The craniosynostoses may be syndromic or non-syndromic. The most common syndromic synostoses include Apert syndrome, Crouzon syndrome (Fig. 2), Pfeiffer syndrome, and Saethre–Chotzen syndrome and are associated with other dysmorphic features. Over 190 congenital syndromes of the head and neck have been identified. The skull and orbital malformations which occur in the different forms of craniosynostosis are given in Table 1.

The American Cleft Palate-Craniofacial Association (ACPA) classification is a simple way to classify the diverse group of craniofacial anomalies:

1. Rare craniofacial clefts using the Tessier classification system
2. Craniosynostosis: (a) Syndromic, (b) Nonsyndromic
3. Atrophy and hypoplasia
4. Neoplasia, hypertrophy, and hyperplasia
5. Unclassified craniofacial deformities

1.2.1 Apert Syndrome

Craniosynostosis causes many of the characteristic facial features of Apert syndrome and is due to genetic mutation to the fibroblast growth factor receptor 2 (FGFR2). Premature fusion of the skull bones prevents the head from growing normally, which leads to a midface hypoplasia (sunken appearance in the middle of the face). The skull morphology is abnormal with elongation of the upper frontal portion of the skull and shortening of the anterior cranial fossa this is called turribrachycephaly with a foreshortened anterior–posterior dimension to the skull and exorbitism.

Ocular features include:

- Exophthalmos due to shallow orbits
- Hypertelorism (wide set eyes)
- Lateral canthal dystopia (down-slanting of palpebral fissures)
- Strabismus (often exotropia)

In addition, patients may have a beaked nose, a wrinkled forehead, cleft palate, missing or crowded teeth, and hearing loss or recurrent ear infections and syndactyly.

Table 1 Skull and orbital malformations in craniosynostosis

Oxycephaly	Multiple synostoses including coronal and sagittal	"Tower skull" (turricephaly alternative term) Compensatory upward movement of the cranium
Brachycephaly	Bilateral coronal suture	Shortened calvarium front to back Upward growth allowed by patent sagittal suture
Acrobrachycephaly	Bilateral coronal with patent anterior fontanelle	Pointed top of the skull Delayed closure of the anterior Fontanelle
Plagiocephaly	Unilateral coronal	Asymmetric deformity Variable depending on extent and location
Scaphocephaly	Interparietal sagittal	Elongated, narrow skull resembling the hull of a ship
Trigonocephaly	Metopic	Triangular frontal area keel-shaped forehead
Triphyllocephaly	Lambdoidal and coronal	"Cloverleaf skull" (Kleeblattschadel) Trilobar skull with cerebral eventration through open sagittal suture and anterior fontanelle

1.2.2 Crouzon Syndrome

Crouzon syndrome is also due to a mutation in the FGFR2 gene (Fig. 2), sharing certain features in common with Apert syndrome with the exception of syndactyly [2]. Crouzon syndrome is considered to be less severe with less asymmetry as compared to Apert syndrome. Cranial vault decompression with reshaping, midfacial and orbital advancement procedures, often in conjunction with a mandibular setback are the most frequent cranio-maxillofacial operations performed for these syndromes.

1.2.3 Pfeiffer Syndrome

Pfeiffer syndrome is caused by a mutation in the FGFR1 or 2 gene and shares some features with Apert syndrome, and is distinguished by a broad thumb and great toe. The craniosynostosis usually causes a very tall forehead and wide, short skull. There is midface hypoplasia with a crescent moon or sunken facial appearance with depressed nasal bridge and beak nose. Decreased growth of the central face can contribute to obstructive sleep apnea and airway concerns.

Ophthalmic findings include

- Shallow orbits
- Hypertelorism
- Down-slanting palpebral fissure
- Midface hypoplasia

1.2.4 Treacher Collins Syndrome

Treacher Collins syndrome is characterised by the classic micrognathia, hypoplastic zygomas with lower eyelid colobomas and is caused by a mutation in the TCOF1, POLR1C, or POLR1D gene. Characteristic eye findings include:

- Hypoplastic zygoma
- Lateral canthal dystopia
- Downward-sloping eyelids
- Pseudocoloboma or true coloboma (usually of the lateral lower eyelid)
- Flattening of the nasofrontal angle
- Underdeveloped or missing eyebrow bones

Additional findings include:

- External ear malformations
- Conductive hearing loss
- Micrognathia with macrostomia
- Abnormal dentition with malocclusion.
- Treacher Collins syndrome

1.2.5 Plagiocephaly and Non-Syndromic Craniosynostosis

Plagiocephaly is a term coined by Virchow to describe the bony abnormality resulting from the unilateral premature closure of the coronal suture, producing a variety of asymmetric deformities, the nature of which depends on the location and extent of synostosis. This can also result in facial asymmetry and relative exophthalmos. Plagiocephaly can also be positional, due to intrauterine position, or acquired in the neonatal period due to torticollis. The treatment for positional plagiocephaly is 'helmet therapy', or placing a wedge under a child's head while sleeping.

1.3 Cephalocoele

Orbital cephalocoele represent the failure of embryonic surface ectoderm to separate from neuroectoderm, resulting in continued intimacy of these developing tissues. A persistent connection between brain tissue, meninges, or the combination of these with orbital contents is broadly termed orbital cephalocoele. More specifically, meningeal herniation is termed meningocoele, while the presence of both brain and meninges is called meningoencephalocoele. The term encephalocoele would apply to the herniation of the brain alone, which in the orbit is usually heterotopic tissue without true connection to the intracranial cavity. Cephalocoele can present with midline deformities, including masses above or below the medial canthus. Rarely, they present at birth with a similar appearance to a lacrimal mucocoele. Figure 3 shows a child with a large orbital encephalocoele, and Fig. 4 an adult with an associated arachnoid cyst.

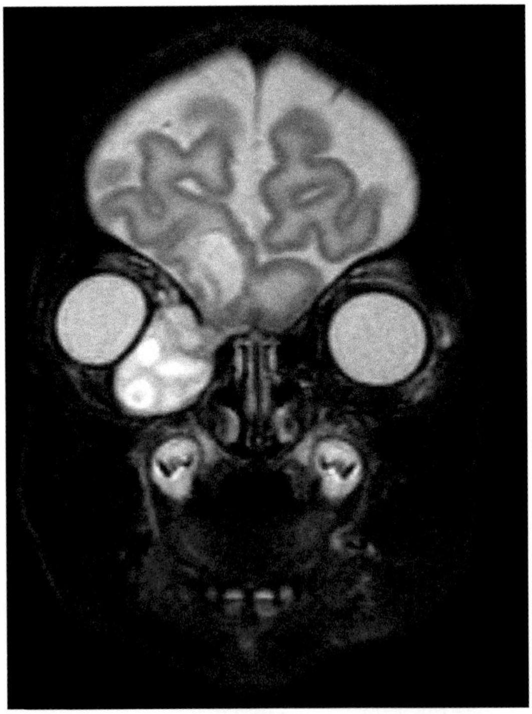

Fig. 3 Orbital encephalocoele. MRI T-2 weighted coronal imaging showing a large right orbital encephalocoele due to a malformation of the fronto-ethmoidal suture. There is right hyperglobus

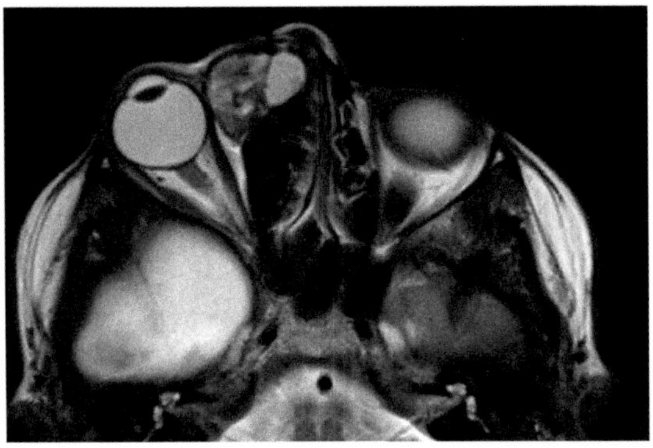

Fig. 4 MRI identifying a large left sided intracranial arachnoid cyst and an associated right fronto-ethmoid encephalocoele extending into the medial aspect of the orbit

1.4 Orbital Choristoma

Orbital choristomas are caused by early separation of ectodermal cells, resulting in an orbital cyst that is classically near to (or entrapped by) a bony suture of the orbit. The word choristoma is from the Greek word χωριστός - choristos - which means separated. This malformation is normal tissue in an abnormal place and classically presents as a superotemporal mass in the lateral eyelid. The different types of choristomas found near the eyes are

- Dermoid cysts
- Epidermoid cysts
- Congenital conjunctival cysts
- Lipodermoid (or dermolipomas)
- Limbal dermoids and epibulbar osseous choristoma
- Phacomatous choristoma (Zimmerman's tumour)

1.4.1 Dermoid Cysts

Orbital dermoid cysts are of ectodermal origin, and can contain skin appendage structures such as hairs. They may also contain tissues that form bone and teeth. Many dermoid cysts are filled with keratin, which over time may leak into the subcutaneous tissue or present as a draining, foul smelling skin fistula. The diagnosis and management of dermoid cysts is greatly aided by the location of their presentation. Lesions located in the upper and outer orbit or eyelid (Fig. 5) are typically firm and mobile under the skin. Such lesions typically do not need to be imaged as they will rarely have deeper bony involvement. Any suspected dermoid lesions that are fixed to the orbit or at another location should warrant concern for intra-orbital, intracranial or intranasal extension (Figs. 6a, b, 7a, b and 8).

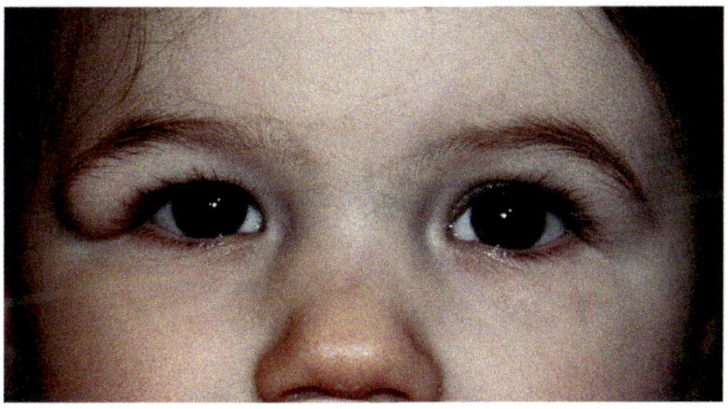

Fig. 5 Periorbital dermoid cyst. The mass is firm and freely mobile in the superotemporal orbital quadrant. This is the most common location for a dermoid cyst

1.4.2 Epidermoid Cyst

Epidermoid cysts are classically fluid-filled and lack the additional ectodermal appendages. They are difficult to distinguish clinically from dermoid cysts. It is best to remove a dermoid cyst or epidermoid cyst during infancy because these lesions can become infected, leak, rupture, or fistulize. Below is a treatment protocol to consider for dermoid cysts.

- Periorbital mass
- Superotemporal—if non-fixed, defer imaging
- Image all mass that are nasal, inferior and fixed to the deeper periosteum
- Imaging modalities to consider
  - Ultrasound—This modality differentiates vascular lesions from cysts, and can be use-

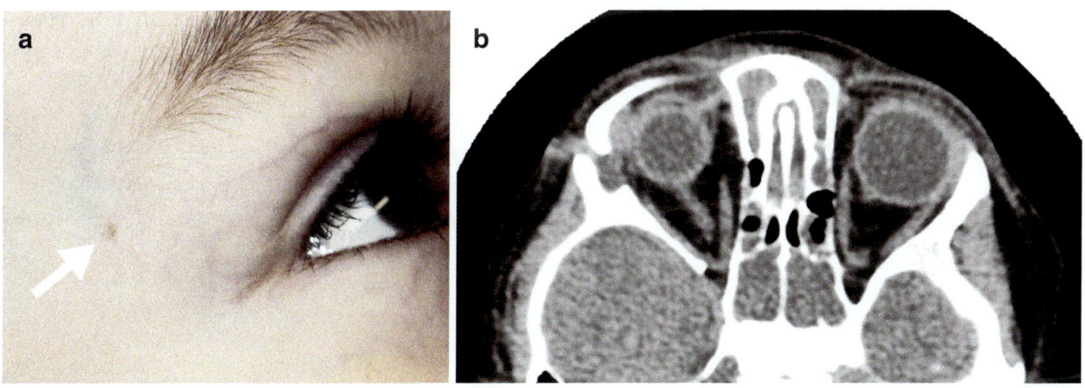

Fig. 6 Dermoid cyst with intra-orbital extension. (**a**) Temporal cutaneous fistula. (**b**) CT axial image showing a bony defect with extension of the choristoma into the orbit

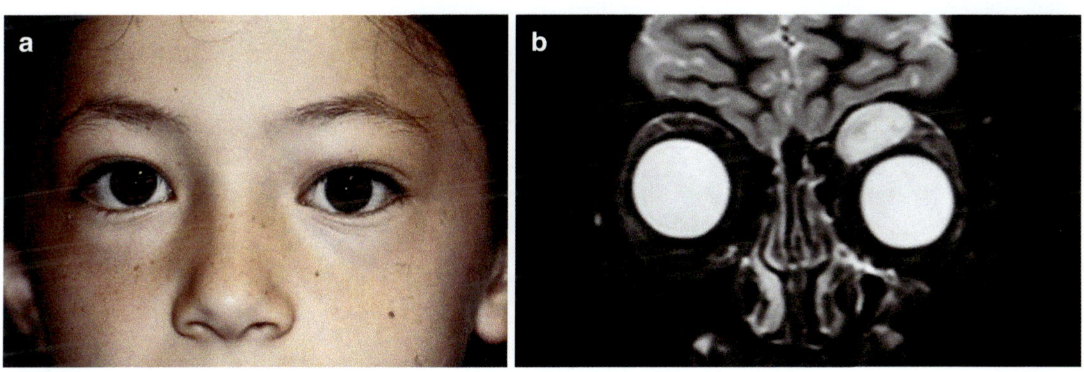

Fig. 7 Orbital dermoid cyst. (**a**) A patient presents with orbital asymmetry. There is relative hypoglobus of the left eye. (**b**) MRI T-2 weighted imaging with a large homogenous mass in the superior orbit

ful when an infantile hemangioma is suspected.
  - CT—This identifies intraosseous involvement of a dermoid cyst, but carries the risk of radiation exposure
  - MRI—This is the safer option when compared to CT but requires more sedation and does not clearly identify the bony orbit.
- Management—consider surgical excision after the age of 6 months

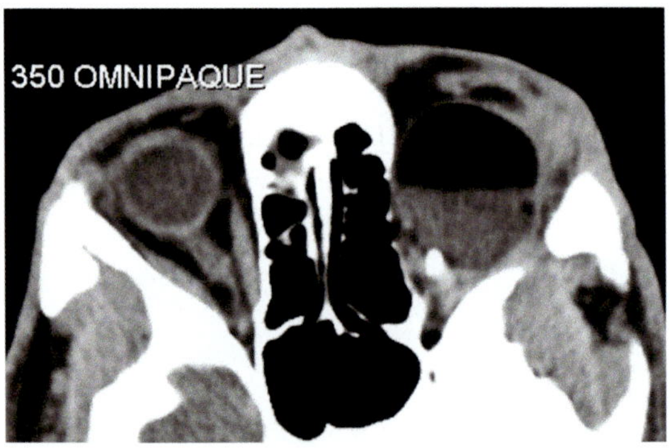

Fig. 8 CT identifying a deep orbital dermoid and internal fluid level due to supernatant oil

1.4.3 Congenital Conjunctival Cyst

Congenital conjunctival cysts of the orbit are rare, presenting with a soft mass in the upper eyelid. These can be anatomically related to the superior rectus muscle or levator palpebrae, (or their common sheath), superior rectus, and superior oblique muscles [3], and therefore require great care in their excision (Fig. 9a, b).

1.4.4 Dermolipoma

Dermolipomas (also referred to as lipodermoids) are choristomas consisting of fat and connective tissue structures and are considered to have further differentiated from their ectodermal origin in contrast to dermoid cysts, which by contrast can contain bone and teeth. These lesions are associated with Goldenhar syndrome and hemifacial microsomia, and can be present in the infero- or supero-temporal peri bulbar region (Figs. 10 and 11). They should be differentiated from herniated or prolapsed orbital fat which, in contrast, is readily reduced posteriorly with gentle pressure over the eyelids.

Dermolipomas can be observed, or excised if they cause evident disfigurement in the primary position [4]. Complete surgical excision is rarely possible as the malformation can be closely asso-

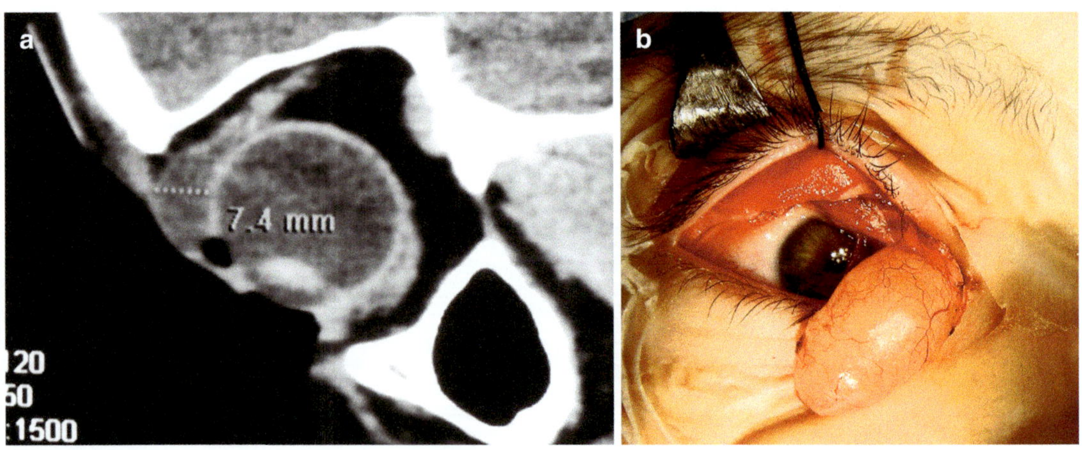

Fig. 9 Orbital conjunctival cyst (lacking dermal structures). (**a**) Sagittal CT identifying lesion. (**b**) Intact excision of lesion via the superior conjunctival fornix

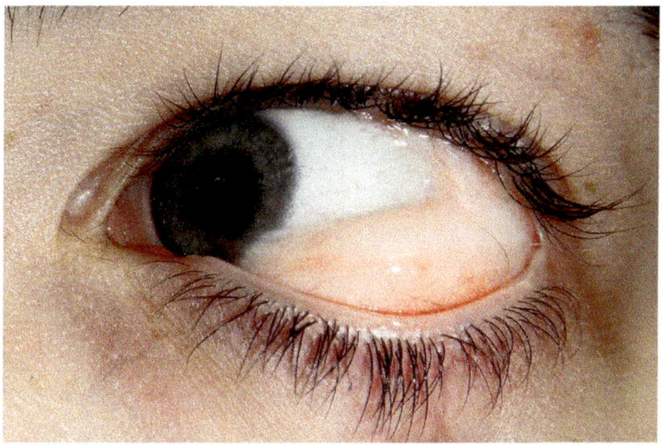

Fig. 10 Peribulbar dermolipoma. A patient with Goldenhar syndrome presents with a right peribulbar lesion. Note the presence of hairs

ciated with deeper orbital structures, including Tenon's capsule, extraocular muscles, sclera, and the lacrimal gland. Partial surgical excision of the visible portion of the malformation including the non-conjunctival epithelium can be performed (Fig. 11); conjunctival reconstruction can be challenging, and post-operative scarring with chronic injection can occur.

1.4.5 Limbal Dermoids

Four variants of limbal dermoids have been described: dermoid (Fig. 12), lipodermoid, complex choristoma, and epibulbar osseous choristoma (Fig. 13) [5]. Most are dermoid, formed of

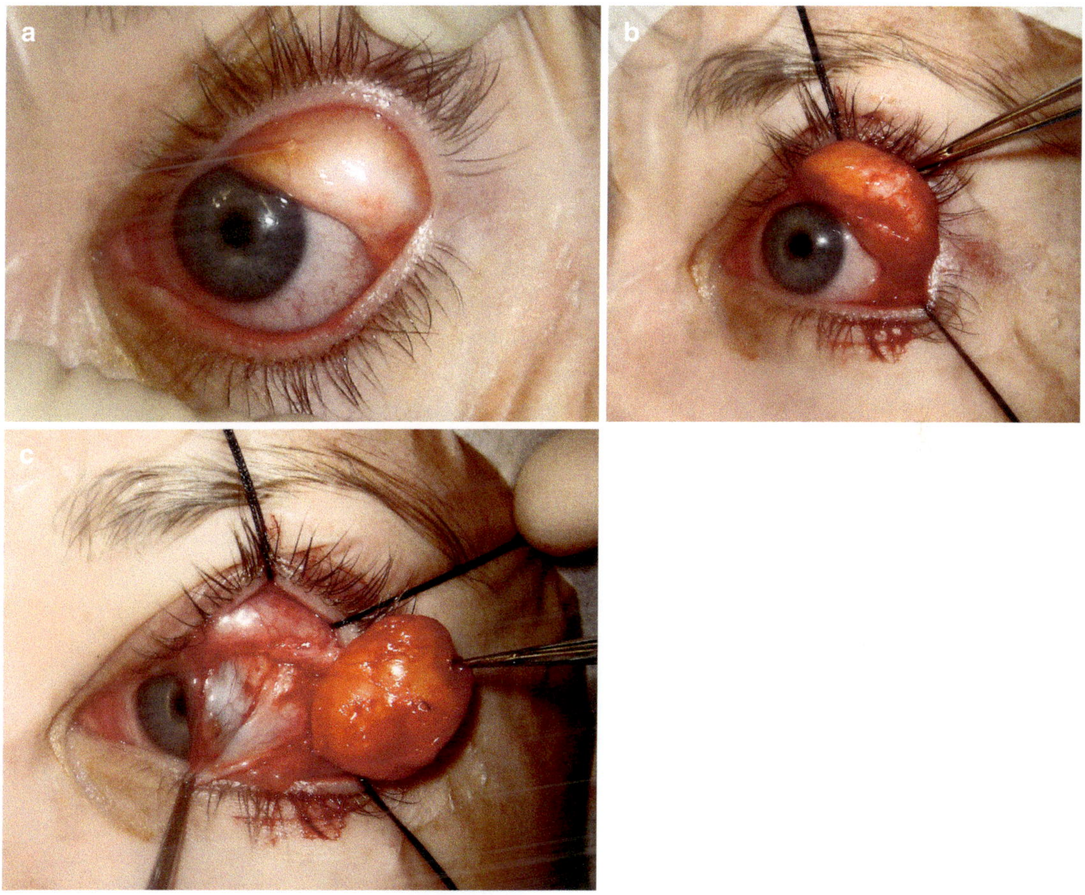

Fig. 11 Excision of left dermolipoma. (**a**) Large superotemporal dermolipoma. (**b**) The island of *abnormal* conjunctiva (but not normal conjunctiva) is excised. (**c**) Careful dissection of the anterior part of the lesion. Note, the lesion lies over the insertion of the lateral rectus muscle, and is continuous with orbital adipose tissue. The lesion is truncated across its base without excessive tissue removal. The conjunctiva is closed horizontally (and not vertically) to avoid post-operative horizontal diplopia

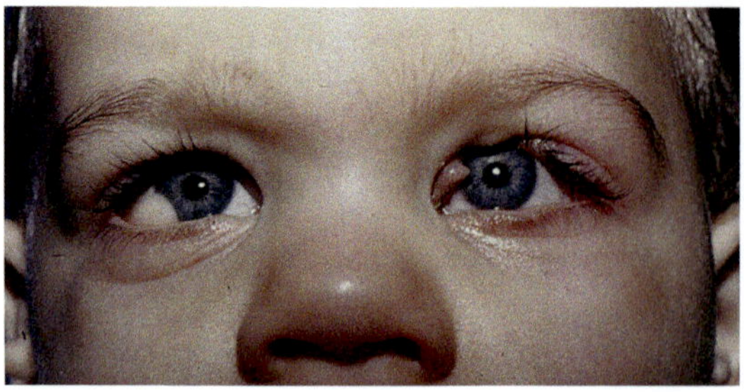

Fig. 12 Patient with Goldenhaur's syndrome: note the presence of a left upper eyelid coloboma, and a right paralimbal dermoid

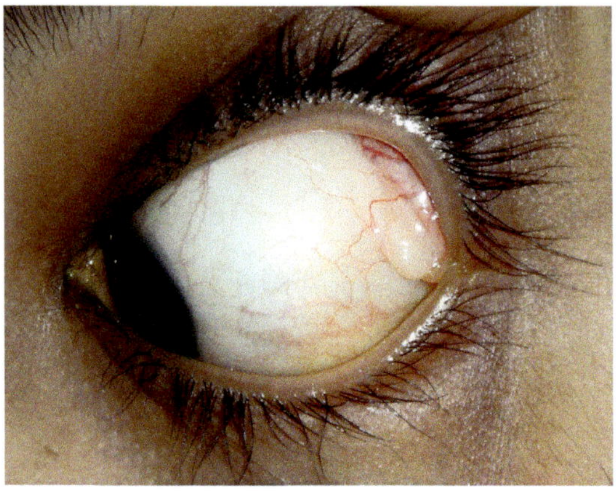

Fig. 13 Parabulbar osseous choristoma: Note, these benign lesions can be noted coincidentally on a skull radiology and mistaken for an orbital or even intraocular foreign body

solid choristoma with a surface epithelium similar to epidermis and dermis. Lipodermoid is usually superficial with an abundance of adipose tissue and fewer adnexal elements. In distinction, complex choristomas contain smooth muscle, lacrimal elements, and neural tissue. Epibulbar osseous choristomas typically present as a supero-temporal subconjunctival nodule with imaging identifying a densely radio-opaque fleck on the sclera, this often being misinterpreted as a parabulbar foreign body [6].

Treatment is frequently conservative, but where they induce astigmatism and risk amblyopia, or are aesthetically unacceptable, surgical excision followed by aggressive amblyopia treatment is advocated. Excision of the dermoid, followed by filling of the residual defect with amniotic membrane and pericardial patch graft with overlying autologous limbal stem cell transplantation has been described [7].

1.4.6 Phacomatous Choristoma

Phakomatous choristoma was first described in 1971 by Zimmerman [8]. A proliferation of ectopic lens tissue, it presents in infancy as an enlarging mass in the medial lower eyelid or orbit, and can masquerade as a dacryocystocoele. Histology identifies lens-type epithelium, with degenerate areas reminiscent of the "bladder-like" or Wedl cells seen in cataract. Pathogenesis remains uncertain, but could include migration of surface ectoderm into the mesoderm of the developing eyelid, 'escape' of developing lens tissue through the closing optic fissure, or that the invaginating ectoderm (which gives rise to the lens) is located in the same area due to form the medial lower eyelid.

Most of the reported cases were isolated findings without ocular or orbital abnormalities, although associated colobomatous hypoplastic optic disc with staphyloma, and severe myopia, have been reported.

2 Microphthalmia/Anophthalmia

Microphthalmia refers to a small malformed eye. Anophthalmia is the absence of an eye (Fig. 14). Most cases of microphthalmia/anophthalmia are caused by sporadic mutations (eg. SOX2, CHX10, PAX gene) or from a malformation

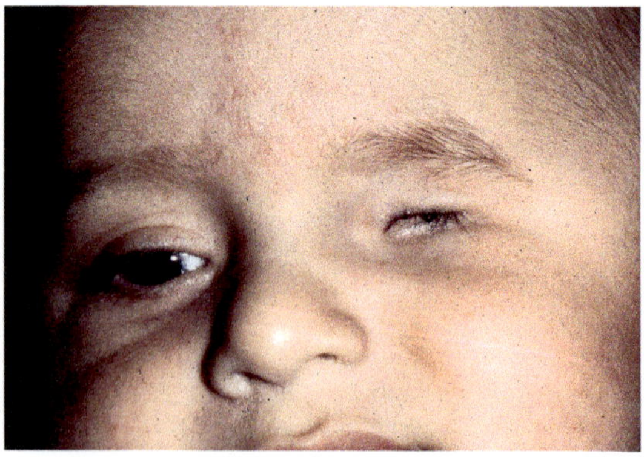

Fig. 14 A child with congenital anophthalmia

within the eye such as a persistent primary hyperplastic primary vitreous.

A microphthalmic eye may be associated with a cyst. This is usually due to a coloboma of the uveal tissue of the eye and can result in overexpansion of the orbit [9]. The management of congenital anophthalmia and microphthalmia is discussed in greater detail in Chapter "Congenital Anophthalmia and Microphthalmia".

- A small or missing eye may result in small orbit with facial asymmetry
- Early intervention is necessary to promote bony growth
- The visual potential of the microphthalmic eye must be assessed as this will determine the kind of intervention
- Orbital expanders and serial conformers both accomplish successful bony expansion when eyelids are present
- An ocularist is a critical member of the care team for each patient
- A genetic evaluation is needed for all microphthalmic and anophthalmic patients
- Abnormalities of the eyelid occurring in association with microphthalmia include eyelid coloboma, decreased horizontal and vertical palpebral fissure length, and decreased conjunctival surface area with relative shortening of the posterior lamellae with or without congenital entropion
- Associated systemic abnormalities may involve the central nervous system, face (cleft lip or palate, hemifacial microsomia, facial hypoplasia, micrognathia), skeletal system (anomalous limbs), ear (pre-auricular skin tags, deafness), heart (ventricular septal defects, tetralogy of Fallot, coarctation of the aorta), genito-urinary system, and gastrointestinal system

3 Vasculature Malformations of the Orbit

Vascular malformations of the orbit occur during embryogenesis and may be present at birth or during childhood due to expansion of the vascular or lymphatic spaces. The International Society for the Study of Vascular Anomalies (ISSVA) modified their classification system in 2018 and describes the type of each malformation based on the vessel type [10]. These can occur as isolated malformations (such as venous or arterial) or as a combined lesion (such as lymphatic and venous - now referred to as lymphatico-venous malformation and previously referred to as lymphangioma). The diagnosis and management of vascular anomalies of the orbit is discussed in greater detail in Chapter "Orbital Vascular Anomalies and Vascular Tumours".

- Orbital lymphangioma is now referred to as 'lymphatico-venous malformation' (LVM, Fig. 15). These lesions can manifest in childhood with gradually progressive proptosis and periorbital swelling. Spontaneous intralesional haemorrhage or venous thrombosis can cause acute proptosis with marked pain and compressive optic neuropathy. They are also associated with ipsilateral conjunctival, episcleral, facial, hard and soft palate disease, and intracranial vascular anomalies.
- LVM may be predominantly microcytic with vascular spaces under 10 mm in diameter, or macrocystic with vascular spaces over 10 mm in diameter.
- In general, microcystic lesions within the orbit are most amenable to sclerotherapy proce-

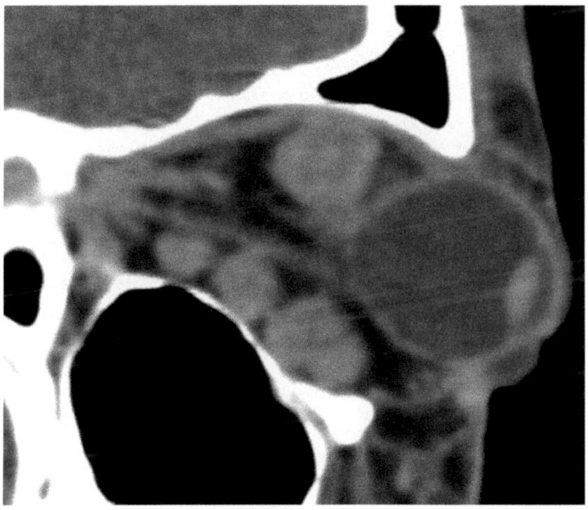

Fig. 15 Orbital lymphatico-venous malformation: Computed tomography (CT) identifies multiple non-enhancing lobulated lesions causing proptosis

dures under guidance, this performed by an interventional radiologist.

- Sclerosing agents include bleomycin, doxycycline, and sodium tetradecyl.
- MRI imaging is critical in the diagnosis of vascular malformations
- Interventions can be deferred for cases of disfigurement, pain or when impacting a patient's vision
- PIK3CA-related disorders include vascular malformations and overgrowth of various tissues that are caused by postzygotic, somatic variants in the gene encoding phosphatidylinositol-3-kinase (PI3K) catalytic subunit alpha. These mutations result in activation of the PI3K/AKT/mTOR signalling pathway.
- Vascular lesions positive for the PIK3CA mutation can respond to rapamycin (sirolimus) therapy.
- Microcystic LVM lesions can be treated empirically with rapamycin or biopsied first to confirm the PIK3CA mutation before treatment.

Capillary malformations (CM) present as a large spectrum of anomalies:

- Naevus simplex/salmon patch, "angel kiss", "stork bite"
- Cutaneous and/or mucosal CM (also known as "port-wine" stain)
- Nonsyndromic CM
- CM with CNS and/or ocular anomalies (Sturge-Weber syndrome)

It can be clinically difficult to differentiate a port-wine stain, nevus simplex, and segmental infantile hemangioma. While naevus simplex and infantile hemangioma will eventually fade, a port-wine stain will not (Fig. 16).

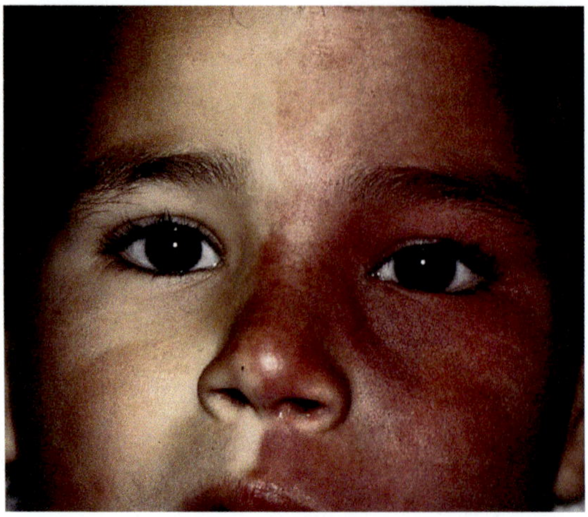

Fig. 16 Cutaneous capillary malformation (also known as "port-wine" stain)

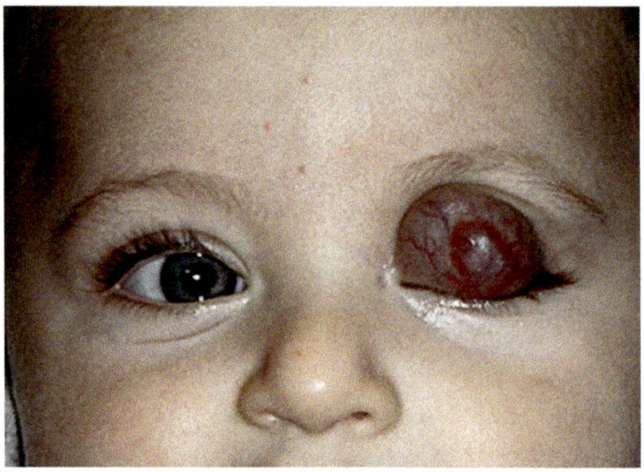

Fig. 17 Large upper eyelid capillary haemangioma associated causing amblyopia: urgent treatment with beta-blockade is indicated

3.1 Tumours of the Orbit

The diagnosis and management of tumours in and around the orbit are discussed in detail in other chapters of this section. Infantile hemangioma is the most common tumour of infancy but is rarely visible at birth.

- The history of presentation is critical: not present at birth, but typically appearing days to weeks after birth (Figs. 17 and 18) [11].
- Rapid growth until 10 months of age with slow involution over the next 5–9 years which may or may not be complete [11].
- They be difficult to distinguish from other vascular tumours such as malformations on MRI and CT imaging modalities, however with contrast and fat suppression on MR the lesion is better delineated
- Orbital ultrasound with doppler flow studies can differentiate these from other vascular

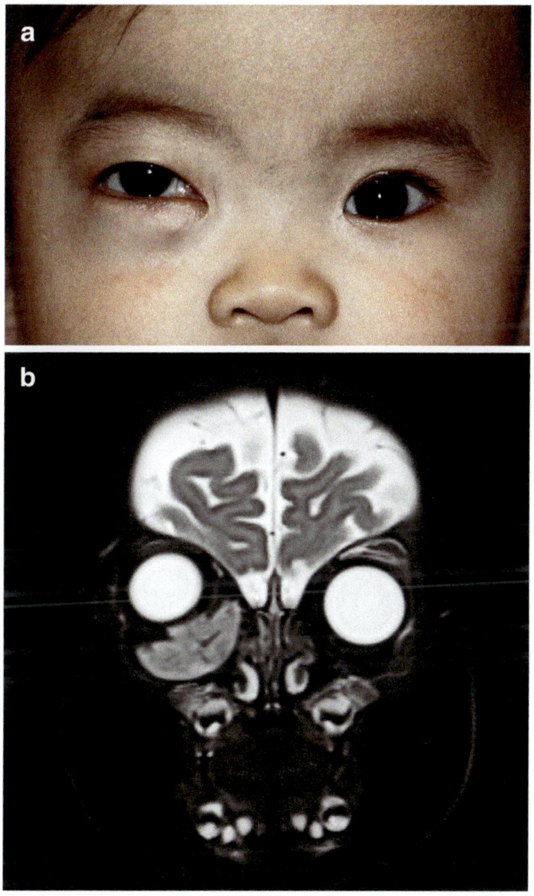

Fig. 18 Orbital infantile haemangioma. (**a**) 5 month-old present with a right orbital mass and superior globe displacement. (**b**) MRI T-2 weighted imaging showing a large mass in the inferior orbit with superior globe displacement. There are flow voids within the lesion consistent with an infantile hemangioma

tumours, obviating the need for more expensive and time-intensive imaging such as MRI

- Note, doppler ultrasonography will often identify internal blood flow in CM as high as 1 m/s (Fig. 19).

Infantile hemangiomas are described clinically as

- Focal
- Multifocal
- Segmental
- Indeterminate

Large facial haemangiomas (> 20 cm^2) are associated with an increased risk of other systemic abnormalities (PHACE syndrome).

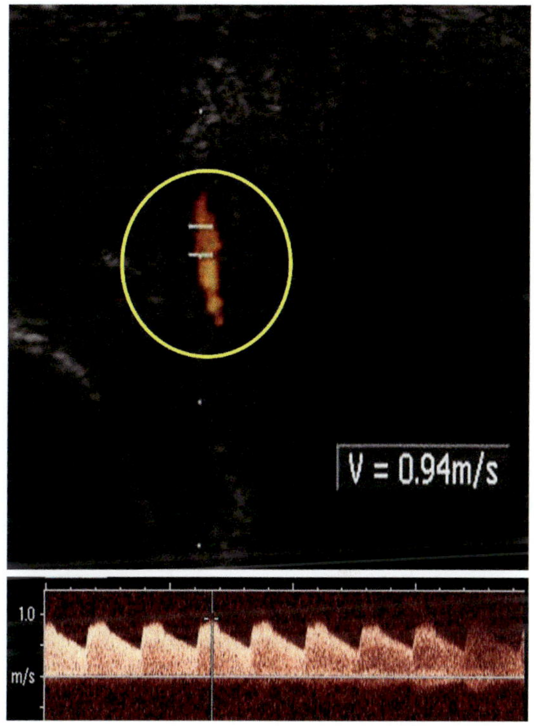

Fig. 19 Spectral Doppler techniques: A region of vessels is selected using a gate (upper image, high-flow vessel identified). A spectrogram of velocity vs. time is plotted, identifying arterial wave forms with velocities as high as 1 m/s

Segmental haemangiomas are large plaque-like patterns of a haemangioma that are associated with PHACE and usually grow in a pattern that follows zones of facial development and not dermatomes.

Infantile haemangiomas are positive for the Glut-1 surface protein. This is useful in distinguishing these lesions from other types of congenital vascular anomalies.

Infantile haemangiomas are usually responsive to oral beta-blockers, but will often require over 12 months of treatment to allow.

Some infantile haemangiomas result in a fibro-fatty infiltration that does not fully involute and warrants surgical debulking or liposuction.

All other tumours of the orbit are rare and warrant urgent imaging (such as in orbital teratomas or rhabdoid tumours).

- MRI imaging of the orbit is critical to diagnose orbital tumours
- CT imaging has a less helpful role in diagnosing soft tissue lesions
- Diffusion weighted imaging (DWI) on MRI modality is critical to diagnose suspected malignant lesions.
- Orbital dermoid cysts can restrict diffusion on the apparent diffusion coefficient sequence on DWI imaging and can mimic a malignancy.

References

1. Naran S, Spadola MF, Storm PB, Bartlett SP. Oculoplastic considerations in pediatric craniofacial surgery. In: Katowitz JA, Katowitz WR, editors. Pediatric oculoplastic surgery. 2nd ed. Cham: Springer; 2018.
2. Stavropoulos D, Tarnow P, Mohlin B, Kahnberg KE, Hagberg V. Comparing patients with Apert and Crouzon syndromes—clinical features and cranio-maxillofacial surgical reconstruction. Comparative study. Swed Dent J. 2012;36:25–34.
3. Wilde C, Vahdani K, Thaung C, Rose GE. Congenital conjunctival cysts of the orbit. Ophthal Plast Reconstr Surg. 2022;38:280–2.
4. Vahdani K, Rose GE. The presentation and surgical treatment of peribulbar dermolipomas. Ophthal Plast Reconstr Surg. 2021;37:226–9.
5. Zhong J, Deng Y, Zhang P, Li S, Huang H, Wang B, Zhang H, Peng L, Yang R, Xu J, Yuan J. New grading system for Limbal dermoid: a retrospective analysis of 261 cases over a 10-year period. Cornea. 2018;37:66–71.
6. Verity DH, Rose GE, Uddin JM, Adams GG, Luthert P. Epibulbar osseous choristoma: benign pathology simulating an intraorbital foreign body. Orbit. 2007;26:29–32.
7. Abdulmannan DM. Successful management of limbal dermoid in infancy and childhood: a case series. Cureus. 2022;14:e22835.
8. Zimmerman LE. Phakomatous choristoma of the eyelid. A tumor of lenticular anlage. Am J Ophthalmol. 1971;71:169–77.
9. Revere K, Katowitz JA, Nazemzadeh M, Katowitz W. Management of the microphthalmic orbit. In: Katowitz JA, Katowitz WR, editors. Pediatric oculoplastic surgery. 2nd ed. Cham: Springer; 2018.
10. Kunimoto K, Yamamoto Y, Jinnin M. ISSVA classification of vascular anomalies and molecular biology. Int J Mol Sci. 2022;23:2358.
11. Verity DH, Restorie M, Rose GE. The natural history of blood velocity and lesion size in infantile orbital capillary haemangiomata. Eye. 2006;20:1228–37.

Orbital Rhabdomyosarcoma

Peerooz Saeed, William Rocamora Katowitz,
Lelio Baldeschi, and Lama Jurdy

Key Messages

- Rhabdomyosarcoma (RMS) is the most common soft-tissue sarcoma of the head and neck in childhood. It comprises 4% of all paediatric malignancies, with 10% of all cases occurring in the orbit, and is one of the few life-threatening diseases that present first to the ophthalmologist.
- A detailed history is essential in any child under 2 years of age presenting with an orbital mass and suspected to have orbital RMS. Imaging plays an important role, and biopsy should be performed if RMS is suspected based on clinical and radiological findings.
- RMS is divided into three histological subgroups: pleomorphic, embryonal, and alveolar. Most orbital RMS are of the embryonal subtype; the pleomorphic subtype occurs almost exclusively in adults.
- With the introduction of surgery combined with adjuvant chemotherapy and radiotherapy in cooperative group trials, survival has improved to around 90%. There is no known benefit to debulking over biopsy alone, and patients with primary orbital RMS fare well regardless of the extent of the initial resection. This finding has shifted the surgical approach from maximal excisional biopsy and debulking to incisional biopsy.
- Radiation technologies which are currently used for RMS include proton beam radiotherapy, intensity modulated radiotherapy (IMRT), 3-D conformational radiotherapy and implant brachytherapy. All aim to minimise the radiation dose to normal tissue.

P. Saeed (✉)
Orbital Centre, Department of Ophthalmology, Amsterdam University Medical Center, Amsterdam, The Netherlands
e-mail: p.saeed@amsterdamumc.nl

W. R. Katowitz
Division of Ophthalmology, The Children's Hospital of Philadelphia, Philadelphia, PA, USA

L. Baldeschi
Department of Ophthalmology, Catholic University of Louvain, Academic Hospital Saint Luc, Brussels, Belgium

L. Jurdy
Orbital Center—Amsterdam University Medical Center, Amsterdam, The Netherlands

1 Introduction, General Characteristics, and Epidemiology

Rhabdomyosarcoma (RMS) is a highly malignant tumour in which the tissue of origin is pluripotent mesenchyme [1]. It is the most common soft-tissue sarcoma of the head and neck in childhood and comprises 4% of all paediatric malignancies, with 10% of all cases occurring in the orbit [1, 2]. Most of these tumours occur in the

F. M. Quaranta Leoni et al. (eds.), *Oculoplastic, Lacrimal and Orbital Surgery*,
https://doi.org/10.1007/978-3-031-39638-0_15

first decade of life, [3] however RMS has been reported from birth to the eighth decade [1, 4, 5].

The incidence of malignant orbital tumours in general has been increasing [6]. Turner et al. in a study of population based incidence and survival in head and neck RMS reported an annual percentage increase of 1.16% and a statistically unchanged 5-year survival over the past 30 years despite advances in treatment modalities, although other studies have reported improved survival [3, 7]. Relative survival (RS) was more dependent on the extent of disease at presentation, rather than primary site, and it was noted that most orbital RMS tumours (60.6%) presented with localised disease and consequently had a 5-year survival of about 84.3%, which was more favourable when compared with other sites in the head and neck [3, 8]. Other factors positively influencing survival were younger age (<10 years), female sex and embryonal subtype (the most common in the orbit) [1, 4, 8–10].

Orbital RMS is one of the few life-threatening diseases that present first to the ophthalmologist. A prompt diagnosis and treatment can be life-saving, and knowledge of the clinical, histopathological, and radiographic features as well as the more recent advances in the management of this entity is essential [2].

2 Clinical Features

Patients with orbital RMS usually present with acute or subacute exophthalmos and/or eyeball dystopia developing rapidly over days to weeks (80–100%). Eyeball dystopia is usually downward and outward because two-thirds of these tumours are supero-nasal [1, 2, 4].

Metastatic spread of orbital RMS is uncommon, however if left untreated RMS has a propensity to metastasize to the lung, bone and bone marrow mainly via haematogenous spread. Locally, orbital RMS can invade the orbital bones and can extend intracranially [2]. Metastatic orbital RMS has an unfavourable prognosis when compared to localised disease; however, in a joint European-North American pooled analysis, a primary orbital site proved to have a favourable prognosis [1, 2, 11, 12].

3 Diagnosis

A detailed history is essential in any child under 2 years of age and presenting with an orbital mass, and suspected to have orbital RMS [2]. The ophthalmologist should specifically ask about pain, visual decrease or loss, symptoms of sinusitis, and should also keep in mind possible misleading presentations such as rapidly progressing alterations of eyelids, conjunctiva or caruncle [1, 2, 13].

The history will help exclude other differential diagnoses, particularly other causes of exophthalmos/eyeball dystopia in children, such as orbital cellulitis, lymphangioma, idiopathic orbital inflammation, dermoid cyst, haemangioma, Langerhans cell histiocytosis (eosinophilic granuloma), sarcomas, metastatic neuroblastoma, and lymphoma [2]. Imaging also plays an important role in the differentiation of these conditions. Biopsy should be performed if RMS is suspected based on clinical and radiological findings [2].

4 Imaging

Orbital RMS is usually extraconal (37–87%) or both intra- and extraconal (13–47%), and more commonly superonasal in location, especially for embryonal subtype (inferior location is more common for alveolar subtype) [4, 9, 14–16]. The mass is usually close to extraocular muscles, but there is no enlargement of the muscle belly [9]. In early stages the tumour is well circumscribed, but in later stages, where there is pseudo capsular invasion, the borders are irregular [2]. There may be some bone deformity, but frank bone destruction with bone involvement is rare, and the diagnosis in this case will change from orbital to parameningeal RMS [15]. The tumour may show area of haemorrhage and cyst formation [2].

4.1 Ultrasound (US)

US findings are neither specific for orbital RMS nor sensitive for detecting parameningeal spread, and US penetration into deeper tissues is limited; hence reports on US findings in orbital tumours are limited [9, 15, 17]. It mainly appears as a well-circumscribed, heterogeneous, irregular mass with low to medium echogenicity on US and a variable intratumoral vascular flow pattern on Doppler US [9, 17]. A "pseudocystic" appearance has been reported as characteristic, and that is thought to be due to spindle cells in embryonal RMS which have abundant cytoplasm and are separated loosely by oedematous fluid [18].

4.2 Computed Tomography (CT) and Magnetic Resonance Imaging (MRI)

CT and MRI are important for the pre-operative evaluation, staging, and follow-up of orbital RMS. CT is important for the detection of bone involvement, and MRI is important for better spatial resolution, soft-tissue contrast, and detection of intracranial spread [6, 9, 14]. Both are also used for post-treatment follow up: CT shows change in bone involvement, and MRI shows residual or recurrent disease [4, 6, 14, 15]. However, exposure to ionising radiation may theoretically induce a second potentially fatal cancer in children who have already manifested a tendency to harbour cancer, and MRI is the preferred imaging modality during follow up [19].

On CT, orbital RMS appears as a well-circumscribed, homogenous, soft tissue mass that is isodense as compared to muscles, without bone destruction in earlier stages, but with invasion of surrounding structures and calcification in more advanced cases where there is destruction of the adjacent bone [2, 4, 9, 14, 16, 20]. A heterogeneous appearance is possible in the event of focal haemorrhage or necrosis, and there is moderate to marked general enhancement with intravenous contrast [1, 2, 4, 9, 16]. A common finding is eyelid thickening, regardless of eyelid involvement, and a less common finding is a cavitated mass with ring-like enhancement [9, 14].

On MRI, the tumour appears isointense with respect to extraocular muscles and hypointense with respect to orbital fat on T1-weighted images, and hyperintense (with respect to both orbital fat and extraocular muscles) on T2-weighted images [4, 16, 20]. Increased signal on T1 and T2 is seen in focal areas of chronic haemorrhage [1]. The globe may be distorted or displaced but rarely invaded [9]. Visualisation is best with gadolinium, (moderate to marked enhancement), and fat suppression for better delineation [2]. Pre- and post-contrast comparison is useful to best detect intracranial and adjacent paranasal sinus invasion (Fig. 3) [14].

Diffusion-weighted imaging (DWI) is an MR imaging technique that gives information about normality of proton and water diffusion through tissue characterised by DWI and ADC (Apparent Diffusion Coefficient) values, respectively [21]. Because of high cellular density, malignant tumours usually have restricted diffusion. Lope et al. studied the usefulness of DWI in identifying characteristics of orbital tumours to aid radiographic diagnosis [21]. They found that RMS was predominantly restricted on DWI/ADC, which was especially helpful in differentiating it from haemangioma, (which has increased DWI/ADC) since the two exhibit a similar appearance on T1 and T2 sequences [21].

4.3 Nuclear Imaging

Bone scintigraphy is being used in the work-up particularly for the detection of osteoblastic metastases [14].

Some studies have demonstrated that PET-CT is better at detecting bone and lymph node metastasis than CT and US; however whole body MRI is being advocated (sensitivity 97.5%, specificity 99.4%) as superior to PET-CT (sensitivity 90%, specificity 100%) [14, 15, 22]. It is still unclear whether PET-CT or whole body MRI should be used routinely because of lack of clinical trials aimed at RMS, however, they can be contemplated in cases with increased metastatic risk [14].

5 Biopsy

RMS is the most common biopsied malignant orbital tumour in a child, and it is important in terms of establishing diagnosis and determining prognosis [2, 23]. The biopsy can be incisional or excisional, based on clinical and imaging finding.

Fine needle aspiration is less useful because the limited amount of tissue obtained is usually insufficient for pathological diagnosis [1]. Moreover, based on cytology only, it might be difficult to differentiate the embryonal from the alveolar type if reverse transcriptase PCR is not performed. This latter text shows a 2–13 translocation in the alveolar type.

The Authors advise incisional biopsy, as opposed to excisional, to avoid dissemination of tumour cells into the adjacent healthy tissue.

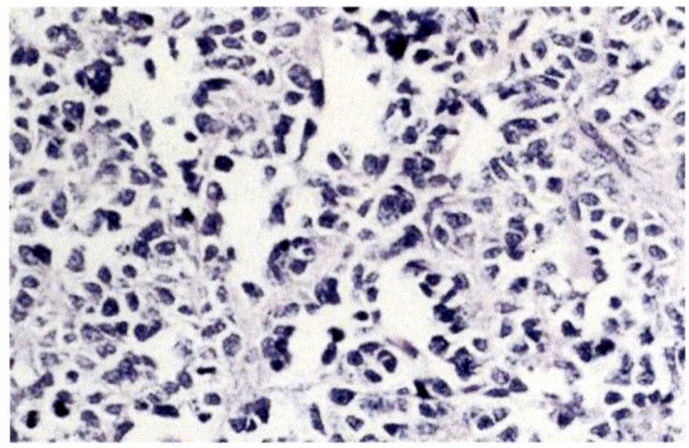

Fig. 2 Alveolar orbital RMS. The cells are large, with abundant eosinophilic cytoplasm and round to polygonal in shape with vesicular nuclei, which are a diagnostic feature of alveolar type as opposed to embryonal

6 Pathology

RMS was believed to arise from extraocular muscles, but now it is thought that it originates from pluripotent mesenchymal cells that differentiate into skeletal muscle [2, 9, 20]. Some cases may be related to prior radiation therapy [2].

RMS is divided into three histological subgroups: pleomorphic, embryonal, and alveolar. Most orbital RMS are of the embryonal subtype; the pleomorphic subtype occurs almost exclusively in adults (median age: sixth decade) [2].

The embryonal subtype (Fig. 1) comprises 50–70% of orbital RMS. Frequently seen cells are bipolar cells with tapered cytoplasmic processes, and less commonly seen cells are "tadpole-like" with long cytoplasmic extensions. The cells are usually arranged in a pattern of interlacing fascicle [9]. Cross-striations (which are bundles of actin and myosin filaments) in the cytoplasm may be visible with Masson trichrome or phosphotungstic acid–hematoxylin stains [2, 9, 20].

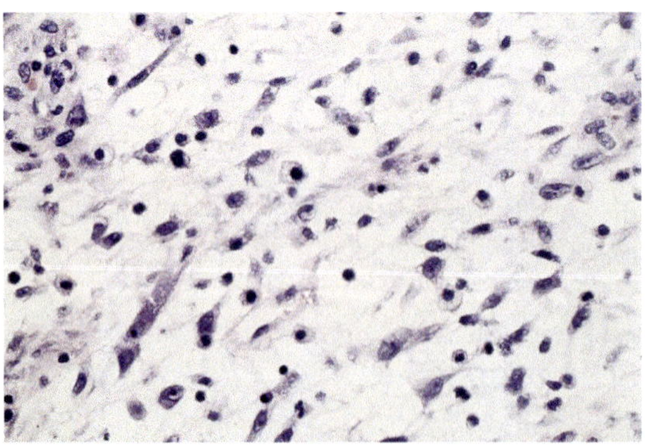

Fig. 1 Embryonal orbital RMS. There are elongated to round spindle cells with features of skeletal muscle in different stages of embryogenesis with a highly eosinophilic cytoplasm and hyperchromatic nuclei

The alveolar type (Fig. 2) (20–30% of orbital RMS) is characterised by ill-defined aggregates of poorly differentiated malignant cells that are loosely arranged and separated into irregular ovoid spaces by thin fibrovascular septa in an alveolar pattern which is absent in the "solid" form [2, 9, 20, 24]. This type has a poor prognosis, and any focus of alveolar morphology is sufficient to classify the tumour as alveolar RMS [24].

The botryoid subtype seems to be a variant of the embryonal type that assumes a papillary configuration [2].

Distinction among the different subtypes of RMS is important and can be aided by immunohistochemical staining and cytogenetic studies [24].

7 Immunohistochemistry

Immunohistochemical studies constitute the main approach to diagnosis. The markers typically found in RMS include antibodies against desmin (90%), muscle-specific actin, myoD1 (71–91%) and myoglobin [2, 23, 25–28]. Myogenin (90%) is expressed more in the alveolar than in the embryonal type [24–26, 28, 29]. Vimentin and desmin are usually positive but less specific since they can be positive in other tumours with skeletal muscle differentiation [2, 25, 30].

Myogenin and MyoD1 are myogenic transcriptional regulators that are expressed early in skeletal muscle differentiation (earlier than desmin, actin, myoglobin and myosin) [25].

8 Electron Microscopy

It is not routinely used for diagnosis of RMS, but may be helpful if histopathologic diagnosis is uncertain by demonstrating parallel arrays of thick myosin filaments [2].

9 Genetics

RMS has been noted to occur more commonly in certain familial syndromes like Li-Fraumeni familial cancer syndrome (associated with p53 mutation), neurofibromatosis, Noonan, Beckwith–Wiedemann and Costello syndromes which suggest a possible genetic contribution to RMS [2, 24, 31–33].

The most common cytogenetic finding in alveolar RMS is a t(2;13)(q35–37;q14) translocation resulting in a transcript composed of 5′ PAX3 sequences fused to 3′ FKHR sequences, and another translocation found in a subset of alveolar RMS is t(1;13)(p36;q14) [24, 26]. One of these two fusion genes is usually found in most alveolar RMS [24, 26]. The detection of PAX3-FKHR fusion protein indicates an unfavourable variant of alveolar RMS, whereas the PAX7-FKHR fusion protein indicates a relatively favourable variant [10, 34].

p53 in RMS varies in a different series ranging from 5% to 44% of cases; CDK4 (cyclin-dependent kinase 4) is also a cell cycle control gene reported to be positive in about 80% of alveolar RMS [25, 26]. C-erbB2 expression is reported to be positive in 60% of cases of RMS [25]. In a study by Andrade et al., the investigators found p53 to be positive in 13.8%, CDK4 in 34.5%, C-erbB2 in 70.4% and FAS in 31% of cases [25].

Chan et al. reported hypermethylation of three tumour suppressor genes (HIN-1, RB1, and CDX-1) in a patient with alveolar RMS, in addition to HIC-1 (present in 100% of studied alveolar RMS cases) [35]. This is important especially due to the absence of MyoD1 methylation in this patient, knowing that it is present in 91% of embryonal RMS [35]. This can thus play a role in differentiating embryonal and alveolar RMS, although further studies are warranted to make definitive conclusions (Fig. 3).

Staibano et al. studied DNA ploidy and immunohistochemical expression of p53 (tumour suppressor gene), bcl-2 (protooncogene), MDR-1 (multidrug resistance protein) and MIB1 (Ki67; cell proliferation associated protein) in the prognostic evaluation of orbital RMS [7, 26]. They divided their findings into two groups:

- Good prognosis (relapse free)
- Poor prognosis (relapsing RMS requiring more aggressive therapeutic protocols).

Their results showed that the cases of tetraploid and/or multiploid RMS overexpressing p53 and MDR-1 were characterised by a worse prognosis;

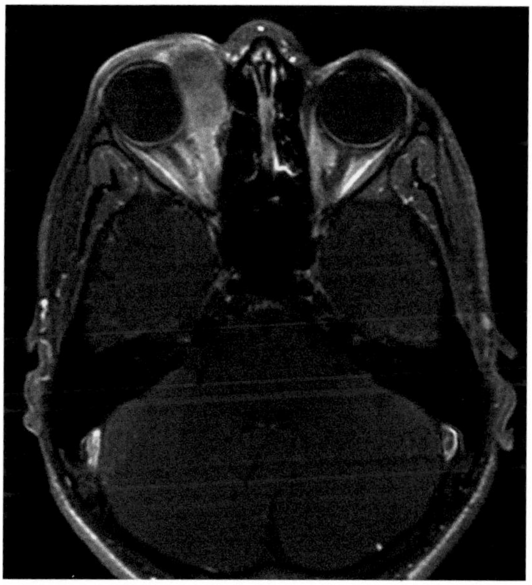

Fig. 3 MRI with T1 weighted images of orbits and the brain shows a large intraorbital mass with local invasion of the lamina papyracea with no intracranial extension

whereas tumours with a good prognosis showed hyperexpression of MIB1 and absence of mutated p53 expression [7, 36]. No difference was found with respect to bcl-2 expression [7].

It is worth noting that the point mutations of p53 as related to recurrence/progression/worse prognosis is still controversial in the literature [25, 31].

These findings, and further studies, can prove useful for subtyping RMS and tailoring treatment protocols [7].

10 Management

The guidelines regarding management of RMS have been introduced by the North American Intergroup Rhabdomyosarcoma Study Group (IRSG) and European cooperative groups—International Society of Pediatric Oncology-Malignant Mesenchymal Tumour Committee (SIOP-MMT), Cooperative Weichteilsarkom Study Group (CWS) and Italian Cooperative Group (ICG) [2]. Prior to that, overall survival (OS) was about 25–30% (with the historically recommended treatment being exenteration up to the late 1960's). With the introduction of surgery combined with adjuvant chemotherapy as well as radiotherapy in cooperative group trials, OS improved to around 90% [1, 4, 10, 15, 37–40].

Although the IRSG is directed at RMS in general, some investigators have retrieved data that pertains only to orbital RMS [2, 41]. The IRSG conclusions represent the American school of thought, whereas the findings SIOP-MMT, CWS and ICG represent the European school of thought [2, 42, 40].

The diagnosis of orbital RMS is made based on histopathologic findings following excisional or incisional biopsy [2]. Some surgeons believe that an incisional biopsy is sufficient (European protocol) since adequate margins cannot be reached and orbital RMS has a good prognosis following radiation and chemotherapy, regardless of amount of tissue excised [43].

Others believe that complete excision or maximal debulking decrease the tumour burden and facilitate subsequent medical treatment [2]. In a pooled analysis of 306 patients with orbital RMS treated according to international protocols (IRSG, SIOP-MMT, CWS, and ICG) in the period 1978–1992, 222/306 (72%) of patients underwent an initial incisional biopsy of tumours that were considered unresectable [40]. A partial excision was achieved by an initial surgery in 75/306 patients (25%), and in only 9/306 patients (3%) an initial oncological radical excision could be performed. Although the initial surgical approach differed between cooperative groups, with the percentage of patients starting therapy after biopsy only varying from 82% (IRSG) to 46% (ICG), this had no impact on prognosis.

Following biopsy, staging for orbital RMS is done according to the IRS post-surgical staging system [22, 44–46].

- Group I: localised disease, completely resected (excisional biopsy)
- Group II: microscopic disease remaining after biopsy
- Group III: gross residual disease remaining after biopsy
- Group IV: distant metastasis present at onset

This classification is useful in terms of treatment, stratification and prognosis [2, 44].

Decision-making for management is based on histopathologic confirmation, genetic testing, as well as staging of orbital RMS, which is done by reviewing imaging (MRI of primary tumour, chest-CT, Tc bone scan), pathology, and further work-up for metastases (bilateral bone marrow punctures and trephines) [1].

Current management includes surgery, irradiation and chemotherapy depending on the stage [1, 2, 47–49].

- Group I is treated with chemotherapy only: VA (vincristine and actinomycin).
- Group II is treated with a combination of chemotherapy (VA and cyclophosphamide; VAC) and radiotherapy (36 Gy).
- Group III is treated with a combination of chemotherapy (VAC) and radiotherapy (45 Gy).
- Group IV is treated with a combination of intensive chemotherapy and radiotherapy.

Patients having a higher risk of relapse also receive cyclophosphamide based on the IRSGIII and IV [12, 49]. Details regarding the different possible chemotherapeutic regimens depending on the risk is beyond the scope of this article but have been reported in the literature [47, 49, 50, 51].

The current European paediatric Soft tissue sarcoma Study Group (EpSSG) protocol (EpSSG-RMS-2005) proposes the following treatment strategy: [42, 52]

- Group I: chemotherapy consisting of VA.
- Groups II and III: chemotherapy VA with ifosfamide added in the first four courses; when in complete remission after three chemotherapy courses policy is to either leave out radiotherapy but add more ifosfamide, or add radiotherapy (36 Gy) and leave out further ifosfamide. Those not in complete remission after induction chemotherapy get radiotherapy (45 Gy) without further ifosfamide.
- Group IV: intensified chemotherapy regimen (IVA and doxorubicin) followed by 1 year of maintenance chemotherapy and radiotherapy to all involved sites (when possible).

A pooled analysis on 306 orbital RMS patients according to European and North American protocols showed 10 year EFS to be significantly better for patients receiving RT as part of their initial treatment compared to those who did not (82 v 53%), however confirmed no statistical difference in OS (87 v 86%), taking advantage of a favourable 'salvage gap' with rescue utilising further treatment [40].

SIOP group data from that analysis showed that up to 40% of patients with an orbital localization could be treated successfully without the use of RT and without disadvantage to the survival of the whole group. However, the total burden of therapy must be considered, as those who relapsed not only received RT as part of their second therapy but also needed additional chemotherapy [40].

Breneman et al. reported no change in prognosis with reduced doses of radiotherapy with the addition of a moderate cumulative dose of cyclophosphamide [31]. No specific guidelines concerning radiotherapy were specified apart from the use of brachytherapy whenever possible [31, 53].

Brachytherapy has been used for local treatment in the Amsterdam University Medical Center since 1991 [15]. The **AMORE** protocol is a novel technique for the treatment of unresectable head and neck RMS [55]. This protocol has since been followed for orbital RMS with the only remark that reconstruction is often not needed at the orbital site [53, 54]. It consists of **A**blative surgery, **MO**ulage technique brachytherapy, and surgical **Re**construction, and targets residual tumour mass [15, 55]. (Figs. 4, 5, and 6).

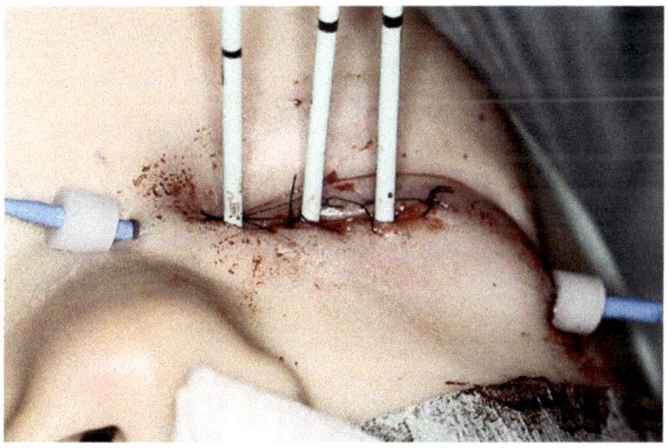

Fig. 4 A 1-year old child treated with brachytherapy applied to the tumour area with a high active Iridium-192 source, after chemotherapy and excision of residual tumour

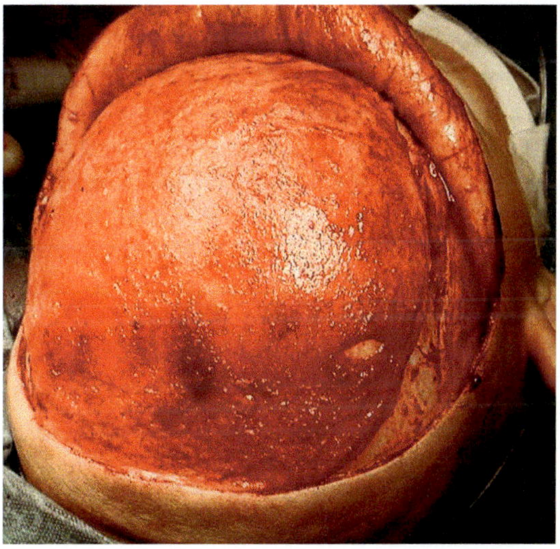

Fig. 5 Galea flap attached to a calvarial bone as a vascular flap for the reconstruction of orbit after brachytherapy

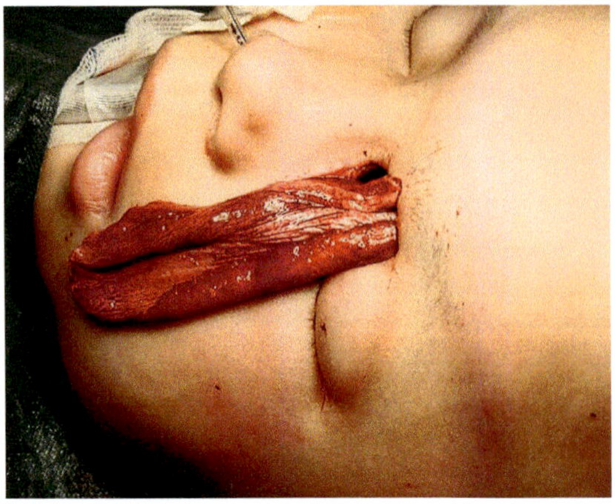

Fig. 6 Galea flap attached to a calvarial bone, brought together to the orbit to reconstruct the medial orbital wall and the orbital floor

After diagnosis and staging, chemotherapy is given according to the European protocol, and imaging is repeated to look for residual disease [15]. The aim of this protocol is to maximise local treatment and to avoid external beam radiotherapy (EBRT). Ablative surgery is performed as conservatively as possible with an effort not to sacrifice important tissue at the expense of possible microscopic remnants - which will be amenable to the brachytherapy which is initiated directly post-surgery [15, 55]. Brachytherapy has advantages over EBRT including a reduction in the treatment time and a focused dose delivery to the tumour bed and rapid fall-off of the dose beyond the treatment volume, sparing surrounding tissues and reducing morbidity, allowing organ preservation and bone growth, and potentially improving the functional and cosmetic outcome [55].

11 Radiotherapy

Radiation is usually in the range of 3600–5040 cGy over 4–5 weeks, and in the case of parameningeal extension the region of extension is irradiated +2 cm [1, 2, 52].

The main goal in novel management options is to maintain excellent survival while reducing the late side effects of treatment [58]. All of this has prompted enthusiasm for no or reduced-dose radiotherapy in low-risk RMS [2, 14, 31, 41, 48, 49, 56] and for new technologies in radiation oncology including proton beam radiotherapy, intensity modulated radiotherapy (IMRT), 3-D conformational radiotherapy and implant brachytherapy, all with the goal to minimise dose to normal tissue [15, 22, 43, 57, 58].

11.1 Intensity Modulated Radiotherapy (IMRT)

Wolden et al. studied IMRT for head-and-neck RMS where they used a smaller margin (1.5 cm as opposed to the standard 2 cm in IRSG protocols) made possible by using imaging (CT, PET, MR) in radiotherapy planning [59]. They concluded that IMRT with image fusion achieved excellent local control (in cases that did not have alveolar histology) with minimal dose reaching adjacent tissue when dose-limiting structures are adjacent to the tumour [10, 36, 59].

Hein et al. focused on the possibility of organ-sparing (particularly lens-sparing) irradiation in children with orbital RMS by using IMRT as opposed to 3D conformational photon radiotherapy [60]. They concluded that although IMRT resulted in a reduced dose to the lens (in treating tumours in retrobulbar and lateral positions) and ipsilateral lacrimal gland, no significant difference was noted for the ipsilateral retina and optic nerve, and more importantly, it resulted in an expanded volume of the brain receiving low dose radiation as compared to 3D conformational radiotherapy [60].

11.2 Fractionated Proton Radiotherapy

Yock et al. reported results on using fractionated proton radiotherapy as superior over 3D conformational photon radiotherapy for orbital RMS; they concluded that proton therapy achieves excellent tumour coverage at the same time, as it reduces radiation to the adjacent normal tissue like the brain, pituitary, hypothalamus, temporal lobes, and ipsilateral and contralateral orbital structures [10, 36, 54, 61]. Proton irradiation has excellent potential for conformal treatment to normal tissue that is better than 3D conformal radiation and perhaps even IMRT- which although advanced in tumour targeting as compared to 3D conformational photon irradiation- does distribute low dose to normal tissue: a disadvantage in a paediatric population with excellent survival that is more prone to secondary malignancies and growth retardation [60, 61].

11.3 Intensity-Modulated Brachytherapy (IMBT)

Perioperative IMBT has also been studied, and in cases of refractory orbital RMS was found to improve local tumour control and quality of life [62].

11.4 Brachytherapy

Brachytherapy offers a high dose to the tumour bed with a low dose to the surrounding tissues and can be considered in cases where radiotherapy is necessary and brachytherapy characteristics fit (single masses <3 cm at presentation, with a calculated cellularity of $\times 10^5$); although there are no conclusive clinical data available yet, the findings after IMRT might seem to be less favourable than those of brachytherapy [53, 54].

Following SIOP guidelines, Blank et al. have reported the use of brachytherapy instead of EBRT as part of the treatment of orbital RMS [54]. The side effects were found to be very low and not clinically significant. They thus concluded that surgery followed by brachytherapy can be considered when there is no residual intracranial extension of the tumour after chemotherapy, macroscopic tumour removal is feasible, and when EBRT is expected to be harmful to eye structures [54].

11.5 Side Effects of Radiotherapy

Many complications can arise from treatment with EBRT, including cataract (55%), dry eyes (36%), orbital hypoplasia (24%), ptosis (9%), radiation retinopathy (90%), facial asymmetry secondary to bone hypoplasia, keratoconjunctivitis, lacrimal duct stenosis, dental defects, growth retardation (in case of incidental irradiation of the pituitary) and secondary neoplasms such as osteogenic sarcoma, lymphoblastic leukaemia and melanoma [1, 2, 41, 57, 58, 63].

Although brachytherapy is not free of side effects, it is less toxic than EBRT, especially with respect to orbital hypoplasia [54, 53, 57]. The side effects of brachytherapy can include cataract, radiation retinopathy, dryness, ptosis, all of which are relatively mild and/or amenable to treatment [54].

12 Evaluation of Metastatic Disease

Work-up for metastatic disease should include chest-CT, Tc bone scan, and bone marrow punctures and trephines. Staging combines TNM (tumour, nodes, metastasis), which includes clinical features, histological grade, and the clinical grouping classification for RMS by the IRSG [14, 25]. A pooled analysis of 788 metastatic patients treated according to international cooperative group protocols (IRSG/COG, SIOP-MMT, ICG) in the time period 1984–2000 revealed that 3-year event free survival (EFS) was significantly and adversely influenced by age ($\leq$1 or $\geq$10 years), location of the primary tumour at an unfavourable site (defined as extremity and "other" sites, the latter predominantly meaning trunk, excluding bladder and prostate), presence of three or more sites of metastatic disease, and the presence of bone or bone marrow involvement. EFS was 50% for patients with zero adverse factors and was respectively 42%, 18%, 12%, and 5% in patients with one, two, three, or four factors [12].

13 Recurrence

Recurrence of orbital RMS can occur in about 17% of cases at a median time of 18 months, with 92% of these cases being local and 8% at distant sites [14, 64]. There are no clear guidelines for treatment in cases of recurrence. Possible options include debulking in addition to chemotherapy, additional EBRT, brachytherapy; and if all fails, exenteration is the remaining option [2, 37, 42, 47].

14 Follow-Up

Follow-up of patients post treatment for orbital RMS is essential to look for late side-effects of radiotherapy, recurrence and secondary tumours. Radiological follow up with MRI is specified in cooperative group protocols and will generally start at 3 month intervals, with decreasing frequency until 5 years after treatment. Initially, ocular examination is suggested every 3–4 months, and after the first year every 4–6 months for several years and then yearly; periodic imaging is performed depending on the clinical findings [1, 2, 15, 42, 63].

15 Prognosis

Orbital RMS has a good prognosis because of the favourable anatomic location, (symptoms apparent at an early stage allowing early diagnosis), favourable histology and biology (80% embryonal) and possibly patient age [2, 37]. Embryonal subtype RMS has a 94% 5-year survival (versus 74% for alveolar subtype) [2]. Overall survival is excellent for groups I, II and III (92% at 5 years and 87% at 10 years) [1, 14, 25]. Survival after relapse is dependent on age at initial presentation, histology, IRS clinical group, nodal-stage, and previous chemotherapy and radiotherapy [65, 66].

16 Conclusions

Orbital RMS is one of the few life-threatening diseases that presents first to the ophthalmologist; therefore, prompt diagnosis and treatment can be life-saving. The knowledge of the clinical, histopathological, and radiographic features as well as the more recent advances in the management of this entity is necessary, and a multidisciplinary approach for the treatment of orbital RMS is essential.

A controversy exists about complete resection of RMS in the orbit, debulking, or incisional biopsy. There is a concern driven by the radiation oncologists, especially in the setting of proton beam therapy that having some or most of a tumour to irradiate near the eye is optimal over microscopic disease [67]. This is to decrease the incidence of radiation induced cataract, uveitis and keratitis [68, 69]. No benefit to debulking over biopsy alone was found in group III RMS [70]. Other authors showed that patients with primary orbital RMS localised to the orbit (clinical group II or III) fared well regardless of the extent of the initial resection, and this finding has shifted the surgical approach from maximal excisional biopsy and debulking to incisional biopsy [71].

References

1. Jurdy L, Merks JH, Pieters BR, Mourits MP, Kloos RJ, Strackee SD, Saeed P. Orbital rhabdomyosarcomas: a review. Saudi J Ophthalmol. 2013;27:167–75.
2. Shields JA, Shields CL. Rhabdomyosarcoma: review for the ophthalmologist. Surv Ophthalmol. 2003;48:39–57.
3. Turner JH, Richmon JD. Head and neck rhabdomyosarcoma: a critical analysis of population-based incidence and survival data. Otolaryngol Head Neck Surg. 2011;145:967–73.
4. Conneely MF, Mafee MF. Orbital rhabdomyosarcoma and simulating lesions. Neuroimaging Clin N Am. 2005;15:121–36.
5. Koopman JH, van der Loo M, van Dijk MR, Bijlsma WR. Incidence of primary malignant orbital tumours in The Netherlands. Eye (Lond). 2011;25:461–5.

6. Staibano S, Franco R, Tranfa F, Mezza E, Lo ML, Strianese D. Orbital rhabdomyosarcoma: relationship between DNA ploidy, p53, bcl-2, MDR-1 and Ki67 (MIB1) expression and clinical behavior. Anticancer Res. 2004;24:249–57.
7. Crist WM, Garnsey L, Beltangady MS, Gehan E, Ruymann F, Webber B. Prognosis in children with rhabdomyosarcoma: a report of the intergroup rhabdomyosarcoma studies I and II. Intergroup rhabdomyosarcoma committee. J Clin Oncol. 1990;8:443–52.
8. Chung EM, Smirniotopoulos JG, Specht CS, Schroeder JW, Cube R. From the archives of the AFIP: pediatric orbit tumors and tumorlike lesions: nonosseous lesions of the extraocular orbit. Radiographics. 2007;27:1777–99.
9. Terezakis SA, Wharam MD. Radiotherapy for rhabdomyosarcoma: indications and outcome. Clin Oncol (R Coll Radiol). 2013;25:27–35.
10. Breneman JC, Lyden E, Pappo AS, Link MP, Anderson JR, Parham DM. Prognostic factors and clinical outcomes in children and adolescents with metastatic rhabdomyosarcoma—a report from the intergroup rhabdomyosarcoma study IV. J Clin Oncol. 2003;21:78–84.
11. Schworm HD, Boergen KP, Stefani FH. The initial clinical manifestations of rhabdomyosarcoma. Ophthalmologe. 1995;92:362–5.
12. Rao AA, Naheedy JH, Chen JY, Robbins SL, Ramkumar HL. A clinical update and radiologic review of pediatric orbital and ocular tumors. J Oncol. 2013;2013:975908.
13. Freling NJ, Merks JH, Saeed P, Balm AJ, Bras J, Pieters BR. Imaging findings in craniofacial childhood rhabdomyosarcoma. Pediatr Radiol. 2010;40:1723–38.
14. Sohaib SA, Moseley I, Wright JE. Orbital rhabdomyosarcoma-the radiological characteristics. Clin Radiol. 1998;53:357–62.
15. Neudorfer M, Leibovitch I, Stolovitch C, Dray JP, Hermush V, Nagar H. Intraorbital and periorbital tumors in children-value of ultrasound and color Doppler imaging in the differential diagnosis. Am J Ophthalmol. 2004;137:1065–72.
16. Boparai MS, Dash RG. Clinical, ultrasonographic and CT evaluation of orbital rhabdomyosarcomas with management. Indian J Ophthalmol. 1991;39:129–31. [PubMed] [Google Scholar]
17. Karcioglu ZA, Hadjistilianou D, Rozans M, DeFrancesco S. Orbital rhabdomyosarcoma. Cancer Control. 2004;11:328–33.
18. Lope LA, Hutcheson KA, Khademian ZP. Magnetic resonance imaging in the analysis of pediatric orbital tumors: utility of diffusion-weighted imaging. J AAPOS. 2010;14:257–62.
19. Malempati S, Hawkins DS. Rhabdomyosarcoma: review of the Children's oncology group (COG) soft-tissue sarcoma committee experience and rationale for current COG studies. Pediatr Blood Cancer. 2012;59:5–10.
20. Viswanathan S, George S, Ramadwar M, Shet T, Arora B, Laskar S. Extraconal orbital tumors in children—a spectrum. Virchows Arch. 2009;454:703–13.
21. Passmore LM, Myers P, Gilbert-Barness E. Pathology teach and tell: solid variant alveolar rhabdomyosarcoma of the orbit. Fetal Pediatr Pathol. 2006;25:51–7.
22. Andrade CR, Takahama JA, Nishimoto IN, Kowalski LP, Lopes MA. Rhabdomyosarcoma of the head and neck: a clinicopathological and immunohistochemical analysis of 29 cases. Braz Dent J. 2010;21:68–73.
23. Constine LS, Marcus RB Jr, Halperin EC. The future of therapy for childhood rhabdomyosarcoma: clues from molecular biology. Int J Radiat Oncol Biol Phys. 1995;32:1245–9.
24. Tapscott SJ, Thayer MJ, Weintraub H. Deficiency in rhabdomyosarcomas of a factor required for MyoD activity and myogenesis. Science. 1993;259:1450–3.
25. Sun XL, Zheng BH, Li B, Li LQ, Soejima K, Kanda M. Orbital rhabdomyosarcoma. Immunohistochemical studies of seven cases. Chin Med J (Engl). 1990;103:485–8.
26. Cintorino M, Vindigni C, Del Vecchio MT, Tosi P, Frezzotti R, Hadjistilianou T. Expression of actin isoforms and intermediate filament proteins in childhood orbital rhabdomyosarcomas. J Submicrosc Cytol Pathol. 1989;21:409–19.
27. Felix CA, Kappel CC, Mitsudomi T, Nau MM, Tsokos M, Crouch GD. Frequency and diversity of p53 mutations in childhood rhabdomyosarcoma. Cancer Res. 1992;52:2243–7.
28. Jung A, Bechthold S, Pfluger T, Renner C, Ehrt O. Orbital rhabdomyosarcoma in Noonan syndrome. J Pediatr Hematol Oncol. 2003;25:330–2.
29. Thavaraj V, Sethi A, Arya LS. Incomplete Beckwith–Wiedemann syndrome in a child with orbital rhabdomyosarcoma. Indian Pediatr. 2002;39:299–304.
30. Chan WM, Liu DT, Pang CP, Lam DS, To KF, Choi PC. Pediatric malignancies. Case 1: hypermethylation in orbital alveolar rhabdomyosarcoma. J Clin Oncol. 2005;23:4790–1.
31. Wolden SL, Wexler LH, Kraus DH, Laquaglia MP, Lis E, Meyers PA. Intensity-modulated radiotherapy for head-and-neck rhabdomyosarcoma. Int J Radiat Oncol Biol Phys. 2005;61:1432–8.
32. Raney B, Huh W, Hawkins D, Hayes-Jordan A, Million L, Rodeberg D. Outcome of patients with localized orbital sarcoma who relapsed following treatment on intergroup rhabdomyosarcoma study group (IRSG) protocols-III and -IV, 1984–1997: a report from the children's oncology g. Pediatr Blood Cancer. 2013;60:371–6.
33. Ashton N, Morgan G. Embryonal sarcoma and embryonal rhabdomyosarcoma of the orbit. J Clin Pathol. 1965;18:699–714.
34. Van Rijn RR, Wilde JC, Bras J. Imaging findings in non craniofacial childhood rhabdomyosarcoma. Pediatr Radiol. 2008;38:617–34.

35. Raney RB, Anderson JR, Kollath J, Vassilopoulou-Sellin R, Klein MJ, Heyn R. Late effects of therapy in 94 patients with localized rhabdomyosarcoma of the orbit: report from the intergroup rhabdomyosarcoma study (IRS)-III, 1984–1991. Med Pediatr Oncol. 2000;34:413–20.
36. Orbach D, Rey A, Oberlin O, Sanchez de Toledo J, Terrier-Lacombe MJ, van Unnik A. Soft tissue sarcoma or malignant mesenchymal tumors in the first year of life: experience of the International Society of Pediatric Oncology (SIOP) malignant mesenchymal tumor committee. J Clin Oncol. 2005;23:4363–71.
37. Olivier PN, Calvo JM, Abelairas Gómez JM. Orbital rhabdomyosarcoma: difficulties with European treatment protocol. Arch Soc Esp Oftalmol. 2005;80:331–8.
38. Raney RB, Maurer HM, Anderson JR, Andrassy RJ, Donaldson SS, Qualman SJ. The intergroup rhabdomyosarcoma study group (IRSG): major lessons from the IRS-I through IRS-IV studies as background for the current IRS-V treatment protocols. Sarcoma. 2001;5:9–15.
39. Wharam MD, Hanfelt JJ, Tefft MC, Johnston J, Ensign LG, Breneman J. Radiation therapy for rhabdomyosarcoma: local failure risk for clinical group III patients on intergroup rhabdomyosarcoma study II. Int J Radiat Oncol Biol Phys. 1997;38:797–804.
40. Shields CL, Shields JA, Honavar SG, Demirci H. Primary ophthalmic rhabdomyosarcoma in 33 patients. Trans Am Ophthalmol Soc. 2001;99:133–43.
41. Wolden SL, Anderson JR, Crist WM, Breneman JC, Wharam MD Jr, Wiener ES. Indications for radiotherapy and chemotherapy after complete resection in rhabdomyosarcoma: a report from the intergroup rhabdomyosarcoma studies I to III. J Clin Oncol. 1999;17:3468–75.
42. Schoot RA, Saeed P, Freling NJ, Blank LE, Pieters BR, van der Grient JN, Strackee SD, Bras J, Caron HN, Merks JH, Amsterdam Head and Neck Working Group on Childhood Tumors. Local resection and brachytherapy for primary Orbital rhabdomyosarcoma: outcome and failure pattern analysis. Ophthal Plast Reconstr Surg. 2016;32:354–60.
43. Raney RB, Walterhouse DO, Meza JL, Andrassy RJ, Breneman JC, Crist WM. Results of the intergroup rhabdomyosarcoma study group D9602 protocol, using vincristine and dactinomycin with or without cyclophosphamide and radiation therapy, for newly diagnosed patients with low-risk embryonal rhabdomyosarcoma: a report from the soft tissue sarcoma committee of the children's oncology group. J Clin Oncol. 2011;29:1312–8.
44. Ruymann FB, Vietti T, Gehan E. Cyclophosphamide dose escalation in combination with vincristine and actinomycin D (VAC) in gross residual sarcoma: a pilot study without hematopoietic growth factor support evaluating toxicity and response. J Pediatr Hematol Oncol. 1995;17:331–7.
45. Arndt C, Tefft M, Gehan E. A feasibility, toxicity, and early response study of etoposide, ifosfamide, and vincristine for the treatment of children with rhabdomyosarcoma: a report from the intergroup rhabdomyosarcoma study (IRS) IV pilot study. J Pediatr Hematol Oncol. 1997;19:124–9.
46. Blank LE, Koedooder K, van der Grient HN, Wolffs NA, van de Kar M, Merks JH. Brachytherapy as part of the multidisciplinary treatment of childhood rhabdomyosarcomas of the orbit. Int J Radiat Oncol Biol Phys. 2010;77:1463–9.
47. Breneman J, Meza J, Donaldson SS, Raney RB, Wolden S, Michalski J. Local control with reduced-dose radiotherapy for low-risk rhabdomyosarcoma: a report from the children's oncology group D9602 study. Int J Radiat Oncol Biol Phys. 2012;83:720–6.
48. Tyl JW, Blank LE, Koornneef L. Brachytherapy in orbital tumors. Ophthalmology. 1997;104:1475–9.
49. Buwalda J, Schouwenburg PF, Blank LE, Merks JH, Copper MP, Strackee SD. A novel local treatment strategy for advanced stage head and neck rhabdomyosarcomas in children: results of the AMORE protocol. Eur J Cancer. 2003;39:1594–602.
50. Forstner D, Borg M, Saxon B. Orbital rhabdomyosarcoma: multidisciplinary treatment experience. Australas Radiol. 2006;50:41–5.
51. Regine WF, Fontanesi J, Kumar P, Zeitzer K, Greenwald C, Bowman L. A phase II trial evaluating selective use of altered radiation dose and fractionation in patients with unresectable rhabdomyosarcoma. Int J Radiat Oncol Biol Phys. 1995;31:799–805.
52. Abramson DH, Fass D, McCormick B, Servodidio CA, Piro JD, Anderson LL. Implant brachytherapy: a novel treatment for recurrent orbital rhabdomyosarcoma. J AAPOS. 1997;1:154–7.
53. Hein PA, Gladstone DJ, Bellerive MR, Hug EB. Importance of protocol target definition on the ability to spare normal tissue: an IMRT and 3D-CRT planning comparison for intraorbital tumors. Int J Radiat Oncol Biol Phys. 2005;62:1540–8.
54. Yock T, Schneider R, Friedmann A, Adams J, Fullerton B, Tarbell N. Proton radiotherapy for orbital rhabdomyosarcoma: clinical outcome and a dosimetric comparison with photons. Int J Radiat Oncol Biol Phys. 2005;63:1161–8.
55. Strege RJ, Kovács G, Meyer JE, Holland D, Claviez A, Mehdorn MH. Perioperative intensity-modulated brachytherapy for refractory orbital rhabdomyosarcomas in children. Strahlenther Onkol. 2009;185:789–98.
56. Yip CC, Kersten RC, McCulley TJ, Ballard ET, Kulwin DR. Osteogenic sarcoma after orbital radiation rhabdomyosarcoma. Ophthalmology. 2003;110:1996–9.
57. Shields CL, Shields JA, Honavar SG, Demirci H. Clinical spectrum of primary ophthalmic rhabdomyosarcoma. Ophthalmology. 2001;108:2284–92.
58. Warrier AR, Syriac S, Rathnam KK. Late recurrence in orbital rhabdomyosarcoma: complete remission after multimodality management. J Cancer Res Ther. 2010;6:307–9.

59. Sultan I, Qaddoumi I, Yaser S, Rodriguez-Galindo C, Ferrari A. Comparing adult and pediatric rhabdomyosarcoma in the surveillance, epidemiology and end results program, 1973 to 2005: an analysis of 2,600 patients. J Clin Oncol. 2009;27:3391–7.
60. Oberlin O, Rey A, Lyden E, Bisogno G, Stevens MC, Meyer WH. Prognostic factors in metastatic rhabdomyosarcomas: results of a pooled analysis from United States and European cooperative groups. J Clin Oncol. 2008;26:2384–9.
61. Paterson A, Frush DP, Donnelly LF. Helical CT of the body: are settings adjusted for pediatric patients? AJR Am J Roentgenol. 2001;176:297–301.
62. Missiaglia E, Williamson D, Chisholm J, Wirapati P, Pierron G, Petel F. PAX3/FOXO1 fusion gene status is the key prognostic molecular marker in rhabdomyosarcoma and significantly improves current risk stratification. J Clin Oncol. 2012;30:1670–7.
63. Oberlin O, Rey A, Anderson J, Carli M, Raney RB, Treuner J. Treatment of orbital rhabdomyosarcoma: survival and late effects of treatment–results of an international workshop. J Clin Oncol. 2001;19:197–204.
64. Maurer HM, Beltangady M, Gehan EA, Crist W, Hammond D, Hays DM. The intergroup rhabdomyosarcoma study-IA final report. Cancer. 1988;61:209–20.
65. Chisholm JC, Marandet J, Rey A, Scopinaro M, de Toledo JS, Merks JH. Prognostic factors after relapse in nonmetastatic rhabdomyosarcoma: a nomogram to better define patients who can be salvaged with further therapy. J Clin Oncol. 2011;29:1319–25.
66. Mazzoleni S, Bisogno G, Garaventa A, Cecchetto G, Ferrari A, Sotti G. Outcomes and prognostic factors after recurrence in children and adolescents with nonmetastatic rhabdomyosarcoma. Cancer. 2005;104:183–90.
67. Meza JL, Anderson J, Pappo AS, Meyer WH. Analysis of prognostic factors in patients with nonmetastatic rhabdomyosarcoma treated on intergroup rhabdomyosarcoma studies III and IV: the Children's Oncology group. J Clin Oncol. 2006;24:3844–51.
68. Hug EB, Adams J, Fitzek M, De Vries A, Munzenrider JE. Fractionated, three-dimensional, planning-assisted proton-radiation therapy for orbital rhabdomyosarcoma: a novel technique. Int J Radiat Oncol Biol Phys. 2000;47:979–84.
69. Gandhi PD, Fleming JC, Haik BG, Wilson WM. Ophthalmic complications following treatment of paranasal sinus rhabdomyosarcoma in comparison to orbital disease. Ophthal Plast Reconstr Surg. 2011;27:241–6.
70. Cecchetto G, Bisogno G, DeCort IF, et al. Biopsy or debulking surgery as initial surgery for locally advanced rhabdomyosarcomas in children the experience of the Italian cooperative group studies. Cancer. 2007;110:2561–7.
71. Raney RB, Maurer HM, Anderson JT, Andrassy RJ, Donaldson SS, Qualman DJ, Wharam MD, Wiener ES, Crist WM. The intergroup rhabdomyosarcoma study group (IRSG): major lessons from the IRS-I through IRS-IV studies as background for the current IRS-V treatment protocols. Sarcoma. 2001;5:9–15.

Orbital Infections

Aaron Jamison, Adriana Iuliano, Gijsbert J. Hötte, and Raman Malhotra

Key Messages

- Orbital infections account for the majority of primary intraorbital disease processes, and sinusitis is the most common aetiology. Systemic conditions which predispose to orbital infection include diabetes, septicaemia, malignancy, and immunosuppression.
- Clinical signs and symptoms include superficial inflammatory changes, proptosis, limitation of extraocular motility, and visual loss. Causative agents are most commonly bacteria, with fungi, viruses, and parasites seen less frequently.
- Imaging (CT and/or MRI) is complementary in certain cases. Differential diagnosis of imaging abnormalities includes inflammatory and granulomatous diseases, and orbital tumours.
- Morbidity and mortality associated with the condition have declined with advances in diagnostic and therapeutic options; however, orbital infection can still lead to serious sight- and life-threatening complications.
- Prompt diagnosis and treatment are crucial. Antibiotic coverage and surgical intervention when needed have benefitted patients and changed the disease prognosis. Indications for surgical drainage should be based on clinical and radiological findings. Loss of vision, an unresponsive pupil or a densely packed orbit are indications for immediate surgical drainage.

1 Orbital Cellulitis

Orbital cellulitis (or postseptal cellulitis) is a serious, potentially sight-threatening and rarely, life-threatening ophthalmic emergency due to infection of the soft tissues behind the orbital septum. Although it may occur at any age, it is most commonly seen in children. Preseptal cellulitis (also referred to as periorbital cellulitis) is an infection of the eyelid and surrounding skin but anterior to the orbital septum, and does not invade the intraorbital structures. Preseptal cellulitis is often caused by an external focus of infection (e.g., a wound) but may occur due to an

A. Jamison
Department of Ophthalmology, NHS Greater Glasgow and Clyde, Glasgow, Scotland, UK

A. Iuliano (✉)
Orbital Unit, University of Naples Federico II, Naples, Italy
e-mail: adriana.iuliano@unina.it

G. J. Hötte
Department of Oculoplastic, Orbital and Lacrimal Surgery, The Rotterdam Eye Hospital, Rotterdam, The Netherlands

R. Malhotra
Corneoplastic Unit, Queen Victoria Hospital, East Grinstead, UK

F. M. Quaranta Leoni et al. (eds.), *Oculoplastic, Lacrimal and Orbital Surgery*, https://doi.org/10.1007/978-3-031-39638-0_16

infection that extends from the nasal sinuses or teeth. Orbital cellulitis usually occurs due to local extension from a concurrent sinusitis, implantation (caused by periorbital trauma) or haematogenous spread from a distant site [1].

1.1 Childhood Orbital Cellulitis

Orbital infection is twice as common in boys, occurring at a mean age of 7 years [2]. In those aged under 5 years, ethmoid sinusitis is the most common source, causing a pre-septal cellulitis more commonly than orbital cellulitis [3]. A wide range of pathogens may cause orbital infection in children, although the most common are α- or non-haemolytic streptococci, Group A β-haemolytic streptococci, Staphylococcus aureus and Haemophilus influenzae. Streptococcal infection is age related, with younger children more likely to present with infection from Streptococcus pneumoniae and older children from group A streptococcus. Additionally, Streptococcus milleri, Streptococcus viridians, and Streptococcus anginosus are the most commonly identified organisms [4]. Haemophilus infection is less common following H. influenzae type b vaccination [5, 6]. Anaerobic organisms, such as Peptostreptococcus, Bacteroides sp., and Fusobacterium necrophorum, less commonly cause orbital infection, but are associated with higher morbidity [7]. In those undergoing abscess or sinus drainage, two-thirds achieve positive cultures, while one-third of these demonstrate polymicrobial infection.

1.1.1 Clinical Features

Clinical history taking should be careful and include questioning regarding history of fever, sinusitis, upper respiratory tract infection and periorbital trauma. The hallmarks of orbital infection are periorbital pain, heat, redness and swelling. Preseptal cellulitis is characterised by the presence of lid oedema and redness, but an otherwise normal ocular examination. Orbital (or postseptal) cellulitis features include chemosis, proptosis, an orbital inflammation line (corresponding to the underlying arcus marginalis), reduced eye movements and loss of vision, forming a spectrum from very subtle early features to fully established orbital cellulitis [8]. In the most severe cases, orbital apex syndrome, cavernous sinus thrombosis, and even meningitis (indicating intracranial spread) may occur.

1.1.2 Investigation

Imaging should not delay the acute management of suspected orbital cellulitis [9]. Contrast-enhanced computed tomography (CT) may help detect sinus disease and the presence of subperiosteal/orbital abscess, while magnetic resonance imaging (MRI) is better suited to the identification of cavernous sinus and intracranial extension. Haematological, microbiological and ultrasound investigations rarely contribute significantly to the diagnosis, and have the potential to delay the initiation of treatment.

1.1.3 Management

Mild preseptal cellulitis can be managed with oral antibiotics ± a topical decongestant on an outpatient basis [10]. Choice of antibiotic should be based on local and national antimicrobial guidelines, although in general it should cover pathogens that most commonly cause acute sinusitis (S. pneumoniae, H. influenzae, M. catarrhalis, S. pyogenes), S. aureus and anaerobes [1]. Simple oral analgesia (paracetamol or ibuprofen) may also be of benefit.

If moderate or severe cellulitis is present, or if the child is unable to tolerate/absorb oral antibiotics, then admission for intravenous (IV) antibiotics and ENT/ophthalmology review is advised. Neuroimaging should be considered if there has been no improvement after 48 h of IV treatment, and sinus drainage to remove the reservoir of infection should be considered in patients with poor response to IV antibiotics and a collection detected on imaging.

Indication for Imaging (After Starting Empiric Antibiotic Therapy)

Contrast enhanced CT orbit, sinuses and brain if:

- CNS involvement/focal neurology/meningism
- Unable to examine eye/open eyelids

- Clinical signs of post-septal (orbital) cellulitis
- Clinical progression despite 24 h treatment or no improvement after 48 h
- Continued pyrexia after 48 h IV antibiotics [10].

Orbital cellulitis should also be managed with IV antibiotics and topical decongestants as an inpatient. ENT and ophthalmology teams should be closely involved, with ophthalmology reviews providing regular visual assessment and the ENT team considering the need for surgical drainage at each stage.

Most cases of isolated 'group 1' cellulitis (preseptal cellulitis, see Chandler's classification under Adult orbital cellulitis) can be treated conservatively with antibiotics. Surgical drainage is rarely necessary. Wong et al. reviewed 15 retrospective studies related to the management of paediatric preseptal cellulitis, evaluating a total of 1083 paediatric patients, and pointed out that the vast majority of studies report surgery and/or procedure rates ranging from 0% to 11% [11].

1.1.4 Indications for Early Surgical Drainage of Subperiosteal Abscess

Van der Veer et al. studied the occurrence of true orbital abscess formation in orbital cellulitis: although the terms abscess and empyema are often used synonymously, they are in fact distinct entities. An abscess is a collection of pus and bacteria surrounded by a wall created by the bacteria through which antibiotics can hardly penetrate and therefore surgery is required to open the abscess and evacuate pus. In contrast, an empyema is a collection of pus and bacteria in a preexisting anatomical space to which antibiotics can penetrate relatively easily. From a theoretical point of view, the approach of an orbital empyema therefore could be less invasive than treatment of an abscess [12]. While orbital abscesses are usually drained through an anterior approach, the subperiosteal abscess (at least the medial subperiosteal abscess, which is the most frequent location) is often drained through an endonasal approach.

Wong et al. reviewed 16 retrospective studies of 12,824 patients with paediatric orbital (post-septal) cellulitis and confirmed a higher likelihood than the adult population of requiring surgical intervention, up to 23% [11]. They state the widely held view that most commonly younger age is associated with greater success with conservative management, and/or less complications from surgery. The exact age cutoff ranges from 2 to 9 years old, and 9 years as a cut off was the most commonly studied in the literature and most clinically significant [11]. It appears that patients older than 9 years of age are at a higher risk of developing early abscesses, requiring surgical drainage.

The Garcia and Harris treatment algorithm is considered the current guide as to the indications for surgical intervention in orbital cellulitis [13]. The authors suggest that surgical intervention is indicated in one or more of the following criteria:

Indication for Surgical Intervention in Orbital Cellulitis

- Children older than 9 years of age
- presence of frontal sinusitis
- non-medial location of subperiosteal abscess or large subperiosteal abscess
- suspicion of anaerobic subperiosteal infection (e.g. presence of gas within the abscess seen on CT imaging)
- recurrence of subperiosteal abscess after previous drainage
- evidence of chronic sinusitis
- acute optic nerve or retinal compromise and infection of dental origin

Intravenous to oral switch should be considered when the child is clinically improving and apyrexial, with the aim to provide a total (IV and oral) antibiotic course of 14 days—although longer courses will be required in the cases of CNS complication and poor response.

1.2 Adult Orbital Cellulitis

In adults, orbital cellulitis may occur as a result of various different mechanisms, although 60–70% of cases are associated with sinus disease (particularly of the ethmoid air cells). Other important sources of infection include direct trauma to the periocular region (± the presence of a foreign body), dental infections, and posterior extension of infection through the orbital septum (e.g., from dacryocystitis) [14–18].

Orbital cellulitis is a sight-, and sometimes, life-threatening condition, with the potential to cause meningitis and cavernous sinus thrombosis (due to posterior extension), abscess formation, septicaemia, and even death. Subperiosteal abscess can occur as a result of direct extension from an infected sinus, or due to local haematogenous spread through the valveless veins crossing from the sinuses to the orbit [1]. Involvement of the more posterior sphenoid sinus may lead to orbital apex syndrome with early visual loss [19].

Gram-positive bacteria—commonly Staphylococcus aureus and Streptococcus species (in particular *Streptococcus pneumoniae*)—are currently the most common causative organisms found in patients presenting with orbital cellulitis [4, 20]. Polymicrobial infections of both aerobic and anaerobic bacteria are common in those aged over 15 years, in contrast to younger children.

Of note, patients with orbital cellulitis caused by Strep. milleri (of which there are three distinct species: S. intermedius; S. constellatus; and S. anginosis) are particularly likely to develop subperiosteal and orbital abscesses requiring early surgical drainage and even multiple drainage procedures in addition to longer-duration antibiotic therapy [21]. The organisms form tiny colonies in culture, and require microaerophilic conditions. Over the last two decades, improved culture techniques have increasingly recognised these organisms as pathogens. They are characterised by a tendency for invasive pyogenic infections with abscess formation [22]. Whiley et al. studied the associations of *S. intermedius, S. constellatus*, and *S. anginosus* with clinical infections and sites of isolation in 153 clinical isolates and showed that *S. intermedius* was associated with abscesses of the brain and liver, while both S. anginosus and S. constellatus were isolated from a wider range of sites and infections [23].

Orbital cellulitis due to the Strep. milleri group of organisms is rare. In a recent large multicentre UK prospective study of patients requiring inpatient treatment for preseptal or orbital cellulitis secondary to sinonasal infections, conducted over a 12-month period at eight centres, Mahalingam et al. recruited 143 patients, and presented data on 103 patients [24]. Of the cases that were culture-positive, the most common organisms grown were gram-positive cocci, including *Staphylococcus aureus*, *Streptococcus pyogenes*, and *Streptococcus pneumoniae*. No cases of Streptococcus Milleri group organisms were identified. In contrast, when considering publications reporting cases of orbital cellulitis with early subperiosteal abscess occurrence, it commonly features as a pathogen. In a review of patients under 18 years of age with sinusitis-related subperiosteal abscess treated from 2002 to 2012, Liao and Harris identified nine of the total 41 cases in that period were due to *Streptococcus anginosus* or *Streptococcus milleri* (*Strep. milleri* group) [25]. Analysis of these cases revealed the presence of either a large medial or superior subperiosteal abscess, all requiring emergency or immediate drainage. Despite early IV antibiotics, occurrence of early onset and recurrent subperiosteal abscess, typically within a week appears very high.

1.2.1 Clinical Features

The clinical history should include history of soft tissue/orbital injury, previous ENT pathology/sinusitis, and any systemic illness signposting a distant infective source (e.g., upper respiratory tract infection).

Clinical examination should be targeted to identify the location of orbital infection (preseptal vs. orbital), and the severity of inflammation present. Both preseptal and orbital cellulitis may present with the four cardinal signs of inflammation—pain, heat, redness and swelling—although post-septal infections are often associated with chemosis, reduced eye movements, proptosis, visual loss, and general malaise. As for childhood orbital cellulitis, there may be a visible orbital inflammation line, which corresponds to the underlying arcus marginalis.

Historically, Chandler's classification of orbital complications of acute sinusitis has been used, based on their location and severity [4]. These complications are classified as groups in order to help define severity of disease and an approach to management, but importantly, they do not always represent stages or necessarily reflect a mode of progression of disease in all cases.

Chandler's classification of orbital complications of acute sinusitis:

Group 1—preseptal cellulitis;
Group 2—orbital cellulitis;
Group 3—subperiosteal abscess, in which purulent material collects in the orbital cavity in the subperiosteal space between the bony walls of the orbit and the periorbita;
Group 4—intraorbital abscess (a purulent collection inside the orbit, within the orbital tissue);
Group 5—cavernous sinus thrombosis (CST).

1.2.2 Investigation

Thin-slice CT imaging with contrast is helpful in measuring the extent of disease, and is the investigation of choice (Fig. 1). CT may also detect the presence of abscess (although abscesses may not be detected by CT imaging), or foreign body [26, 27]. Thin-slice MRI with fat suppression is advised in cases where intracranial spread/abscess are suspected (Fig. 2) [28].

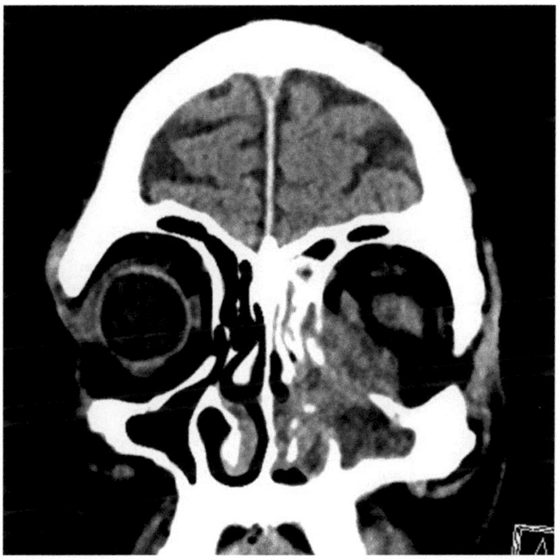

Fig. 1 Coronal CT scan of a patient with infection of left maxillary sinus, nose and left orbit (orbital cellulitis)

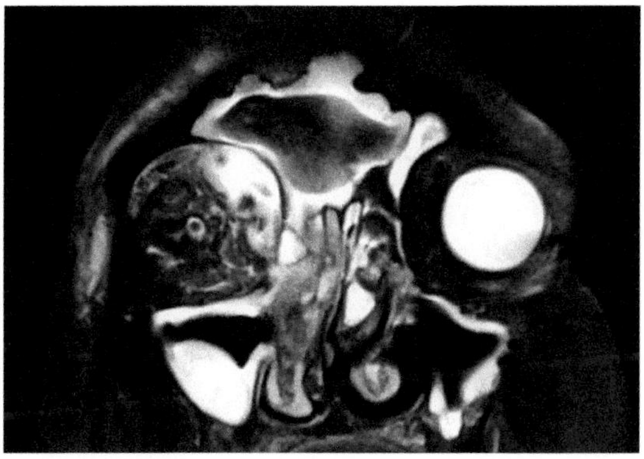

Fig. 2 Right coronal MRI scan of a patient with orbital cellulitis and infection of paranasal sinuses

1.2.3 Management

Exclusively preseptal cellulitis can often be managed on an outpatient basis with oral antibiotics, with a higher threshold for admission than for childhood preseptal cellulitis. However, where there is any sign of orbital or systemic disease, immediate admission and high-dose, broad-spectrum IV antibiotics are required in order to reduce the risk of significant irreversible visual loss [9]. An empirical approach such as IV 1.5 g cefuroxime three times daily combined with IV 500 mg metronidazole provides broad-spectrum cover until blood culture results and microbiologist's advice can be obtained. Vancomycin may be more effective in regions where the incidence of community-acquired methicillin-resistant staphylococcal infection is greater [29].

Joint care with ENT is essential where there is co-existing sinus or ear disease. A nasal decongestant should also be prescribed due to the prevalence of associated sinus inflammation in these patients, which may aid sinus drainage as well as, potentially, the drainage of any associated subperiosteal abscess (Fig. 3a, b) [30].

Steroids may promote recovery in patients with orbital cellulitis, although their use is generally not advised due to the risk of deterioration in patients with fungal disease or immunosuppression. They may be considered in patients who have confirmed bacterial infection on microbiological test and have shown definite clinical improvement on medical treatment [31].

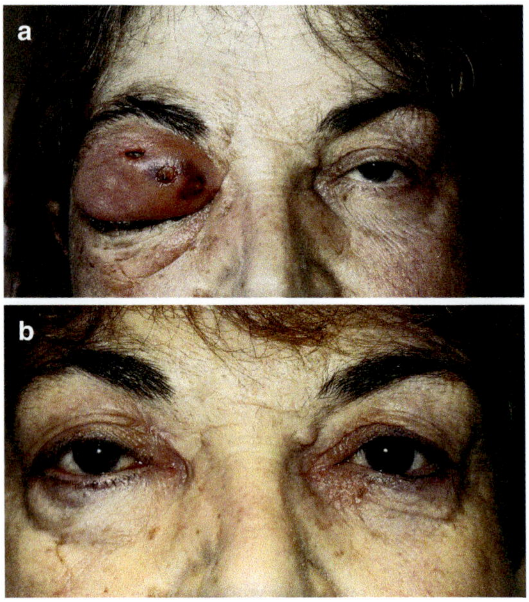

Fig. 3 (**a**) Clinical presentation of a patient with a right orbital abscess. (**b**) Resolution after antibiotic therapy and surgical drainage

Whilst most adults with orbital cellulitis improve with medical measures only, the need for surgical drainage must be considered regularly.

The presence of an abscess is itself not an indication for surgical drainage, although intervention becomes necessary when there is poor response to antibiotic management [1, 32]. Medial collections may be reached via a trans/retro-caruncular approach or medial skin crease approach. Superior and superolateral collections should be amenable to a standard skin crease approach, while inferior and inferolateral collections likely require a transconjunctival inferior forniceal approach or tear-trough approach. Following acquisition of a microbiology specimen, the subperiosteal space should be irrigated with saline, and a sutured corrugated drain placed in this space and left in situ for 2–3 days to promote maximal drainage.

2 Other Bacterial Orbital Infections

2.1 Necrotising Fasciitis

Necrotising fasciitis is a rapidly progressive infection of the subcutaneous facial planes, caused by group A β-haemolytic Streptococcus (GAS) in two-thirds of cases. Other bacteria have been isolated in necrotising fasciitis—group G β-haemolytic Streptococcus (GGS), Staphylococcus aureus, *Escherichia coli*, pseudomonas, Enterobacter, Klebsiella, Proteus, Bacteroides, Clostridium, and *Moraxella catarrhalis*—although it is unclear whether these are primary infections, or arise as a result of primary GAS infection [33–35].

Periocular necrotising fasciitis is an ophthalmic emergency, requiring immediate treatment with IV antibiotics and debridement. Inflammation may spread from the fibrofatty fascial tissue planes in the eyelid to the fibrous septae of the orbit. Marked subsequent perivasculitis can lead to ophthalmic or central retinal artery thrombosis and visual loss [36].

2.1.1 Clinical Features

Periocular necrotising fasciitis is often bilateral, painful, and associated with violaceous (violet-coloured) skin discolouration, vesicle formation and frank necrosis. GAS, a commensal organism, may also cause pharyngitis, pyoderma (impetigo), pneumonia, meningitis and puerperal sepsis, and so GAS-related necrotising fasciitis may present with these features concomitantly [37].

2.1.2 Investigation

Necrotising fasciitis must be diagnosed on clinical findings, in order to expedite the prompt initiation of treatment. Tissue biopsy, if it were performed, would demonstrate extensive subcutaneous and fascial necrosis.

2.1.3 Management

Suspected necrotising fasciitis of the periorbita and orbit is a true ophthalmic emergency, requiring prompt diagnosis and immediate treatment with extensive debridement of the necrotic subcutaneous tissue and high-dose IV penicillin and clindamycin [33–36]. Repeated debridement is required if there is any evidence of disease progression. Failure to control the rapid progression of necrotising fasciitis can lead, over the course of hours to days, to septicaemia, multi-organ failure, and death in a quarter of patients [38].

2.2 Mycobacterium

Atypical mycobacterium and *Mycobacterium hominis* rarely infect the orbit, but when they do, can involve any of the periorbital and orbital tissues, including even the periosteum and bony walls [39–44]. Such infections can occur at any age, and in the absence of pulmonary disease [41, 45].

2.2.1 Clinical Features

Mycobacterial orbital infections are often associated with a 'cold' orbital abscess, a discharging cutaneous sinus, and even sphenoidal osteomyelitis causing optic neuritis [46]. They can also extend into the adjacent sinuses or intracranial cavity [40, 47].

3 Fungal Orbital Infections

Fungal infections of the orbit are rare, but should be considered in the immunocompromised patient. Fungi, which are commonplace in the environment, reach the orbit via the sinuses. Organisms that have been implicated in orbital infection include the Phycomycetes (*Mucor* and *Rhizopus* spp.) and Ascomycetes (Aspergillus spp.)—both discussed below—in addition to Blastomycetes, *Sporothrix* spp. and Phaeohyphomycosies (*Bipolarina* spp.) [48–51].

3.1 Phycomycetes

Mucoris—a subset of the class Phycomycetes, and a genera of the order Mucorales—are ubiquitous spores which can cause disease in debilitated patients due to their ability to invade blood vessels (angioinvasive), causing endothelial damage, ischaemia and necrosis [52, 53]. Predisposing factors include pre-existing uncontrolled diabetes mellitus, solid malignancies, haematological malignancies associated with neutropenia, extensive burns, and haemochromatosis [54, 55].

Half of all patients with *mucoris* infection develop rhino-orbital-cerebral mucormycosis, which originates in the nasal passage, then the maxillary and ethmoid sinuses, before extending into the orbit [53, 56, 57]. The incidence of mucormycosis is increasing with the increasing number of immunocompromised patients, although infection may, rarely, occur in immunocompetent patients [58–60]. Intracranial extension, if present, occurs via the orbital roof and the orbital apex, through the cribiform plate [52, 56].

3.1.1 Clinical Features

The signs of orbital involvement in *mucormycosis* include proptosis, reduced eye movements, reduced visual acuity, loss of trigeminal sensation, and the presence of a relative afferent pupillary defect [61]. Orbital apex involvement is suggested by the presence of internal and external ophthalmoplegia, blepharoptosis and periorbital paraesthesia [52].

Systemic features include general malaise, fever, sinusitis, pharyngitis, nasal discharge, anosmia, and facial pain and paraesthesia. The necrotic black nasal or oral *eschar* classically associated with mucormycosis is a late finding, and may be absent.

3.1.2 Investigation

Blood tests are generally unhelpful, although may identify a raised erythrocyte sedimentation rate or white blood cell count [61]. Tissue specimens, if obtained, demonstrate broad hyposeptate hyphae with irregular branching, and when these are folded, give a unique "twisted ribbon" pattern [62].

CT and MRI imaging are useful in identifying the extent of disease (Fig. 4). Mucosal thickening, bony destruction and venous filling defects (which suggest a thrombosis) are detectable with CT, while MRI of the sinuses may identify loss of the sinus cavity [63, 64].

3.1.3 Management

The mainstays of treatment are prompt wide debridement of devitalised tissue and antifungal therapy (Fig. 5) [65]. Lipid formulations of amphotericin B (LFAB, 3–10 mg/kg/day)—a fungistatic agent effective against most yeasts and moulds—are the most common choice, although the use of posaconazole and isavuconazole have also been reported [66–70].

Repeated tissue debridement may be required, with the potential for extensive tissue removal.

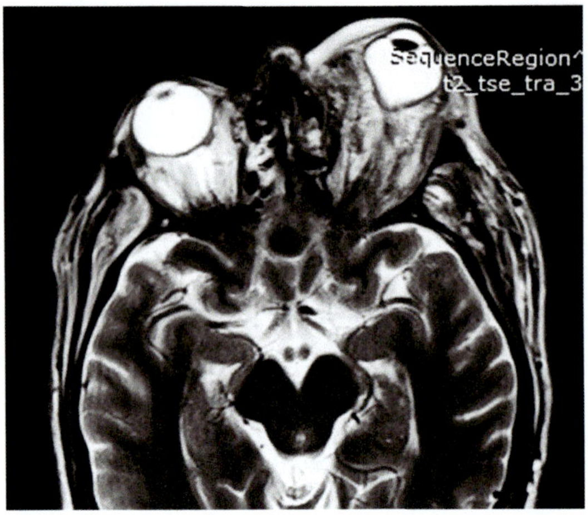

Fig. 4 Left orbital mucormycosis (MRI-imaging). Note the extensive soft tissue swelling, the exophthalmos and globe deformity

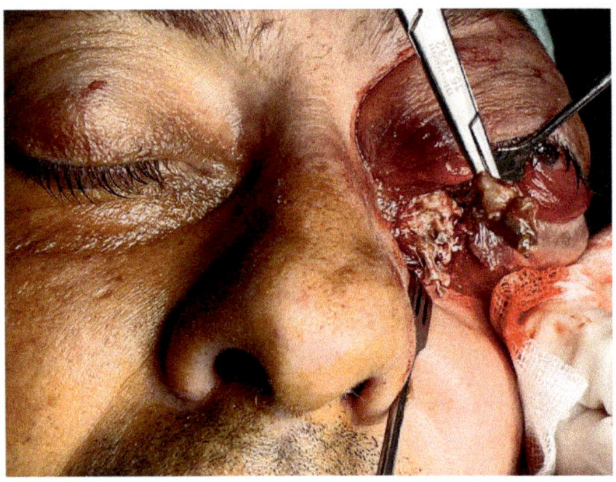

Fig. 5 Left orbital mucormycosis (surgical drainage and removal of inflamed tissue)

Orbital exenteration is often necessary in posterior disease, but may not be required for more anterior disease [53, 71–73].

Rhino-orbital-cerebral mucormycosis (ROCM) previously had a very poor prognosis—due to both the aggressive profile of *Mucor* and frequently delayed diagnosis—with an overall survival rate of 10%. However, with the introduction of LFAB antifungal treatment, survival rates have risen to 70%.

ROCM has significantly increased due to the COVID 19 pandemic. COVID-19 may be the predisposing factor for mucormycosis especially in individuals with diabetes and increased usage of steroids [74]. Patients with diabetes and hyperglycemia often have an inflammatory state that could be potentiated by the activation of antiviral immunity to SARS-CoV2, which might favour secondary infections [75]. In these cases, treatment needs a multimodality approach with antifungals and surgical debridement with careful surveillance for good outcome. According to a recent study, despite surgical debridement and antifungal therapy, 5.8% of affected patients died from mucormycosis [74]. Moreover, a substantial proportion of patients who survive have life changing morbidities, with loss of vision in 46% of survivors [75].

3.2 Ascomycetes

Aspergillus—a ubiquitous fungus which survives by absorbing decaying organic material (saprophytic)—may cause sinus infection [76, 77]. In immunocompetent individuals, this usually takes the form of *non-invasive* disease, with allergic sinusitis or sinonasal fungal ball (aspergilloma) [78, 79]. *Invasive* disease generally occurs in immunocompromised patients—often with coexisting haematological disease such as leukemia, lymphoma or HIV infection—and rarely occurs in healthy individuals [80–82]. *Invasive* disease may be associated with arteritis (and secondary thrombosis and aneurysm formation), and often posterior extension from the orbit to the cavernous sinus and brain, with a 28% mortality rate despite treatment [83, 84].

3.2.1 Clinical Features

Aspergillus infections are often slowly progressive, in contrast to disease caused by *Mucor* and *Rhizopus*. Orbital involvement often presents with gradually progressive proptosis, although visual loss may occur due to chronic fibrosing granulomatous disease of the sinuses [85]. In cases of isolated sphenoid sinus disease, optic neuritis may occur, leading to visual loss, without any actual orbital involvement (or proptosis) [86].

3.2.2 Investigation

Tissue histology demonstrates a typical pattern of branching septate hyphae (with Gomori methenamine silver and periodic acid Schiff stains).

CT imaging typically demonstrates a hyperdense mass which may be expanding or destroying the paranasal sinuses, or extending into the cranium. On MRI, *Aspergillus* lesions are T1-isointense and T2-hypointense.

3.2.3 Management

The successful treatment of orbital aspergillosis, once again, relies on prompt diagnosis (which requires an already high degree of clinical suspicion), extensive debridement of the infected tissues, and intensive antifungal treatment. IV LFAB treatment is the most common choice, although flucytosine, itraconazole and voriconazole have all been used with success [87–91]. Despite such intensive treatment, almost one-third of all cases prove ultimately fatal, increasing to 66–100% in (usually debilitated) patients who develop intracerebral aspergillosis [92].

4 Parasitic Orbital Infections

4.1 Echinococcus

Echinococcus granulosus, which causes hydatid disease, predominantly occurs in agricultural regions of the Mediterranean, Middle East, Southeast Asia, Australia, New Zealand and South America [93, 94]. These parasites live in the intestinal tract of dogs. They release their eggs in the dog's faeces, which are then ingested by an intermediate host (such as a cow or sheep) and hatch in the livestock's gut. These hydatid cysts then disseminate via the bloodstream throughout the intermediate host, and when these tissues are ingested by the final host (humans) they reach the final larval stage [95].

Hydatid disease tends to affect the liver and lungs most commonly, with less than 1% of cases involving the orbit [95–97]. However, in endemic areas, hydatid disease can still account for a quarter of all cystic orbital lesions [98–100].

4.1.1 Clinical Features

Orbital hydatid disease usually presents in patients under the age of 20, with slowly progressive, painless proptosis and extraocular motility restriction (due to a solitary intraconal lesion) [95, 99, 101].

4.1.2 Investigation

Ultrasonography may identify a well-circumscribed cystic orbital structure. CT imaging may demonstrate a cyst with aqueous-like density and a contrast-enhancing rim. Serological testing is usually unreliable, as the parasite generally remains encysted [95, 102].

4.1.3 Management

Surgical excision has traditionally been the mainstay of treatment. In around half of cases, the ovoid orbital lesion is normally found to be surrounded by an adventitious fibrous membrane [95, 101]. Albendazole may also play a role in the treatment of orbital hydatid disease—either alone, or in combination with surgery [102].

4.2 Microfilaria

Dirofilaria—a parasitic worm that generally infests domestic and wild animals—may rarely use an insect vector (Culex and Aedes mosquitoes) to infect humans [103, 104]. In these cases, patients may present with subconjunctival, intraocular, periorbital and even extraocular muscle infestation. Common signs include chemosis and proptosis. Treatment is generally by surgical excision.

4.3 Cysticercosis

Cysticercosis is a potentially fatal infection which is more common in areas with poor sanitation, such as South America, sub-Saharan Africa and regions of Asia. It is caused by the parasite *Taenia solium*, which can be found in raw pork, and if ingested, hatch in the stomach and release larvae which spread via the blood throughout the body [105–107]. Cysticercosis of the eye (ocular cysticercosis) makes up around 75–85% of cysticercosis cases worldwide, although orbital disease forms only a small percentage of these [108].

4.4 Ophthalmomyiasis

Botfly larvae infestation, known as myiasis, affects the eyes (ophthalmomyiasis) in 5% of all cases, with larval invasion of the periorbita, conjunctiva or cornea [109, 110]. The most common culprits are the sheep botfly *Oestrus ovis* and the human botfly *Diptera hominis*. Interestingly, several reports have suggested a link between ophthalmomyiasis and pre-existing periocular ulcerative skin cancers [111, 112].

Ophthalmomyiasis leads to significant tissue destruction, which is associated with pain, while patients may notice itching or even a sensation of tissue movement due to the moving larvae.

Treatment is by surgical excision, although this is technically challenging due to the presence of numerous small spicules on the surface of the organism.

References

1. Hamed-Azzam S, AlHashash I, Briscoe D, Rose G, Verity DH. Common orbital infections—state of the art: Part I. J Ophthalmic Vis Res. 2018;13:175–82.
2. Nageswaran S, Woods C, Benjamin D, Givner LB, Shetty A. Orbital cellulitis in children. Pediatr Infect Dis J. 2006;25:695–9.
3. Ferguson MP, McNab AA. Current treatment and outcome in orbital cellulitis. Aust N Z J Ophthalmol. 1999;27:375–9.
4. Tsirouki T, Dastiridou AI, Ibánez Flores N, Cerpa JC, Moschos MM, Brazitikos P, Androudi S. Orbital cellulitis. Surv Ophthalmol. 2018;63:534–53. Epub 2017 Dec 15.
5. Barone SR, Aiuto LT. Periorbital and orbital cellulitis in the Haemophilus influenzae vaccine era. J Pediatr Ophthalmol Strabismus. 1997;34:293–6.
6. Ambati BK, Ambati J, Azar N, Stratton L, Schmidt EV. Periorbital and orbital cellulitis before and after the advent of Haemophilus influenzae type B vaccination. Ophthalmology. 2001;108:1514–5.
7. Partamian LG, Jay WM, Fritz KJ. Anaerobic orbital cellulitis. Ann Ophthalmol. 1983;15:123–6.
8. Rubin SE, Slavin ML, Rubin LG. Eyelid swelling and erythema as the only signs of subperiosteal abscess. Br J Ophthalmol. 1989;73:576–8.
9. Rose GE. Suspicion, speed, sufficiency and surgery: keys to the management of orbital infection. Orbit. 1998;17:223–6.
10. BSAC/BOPSS Guideline. https://bsac.org.uk/paediatricpathways/preseptal-orbital-cellulitis.php.
11. Wong SJ, Levi J. Management of pediatric orbital cellulitis: a systematic review. Int J Pediatr Otorhinolaryngol. 2018;110:123–9. Epub. 2018 May.
12. Van der Veer EG, van der Poel NA, de Win MM, Kloos RJ, Saeed P, Mourits MP. True abscess formation is rare in bacterial orbital cellulitis; consequences for treatment. Am J Otolaryngol. 2017;38:130–4.
13. Garcia GH, Harris GJ. Criteria for nonsurgical management of subperiosteal abscess of the orbit: analysis of outcomes 1988-1998. Ophthalmology. 2000;107:1454–6.
14. Smith AT, Spencer JT. Orbital complications resulting from lesions of the sinuses. Ann Otol Rhinol Laryngol. 1948;57:5–27.
15. Clary R, Weber AL, Eavey R, Oot RF. Orbital cellulitis with abscess formation caused by sinusitis. Ann Otol Rhinol Laryngol. 1988;97:211–2.
16. Bergin DJ, Wright J. Orbital cellulitis. Br J Ophthalmol. 1986;70:174–8.
17. Jackson K, Baker SR. Periorbital cellulitis. Head Neck Surg. 1987;9:227–34.
18. Bullock JD, Fleishman JA. Orbital cellulitis following dental extraction. Trans Am Ophthalmol Soc. 1984;87:111–33.
19. Slavin ML, Glaser JS. Acute severe irreversible visual loss with sphenoethmoiditis "posterior" orbital cellulitis. Arch Ophthalmol. 1987;105:345–8.
20. Williams KJ, Allen RC. Paediatric orbital and periorbital infections. Curr Opin Ophthalmol. 2019;30:349–55.
21. Ball JL, Malhotra RM, Leong P, Bacon AS. The importance of recognising Streptococcus milleri as a cause of orbital cellulitis. Eye. 2000;14:814–5.
22. Gossling J. Occurrence and pathogenicity of the Streptococcus milleri group. Rev Infect Dis. 1988;10:257–85.
23. Whiley RA, Beighton D, Winstanley TG, Fraser HY, Hardie JM. Streptococcus intermedius, Streptococcus constellatus, and Streptococcus anginosus (the Streptococcus milleri group): association with different body sites and clinical infections. J Clin Microbiol. 1992;30:243–4.
24. Mahalingam S, Hone R, Lloyd G, Grounds R, Shamil E, Wong G, Al-Lami A, Pervez A, Rudd J, Poon JS, Riley P, Hopkins C. The management of periorbital cellulitis secondary to sinonasal infection: a multicenter prospective study in the United

Kingdom. Int Forum Allergy Rhinol. 2020;10:726. [Epub ahead of print].
25. Liao JC, Harris GJ. Subperiosteal abscess of the orbit: evolving pathogens and the therapeutic protocol. Ophthalmology. 2015;122:639–47.
26. Weber AL, Mikulis DK. Inflammatory disorders of the periorbital sinuses and their complications. Radiol Clin North Am. 1987;25:615–30.
27. Hodges E, Tabbara KF. Orbital cellulitis: review of 23 cases from Saudi Arabia. Br J Ophthalmol. 1989;73:205–8.
28. Hartstein ME, Steinvurzel MD, Cohen CP. Intracranial abscess as a complication of subperiosteal abscess of the orbit. Ophthal Plast Reconstr Surg. 2001;17:395–7.
29. Yen MT. Current techniques for the management of orbital cellulitis. Tech Ophthalmol. 2006;4:45–9.
30. Benninger MS, Anon J, Mabry RL. The medical management of rhinosinusitis. Otolaryngol Head Neck Surg. 1997;117:S41–9.
31. Yen MT, Yen KG. Effect of corticosteroids in the acute management of pediatric orbital cellulitis with subperiosteal abscess. Ophthal Plast Reconstr Surg. 2005;21:363–6.
32. Gold SC, Arrigg PG, Hedges TR. Computerized tomography in the management of acute orbital cellulitis. Ophthalmic Surg. 1987;18:753–6.
33. Headley AJ. Necrotizing soft tissue infections: a primary care review. Am Fam Physician. 2003;15:323–8.
34. Childers BJ, Potyondy LD, Nachreiner R, Rogers FR, Childers ER, Oberg KC, Hendricks DL, Hardesty RA. Necrotizing fasciitis: a fourteen-year retrospective study of 163 consecutive patients. Am Surg. 2002;68:109–16.
35. Brittain CJ, Penwarden A, Mearza A, Verity D. Moraxella as a cause of necrotizing fasciitis of the eyelid. Eye. 2006;20:1312–4.
36. Elner VM, Demirci H, Nerad JA, Hassan AS. Periocular necrotizing fasciitis with visual loss pathogenesis and treatment. Ophthalmology. 2006;113:2338.
37. Currie BJ. Group a streptococcal infections of the skin: molecular advances but limited therapeutic progress. Curr Opin Infect Dis. 2006;19:132–8.
38. Costet-Fighiera C, Lagier J, Bastiani-Griffet F, Bernard E, Gastaud P. Necrotizing fasciitis of the eyelids and orbit: a life-threatening ophthalmological emergency. J Fr Ophtalmol. 2002;25:375–8.
39. Levine RA. Infection of the orbit by an atypical *mycobacterium*. Arch Ophthalmol. 1969;82:608–10.
40. Sen DK. Tuberculosis of the Orbita and lacrimal gland: a clinical study of 14 cases. J Pediatr Ophthalmol Strabismus. 1980;17:232–8.
41. Khali M, Lindley S, Matouk E. Tuberculosis of the orbit. Ophthalmology. 1985;92:1624–7.
42. Oakhill A, Shah KJ, Thompson AG, et al. Orbital tuberculosis in childhood. Br J Ophthalmol. 1982;66:396–7.
43. Helm CJ, Holland GN. Ocular tuberculosis. Surv Ophthalmol. 1993;38:229–56.
44. Sardana K, Koranne RV, Langan U, Sharma RC, Bhatnagar SK. Ocular scrofuloderma with unilateral proptosis. J Dermatol. 2002;29:232–4.
45. van Assen S, Lutterman JA. Tuberculous dacryoadenitis: a rare manifestation of tuberculosis. Neth J Med. 2002;60:327–9.
46. Das JC, Singh K, Sharma P, Singla R. Tuberculous osteomyelitis and optic neuritis. Ophthalmic Surg Lasers Imaging. 2003;34:409–12.
47. Aggarwal D, Suri A, Mahapatra AK. Orbital tuberculosis with abscess. J Neuroophthalmol. 2002;22:208–10.
48. Vida L, Moel SA. Systemic north American blastomycosis with orbital involvement. Am J Ophthalmol. 1974;77:240–2.
49. Jakobiec FA, Jones IS. Orbital inflammations. In: Duane TD, editor. Clinical ophthalmology. Philadelphia: JB Lippincott; 1988.
50. Streeten BW, Rabuzzi DD, Jones DB. Sporotrichosis of the orbital margin. Am J Ophthalmol. 1974;77:750–5.
51. Maskin SL, Fetchick RJ, Leone CR Jr, et al. *Bipolaris hawaiiensis*-caused phaeohyphomycotic orbitopathy. Ophthalmology. 1989;96:175–9.
52. Bray WH, Giangiacomo J, Ide CH. Orbital apex syndrome. Surv Ophthalmol. 1987;32:136–40.
53. Kohn R, Hepler R. Management of limited rhino-orbital mucormycosis without exenteration. Ophthalmology. 1985;92:1440–4.
54. McNab AA, McKelvie P. Iron overload is a risk factor for zygomycosis. Arch Ophthalmol. 1997;115:919 21–921.
55. Hamed-Azzam S, AlHashash I, Briscoe D, Rose G, Verity DH. Rare orbital infections—state of the art: Part II. J Ophthalmic Vis Res. 2018;13:183–90.
56. Schwartze GM, Kilgo GR, Ford CS. Internal ophthalmoplegia resulting from acute orbital phycomycosis. J Clin Neuroophthalmol. 1984;4:105–8.
57. Hosseini SM, Borghei P. Rhinocerebral mucormycosis: pathways of spread. Eur Arch Otorhinolaryngol. 2005;262:932–8.
58. Garcia-Diaz JB, Palau L, Pankey G. Resolution of rhinocerebral zygomycosis associated with adjuvant administration of granulocyte-macrophage colony-stimulating factor. Clin Infect Dis. 2001;32:e166–70.
59. Georgopoulou S, Kounougeri E, Katsenos C, Rizos M, Michalopoulos A. Rhinocerebral mucormycosis in a patient with cirrhosis and chronic renal failure. Hepatogastroenterology. 2003;50:843–5.
60. Fairley C, Sullivan TJ, Bartley P, Allworth T, Lewandowski R. Survival after rhino-orbital-cerebral mucormycosis in an immunocompetent patient. Ophthalmology. 2000;107:555–8.
61. Ferry AP, Abedi S. Diagnosis and management of rhino orbito cerebral mucormycosis (phycomycosis). Ophthalmology. 1983;90:1096–104.

62. Virmani R, Connor DH, McAllister HA. Cardiac mucormycosis: a case report of five patients and review of 14 previously reported cases. Am J Clin Pathol. 1982;78:42–7.
63. Gamba JL, Woodruff WW, Djang WT, et al. Craniofacial mucormycosis: assessment with CT. Radiology. 1986;160:207–12.
64. Press GA, Weindling SM, Hesselink JR, et al. Rhinocerebral mucormycosis: MR manifestations. J Comput Assist Tomogr. 1988;12:744–9.
65. Petrikkos G, Skiada A, Sambatakou H, et al. Mucormycosis: ten-year experience at a tertiary-care center in Greece. Eur J Clin Microbiol Infect Dis. 2003;22:753–6.
66. Sorensen J, Becker M, Porto L, Lambrecht E, Schuster T, Beske F, Rickerts V, Klingebiel T, Lehrnbecher T. Rhinocerebral zygomycosis in a young girl undergoing allogeneic stem cell transplantation for severe aplastic anaemia. Mycoses. 2006;49:31–6.
67. Greenberg RN, Mullane K, van Burik JA, et al. Posaconazole as salvage therapy for zygomycosis. Antimicrob Agents Chemother. 2006;50:126–33.
68. Simmons JH, Zeitler PS, Fenton LZ, Abzug MJ, Fiallo-Scharer RV, Klingensmith GJ. Rhinocerebral mucormycosis complicated by internal carotid artery thrombosis in a pediatric patient with type 1 diabetes mellitus: a case report and review of the literature. Pediatr Diabetes. 2005;6:234–8.
69. Sun QN, Fothergill AW, McCarthy DI, et al. In vitro activities of posaconazole, itraconazole, voriconazole, amphotericin B and fluconazole against 37 clinical isolates of Zygomycetes. Antimicrob Agents Chemother. 2002;46:1581–2.
70. van Burik JA, Hare RS, Solomon HF, et al. Posaconazole is effective as salvage therapy in zygomycosis: a retrospective summary of 91 cases. Clin Infect Dis. 2006;42:e61–5.
71. Pelton RW, Peterson EA, Patel BCK, Davis K. Successful treatment of rhino-orbital mucormycosis without exenteration: the use of multiple treatment modalities. Ophthal Plast Reconstr Surg. 2001;17:62–6.
72. Nithyanandam S, Jacob MS, Battu RR, Thomas RK, Correa MA, D'Souza O. Rhino-Orbito-Cerebral Mucormycosis. A retrospective analysis of clinical features and treatment outcomes. Indian J Ophthalmol. 2003;51:231–6.
73. Songu M, Unlu HH, Gunhan K, Ilker SS, Nese N. Orbital exenteration: a dilemma in mucormycosis presented with orbital apex syndrome. Am J Rhinol. 2008;22:98–103.
74. Vadivel S, Gowrishankar M, Vetrivel K, Sujatha B, Navaneethan P. Rhino orbital cerebral mucormycosis in Covid-19 crisis. Indian J Otolaryngol Head Neck Surg. 2023;75:1014–20. Epub ahead of print.
75. Hoenigl M, Seidel D, Carvalho A, Rudramurthy SM, Arastehfar A, Gangneux JP, Nasir N, Bonifaz A, Araiza J, Klimko N, Serris A, Lagrou K, Meis JF, Cornely OA, Perfect JR, White PL, Chakrabarti A, ECMM and ISHAM collaborators. The emergence of COVID-19 associated mucormycosis: a review of cases from 18 countries. Lancet Microbe. 2022;3:e543–52.
76. Seif SR, Choo PH, Carter SR. Role of local amphotericin B therapy for sino-orbital fungal infections. Ophthal Plast Reconstr Surg. 1999;15:28–32.
77. Abzug MJ, Walsh TJ. Interferon-gamma and colony-stimulating factors as adjuvant therapy for refractory fungal infections in children. Pediatr Infect Dis J. 2004;23:769–73.
78. Luna JD, Ponssa XS, Rodriguez SD, Luna NC, Juarez CP. Intraconal amphotericin B for the treatment of rhino-orbital mucormycosis. Ophthalmic Surg Lasers. 1996;27:706–8.
79. Kargi S, Kargi AE, Akduman D, Hanioglu S. Invasive fungal sinusitis. Plast Reconstr Surg. 2004;113:1067–9.
80. Gulen H, Erbay A, Gulen F, Kazanci E, Vergin C, Demir E, Tanac R. Sinopulmonary aspergillosis in children with hematological malignancy. Minerva Pediatr. 2006;58:319–24.
81. Levin LA, Avery R, Shore J, et al. The spectrum of orbital aspergillosis: a clinicopathological review. Surv Ophthalmol. 1996;41:142–54.
82. Johnson TE, Casiano RR, Kronish JW, Tse DT, Meldrum M, Chang W. Sino-orbital aspergillosis in acquired immunodeficiency syndrome. Arch Ophthalmol. 1999;117:57–64.
83. Yumoto E, Kitani S, Okomura H, Yanagihara N, et al. Sino-orbital aspergillosis associated with total ophthalmoplegia. Laryngoscope. 1985;95:190–2.
84. Siddiqui A, Shah A, Bashir S. Craniocerebral aspergillosis of sinonasal origin in immunocompetent patients: clinical spectrum and outcome in 25 cases. Neurosurgery. 2004;55:602–13.
85. Mauriello JA Jr, Yepez N, Mostafavi R, Barofsky J, Kapila R, Baredes S, Norris J. Invasive rhinosino-orbital aspergillosis with precipitous visual loss. Can J Ophthalmol. 1995;30:124–30.
86. Nielsen EW, et al. Aspergillosis of the sphenoid sinus presenting as orbital pseudotumor. Otolaryngol Head Neck Surg. 1983;91:699–703.
87. Steinbach WJ, Stevens DA, Denning DA. Combination and sequential antifungal therapy for invasive aspergillosis: review of published in vitro and in vivo interactions and 6281 clinical cases from 1966 to 2001. Clin Infect Dis. 2003;37:S188–224.
88. Walsh TJ, Goodman JL, Pappas P, et al. Safety, tolerance, and pharmacokinetics of high-dose liposomal amphotericin B (AmBisome) in patients infected with aspergillus species and other filamentous fungi: maximum tolerated dose study. Antimicrob Agents Chemother. 2001;45:3487–96.
89. Herbrecht R, Denning DW, Patterson TF, et al. Voriconazole versus amphotericin B for primary therapy of invasive aspergillosis. N Engl J Med. 2002;347:408–15.

90. O'Doherty M, Hannan M, Fulcher T. Voriconazole in the treatment of fungal osteomyelitis of the orbit in the immunocompromised host. Orbit. 2005;24:285–9.
91. Parsonage MJ, Stafford ND, Lillie P, Moss PJ, Barlow G, Thaker H. Oral voriconazole for invasive fungal skull base infection. J Laryngol Otol. 2009;1-4:1010–3.
92. Denning DW. Therapeutic outcome in invasive aspergillosis. Clin Infect Dis. 1996;23:608–15.
93. Akhan O, Dincer A, Gokoz A, et al. Percutaneous treatment of abdominal hydatid cysts with hypertonic saline and alcohol: an experimental study in sheep. Invest Radiol. 1993;28:121–7.
94. Basset D, Girou C, Nozais IP, D'Hermies F, Hoang C, Gordon R, D'Alessandro A. Neotropical echinococcosis in Suriname: Echinococcus oligarthrus in the orbit and Echinococcus vogeli in the abdomen. Am J Trop Med Hyg. 1998;59:787–90.
95. Morales AG, Croxatto JO, Crovetto L, et al. Hydatid cysts of the orbit: a review of 35 cases. Ophthalmology. 1988;95:1027–32.
96. Xiao A, Xueyi C. Hydatid cysts of the orbit in Xinjiang: a review of 18 cases. Orbit. 1999;18:151–5.
97. Abbassioun K, Amirjamshidi A. Diagnosis and Management of Hydatid Cyst of the central nervous system: part 2: hydatid cysts of the skull, orbit, and spine. Neurosurg Q. 2001;11:10–6.
98. Belmekki M, El Bakkali M, Abdellah H, et al. Epidemiologie des processus orbitaires chez l'enfant. A propos de 54 cas. J Fr Ophthalmol. 1999;22:394–8.
99. Gomez Morales A, Croxatto JO, Crovetto L, et al. Hydatid cysts of the orbit. A review of 35 cases. Ophthalmology. 1988;95:1027–32.
100. Talib H. Orbital hydatid disease in Iraq. Br J Surg. 1972;59:391–4.
101. Kars Z, Kansu T, Ozcan OE, et al. Orbital echinococcosis: report of two cases studied by computerized tomography. J Clin Neuroophthalmol. 1982;2:197–9.
102. Senyuz OF, Yesildag E, Celayir S. Albendazole therapy in the treatment of hydatid liver disease. Surg Today. 2001;31:487–91.
103. Angunawela RI, Ataullah S, Whitehead KJ, Sullivan TJ, Rosser P. Dirofilarial infection of the orbit. Orbit. 2003;22:41–6.
104. Strianese D, Martini A, Molfino G, Falabella L, Tranfa F. Orbital dirofilariasis. Eur J Ophthalmol. 1998;8:258–62.
105. Pushker N, Bajaj MS, Balasubramanya R. Disseminated cysticercosis involving orbit, brain and subcutaneous tissue. J Infect. 2005;51:245–8.
106. Gulliani BP, Dadeya S, Malik KPS, JainDC. Bilateral cysticercosis of the optic nerve. J Neuroophthalmol. 2001;21:217–8.
107. Walrath JD, Lalin SC, Leib ML. Cysticercosis isolated to the orbit. Ophthal Plast Reconstr Surg. 2003;19:243–4.
108. Auzemery A, Andriantsimahavandy A, Esterre P, Bouat C, Boitte JP, Huguet P. Ocular cysticercosis. Medecine tropicale: revue du Corps de sante colonial. 1995;55:429–33.
109. Wilhelmus K. Myiasis palpebrarum. Am J Ophthalmol. 1986;101:496–7.
110. Devoto MH, Zaffaroni MC. Orbital myiasis in a patient with a chronically exposed hydroxyapatite implant. Ophthal Plast Reconstr Surg. 2004;20:395–6.
111. Yeung JC, Chung CF, Lai JS. Orbital myiasis complicating squamous cell carcinoma of eyelid. Hong Kong Med J. 2010;16:63–5.
112. Abalo-Lojo JM, López-Valladares MJ, Llovo J, Garcia A, Gonzalez F. Palpebro-orbital myiasis in a patient with basal cell carcinoma. Br J Ophthalmol. 2009;19:683–5.

Idiopathic Orbital Inflammation

Ilse Mombaerts, Peerooz Saeed,
and Rachel Kalmann

Key Messages

- Idiopathic orbital inflammation (IOI) is characterised by a soft tissue mass or enlarged structure featuring nonspecific orbital inflammation of unknown origin.
- In a clinicoradiological context suggesting IOI, lesions of the lacrimal gland and orbital fat require biopsy to confirm diagnosis and exclude other disorders.
- Idiopathic orbital myositis may be diagnosed based on corticosteroid responsiveness.
- Treatment options include surgical debulking, anti-inflammatory, immunomodulating or biological drugs, and radiation therapy.

1 Introduction

Idiopathic orbital inflammation (IOI), formerly called *orbital pseudotumor*, is a term applied to an orbit-specific disorder characterised by a mass or enlarged orbital soft tissue structure consisting of nonspecific inflammation without identifiable local or systemic cause [1]. Based on the involvement of the orbital structure, IOI is categorized as *idiopathic dacryoadenitis* (lacrimal gland), *idiopathic orbital myositis* (extraocular muscle(s)), or *diffuse IOI* (orbital fibrofatty matrix or multiple structures). *Sclerosing IOI* is a distinct variant of IOI where dense fibrous tissue predominates [2].

2 Pathogenesis

The etiology and pathogenesis of IOI are poorly understood. Based on its heterogeneous clinical presentation and course, it is believed that IOI may represent an inflammatory process rather than a specific disease [3]. A subclinical infection or an immune response secondary to infection has been postulated [4]. The infection theory is supported by the detection of an aberrant cell-mediated type 1 helper T cell (T_H1) pathway, particularly observed in patients with sclerotic idiopathic dacryoadenitis, and Toll-like receptors of the innate immune system [5–7]. Also, there is genetic evidence for the presence of Epstein-Barr virus in some cases of nonsclerotic IOI [8]. T_H2-B cell humoral immunity has been implicated in the pathogenesis of nonsclerotic idiopathic dacryadenitis [5]. Mast cells have been linked to fibrogenesis in IOI, with evidence for a role of

I. Mombaerts (✉)
Department of Ophthalmology, University Hospitals Leuven, Leuven, Belgium
e-mail: Ilse.mombaerts@uzleuven.be

P. Saeed
Orbital Center, Department of Ophthalmology, Amsterdam University Medical Center, Amsterdam, The Netherlands

R. Kalmann
Department of Ophthalmology, University Medical Center Utrecht, Utrecht, The Netherlands

F. M. Quaranta Leoni et al. (eds.), *Oculoplastic, Lacrimal and Orbital Surgery*,
https://doi.org/10.1007/978-3-031-39638-0_17

fibrocytes, which have features of both immune cells and fibroblasts [9, 10]. Nearly half of the specimens of presumed IOI share gene expression profiling with granulomatosis with polyangiitis (GPA), and, a small subset of idiopathic dacryoadenitis with sarcoidosis, suggesting that these patients may have a limited form of GPA or sarcoidosis, which underscores the weak concept of a diagnosis of IOI [11–13].

Discrete serological similarities between IOI and orbital lymphoma have been documented. Serum analysis with immunophenotyping using flow cytometry shows similar micro RNAs (miRNA) and peripheral blood mononuclear cells (PBMC) profiles of IOI and lymphoma [14, 15]. Compared to orbital lymphoma, IOI exhibits a decreased conventional dendritic cell (cDC) type-2 population [15]. These cells also are implicated in other inflammatory disorders such as uveitis [16].

There is a well-reported concurrence of IOI with rheumatologic and auto-immune diseases, implying an immune-mediated mechanism and suggesting a genetic predisposition or dysregulated immune system [17–19]. Some authors consider the presence of IOI in children as a possible precursor of systemic inflammatory disease [20]. The intake of aminobisphosphonates has been associated with IOI [21]. However, when a causal agent or associated local or systemic disease is found in a patient with presumed IOI, the diagnosis of IOI should—by definition—be abandoned. These orbital conditions likely represent a distinct entity rather than IOI. In this way, a substantial number of cases of myositic IOI have been retrospectively reclassified as Crohn's or ulcerative colitis orbital myositis, and of sclerosing IOI as Immunoglobulin G4 (IgG4)-related disease [22–24]. With advancement of novel diagnostics and insights, underlying disease will be increasingly identified, eventually causing fewer cases recognized as "true IOI".

3 Demographics

Any age group can be affected, with a peak incidence at the sixth decade of life in idiopathic dacryoadenitis and at the fourth decade in idiopathic orbital myositis. Although there is no absolute age limit, young (<10 years) and old (>75 years for nonmyositic IOI, and >60 years for myositic IOI) patients are rarely affected by IOI and should be strongly considered as suffering from another disease [4, 25]. IOI is slightly more prevalent in females, and there are no racial preferences. Although a causal relationship has not been established, idiopathic orbital myositis may arise during or after pregnancy [26]. The prevalence of IOI, without anatomical specification, is reportedly associated with lower socio-economic status and higher body mass index [27]. Bilateral involvement is less common in IOI and strongly suggests underlying systemic disease [25].

4 Clinical Presentation

Depending on the orbital tissue(s) involved, degree of inflammation, associated fibrosis, and mass effect, symptoms of IOI vary and can include proptosis, double vision and limited eye motility, pain, eyelid swelling, redness and ptosis, corneal dryness, and optic nerve dysfunction. The onset of presentation is typically acute (within days) or subacute (within weeks), with a subsequent slow rate of progression.

5 Orbital Subtypes

The orbital structures on imaging most commonly involved are the lacrimal gland, extraocular muscle(s) and intra- or extraconal orbital fat. Optic nerve sheath infiltration rarely occurs.

5.1 Idiopathic Dacryoadenitis

Idiopathic dacryoadenitis is characterized by acute to subacute onset of upper eyelid swelling, ptosis and redness, and, in 70% of cases, associated with pain which varies from discomfort and tenderness, to severe pain in the periorbital region (Fig. 1) [28, 29]. Half of patients with idiopathic dacryoadenitis present with a dry eye and 20% with episcleritis in the superolateral quadrant

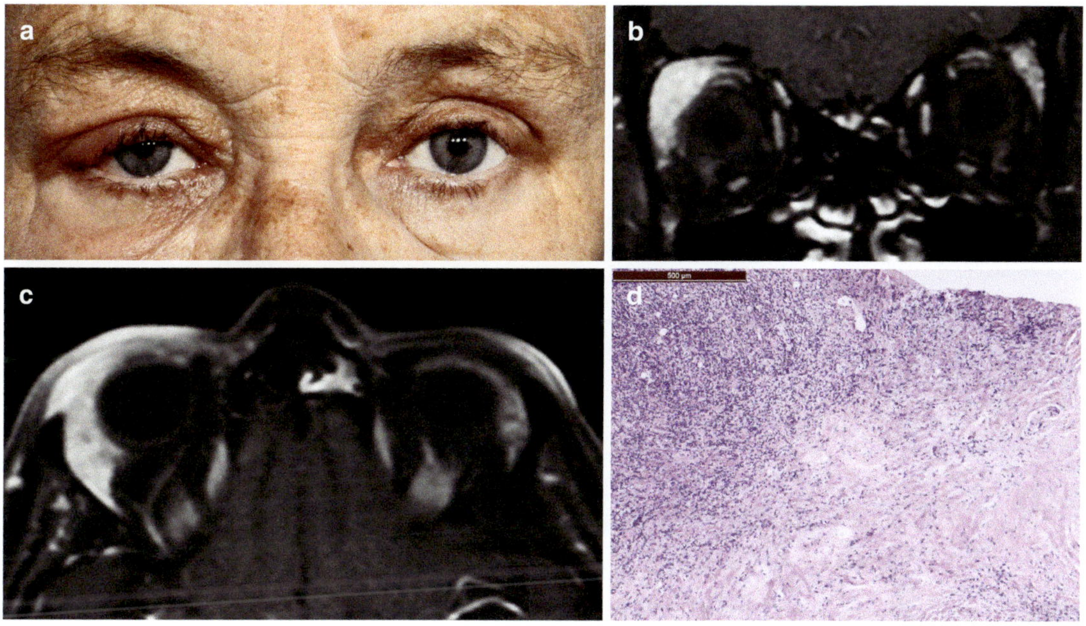

Fig. 1 (**a**) Patient with idiopathic dacryoadenitis of the right side. (**b**, **c**) Orbital MRI demonstrating a well-defined enlarged lacrimal gland with homogeneous enhancement, reaching but not invading the lateral rectus muscle. Histopathological analysis showing IgG4-negative lymphoplasmacytic infiltration with a few lymphoid follicles. (H&E, original magnification ×50)

[29]. Most commonly one gland is affected. Bilateral involvement, either concurrently or sequentially, occurs in 16-20% of cases [28, 29].

5.2 Idiopathic Orbital Myositis

Idiopathic orbital myositis typically presents with acute or subacute onset of conjunctival redness, eyelid swelling, orbital pain, diplopia, and mild proptosis [19]. The feature of acute onset of severe orbital pain distinguishes idiopathic orbital myositis from thyroid-associated orbitopathy (TAO). Pain is typically exacerbated on eye movement. The involved muscle can be clinically identified by episcleral redness at the site of its insertion. The eye motility is limited due to a weakened muscle (most commonly), restricted muscle, or both [23]. Bilateral myositis, either synchronous or metachronous, accounts for 20–50% of cases [19, 23].

Any extraocular muscle can be affected, but more commonly one or more horizontal rectus muscle(s) are involved. Idiopathic myositis tends to relapse, in which case the same or contralateral muscle is commonly affected [19]. When different muscles become involved, it is referred to as *migratory idiopathic orbital myositis* [30].

5.3 Diffuse Idiopathic Orbital Inflammation

Symptoms of diffuse IOI vary according to the structures involved. It often presents with orbital pain, double vision, proptosis, eyelid swelling, and, in orbital apex involvement, compressive optic neuropathy. Diffuse IOI is commonly sclerotic on histology and involves the superolateral, mid-, or apical/posterior orbit, of which 25% extend outside the orbit [31].

6 Diagnostic Evaluation

Given the variability of the clinical phenotype and lack of pathognomonic features, diagnosing IOI is difficult. An algorithm for diagnosis of IOI

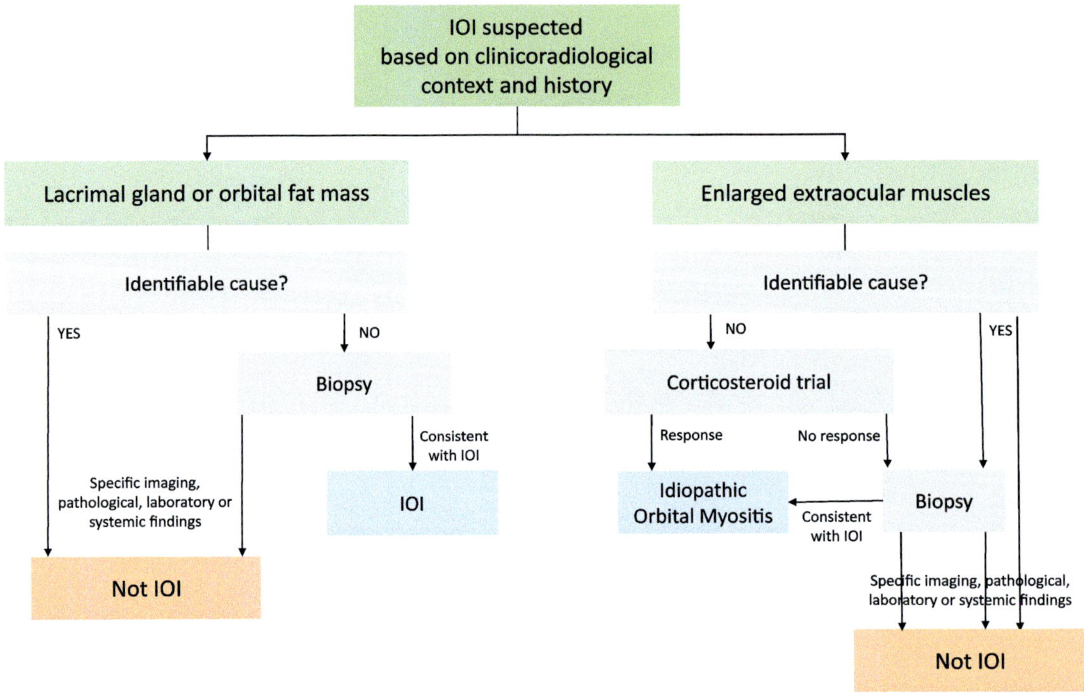

Fig. 2 Algorithm for diagnosis of IOI

is shown in Fig. 2. The presentation of IOI may overlap that of other diseases, in particular lymphoproliferative orbital lesions. Hence, a diagnosis of IOI should be supported by tissue biopsy [32]. Biopsy may be deferred where surgical morbidity is expected to be high, such as in mass lesions confined to the orbital apex or around the optic nerve. In idiopathic orbital myositis, a prompt response to high-dose corticosteroids is considered typical [25].

6.1 Imaging

Orbital computed tomography (CT) and magnetic resonance imaging (MRI) are essential in the evaluation of IOI. MRI is superior to CT in evaluating soft tissues, like optic nerve, orbital fat, muscles and lacrimal gland. The lesions enhance with contrast, and, on MRI, may display bright fat-suppressed T2-weighted image signals depending on the amount of tissue oedema. New MRI protocols such as diffusion-weighted (DWI) and dynamic contrast-enhanced (DCE) MRI may help distinguishing malignant from benign lesions, in particular high-grade lymphoma from inflammation and reactive lymphoid hyperplasia, although features of diseases may overlap [33–35].

Idiopathic dacryoadenitis is marked by a diffuse enlargement of the orbital and palpebral lobe of the gland, which appears as almond- or bean-shaped. The glandular mass may extend into the surrounding orbital fat, lateral and superior rectus muscle, or upper eyelid [29]. Idiopathic orbital myositis is featured by diffuse and smooth enlargement of one or several extraocular muscles, with the horizontal recti being most commonly affected. Other orbital structures are not affected. In addition to muscle belly enlargement, anterior tendon thickening occurs in approximately half of the cases. The feature of tendon enlargement, however, is not pathognomonic nor conclusive for a diagnosis of idiopathic myositis, as it can also be present in orbital lymphoproliferative disease, orbital giant cell myositis, TAO and paraneoplastic orbital myositis [36–38]. The presence of focal, nodular or heterogeneous enlargement of an extraocular muscle is not typical of idiopathic orbital myositis and raises concern about malignancy.

Diffuse IOI presents as an ill-defined infiltrative mass incorporating several orbital structures, often localized in the superolateral orbit [39, 40]. Spread may occur outside the orbit, via the superior orbital fissure into the cavernous sinus and middle cranial space, or via the inferior orbital fissure into the pterygopalatine and infratemporal fossa [41]. In 36% of cases, extra-orbital extension is associated with bone changes, such as erosion, destruction, sclerosis or remodelling [41]. The association of bony and mucosal changes of the adjacent paranasal sinuses, however, should raise suspicion of other causes such as GPA, lymphoproliferative tumors, malignancy and IgG4-RD.

The use of Zirconium-89-labelled (^{89}Zr)-rituximab positron emission tomography (PET-CT) has been studied in therapy refractory IOI [42]. Lacrimal gland and diffuse IOI lesions showed strong uptake of ^{89}Zr-rituximab, while myositic and apical IOI lesions exhibited low to moderate uptake [42]. Further research is required to define the value of ^{89}Zr-rituximab PET-CT in the diagnosis (to guide biopsy taking) and treatment (to predict response to rituximab) in IOI and other B-cell orbital lesions alike.

6.2 Laboratory Testing

In patients with suspected IOI, inflammatory and auto-immune markers are used to identify sarcoidosis, GPA, Sjögren's disease, IgG4-RD and TAO as possible cause of the orbital inflammatory condition [25, 43]. A comprehensive laboratory panel includes:

- White blood cell count with differential, platelet count, calcium, liver function
- Erythrocyte sedimentation rate, C-reactive protein
- Anti-neutrophil cytoplasmic antibody/proteinase-3, IgG, IgG2, IgG4, angiotensin-converting enzyme, lysozyme
- *In solitary lacrimal gland involvement*

Add anti-Ro (Sjögren syndrome-A), anti-La (Sjögren syndrome-B), rheumatoid factor, anti-cyclic citrullinated peptide antibody, anti-citrullinated protein antibody, antinuclear antibody titer and pattern

- *In solitary extraocular muscles involvement*

Add triiodothyronine (T_3), thyroxine (T_4), thyroid-stimulating hormone, thyroid-stimulating hormone receptor antibody.

Serological tests in IOI and other inflammatory orbital lesions, however, have limited value. Inflammatory markers reflect inflammation disregarding the etiology. Biomarkers and auto-antibodies are associated with burden of disease, and thus results can be false-negative when the disease is limited to the orbit only or has mild activity, and they also confer a likelihood of false-positive results [25, 44].

6.3 Known History of Orbital-related Systemic Disease

The diagnosis of IOI is unlikely in patients with a known history of systemic disease such as sarcoidosis, GPA, Sjögren's disease, IgG4-RD, lymphoproliferative and histiocytic disorders, xanthogranulomatous disease, and malignant and metastatic disease. This exclusion criterion is less strict in co-existing thyroid disease, as comorbidity of IOI with TAO is possible [45]. In the absence of clinical evidence of systemic disease, an internal medicine work-up is not routinely performed but can be useful in selected cases.

6.4 Tissue Biopsy

Tissue biopsy is a critical diagnostic step in IOI lesions of the lacrimal gland and orbital fat, primarily to exclude other causes [46, 47]. Adequate (i.e., large) and representative (i.e., from various involved sites and depths) tissue specimens are obtained by open biopsy [48]. Corticosteroids or other immunosuppressants should ideally be stopped two weeks prior to biopsy to ensure lymphocytic representivity of the specimen [25]. The lesion is accessed through a bone- and canthal-sparing transconjunctival, lateral canthotomy or transcutaneous orbitotomy, which are minimally invasive procedures and can often be performed under local anesthesia [48, 49]. Fine needle aspiration biopsy is less suitable as it entails a low diagnostic yield in lesions solid in consistency—as in IOI -, and does not allow assessment of the complete morphological picture. Biopsy may be deferred where surgical morbidity is expected to be high, such as in mass lesions confined to the orbital apex or surrounding the optic nerve.

In typical idiopathic orbital myositis, biopsies are not routinely taken. Atypical myositic cases, on the other hand, are suspected of other distinct disease and may warrant muscle biopsy after exclusion of TAO [50]. Atypical cases include the absence of pain, slow onset of symptoms, all extraocular muscles affected, focal, nodular or inhomogeneous muscle enlargement, extremely enlarged single muscle, other orbital structures involved, history of primary or secondary malignancy, and unresponsiveness to corticosteroids [50].

6.5 Histopathology

IOI is characterized by a mixed polymorphous infiltrate of small, well-differentiated lymphocytes with T-cells outnumbering the B-cells, plasma cells, and neutrophil and eosinophil granulocytes [1]. Other findings include the presence of histiocytes and macrophages. The infiltrate can be locally organized in lymphoid follicles with reactive germinal centers. Presence of granulomas, granulomatous inflammation, vasculitis, necrosis, and a high number of plasma cells generally excludes the diagnosis of IOI. In the lacrimal gland, varied degrees of destruction of the acini and ductules are observed. In the muscle, rhabdomyolysis with loss of normal striations and degeneration of the myofibers may occur.

Fibrosis is a common histologic feature in IOI and is not associated with duration of the disease. Where fibrosis is highly prominent and the inflammatory infiltrate is paucicellular, sclerosing IOI is considered [51]. The finding of sclerosing orbital inflammation should prompt investigation for systemic IgG4-related disease [22, 52]. The finding of fibrosis, lymphoplasmacytic infiltration and atrophy of the lacrimal gland, however, should not be confused with the intrinsic connective tissue and immunoarchitecture, and involutional atrophy of respectively a normal and ageing lacrimal gland [47].

For reason of overlapping histopathological features between IOI, IgG4-RD and lymphoproliferative disease, ancillary testing with immunohistochemistry, immunophenotyping and gene rearrangement analysis may be required [48, 53]. In IOI, tissue plasma cell IgG4-positivity is not a prominent finding. With a ratio of IgG4-positive to IgG-positive plasma cells of 40% or less, up to 30 IgG4-positive cells/high power field may be present in IOI [25]. Notably, similar tissue IgG4 positivity can be present in auto-immune and other orbital inflammatory disorders unrelated to IgG4-RD, including GPA [54]. There is limited evidence that tissue IgG2-positive plasma cells, along with serum IgG2, could represent more specific diagnostic parameters for IgG4-RD [55]. Gene expression profiling can further discriminate IOI from limited GPA, which is experimentally but not routinely performed [4].

6.6 The Corticosteroid Trial

Patients with orbital inflammatory disease may show dramatic improvement of the signs and symptoms within 48 hours after systemic administration of prednisolone at an initial dose of 1 mg/kg/day, referred to as *the corticosteroid trial* [56]. Myositic IOI is characterized by such a dramatic response, rendering the trial diagnostic [23, 25]. In nonmyositic IOI, however, the trial confers a low positive predictive value, with only 44–79% of cases responding, and a poor diagnostic specificity because a response is observed in several conditions with an inflammatory component, amongst which B- and T-cell lymphoma, metastatic disease, fungal infection, GPA, IgG4-RD, and sarcoidosis [32, 39, 47, 57, 58].

Regrettably, the clinical practice of a corticosteroid trial without biopsy or adequate investigation has introduced delays in a definitive diagnosis of these conditions. While the trial may secure a diagnosis of IOI lesions limited to the extraocular muscles and orbital apex, the possibility of another diagnosis remains a point of vigilance [25, 59].

7 Treatment

Treatment of IOI is tailored to severity and progression of disease to prevent damage and fibrosis of the orbital structures, and to minimize morbidity, such as pain, double vision, and optic nerve dysfunction. Therapeutic strategies depend on the orbital structures involved, and include surgical debulking, non-steroidal anti-inflammatory drugs, corticosteroids, radiation therapy, and immunomodulating and biologic agents. In selected cases of IOI with mild disease and low morbidity, nonsteroidal anti-inflammatory drugs and simple observation may be a preferred first approach [3, 19]. Early treatment is generally required to relieve inflammatory symptoms, prevent recurrence and ultimately protect orbital tissue from scarring.

Recurrence of symptoms following treatment occurs between 38–52% of patients, particularly in diffuse and myositic IOI [57, 58, 60]. Within the spectrum of treatment modalities, involvement of extraocular muscles on imaging is identified as the only significant risk factor associated with recurrence of IOI [4]. Notably, it is essential to distinguish lack or poor response from rebound of symptoms owing to an inappropriate regimen (i.e., too low dosage, too quick taper) of corticosteroids.

7.1 Surgical Debulking

Surgical debulking is part of the diagnostic biopsy procedure for lesions located in the lacrimal gland and orbital fat of the anterior and mid-orbit. Generous biopsies are taken and fibrotic tissue is removed with sparing of the critical structures. In idiopathic dacryoadenitis, debulking is therapeutically successful in 74% of cases, with a recurrence rate of 8% [29]. Debulking may be the only effective measure in recalcitrant IOI with residual fibrosis [31, 39].

An approach using a bone- and canthal-sparing minimally invasive orbitotomy technique limits the surgical morbidity [61]. However lesions located in the orbital apex or close to the optic nerve entail an increased risk of damage to vital structures. Local corticosteroids can be administered at the end of the surgical intervention. After initial increase of oedema, gradual relief of symptoms can be anticipated within two months post-operatively.

7.2 Corticosteroids

High-dose (60–80 mg) systemic corticosteroids initially relieve clinical symptoms in most myositic cases and in about 80% of nonmyositic nonsclerotic cases, and are useful in 92% of cases with combined compressive optic neuropathy [57]. Following initial high dose, corticosteroid administration should be tapered off gradually over the course of several months. Approximately half of cases relapse on tapering or ceasing, implicating a 37% efficacy to corticosteroids as a long-term cure [57, 58]. In sclerosing IOI, corticosteroids are less effective with only 33% of cases responding [39].

There is no difference in outcome and morbidity in administration of intravenous methylprednisolone followed by oral prednisolone versus oral prednisolone alone [62]. To reduce side-effects from systemic use, intralesional corticosteroids can be used for lesions localized in the anterior orbit, such as the lacrimal gland [63, 64].

7.3 Radiation Therapy

External beam radiation, in doses between 20 and 30 Gray, has been demonstrated with modest efficacy as a second-line adjunctive therapy in IOI lesions which are cortico-dependent, fail to respond to corticosteroids, or recur [65]. In non-myositic nonsclerotic IOI, symptoms improve in 75–85% of cases, with local control in 63% of cases at 5 years and 53% at 10 years, and 45% of cases achieving complete discontinuation of corticosteroids [66, 67]. On the other hand, sclerotic and myositic cases display low radiosensitivity, with, in the latter group, radiation merely delaying the next recurrence [2, 19, 39].

7.4 Immunomodulatory Drugs Other than Corticosteroids

Nonspecific immunosuppressive or conventional disease-modifying antirheumatic drugs and newer specific biologic agents are employed as second- and third-line therapy to control the inflammatory process in cortico-dependent and recalcitrant IOI, with varying degrees of success. They should be given for prolonged times. Overall, there is limited scientific evidence of the outcome with such immunomodulatory drugs and biologicals as it is difficult to assure that all reported cases met the diagnostic criteria of IOI.

The antimetabolite methotrexate is reportedly moderately successful and well-tolerated as corticosteroid-sparing agent in IOI [68, 69]. In view of anticipated recurrent disease with corticosteroid treatment, some authors routinely start methotrexate concomitantly [4]. Small case series report response to mycophenolate mofetil (antimetabolite), cyclosporin-A (T-cell inhibitor), azathioprine (antimetabolite), and cyclophosphamide (alkylating agent) [68].

Of the biologics, rituximab (B-cell inhibitor) and infliximab (anti-tumor necrosis factor-alpha agent) have anti-inflammatory potential in cases with severe, recurrent or recalcitrant to corticosteroids and methotrexate disease [18]. There is anecdotal evidence of clinical benefit with adalimumab (anti-tumor NF monoclonal antibody), tocilizumab (anti-interleukin-6 receptor monoclonal antibody) and daclizumab (anti-interleukin-2 monoclonal antibody) [4].

Of all these agents, it appears that methotrexate and rituximab are the most frequently used in IOI. In view of their systemic toxicity profile, and the costs inherent in newer biologic agents, these drugs are reserved as third-line strategy for IOI lesions with a severe and deteriorating pattern, such as sclerosing IOI and the association with optic nerve dysfunction. In addition, it should be noted that these drugs are also successfully used for other orbital inflammatory and lymphoproliferative lesions, hence a therapeutic response not delivering any diagnostic certainty [70, 71].

8 Conclusion

IOI is a heterogeneous disease with an unknown natural course and unpredictable outcome. The diagnosis of IOI is one of exclusion, for the clinician, radiologist and pathologist. An adequate response to a trial of systemic corticosteroids as sole evidence is not diagnostic for IOI lesions involving the lacrimal gland or orbital fat, but may be sufficient for idiopathic orbital myositis. It should be emphasized that IOI is not a sound long-term diagnosis. When new findings manifest, diagnostic re-evaluation is necessary for the possibility of other distinct—possibly systemic—disease.

Treatment depends on orbital structures affected and is tailored to severity and progression of disease. Surgical debulking following the biopsy procedure, or non-steroidal anti-inflammatory drugs, can be efficacious as first-line treatment in selected cases. In view of the high recurrence rate, corticosteroids are less attractive as first choice therapy but remain useful in patients with significant morbidity where the muscles and optic nerve are involved. Although evidence is limited, additional treatment options comprise radiation therapy and other immunomodulators in severe refractory, progressive or recurrent disease.

References

1. Mombaerts I, Goldschmeding R, Schlingemann RO, Koornneef L. What is orbital pseudotumor? Surv Ophthalmol. 1996;41:66–78.
2. Rootman J, McCarthy M, White V, Harris G, Kennerdell J. Idiopathic sclerosing inflammation of the orbit. A distinct clinicopathologic entity. Ophthalmology. 1994;101:570–84.
3. Harris GJ. Idiopathic orbital inflammation: a pathogenetic construct and treatment strategy: The 2005 ASOPRS Foundation Lecture. Ophthal Plast Reconstr Surg. 2006;22:79–86.
4. Lee MJ, Planck SR, Choi D, et al. Non-specific orbital inflammation: current understanding and unmet needs. Prog Retin Eye Res. 2021;81:100885.
5. Guo J, Qian J, Zhang R. Histopathology and immunohistochemical profile in idiopathic dacryoadenitis. Curr Eye Res. 2012;37:365–71.
6. Wladis EJ, Iglesias BV, Adam AP, Nazeer T, Gosselin EJ. Toll-like receptors in idiopathic orbital inflammation. Ophthal Plast Reconstr Surg. 2012;28:273–6.
7. Wladis EJ, Iglesias BV, Gosselin EJ. Characterization of the molecular biologic milieu of idiopathic orbital inflammation. Ophthal Plast Reconstr Surg. 2011;27:251–4.
8. Ren MW, Du Y, Ren S, Tang CY, He JF. Epstein-Barr virus-encoded small RNAs in idiopathic orbital inflammatory pseudotumor tissues: a comparative case series. Int J Ophthalmol. 2017;10:1268–72.
9. Lee BJ, Atkins S, Ginter A, Elner VM, Nelson CC, Douglas RS. Increased CD40+ fibrocytes in patients with idiopathic orbital inflammation. Ophthal Plast Reconstr Surg. 2015;31:202–6.
10. Yan J, Li Y, Qiu H, et al. Immunohistochemical study of the presence of mast cells in idiopathic orbital inflammatory pseudotumor: possible role of mast cells in the course of its pathogenesis. Int Ophthalmol. 2007;27:235–9.
11. Rosenbaum JT, Choi D, Harrington CA, et al. Gene expression profiling and heterogeneity of nonspecific orbital Inflammation affecting the lacrimal gland. JAMA Ophthalmol. 2017;135:1156–62.
12. Rosenbaum JT, Choi D, Wilson DJ, et al. Orbital Disease Consortium. Molecular diagnosis of orbital inflammatory disease. Exp Mol Pathol. 2015;98:225–9.
13. Rosenbaum JT, Choi D, Wilson DJ, et al. Orbital pseudotumor can be a localized form of granulomatosis with polyangiitis as revealed by gene expression profiling. Exp Mol Pathol. 2015;99:271–8.
14. Laban KG, Kalmann R, Bekker CPJ, et al. A pan-inflammatory microRNA-cluster is associated with orbital non-Hodgkin lymphoma and idiopathic orbital inflammation. Eur J Immunol. 2020;50:86–96.
15. Laban KG, Rijken R, Hiddingh S, et al. cDC2 and plasmacytoid dendritic cells diminish from tissues of patients with non-Hodgkin orbital lymphoma and idiopathic orbital inflammation. Eur J Immunol. 2020;50:548–57.
16. Chen P, Denniston A, Hannes S, et al. Increased CD1c+ mDC1 with mature phenotype regulated by TNFα-p38 MAPK in autoimmune ocular inflammatory disease. Clin Immunol. 2015;158: 35–46.
17. Culver EL SJ, Frith P, Travis SP. Recurrent posterior scleritis and orbital myositis as extra-intestinal manifestations of Crohn's disease: case report and systematic literature review. J Crohns Colitis. 2008;2:337–42.
18. Garrity JA, Coleman AW, Matteson EL, Eggenberger ER, Waitzman DM. Treatment of recalcitrant idiopathic orbital inflammation (chronic orbital myositis) with infliximab. Am J Ophthalmol. 2004;138:925–30.
19. Mombaerts I, Koornneef L. Current status in the treatment of orbital myositis. Ophthalmology. 1997;104:402–8.
20. Tsukikawa M, Lally SE, Shields CL, et al. Idiopathic orbital pseudotumor preceding systemic inflammatory disease in children. J Pediatr Ophthalmol Strabismus. 2019;56:373–7.
21. Keren S, Leibovitch I, Ben Cnaan R, et al. Aminobisphosphonate-associated orbital and ocular inflammatory disease. Acta Ophthalmol. 2019;97:e792–9.
22. Andrew NH, Sladden N, Kearney DJ, Selva D. An analysis of IgG4-related disease (IgG4-RD) among idiopathic orbital inflammations and benign lymphoid hyperplasias using two consensus-based diagnostic criteria for IgG4-RD. Br J Ophthalmol. 2015;99:376–81.
23. McNab AA. Orbital myositis: a comprehensive review and reclassification. Ophthalmic Plast Reconstr Surg. 2020;36:109–17.
24. Sa HS, Lee JH, Woo KI, Kim YD. IgG4-related disease in idiopathic sclerosing orbital inflammation. Br J Ophthalmol. 2015;99:1493–7.
25. Mombaerts I, Bilyk JR, Rose GE, et al. Consensus on diagnostic criteria of idiopathic orbital inflammation using a modified Delphi approach. JAMA Ophthalmol. 2017;135:769–76.
26. Jakobiec FA, Syed ZA, Stagner AM, et al. Orbital inflammation in pregnant women. Am J Ophthalmol. 2016;166:91–102.
27. Bijlsma WR, van Gils CH, Paridaens D, Mourits MP, Kalmann R. Risk factors for idiopathic orbital inflammation: a case-control study. Br J Ophthalmol. 2011;95:360–4.
28. Andrew NH, Kearney D, Sladden N, et al. Idiopathic dacryoadenitis: clinical features, histopathology, and treatment outcomes. Am J Ophthalmol. 2016;163:e141.
29. Mombaerts ICJ, Chanlalit W, Garrity JA. Surgical debulking for idiopathic dacryoadenitis: a diagnosis and a cure. Ophthalmology. 2014;121:603–9.

30. Avni-Zauberman N, Tripathy D, Rosen N, Ben Simon GJ. Relapsing migratory idiopathic orbital inflammation: six new cases and review of the literature. Br J Ophthalmol. 2012;96:276–80.
31. Pemberton JD, Fay A. Idiopathic sclerosing orbital inflammation: a review of demographics, clinical presentation, imaging, pathology, treatment, and outcome. Ophthal Plast Reconstr Surg. 2012;28:79–83.
32. Mombaerts I, Rose GE, Garrity JA. Orbital inflammation: biopsy first. Surv Ophthalmol. 2016;61:664–9.
33. Fatima Z, Ichikawa T, Ishigame K, et al. Orbital masses: the usefulness of diffusion-weighted imaging in lesion categorization. Clin Neuroradiol. 2014;24:129–34.
34. Hu H, Xu XQ, Liu H, et al. Orbital benign and malignant lymphoproliferative disorders: differentiation using semi-quantitative and quantitative analysis of dynamic contrast-enhanced magnetic resonance imaging. Eur J Radiol. 2017;88:88–94.
35. Sun B, Song L. Orbital malignant lesions in adults: multiparametric MR imaging. Jpn J Radiol. 2017;35:454–62.
36. Ben Simon GJ, Syed HM, Douglas R, McCann JD, Goldberg RA. Extraocular muscle enlargement with tendon involvement in thyroid-associated orbitopathy. Am J Ophthalmol. 2004;137:1145–7.
37. Harris GJ, Murphy ML, Schmidt EW, Hanson GA, Dotson RM. Orbital myositis as a paraneoplastic syndrome. Arch Ophthalmol. 1994;112:380–6.
38. Mombaerts I, Tousseyn T, Van Limbergen E, Demaerel P. Clinically recognizing enlarged extraocular muscles from lymphoid origin. Ophthalmology. 2015;122:217–8.
39. Hsuan JD, Selva D, McNab AA, et al. Idiopathic sclerosing orbital inflammation. Arch Ophthalmol. 2006;124:1244–50.
40. Yuen SJ, Rubin PA. Idiopathic orbital inflammation: distribution, clinical features, and treatment outcome. Arch Ophthalmol. 2003;121:491–9.
41. Zborowska B, Ghabrial R, Selva D, McCluskey P. Idiopathic orbital inflammation with extraorbital extension: case series and review. Eye (Lond). 2006;20:107–13.
42. Laban KG, Kalmann R, Leguit RJ, de Keizer B. Zirconium-89-labelled rituximab PET-CT in orbital inflammatory disease. EJNMMI Res. 2019;9:1–7.
43. Srinivasan A, Kleinberg TT, Murchison AP, Bilyk JR. Laboratory investigations for diagnosis of autoimmune and inflammatory periocular disease: Part II. Ophthal Plast Reconstr Surg. 2016;32:321–8.
44. Rabinowitz MP, Halfpenny CP, Bedrossian EH Jr. The frequency of granulomatous lacrimal gland inflammation as a cause of lacrimal gland enlargement in patients without a diagnosis of systemic sarcoidosis. Orbit. 2013;32:151–5.
45. Bijlsma WR, Kalmann R. Idiopathic orbital inflammation and Graves ophthalmopathy. Arch Ophthalmol. 2010;128:131–2.
46. Luemsamran P, Rootman J, White VA, Nassiri N, Heran MKS. The role of biopsy in lacrimal gland inflammation: a clinicopathologic study. Orbit. 2017;36:411–8.
47. Mombaerts I. The many facets of dacryoadenitis. Curr Opin Ophthalmol. 2015;26:399–407.
48. Mombaerts I, Ramberg I, Coupland SE, Heegaard S. Diagnosis of orbital mass lesions: clinical, radiological, and pathological recommendations. Surv Ophthalmol. 2019;64:741–56.
49. Hamed-Azzam S, Verity DH, Rose GE. Lateral canthotomy orbitotomy: a rapid approach to the orbit. Eye (Lond). 2018;32:333–7.
50. Mombaerts I, Rose GE, Verity DH. Diagnosis of enlarged extraocular muscles: when and how to biopsy. Curr Opin Ophthalmol. 2017;28:514–21.
51. McCarthy JM, White VA, Harris G, et al. Idiopathic sclerosing inflammation of the orbit: immunohistologic analysis and comparison with retroperitoneal fibrosis. Mod Pathol. 1993;6:581–7.
52. Winn BJ, Rootman J. Sclerosing orbital inflammation and systemic disease. Ophthal Plast Reconstr Surg. 2012;28:107–18.
53. Deshpande VZY, Chan JK, et al. Consensus statement on the pathology of IgG4-related disease. Mod Pathol. 2012;25:1181–92.
54. Wong AJ, Planck SR, Choi D, et al. IgG4 immunostaining and its implications in orbital inflammatory disease. PLoS One. 2014;9:e109847.
55. Chan ASY, Mudhar H, Shen SY, et al. Serum IgG2 and tissue IgG2 plasma cell elevation in orbital IgG4-related disease (IgG4-RD): potential use in IgG4-RD assessment. Br J Ophthalmol. 2017;101:1576–82.
56. Glass LRD, Freitag SK. Orbital inflammation: corticosteroids first. Surv Ophthalmol. 2016;61:670–3.
57. Mombaerts I, Schlingemann RO, Goldschmeding R, Koornneef L. Are systemic corticosteroids useful in the management of orbital pseudotumors? Ophthalmology. 1996;103:521–8.
58. Swamy BN, McCluskey P, Nemet A, et al. Idiopathic orbital inflammatory syndrome: clinical features and treatment outcomes. Br J Ophthalmol. 2007;91:1667–70.
59. Bijlsma WR, Elbert NJ, Kalmann R. The role of biopsy in diagnosing patients suspected of idiopathic orbital inflammation. Curr Eye Res. 2012;37:251–3.
60. Young SM, Chan ASY, Jajeh IA, et al. Clinical features and treatment outcomes of orbital inflammatory disease in Singapore: a 10-year clinicopathologic review. Ophthalmic Plast Reconstr Surg. 2017;33:182–8.
61. Jacobs SM, McInnis CP, Kapeles M, Chang SH. Incidence, risk factors, and management of blindness after orbital surgery. Ophthalmology. 2018;125:1100–8.
62. Bijlsma WR, Paridaens D, Kalmann R. Treatment of severe idiopathic orbital inflammation with intravenous methylprednisolone. Br J Ophthalmol. 2011;95:1068–71.
63. Leibovitch I, Prabhakaran VC, Davis G, Selva D. Intraorbital injection of triamcinolone acetonide in patients with idiopathic orbital inflammation. Arch Ophthalmol. 2007;125:1647–51.

64. Reggie S, Neimkin M, Holds J. Intralesional corticosteroid injections as treatment for non-infectious orbital inflammation. Orbit. 2018;37:41–7.
65. Lee JH, Kim YS, Yang SW, et al. Radiotherapy with or without surgery for patients with idiopathic sclerosing orbital inflammation refractory or intolerant to steroid therapy. Int J Radiat Oncol Biol Phys. 2012;84:52–8.
66. Mokhtech M, Nurkic S, Morris CG, Mendenhall NP, Mendenhall WM. Radiotherapy for orbital pseudotumor: The University of Florida experience. Cancer Invest. 2018;36:330–7.
67. Prabhu RS, Kandula S, Liebman L, et al. Association of clinical response and long-term outcome among patients with biopsied orbital pseudotumor receiving modern radiation therapy. Int J Radiat Oncol Biol Phys. 2013;85:643–9.
68. Carruth BP, Wladis EJ. Inflammatory modulators and biologic agents in the treatment of idiopathic orbital inflammation. Curr Opin Ophthalmol. 2012;23:420–6.
69. Smith JR, Rosenbaum JT. A role for methotrexate in the management of non-infectious orbital inflammatory disease. Br J Ophthalmol. 2001;85:1220–4.
70. Detiger SE, Karim AF, Verdijk RM, van Hagen PM, van Laar JAM, Paridaens D. The treatment outcomes in IgG4-related orbital disease: a systematic review of the literature. Acta Ophthalmol. 2019;97:451–9.
71. Suhler EB, Lim LL, Beardsley RM, et al. Rituximab therapy for refractory orbital inflammation: results of a phase 1/2, dose-ranging, randomized clinical trial. JAMA Ophthalmol. 2014;132:572–8.

IgG4-Related Orbital Disease

Dion Paridaens, Robert M. Verdijk,
and Gustavo Savino

Key Messages

- IgG4-RD is a systemic fibro-inflammatory disease
- IgG-RD may primarily present in the orbit and periorbital tissues
- The diagnostic gold standard is histology
- In IgG4-ROD glucocorticoids are the first choice of treatment

1 Introduction

IgG4 related disease (IgG4-RD) is a systemic fibro-inflammatory disease leading to tumour-like infiltrations potentially affecting all parts of the human body [1]. The pathophysiological mechanism of IgG4-RD is still unclear, but fibrosis, which may lead to irreversible organ damage, is the hallmark of this disease making early recognition and therapy critical [2]. IgG4-RD is increasingly recognized as part of the spectrum of orbital diseases (IgG4-ROD) [3–5]. IgG4-RD may primarily present in the orbit and periorbital tissue (Fig. 1).

D. Paridaens (✉)
Department of Oculoplastic, Orbital and Lacrimal Surgery, The Rotterdam Eye Hospital and Erasmus Medical Center, Rotterdam, The Netherlands
e-mail: d.paridaens@oogziekenhuis.nl; a.paridaens@erasmusmc.nl

R. M. Verdijk
Department of Pathology, Section Ophthalmic Pathology, Erasmus MC & the Rotterdam Eye Hospital, Rotterdam, The Netherlands

Department of Pathology, Leiden University Medical Center, Leiden, The Netherlands

G. Savino
Department of Ophthalmology, Fondazione Policlinico Universitario A. Gemelli IRCCS, Rome, Italy

F. M. Quaranta Leoni et al. (eds.), *Oculoplastic, Lacrimal and Orbital Surgery*,
https://doi.org/10.1007/978-3-031-39638-0_18

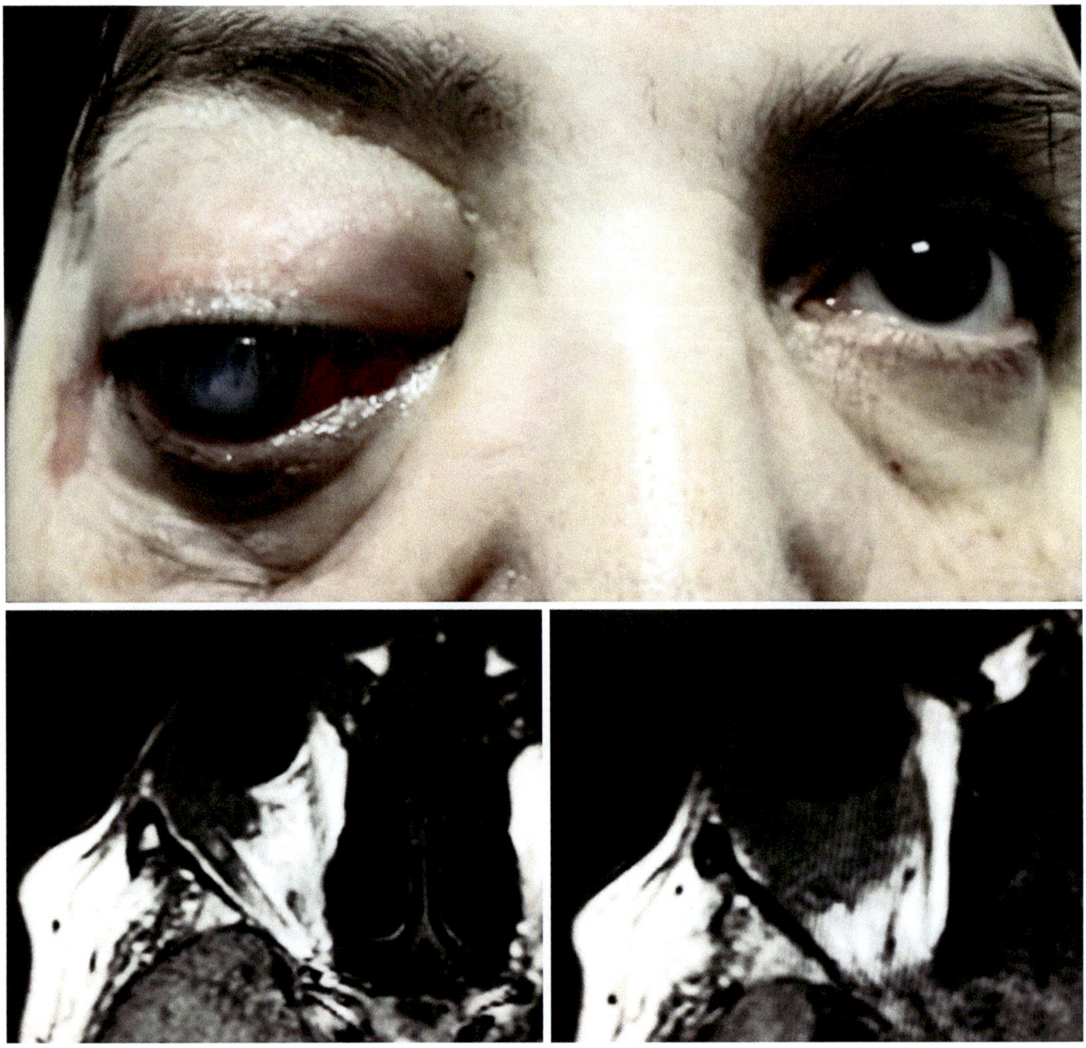

Fig. 1 Fifty-six year old woman with severe right proptosis and corneal damage. Magnetic resonance imaging: retrobulbar right orbital IgG4 infiltration involving the lacrimal gland and the lateral rectus

2 Clinical Presentation

IgG4-ROD mimics many infectious, inflammatory and malignant disorders. The clinical presentation of IgG4-ROD can vary depending on the involved orbital structures. Patients mostly present with proptosis or painless periorbital/eyelid swelling, diplopia, lacrimal complaints, or, less frequently, myositis, scleritis, bone lesions, perineuritis or uveitis [6–10]. Some patients show involvement of only a single organ like in isolated orbital IgG4-related disease. IgG4-ROD mostly affects men and occurs in middle-aged patients [6], although pediatric presentations have been observed [11, 12].

3 Diagnosis

Histopathologically, IgG4-R(O)D is characterized by tumour-like lesions, lymphoplasmacytic infiltrate enriched with IgG4-positive plasma cells, storiform fibrosis and obliterative phlebitis [13, 14]. The obliterative phlebitis is often absent in the periorbital specimen [13].

The exclusion of alternative histopathological diagnoses such as sarcoidosis, granulomatosis with polyangiitis, xanthogranuloma or lymphoma is an important aspect in the histopathological diagnosis of IgG4-ROD. Serum IgG4 is often elevated, however, histologically proven cases may have normal serum IgG4 concentrations [15]. The diagnostic gold standard is histology, however, serum IgG4 and the clinical presentation may be supportive in establishing the diagnosis [14–17] (Figs. 2 and 3).

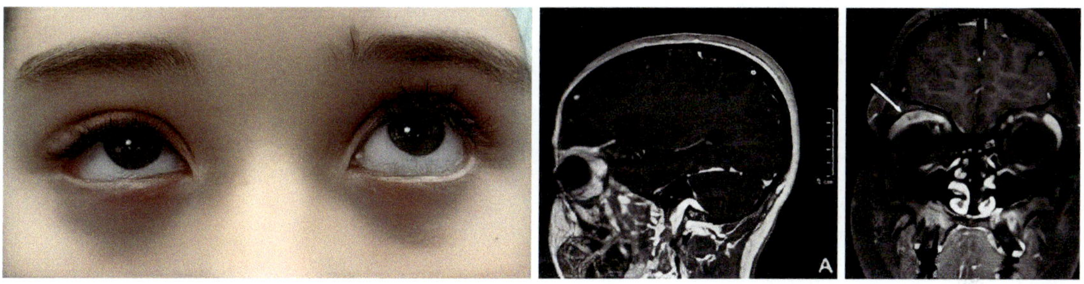

Fig. 2 Ten-year old child with mild ptosis, S-shaped eyelid, and vertical strabismus in upward gaze in the right eye. Magnetic resonance imaging (sagittal T1-weighted): hypointense superior mass involving the lacrimal gland and the superior rectus/levator complex with posterior extension (*arrow*)

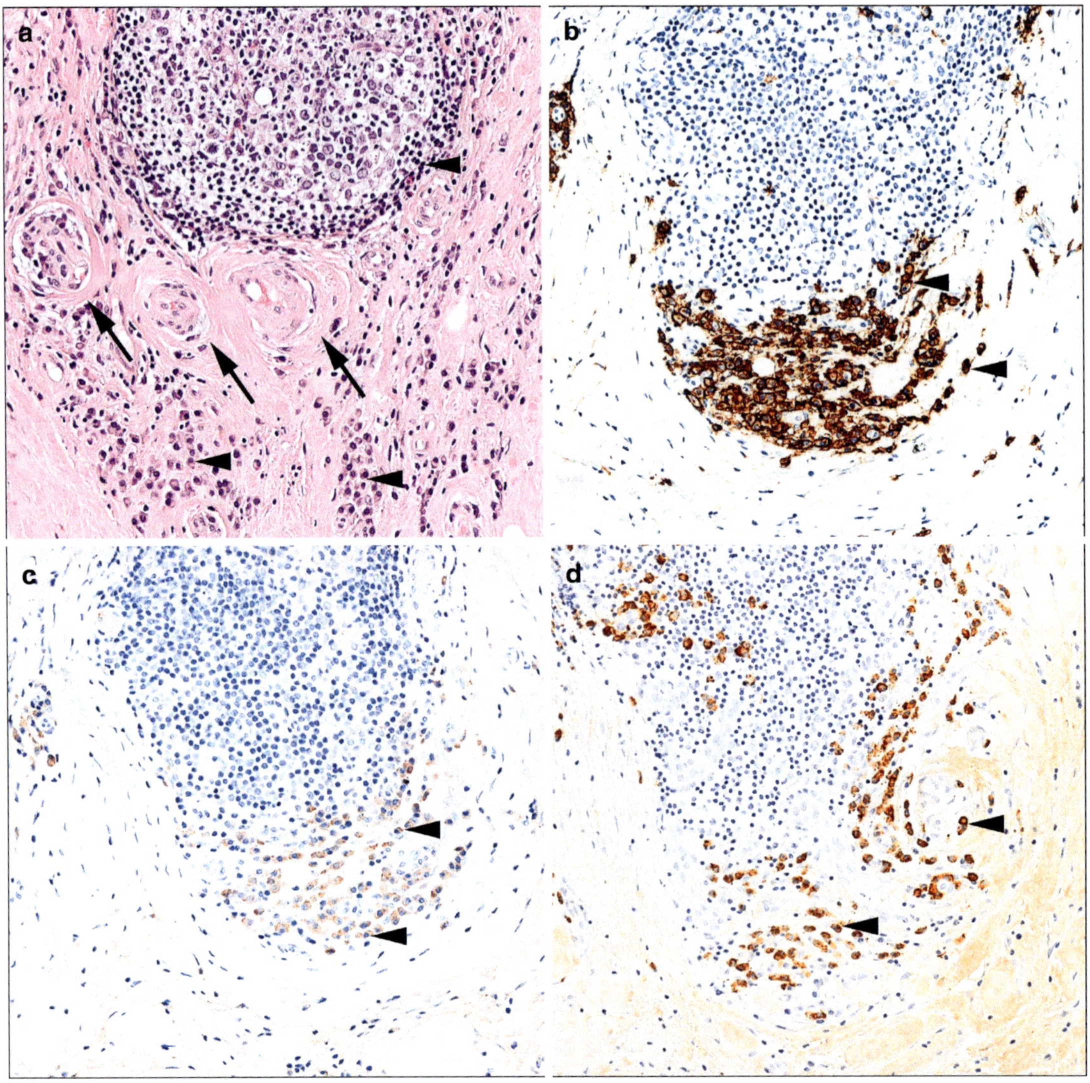

Fig. 3 Histopathology. (**a**) Dense, fibrous, pleomorphic cellular infiltrate (plasma cells and lymphocytes) (*arrowheads*), with characteristic reactive storiform fibrosis (*arrows*) (Hematoxylin and eosin, 200×); (**b**) Plasma cells stained by CD138 (*arrowheads*) (immunostain CD138, 200×), (**c**) IgG immunoreactive plasma cells (*arrowheads*) (immunostain 200×), (**d**) IgG4 immunoreactive plasma cells (*arrowheads*) (immunostain 200×)

4 Radiological Features of IgG-ROD

On CT or MRI, the primary radiological features are lacrimal gland and/or extraocular muscle enlargement, with a preference for the lateral rectus muscle. The anterior tendon is spared in the majority of IgG4-ROD cases. In addition, signs of orbital fat inflammation, infra- and/or supraorbital nerve enlargement and paranasal sinus disease may be present [18].

5 Differential Diagnosis

The differential diagnosis includes other causes of inflammation (infectious and autoimmune) and malignancy (especially in unilateral disease).

For treatment as well as for work-up, it is important to differentiate IgG4-ROD from idiopathic orbital inflammation (IOI). IOI is a heterogeneous group of non-specific, non-infectious orbital inflammatory disease without an underlying specific systemic or local cause. It is a diagnosis of exclusion after evaluating other causes of orbital disease. Multiple retrospective case series have revealed IgG-ROD to be present in 5–45% of cases earlier diagnosed as IOI [19–21]. Other orbital inflammatory conditions such as eosinophilic angiocentric fibrosis or seronegative granulomatosis with polyangiitis are now recognized as part of IgG4-ROD as well [22, 23]. Therefore, in IOI, immunohistochemical examination of the material regarding IgG4-mediated disease should always be performed.

6 First-line Treatment

When diagnosed with IgG4-ROD, therapy may be necessary to avoid organ damage due to fibrosis. Untreated disease may also lead to secondary amyloidosis making prompt treatment critical [24].

In IgG4-ROD glucocorticoids are the first choice of treatment. Although steroid therapy is generally effective in reducing the size of the lesion in IgG4-ROD, recurrences frequently occur after cessation of steroids. IgG4-ROD may in some cases remain dormant for many years and may then re-occur with a very similar clinical presentation [25].

7 Second-line Treatment

Initiating second-line treatment is challenging [14, 26]. Due to the heterogeneity of this disease the treatment is often tailor made and shall thus differ per individual patient. Personal preferences of treating physicians may further influence the choice of treatment. DMARDs such as azathioprine, methotrexate and mycophenolate mofetil may be indicated when there is recurrence of the disease after tapering glucocorticoids but the efficacy for each may be less than 50% [14, 26]. Based on our experience and a review of the literature [27, 28], we therefore suggest the following treatment strategy in IgG4-ROD: (1) Glucocorticoids are the preferred first-line systemic treatment of IgG4-ROD. The initial glucocorticoid dose is prednisolone 0.5–1 mg/kg/day (2). In severe refractory or vision threatening disease, rituximab of 2 × 1 g with 2 weeks in between combined with glucocorticoids tapered in 3 months is started. When indicated, a high dose of glucocorticoid pulse therapy (1 g, 1–3 days intravenously) can be used as an induction strategy. Rituximab initiation will be followed every 6 months for the duration of 2 years. When refractory, cyclophosphamide treatment can be initiated (3). In less severe cases, mycophenolate mofetil or infliximab can be considered as maintenance or steroid-sparing therapy [27]. Consider radiotherapy or surgery in localised refractory disease in patients with compressive optic neuropathy or proptosis. The dose of radiotherapy is usually ranged between 20 and 30 Gy in 10–15 fractions [27].

References

1. Brito-Zeron P, Bosch X, Ramos-Casals M, Stone JH. IgG4-related disease: advances in the diagnosis and treatment. Best Pract Res Clin Rheumatol. 2016;30:261–78.
2. Heeringa JJ, Karim AF, van Laar JAM, Verdijk RM, Paridaens D, van Hagen PM, et al. Expansion of blood IgG4(+) B, TH2, and regulatory T cells in patients with IgG4-related disease. J Allergy Clin Immunol. 2018;141:1831–43.e10.
3. Andrew N, Kearney D, Selva D. IgG4-related orbital disease: a meta-analysis and review. Acta Ophthalmol. 2013;91:694–700.
4. Wallace ZS, Deshpande V, Stone JH. Ophthalmic manifestations of IgG4-related disease: single-center experience and literature review. Semin Arthritis Rheum. 2014;43:806–17.
5. Ebbo M, Patient M, Grados A, Groh M, Desblaches J, Hachulla E, et al. Ophthalmic manifestations in IgG4-related disease: clinical presentation and response to treatment in a French case-series. Medicine (Baltimore). 2017;96:e6205.
6. Karim AF, Verdijk RM, Guenoun J, van Hagen PM, van Laar JA. An inflammatory condition with different faces: immunoglobulin G4-related disease. Neth J Med. 2016;74:110–5.

7. Verhoekx JSN, Karim AF, van Laar JAM, Verdijk RM, Paridaens D. The tarsal plate manifestation of IgG4-related disease. Int Ophthalmol. 2019;39:1613–5.
8. Savino G, Midena G, Tartaglione T, Milonia L, Caputo CG, Grimaldi G. Clinical-radiological patterns and histopathological outcomes in non-thyroid extraocular muscle enlargement: retrospective case series and current concepts. Ophthal Plast Reconstr Surg. 2020;36:284–91.
9. Karim F, de Hoog J, Paridaens D, Verdijk R, Schreurs M, Rothova A, et al. IgG4-related disease as an emerging cause of scleritis. Acta Ophthalmol. 2017;95:e795–e6.
10. Detiger SE, Karim F, Monserez D, Verdijk R, van Hagen M, Paridaens D, et al. IgG4-related disease of skull base: case series of 3 patients with headache. World Neurosurg. 2020;134:536–9.
11. Savino MG, Campana MA, Petrone MG, Grimaldi MG, Murchison AP. In search of a disease. Surv Ophthalmol. 2017;62:716–21.
12. Karim F, Loeffen J, Bramer W, Westenberg L, Verdijk R, van Hagen M, et al. IgG4-related disease: a systematic review of this unrecognized disease in pediatrics. Pediatr Rheumatol Online J. 2016;14:18.
13. Deshpande V, Zen Y, Chan JK, Yi EE, Sato Y, Yoshino T, et al. Consensus statement on the pathology of IgG4-related disease. Mod Pathol. 2012;25:1181–92.
14. Khosroshahi A, Wallace ZS, Crowe JL, Akamizu T, Azumi A, Carruthers MN, et al. International consensus guidance statement on the management and treatment of IgG4-related disease. Arthritis Rheumatol. 2015;67:1688–99.
15. Carruthers MN, Khosroshahi A, Augustin T, Deshpande V, Stone JH. The diagnostic utility of serum IgG4 concentrations in IgG4-related disease. Ann Rheum Dis. 2015;74:14–8.
16. Xu WL, Ling YC, Wang ZK, Deng F. Diagnostic performance of serum IgG4 level for IgG4-related disease: a meta-analysis. Sci Rep. 2016;6:32035.
17. Su Y, Sun W, Wang C, Wu X, Miao Y, Xiong H, et al. Detection of serum IgG4 levels in patients with IgG4-related disease and other disorders. PLoS One. 2015;10:e0124233.
18. Tiegs-Heiden CA, Eckel LJ, Hunt CH, Diehn FE, Schwartz KM, Kallmes DF, Salomão DR, Witzig TE, Garrity JA. Immunoglobulin G4-related disease of the orbit: imaging features in 27 patients. AJNR Am J Neuroradiol. 2014;35:1393–7.
19. Sato Y, Ohshima K, Ichimura K, Sato M, Yamadori I, Tanaka T, et al. Ocular adnexal IgG4-related disease has uniform clinicopathology. Pathol Int. 2008;58:465–70.
20. Deschamps R, Deschamps L, Depaz R, Coffin-Pichonnet S, Belange G, Jacomet PV, et al. High prevalence of IgG4-related lymphoplasmacytic infiltrative disorder in 25 patients with orbital inflammation: a retrospective case series. Br J Ophthalmol. 2013;97:999–1004.
21. Van Tilburg A, Breijer A, Paridaens AD, Vann den Bosch W, Simonsz HJ, Bleyen I, et al. Frequency of IgG4-positive plasma cells in idiopathic orbital inflammation (ESP Abstracts 2014). Virchovs Arch. 2014;465:S34.
22. Karim AF, Verdijk RM, Nagtegaal AP, Bansie R, Paridaens D, van Hagen PM, et al. To distinguish IgG4-related disease from seronegative granulomatosis with polyangiitis. Rheumatology (Oxford). 2017;56:2245–7.
23. Deshpande V, Khosroshahi A, Nielsen GP, Hamilos DL, Stone JH. Eosinophilic angiocentric fibrosis is a form of IgG4-related systemic disease. Am J Surg Pathol. 2011;35:701–6.
24. Karim F, Clahsen-van Groningen M, van Laar JA. AA Amyloidosis and IgG4-related disease. N Engl J Med. 2017;376:599–600.
25. Heidari P, Verdijk RM, van den Bosch WA, Paridaens D. Biopsy-proven recurrence of unilateral IgG4-related orbital inflammation after 20 years. Orbit. 2014;33:388–91.
26. Della-Torre E, Stone JH. "How I manage" IgG4-related disease. J Clin Immunol. 2016;36:754–63.
27. Detiger SE, Karim AF, Verdijk RM, van Hagen PM, van Laar JAM, Paridaens D. The treatment outcomes in IgG4-related orbital disease: a systematic review of the literature. Acta Ophthalmol. 2019;97:451–9.
28. Karim F, Paridaens D, Westenberg LE, Guenoun J, Verdijk RM, van Hagen PM, et al. Infliximab for IgG4-related orbital disease. Ophthal Plast Reconstr Surg. 2017;33:S162–5.

Orbital and Adnexal Lymphoproliferative Lesions

Robert M. Verdijk and Ronald O. B. de Keizer

Key Messages

- Orbital and adnexal lymphoproliferative lesions (OAL) may present as bilateral slowly progressive painless masses in up to half of the cases.
- A biopsy is required for diagnosis; FNAB is contraindicated.
- Multimodal histopathological, immunophenotyping, and molecular genetic investigations are needed to precisely diagnose and classify lymphoproliferative tumours of the OA.
- The eyelids show the highest proportion of secondary lymphoma involvement.
- Primary OAL should be staged according to the TNM classification devised for OAL.

R. M. Verdijk (✉)
Department of Pathology, Section Ophthalmic Pathology, Erasmus MC & the Rotterdam Eye Hospital, Rotterdam, The Netherlands

Department of Pathology, Leiden University Medical Center, Leiden, The Netherlands
e-mail: r.verdijk@erasmusmc.nl

R. O. B. de Keizer
Department of Oculoplastic, Orbital and Lacrimal Surgery, The Rotterdam Eye Hospital, Rotterdam, The Netherlands

1 Introduction

Ocular adnexal lymphoproliferative disease (OALD) is a general term for the spectrum of lymphoproliferative tumours of the ocular adnexa (OA). The OA comprise the eyelids, conjunctiva, lacrimal apparatus, and orbital soft tissues. Benign OALD is a reactive lymphoid hyperplasia (RLH) of polyclonal small B cells and T cells. Any type of lymphoma can involve the OA. Malignant lymphomas are classified according to the presumed cell of origin as defined by the World Health Organization (WHO) Classification of Tumours of Haematopoietic and Lymphoid Tissues [1], of which the updated fifth edition is yet to be published at the time of writing this chapter. Lymphomas can be divided into two major groups: Hodgkin lymphoma and non-Hodgkin lymphoma (NHL). Because Hodgkin disease of the OA is extremely rare, it will not be discussed here. Primary ocular adnexal lymphoma (OAL) is defined as a lymphoma of the OA without evidence of concurrent systemic lymphoma and no prior history of lymphoma. Primary OAL should be staged according to the TNM classification devised for OAL (Table 1) because the TNM-based staging system better predicts outcome in OAL than the Ann Arbor system [2].

F. M. Quaranta Leoni et al. (eds.), *Oculoplastic, Lacrimal and Orbital Surgery*,
https://doi.org/10.1007/978-3-031-39638-0_19

Table 1 TNM staging system for OAL (adapted from reference [2])

Primary Tumor (T)

TX Lymphoma extent not specified

T0 No evidence of lymphoma

T1 Lymphoma involving the conjunctiva alone without orbital involvement

- T1a Bulbar conjunctiva only
- T1b Palpebral conjunctiva ± fornix ± caruncle
- T1c Bulbar and nonbulbar conjunctival involvement
- T2 Lymphoma with orbital involvement ± any conjunctival involvement
- T2a Anterior orbital involvement but no lacrimal grand involvement ± conjunctival disease
- T2b Anterior orbital involvement with lacrimal gland involvement ± conjunctival disease
- T2c Posterior orbital involvement ± conjunctival involvement ± any extraocular muscle involvement
- T2d Nasolacrimal drainage system involvement ± conjunctival involvement but not including nasopharynx

T3 Lymphoma with preseptal eyelid involvement ± orbital involvement ± any conjunctival involvement

T4 Orbital adnexal lymphoma extending beyond orbit to adjacent structures, such as bone and brain

- T4a Involvement of nasopharynx
- T4b Osseous involvement (including periosteum)
- T4c Involvement of maxillofacial, ethmoidal, frontal sinuses
- T4d Intracranial spread

Lymph Node Involvement (N)

NX Involvement of lymph nodes not assessed

N0 No evidence of lymph node involvement

N1 Involvement of ipsilateral regional lymph nodes

N2 Involvement of contralateral or bilateral regional lymph nodes

N3 Involvement of peripheral lymph nodes not draining ocular adnexal region

N4 Involvement of central lymph nodes

Distal metastasis (M)

MX Dissemination of lymphoma not assessed

M0 No evidence of involvement of other extranodal sites

M1 Lymphomatous involvement in other organs recorded either at first diagnosis or subsequently

- M1a Noncontiguous involvement of tissues or organs external to the ocular adnexa (e.g., parotid gland, submandibular gland, lung, liver, spleen, kidney, breast)
- M1b Lymphomatous involvement of the bone marrow

M1c Both M1 and M1b involvement

2 Clinical Presentation and Evaluation

Most patients with OAL complain of a slowly progressive and painless mass. Pain can, however, be a symptom and is mostly mild. When the patient primarily presents with a painful mass, the ophthalmologist must rule out other diseases (specific orbital inflammations like IgG4 related orbital disease, sarcoidosis, granulomatosis with polyangiitis and Sjogren disease). Ophthalmic evaluation in OAL typically shows a so-called salmon patch, a fleshy pink mass of the conjunctiva (Fig. 1). Anterior orbital masses including lacrimal gland OAL will present with an eyelid swelling. OAL in an extraocular muscle presents with proptosis, double vision and/or with ptosis. Patients may have an history of systemic lymphoma, leukaemia or autoimmune disease [3]. On clinical examination both eyes are inspected carefully as the more common AOL types can be bilateral in up to half of the cases [4].

It is advised to do a work-up of the blood including: red and white blood cell count with differential, platelet count, kidney- and liver function tests. As the above described autoimmune and inflammatory diseases are in the differential diagnosis general inflammation markers such as sedimentation rate and C-reactive protein may be tested as well.

Masses can be evaluated with computed tomography and/or magnetic resonance imaging (MRI) with contrast enhancement. OAL are

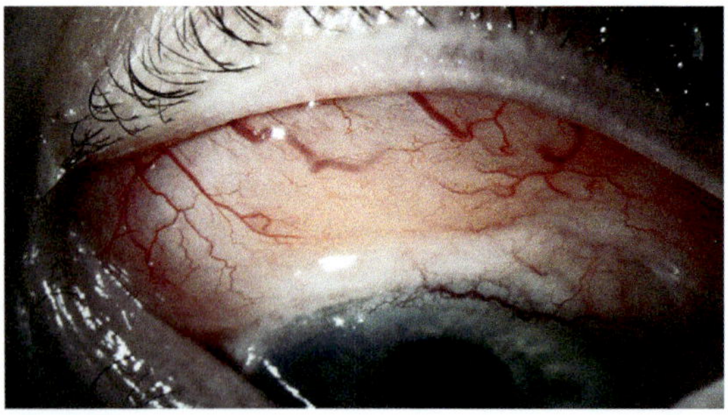

Fig. 1 Salmon patch. The right superior temporal quadrant of the conjunctiva shows the typical salmon colored swelling of conjunctival lymphoma

mostly iso- or hyperintense on T2 weighted images in MRI. OAL has more diffusion restriction compared to inflammatory lesions in diffusion weighted mating on MRI [3, 5–8].

Fine needle aspiration is contraindicated in OAL diagnosis as the aspirated materials lose the architecture needed for classification. Therefore, an incisional biopsy is required [9, 10]. In close collaboration with your pathology department we advise to send (at least a part) of the biopsied material fresh on a wet gauze to enable a combination of histopathology and flow cytometric evaluation. Molecular studies, these days, can be performed on formalin fixed paraffin embedded tissue. In general, biopsies taken from the conjunctiva and eyelid have a low risk of complications, but deep apical biopsies pose the risk of vision loss [11].

It is advised to discuss complex cases in a multidisciplinary team with at least an experienced neuroradiologist, orbital surgeon and ophthalmic pathologist. In selected cases a neurosurgeon, ENT specialist and maxillofacial surgeon are advised to join the orbital team. After diagnosis, a haematologist-oncologist and radiotherapist should be consulted for therapeutic planning. It is advised to discuss and annotate the diagnosis and therapeutic options in a tumour board meeting [12].

3 Regional Aspects

The orbital bone and (peri-) ocular connective tissues are derived from neural crest cells (i.e., mesectoderm not mesoderm). Although the lacrimal gland arises from a thickening of the ectoderm of the superior conjunctival fornix, the mesenchymal cells that surround the point of epithelial budding are also of neural crest origin. This exceptional mesenchymal environment can be expected to be of relevance to the specific etiologic, molecular genetic, and clinical features of OAL that, as will be discussed below, differ from other extranodal NHL.

In the non diseased lacrimal gland, IgA-producing plasma cells account for approximately 50% of all lymphoid cells. T cells, representing the second most common cell type, are located predominantly in small lymphocytic foci and singly in the stroma of the lacrimal gland. Conjunctival lymphoid tissue can be observed in the healthy palpebral conjunctiva, more pronounced in the upper than in the lower lid. It occurs both as diffuse lymphocytes and IgA-producing plasma cells located in the substantia propria. Additionally, approximately 60% of non diseased conjunctival sacs have organised lymphoid accumulations in the substantia propria. The epithelium of the lacrimal gland tubules and acini, along with the conjunctival crypts, expresses lysozyme and the IgA secretory component. The conjunctiva and lacrimal gland thus belong to the mucosa-associated lymphoid (MALT) system, also called eye-associated lymphoid tissue (EALT). Lymphocytes recirculate to the EALT via high endothelial venules (inflow) and lymph vessels (outflow) through a complex interplay of chemokines, chemokine receptors, and integrins. The non-conjunctival side of the eyelids contains dispersed inflammatory cells, mainly CD4-positive T cells, macrophages, and dendritic cells of the skin. The skin of the eyelids contains lymph vessels, comparable to skin at other sites. In contrast to the eyelid, conjunctiva, and lacrimal gland, the soft tissues of the orbit and its contents have long been considered extralymphatic sites that do not contain lymph vessels or lymphoid cells in a healthy state. However, transient expression of lymphatic markers has been documented in retrobulbar intraconal orbital vasculature during fetal and early neonatal development. The orbit may, therefore, be proposed to possess a full range of lymphatic plasticity that may be activated in the diseased state.

Apart from the genetic changes described below, the development and progression of B-NHL is also known to depend on interactions with the tumour microenvironment that are mediated/directed by chemokines, chemokine receptors, and integrins. The expression profile of motility and adhesion molecules in OAL have recently been described to differ from that in lymphomas of the secondary lymphoid organs [13]. These findings suggest that the malignant cells in OAL likely undergo a dynamic process of trafficking involving egress into the blood and homing back to the extranodal tissues where an element of retention may occur.

4 Epidemiology

OALD includes benign and malignant disease such as RLH [14] and OAL based on histopathology, immunophenotype, and molecular features. OAL represents malignant lymphoid neoplasms, which can develop as primary or secondary tumour manifestations. One to two percent of all lymphomas and approximately 8% of all extranodal lymphomas arise in the OA and the incidence is increasing [15]. In Europe there is a consistent overall increase in incidence of NHL. An estimated 5% of NHL patients develop secondary OA involvement during the course of their disease. Lymphoid tumours comprise 10% to more than 20% of orbital mass lesions in different series, and lymphoma is the most common orbital malignancy [16]. Likewise, lymphomas involving the conjunctiva are relatively common [17]. Ocular adnexal lymphoma is primarily a disease of older adults (peak age 65 years) with a slight female preponderance.

To gain insight into the relative frequencies of the types and location of biopsied OA lymphoid disease, the diagnoses and location of 343 consecutive OALD lesions diagnosed between 1987 and 2021 in the department of pathology of the Erasmus MC University Medical Center were evaluated (Table 2). In this series the most frequent OA presentation was in the orbit, 36%; fol-

Table 2 Diagnosis, anatomic localization and frequency of tumor in 343 consecutive patients with histopathologically confirmed ocular adnexal lymphoproliferative tumor (updated from reference [18])

	Orbit		Conj		Lacr		Eyelid		All				
	Pr	Sec	Pr	Sec	Pr	Sec	Pr	Sec	Pr	Sec	All	%	% l
RLH	10	0	11	0	28	0	3	0	52	0	52	15	na
MALT	na	1	55	1	16	2	0	2	71	6	77		
ENMZL	46	7	0	3	0	0	8	1	54	11	65		
Subtotal MALT+ENMZL									125	17	142	41	48
Follicular	15	10	9	3	5	4	5	2	34	19	53	15	18
DLBCL	13	4	0	0	6	1	1	2	20	7	27	8	9
Mantle	3	6	4	3	2	5	3	6	12	20	32	9	11
CLL/SLL	2	1	1	3	3	3	2	3	8	10	18	5	6
Lymphopl	3	1	0	1	0	1	0	1	3	4	7	2	2
Burkitt	1	0	0	0	0	0	0	0	1	0	1	<1	<1
Pr cut follicle	0	0	0	0	0	0	0	1	0	1	1	<1	<1
Pr cut DLBCL	0	0	0	0	0	0	0	1	0	1	1	<1	<1
Myc fungoides	0	0	0	0	0	0	0	1	0	1	1	<1	<1
Pr cut anapl	0	0	0	0	0	0	1	1	1	1	2	<1	<1
T cell NOS	0	2	0	0	0	0	0	0	0	2	2	<1	<1
Lymph papul	0	0	0	0	0	0	0	2	0	2	2	<1	Na
T cell hyperpl	0	0	0	0	0	0	1	0	1	0	1	<1	Na
NK/T cell	0	0	0	1	0	0	0	0	0	1	1	<1	<1
Subtotal (%)	93 (74)	32 (26)	80 (84)	15 (16)	60 (83)	16 (17)	24 (51)	23 (49)	257 (75)	86 (25)	343	100	100
Total (%)	125 (36)		95 (28)		76 (22)		47 (14)						

Conj conjunctiva, *Lacr* lacrimal apparatus, *Pr* primary, *Sec* secondary, *l* lymphoma, *RLH* reactive lymphoid hyperplasia, *MALT* MALT lymphoma, *ENMZL* extra nodal marginal zone lymphoma, *Follicular* follicular lymphoma, *DLBCL* diffuse large B cell lymphoma, *Mantle* mantle cell lymphoma, *SLL* small lymphocytic lymphoma, *CLL* chronic lymphocytic leukemia, *Lymphopl* lymphoplasmacytic lymphoma, *Burkitt* Burkitt lymphoma, *Pr cut follicle* primary cutaneous follicle center lymphoma, *Pr cut DLBCL* primary cutaneous diffuse large B cell lymphoma, *Myc fungoides* mycosis fungoides, *Pr cut anapl* Primary cutaneous anaplastic large cell lymphoma, *T cell NOS* Peripheral T-cell lymphoma NOS, *Lymph papul* lymphomatoid papulosis, *T cell hyperpl* T cell hyperplasia, *NK/T cell* NK/T cell lymphoma, *Na* not applicable

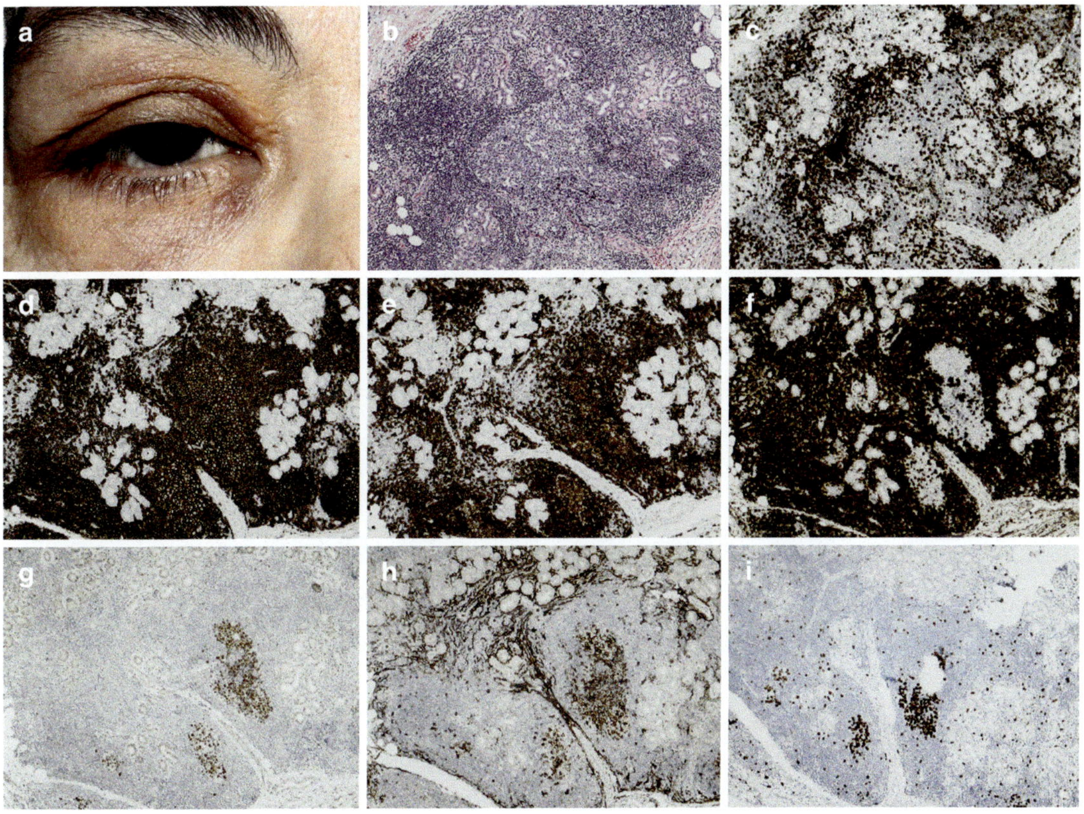

Fig. 2 Reactive lymphoid hyperplasia of the lacrimal gland. (**a**) Swelling of the right lacrimal gland. (**b**) Atrophic acini and ductuli of the lacrimal gland with a dense follicular infiltration of lymphoid cells, hematoxylin and eosin stain (H&E). (**c**) CD3 stains T-cell in the interfollicular areas. (**d**) CD20 stains the B-cells concentrated in the follicular areas. (**e**) CD79a stains the B-cells. (**f**) BCL2 remains negative central in the follicular areas. (**g**) BCL6 stains positive central in the follicular areas. (**h**) CD10 stains positive central in the follicular areas. (**i**) Ki-67 shows a high proliferation fraction in the reactive follicles, whereas in most small cell lymphomas the proliferation fraction is low. All histopathological images are at an original magnification of ×100

lowed by conjunctiva, 28%; lacrimal apparatus, 22%; and eyelid, 14%. These updated figures do not differ significantly from earlier published reviews [19].

Reactive lymphoid hyperplasia is diagnosed in about 16% of OALD (Fig. 2). The most frequent primary OAL diagnosis is extranodal marginal zone lymphoma (ENMZL) in 42% of all lymphoid lesions and 62% of all primary OAL (Table 2, Fig. 3). The highest frequency of ENMZL/MALT lymphoma is observed in the conjunctiva in 70% of all primary lymphoid conjunctival lesions. Primary marginal zone lymphomas of the orbit (50%) should be designated ENMZL, as no MALT tissue is supposedly involved in the genesis of these lesions. One case of gastric MALT lymphoma secondarily involved the orbit, but the conjunctiva and lacrimal gland may also show secondary involvement of distant MALT lymphoma (Table 2) [20]. The different OA structures show a distinctly different disease spectrum. The eyelids show the highest proportion of secondary lymphoma involvement (49% of all eyelid lymphoproliferative lesions), and this probably also explains the most varied list of 13 different diagnostic entities, including T-cell lymphoma (Table 2). This seems to separate eyelid lymphoid lesions clearly from the other ocular adnexa. For the conjunctiva, lacrimal apparatus, and orbit there is approximately 80% primary lymphoid lesions and 20% secondary involvement (Table 2) [20].

The second most frequent primary OAL diagnosis is follicular lymphoma (FL, Fig. 4), 17% of all OAL, closely followed by diffuse large B-cell lymphoma (DLBCL, Fig. 5) at 10%. Mantle cell lymphoma was diagnosed in 4% of primary lesions. Other primary diagnoses are small lymphocytic lymphoma, 4%; lymphoplasmacytic lymphoma, 2%; and 1 case of Burkitt lymphoma. Almost all (90%) ENMZL are primary OAL [20]. The most common secondary lymphoma subtype is mantle cell lymphoma with 22% of all secondary lymphomas, followed by ENMZL (including MALT lymphoma), 17%; chronic lymphocytic leukaemia (CLL), 16%; FL, 14%; DLBCL, 11%; and lymphoplasmacytic lymphoma, 6%. Other secondary lymphoma diagnoses are given in Table 2.

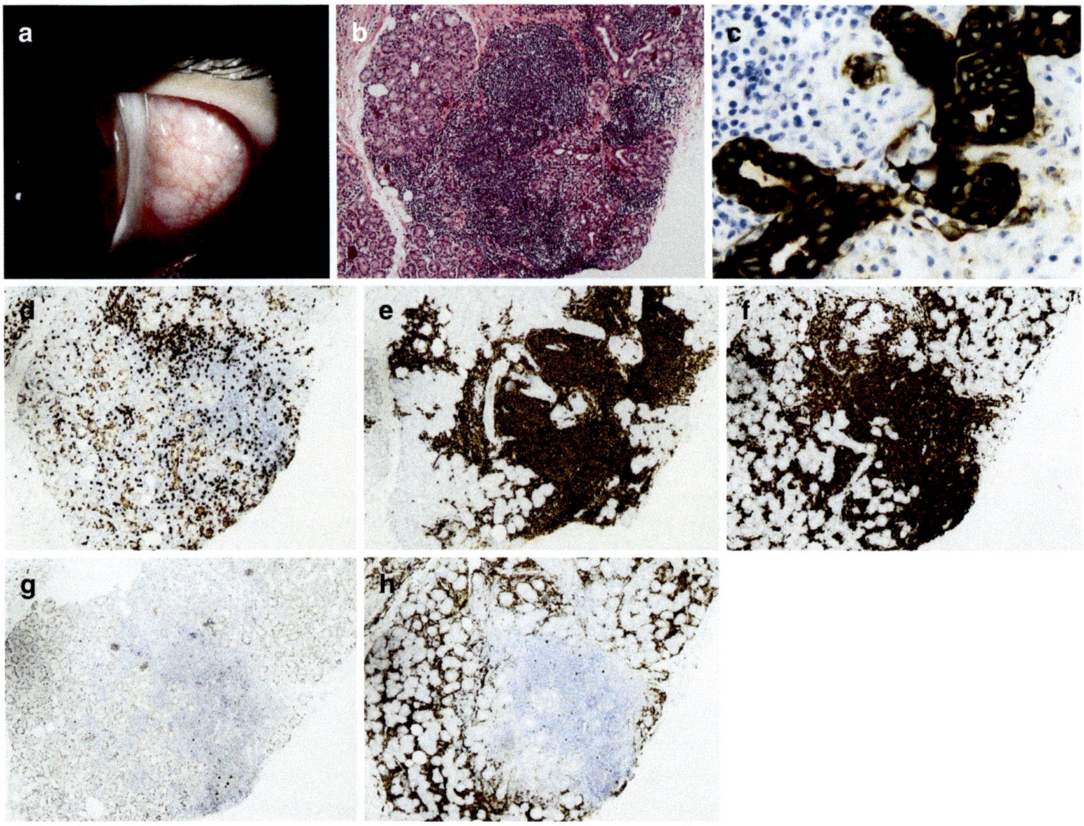

Fig. 3 Extranodal marginal zone lymphoma (MALT lymphoma) of the lacrimal gland. (**a**) Swelling of the left lacrimal gland. (**b**) Acini and ductuli infiltrated by a nodular lymphocytic mass (H&E). (**c**) Keratin positive acini are destroyed by lymphocyte infiltration giving rise to lymphoepithelial lesions. (**d**) CD3 stains few reactive T-cells. (**e**) CD20 massively stains the lymphoid infiltrate. (**f**) BCL2 is activated in all infiltrating B-cells. (**g**) No expression of BCL6, no follicular B-cells are present. (**h**) Absence of staining for CD10 also shows the lack of follicular differentiation. (**i**) B-cell receptor rearrangement studies show a monoclonal rearrangement. Original magnification of panel C is ×630. All other histopathological images are at an original magnification of ×100

i

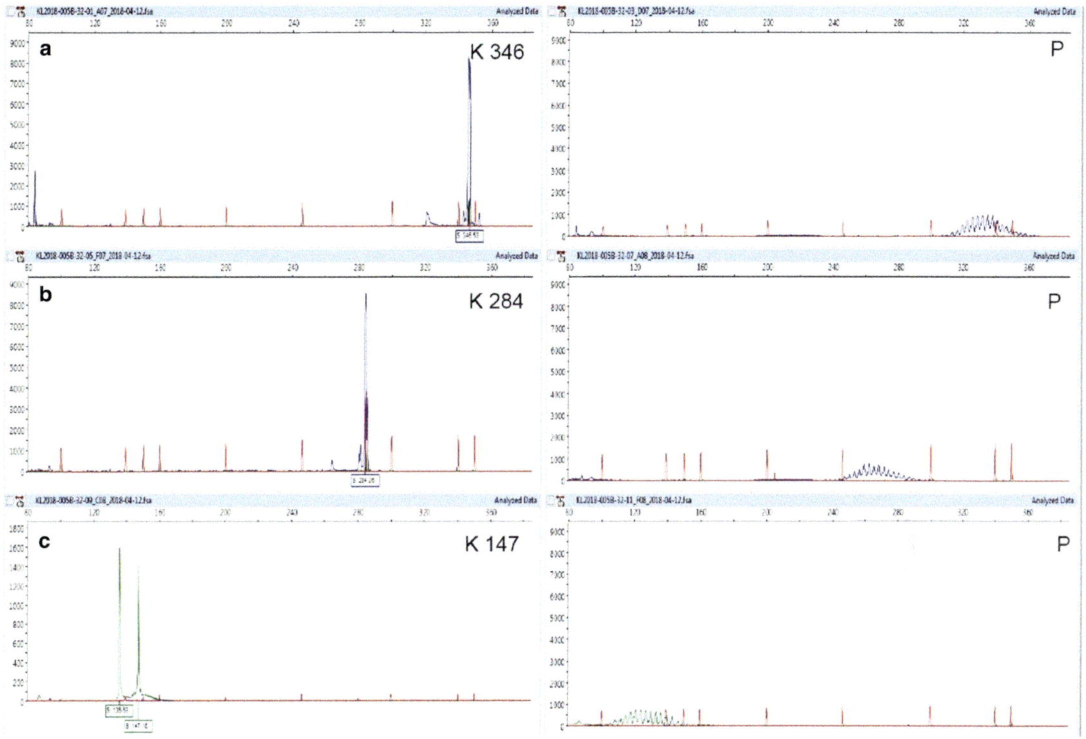

Fig. 3 (continued)

5 Reactive Lymphoid Hyperplasia

Reactive lymphoid hyperplasia is diagnosed in about 16% of OALD and is most common in the lacrimal gland (48% of all primary lymphoid lesions of the lacrimal gland, Table 2). The diagnosis of RLH is made based on morphology (Fig. 2) in the absence of a monotypic B cell population by immunohistochemistry (Fig. 2b–h) or preferably by exclusion of a monoclonal B cell population by flow cytometry and/or molecular techniques. No lymphoepithelial lesions should be present. It is widely recognized that the generally hypocellular lymphoid cell-poor orbital pseudotumors (idiopathic orbital inflammation) and RLH represent distinct entities [14]. Reactive lymphoid hyperplasia comprises 2% of all lesions of the orbit, representing 7% of all inflammatory lesions [16]. With the advent of multimodal lymphoma diagnostics, including flow cytometry and molecular testing, there has been a shift in diagnostic patterns with previously thought benign RLH being reclassified as ENMZL [14]. The designation of atypical lymphoid hyperplasia may be used for indeterminate lesions where the amount of tissue available or the combined results of flow cytometric or molecular investigations are inconclusive. The use, however sparse, of this diagnostic category can guide management and follow-up. Reactive lymphoid hyper-

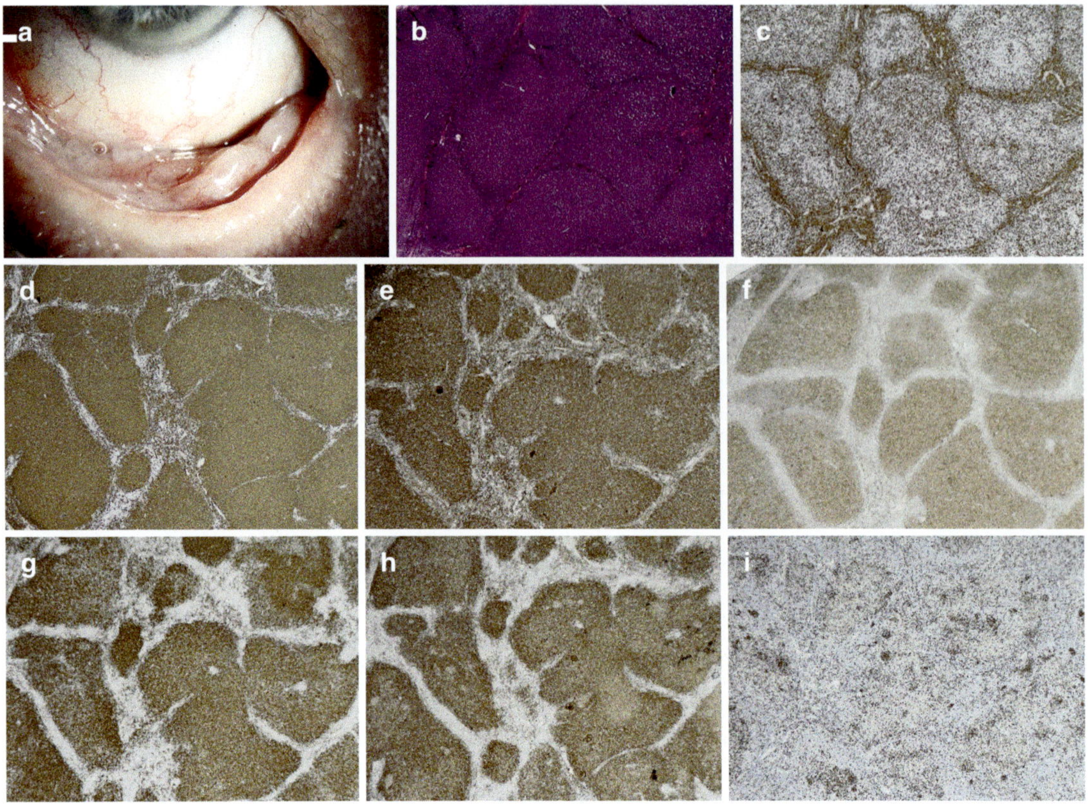

Fig. 4 Follicular lymphoma of the conjunctiva. (**a**) Serpentine salmon colored swelling of the left lower conjunctiva. (**b**) Dense follicular lymphoid infiltration. (**c**) CD3 stains few reactive T-cells. (**d**) Cd20 massively stains the B-cells. (**e**) All B-cells show BCL2 activation. (**f**) All B-cells stain positive for BCL6 a follicular marker. (**g**) All B-cells stain positive for CD10 a follicular marker. (**h**) CD23 shows a massive expansion of follicular dendritic cells. (**i**) Ki-67 only shows a low proliferation fraction. All histopathological images are at an original magnification of ×25

plasia may mimic early IgG4-related disease and has been documented in single cases to develop into the typical sclerotic lesions of this disease over a period of 20 years [21]. Immunohistochemical staining for IgG and IgG4 is therefore recommended in all cases of RLH.

6 ENMZL/MALT Lymphoma

The deep orbital tissue is not considered lymphoid tissue, whereas the lacrimal gland, the conjunctiva, and the lacrimal sac are considered as functional MALT [22, 23]. Ophthalmologists and ophthalmic pathologists therefore should know that MALT lymphoma is not synonymous with ENMZL and is characterised by mucosal location and lymphoepithelial lesions. Extranodal marginal zone lymphoma may arise in MALT or reactive tertiary lymphoid tissue acquired through chronic antigenic stimulation because of persistent inflammation or infection as exemplified by Helicobacter pylori infection in patients with gastric MALT lymphoma. Likewise, Chlamydia psittaci infection has been associated with ENMZL of OA [24]. C. psittaci is living and infective both in conjunctival tissue and peripheral blood mononuclear cells. In vitro isolation of this microorganism from patients with ENMZL of OA fulfils Koch's second postulate, enhancing the specific relationship between C. psittaci and lymphomagenesis in this anatomical region. However, epidemiologic studies analysing association between C. psittaci and OA MALT lym-

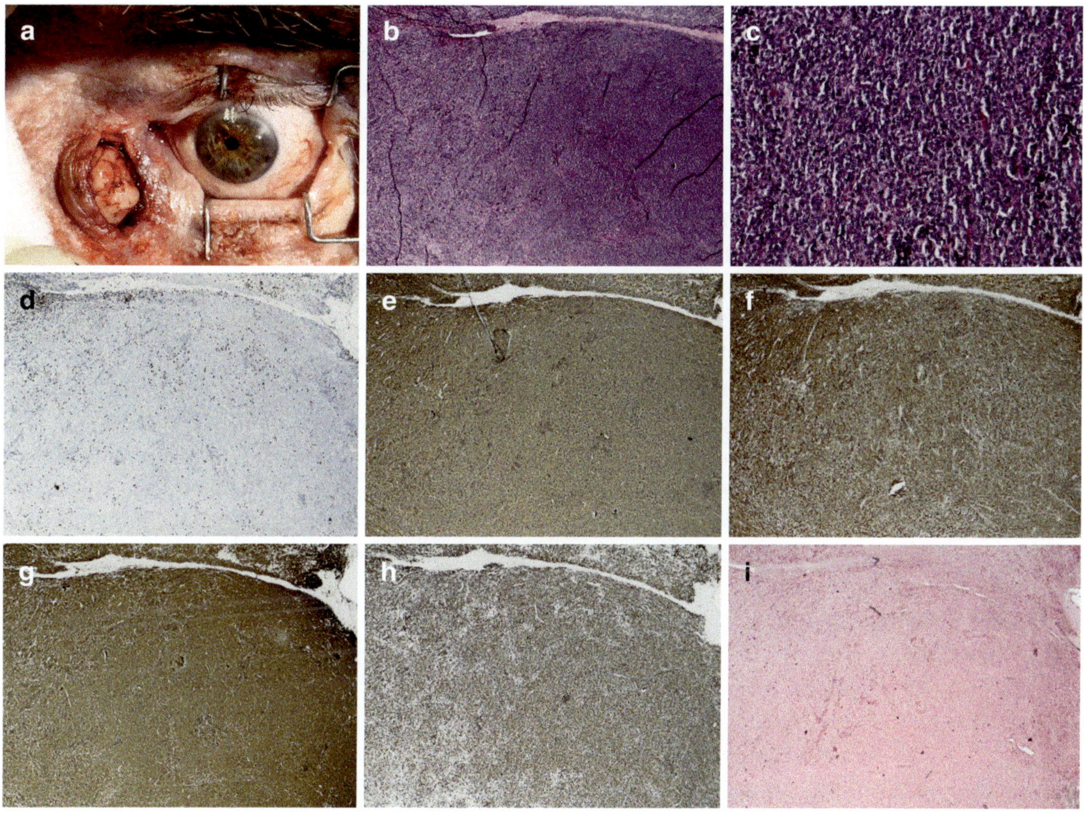

Fig. 5 Diffuse large B-cell lymphoma of the lacrimal sac. (**a**) Intra-operative image of the swelling of the lacrimal sac. (**b**) Hematoxylin and eosin stain shows a massive lymphoid infiltration. (**c**) Higher magnification shows large cells with pleomorphic nuclei. (**d**) CD3 shows few reactive T-cells. (**e**) CD20 shows a massive positive staining of B-Cells. (**f**) All the B-cells stain positive for CD10 a follicular differentiation marker. (**g**) All B-cells show activation of BCL2. (**h**) Ki-67 shows an extremely high proliferation fraction. (**i**) In situ hybridization for Epstein Barr Virus specific DNA is negative. Original magnification of panel C is ×200. All other histopathological images are at an original magnification of ×25

phoma demonstrated marked geographic and methodical differences [25]. Gastric H. pylori positivity has been documented in 32% of ENMZL of OA patients; none of these patients responded with lymphoma regression upon H. pylori eradication therapy [26]. Direct infection of the orbit by H. pylori has been suggested but appears highly implausible. Extranodal marginal zone lymphoma has consistently been associated with several autoimmune disorders. The exact mechanism of lymphomagenesis in the context of autoimmunity is largely unexplained. An interesting association has occasionally been observed between IgG4-related disease and ENMZL of the OA [27]. On the other hand, documented long-term IgG4-related disease does not necessarily develop into lymphoma [21].

ENMZ of the OA can be solitary or multicentric, unilateral or bilateral. Dissemination can occur to ipsilateral and/or contralateral regional lymph nodes and to more distant sites. Clinical features are of a space-occupying mass that is painful in less than 10% of patients. Few patients have B symptoms such as fever, night sweats, or weight loss. The duration of symptoms at presentation ranges from a few months to 3 years. A resection or biopsy yields white to salmon pink fleshy tissue.

OA MALT/ENMZL (Fig. 3) are composed of small- to medium-sized cells with round or indented nuclei, clumped chromatin, inconspicuous nucleoli, and inconspicuous to moderately abundant cytoplasm (Fig. 3b). Other than lymphoepithelial lesions more easily identified using keratin stain (Fig. 3c), marginal zone involvement (Figs. 3d–h), and follicular colonisation (BCL2 positive staining of the follicle, Fig. 3f), most of the findings are rather nonspecific for distinction from other small B lymphomas. Plasmacytoid differentiation is frequent in ENMZL of OA. Extranodal marginal zone lymphoma of OA lack specific markers of other small-cell lymphomas and are positive for B lineage markers (Fig. 3e) and BCL2 (Fig. 3f). There is a low proliferation rate. In current practice, there is no distinctive positive immunological marker for ENMZL1: they are negative for CD23, CD5, BCL6 (Fig. 3g), CD10 (Fig. 3h), and CyclinD1. At a molecular level there is clonal rearrangement of immunoglobulin heavy chain and light chain (Fig. 3i), which is essential to make the distinction between RLH and lymphoma.

On the genetic and molecular level different mechanisms can be observed in ENMZL of OA; aneuploidy, translocations, deletions, and mutations mostly affect or target genes encoding for regulators of NF-κB. Trisomy of chromosomes 3, 12, and 18 are frequent in all ENMZL, but gain of chromosome 6, including trisomy, is more specific for ENMZL of OA [28]. Translocations occur relatively infrequently in ENMZL of OA when compared with MALT lymphoma at other sites [28, 29]. Extranodal marginal zone lymphoma of OA translocations may include t(11, 19)(q21;q21) in 0–15%, t(14, 19)(q32;q21) in 0–38%, t(1, 14)(p22;q32) in 0–3%, and t(3, 14)(p13;q32) in 0–20% (reviewed by Zhu et al28), along with 1 published case each of t(6, 14)(p21.1;q32.3), t(14, 18)(q32.33;p13.1), and t(5, 11)(q33;p11.2). These translocations target the MALT1, BCL10, or FOXP1 genes. The different incidence of the translocations in MALT-type lymphomas from distinct geographic and anatomical sites is probably linked to specific prelymphomatous conditions (geographical, environmental, embryonic/developmental, or other unknown conditions) that influence neoplastic transformation. TNFAIP3, a tumor suppressor, is inactivated by promoter methylation, mutations, and/or deletions in about 15–30% of ENMZL of OA [30]. Deletion of chromosome 6q23 affects the A20 gene [28], which may also be mutated [29] and is affected in about 30% of ENMZL of OA cases. Activating mutations of MYD88, a factor physiologically linking toll-like receptor signaling to NF-κB activation, have been described in about 0–7% of the cases along with occasional mutations in the BIRC3 and PRDM1 genes, all affecting the NF-κB pathway. In case of MYD88 L265P mutation, a lymphoplasmacytic lymphoma (morbus Waldenström) should be considered because 80–90% of lymphoplasmacytic lymphoma harbour this mutation [31]. Mutations in MYD88 have reportedly been associated with an inferior disease-free survival in ENMZL of OA [30]. MicroRNA expression patterns have also been described to relate to the NF-κB pathway in ENMZL of OA [32]. The updated WHO Classification of Tumours of Haematopoietic and Lymphoid Tissues is not expected to pose any changes in ENMZL diagnosis and classification [33].

In some cases, incisional biopsy or surgical resection may serve as therapy for ENMZL of OA; however, attempts for complete resection should not be made because this does not influence survival and can lead to severe complications. A “wait and watch” strategy can be safely proposed for elderly or frail patients with little symptoms. Recently, the effectiveness of primary antibiotic treatment of ENMZL of OA directed at eradication of C. psittaci was reviewed [34]. The median follow-up for these studies was 25 months, and both C. psittaci—positive and C. psittaci—negative patients responded. Complete remission (CR) was achieved in 18% of patients out of 131 patients reported. The combined numbers of CR and partial remission (PR) account for an overall remission rate of 45% ENMZL of OA. Although lacking long-term follow-up information, these results do not seem inferior to the outcome reported for chemotherapy and radiotherapy, suggesting that upfront doxycycline is a reasonable and effective treatment proposal for patients with stage I C. psittaci—positive ENMZL of OA before considering more aggressive strategies [35]. Resistance to C. psittaci eradication has not been described to be related to MALT1 translocation. Most OAL are localised (stage I) at presentation, and radiation therapy provides excellent local control [36], with 4-year relapse rates of 20–25%. However, 45% of patients develop late sequelae of radiation therapy (especially cataract) and 25% of patients experience side effects WHO grade 3–4. For more advanced disease stages, chemotherapy with chlorambucil with or without prednisolone yields excellent response rates with a 5-year relapse free survival of 60%. The use of upfront additional anthracycline-based chemotherapy does not show clinical advantages. The use of rituximab as a single agent is associated with short-lived responses [37]. Intralesional injections with rituximab or interferon alpha may be safe and active strategies for conjunctival MALT lymphomas, but long-term results remain to be confirmed [37, 38].

7 Follicular Lymphoma

For patients with FL of the ocular adnexa (OAFL), no etiologic or predisposing factors have been identified. However, low numbers of t(14;18)-positive B cells can be detected in healthy individuals [39], and these B cells are reported to have biological features that are closely associated with the pathogenesis of the disease. What used to be called in situ follicular lymphoma is proposed to be renamed in situ follicular neoplasia in the updated WHO classification using the same criteria [33]. OAFL occurs most frequently in the orbit and conjunctiva but may involve all ocular adnexa (Table 2) [40]. Clinical features are of a space-occupying mass that is painful in over 20% of patients39 (Fig. 4). Patients generally do not present with B symptoms. The duration of symptoms at presentation ranges from 1 month to 9 years [40]. Follicular lymphoma can present as primary ocular adnexal disease and secondary involvement is found in about one third of cases; it may be bilateral in up to 20% of cases [40]. Dissemination of OAFL mainly occurs to the regional lymph nodes and the salivary glands and may involve distant lymph nodes. Follicular lymphoma can transform to DLBCL in 3% of cases.

Follicular lymphoma is composed of uniform, densely packed follicles, which may coalesce, simulating diffuse areas (Fig. 4b). The follicular population is uniformly atypical. Small cells (centrocytes) have cleaved, indented, angulated nuclei; large cells (blastic centrocytes) may be cleaved or noncleaved. In addition, variable large cells (centroblasts and immunoblasts) with vesicular nuclei containing 1 or 2 nucleoli, often adjacent to the nuclear membrane, can be found. Mitotic figures are less frequent in grade 1 and grade 2 FL than in RLH; however, grade 3 FL may have a high mitotic rate. In general the prognosis of FL supposedly worsens with greater proportions of centroblasts. Follicular lymphoma grading is performed by estimating the average number of centroblasts per high power field (HPF) in 10 neoplastic follicles (grade 1, 0–5 centroblasts per high-power field; grade 2, 6–15 centroblasts per high-power field; grade 3A, >15 centroblasts per high-power field)1; grade 3B also contains more than 15 centroblasts but in addition the centroblasts form coalescent tumour areas without centrocytes. Because of the small size of the ophthalmic biopsies, formal grading is not always possible. Grades may be reported as low grade (1, 2) and high grade (3A and 3B). In some institutions distinction is made between grade 3A and 3B for therapeutic strategy reasons. The interfollicular zone is typically composed of small reactive T-cells (Figs. 4c). Follicular lymphoma is positive for B-cell markers like CD79a (Fig. 4d) are BCL2, BCL6 and CD10 positive in 85% of cases (Fig. 4e–g). Positive staining for BCL2 is quite specific versus pre-existent secondary germinal centres (Fig. 4e). CD10 expression distinguishes this entity from other mature small B lymphomas. Follicular lymphoma also stains positive for BCL6 (Fig. 4f) and show expansion, demarcated by follicular dendritic cell meshworks that stain positive for CD21, CD23 (Fig. 4h), and CD35. However, these meshworks are usually compact and intact instead of demonstrating a more ragged aspect as in marginal zone lymphoma and mantle cell lymphoma. OAFL grade 1–2 shows a low Ki-67 staining (Fig. 4i).

On the genetic level t(14;18) translocation has been recognized as a genetic hallmark of FL, but additional genetic aberrations are required for the development of FL. Cytogenetic analyses of FL samples have revealed that they contain 4–6 additional genomic alterations on average, and 6q-, trisomy 7, trisomy 12, der (19), and + X are frequently observed. On the basis of the fluorescent in situ hybridization (FISH) results, 76% of all OAFL test t(14;18)-positive [40]. This genetic aberration results in the constitutive expression of BCL2 and confers a survival advantage to B cells. Recently, additional recurrent gene aberrations such as TNFRSF14, EPHA7, EZH2, CREBBP, EP300, MLL2, and MEF2B have been identified in FL at large [41]. Many of these mutations have been confirmed in OAFL [42]. Thus, unlike ENMZL, multiple pathways are involved in lymphomagenesis of FL. This is assumed to constitute a major reason for the clinical heterogeneity of the disease. A new prognostic model integrating gene mutations with clinical parameters has been proposed, but, although conceptually interesting, requires validation [43]; in particular, relevance for OAFL needs to be established for the most prognostically important genes, ARID1A and TP53. Whether mutational analysis should be performed routinely for diagnostic, prognostic, or therapeutic purposes and whether it should be integrated with other pathological and clinical prognostic factors remains to be determined. The updated WHO Classification of Tumours of Haematopoietic and Lymphoid Tissues has newly defined paediatric-type FL as a localised clonal proliferation with excellent prognosis where a conservative therapeutic approach may be sufficient [33]. This new entity is of limited relevance to OAFL because it occurs in children and young adults, rarely in older individuals. The molecular genetic hallmarks of this new entity are the absence of BCL2, BCL6, and MYC rearrangements.

Most patients with OAFL stage I/II disease are treated with radiotherapy (usual dosage 30 Gy), which results in an 85% local disease control rate [40]. Distant relapse occurs in 6–50% of patients at a median follow-up of 7 years, and there is a 10-year OS rate of 83%. Interestingly, a significantly better disease-specific survival was found for patients with primary OAFL treated with radiotherapy only compared with patients receiving radiotherapy plus chemotherapy [40]. For stage III–IV OAFL, systemic chemotherapy is indicated following standard regimens currently used for nodal disease. Anthracycline-based regimens such as cyclophosphamide, vincristine, and prednisone or chlorambucil/cyclophosphamide, hydroxydaunorubicin, vincristine, and prednisone combined with rituximab (R-CVP or R-CHOP) are suitable for treating these patients. The overall median progression-free survival from the date of diagnosis was 5.3 years in a recent multicenter trial. The overall survival rates at 10 and 20 years were 60% and 15% (median overall survival, 11 years), respectively, for the entire patient group, whereas the 10- and 20-year disease-specific survival rates were 69 and 29% (median disease-specific survival, 20 years), respectively. The disease-specific survival was not different in patients with primary, disseminated, and relapsed OAFL [40].

8 Diffuse Large B-Cell Lymphomas

Diffuse large B-cell lymphomas may evolve de novo or may be the result of transformation of a less aggressive lymphoma, most commonly follicular lymphoma. Risk factors include AIDS, organ transplantation, hereditary immunodeficiency syndromes, and autoimmune disease. Diffuse large B-cell lymphomas in the OA region are primary in two thirds of cases, but in one third are the result of secondary involvement of systemic disease (Table 2). Diffuse large B-cell lymphoma is the third most common lymphoma subtype occurring in the ocular adnexa (Table 2) [44]. Patients usually present with a rapidly expanding tumour mass that is often unilateral and located mainly in the orbit, but may involve the lacrimal drainage system as well (Fig. 5). Thirty percent of patients experience pain or irritation. Patients may experience B symptoms.

Diffuse large B-cell lymphomas show diffuse effacement of normal architecture and are composed of large non cohesive cells, which make up over 50% of the population or are present in confluent foci. The usual appearance is large vesicular nuclei with multiple irregular eosinophilic nucleoli (Fig. 5b, c). Usually there are few reactive T cells (Fig. 5d). Diffuse large B-cell lymphomas positive for CD20 (Fig. 5e); however, in biopsies taken after treatment with rituximab this marker may be negative and alternative B cell markers such as CD79a and PAX5 should be employed. A high proliferation index with high expression of Ki-67 is observed (Fig. 5h).

Genome-wide expression profiling has revealed a number of features associated with an unfavourable clinical outcome. According to similarities to the putative cell of origin, OA DLBCL can be largely divided into two different groups: germinal centre B-cell-like (GCB) DLBCL and activated B-cell-like (ABC) DLBCL [45]; however, 15–30% of DLBCL cannot be classified definitively. Further investigations have revealed different activation pathways for the respective subtypes. Activated B-cell-like DLBCL have a poorer overall survival compared with GCB-DLBCL and respond less effectively to chemotherapy. Different immunohistochemical marker combinations can aid in discrimination between ABC-DLBCL and GCB-DLBCL. Several of these algorithms have been demonstrated to be predictive of survival. The most widely known "Hans classifier" composed of CD10 (Fig. 5f), MUM1, and BCL6 protein expression can divide DLBCL into GCB-DLBCL and ABC-DLBCL with about 80% concordance with the molecular classification. A combination of five immunohistochemical markers—GCTE1, CD10, BCL6, MUM1, and FOXP1—can achieve about 90% concordance with the molecular results, whereas others using either 3 or 5 markers have been proposed but have not been widely tested on independent patient cohorts. All these algorithms have been shown to have a high concordance [46]. The better understanding of the molecular pathogenesis of these two subgroups has led to the investigation of more specific therapeutic strategies to mitigate the worse outcome among those with ABC/non-GCB type DLBCL reported in most studies; prospective trials are ongoing to determine whether these therapies should be incorporated into clinical practice. For this reason, the revised WHO classification will require the identification of these 2 DLBCL subtypes [33].

The revised WHO classification also focuses on MYC alterations in DLBCL. MYC is rearranged in 5–15% of DLBCL, not otherwise specified (NOS) and is often associated with BCL2 and/or, less frequently, BCL6 translocation in the "double-hit" or "triple-hit" lymphomas that are included in the updated WHO classification in the new category of high-grade B-cell lymphoma (HGBL), with rearrangements of MYC and BCL2 and/or BCL6 [33]. MYC protein expression is detected in a higher proportion of DLBCL (30–50%) and is associated with protein expression of BCL2 in 20–35% of cases. Often these tumours do not carry MYC/BCL2 chromosomal alterations and have been named "double-expressor lymphoma." A cutoff of 40% MYC-expressing cells can be used to define these cases. For BCL2 expression a cutoff of 50% is recommended (Fig. 5g). Double expression of MYC and BCL2 proteins without gene aberrations should be considered a prognostic indicator in DLBCL, NOS but will not be assigned a separate category [33]. All large B-cell lymphomas with MYC and BCL2 and/or BCL6 rearrangements need to be designated HGBL, with MYC and BCL2 and/or BCL6 rearrangements. Other cases that appear blastoid or cases intermediate between DLBCL and Burkitt lymphoma, but which lack a MYC and BCL2 and/or BCL6 rearrangement, should be designated HGBL, NOS. A consensus has not yet been reached to provide specific guidelines as to which large B-cell lymphomas should have fluorescence in in situ hybridization studies [33]. Testing for MYC, BCL2, and BCL6 rearrangements should always be contemplated in NOS cases and cases with a GCB phenotype. Diffuse large B-cell lymphomas with high-grade morphology or cases with more than 40% MYC-positive cells should also be tested for MYC, BCL2, and BCL6 rearrangements.

Epstein-Barr virus (EBV)–positive DLBCL generally occurs in immunocompetent patients over 50 years old and have a worse prognosis than EBV-negative tumours. Epstein-Barr virus–positive DLBCL has also been recognized in younger patients who have a better survival. This new information has led to the proposal of a new entity of EBV-positive DLBCL, NOS [33].

In summary, current state-of-the-art diagnosis of DLBCL requires testing for determination of the subtype of DLBCL by molecular or immunohistochemical testing for ABC- or GCB-DLBCL. In cases of GCB-DLBCL or DLBCL, NOS additional testing for MYC and BCL2 immunohistochemistry and FISH is advisory. In ABC-DLBCL at least immunohistochemical testing for BCL2 and MYC expression is recommended, as positive cases indicate a worse prognosis. Epstein-Barr virus status can most reliably be determined by EBV-encoded RNA (EBER)-FISH (Fig. 5i).

The International Prognostic Index has been developed as a clinical tool for predicting outcome in DLBCL. Negative prognostic factors are an age at the time of diagnosis over 60 years, Ann Arbor stage III or higher, the involvement of more than 1 extranodal sites, elevated LDH serum level, and poor performance status. The treatment results of DLBCL have greatly improved with the introduction of the CHOP chemotherapy scheme and have further improved with the addition of rituximab (R-CHOP) to a 5-year OS of 60%. For patients younger than 60 years of age and with a high-risk profile, the addition of etoposide shows an improved outcome (R-CHOEP).

9 Conclusions

Any type of lymphoma can involve the OA. Multimodal histopathological, immunophenotyping, and molecular genetic investigations are therefore essential to precisely diagnose and classify lymphoproliferative tumours of the OA and are important for identifying potential therapeutic targets and prognostic factors. Therefore, an incisional biopsy is required. Immunophenotyping can be performed using flow cytometry and immunohistochemistry. Flow cytometry is a rapid, quantitative procedure and allows multiple antigens to be evaluated on the same cell simultaneously, which aids in the identification of clonal lymphocyte populations. Flow cytometry can only be performed on fresh (i.e. non fixated) biopsy material. Immunohistochemistry requires more time to perform and quantitation is more subjective, but it allows for correlation of antigen expression with cytoarchitecture and cytomorphology required for exact classification. Molecular genetic investigations may reveal additional diagnostic, prognostic, and potentially therapeutic relevant markers. A cohesive report based on clinical, radiological, pathologic immunologic, and molecular genetic investigations is the ultimate goal. Ideally the results of all these investigations should be discussed in a multidisciplinary tumour board for an integrated diagnosis and management proposal.

References

1. Swerdlow SH, Campo E, Harris NL, Jaffe ES, Pileri SA, Stein H, Thiele J. WHO classification of tumours of haematopoietic and lymphoid tissues. Revised 4th ed. Lyon: IARC; 2016.
2. Rath S, Connors JM, Dolman PJ, Rootman J, Rootman DB, White VA. Comparison of American Joint Committee on Cancer TNM-based staging system (7th edition) and Ann Arbor classification for predicting outcome in ocular adnexal lymphoma. Orbit. 2014;33:23–8.
3. Laban K. Clinical and molecular aspects of orbital inflammation and lymphoma. Ophthalmology. Ridderkerk: Utrecht University Repository; 2020. p. 186.

4. Lee GI, Oh D, Kim WS, Kim SJ, Ko YH, Woo KI, Kim YD, Ahn YC. Low-dose radiation therapy for primary conjunctival marginal zone B-cell lymphoma. Cancer Res Treat. 2018;50:575–81.
5. Akansel G, Hendrix L, Erickson BA, Demirci A, Papke A, Arslan A, Ciftci E. MRI patterns in orbital malignant lymphoma and atypical lymphocytic infiltrates. Eur J Radiol. 2005;53:175–81.
6. Haradome K, Haradome H, Usui Y, Ueda S, Kwee TC, Saito K, Tokuuye K, Matsubayashi J, Nagao T, Goto H. Orbital lymphoproliferative disorders (OLPDs): value of MR imaging for differentiating orbital lymphoma from benign OPLDs. AJNR Am J Neuroradiol. 2014;35:1976–82.
7. Sepahdari AR, Aakalu VK, Setabutr P, Shiehmorteza M, Naheedy JH, Mafee MF. Indeterminate orbital masses: restricted diffusion at MR imaging with echo-planar diffusion-weighted imaging predicts malignancy. Radiology. 2010;256:554–64.
8. Purohit BS, Vargas MI, Ailianou A, Merlini L, Poletti PA, Platon A, Delattre BM, Rager O, Burkhardt K, Becker M. Orbital tumours and tumour-like lesions: exploring the armamentarium of multiparametric imaging. Insights Imaging. 2016;7:43–68.
9. Mombaerts I, Rose GE, Verity DH. Diagnosis of enlarged extraocular muscles: when and how to biopsy. Curr Opin Ophthalmol. 2017;28:514–21.
10. Mombaerts I, Ramberg I, Coupland SE, Heegaard S. Diagnosis of orbital mass lesions: clinical, radiological, and pathological recommendations. Surv Ophthalmol. 2019;64:741–56.
11. Jacobs SM, McInnis CP, Kapeles M, Chang SH. Incidence, risk factors, and management of blindness after orbital surgery. Ophthalmology. 2018;125:1100–8.
12. Specchia ML, Frisicale EM, Carini E, Di Pilla A, Cappa D, Barbara A, Ricciardi W, Damiani G. The impact of tumor board on cancer care: evidence from an umbrella review. BMC Health Serv Res. 2020;20:73.
13. Middle S, Coupland SE, Taktak A, Kidgell V, Slupsky JR, Pettitt AR, Till KJ. Immunohistochemical analysis indicates that the anatomical location of B-cell non-Hodgkin's lymphoma is determined by differentially expressed chemokine receptors, sphingosine-1-phosphate receptors and integrins. Exp Hematol Oncol. 2015;4:10.
14. Turbiner Geyer J, Knowles DM. Malignant lymphomas and lymphoid hyperplasias that occur in the ocular adnexa (orbit, conjunctiva and eyelids). In: Knowles DM, editor. Neoplastic hematopathology. 3rd ed. Philadelphia: Lippincott Williams & Wilkins; 2013. p. 1304.
15. Sjo LD, Ralfkiaer E, Prause JU, Petersen JH, Madsen J, Pedersen NT, Heegaard S. Increasing incidence of ophthalmic lymphoma in Denmark from 1980 to 2005. Invest Ophthalmol Vis Sci. 2008;49:3283–8.
16. Verdijk RM, Pecorella I, Mooy C. The orbit, including the lacrimal gland and lacrimal drainage system. In: Heegaard S, Grossniklaus HE, editors. Eye pathology: an illustrated guide. 1st ed. Berlin: Springer; 2015. p. 547–732.
17. Kirkegaard MM, Coupland SE, Prause JU, Heegaard S. Malignant lymphoma of the conjunctiva. Surv Ophthalmol. 2015;60:444–58.
18. Verdijk RM. Lymphoproliferative tumors of the ocular adnexa. Asia Pac J Ophthalmol (Phila). 2017;6:132–42. PMID: 28399341.
19. Verdijk RM. An update of ocular adnexal lymphomas. Diagn Histopathol. 2015;21:26–33.
20. Ferry JA, Fung CY, Zukerberg L, Lucarelli MJ, Hasserjian RP, Preffer FI, Harris NL. Lymphoma of the ocular adnexa: a study of 353 cases. Am J Surg Pathol. 2007;31:170–84.
21. Heidari P, Verdijk RM, van den Bosch WA, Paridaens D. Biopsy-proven recurrence of unilateral IgG4-related orbital inflammation after 20 years. Orbit. 2014;33:388–91.
22. Wieczorek R, Jakobiec FA, Sacks EH, Knowles DM. The immunoarchitecture of the normal human lacrimal gland. Relevance for understanding pathologic conditions. Ophthalmology. 1988;95:100–9.
23. Knop N, Knop E. Conjunctiva-associated lymphoid tissue in the human eye. Invest Ophthalmol Vis Sci. 2000;41:1270–9.
24. Ferreri AJ, Guidoboni M, Ponzoni M, De Conciliis C, Dell'Oro S, Fleischhauer K, Caggiari L, Lettini AA, Dal Cin E, Ieri R, Freschi M, Villa E, Boiocchi M, Dolcetti R. Evidence for an association between Chlamydia psittaci and ocular adnexal lymphomas. J Natl Cancer Inst. 2004;96:586–94.
25. Collina F, De Chiara A, De Renzo A, De Rosa G, Botti G, Franco R. Chlamydia psittaci in ocular adnexa MALT lymphoma: a possible role in lymphomagenesis and a different geographical distribution. Infect Agent Cancer. 2012;7:8.
26. Ferreri AJ, Ponzoni M, Viale E, Guidoboni M, Conciliis CD, Resti AG, Politi L, Lettini AA, Sacchetti F, Dognini G, Dolcetti R, Doglioni C. Association between Helicobacter pylori infection and MALT-type lymphoma of the ocular adnexa: clinical and therapeutic implications. Hematol Oncol. 2006;24:33–7.
27. Nakayama R, Matsumoto Y, Horiike S, Kobayashi S, Nakao R, Nagoshi H, Tsutsumi Y, Nishimura A, Shimura K, Kobayashi T, Uchiyama H, Kuroda J, Taki T, Inaba T, Nishida K, Yokota S, Yanagisawa A, Taniwaki M. Close pathogenetic relationship between ocular immunoglobulin G4-related disease (IgG4-RD) and ocular adnexal mucosa-associated lymphoid tissue (MALT) lymphoma. Leuk Lymphoma. 2014;55:1198–202.
28. Chanudet E, Ye H, Ferry J, Bacon CM, Adam P, Muller-Hermelink HK, Radford J, Pileri SA, Ichimura K, Collins VP, Hamoudi RA, Nicholson AG, Wotherspoon AC, Isaacson PG, Du MQ. A20 deletion is associated with copy number gain at the TNFA/B/C locus and occurs preferentially in translocation-negative MALT lymphoma of the ocular adnexa and salivary glands. J Pathol. 2009;217:420–30.

29. Zhu D, Ikpatt OF, Dubovy SR, Lossos C, Natkunam Y, Chapman-Fredricks JR, Fan YS, Lossos IS. Molecular and genomic aberrations in Chlamydophila psittaci negative ocular adnexal marginal zone lymphomas. Am J Hematol. 2013;88:730–5.
30. Johansson P, Klein-Hitpass L, Grabellus F, Arnold G, Klapper W, Pfortner R, Duhrsen U, Eckstein A, Durig J, Kuppers R. Recurrent mutations in NF-kappaB pathway components, KMT2D, and NOTCH1/2 in ocular adnexal MALT-type marginal zone lymphomas. Oncotarget. 2016;7:62627–39.
31. Treon SP, Xu L, Yang G, Zhou Y, Liu X, Cao Y, Sheehy P, Manning RJ, Patterson CJ, Tripsas C, Arcaini L, Pinkus GS, Rodig SJ, Sohani AR, Harris NL, Laramie JM, Skifter DA, Lincoln SE, Hunter ZR. MYD88 L265P somatic mutation in Waldenstrom's macroglobulinemia. N Engl J Med. 2012;367:826–33.
32. Hother C, Rasmussen PK, Joshi T, Reker D, Ralfkiaer U, Workman CT, Heegaard S, Ralfkiaer E, Gronbaek K. MicroRNA profiling in ocular adnexal lymphoma: a role for MYC and NFKB1 mediated dysregulation of microRNA expression in aggressive disease. Invest Ophthalmol Vis Sci. 2013;54:5169–75.
33. Swerdlow SH, Campo E, Pileri SA, Harris NL, Stein H, Siebert R, Advani R, Ghielmini M, Salles GA, Zelenetz AD, Jaffe ES. The 2016 revision of the World Health Organization classification of lymphoid neoplasms. Blood. 2016;127:2375–90.
34. Kiesewetter B, Raderer M. Antibiotic therapy in non gastrointestinal MALT lymphoma: a review of the literature. Blood. 2013;122:1350–7.
35. Zucca E, Bertoni F. The spectrum of MALT lymphoma at different sites: biological and therapeutic relevance. Blood. 2016;127:2082–92.
36. Uno T, Isobe K, Shikama N, Nishikawa A, Oguchi M, Ueno N, Itami J, Ohnishi H, Mikata A, Ito H. Radiotherapy for extranodal, marginal zone, B-cell lymphoma of mucosa-associated lymphoid tissue originating in the ocular adnexa: a multi institutional, retrospective review of 50 patients. Cancer. 2003;98:865–71.
37. Savino G, Battendieri R, Gari M, Caputo CG, Laurenti L, Blasi MA. Long-term outcomes of primary ocular adnexal lymphoma treatment with intraorbital rituximab injections. J Cancer Res Clin Oncol. 2013;139:1251–5.
38. Blasi MA, Tiberti AC, Valente P, Laguardia M, Sammarco MG, Balestrazzi A, Larocca LM, Balestrazzi E. Intralesional interferon-alpha for conjunctival mucosa-associated lymphoid tissue lymphoma: long-term results. Ophthalmology. 2012;119:494–500.
39. Limpens J, Stad R, Vos C, de Vlaam C, de Jong D, van Ommen GJ, Schuuring E, Kluin PM. Lymphoma-associated translocation t(14,18) in blood B cells of normal individuals. Blood. 1995;85:2528–36.
40. Rasmussen PK, Coupland SE, Finger PT, Graue GF, Grossniklaus HE, Honavar SG, McKelvie P, Mulay K, Prause JU, Ralfkiaer E, Sjo LD, Heegaard S. Ocular adnexal follicular lymphoma: a multicenter international study. JAMA Ophthalmol. 2014;132:851–8.
41. Kishimoto W, Nishikori M. Molecular pathogenesis of follicular lymphoma. J Clin Exp Hematop. 2014;54:23–30.
42. Cani AK, Soliman M, Hovelson DH, Liu CJ, McDaniel AS, Haller MJ, Bratley JV, Rahrig SE, Li Q, Briceno CA, Tomlins SA, Rao RC. Comprehensive genomic profiling of orbital and ocular adnexal lymphomas identifies frequent alterations in MYD88 and chromatin modifiers: new routes to targeted therapies. Mod Pathol. 2016;29:685–97.
43. Pastore A, Jurinovic V, Kridel R, Hoster E, Staiger AM, Szczepanowski M, Pott C, Kopp N, Murakami M, Horn H, Leich E, Moccia AA, Mottok A, Sunkavalli A, Van Hummelen P, Ducar M, Ennishi D, Shulha HP, Hother C, Connors JM, Sehn LH, Dreyling M, Neuberg D, Moller P, Feller AC, Hansmann ML, Stein H, Rosenwald A, Ott G, Klapper W, Unterhalt M, Hiddemann W, Gascoyne RD, Weinstock DM, Weigert O. Integration of gene mutations in risk prognostication for patients receiving first-line immunochemotherapy for follicular lymphoma: a retrospective analysis of a prospective clinical trial and validation in a population-based registry. Lancet Oncol. 2015;16:1111–22.
44. Rasmussen PK. Diffuse large B-cell lymphoma and mantle cell lymphoma of the ocular adnexal region, and lymphoma of the lacrimal gland: an investigation of clinical and histopathological features. Acta Ophthalmol. 2013;91:1–27.
45. Alizadeh AA, Eisen MB, Davis RE, Ma C, Lossos IS, Rosenwald A, Boldrick JC, Sabet H, Tran T, Yu X, Powell JI, Yang L, Marti GE, Moore T, Hudson J Jr, Lu L, Lewis DB, Tibshirani R, Sherlock G, Chan WC, Greiner TC, Weisenburger DD, Armitage JO, Warnke R, Levy R, Wilson W, Grever MR, Byrd JC, Botstein D, Brown PO, Staudt LM. Distinct types of diffuse large B-cell lymphoma identified by gene expression profiling. Nature. 2000;403:503–11.
46. Hwang HS, Park CS, Yoon DH, Suh C, Huh J. High concordance of gene expression profiling-correlated immunohistochemistry algorithms in diffuse large B-cell lymphoma, not otherwise specified. Am J Surg Pathol. 2014;38:1046–57.

Histiocytic Disease of the Orbit

David H. Verity, Kaveh Vahdani, and Geoffrey E. Rose

Key Messages

- LCH is the most common of the histiocytoses.
- LCH represents a spectrum of overlapping diseases characterised by abnormal accumulation of histiocytic cells, encompassing the classic triad of eosinophilic granuloma, Hand–Schüller–Christian syndrome and Letterer–Siwe syndrome.
- Modern classification describes LCH by extent (unifocal or multifocal) and organ involvement (unisystem or multisystem).
- Debate continues as to whether LCH is a reactive disease with abnormal LC clonal proliferation, or a true neoplasm.
- Histology identifies characteristic large Langerhans cells containing Birbeck granules (cytoplasmic inclusion bodies).

Systemic immunosuppression with targeted molecular treatment or cytotoxic drugs is indicated in cases of local recurrence or disseminated disease.

D. H. Verity (✉) ·
Adnexal Service, Moorfields Eye Hospital, London, UK

St John of Jerusalem Eye Hospital Group, London, UK
e-mail: david.verity@nhs.net

K. Vahdani · G. E. Rose
Adnexal Service, Moorfields Eye Hospital, London, UK

The histiocytic disorders are caused by an abnormal accumulation of cells of the mononuclear phagocytic system (MPS), which are derived from bone marrow stem cells and consist of dendritic cells and macrophages. While the term 'histiocyte' refers to a connective tissue macrophage, the histiocytic disorders encompass proliferations of both dendritic cells and macrophages of different origins; thus, the term 'histiocytosis' has been adopted universally to describe an aberrant accumulation of either of the mononuclear phagocytes.

Historically, distinguishing these diverse but related diseases has been difficult due to the overlap at both the clinical and cellular level. Following a systematic reclassification in 1997, two broad groups have emerged: 'benign' diseases with varying biological behaviour, and those classified as 'malignant', with abnormal dendritic cell and monocyte accumulations in each group [1]. For a comprehensive review covering aetiology and systemic features of benign and malignant histiocytic disease, the reader is referred to an overview of the subject [2].

The two major benign disorders of the MPS are Langerhans cell histiocytosis (LCH) and hemophagocytic lymphohistiocytosis (HLH); the remaining diverse nonmalignant disorders are grouped together under the term non-LCH. This chapter reviews the histiocytic disorders of varying biological behaviour which present in the orbit, encompassing both LCH and non-LCH (Table 1). In addition, distinct clinical entities in which histiocytic cells are prominent, but not thought to be pathological—such

F. M. Quaranta Leoni et al. (eds.), *Oculoplastic, Lacrimal and Orbital Surgery*,
https://doi.org/10.1007/978-3-031-39638-0_20

Table 1 Orbital diseases caused by a pathological tissue accumulation of histiocytes

1. Dendritic cell origin
   (i) Langerhans cell histiocytosis (LCH) (previously encompassing eosinophilic granuloma, Hand–Schüller–Christian syndrome, and Letterer–Siwe syndrome)
   (ii) Non-Langerhans cell histiocytoses (non-LCH)
      i. Juvenile xanthogranuloma
      ii. Idiopathic xanthogranuloma in the adult
         1. Adult-onset xanthogranuloma (AOX)
         2. Necrobiotic xanthogranuloma (NXG)
         3. Erdheim–Chester disease (E-CD)
2. Monocyte/macrophage origin
   (i) Sinus histiocytosis with massive lymphadenopathy (Rosai–Dorfman disease)

Table 2 Orbital diseases characterized by a predominance of histiocytic cells

1. Sarcoidosis
2. Pseudorheumatoid nodules
3. Primary intraosseous histiocytic lesions
   (a) Giant cell reparative granuloma of bone
   (b) Giant cell tumor of bone
   (c) Aneurysmal bone cyst
4. Orbital reactions to blood and its break down products
   (a) Haematic pseudocyst
   (b) Cholesterol granuloma
   (c) Cholesteatoma
5. Tuberous xanthoma
6. Giant cell polymyositis
7. Orbital foreign body reaction

as sarcoidosis, cholesterol granuloma, and orbital foreign body reactions—are also discussed (Table 2). This chapter does *not* cover malignant histiocytic disorders, such as histiocytic sarcoma and the monocytic leukaemias, nor does it describe granulomatous processes in response to mycobacteria, fungi, and other pathogens.

1 Langerhans Cell Histiocytosis

The term 'Langerhans cell histiocytosis' (LCH) was proposed by Lichtenstein in 1953 to include the triad of eosinophilic granuloma, Hand–Schüller–Christian syndrome, and Letterer–Siwe syndrome [3]. These three related disorders share clinical and histological features, and are best regarded as one entity covering a spectrum of clinical severity. Currently, the term eosinophilic granuloma is frequently used for both unifocal and multifocal masses, and the two eponymous terms for disseminated disease are no longer used. Because the predominant histiocyte within the characteristic lesions is the Langerhans cell (LC), the contemporary term 'Langerhans cell histiocytosis' was adopted in 1987 [4, 5].

1.1 Aetiology

Despite original descriptions of LCH a century ago, the aetiology remains poorly understood, although recent studies implicate clonal proliferation of phenotypically abnormal LCs. LCH cells express a variety of cell surface and cytoplasmic markers not expressed on normal histiocytes, suggesting an arrested state of cellular maturation. Selectin and integrin adhesion molecules are both upregulated by LCH cells, which may account for the occurrence of these lesions at sites where LC are not usually encountered, such as bone [6]. However, whether these differences represent a reactive, immune-dysregulatory process to an environmental trigger, or a primary neoplastic disorder, remains unknown.

1.2 Pathogenesis

Technical advances in genomics have led to an increased understanding of LCH biology [7–9], with somatic mutations of the mitogen-activated protein kinase (MAPK) signalling pathway being thought to play a key role in the pathogenesis of LCH. MAPK activation facilitates formation of LCH lesions through differentiation of precursor cells towards Langerhans-cell (LC) phenotype. It also contributes to impaired migration and increased resistance of these LC cells to apoptosis, leading to accumulation of pathological dendritic-cells and the formation of an immune infiltrate, the latter resulting in local and systemic inflammation [7, 10]. In one study, an activating somatic MAPK mutation was found in over 85% of cases [11].

Several studies have confirmed the presence of *BRAF* ^{V600E} mutation in a majority of LCH lesions [8, 9, 12–14], the mutated proteins having elevated kinase activity that leads to MAPK pathway activation [15]. Other activating mutations in *BRAF*—including in-frame deletions, fusions, and duplications—have been reported in LCH lesions [11, 14, 16–19]. Moreover, activating somatic mutations in receptor tyrosine kinase genes (*ERBB3*), *NRAS*, *KRAS*, *ARAF* and *MAP 2K1* have also been identified in adults with LCH lesions [14, 17, 20, 21]. These recent discoveries have opened the doors to more targeted therapies in future.

The extent and severity of disease is considered to be determined by the stage of differentiation in which the myeloid cell acquires activating MAPK somatic mutations [7]. Based on this model of "misguided myeloid differentiation", high-risk multisystem disease arises from self-renewing stem (or progenitor) cells from bone marrow, whereas low-risk multisystem LCH arises from committed dendritic cell precursors or monocytes, and solitary low-risk lesions arise from mutation in a local dendritic cell precursor [7].

1.3 General Clinical Features

LCH arises most commonly from 1 to 3 years of age, with an annual incidence of between four and five cases per million [22]. The commonest variant is eosinophilic granuloma (70% of cases) which occurs in older children and young adults and carries the most favourable prognosis. However, because of the risk of dissemination, and with the differential diagnosis including non-LCH diseases with systemic involvement, (such as Erdheim- Chester disease (E–CD)), a thorough systemic evaluation and close follow-up are required in all cases [23] (Table 3).

The chronic forms of LCH (Hand–Schüller–Christian syndrome, and multifocal eosinophilic granuloma) have not been reported in infants, usually occurring in children, and, very rarely, in adults. There are typical clinical sites of disease (Table 4), which often follows a protracted course although aggressive bursts of progression may also occur [24].

Table 3. Staging investigations in biopsy-proven cases of LCH

Full blood count, liver function tests, coagulation studies
Chest radiography
Skeletal survey and bone scan
Bone marrow examination
Urine specific gravity
MRI to exclude asymptomatic CNS involvement

Table 4 Systemic involvement in disseminated LCH

1. Bone masses
   - Skull, femur, pelvis, tibia, scapula, jaw, humerus
   - Well-defined lytic lesions with, or without, sclerosis
2. Skin lesions in up to 80%
   - Seborrhoeic-like papules, scaly eruptions
3. Central nervous system involvement
   - Secondary diabetes insipidus, growth retardation, thyroid hormone deficiency
4. Peripheral infiltration
   - Peripheral and central lymph nodes, bone marrow, peripheral blood, liver, spleen, lung, gastrointestinal tract

The rare, but most acute and aggressive variant of LCH (Letterer–Siwe syndrome) afflicts children younger than 3 years of age, and is associated with marked constitutional symptoms and mucocutaneous involvement. Most patients deteriorate rapidly, with progressive involvement of bone marrow or vital organs, and death may occur within a few years of disease onset.

1.4 Orbital Disease

LCH is uncommon and accounts for less than 1% of orbital lesions [6, 25, 26]. Among patients with a diagnosis of LCH, orbital involvement occurs in up to 24%, with the highest prevalence in eosinophilic granuloma [25–28]. Clinical features in one series included proptosis (uni- or bilateral), ptosis, papilledoema, optic atrophy, and seventh nerve palsy (in decreasing frequency) [26]. Proptosis may be severe and globe luxation has been reported [29]. Neuro-ophthalmic complications are rare [26], but a case of cavernous sinus syndrome has been reported [30]. Intraocular involvement is also rare, being asso-

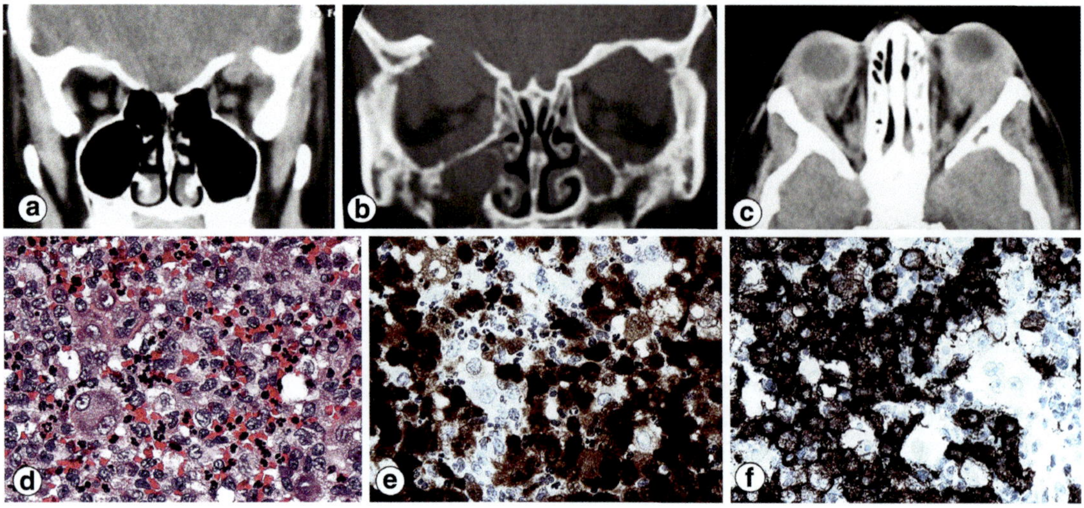

Fig. 1 Langerhans cell histiocytosis (LCH). (**a–c**) CT imaging identifying chronic lytic lesions in the superior orbit. (**d–f**) LCH histopathology: (**d**) High-power photomicrograph showing sheets of Langerhans cells with large folded and grooved nuclei admixed with eosinophils and neutrophils. H&E 400 μ. (**e**) Langerhans cells showing nuclear and cytoplasmic staining for S100. Immunoperoxidase stain. (**f**) Langerhans cells displaying strong membrane immunoreactivity with CD1a. Immunoperoxidase stain

ciated with more aggressive, subacute granulomatous disease in infants [26].

Orbital involvement is common in chronic LCH, and rare in the acute, disseminated forms. Lytic lesions have a distinct predilection for the superotemporal rim of the orbit (Fig. 1a–c) [31–33]. An inflammatory response may ensue when the orbital soft tissues are invaded, which clinically can mimic dacryoadenitis, but where orbital soft tissues are involved without bone destruction, other lesions containing eosinophils (such as granulocytic sarcoma and paediatric idiopathic orbital inflammation) must be excluded [33, 34]. Computed tomography (CT) imaging identifies the bony changes in LCH, which, in an advanced stage, may include a lytic lesion of the orbital wall with enlargement beyond the diploë and extension through the periorbita. Magnetic resonance imaging (MRI) is valuable in assessing intracranial extension of disease, providing better soft tissue definition than CT.

Table 5 Histological features of LCH

- Light microscopy
  - Sheets of Langerhans cells containing large ovoid, indented, grooved or folded nuclei with fine chromatin, inconspicuous nucleoli and thin nuclear membranes
  - Variable numbers of eosinophils, occasionally as eosinophilic microabscesses with necrosis in early lesions
  - Variable numbers of neutrophils, plasma cells, lymphocytes and multinucleated giant cells
  - Fibrosis and vacuolated cells containing accumulated cholesterol (foam cells) in older lesions
- Immunological studies
  - Cell surface markers: CD1a, S100, HLA-DR, CD207 (Langerin)
  - Extracellular deposition of eosinophil core granule protein (major basic protein), which may have a pathogenic role [33]
- Electron microscopy
  - Birbeck granule of Langerhans cells (caused by the presence of CD207 (Langerin) which results in membrane superimposition)

1.5 Histopathological Features

Macroscopically, LCH lesions are soft, friable, haemorrhagic and tan-yellow. Histological examination of all forms of LCH identifies common features (Table 5), but differentiation of unifocal from multifocal disease, and acute from chronic disease, is not possible on the basis of a single biopsy. Because haemorrhage often occurs within the lesions, hemosiderin-laden macrophages are also observed.

Various ultrastructural and immunohistochemical studies have demonstrated that the abnormal proliferation of histiocytes in LCH is derived from LCs [23, 35, 36]. Ultrastructural studies identify the characteristic cytoplasmic Birbeck granule of LCs (racket body, Birbeck's granule, Langerhans granule, or X body) (see Fig. 1d–f) [33, 37, 38], although these structures may be present in as few as 2% of all histiocytes within pathological specimens [36]. Other confirmatory markers include CD1a, a cell surface and cytoplasmic marker, and S100 protein [39, 40]. However, the current gold standard for a diagnosis of LCH is a lesion which is morphologically appropriate for LCH, displays cellular expression of CD1a and CD207 (Langerin) and electron microscopic demonstration of Birbeck granules. Finally, the multinucleated giant cells contain abundant mitochondria and profiles of smooth-surfaced endoplasmic reticulum but do not contain Langerhans granules. It should be noted that the stage of the disease may markedly affect both the histopathology and imaging studies; early proliferating lesions show a higher number of LCH cells with a lytic picture on imaging. Thus, the differential diagnosis in early LCH includes Ewings' sarcoma, osteosarcoma, neuroblastoma in children, and, in adults, metastatic disease.

1.6 Prognosis and Management

In general, the prognosis in LCH improves with age, being most favourable for isolated lesions without systemic involvement—for example, an isolated eosinophilic granuloma in a young adult. Conversely, features carrying a poor prognosis include bone marrow involvement, pulmonary dysfunction or respiratory failure and absence of osteolytic lesions [35]. The Letterer–Siwe variant has the worst prognosis which, despite chemotherapy, has a 5-year survival of only 50%.

Although spontaneous clinical remissions have been reported (probably due to progressive replacement of the lesion by fibrosis [41]), local intervention is the currently-favoured treatment for solely orbital LCH; systemic treatment is reserved for incomplete response, local reactivation, or the appearance of lesions elsewhere (Table 6) [42].

Table 6 Treatment options in LCH

Intervention	Indication
Conservative	Localized, asymptomatic disease
Local surgery	Localized, symptomatic disease, cosmetic disfigurement
Low-dose radiation therapy	Risk of fracture or functional impairment
Intralesional steroid	Recurrent, superficial lesions
Systemic chemotherapy	Recurrence after local surgery, disseminated systemic disease

Biopsy, subtotal curettage, and intralesional corticosteroid injections can result in a favourable outcome in solely orbital disease [43–45], and prompt resolution has also been reported after intralesional corticosteroid injections in both extraorbital and orbital lesions [45–48]. Intralesional injection of Interferon-α2b has also been shown to be effective in a small series of patients with orbital eosinophilic granuloma [49].

Treatment for lesions localised to non-weight-bearing bones is usually conservative, but can involve limited surgery or curettage, although even with surgical removal up to one-third of cases recur [50]. Low-dose fractionated radiotherapy (400–800 cGy) is effective, particularly for lesions in surgically-inaccessible areas or in sites associated with high surgical morbidity [33, 50–52]. Systemic corticosteroids should be considered for disseminated disease, with addition of chemotherapeutic agents if the response to steroids is inadequate [23, 26, 35, 53–55]. When frontline chemotherapy fails, other treatment options including nucleoside analogues (such as cladribine), bone marrow transplantation or immunoglobulin therapy play a role [56–59].

MAPK-pathway targeted therapy, with vemurafenib, has shown promising responses in early trials for adults with multifocal LCH or Erdheim–Chester disease (E-CD) [60–63]. Vemurafenib has also been used in orbital E-CD with good response documented in early case reports [64, 65]. Several reports have also supported a potential benefit of mitogen-activated protein/extracellular signal-regulated kinase kinase (MEK) inhibitors (such as cobimetinib or trametinib) in treating E-CD [14, 21, 60, 66]. However, the potential of cure with targeted therapy is uncertain, and disease relapse has been observed in a significant proportion of cases after cessation of therapy [61]. Future studies will determine the safety and efficacy of MAPK-inhibitor as monotherapy, or in combination with standard chemotherapy.

mTOR inhibitors (such as sirolimus and everolimus), which are used to treat a variety of inflammatory and neoplastic conditions, have also been shown to be effective as monotherapy for E-CD and induced responses regardless of BRAF mutation status, representing a viable alternative to conventional E-CD treatments [67].

2 Non-Langerhans Cell Histiocytoses

Several diseases cause xanthomatous deposits in the periorbital area (Table 7). Although necrobiosis lipoidica tends to affect the pretibial areas in diabetic patients, it can also produce xanthomatous lesions in the periorbital region [68, 69]. Other conditions with similar histopathologic findings include granuloma annulare, subcutaneous rheumatoid nodules, and pseudorheumatoid nodules, and these disorders can be distinguished on clinical examination.

Table 7 Differential diagnosis for xanthomatous deposits in the periorbital area

Xanthelasma (xanthoma planum)
Xanthoma tuberosum
Generalized normolipemic xanthoma
Xanthomas associated with hyperlipidemia
Adult-onset xanthogranuloma
Juvenile xanthogranuloma (JXG)
Necrobiosis lipoidica
Necrobiotic xanthogranuloma
Erdheim–Chester disease

3 Juvenile Xanthogranuloma

Juvenile xanthogranuloma (JXG), an idiopathic non-LCH, is a benign proliferative disorder which typically affects the skin, with ocular disease being the most common extracutaneous manifestation. Eye disease manifests as a xanthogranulomatous infiltration of the iris, and primary orbital involvement is rare; in such patients the typical cutaneous lesions are usually absent. Orbital JXG has been reported in infants under 1 year of age, with a second age peak in adults [70–72]. Such patients present with a mass, or proptosis, the differential diagnosis including other tumours (such as capillary haemangioma, rhabdomyosarcoma, fibrosarcoma, dermoid and teratoma), idiopathic orbital inflammation, and LCH (Fig. 2a).

Of 174 cases of JXG, Dehner described three patients with orbital involvement, either directly or by extension from the paranasal sinuses and nasal cavity with irregular bony destruction [70]. In one patient multiple visceral lesions were also present, but none had cutaneous disease. Zimmerman reported five patients with orbital involvement, four of whom similarly had no skin involvement [73]. In three cases, the lesion was present at birth, and occurred within 3 months of age in the other cases. Miszkiel et al. report a child with progressive proptosis from the age of 2½, in whom CT identified a large posteromedial soft tissue density mass with inferior displacement of the globe; at surgery a fatty mass above the lateral rectus muscle and lacrimal gland was removed, with histology identifying giant cells, histiocytes, and an abundance of intracytoplasmic and extracytoplasmic fat globules [72]. Schwartz et al. reported a patient with congenital macronodular juvenile xanthogranuloma affecting the eyelids and anterior orbit [74]. Finally, Shields and coworkers describe a newborn child with a congenital superonasal orbital and presep-

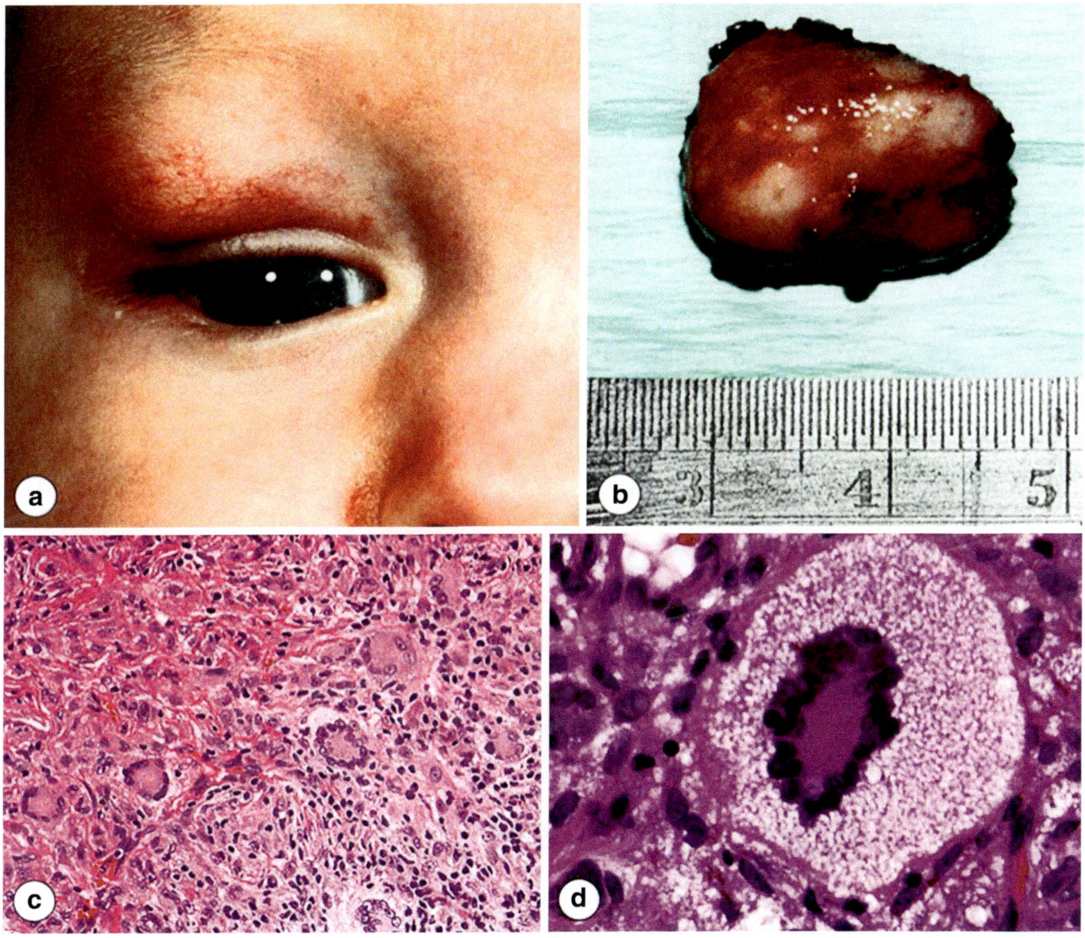

Fig. 2 Juvenile xanthogranuloma: (**a**) Primary orbital involvement in a child of one year of age who presented with proptosis. (**b**) Per-operative view of excised lesion. (**c**) Histology reveals numerous mononuclear histiocytes with several Touton giant cells and a minor population of lymphocytes. H&E 200 μ. (**d**) High-power photomicrograph of a typical Touton giant cell showing a ring of nuclei around an eosinophilic central and foamy outer cytoplasm. H&E 600 μ

tal mass, with a biopsy identifying histiocytes and Touton giant cells compatible with JXG. This patient had no evidence for peripheral features of JXG [75].

The diagnosis of JXG rests on tissue biopsy, although cutaneous lesions are not pathognomonic, and are absent in 5% or more of cases. Characteristic microscopic features include sheets of histiocytes and Touton giant cells are present in up to 85% of cases (Fig. 2a–d). The background stroma is composed of lymphocytes, plasma cells, and occasional eosinophils admixed with the mononucleated polygonal and rarely spindled histiocytes. Immunohistochemically, the histiocytes are positive for CD68, FXIIIa, fascin and HLA-DR. In contrast to LCH, JXG is considered to be derived from dermal dendrocytes which are negative for S100, CD1a, and reveal no Birbeck granules ultrastructurally.

JXG is typically a benign disorder, with most lesions resolving spontaneously, although complications of intraocular disease should be treated on their own merit. Symptomatic patients with unresectable extracutaneous disease may be treated with systemic steroid, chemotherapy, and/or radiotherapy. Orbital cases with residual, symptomatic lesion may be managed with systemic corticosteroids or low-dose radiotherapy where a large mass threatens either ocular structures or visual development.

4 Idiopathic Xanthogranuloma in Adults

4.1 Adult-Onset Xanthogranuloma

The characteristic appearance of adult-onset xanthogranuloma (AOX) is diffuse, yellow plaque-like masses in the eyelids, and the diagnosis is confirmed by tissue biopsy, with pre-operative CT to determine the extent of orbital disease (Figs. 3b, c and 4b, e). These patients should be screened for the known associations with this disease; namely, hepatosplenomegaly, blood dyscrasias, and lymphoproliferative malignancies.

Miszkiel et al. describe nine cases of orbital xanthogranuloma, eight of whom were adult patients; among the adults, the mean age at onset of symptoms was 41.2 years (range 19–62) [72]. All patients had soft tissue swelling within the lid, with yellow plaques within the subcutaneous tissue or conjunctiva present in all but two patients. Imaging identified an infiltrative mass with poorly defined margins predominantly involving the preseptal soft tissues in all patients. All showed orbital infiltration with posterior extension around the globe and extraocular muscle involvement, and lacrimal gland infiltration was present in five. Bilateral disease was present in three cases, and all but one had evidence for proptosis on radiological examination.

Periorbital xanthogranuloma is primarily a histological diagnosis, with characteristic features including a prominent infiltrate of xanthoma cells (lipid-laden macrophages) in the dermis extending deep into the subcutis (Fig. 3a–e). Variable numbers of lymphocytes may be present and often numerous foreign body and Touton-type giant cells are present. In the necrobiotic form (*vide infra*), there are areas of hyaline necrobiosis characterised by collagen degeneration.

The aetiology of periorbital xanthogranuloma remains uncertain. The association with a diverse range of systemic abnormalities, including eosinophilia, raised immunoglobulins (Igs), psoriasis, thyroid disease and lymphoid hyperplasia impli-

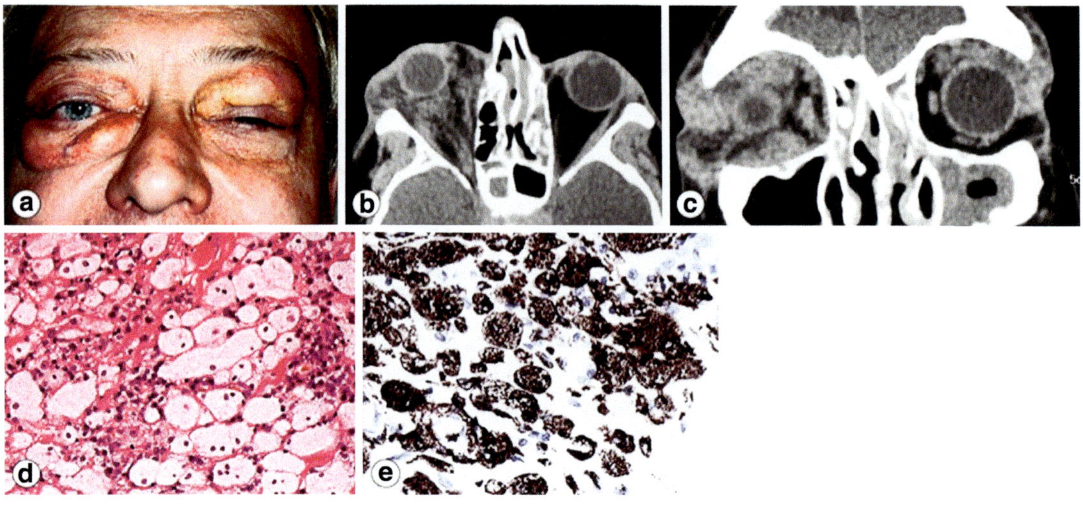

Fig. 3 Adult-onset xanthogranuloma: (**a**) A 43-year-old male was investigated for recurrent swelling of the right upper and lower lids, 3 mm of right-sided proptosis and reduced upgaze. He underwent several debulking procedures, and, 5 years after presentation, began to develop a similar lesion in the left upper lid. His general health over a 10-year follow-up period remained good. A full blood count revealed a slight eosinophilia but was otherwise normal. (**b, c**) A repeat CT, performed 3 years after initial presentation, identified a diffuse mass in the right orbit, extending from the region of the lacrimal gland into the superior orbit, with similarly poorly-defined tissue in the inferior and medial quadrants of the orbit. The optic nerve sheath is thickened, and the extraocular muscles enlarged. Disease was also identified in the superior left orbit. (**d**) Histology identifies numerous foam cells (histiocytes with ingested lipid) displaying abundant finely vacuolated cytoplasm. H&E 400 μ. (**e**) CD68 immunoreactivity in the foamy histiocytes. Immunoperoxidase stain

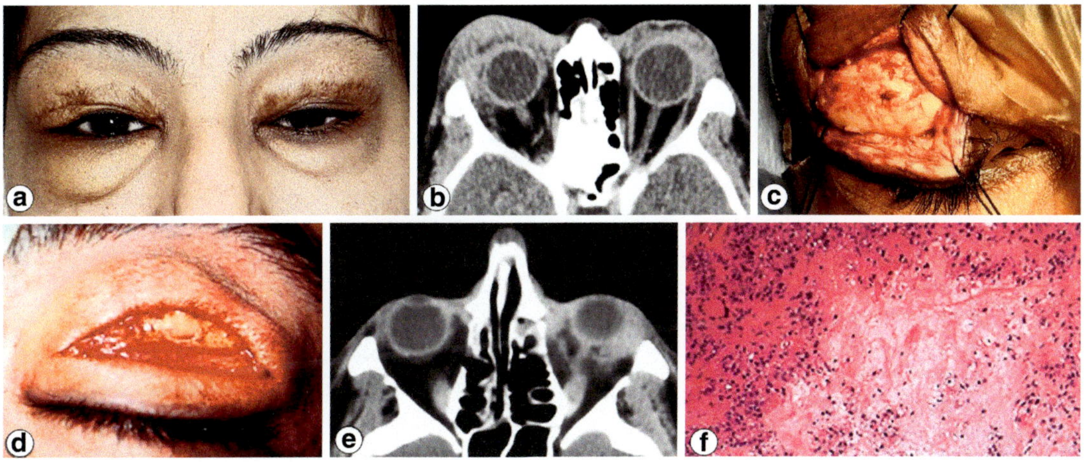

Fig. 4 Adult onset asthma and periocular xanthogranuloma (AAPOX) (**a–c**): (**a**) A 43-year old female with a 7 year history of bilateral yellow upper lid swelling. (**b**) Axial CT showing asymmetrical bilateral preseptal heterogeneous soft tissue swelling, extending into the orbit and contiguous periorbital tissue with enlargement of the lacrimal glands. (**c**) Intra-operative appearance of the lesion, with subsequent histopathologic examination revealing compact fibrofatty tissue with a heavy infiltrate of xanthoid cells including Touton giant cells and lymphoid follicles suggestive of xanthogranuloma. Necrobiotic xanthogranuloma (**d–f**): (**d**) A 46-year-old male underwent biopsy of a gradually enlarging lesion in the left upper eyelid. A per-operative view shows a waxy xanthomatous mass in the eyelid extending into the anterior orbit. (**e**) CT identifies extension of lesion into the anterior half of orbit. (**f**) Histology identifies central zones of necrobiotic collagen surrounded by a granulomatous infiltrate of histiocytes and a Touton giant cell. H&E 100 μ

cates an immunological mechanism [76–79]. Bullock and colleagues suggested that a reaction between serum Igs and tissue lipids results in the deposition of immune complexes leading to a foreign body giant cell reaction in the tissues [80], although the tendency for disease to occur around the periorbita remains unexplained.

Untreated periorbital xanthogranuloma tends to progress, and the response to various forms of treatment—which include surgical debulking, radiotherapy, systemic and intralesional steroids, and cytotoxic agents—is variable. Elner et al. reported a favourable response to intralesional triamcinolone injection in patients with AOX and necrobiotic xanthogranuloma (NXG) [81]. Their protocol consisted of injections of 20–40 mg (40 mg/mL) in sites of nodularity to a total dose of 120 mg, with repeated injections at 1–6 month intervals until disappearance of the nodules. The authors report a good response in all patients, without complications, to an average follow-up of 52 months.

4.2 Necrobiotic Xanthogranuloma (NXG)

NXG is a rare disorder, first described by Kossard and Winkelmann in 1980 [82], which generally affects patients in the fifth and sixth decades of life. The yellow-red skin nodules most commonly affect the eyelid and periorbital area, flexural extremities and trunk [83], and is associated with multiple organ involvement and haematological abnormalities (Table 8), and long-term follow-up is therefore required [84].

The periorbital region is the most common area of presentation (Fig. 4a–c), but a variety of ocular lesions may occur in NXG (Table 9) [85]. Periorbital involvement appears as painless waxy xanthomatous lesions, deeper violaceous plaques, or flesh-coloured nodules which may ulcerate and scar; these lesions may extend into the anterior orbit, with more posterior masses presenting with proptosis [83]. Severe lid involvement may

Table 8 Associated clinical features of NXG

Hematological abnormalities
- Raised erythrocyte sedimentation rate
- Monoclonal proteinemia in over 75% (k or l) [79]
- Neutropenia
- Hypocomplementemia
- Cryoglobulinemia
- Hyperlipidemia

Systemic associations
- Lymphoproliferative disorders
  - Multiple myeloma
  - Hodgkin lymphoma
  - Non-Hodgkin lymphoma
- Vital organ involvement (cerebral, pulmonary, and myocardial lesions)

Table 9 Ocular features of NXG

- Periorbital nodules
- Episcleritis
- Uveitis
- Keratitis
- Cellulitis
- Proptosis

be complicated by ptosis or, where there is scarring, lagophthalmos and secondary corneal exposure. Disease tends to recur or even increase in severity after incisional biopsy or surgical debulking, and in some cases, NXG may present with a non-healing surgical incision.

Microscopically, there are large areas of eosinophilic collagen degeneration, or necrobiosis, separating granulomatous masses comprising foamy histiocytes, numerous Touton and foreign body type giant cells and lesser numbers of lymphocytes (Fig. 4d–f). Involvement of the skin from the dermis through the subcutis is common, occasionally with an apparent "Touton cell panniculitis." Lymphoid nodules, foci of plasma cells, and cholesterol clefts may also be noted. The histiocytes and giant cells fail to show significant S100 protein immunohistochemical staining, confirming their non-Langerhans origin, but consistently stain with lysozyme and CD68 [84].

The aetiology of NXG, and the roles of serum Igs and lipids, remain unknown. Of the pathways proposed, one suggests that a lipid–serum Ig complex is deposited in the skin, exciting a giant cell foreign body reaction [80]. A second hypothesis is that the Fc portion of IgG is recognised as an antigen by tissue macrophages and a third that the paraprotein is functionally similar to a lipoprotein, causing direct stimulation of tissue histiocytes [86].

Table 10. Treatment regimens for NXG

- Excision
- Local corticosteroid injection
- Systemic corticosteroid
- Plasmapheresis
- Chemotherapy—methotrexate, azathioprine, melphalan, chlorambucil, cyclophosphamide, nitrogen mustard, interferon a-2b
- Radiotherapy

Various forms of intervention have been described for NXG (Table 10). Ugurlu et al. report their experience with a cohort of 26 patients of whom 21 had adnexal lesions, the majority of whom (90%) had bilateral disease [85]. Findings included ptosis (six), restricted ocular motility (four), proptosis (three), episcleritis (one), and keratitis (one). Chemotherapy was the most common form of treatment, with improvement documented in 59% of patients. The response to radiotherapy (1500–2400 cGy) in three patients was variable, with no response in two, a response in one, and a response in both patients receiving both radiotherapy and chemotherapy. Due to a high rate of recurrence after surgical debulking (42%), some authors suggest that surgery should be delayed, and that patients should be monitored throughout life for haematological malignancies which may not become apparent for many years.

4.3 Erdheim–Chester Disease (E–CD)

E-CD is rare lipogranulomatous disorder which typically presents with chronic and progressive bone pain between the fourth and fifth decades of life, although the clinical spectrum ranges from asymptomatic infiltration to fulminant organ failure [87–93]. The characteristic radiological findings are bilateral, and symmetrical, osteolytic and sclerotic changes of the diaphyses and metaphyses of the long bones, with technetium (^{99}Tc) studies identifying radionuclide uptake in areas of bony abnormality. These radiological findings allow differentiation of E-CD from LCH, in which the skeletal lesions are osteolytic and very rarely located on long bones [90, 94].

E-CD is characterised by a widespread infiltration by foamy, lipid-laden, non-Langerhans histiocytes. These cells are identical to those in JXG on both morphological and immunohistochemical grounds, with some authorities considering E-CD to be a variant of JXG with chiefly osseous and major organ involvement. Biopsy of orbital lesions identifies fibrosing xanthogranulomas with xanthomatous histiocytes predominantly containing cholesterol, fibrotic changes with collagen deposition, and Touton giant cells. Unlike LCH, the histiocytes do not stain for S100 protein, and Birbeck granules are not identified on electron microscopy (EM) [95]. Mononuclear inflammatory cells are encountered within the sheets of xanthoma cells, the latter having small central nuclei and abundant vacuolated pale cytoplasm due to lipid loss during routine paraffin embedding. In contrast to NXG, no necrobiotic foci are found in E-CD.

Over half of patients with E-CD have extraskeletal features, which, unlike the skeletal radiographic changes, can occur in various other histiocytic diseases (Table 11). Ocular involvement is typically bilateral and includes eyelid xanthogranulomas, which tend to be more indurated than the ordinary velvety xanthelasmata, and proptosis secondary to retrobulbar soft tissue (Fig. 5a, b) [96–99]. In 1996, Veyssier-Belot et al. summarised all 52 cases in the literature

Table 11 Extraskeletal involvement in E-CD

Ocular	Bilateral eyelid xanthogranuloma, retrobulbar soft tissue lesions
Skin	Pruritic rash, xanthelasma, periorbital xanthoma
Lung	Pleural effusion, pulmonary fibrosis
Heart	Cardiac failure, pericardial infiltration
CNS	Diabetes insipidus, ataxia, behavioral disorders, paraplegia
Abdomen	Retroperitoneal xanthogranuloma or fibrosis (causing renal or ureteric obstruction)

since 1983, when Alper and colleagues reported the first two orbital cases [95], and proptosis was reported in over a quarter of patients [90]. Orbital disease is frequently bilateral, usually intraconal, unlike other xanthogranulomatous diseases which tend to be extraconal (with the exception of sinus histiocytosis with massive lymphadenopathy - SHML), and may progress to ophthalmoplegia and compressive optic neuropathy. Because of the severity of systemic disease in E-CD, all patients presenting with periorbital histiocytic features should undergo systemic screening outlined in Table 3.

The aetiology of E-CD remains unknown. Most reported cases of E-CD do not show clonal cytogenetic abnormality, and cannot therefore be considered to be truly neoplastic. However, the association between E-CD and various immunological diseases, and to diseases linked to T-cell dysfunction—such as asthma, Hashimoto thyroiditis and idiopathic thrombocytopenia [77, 100–102],—implicates an abnormal interaction between T cells and macrophages. Supporting evidence comes from a rare histiocytic disease known as the macrophage activation syndrome (MAS) in which macrophages invade and engulf haematopoietic cells in the bone marrow. MAS is thought to be a manifestation of dysfunctional natural killer cells or cytotoxic T-lymphocytes, resulting in uncontrolled macrophage activation, and it is of interest that associations have been reported between MAS and both LCH and E-CD [103–105].

The optimum treatment of E-CD is uncertain due to the rarity of the disease, variation in the natural history, and the lack of adequately designed trials. Systemic corticosteroids may ameliorate orbital and extraorbital disease [105], and systemic disease has been managed with chemotherapeutic drugs, including the vinca alkaloids, anthracyclines, cyclophosphamide [91, 92], and mycophenolate mofetil [93], often in association with prednisolone. There is a scarcity of data on the ophthalmic results of targeted therapies such as MEK inhibitors, IL-1 and TNF-a blockers, and mTOR inhibitors, however these have been associated with high rates of systemic clinical and radiological improvement

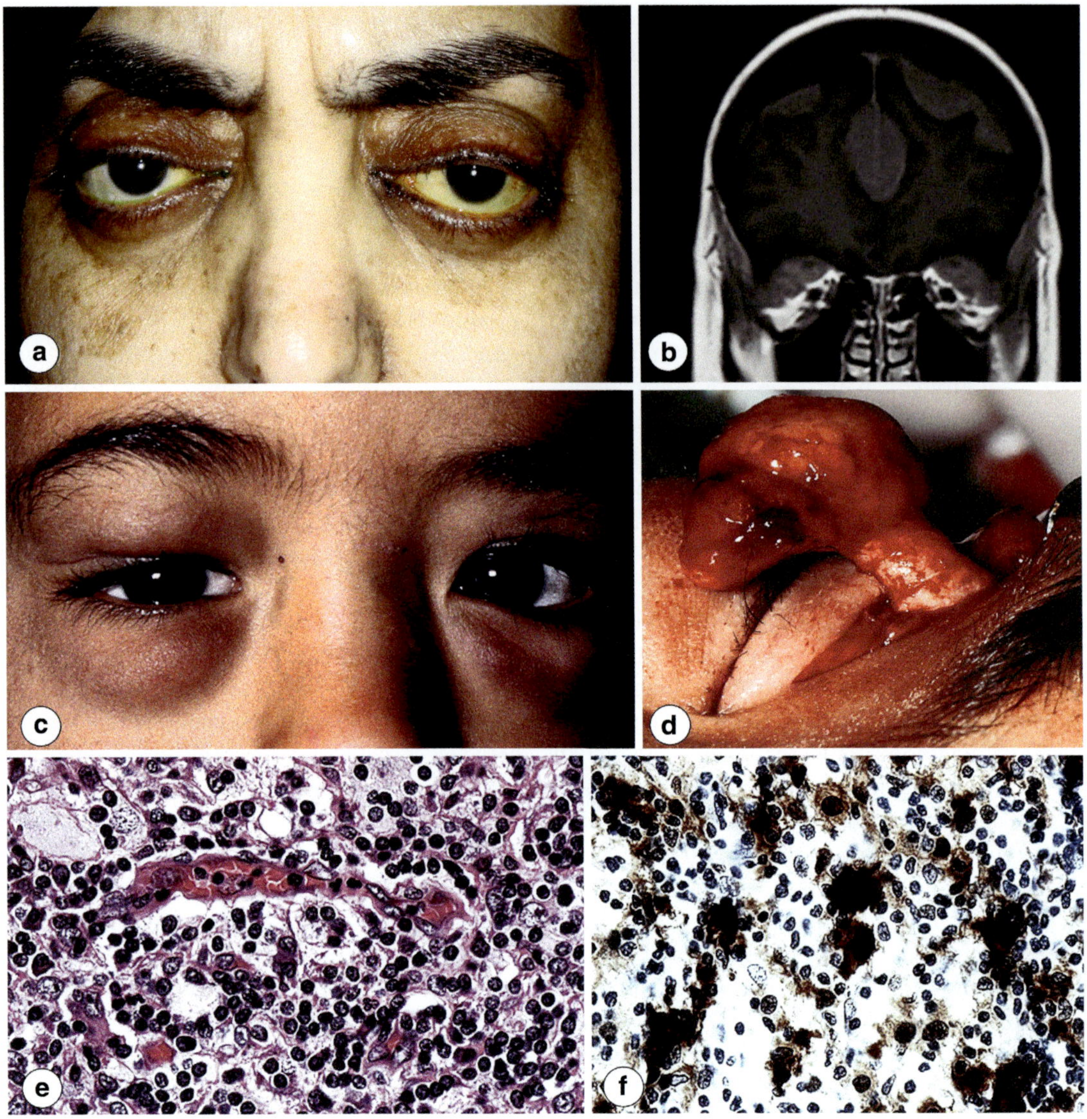

Fig. 5 Erdheim-Chester disease (E-CD) (**a**, **b**): (**a**) a 47-year-old female presented with 3 years of bilateral progressive proptosis and lid swelling. She had good visual function, but a global reduction of ocular motility and 8–10 mm of exophthalmos on each side. (**b**) MRI shows bilateral hypointense superior orbital infiltrates, parafalcine and similar dural- soft tissue masses. Subsequent systemic work-up revealed evidence of retroperitoneal fibrosis, giving rise to hydronephrosis and peri-aortitis, as well as multiple lytic and sclerotic skeletal lesions. Orbital biopsy showed extensive infiltrate with a predominantly xanthoid histiocytic component. Touton giant cells were not present. Immunohistochemistry identified no immunoreactivity for s-100, but extensive staining for cd68; appearances were suggestive of E-CD. Treatment with systemic steroids and interferon-alfa resulted in improvement of symptoms and signs. Sinus histiocytosis with massive lymphadenopathy (Rosai–Dorfman syndrome) (**c**–**f**): (**c**) A 9-year-old child presented with a 16-month history of bilateral upper and lower lid fullness, identified at surgery (**d**) as pedunculated firm rubbery fibrofatty lesions. (**e**) Microscopy shows an infiltrate of lymphocytes and plasma cells and pale staining histiocytes showing emperipolisis. H&E 400 μ. (**f**) The histiocytes are immunoreactive for S-100 immunoperoxidase stain

[67, 106]. The prognosis for E-CD is however, the most dismal of all the histiocytic diseases. In the report by Veyssier-Belot et al., 22/37 (57%) died within the mean follow-up period of 2.7 years (range: 3–120 months), and, in 8/37 cases (22%), death occurred within 6 months of diagnosis [90].

4.4 Sinus Histiocytosis with Massive Lymphadenopathy (Rosai–Dorfman Syndrome)

Sinus Histiocytosis with Massive Lymphadenopathy (SHML) is a rare idiopathic disease characterised by massive tissue infiltration by S100 positive histiocytes. Bilateral painless cervical lymphadenopathy occurs in over 80% of patients, and is associated with systemic upset, fever, malaise, weight loss, and night sweats [107]. Extranodal disease occurs in 43% and commonly involves the respiratory tract, visceral organs, skin, bone, central nervous system (CNS), genitourinary tract and orbit [108–111]. Although SHML does occur in children [112], the disease typically presents early in adult life with a mean age at diagnosis of 20.6 years [113]; patients presenting with isolated intracranial disease are typically older (mean 37.5 years) [114]. Disease limited to the skin, without nodal or systemic involvement, is a recognized variant but is uncommon (cutaneous Rosai–Dorfman disease (CRD)) [115].

Adnexal involvement in SHML occurs in ~10% of patients [116]. Lesions may be restricted to epibulbar areas or the lid, or may involve the intraconal or extraconal space, presenting with progressive proptosis (Fig. 5c, d) [117–122]. Systemic manifestations with ocular disease were originally reported as mild, but a recent review of seven patients with periocular disease suggested the converse; in this series, one patient with bilateral eyelid masses developed testicular, pulmonary, and retroperitoneal disease, another with an asymptomatic eyelid mass had pulmonary nodules, and a third with proptosis due to bilateral orbital masses developed multifocal intracranial disease [123]. Based on these observations, the authors recommend that all patients with a diagnosis of SHML should undergo a thorough systemic evaluation, this including imaging of the abdomen, chest, and CNS.

The histology of SHML lesions reveals abundant fibrous tissue, with low-power microscopic examination showing pale-staining areas containing histiocytes subdivided by trabeculae of connective tissue. The histiocytes form sheets of cells and may contain engulfed erythrocytes (erythrophagocytosis), plasma cells, or lymphocytes (emperipolesis, lymphophagocytosis) (Fig. 5e, f). Emperipolesis is not unique to SHML, but is considered diagnostic where histiocytes express S100 positivity in the appropriate clinical setting. Mature lymphocytes are also scattered throughout the lesion, sometimes demonstrating follicular organisation. In lymph nodes, the histiocytes are distinctively localised along the sinus channels, in both subcapsular and central medullary regions. In the absence of lymph nodes in the orbit, the affected areas contain randomly dispersed lymphocytes and histiocytes, without an organised topography. Ultrastructural studies have failed to demonstrate the cytoplasmic inclusions typical of Langerhans cells, suggesting that this lesion has a histiocytic heritage that is distinct from eosinophilic granuloma [124, 125]; the cells, however, are S100-positive but OKT6-negative.

Although SHML is self-limiting, patients can suffer relapses and remissions over many years, and death—due to vital organ compression, immunologic abnormalities (Table 12), or infections—occurs in ~7% [108]. Current recommendations for treatment include airway obstruction secondary to massive adenopathy, sudden

Table 12 Immunologic abnormalities associated with SHML

- Autoimmune joint disease
- Coombs-positive anemia
- Systemic amyloidosis
- Wiskott–Aldrich syndrome
- Immunologic pancytopenia
- Asthma
- Glomerulonephritis
- Nephrotic syndrome
- Anti-factor VIII antibodies

enlargement of nodes, and vital organ compression. High-dose corticosteroids are the first line of treatment, but life-threatening lesions may require surgery or emergency radiotherapy [126]. Surgical resection of anterior periorbital lesions and intracranial lesions attached to the dura is successful in most cases, and excision of lesions in CRD may be indicated for aesthetic reasons alone. Chemotherapy may be valuable in managing optic neuropathy due to severe orbital disease [121] and in life-threatening systemic disease [2].

5 Orbital Disease Characterised By a Predominance of Histiocytic Cells

5.1 Sarcoidosis

5.1.1 Introduction

Sarcoidosis is a systemic disease characterised by non-caseating granulomas and occurs most commonly in adults under the age of 40. The disease is more common, and severe, among African-Americans, in whom the age-adjusted annual incidence rate (35.5 per 100,000) is up to threefold higher than among Caucasians [127].

5.1.2 Histology

The histology of a sarcoid granuloma is characterised by epithelioid cells arranged concentrically around multinucleated giant cells which may contain cytoplasmic inclusions (asteroid bodies and Schaumann bodies). Where mononuclear inflammatory cells are sparse or absent, the term 'naked granuloma' is used. No specific ultrastructural features have been described, except that the histiocytes lack Langerhans granules or other inclusions. T-cell subsets are distributed in a zonal fashion within the granulomas, with helper T-cells located preferentially in the central areas and suppressor T-cells located at the periphery, thus suggesting a role for the latter in containing the outward extension of the granulomas.

5.1.3 Aetiology

The aetiology of sarcoidosis is unknown. Lesions are associated with an accumulation of CD4+ T-cells and a TH1 immune response, and current opinion is that specific inhalation triggers promote an abnormal CD4+ response in genetically susceptible individuals [128, 129]. Disease transmission by cardiac and bone marrow transplantation [130], and reports of community outbreaks [131], both support a transmissible trigger for disease. Heritable factors may also be relevant: familial clustering is well recognized [127], and recent high-resolution molecular typing studies have confirmed an association with an allelic variation at the HLA-DRB1 locus within the human major histocompatibility complex (MHC) on chromosome 6p [132]. However, genetic influences may vary according to ethnic background: among an African-American population, a recent genome-wide, sibling-pair multipoint analysis identified linkage with chromosome 5q11, as well as with five other chromosomes, implicating numerous genetic influences on the disease [133].

Activated CD4+ T-cell subsets are known to accumulate in pulmonary lesions, and among Scandinavian patients positive for HLA-DRB3*0101 and DRB1*0301, expression of such T-cell subsets in the lungs is significantly raised [134]. Since T-cell activation by antigen presenting cells is restricted by HLA type, these observations suggest that certain HLA types predispose to inappropriate antigen presentation and T-cell expansion, with subsequent granuloma formation. Further evidence for heritable influences on T-cell activation come from the recent report of a strong association between a point mutation within the gene butyrophilin-like 2 (BTNL2) on chromosome 6p21 and sarcoidosis [135]. BTNL2 belongs to the Ig superfamily and may have a role as a co-stimulatory molecule in T-cell activation. Sarcoidosis may therefore be due to an upregulated T cell response in genetically predisposed individuals to an inhaled, as yet undefined, trigger [129, 136]. However, the propensity for sarcoidosis in certain extrapulmonary sites—such as the eye, orbit and skin—remains entirely unexplained.

5.1.4 Ocular Disease

Lesions affecting the visual pathway occur in a quarter of patients, being the second most commonly affected system after the lungs [128]. Anterior uveitis is the most common feature of ocular disease, occurring in 85% of patients, while posterior segment inflammation is the commonest cause of visual morbidity. The most frequent adnexal finding is lacrimal gland disease, which is typically bilateral (Fig. 6a–c) [137–140]. Although fewer than 15% of patients with systemic sarcoidosis have clinically detectable lacrimal gland enlargement [21], Ga scanning identifies increased activity in up to 80% of glands [141].

Sarcoid lesions of the orbit may present in the fibroadipose tissue, extraocular muscles [142, 143], and orbital apex [142–144], and granulomas may also occur within the optic nerve, chiasm, and more posterior visual pathways [145]. Adnexal disease outside the lacrimal gland is usually unilateral [146]. The presenting features of orbital disease depend upon the location, and include pain, lid swelling, globe displacement, proptosis, and, less commonly, diplopia and ptosis. Apical granulomas may present with subacute visual loss and ophthalmoplegia, and be clinically and radiologically indistinguishable from other causes of apical inflammation.

True orbital sarcoidosis is defined as an idiopathic non-caseating granulomatous lesion in the orbit in the context of systemic sarcoidosis, and patients presenting with isolated orbital lesions should undergo systemic assessment [144, 148, 149]. Rare cases of isolated orbital involvement do, however, occur—typically in women in late middle age. Some authors consider these to be cases of isolated idiopathic granulomatous orbital inflammation (rather than true sarcoidosis) [150, 151], and emphasises that other causes of granuloma formation (such as retained foreign body, granulomatosis with polyangitis, and mycobacterial infection) should be excluded before a diagnosis of sarcoidosis is made.

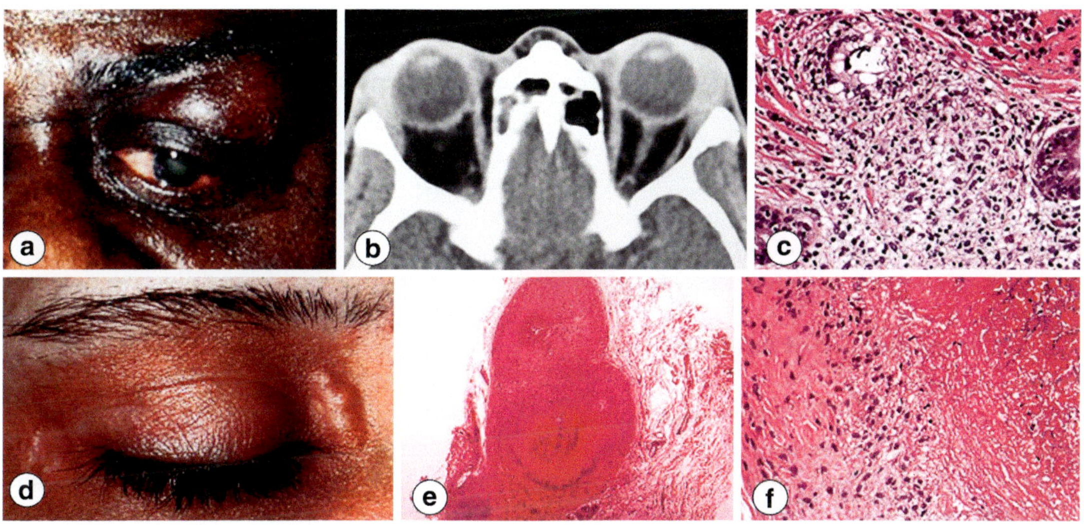

Fig. 6 Sarcoidosis (**a–c**): (**a**) A 55-year-old Afro-Caribbean male presented with pain and swelling in the superotemporal quadrant of the orbit. (**b**) CT identified bilateral lacrimal gland enlargement. (**c**) A lacrimal gland biopsy was performed, and histology identified granulomatous changes in the lacrimal gland, comprising epithelioid histiocytes, giant cells, and calcified Schaumann bodies. H&E 400 μ. Subcutaneous granuloma annulare (**d–f**): (**d**) Subcutaneous nodules in the medial canthal region (**e**) Low-power view of subcutaneous granulomatous nodules showing palisaded histiocytes surrounding central necrobiotic areas. H&E 20 μ. (**f**) The edge of a granuloma showing palisaded histiocytes (*left*) and the hyaline degeneration of collagen in the necrobiotic center (*right*). H&E 200 μ

5.1.5 Investigation

Several investigations support a diagnosis of sarcoidosis, but all lack specificity (these include serum angiotensin-converting enzyme (ACE), lysozyme, and urine and serum calcium levels). Radiographic evidence of hilar or paratracheal lymph node enlargement, or parenchymal involvement, is evident in ~90% of patients [128]. Gallium scintigraphy, although nonspecific, is highly sensitive, identifying uptake over the orbits, parotid glands, and lungs, and if taken in concert with serum ACE, specificity levels approaching 100% have been reported [152]. Transbronchial biopsy is positive in 90% of all cases with pulmonary sarcoidosis, and in half where there is clinical evidence for extrapulmonary disease in the presence of a normal chest radiograph.

In lacrimal gland disease, CT imaging identifies a wedge-shaped lesion, often extending beyond the superotemporal rim of the orbit due to superimposition of the enlarged palpebral and orbital lobes [138]. Both lacrimal gland and extraocular muscle lesions are isointense relative to muscle on T1-weighted MRI and hypointense on T2-weighted images, with homogeneous enhancement [147].

Sarcoidosis is a tissue diagnosis and, if orbital disease is suspected, biopsy of a conjunctival nodule or enlarged lacrimal gland is indicated; biopsy of the orbital lobe of the lacrimal gland is performed through the skin crease of the upper eyelid, as palpebral lobe biopsy is likely to be negative, and risks injury to the secretory ductules.

5.1.6 Management of Adnexal Disease

Eyelid and conjunctival granulomas typically respond to topical treatment [153], although, in resistant cases, intralesional corticosteroid administration is usually beneficial and can periodically be repeated. Spontaneous resolution of orbital lesions is rare and systemic corticosteroid therapy is the mainstay of treatment, with initial prednisone doses in the range of 60–100 mg/day. Although improvement can occur within days, typically a response is seen over a few weeks, although recurrence after cessation of treatment is common. In acute systemic disease and sarcoid uveitis, methotrexate is useful as a steroid-sparing agent [154, 155], and anti-tumor necrosis factor (TNF) agents may play a role in complicated systemic disease [156], but the value of these agents in orbital disease remains unknown.

5.2 Subcutaneous Granuloma Annulare

Subcutaneous granuloma annulare (SGA) typically occur in healthy children on the extremities and scalp, and may rarely occur in healthy young to middle-aged adults [157–160, 168]. Histologically, deep dermal nodules are characterised by stellate areas of necrobiotic epithelioid granulomata separated by collagen bundles and occasionally surrounded by palisading arrays of reactive histiocytes and fibroblasts. Occasionally, eosinophils and multinucleated giant cells are present. Connective tissue mucins can be identified within the necrobiotic areas as thin basophilic strands which can be highlighted with histochemical stains such as alcian blue. Although perivascular aggregates of lymphocytes may suggest a focal arteritis, the histological picture is distinct to that of other clinically similar lesions seen in systemic lupus erythematosus, rheumatoid arthritis, and necrobiosis lipoidica diabeticorum [161].

SGA is reported much less commonly in the periocular skin near the orbital rim [161–164], with a history of preceding trauma in up to a quarter of cases (Fig. 6d–f) [165, 166]. Lesions are often misdiagnosed as molluscum contagiosum, basal cell carcinoma, pilomatrixoma, neurofibroma, sarcoidosis, or syringoma. Lesions are usually in the lateral upper eyelid and outer canthal region and may be multiple, occasionally with a ‘cystic’ consistency. By definition, there is no association with rheumatoid fever, rheumatoid arthritis, or systemic disease. Lesions are managed with simple excision, but local recurrences can occur in a fifth of cases [162, 167].

The lesions of SGA may resolve spontaneously, albeit in some cases over many years or decades [166, 167], and excisional biopsy is indicated for diagnostic purposes [167]. Topical and intralesional steroid can be used to reduce the size of these lesions [169, 170].

6 Primary Intraosseous Histiocytic Lesions

6.1 Giant Cell Granuloma of Bone

Thought to be related to trauma or intraosseous haemorrhage, this benign lesion usually originates in flat bones of the skull and mandible and predominantly affects patients between the ages of 10 and 25 years [171–173]. However, since a history of antecedent trauma is unusual, the preferred term is giant cell granuloma (GCG) of bone. Giant cell granuloma of the orbit is rare, and usually occurs in young adults [174], although it has also been reported in an elderly female patient [175]. Histopathologically, these granulomas display a zonal pattern, with areas of haemorrhage, fibroblastic proliferation and osteoclast-like multinucleated giant cells. The giant cells are usually found at the periphery of haemorrhagic areas but may be distributed throughout the lesion. The most consistent histological features of this lesion are collagenised, fibrous connective tissue with osteoid formation, evidence of stromal haemorrhage, and a zonal clustering of giant cells [176].

Although spontaneous resolution of GCG may occur, rapid clinical progression suggests sudden haemorrhage within the lesion. Definitive treatment consists of surgery [174], but subsequent recurrence occurs in up to 15% of cases [173, 177]. Radiotherapy can play a role in resistant cases, but carries a risk of malignant transformation [177].

6.2 Giant Cell Tumour of Bone

Giant cell tumour (GCT) of bone is a rare, slowly progressive, primary neoplasm typically involving the epiphyses of the long bones, and those very rare lesions affecting the skull tend to involve the sphenoid and temporal bones [178]. The lesion is benign in 90% of cases, but may be locally aggressive [179]. It occurs later than GCG—between the third and fifth decades of life (Table 13)—but may otherwise be difficult to distinguish from GCG on clinical grounds [178]. CT findings are nonspecific, identifying an expanding lesion causing bony erosion, with homogenous intravenous contrast enhancement. In contrast to GCG, histological examination of GCT of bone reveals a uniform distribution of mononuclear polygonal cells admixed with osteoclast-like giant cells. The giant cells are usually larger, more rounded, and contain a greater number of nuclei. The mononuclear cells are now considered to be the neoplastic component and are thought to arise from primitive mesenchymal stromal cells. New bone formation within the tumour is rare and haemorrhage is less prominent. Unlike GCG, GCT has a high local recurrence rate and may metastasise without cytologically malignant features. However, with wide surgical resection margins, recurrence rates have fallen to ~7% [180]. Radiotherapy may play a role in recurrent cases, but, as with GCG, carries a risk of malignant transformation.

Table 13 Clinical and histological comparison of GCG of bone and GCT of bone

	Giant cell granuloma	Giant cell tumor
Typical age of onset	First–third decade	Third–fourth decade
Giant cell distribution	Zonal	Uniform
Hemorrhage within the lesion	+	+/−
New bone formation	++	−
Malignancy	0%	5–10%
Local recurrence or metastasis	Nil (benign)	7%

6.3 Aneurysmal Bone Cyst

Aneurysmal bone cyst (ABC) was first described by Jaffe and Lichtenstein in 1942 as "peculiar blood-containing cysts of large size" [181]. These uncommon benign lesions are expansile and lead to bony lysis, the term 'aneurysmal' referring to the remodelled, or ballooned, bony contour seen on CT imaging. ABC develops in childhood or early adulthood [182], and a history of antecedent pathology or trauma is present in a third of patients [183]. Pain and swelling are the main symptoms and lesions can occur throughout the skeleton, although they usually affect the metaphyses of long bones. Skull involvement occurs in less than 1% of all cases, and reports of orbital involvement are limited to small series [184–188]. Most patients present with proptosis, which can be precipitous due to rapid expansion of the lesion from intralesional haemorrhage.

ABC may arise de novo (primary ABC), or occur in association with other bone lesions (secondary ABC) such as fibrous dysplasia, GCT, non-ossifying fibroma, chondroblastoma, osteosarcoma, and fibromyxoma [188–190]. Primary bone lesions (including venous thrombosis, arteriovenous communication) lead to ABC formation as a result of locally elevated venous pressure, while trauma results in faulty bone formation and organisation of haemorrhage. Fibrous dysplasia has been associated with aneurysmal bone cyst possibly because of mechanical closure of venous outflow in affected areas. However, such structural changes may be genetically influenced, since cytogenetic studies indicate that transcriptional oncogene upregulation on chromosome 17p13 may play a role in patients with ABC [191].

The radiological appearance of ABC may suggest the diagnosis, the affected bone often having a 'blown-out' appearance (Fig. 7a, b). Several radiological phases have, however, been identi-

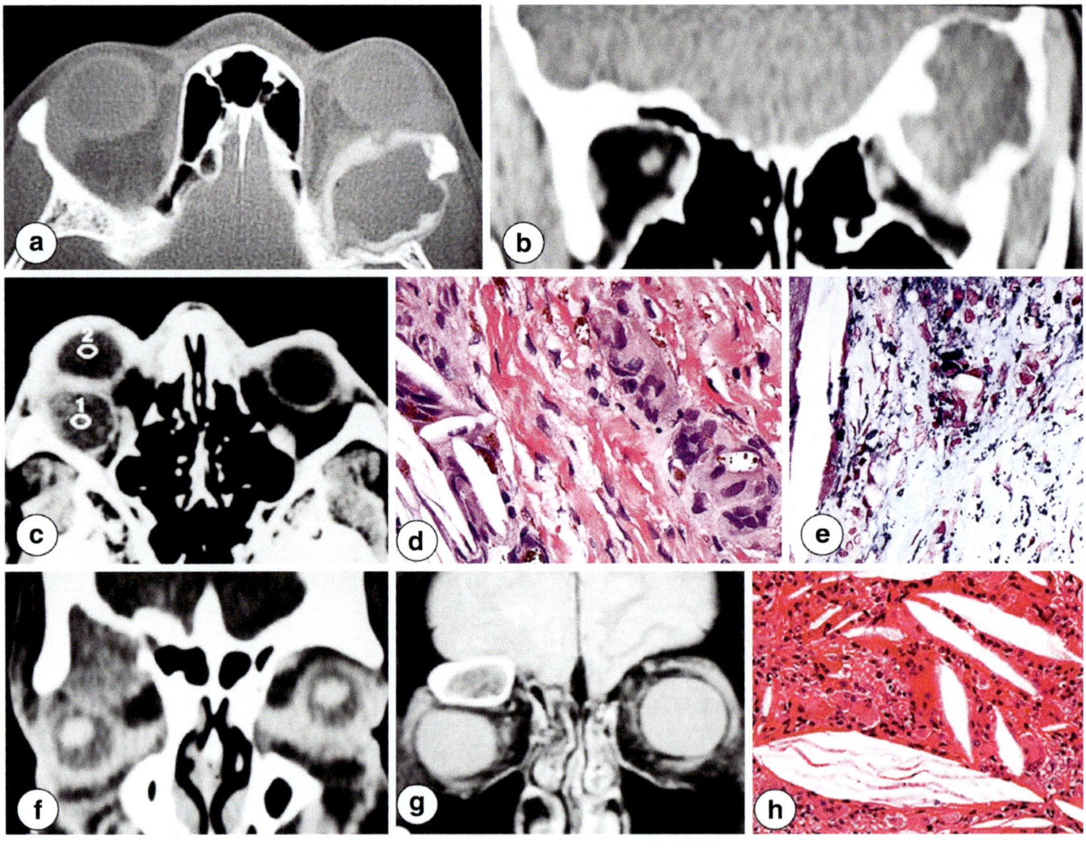

Fig. 7 Aneurysmal bone cyst: (**a, b**) A 19-year-old female developed increasing prominence of the left eye over 4 months, presenting with 8 mm of left proptosis and 3 mm of hypoglobus. CT scan identified an intradiploeic mass arising from the left lateral orbital margin and roof, with associated proptosis, and medial bowing of the optic nerve sheath. Haematic pseudocyst (**c–e**): A 35-year-old man with an orbital mass 2 weeks after blunt trauma to the right eye. (**c**) CT shows a well-circumscribed, cystic orbital mass (1) displacing the globe anteriorly (2). (**d**) Histopathology from a second case: high-power photomicrograph of the fibrous cyst wall containing multinucleated giant (foreign body type) cells, cholesterol clefts and golden-brown hemosiderin pigment. H&E 400 μ. (**e**) Hemosiderin granules staining for iron with Perl's Prussian blue 400 μ. Cholesterol granuloma (**f–h**): A 36-year-old male presented with a 2-week history of ocular asymmetry, examination revealing 2 mm of right hypoglobus and a fullness in the right brow. (**f, g**) Imaging identified an expansile mass expanding the right orbital roof and depressing the globe. The patient proceeded to curettage of the lesion. (**h**) Histology revealed numerous cholesterol clefts surrounded by histiocytes and occasional multinucleated (foreign body-type) giant cells. H&E 100 μm

fied, including osteolysis, rapid growth, stabilisation, and healing with progressive ossification. CT reveals a destructive lesion with a delicate trabeculated appearance surrounding a central cavity [183], and fluid levels may be seen in a third of cases, with dependent layers being more attenuated. MRI also indicates the presence of blood-breakdown products with an intense signal in T1-weighted images. CT and MRI may reveal an associated primary lesion in cases of secondary ABC.

Histologically, ABC is characterised by the presence of large blood-filled cystic spaces separated by fibrous septa which contain spindled fibroblasts, inflammatory cells, and osteoclast-like multinucleated giant cells. The giant cells are typically found lining the haemorrhagic cystic spaces. Osteoid formation occurs, often with osteoblastic rimming, and occasionally has a basophilic appearance. The solid variant, which lacks cystic spaces, is morphologically similar to giant cell granuloma. Treatment is usually with curettage alone; radiotherapy has been advocated for recurrent lesions.

7 Orbital Reactions to Blood and its Breakdown Products

The terminology to describe an accumulation of blood and blood-breakdown products has been confusing.

- Ecchymosis. The diffuse extravasation of fresh blood throughout tissues and tissue planes.
- Haematoma. A focal collection of blood, which may be delimited by surrounding fascial and periorbital membranes. In the orbit, most hematomas occur subperiosteally after trauma but rarely may develop within the soft tissues of the orbit itself.
- Blood cyst. A collection of blood in a pre-existing lesion with a distinct lining (e.g., dermoid cyst, cavernous haemangioma, lymphangioma), these lesions being sometimes referred to as chocolate cysts. Blood cysts are usually intraconal in location. When associated with lymphangioma, they typically occur in patients younger than 10 years, but those associated with cavernous haemangioma are usually found in patients in the second to fourth decades.
- Cholesterol granuloma. Intraosseous idiopathic or post-traumatic granuloma formation.
- Haematic pseudocyst. Chronic subperiosteal or intraorbital soft tissue accumulations of blood-breakdown products. These lesions may have a fibrous condensation or pseudocapsule but have no true lining.
- Haematocoele. An inexact term which has been discontinued.

7.1 Haematic Pseudocyst

An orbital haematic pseudocyst is defined as a chronic cystic accumulation of blood-breakdown products, encompassed by a granulomatous reaction, and contained by a fibrous pseudocapsule. Lacking an epithelial or endothelial lining, the structure is correctly termed a pseudocyst. The aetiology is unknown, but associations with blunt orbital trauma, blood dyscrasia, vascular disease, prosthetic orbital floor implants, and spontaneous haemorrhage have all been reported [192–197].

Both haematic pseudocyst and cholesterol granuloma (v.i.) are xanthomatous reactive lesions that are either closely related or the same entity at different stages of development and organisation. However, the term cholesterol granuloma is more aptly applied to intraosseous and predominantly solid lesions, whereas the term haematic pseudocyst suggests a lesion that at least partially contains fluid.

Haematic pseudocysts may occur at any age, with an unexplained male predominance [193], and the presenting picture is usually one of painless proptosis and diplopia over a period of months to years. A less common scenario is that of acute proptosis and visual loss due to optic nerve compression [196]. Treatment of haematic pseudocyst is with surgical curettage.

Haematic pseudocysts often present in the superotemporal orbit and may involve the frontal bone. They have a predilection for the subperiosteal space and may mimic subdural hematoma, although rare intraconal cases have also been reported (Fig. 7c–e) [197, 198]. Low internal reflectivity on B-scan ultrasonography confirms the cystic nature of the lesion, and CT imaging shows a well-defined, non-enhancing extraconal mass often with erosion of the surrounding bone. Due to accumulation of methaemoglobin in the periphery, chronic haematic pseudocysts are, relative to orbital fat, isointense on T1-weighted images and hyperintense on T2-weighted images, although, in the acute phase, the signal characteristics may vary [199, 200].

Microscopically, the haematic pseudocyst has a fibrous pseudocapsule containing neither epithelium or endothelium. Cholesterol clefts, and a granulomatous reaction to blood breakdown products with chronic inflammatory cells, giant cells, lipid-laden histiocytes, and hemosiderin-laden macrophages may be present. Haematoidin bodies or crystals are identified as red-brown birefringent crystals seen among cholesterol clefts. Haematoidin is a haemoglobin-derived pigment closely related to bilirubin, which stains with the Gmelin reaction for bile pigments (and does not stain with Prussian blue) [201]. Haemosiderin in the pseudocyst may react with Prussian blue, which stains for free iron.

The typical subperiosteal position of these lesions in the superior orbit may be a reflection both of the concavity of the superotemporal orbit, and the loose attachment of periosteum to underlying bone. Haematic pseudocysts may form in a similar way to a chronic subdural hematoma: transudation of fluid into the cavity down a hyperosmotic gradient, with repeated haemorrhage from fragile vessels within the pseudocyst wall, or neomembrane, are each considered to play a role. In addition, fibrinolytic activity and the presence of fibrin degradation products within the pseudocyst interfere with normal haemostasis, further promoting haemorrhage into the cavity.

Haematic pseudocysts are likely to be related to trauma, which may be subclinical or forgotten, occurring years to decades earlier. Henderson has described six cases of post-traumatic haematic pseudocysts among a total of 764 orbital lesions managed at the Mayo Clinic between 1948–80 [202]. However, eosinophilic granuloma, venous engorgement (as might occur during heavy exercise or Valsalva manoeuvre), systemic disease (bleeding diatheses, scurvy, rickets, leukaemia) and systemic vascular disease have also been associated with these lesions [193, 203].

7.2 Orbitofrontal Cholesterol Granuloma

Cholesterol granuloma is a rare lesion occurring in young to middle-aged men, encountered in the petrous temporal bone and infrequently in the lacrimal region of the frontal bone (Fig. 7f–h) [204, 205]. The aetiology is unknown, but trauma and secondary intradiploic haemorrhage, with release of cholesterol from blood-breakdown products, is thought to be the cause in many. In others, pre-existing pathology, such as fibrous dysplasia or lytic Paget disease, may predispose to cholesterol deposition [205, 206].

Cholesterol granuloma resembles haematic pseudocyst both clinically and morphologically [207]. Although the diagnosis is usually confirmed on histological grounds, cytological diagnosis of orbital cholesterol granuloma has also been reported [207]. CT imaging typically identifies an extraconal soft tissue mass with a lytic lesion in the superolateral bony orbit which may be associated with erosion of the orbital roof (Fig. 7f). In atypical cases, MRI may be helpful because the lesion has a high signal on both T1 and T2 sequences, suggesting the presence of lipid (Fig. 7g) [208].

Orbitofrontal cholesterol granuloma can present with upper lid fullness, ptosis, proptosis and hypoglobus due to expansion of the granuloma from the frontal bone into the extraperiosteal space of the lacrimal fossa [204, 210]. Rarely, the mass may erode the superolateral orbital roof, with expansion of the granuloma into the cranium [210].

Management of orbital lesions is by drainage and complete removal of granulomatous tissue which may be performed percutaneously via an upper lid skin-crease incision [211], or via lateral orbitotomy [209].

7.3 Cholesteatoma

Cholesteatomas are unusual benign cystic lesions most commonly found in the temporal bone. Primary orbital cholesteatoma originates in the frontal, sphenoidal, and ethmoidal diploë and may extend into neighbouring structures, typically presenting as a painless, slowly enlarging mass without inflammation [212–214]. CT identifies a cystic lesion with sclerotic changes at the edge of the bony defect. On MRI, the lesion appears similar to cholesterol granuloma, having a high signal intensity in T1-weighted images.

These lesions are distinct from dermoid cysts, lacking ectodermal structures such as hair follicles and sebaceous glands, and may be distinguished from cholesterol granulomas on histological grounds. The aetiology is considered to be entrapment of ectodermal remnants during embryonic development of the cranial bones, but secondary cholesteatomas may also develop after trauma or surgery.

The characteristic microscopic feature of this cyst is a capsule lined with hyperkeratotic squamous epithelium, which proliferates exuberantly and may extend outside the cyst lumen. The cyst contents include cholesterol crystals and histiocytes, but eosinophils are absent. In contrast to the management of cholesterol granuloma, simple cavity drainage is inadequate. Unless the cyst lining is completely excised, continuing desquamation of the cyst lining occurs, with expansion of the lesion and erosion of surrounding structures, with an increased risk of carcinomatous degeneration.

8 Giant Cell Polymyositis

Orbital granulomatous giant cell myositis is a rare histological entity, severe and potentially fatal. It is associated with giant cell myocarditis and underlying malignancy, and its description is limited to a few case reports in the literature. Selva et al. reported a 51-year-old woman with a past history of melanoma, who developed a chronic, biopsy proven bilateral orbital granulomatous giant cell myositis which was partially steroid responsive [215]. Kattah et al. reported a 37-year-old with severe bilateral painful proptosis and ophthalmoplegia, with subsequent facial, pharyngeal, laryngeal, and cardiac muscle involvement. She also showed a partial response to immunomodulation (steroids and chemotherapy), but developed a cardiac dysrhythmia and died 18 months after the onset of symptoms [216]. Klein and colleagues reported a 65-year-old woman with a granulomatous orbital myositis who also died of a cardiac arrhythmia; histology of the extraocular muscles showed necrosis and regeneration, with a histiocytic and mononuclear cell infiltration [217]. The histological findings of severe giant cell myocarditis indicated that this case may have been a variant of giant cell polymyositis. Leib et al. report a further case, in which a 22-year-old woman with orbital polymyositis and associated giant cell myocarditis developed cardiogenic shock but survived with parenteral steroids and heart transplantation [218].

These cases identify a form of myositis which is distinct from idiopathic orbital myositis—a more benign inflammatory disease which is typically isolated to the orbit, is steroid responsive, and has a reasonable prognosis [219]. In contrast, giant cell polymyositis is often refractory to immunosuppression and is associated with acute myocardial involvement, with fatal arrhythmias or fulminating congestive heart failure [220]. Histological features include diffuse destruction of muscle fibres with infiltration by histiocytes, lymphocytes, and multinucleated giant cells (Fig. 8a–c). Both polymyositis and dermatomyositis can cause ophthalmoplegia, but granulomatous inflammation with giant cells is not found in the latter [219].

9 Tuberous Xanthoma

Xanthoma is defined as a fibro-fatty change in the skin associated with the formation of yellow or yellowish-brown plaques, nodules or tumours. They may be deposited in a variety of tissues, having different etiologies [220]. Tuberous xanthoma is characterised by numerous slow growing, discrete or grouped, yellowish brown cutaneous nodules.

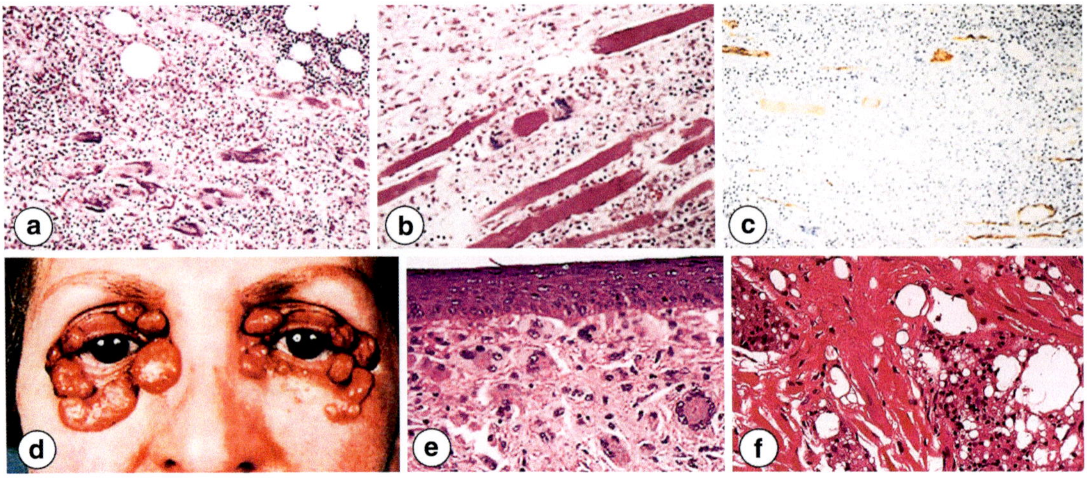

Fig. 8 Giant cell polymyositis (**a–c**): (**a**) Histological examination shows replacement of normal muscle tissue with a chronic inflammatory infiltrate consisting of histiocytes, eosinophils, lymphocytes, and multinucleated giant cells. H&E. (**b**) Higher power shows remnants of degenerated skeletal muscle with giant cells on both sides of one fragment. There is a dense background infiltrate of histiocytic cells and lymphocytes. (**c**) Immunohistochemical staining for muscle-specific actin shows that the small fragments are remnants of degenerated muscle cells (**a–c**, Courtesy of L. E. Zimmerman, MD. Tuberous xanthoma). (**d**, **e**): (**d**) Multiple firm, nontender yellowish nodules of 6 year duration involving upper and lower eyelids bilaterally. (**e**) Microscopic examination shows multinucleated giant cells and histiocytes with a fibrous background (**d**, Courtesy of M. O. M. Tso, MD; **e**, Courtesy of F. Buffam, MD, and J. Rootman, MD). Histology of an orbital lipogranuloma following an industrial grease gun injury: (**f**) histiocytes are seen surrounding variably sized round empty spaces representing dissolved lipids. H&E 400 μ

These lesions occur most frequently in conjunction with a primary or secondary disorder of lipid metabolism, but may also occur in normolipemic patients [221, 222]. They may occur on the eyelid, but are more common on the extensor surfaces in patients with type II or type III hyperlipidemia [223]. The histological picture is one of sheets of lipid-laden histiocytes, cholesterol clefts and multinucleated giant cells, with proliferation of fibroblasts in chronic lesions (Fig. 8d, e). The marked fibrosis observed in long-standing tuberous xanthomas may be related to the fibrogenic properties of extracellular cholesterol, which may extravasate from abnormally permeable blood vessels in these lesions.

10 Orbital Foreign Body Reaction: Lipogranuloma

Orbital lipogranuloma may occur in response to oil from a variety of sources. These include industrial grease gun injuries [224–227], periocular paraffin injection [226, 228], and self-inflicted injection of petroleum jelly [229]. Iatrogenic causes of orbital lipogranuloma include bone wax [230], packing gauzes after sinus surgery [231, 232], and periocular steroid injection [233]. Trauma or inflammation involving lipocytes can lead to extracellular oil and be a further cause of lipogranuloma. Finally, rupture or leakage of a dermoid cyst—or incomplete excision—may also incite a lipogranulomatous reaction.

Histologically, lipogranuloma is distinct from xanthogranuloma, containing histiocytes which surround prominent extracellular collections of lipids (Fig. 8f). In comparison, the histiocytes in a xanthogranuloma have a honeycombed appearance due to numerous intracytoplasmic vacuoles, giving rise to the term foam cells.

References

1. Favara BE, Feller AC, Pauli M, et al. Contemporary classification of histiocytic disorders. Reclassification Working Group of the Histiocytic Society. Med Pediatr Oncol. 1997;29:157.

2. Weitzman S, Maarten ER. Histiocytic disorders of children and adults. Basic science, clinical features and therapy. 1st ed. Cambridge: Cambridge University Press; 2006.
3. Lichtenstein L. Histiocytosis X; integration of eosinophilic granuloma of bone, Letterer-Siwe disease, and Schüller-Christian disease as related manifestations of a single nosologic entity. Arch Pathol. 1953;56:84.
4. Favara BE, Jaffe R. Pathology of Langerhans' cell histiocytosis. Hematol Oncol Clin North Am. 1987;1:75.
5. McClelland J, Pritchard J, Chu AC. Current controversies. Hematol Oncol Clin North Am. 1987;1:147.
6. De Graaf JH, Tamminga RYA, Kamps WA, et al. Expression of cellular adhesion molecules in Langerhans cell histiocytosis and normal Langerhans cells. Am J Pathol. 1995;147:1161.
7. Allen CE, Merad M, McClain KL. Langerhans-cell histiocytosis. N Engl J Med. 2018;379:856–68.
8. Badalian-Very G, Vergilio JA, Degar BA, et al. Recurrent BRAF mutations in Langerhans cell histiocytosis. Blood. 2010;116:1919–23.
9. Rollins BJ. Genomic alterations in Langerhans cell histiocytosis. Hematol Oncol Clin North Am. 2015;29:839–51.
10. Allen CE, Li L, Peters TL, et al. Cell-specific gene expression in Langerhans cell histiocytosis lesions reveals a distinct profile compared with epidermal Langerhans cells. J Immunol. 2010;184:4557–67.
11. Chakraborty R, Burke TM, Hampton OA, et al. Alternative genetic mechanisms of BRAF activation in Langerhans cell histiocytosis. Blood. 2016;128:2533–7.
12. Satoh T, Smith A, Sarde A, et al. B-RAF mutant alleles associated with Langerhans cell histiocytosis, a granulomatous pediatric disease. PloS One. 2012;7:e33891.
13. Sahm F, Capper D, Preusser M, et al. BRAFV600E mutant protein is expressed in cells of variable maturation in Langerhans cell histiocytosis. Blood. 2012;120:e28–34.
14. Diamond EL, Durham BH, Haroche J, et al. Diverse and targetable kinase alterations drive histiocytic neoplasms. Cancer Discov. 2016;6:154–65.
15. Davies H, Bignell GR, Cox C, et al. Mutations of the BRAF gene in human cancer. Nature. 2002;417:949–54.
16. Nelson DS, van Halteren A, Quispel WT, et al. MAP 2K1 and MAP 3K1 mutations in Langerhans cell histiocytosis. Genes Chromosomes Cancer. 2015;54:361–8.
17. Chakraborty R, Hampton OA, Shen X, et al. Mutually exclusive recurrent somatic mutations in MAP 2K1 and BRAF support a central role for ERK activation in LCH pathogenesis. Blood. 2014;124:3007–15.
18. Brown NA, Furtado LV, Betz BL, et al. High prevalence of somatic MAP 2K1 mutations in BRAF V600E-negative Langerhans cell histiocytosis. Blood. 2014;124:1655–8.
19. Héritier S, Hélias-Rodzewicz Z, Chakraborty R, et al. New somatic BRAF splicing mutation in Langerhans cell histiocytosis. Mol Cancer. 2017;16:115.
20. Mourah S, How-Kit A, Meignin V, et al. Recurrent NRAS mutations in pulmonary Langerhans cell histiocytosis. Eur Respir J. 2016;47:1785–96.
21. Lee LH, Gasilina A, Roychoudhury J, et al. Real-time genomic profiling of histiocytoses identifies early-kinase domain BRAF alterations while improving treatment outcomes. JCI Insight. 2017;2:e89473.
22. Nicholson HS, Egeler RM, Nesbit ME. The epidemiology of Langerhans cell histiocytosis. Hematol Oncol Clin North Am. 1998;12:379.
23. Char DH, Ablin A, Beckstead J. Histiocytic disorders of the orbit. Ann Ophthalmol. 1984;16:867.
24. MacCumber MW, Hoffman PN, Wand GS, et al. Ophthalmic involvement in aggressive LCH. Ophthalmology. 1990;97:22.
25. Shields JA. Histiocytic tumors and pseudotumors. In: Shields JA, editor. Diagnosis and management of orbital tumors. Philadelphia: WB Saunders; 1989.
26. Moore AT, Pritchard J, Taylor DSI. LCH: An ophthalmological review. Br J Ophthalmol. 1985;69:7.
27. Oberman HA. Idiopathic histiocytosis: a correlative review of eosinophilic granuloma, Hand-Schüller-Christian disease and Letterer-Siwe disease. J Pediatr Ophthalmol. 1968;5:86.
28. Bray PT. LCH. In: Deeley TJ, editor. Modern radiotherapy and oncology: malignant disease in childhood. London: Butterworth; 1974.
29. Wood CM, Pearson ADJ, Craft AD, et al. Globe luxation in LCH. Br J Ophthalmol. 1988;72:631.
30. Gross FJ, Waxman JS, Rosenblatt MA, et al. Eosinophilic granuloma of the cavernous sinus and orbital apex in an HIV-positive patient. Ophthalmology. 1989;96:462.
31. Baghdassarian SA, Shammas HF. Eosinophilic granuloma of the orbit. Ann Ophthalmol. 1977;9:1247.
32. Feldman RB, Moore DM, Hood CI, et al. Solitary eosinophilic granuloma of the lateral orbital mass. Am J Ophthalmol. 1985;100:318.
33. Jakobiec FA, Trokel SL, Aron-Rosa D, et al. Localized eosinophilic granuloma (Langerhans' cell histiocytosis) of the orbital frontal bone. Arch Ophthalmol. 1980;98:1814.
34. Jakobiec FA, Mottow L. Pediatric orbital pseudotumor. In: Jakobiec FA, editor. Ocular and adnexal tumors. Birmingham: Aesculapius; 1978.
35. Nolph MB, Luikin GA. Histiocytosis X. Otolaryngol Clin North Am. 1982;15:635.
36. Mierau GW, Favara BE, Branman JM. Electron microscopy in LCH. Ultrastruct Pathol. 1982;3:137.
37. Hashimoto K. Langerhans' cell granule: an endocytotic organelle. Arch Dermatol. 1971;104:148.
38. Anemiya T, Yoshida H. Electron microscopic study of the orbital lesion of Hand-Schüller-Christian disease. J Pediatr Ophthalmol. 1977;14:242.
39. Jakobiec FA, Lefkowitch J, Knowles DM II. B-and T-lymphocytes in ocular disease. Ophthalmology. 1984;91:635.

40. Beckstead JH, Woods GS, Turner RR. Histiocytosis-X cells and Langerhans' cells: enzyme histochemical and immunological similarities. Hum Pathol. 1984;15:826.
41. Glover AT, Grove AS Jr. Eosinophilic granuloma of the orbit with spontaneous healing. Ophthalmology. 1987;94:1008.
42. Harris GJ. Langerhans cell histiocytosis of the orbit: a need for interdisciplinary dialogue. Am J Ophthalmol. 2006;141:374.
43. Harris GJ, Woo KI. Eosinophilic granuloma of the orbit: A paradox of aggressive destruction responsive to minimal intervention. Trans Am Ophthalmol Soc. 2003;101:93–103.
44. Singh S, Kaliki S, Reddy Palkonda VA, Naik MN. Langerhans cell histiocytosis of the orbit: A study of eight cases. Oman J Ophthalmol. 2018;11:134–9.
45. Woo KI, Harris GJ. Eosinophilic granuloma of the orbit: Understanding the paradox of aggressive destruction responsive to minimal intervention. Ophthal Plast Reconstr Surg. 2003;19:429–39.
46. Cohen M, Zornoza J, Cangir A, et al. Direct injection of methylprednisolone sodium succinate in the treatment of solitary eosinophilic granuloma of the bone: a report of 9 cases. Radiology. 1980;136:289.
47. Wirtschaffer JD, Nesbit M, Anderson P, et al. Intralesional methylprednisolone for Langerhans' cell histiocytosis of the orbit and cranium. J Pediatr Ophthalmol Strabismus. 1987;24:194.
48. Kindy-Degnan NA, LaFlamme P, Duprat G, et al. Intralesional steroid in the treatment of an orbital eosinophilic granuloma. Arch Ophthalmol. 1991;109:617.
49. Kashkouli MB, Shahrzad S. Intralesional injection of Interferon-α2b in orbital eosinophilic granuloma. Ophthalmic Plast Reconstr Surg. 2016;32:e106–9.
50. Broadbent V, Gadner H. Current therapy for Langerhans cell histiocytosis. Hematol Oncol Clin North Am. 1998;12:327.
51. Harnett AN, Doughty D, Hirst A, et al. Radiotherapy in benign orbital disease. II: Ophthalmic Graves' disease and orbital LCH. Br J Ophthalmol. 1988;72:289.
52. Arceci RJ, Brenner MK, Pritchard J. Controversies and new approaches to treatment of Langerhans cell histiocytosis. Hematol Oncol Clin North Am. 1998;12:339.
53. Favara BE, McCarthy RL, Milerau GW. Histiocytosis X. Hum Pathol. 1983;14:663.
54. Gadner H, Grois N, Arico M, et al. A randomized trial of treatment for multisystem Langerhans' cell histiocytosis. J Pediatr. 2001;138:728.
55. Song A, Johnson TE, Dubovy SR, Toledano S. Treatment of Recurrent Eosinophilic Granuloma With Systemic Therapy. Ophthalmic Plastic Reconstr Surg. 2003;19:140.
56. Donadieu J, Bernard F, van Noesel M, et al. Cladribine and cytarabine in refractory multisystem Langerhans cell histiocytosis: results of an international phase2 study. Blood. 2015;126:1415–23.
57. Bernard F, Thomas C, Bertrand Y, et al. Multi-centre pilot study of 2-chlorodeoxyadenosineand cytosine arabinoside combined chemotherapy in refractory Langerhans cell histiocytosis with haematological dysfunction. Eur J Cancer. 2005;41: 2682–97.
58. Veys PA, Nanduri V, Baker KS, et al. Haematopoietic stem cell transplantation for refractory Langerhans cell histiocytosis: outcome by intensity of conditioning. Br J Haematol. 2015;169:711–8.
59. Gavhed D, Laurencikas E, Akefeldt SO, et al. Fifteen years of treatment with intravenous immunoglobulin in central nervous system Langerhans cell histiocytosis. Acta Paediatr. 2011;100:36–9.
60. Diamond EL, Subbiah V, Lockhart AC, et al. Vemurafenib for BRAF V600-Mutant Erdheim-Chester disease and Langerhans cell histiocytosis: analysis of data from the histology-independent, phase 2, open label VE-BASKET study. JAMA Oncol. 2018;4:384–8.
61. Cohen Aubart F, Emile JF, Carrat F, et al. Targeted therapies in 54 patients with Erdheim-Chester disease, including follow-up after interruption (the LOVE study). Blood. 2017;130:1377–80.
62. Haroche J, Cohen-Aubart F, Emile JF, et al. Dramatic efficacy of vemurafenib in both multisystemic and refractory Erdheim-Chester disease and Langerhans cell histiocytosis harboring the BRAF V600E mutation. Blood. 2013;121:1495–500.
63. Haroche J, Cohen-Aubart F, Emile JF, et al. Reproducible and sustained efficacy of targeted therapy with vemurafenib in patients with BRAF(V600E)-mutated Erdheim-Chester disease. J Clin Oncol. 2015;33:411–8.
64. Gupta A, Yeganeh A, Rootman D, Goldberg R. Vemurafenib (BRAF Inhibitor) therapy for orbital Erdheim-Chester disease. Ophthalmic Plast Reconstr Surg. 2017;33:e138–9.
65. Grumbine FL, Aderman C, Vagefi MR, Kersten RC. Orbital MRI pre- and post-Vemurafenib therapy for Erdheim-Chester disease. Ophthalmic Plast Reconstr Surg. 2015;31:e169.
66. Cohen Aubart F, Emile JF, Maksud P, et al. Efficacy of the MEK inhibitor cobimetinib for wild-type BRAF Erdheim-Chester disease. Br J Haematol. 2018;180:150–3.
67. Pegoraro F, Maniscalco V, Peyronel F, et al. Long-term follow-up of mTOR inhibition for Erdheim-Chester disease. Blood. 2020;135:1994–7.
68. Bowling GB, Wilson JE. Atypical (annular) necrobiosis lipoidica of the face and scalp. Dermatologica. 1967;135:11.
69. Mackey JP. Necrobiosis lipoidica diabeticorum involving scalp and face. Br J Dermatol. 1975;93:729.
70. Dehner LP. Juvenile Xanthogranulomas in the first two decades of life: a clinicopathologic study of 174

cases with cutaneous and extracutaneous manifestations. Am J Surg Pathol. 2003;27:579.
71. Hidayat AA, Mafee MF, Laver NV, Noujaim S. Langerhans' cell histiocytosis and juvenile xanthogranuloma of the orbit. Clinicopathologic, CT, and MR imaging features. Radiol Clin North Am. 1998;36:1229.
72. Miszkiel KA, Sohaib SAA, Rose GE, et al. Radiological and clinicopathologic features of orbital xanthogranuloma. Br J Ophthalmol. 2000;84:251.
73. Zimmerman LE. Ocular lesions of juvenile xanthogranuloma. Am J Ophthalmol. 1965;69:412.
74. Schwartz TL, Carter KD, Judisch GF, et al. Congenital macronodular juvenile xanthogranuloma of the eyelid. Ophthalmology. 1991;98:1230.
75. Shields CL, Shields JA, Buchanon HW. Solitary orbital involvement with juvenile xanthogranuloma. Arch Ophthalmol. 1990;108:1587.
76. Rose GE, Patel BC, Garner A, Wright JE. Orbital xanthogranuloma in adults. Br J Ophthalmol. 1991;75:680.
77. Jakobiec FA, Mills MD, Hidayat AA, et al. Periocular xanthogranulomas associated with severe adult-onset asthma. Trans Am Ophthalmol Soc. 1993;91:99–125; discussion 125-9
78. Karcioglu ZA, Sharara N, Boles T, Nasr AM. Orbital xanthogranuloma: clinical and morphologic features in eight patients. Ophthal Plast Reconstr Surg. 2003;19:372.
79. Hammond MD, Niemi EW, Ward TP, Eiseman AS. Adult orbital xanthogranuloma with associated adult-onset asthma. Ophthal Plast Reconstr Surg. 2004;20:329.
80. Bullock JD, Bartley GB, Cambell RJ, et al. Necrobiotic xanthogranuloma with paraproteinaemia. Case report and a pathogenetic theory. Ophthalmology. 1986;93:1233.
81. Elner VM, Mintz R, Demirci H, Hassan AS. Local corticosteroid treatment of eyelid and orbital xanthogranuloma. Ophthal Plast Reconstr Surg. 2006;22:36.
82. Kossard S, Winkelmann RK. Necrobiotic xanthogranuloma with paraproteinemia. J Am Acad Dermatol. 1980;3:257.
83. Wee SA, Shupack JL. Necrobiotic xanthogranuloma. Dermatol Online J. 2005;11:24.
84. Winkelmann RK, et al. Giant cell granulomatous pulmonary and myocardial lesions in nerobiotic xanthogranuloma with paraproteinemia. Mayo Clin Proc. 1997;72:1028.
85. Ugurlu S, Bartley GB, Gibson LE. Necrobiotic xanthogranuloma: long-term outcome of ocular and systemic involvement. Am J Ophthalmol. 2000;129:651.
86. Rappersberger K, Wrba F, Heinz R, et al. Necrobiotic xanthogranuloma in paraproteinemia [German]. Hautarzt. 1989;40:358.
87. Miller RL, Sheeler LR, Bauer TW, et al. Erdheim-Chester disease: acase report and review of the literature. Am J Med. 1986;80:1230.
88. Sheu S-Y, Wenzel RR, Kersting C, et al. Erdheim-Chester disease: case report with multisystemic manifestations including testes, thyroid, and lymph nodes, and a review of literature. J Clin Pathol. 2004;57:1225.
89. Nagatsuka H, Han PP, Taguchi K, et al. Erdheim-Chester disease in a child presenting with multiple jaw lesions. J Oral Pathol Med. 2005;34:420.
90. Veyssier-Belot C, Cacoub P, Caparros-Lefebvre D, et al. Erdheim-Chester disease, clinical and radiologic characteristics of 59 cases. Medicine (Baltimore). 1996;75:157.
91. Gupta A, Kelly B, McGuigan JE. Erdheim-Chester disease with prominent pericardial involvement: clinical, radiologic, and histologic findings. Am J Med Sci. 2002;324:96.
92. Bourke SC, Nicholson AG, Gibson GJ. Erdheim-Chester disease: pulmonary infiltration responding to cyclophosphamide and prednisolone. Thorax. 2003;58:1004.
93. Jendro MC, Zeidler H, Rosenthal H, et al. Improvement in Erdheim-Chester disease in two patients with sequential treatment with vinblastine and mycophenolate mofetil. Clin Rheumatol. 2004;23:52.
94. Breuil V, Brocq O, Pellegrino C, et al. Erdheim-Chester disease: typical bone features for a rare xanthogranulomatosis. Ann Rheum Dis. 2002; 61:199.
95. Alper MG, Zimmerman LE, LaPiana FG. Orbital manifestations of Erdheim-Chester disease. Trans Am Ophthalmol Soc. 1983;81:64.
96. Shields JA, Shields CL. Clinical spectrum of histiocytic tumors of the orbit. Trans Pa Acad Ophthalmol Otolaryngol. 1990;42:931.
97. Rozenberg I, Wechsler J, Koenig F, et al. Erdheim-Chester disease presenting as malignant exophthalmos. Br J Radiol. 1986;59:173.
98. Palmer FJ, Talley NJ. Erdheim-Chester disease with bilateral exophthalmos and lever cell adenoma. Australas Radiol. 1984;28:305.
99. de Abreu MR, Chung CB, Biswal S, et al. Erdheim-Chester disease: MR imaging, anatomic, and histopathologic correlation of orbital involvement. AJNR Am J Neuroradiol. 2004;25:627.
100. Cruz AA, de Alencar VM, Falcao MF, et al. Association between Erdheim-Chester disease, Hashimoto thyroiditis, and familial thrombocytopenia. Ophthal Plast Reconstr Surg. 2006;22:60.
101. Larché M, Robinson DS, Kay AB. The role of T lymphocytes in the pathogenesis of asthma. J Allergy Clin Immunol. 2003;111:450.
102. Tang WK, Lee KC, Chong LY. Three patients with orbital xanthogranuloma and non-progressive haematological abnormalities. Australas J Dermatol. 2003;44:185.
103. Favara BE, Jaffe R, Egeler RM. Macrophage activation and hemophagocytic syndrome in Langerhans cell histiocytosis: report of 30 cases. Pediatr Dev Pathol. 2002;5:130.

104. Rao RN, Chang CC, Uysal N, et al. Fulminant multisystem non-Langerhans cell histiocytic proliferation with hemophagocytosis: a variant form of Erdheim-Chester disease. Arch Pathol Lab Med. 2005;129:39.
105. Devouassoux G, Lantuejoul S, Chantelain P, et al. Erdheim-Chester disease a primary macrophage cell disorder. Am J Respir Crit Care Med. 1998;157:650.
106. Pegoraro F, Papo M, Maniscalco V, Charlotte F, Haroche J, Vaglio A. Erdheim-Chester disease: a rapidly evolving disease model. Leukemia. 2020;34:2840–57.
107. Rosai J, Dorfman RF. Sinus histiocytosis with massive lymphadenopathy: a benign pseudolymphomatous benign disorder. Cancer. 1970;30:1174.
108. Foucar E, Rosai J, Dorfman RF. The ophthalmologic manifestations of sinus histiocytosis with massive lymphadenopathy. Am J Ophthalmol. 1979;87:354.
109. Lauwers GY, Perez-Atayde A, Dorfman RF, Rosai J. The digestive system manifestations of Rosai-Dorfman disease (sinus histiocytosis with massive lymphadenopathy): review of 11 cases. Hum Pathol. 2000;31:380.
110. Bhandari A, Patel PR, Patel MP. Extranodal Rosai-Dorfman disease with multiple spinal lesions: a rare presentation. Surg Neurol. 2006;65:308.
111. Ture U, Seker A, Bozkurt SU, et al. Giant intracranial Rosai-Dorfman disease. J Clin Neurosci. 2004;11:563.
112. Remadi S, Anagnostopoulou ID, Jlidi R, et al. Extranodal Rosai-Dorfman disease in childhood. Pathol Res Pract. 1996;192:1007.
113. Juskevicius R, Finley JL. Rosai-Dorfman disease of the parotid gland: cytologic and histopathologic findings with immunohistochemical correlation. Arch Pathol Lab Med. 2001;125:1348.
114. Deodhare SS, Ang LC, Bilbao JM. Isolated intracranial involvement in Rosai-Dorfman disease: a report of two cases and review of the literature. Arch Pathol Lab Med. 1998;122:161.
115. Van Zander J. Cutaneous Rosai-Dorfman disease. Dermatol Online J. 2004;10:12.
116. Zimmerman LE, Hidayat AA, Grantham RL, et al. Atypical cases of sinus histiocytosis (Rosai-Dorfman disease) with ophthalmological manifestations. Trans Am Ophthalmol Soc. 1988;86:113.
117. Khan R, Moriarty P, Kennedy S. Rosai Dorfman disease or sinus histiocytosis with massive lymphadenopathy of the orbit. Br J Ophthalmol. 2003;87:105.
118. Marion JR, Geisinger KR. Sinus histiocytosis with massive lymphadenopathy: bilateral orbital involvement spanning 17 years. Ann Ophthalmol. 1989;21:55.
119. Lee-Wing M, Oryschak A, Attariwala G, Ashenhurst M. Rosai-Dorfman disease presenting as bilateral lacrimal gland enlargement. Am J Ophthalmol. 2001;131:677.
120. de Silva D, Joshi N. Rosai-Dorfman disease recurrence with bilateral orbital masses following immunosuppressant therapy. Orbit. 2005;24:51.
121. Goldberg S, Mahadevia P, Lipton M, Rosenbaum PS. Sinus histiocytosis with massive lymphadenopathy involving the orbit: reversal of compressive optic neuropathy after chemotherapy. J Neuroophthalmol. 1998;18:270.
122. Jogai S, Temmim L, Al-Baghli A, Adesina AO. Rosai-dorfman disease presenting as bilateral eyelid swellings. Med Princ Pract. 2006;15:163.
123. Mohadjer Y, Holds JB, Rootman J, et al. The spectrum of orbital Rosai-Dorfman disease. Ophthal Plast Reconstr Surg. 2006;22:163.
124. Sanchez R, Sibley RK, Rosai J. The electron microscopic features of sinus histiocytosis with massive lymphadenopathy: a study of eleven cases. Ultrastruct Pathol. 1981;2:101.
125. Ngendagayo P, Roels H, Quatacker J, et al. Sinus histiocytosis with massive lymphadenopathy in Rwanda: Report of 8 cases with immunohistochemical and ultrastructural studies. Histopathology. 1983;7:49.
126. Pulsoni A, Anghel G, Falcucci P, et al. Treatment of sinus histiocytosis with massive lymphadenopathy (Rosai-Dorfman disease): report of a case and literature review. Am J Hematol. 2002;69:67–71.
127. Rybicki BA, Kirkey KL, Major M, et al. Familial risk ratio of sarcoidosis in African-American sibs and parents. Am J Epidemiol. 2001;153:188.
128. Newman LS, Rose CS, Maier LA. Sarcoidosis. N Eng J Med. 1997;336:1224.
129. Moller DR, Chen ES. Genetic basis of remitting sarcoidosis—triumph of the trimolecular complex? Am J Respir Cell Mol Biol. 2002;27:391.
130. Burke WM, Keogh A, Maloney PJ, et al. Transmission of sarcoidosis via cardiac transplantation. Lancet. 1990;336:1579.
131. Parkes SA, Baker SB, Bourdillon RE, et al. Epidemiology of sarcoidosis in the Isle of Man-1: A case controlled study. Thorax. 1987;42:420.
132. Rossman MD, Thompson B, Frederick M, et al. ACCESS Group.HLA-DRB1*1101: a significant risk factor for sarcoidosis in blacks and whites. Am J Hum Genet. 2003;73:720.
133. Iannuzzi MC, Iyengar SK, Gray-McGuire C, et al. Genome-wide search for sarcoidosis susceptibility genes in African Americans. Genes Immun. 2005;6:509.
134. Grunewald JW, Berlin M, et al. Lung restricted T cell receptor AV2S3+ CD4+ T cell expansions in sarcoidosis patients with a shared HLA-DRb chain conformation. Thorax. 2002;57:348.
135. Valentonyte R, Hampe J, Huse K, et al. Sarcoidosis is associated with a truncating splice site mutation in BTNL2. Nat Genet. 2005;37:357.
136. Lee S, Newman CS, et al. A case control etiologic study of sarcoidosis. Environmental and occupational risk factors. Am J Respir Crit Care Med. 2004;170:1324.
137. Melmon KL, Goldberg JS. Sarcoidosis with bilateral exophthalmos as the initial symptom. Am J Med. 1960;33:158.

138. Jakobiec FA, Yeo JH, Trokel SL, et al. Combined clinical and computed tomographic diagnosis of lacrimal fossa lesions. Am J Ophthalmol. 1982;94:785.
139. Nowinski T, Flanagan J, Ruchman M. Lacrimal gland enlargement in familial sarcoidosis. Ophthalmology. 1983;90:909.
140. Sacher M, Lanzieri CF, Sobel LI, et al. Computed tomography of bilateral lacrimal gland sarcoidosis. J Comput Assist Tomogr. 1984;8:213.
141. Weinreb RN, Yavitz EQ, O'Conner GR, et al. Lacrimal gland uptake of gallium citrate (Ga-67). Am J Ophthalmol. 1981;92:16.
142. Stannard K, Spalton DJ. Sarcoidosis with infiltration of the external ocular muscles. Br J Ophthalmol. 1985;69:562.
143. Simon EM, Zoarski GH, Rothman MI, et al. Systemic sarcoidosis with bilateral orbital involvement: MR findings. AJNR Am J Neuroradiol. 1998;19:336.
144. Segal EI, Tang RA, Lee AG, et al. Orbital apex lesion as the presenting manifestation of sarcoidosis. J Neuroophthalmol. 2000;20:156.
145. Carmody RF, Mafee MF, Goodwin JA, et al. Orbital and optic pathway sarcoidosis: MR findings. AJNR Am J Neuroradiol. 1994;15:775.
146. Collison JMT, Miller NR, Green WR. Involvement of orbital tissues by sarcoid. Am J Ophthalmol. 1986;102:302.
147. Mafee MF, Dorodi S, Pai E. Sarcoidosis of the eye, orbit, and central nervous system. Role of MR imaging. Radiol Clin North Am. 1999;37:73.
148. Faller M, Purohit A, Kennel N, et al. Systemic sarcoidosis initially presenting as an orbital tumour. Eur Respir J. 1995;8:474.
149. Shaikh ZA, Bakshi R, Greenberg SJ. Orbital involvement as the initial manifestation of sarcoidosis: magnetic resonance imaging findings. J Neuroimaging. 2000;10:180.
150. Jakobiec FA, Jones I. Orbital inflammations. In: Jakobiec FA, Jones I, editors. diseases of the orbit. New York: Harper & Row; 1979.
151. Spencer WH. Ophthalmic pathology: an atlas and textbook, vol. 3. Philadelphia: WB Saunders; 1986.
152. Neves RA, Rodrigues A, Power WJ, et al. The value of combined serum angiotensin converting enzyme and gallium scan in the diagnosis of ocular sarcoidosis. In: Nussenblatt RB, Whitcup SM, Caspi RR, Gery I, editors. Advances in ocular immunology. Amsterdam: Elsevier; 1994. p. 353–6.
153. Hall JG, Cohen KL. Sarcoidosis of the eyelid skin. Am J Ophthalmol. 1995;119:100.
154. Baughmann RP, Winget DB, Lower EE. Methotrexate is steroid sparing in acute sarcoidosis: results of a double blind, randomized trial. Sarcoidosis Vasc Diffuse Lung Dis. 2000;17:60.
155. Dev S, McCallum RM, Jaffe GJ. Methotrexate treatment for sarcoid-associated panuveitis. Ophthalmology. 1999;106:111.
156. Yee AM, Pochapin MB. Treatment of complicated sarcoidosis with infliximab anti-tumour necrosis factor-alpha therapy. Ann Intern Med. 2001;135:27.
157. Dutton JJ, Escaravage GK. Periocular subperiosteal deep granuloma annulare in a child. Ophthal Plast Reconstr Surg. 2006;22:141.
158. Barzilai A, Huszar M, Shpiro D, et al. Pseudorheumatoid nodules in adults: a juxta-articular form of nodular granuloma annulare. Am J Dermatopathol. 2005;27:1.
159. Salomon RJ, Gardepe SF, Woodley DT. Deep granuloma annulare in adults. Int J Dermatol. 1986;25:109.
160. Grogg KL, Nascimento AG. Subcutaneous granuloma annulare in childhood: clinicopathologic features in 34 cases. Pediatrics. 2001;107:E42.
161. Ross MJ, Cohen KL, Peiffer RL, et al. Episcleral and orbital pseudorheumatoid nodules. Arch Ophthalmol. 1983;101:418.
162. Rao NA, Font RL. Pseudorheumatoid nodules of the ocular adnexa. Am J Ophthalmol. 1975;79:471.
163. Burnstine MA, Headington JT, Reifler DM, et al. Periocular granuloma annulare, nodular type-Occurrence in late middle age. Arch Ophthalmol. 1994;112:1590.
164. McNeal S, Daw JL. Subcutaneous granuloma annulare. An unusual presentation in the eyelids and scalp. Ann Plast Surg. 2005;55:684.
165. Floyd BB, Brown B, Isaacs H, Minckler DS. Pseudorheumatoid nodule involving the orbit. Arch Ophthalmol. 1982;100:1478.
166. Evans MJ, Blessing K, Gray ES. Pseudorheumatoid nodule (deep granuloma annulare) of childhood: clinicopathologic features of twenty patients. Pediatr Dermatol. 1994;11:6.
167. Felner EI, Steinberg JB, Weinberg AG. Subcutaneous granuloma annulare: a review of 47 cases. Pediatrics. 1997;100:965.
168. Wong GA, Verbov JL. Subcutaneous granuloma annulare of the scalp in a diabetic child. Pediatr Derm. 2002;19:276.
169. Sandwich JT, Davis LS. Granuloma annulare of the eyelid: a case report and review of the literature. Pediatr Derm. 1999;16:373.
170. Cronquist SD, Stashower ME, Benson PM. Deep dermal granuloma annulare presenting as an eyelid tumor in a child, with review of pediatric lesions. Pediatr Dermatol. 1999;16:377.
171. Yoshimura J, Onda K, Tanaka R, Takahashi H. Giant cell reparative granuloma of the temporal bone: neuroradiological and immunohistochemical findings. Neurol Med Chir (Tokyo). 2002;42:510.
172. Scully RE, Mark EJ, McNeely BU. Case records of the Massachusetts General Hospital: Case 10–1984. N Engl J Med. 1984;310:642.
173. Hoopes PC, Anderson RL, Blodi FC. Giant cell (reparative) granuloma of the orbit. Ophthalmology. 1981;88:1361.
174. Mercado GV, Shields CL, Gunduz K, et al. Giant cell reparative granuloma of the orbit. Am J Ophthalmol. 1999;127:485.

175. Pherwani AA, Brooker D, Lacey B. Giant cell reparative granuloma of the orbit. Ophthal Plast Reconstr Surg. 2005;21:463.
176. Wold LE, Dobyns JH, Swee RG, Dahlin DC. Giant cell reaction (giant cell reparative granuloma) of the small bones of the hands and feet. Am J Surg Pathol. 1986;10:491.
177. Hirschl S, Katz A. Giant cell reparative granuloma outside the jaw bone. Hum Pathol. 1974;5:171.
178. Vernet O, Ducrey N, Deruaz JP, et al. Giant cell tumor of the orbit. Neurosurgery. 1993;32:848.
179. Unni KK. Dahlin's bone tumors: general aspects and data on 11,087 cases. 5th ed. Philadelphia: Lippincott-Raven; 1996.
180. Murphey MD, Nomikos GC, Flemming DJ, et al. From the archives of AFIP. Imaging of giant cell tumor and giant cell reparative granuloma of bone: radiologic-pathologic correlation. Radiographics. 2001;21:1283.
181. Jaffe HL, Lichtenstein L. Solitary unicameral bone cyst with emphasis on the roentgen picture, the pathologic appearance and the pathogenesis. Arch Surg. 1942;44:1004.
182. Ronner HJ, Jones IS. Aneurysmal bone cyst of the orbit: a review. Ann Ophthalmol. 1983;15:626.
183. Kransdorf MJ, Sweet DE. Aneurysmal bone cyst: concept, controversy, clinical presentation, and imaging. AJR Am J Roentgenol. 1995;164:573.
184. Senol U, Karaali K, Akyuz M, Luleci E. Aneurysmal bone cyst of the orbit. AJNR Am J Neuroradiol. 2002;23:319.
185. Hino N, Ohtsuka K, Hashimoto M, Sakata M. Radiographic features of an aneurysmal bone cyst of the orbit. Ophthalmologica. 1988;212:198.
186. Bealer LA, Cibis GW, Barker BF. Aneurysmal bone cyst: report of a case mimicking orbital tumour. J Pediatr Ophthalmol Strabismus. 1993;30:199.
187. Dailey R, Gilliland G, McCoy GB. Orbital aneurysmal bone cyst in a patient with renal cell carcinoma. Am J Ophthalmol. 1994;117:643.
188. Yuen V, Jordan DR, Jabi M, Agbi C. Aneurysmal bone cyst associated with fibrous dysplasia. Ophthal Plast Reconstr Surg. 2002;18:471.
189. Lucarelli MJ, Bilyk JR, Shore JW, et al. Aneurysmal bone cyst of the orbit associated with fibrous dysplasia. Plast Reconstr Surg. 1995;96:440.
190. Biesecker JL, Marcove RC, Huvos AG, et al. Aneurysmal bone cysts. Cancer. 1970;26:615.
191. Oliveira AM, Perez-Atayde A, Dal Cin P, et al. Aneurysmal bone cyst variant translocations upregulate USP6 transcription by promoter swapping with the ZNF9, COL1A1, TRAP150, and OMD genes. Oncogene. 2005;24:3419.
192. Pearson PA, Rakes SM, Bullock JD. Clinicopathologic study of hematic cysts of the orbit (Letter). Am J Ophthalmol. 1986;102:804.
193. Milne HL III, Leone CR, Kincaid MC, et al. Chronic hematic cyst of the orbit. Ophthalmology. 1987;94:271.
194. Shapiro A, Tso MOM, Putterman AM, Goldberg MFA. Clinicopathologic study of hematic cysts of the orbit. Am J Ophthalmol. 1986;102:237.
195. Marks MW, Yeatts RP. Hemorrhagic cyst of the orbit as a long term complication of prosthetic orbital floor implant. Plast Reconstr Surg. 1993; 93:856.
196. Amrith S, Baratham G, Khoo CY, et al. Spontaneous hematic cysts of the orbit presenting with acute proptosis: a report of three cases. Ophthalmic Plast Reconstr Surg. 1990;6:273.
197. Travis RC, Murray PI, Moseley IF, et al. Orbital intraconal haematic cysts in young people: computed tomography and magnetic resonance imaging. Br J Radiol. 1989;62:521.
198. Goldberg SH, Sassani JW, Parnes RE. Traumatic intraconal hematic cyst of the orbit. Arch Ophthalmol. 1992;110:378.
199. Kersten RC, Kersten JL, Bloom HR, et al. Chronic hematic cyst of the orbit: Role of magnetic resonance imaging in diagnosis. Ophthalmology. 1988;95:1549.
200. Loeffler M, Hornblass A. Hematic cyst of the orbit. Arch Ophthalmol. 1990;108:886.
201. Shapiro A, Tso MOM, Putterman AM, et al. A clinicopathologic study of hematic cysts of the orbit. Am J Ophthalmol. 1986;102:237.
202. Henderson J, Farrow G. Hematic cyst in orbital tumours. 2nd ed. New York: Thieme Stratton; 1980. p. 107.
203. Bergin DJ, McCord CD, Dutton JJ, et al. Chronic hematic cyst of the orbit. Ophthalmic Plast Reconstr Surg. 1988;4:31.
204. McNab AA, Wright JE. Orbitofrontal cholesterol granuloma. Ophthalmology. 1990;97:28.
205. Karim MM, Inoue M, Hayashi Y, et al. Orbital cholesterol granuloma with destruction of the lateral orbital roof. Jpn J Ophthalmol. 2000;44:179.
206. Miller NR, McCarthy EF, Carter N, et al. Lytic Paget disease as a cause of orbital cholesterol granuloma. Arch Ophthalmol. 1999;117:1084.
207. Parke DW II, Font RL, Boniuk M, et al. 'Cholesteatoma' of the orbit. Arch Ophthalmol. 1982;100:612.
208. Chow LP, McNab AA. Orbitofrontal cholesterol granuloma. J Clin Neurosci. 2005;12:206.
209. Arat YO, Chaudhry IA, Boniuk M. Orbitofrontal cholesterol granuloma: distinct diagnostic features and management. Ophthal Plast Reconstr Surg. 2003;19:382.
210. Selva D, Phipps SE, O'Connell JX, et al. Pathogenesis of orbital cholesterol granuloma. Clin Exp Ophthalmol. 2003;31:78.
211. Selva D, Chen C. Orbitofrontal cholesterol granuloma: percutaneous endoscopic-assisted curettage. Orbit. 2004;23:49.
212. Eisenberg MB, Haddad G, Al-Mefty O. Petrous apex cholesterol granulomas: evolution and management. J Neurosurg. 1997;86:822.

213. Rosca T, Bontas E, Vladescu TG. Clinical controversy in orbitary cholesteatoma. Ann Diagn Pathol. 2006;10:89.
214. Campanella RS, Caldarelli DD, Friedberg SA. Cholesteatoma of the frontal and ethmoid areas. Ann Otol Rhinol Laryngol. 1979;88:518.
215. Selva D, Dolman PJ, Rootman J. Orbital granulomatous giant cell myositis: a case report and review. Clin Exp Ophthalmol. 2000;28:65–8.
216. Kattah JC, Zimmerman LE, Kolsky MP, et al. Bilateral orbital involvement in fatal giant cell polymyositis. Ophthalmology. 1990;97:520.
217. Klein BR, Hedges TR III, Dayal Y, et al. Orbital myositis and giant cell myocarditis. Neurology. 1989;39:988.
218. Leib ML, Odel JG, Cooney MJ. Orbital polymyositis and giant cell myocarditis. Ophthalmology. 1994;101:950.
219. Mombaerts I, Koornneef L. Current status in the treatment of orbital myositis. Ophthalmology. 1997;104:402.
220. Menghini VV, Savcenko V, Olson LJ, et al. Combined immunosuppression for the treatment of idiopathic giant cell myocarditis. Mayo Clin Proc. 1999;74:1221.
221. Cho HR, Lee MH, Haw CR. Generalized tuberous xanthoma with type IV hyperlipoproteinemia. Cutis. 1997;59:315.
222. Critchley M, editor. Butterworths medical dictionary. 2nd ed. Butterworth: London; 1978. p. 1847.
223. Mancuso G, La Regina G, Bagnoli M, et al. 'Normolipidemic' tendinous and tuberous xanthomatosis. Dermatology. 1996;193:27.
224. Wolter JR, Nelson CC. Eyelid lipogranuloma after hydraulic oil injury. Ophthal Plast Reconstr Surg. 1991;7:133.
225. Holds JB, Patrinely JR, Zimmerman PL, et al. Hydraulic orbital injection injuries. Ophthalmology. 1993;100:1475.
226. Goel N, Johnson R, Phillips M, Westra I. Grease gun injuries to the orbit and adnexa. Ophthal Plast Reconstr Surg. 1994;10:211.
227. Gekeler F, Cruz AA, de Paula SA, et al. Intraconal grease-gun injury: a therapeutic dilemma. Ophthal Plast Reconstr Surg. 2005;21:393.
228. Hintschich CR, Beyer-Machule CK, Stefani FH. Paraffinoma of the periorbit-A challenge for the oculoplastic surgeon. Ophthal Plast Reconstr Surg. 1995;11:39.
229. Boynton JR, Searl SS, Heimer JL, et al. Eyelid oleogranulomas caused by petroleum jelly injection. Arch Ophthalmol. 1988;106:550.
230. Katz SE, Rootman J. Adverse effects of bone wax in surgery of the orbit. Ophthal Plast Reconstr Surg. 1996;12:121.
231. Witschel H, Geiger K. Paraffin induced sclerosing lipogranuloma of eyelids and anterior orbit following endonasal sinus surgery. Br J Ophthalmol. 1994;78:61.
232. Rosner M, Kurtz S, Shelah M, Rosen N. Orbital lipogranuloma after sinus surgery. Eur J Ophthalmol. 2000;10:183.
233. Abel AD, Carlson JA, Bakri S, Meyer DR. Sclerosing lipogranuloma of the orbit after periocular steroid injection. Ophthalmology. 2003;110:1841.

Disorders of the Lacrimal Gland

Diego Strianese and Geoffrey E. Rose

Key Messages

- Lacrimal gland diseases fall into one of three main categories: acute or subacute lesions; lesions with a chronic course; well-circumscribed lesions with variable duration of symptoms.
- Acute or subacute lesions are predominantly inflammatory or lymphoproliferative. If there is a short history, particularly with a viral-like illness, treatment with non-steroidal anti-inflammatories provide symptomatic relief in many cases. If symptoms persist, imaging and exploration through an upper eyelid skin-crease incision is appropriate.
- Lesions with a chronic course include most malignant epithelial tumours and chronic sclerosing inflammation of the lacrimal gland. In such cases, the diagnosis should be established by open biopsy or, if readily feasible, intact excision of the abnormal mass.
- Well-defined ovoid masses in the orbital lobe of the gland are likely to be pleomorphic adenoma and need intact excision without prior incisional biopsy.

The suggested surgical approach for lacrimal gland lesions is through an incision in the lateral two-thirds of the upper lid skin-crease, with or without lateral osteotomy, which is required rarely, and should be avoided where there is a possibility of lacrimal gland malignancy.Lacrimal gland swelling constitutes about 5–10% of all orbital masses [1–3]. A good indication of the likely lacrimal gland disease may be derived from the history and clinical features [4–8] and, although rarely pathognomonic, imaging is often strongly suggestive [9–15]. The diagnosis and management of lacrimal gland pathology changed dramatically with the advent of computed X-ray tomography (CT) in 1974, this enabling accurate estimates of size and borders, recognition of intrinsic calcification, and the assessment of expansion or erosion of neighbouring bone—bone erosion and tumour calcification being "red flags" for lacrimal gland malignancy [16]. Soft-tissue characterization improved further with the introduction of magnetic resonance imaging (MRI).

Despite diagnostic improvements, the treatment of lacrimal gland disease remains controversial—particularly for malignant epithelial tumours—and this chapter will discuss such difficulties with the aim of improving the confidence of physicians dealing with lacrimal gland masses. The conditions will be considered in five groups: inflammation, lymphoproliferative disorders, epithelial tumours, metastatic tumours and cystic lesions.

D. Strianese
Orbital Unit, University of Naples Federico II, Naples, Italy

G. E. Rose (✉)
Adnexal Service, Moorfields Eye Hospital, London, UK
e-mail: rose.geoff@googlemail.com

F. M. Quaranta Leoni et al. (eds.), *Oculoplastic, Lacrimal and Orbital Surgery*,
https://doi.org/10.1007/978-3-031-39638-0_21

1 Anatomy and Embryogenesis

Lacrimal gland embryogenesis starts at week 8, with exophytic "budding" of basal epithelium from the upper conjunctiva, and includes both ectoderm, forming the glandular component, and mesoderm that forms the mesenchymal components of the mature gland. Interestingly, pleomorphic adenomas are derived from both mesenchymal and ectodermal elements, whereas epithelial malignancies arise from the cells of ectodermal origin. Circulating lymphocytes are attracted into receptor-laden mesenchymal tissues in late embryogenesis and infancy, and these resident lacrimal gland lymphocytes produce tear-film immunoglobulin-A (IgA), as well as being subject to pathological proliferations later in life.

The size and shape of a pecan, the mature gland lies in an antero-supero-lateral fossa, and has a larger deep "orbital lobe" and a smaller, so-called, "palpebral lobe" that extends antero-inferiorly below the lateral horn of the levator aponeurosis; the lacrimal ductules pass through the palpebral lobe to drain into the supero-lateral conjunctival fornix. Similar to salivary glands, lacrimal glands are multilobulated tubulo-acinar structures, with each acinus releasing serous secretions into short-branched ductules. The acini have two layers of cells within a thin hyaline basement membrane, and surround a central lumen: the basal acinar cells are myoepithelial and the cylindrical secretory cells produce aqueous tears that contain lysozyme and electrolytes.

The lacrimal artery arises from the ophthalmic artery lateral to the optic nerve, and, together with the lacrimal nerve, supplies the gland by passing along the upper border of lateral rectus; venous drainage is through lacrimal vein(s) to the superior ophthalmic vein. The lacrimal nerve carries sensory innervation from the lateral part of the forehead and gland, and provides a pathway for perineural spread of lacrimal gland malignancies into the posterior orbit and cranium. Reflex tearing is mediated through an afferent and efferent pathway: the afferent pathway consists of corneal sensory fibres (carried in the long posterior ciliary nerves), intranasal sensory nerves and olfactory nerves. The efferent pathway arises in the lacrimal nucleus within the ventral pons, from which parasympathetic nerves are carried with the facial nerve to the greater petrosal nerve, and synapse within the sphenopalatine ganglion in the pterygopalatine fossa; postganglionic efferent fibres then enter the orbit through the inferior orbital fissure, form a plexus with sympathetic fibres behind the globe, and mediate lacrimal secretion and myoepithelial contraction.

2 Epidemiology of Lacrimal Gland Masses

There is a wide variation in the reported incidence of lacrimal gland masses, with some series based on general clinics, and others are drawn from tertiary referral centres [1–3]; this sampling bias is compounded by some reports including all lacrimal fossa lesions, whilst others include only biopsy-proven diagnoses. Despite these limitations, however, most lacrimal gland masses are inflammatory, followed by lymphoproliferative diseases and epithelial tumours.

The presenting age varies amongst these various conditions: infective dacryoadenitis is commoner in children, whereas non-infectious inflammation favours young or middle-aged adults. Whilst lymphoma and epithelial tumours can occur at any age, lymphoma is much more frequent after the fifth decade, and epithelial tumours mainly affect young and middle-aged adults. Pleomorphic adenoma (PA), the most common primary lacrimal gland solid tumour, presents at a mean age of 40 years, with a range from 8 to 80 years. Adenoid cystic carcinoma (ACC), the commonest lacrimal gland epithelial malignancy, has a bimodal age distribution—with most patients diagnosed in middle-age, but with a smaller peak in teenagers. Carcinoma ex-PA (CEPA), adenocarcinoma and mucoepidermoid carcinoma (MEC) all present around the age of 50 years. MEC is commoner in women (female/male ratio 3:2) and adenocarcinoma in men, whereas there is no gender predilection for PA, ACC or CEPA. No racial predilection has been reported for lacrimal gland

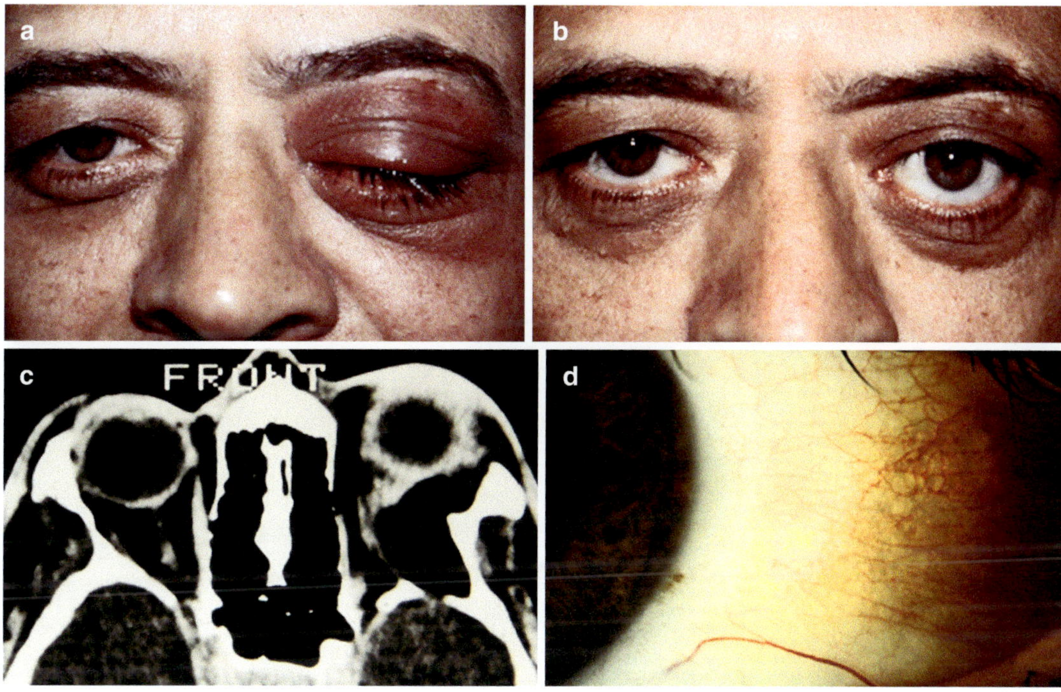

Fig. 1 (**a**) A male presenting with 4 weeks of red and swollen left eyelids, with lacrimal gland tenderness, (**b**) the inflammation settling on oral non-steroidal anti-inflammatories. (**c**) Imaging showed the dacryoadenitis to be secondary to a large sphenoidal wing dermoid cyst. (**d**) Longstanding deep orbital dermoid cysts are associated with chronic leakage of lipid contents, that may be visible as xanthochromic droplets in the lateral subconjunctival space

epithelial tumours. Bilateral epithelial tumours are extraordinarily rare, and bilateral lacrimal gland enlargement usually arises from inflammatory or lymphoproliferative disease [17].

3 Lacrimal Gland Disorders

3.1 Inflammatory Diseases

Dacryoadenitis can result from infection or autoimmune disease. Acute inflammation is generally idiopathic, with an infective agent only rarely identified, whereas chronic dacryoadenitis is usually due to a chronic lymphocytic or granulomatous inflammation that is possibly of autoimmune origin. Chronic relapsing dacryoadenitis can occasionally be secondary to (and the presenting symptom for) a deep orbital dermoid cyst [18]; these dermoid typically present in middle age (Fig. 1a–c), are situated behind the orbital lobe of the gland, and the chronic leakage of lipid may be visible as subconjunctival oil droplets (Fig. 1d) [19].

3.1.1 Infectious Dacryoadenitis

Infectious dacryoadenitis, of viral, bacterial or fungal origin, probably arises by retrograde ductular spread from the conjunctiva, or by direct haematogenous spread, may involve one or both lobes, and about a half of cases are bilateral [20]. In children, infectious dacryoadenitis may occur during mumps, measles, influenza, scarlet fever or erysipelas, whereas in adults it tends to favour diabetes or immuno-deficient patients. Presenting symptoms include pain, epiphora, chemosis, conjunctival injection, mucus discharge, and erythematous swelling of the upper eyelid that often adopts an S-shaped configuration. In children, the oedema may extend into the temple and cheek, in association with enlarged preauricular lymph nodes. Involvement of the orbital lobe is often associated with proptosis and painful eye movements.

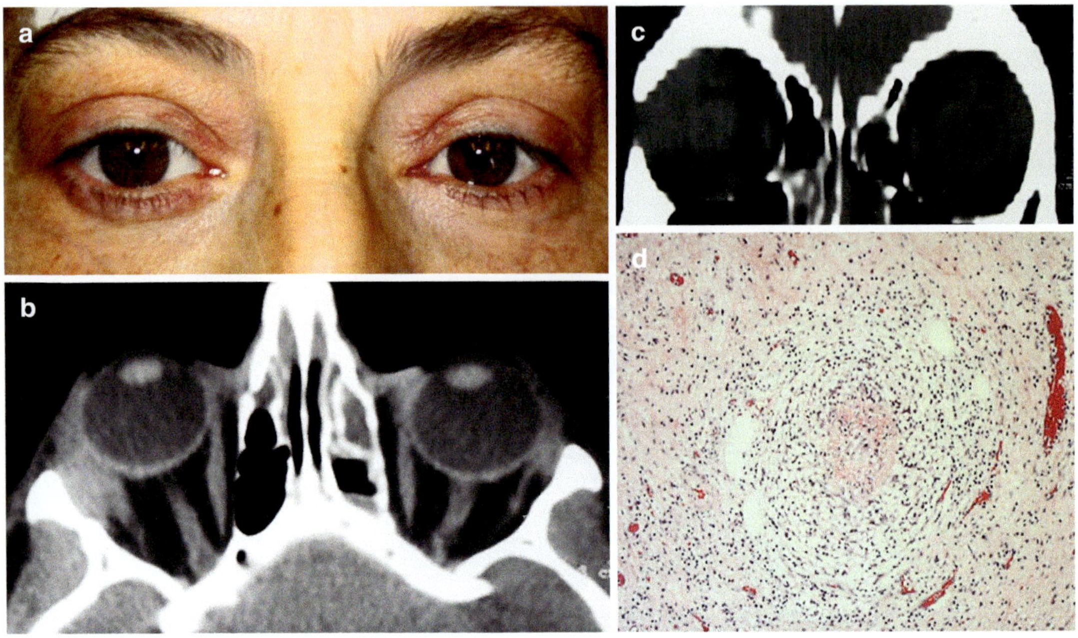

Fig. 2 (**a**) A 45-year-old healthy woman presents with mild chronic swelling her right upper eyelid, and slight orbital ache. (**b**, **c**) CT revealed slight right proptosis due to a moderately swollen lacrimal gland, this having uniform radiodensity and moulding around the globe; there is no bone expansion or erosion, and no intrinsic calcification of the mass. (**d**) Incisional biopsy showed a gland with chronic perivascular lymphocytic infiltration, areas of vascular necrosis, and non-caseating granuloma formation—compatible with active granulomatous polyangiitis

Acute dacryoadenitis is usually self-limited, and cold compresses, steroid ointment and oral anti-pyretics may offer some relief. Systemic antibiotics should be administered if bacterial infection is suspected—with a mucopurulent discharge, history of trauma or systemic bacterial infection; response to treatment should be evident within the first 24–48 h, with a marked resolution of symptoms within a week. Although ultrasonography, CT or MRI may help refine the diagnosis, an incomplete response should prompt a diagnostic biopsy: biopsy-proven chronic infections, such as tuberculous or fungal dacryoadenitis, should be treated with appropriate antibiotics guided by the results of culture, PCR and systemic investigation.

3.1.2 Autoimmune Dacryoadenitis

Autoimmune dacryoadenitis may be unrelated to any systemic condition, or can arise in the setting of named disorders—such as sarcoidosis, Sjögren's syndrome, systemic sclerosis, systemic lupus erythematosus (SLE), eosinophilic granulomatosis with polyangiitis (formerly called Churg-Strauss syndrome), granulomatous polyangiitis (GPA; formerly called Wegener's disease) and microscopic polyangiitis [21–25]. Many cases of sclerosing or fibrotic dacryoadenitis with systemic associations—previously regarded as idiopathic dacryoadenitis—are now thought to be due to immunoglobulin-G4 plasmacytes (IgG4-related disease; IgG4-RD) [26, 27]. With the exception of sclerosing variants that often produce a firm mass, non-infectious dacryoadenitis shares similar clinical features to infectious and may result in diplopia, proptosis, impaired vision and persistent pain (Fig. 2a–d). Although often appearing clinically unilateral, imaging will often suggest bilateral involvement, but cases that are truly unilateral should probably undergo long-term review because of the risk of late contralateral disease. Imaging features range from a well-defined mass to a diffuse infiltrating lesion, the latter resembling malignancy.

If dacryoadenitis persists despite treatment with non-steroidal anti-inflammatory drugs, biopsy should be undertaken prior to corticosteroid or other immunosuppression, particularly in adults where the risk of a malignant lymphoproliferative disorder is higher. A "trial of steroids" is to be strongly discouraged, as a rapid improvement in symptoms and signs (historically taken as confirmatory for inflammation) occurs with inflammation arising from all causes—be it due to infection, "chemical" irritants, tumours, foreign bodies or unknown causes; remember a key mantra, that "Inflammation is a tissue response, and **not** a diagnosis" [28]. Once a tissue diagnosis of subacute lymphocytic dacryoadenitis has been established, most cases will settle with oral corticosteroids tailing over a few weeks.

Specific inflammatory diseases—such as small-vessel vasculitis, sarcoidosis, SLE or Churg-Strauss syndrome—can require specific, individual treatment protocols. GPA, sclerosing dacryoadenitis or IgG4-RD may be more refractory to therapy and need a much slower tailing at the low-dosages (for example, below 10 mg prednisolone daily) over many months, and might also require additional immunosuppressants, such as cyclosporin or mycophenolate, under co-management with internal physicians. Some sclerosing variants of dacryoadenitis, such as IgG4-RD, constitute an unusual subgroup with a tendency to progress after initial immunosuppression, and surgical debulking can be of value in improving orbital function, slowing disease progression, and reducing chronic pain [26, 27].

4 Lymphoproliferative Disease

Lymphoproliferative diseases include benign reactive lymphoid hyperplasia, atypical lymphoproliferative processes, and malignant lymphomas.

Although the incidence of lymphoma appears to be increasing over recent decades [29], primary orbital lymphoma represents ~1% of all non-Hodgkin lymphomas (NHLs) and 8% of extranodal NHLs. Likewise, NHL accounts for ~7% of lacrimal gland masses and ~3% of all tumours in the superotemporal quadrant [1–8]. Whilst orbital structures derived from mucosa—such as the lacrimal gland—contain a standing population of mucosa-associated lymphoid tissue (MALT), most of the orbit lacks lymphatic vessels and is regarded as an extranodal site. In some countries (such as Italy, United States and Japan) a controversial association has been reported between orbital lymphoma and various infections, such as Hepatitis B or C, Epstein-Barr virus or *Chlamydia psittaci*. The variable prevalence of these infections, together with different environmental and genetic factors, could explain conflicting evidence [30–32].

Most patients with lacrimal gland lymphomas present at over 60 years of age, usually with a slowly-progressive, non-tender enlargement of one or both glands, this causing hypoglobus, proptosis and an S-shaped upper lid deformity; about 10–15% of orbital NHLs are bilateral [33, 34]. Occasionally NHL will present with acute inflammation or a slow, sclerosing disease. On CT, lacrimal gland lymphoma appears as a rather homogeneous glandular enlargement, often moulding around the globe, and on MRI it is usually T1- and T2-isointense compared with extraocular muscles, with only moderate contrast enhancement on CT or MRI (Fig. 3a–d). Extranodal marginal zone B-cell lymphoma ("MALToma") is the commonest variant, but others include diffuse large B-cell lymphoma and follicular lymphoma; other, much rarer types include mantle cell lymphoma, chronic lymphocytic leukaemia and lymphoplasmacytic lymphomas.

Localised, Stage I lymphoma is usually treated with radiotherapy (RT)—traditionally 20–24 Gy fractionated dosage—but recent years have seen the use of low-doses (2 × 2Gy) for MALT and follicular lymphomas, with good short-term disease control [35]. Systemic and high-grade lymphomas, such as diffuse large B-cell lymphoma, require a combination of slightly higher dosage radiotherapy (for example, 35 Gy) and chemotherapy. More recent therapies have included the use of biologic agents, such as anti-CD20 antibodies, either given systemically or as local injections [36].

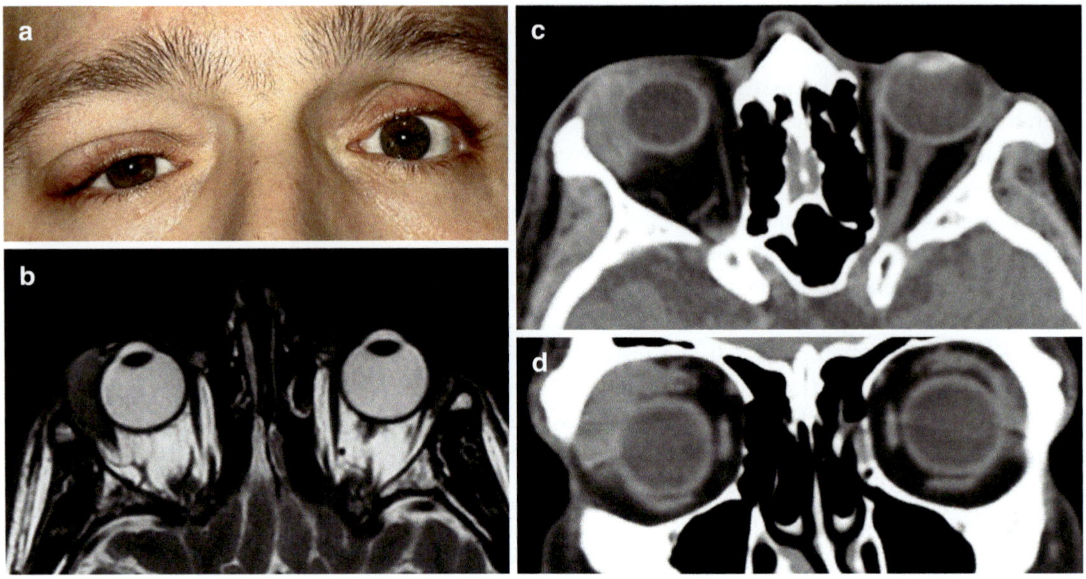

Fig. 3 (**a**) Right lacrimal gland lymphoma presenting with subacute painless swelling of the upper eyelid, resulting in an S-shaped contour; he also had mild diplopia on extreme abduction and infero-medial displacement of the right globe. (**b–d**) A well-defined, homogeneous right lacrimal gland mass, moulding around the globe and displacing the globe and lateral rectus infero-medially. The mass is iso-intense with brain on T2 sequence (**b**)

4.1 Epithelial Tumours

Epithelial tumours are the third most common lacrimal gland masses and include both benign and malignant neoplasms [37–41].

4.1.1 Pleomorphic Adenoma (Benign Mixed Tumour)

Being about half of all lacrimal gland epithelial tumours in most series, pleomorphic adenoma (PA) is the commonest epithelial tumour and has a peak incidence in the fourth and fifth decades [42]. As most PAs involve the orbital lobe, they usually present as a slowly-progressive, painless inferonasal globe displacement and upper lid fullness (Fig. 4a–d), although atypical presentations—such as pain or inflammatory signs—have also been reported. Because of the slow growth, symptom duration can vary from a month to more than 5 years. So-called "palpebral" PAs are relatively rare, are distinct from true PAs within the orbital lobe, and almost always arise within the preseptal eyelid tissues rather than in the "palpebral lobe" of the lacrimal gland [43, 44].

Lacrimal gland PAs present as a well-circumscribed oval lesion on imaging, with variable CT attenuation (or MRI signal) because of disparate composition and cellularity within the lesion—highly cellular regions appearing homogeneous, whereas less cellular areas are inhomogeneous due to the mixture of stroma, cystic degeneration, necrosis, or serous or mucinous collections. Calcification is infrequent, and more suggestive of carcinoma [16, 42]. On MRI, the cellular areas of tumour usually have intermediate T1 and high T2 signal intensities [9–12], and marked peripheral enhancement around a dark centre suggests possible infarction, with a higher risk of carcinoma ex-pleomorphic adenoma [45].

PA contains proliferation of both epithelial and mesenchymal components: the epithelium forms ducts with surrounding myoepithelium, and some closely-associated non-ductal cells that may have spindle, round, stellate, plasmacytoid,

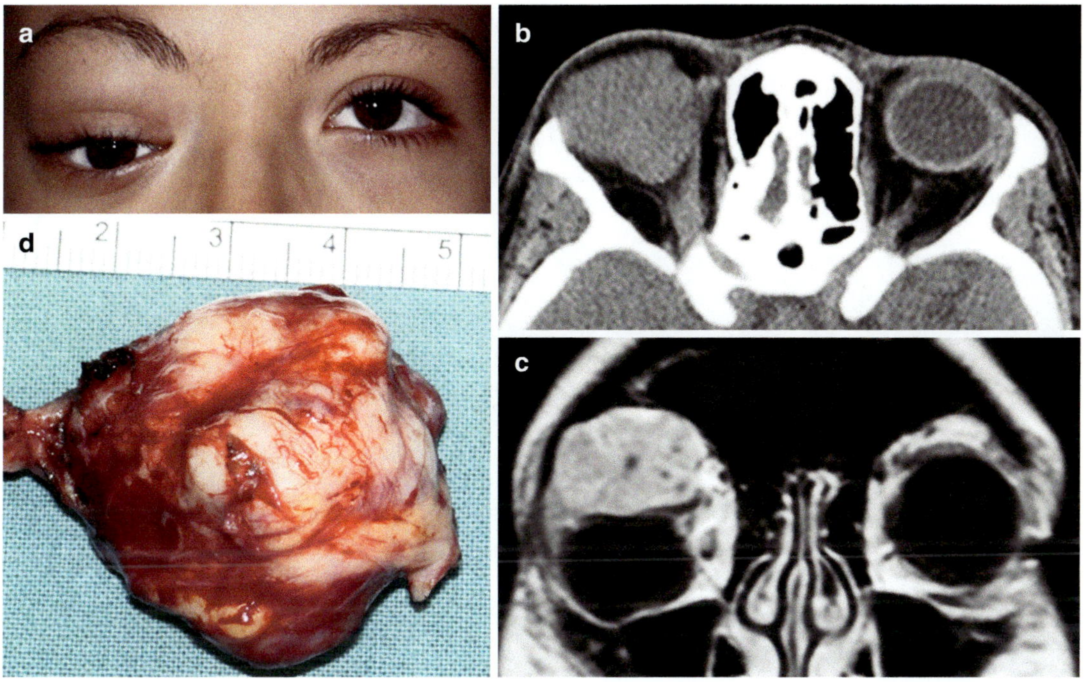

Fig. 4 (**a**) Longstanding marked right hypoglobus due to a painless lacrimal gland mass, the patient not having any diplopia. (**b**, **c**) The well-defined, ovoid mass associated with marked expansion of the orbital roof and globe indentation made pleomorphic adenoma the favoured pre-operative diagnosis; this diagnosis was also compatible with the variable signal within the mass. (**d**) The mass was excised intact, without prior incisional biopsy, and shows the characteristic firm mass and bosselation of this benign tumour

oncocytoid, polygonal and clear forms; squamous metaplasia occurs rarely. The epithelial component lies within a myxomatous mesenchyme, this usually showing various degrees of myxoid, hyaline, cartilaginous or osseous differentiation. Multifocal and multinodular growth patterns are said to have an increased risk of recurrence. Pleomorphic adenomas often show genetic abnormalities, particularly affecting the PLAG1 and HMGA2 genes [46, 47].

Intact excision is mandatory for PA [42], with effectively complete cure [48]. Preservation of the palpebral lobe is generally possible during surgery, this significantly reducing the rate of post-operative dry eye [42], although reflex/emotional tearing is usually abolished due to glandular denervation. Most orbital lobe tumours can be excised intact without lateral osteotomy [49] although, if required, this can be readily performed to facilitate intact excision. It has been suggested that fine-needle aspiration biopsy (FNAB) carries minimal risk of seeding of PA [50] but, realistically any tumour disruption (be it FNAB, wide-bore or open biopsy) carries a not insignificant risk of tumour recurrence and is probably unjustified [51]. Although intact tumour removal will rarely lead to excision of non-neoplastic masses [51], with contemporary imaging there is no cogent reason for pre-operative or intra-operative biopsy: where a well-defined mass turns out to not be PA after intact excision, it is generally carcinoma ex-pleomorphic adenoma (malignant mixed tumour), or else severe chronic inflammation or lymphoma without any residual functioning acini.

The prognosis for PA depends on the risk of recurrence or malignant transformation. The 5-year recurrence rate is negligible for completely excised lesions [48], but is reported to be as high as 30% for incompletely excised tumours [40]. One multicentre study recorded no cases of malignancy arising within recurrent PAs [38], but

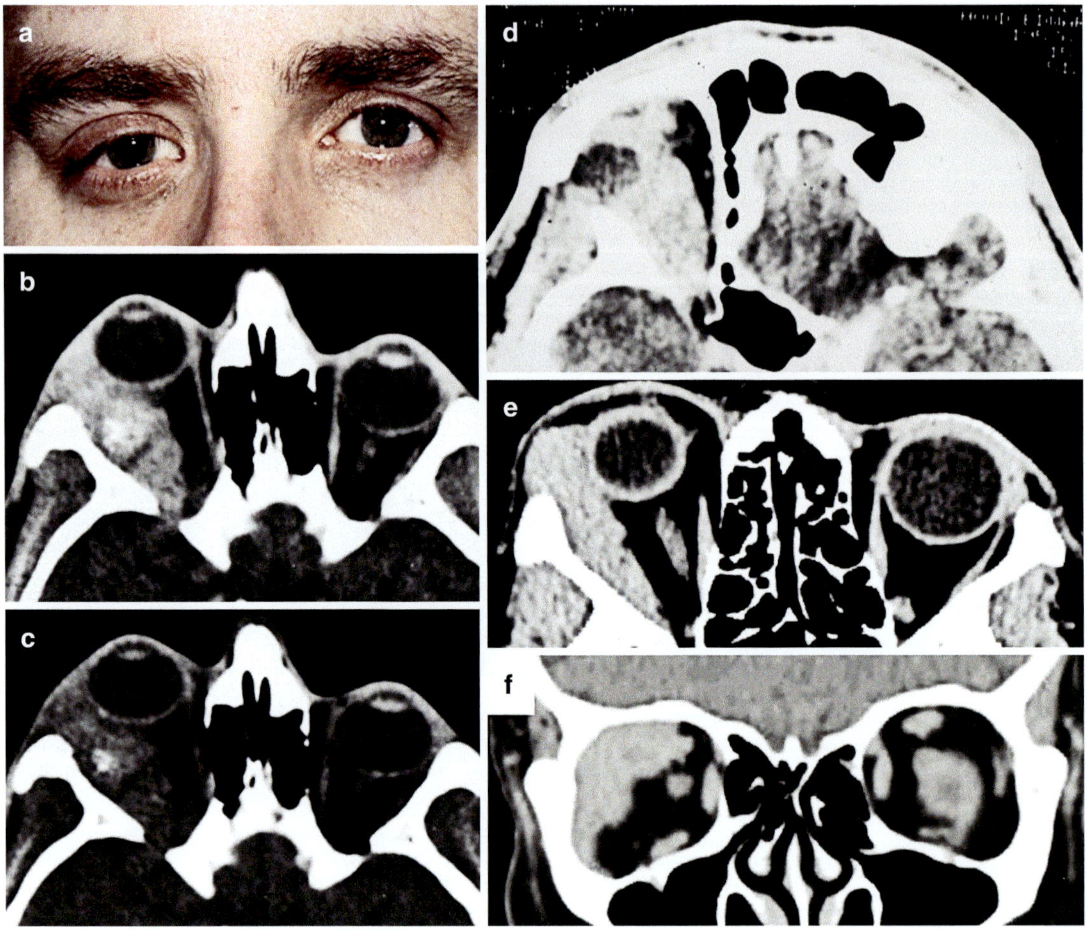

Fig. 5 (**a**) A young man presented with a short history of right lacrimal gland ache and a swollen and red upper eyelid. (**b**) CT showed right proptosis due to a mass extending back to the right superior orbital fissure, (**c**) with some fine calcification in the mass—this scenario being commonest with lacrimal gland carcinoma. (**d**) Advanced lacrimal gland carcinoma may erode the lateral orbital wall and show areas of necrosis in the centre of the tumour, as in this right-sided malignancy. (**e**, **f**) The "Wedge Sign": aggressive lacrimal gland diseases tends to spread posteriorly towards the orbital apex to form a wedge—this tissue growth often respecting the intermuscular septum between the lateral and superior rectus muscles (**f**). The example here is due to adenoid cystic carcinoma of the lacrimal gland

this complication has been reported in ~10% by 20 years after primary treatment [40]. A recent study has estimated the risk of transformation from PA to carcinoma ex-pleomorphic adenoma to rise by 1.04 per year, this risk rising from zero in the first two decades of life to ~28% by the ninth and tenth decades [52].

4.1.2 Adenoid Cystic Carcinoma

Adenoid cystic carcinoma (ACC) can arise at many sites (such as breast, skin, vulva or prostate), but most commonly affects the head-and-neck, with ACC being the commonest epithelial malignancy of the lacrimal gland. Lacrimal gland ACC presents at a considerably younger age than PA (even in childhood), and with a female predominance [16]. The presenting symptoms and signs are those of PA, but with a shorter history and often with pain (Fig. 5a) [16, 42]—the pain (and occasional fronto-temporal hypoesthesia) probably being due to early invasion of sensory nerves. Imaging usually reveals a somewhat ill-defined lacrimal gland mass with erosion of neighbouring cortical bone and often flecked calcification within the tumour (Fig. 5b–d) [16]. Unlike PAs, lacrimal gland malignancy will often show the "wedge sign"—where the tumour forms a wedge along the extraconal space, towards the superior orbital fissure, whilst often macroscopically respecting the intermuscular septum between the superior and lateral recti (Fig. 5e, f) [53].

ACC has three main histological subtypes: The "classical" and commonest pattern has a cribriform arrangement of tumour cells, the "tubular" variant has glands with a single lumen, and the solid ("basaloid") pattern has predominantly epithelial differentiation with high-grade features, and is associated with a higher proliferation rate, more aggressive nature, and the worst prognosis [38, 41]. ACC is generally characterised by a bidirectional differentiation of myoepithelial and epithelial cells, and the poor prognosis for basaloid ACC has been attributed to a lack of myoepithelial differentiation. Epithelial cells display cytostaining with CK7, CD117, epithelial membrane antigen (EMA), CK14, CK8/18 and CAM5.2, whilst myoepithelial cells express CK5/6, S100, P63, smooth muscle actin (SMA) and calponin. S100 proteins—a group of calcium-binding proteins—were initially considered unique to the nervous system, but are now recognised as being expressed in other tissues, such as myoepithelium (seen in ACC), cartilage or fat. Whilst investigated mainly in salivary gland tumours, most ACCs show a wide spectrum of genomic aberrations, that particularly affect the MYB and NFIB pathways, and anomalies of molecular control mechanisms [54–60].

ACC is a relatively slow-growing tumour with a propensity for late recurrence and metastasis, and this renders treatment controversial as studies with short follow-up can be misleading. Whilst surgical resection remains the mainstay for local control of disease it is now recognised that—with the propensity for perineural and intravascular spread—orbital exenteration (and bone resection) is probably <u>not</u> curative [61–64]. Indeed, exenteration might actually worsen the prognosis by "seeding" tumour into cranial diploe [61], and this technique should probably be reserved only as palliation for patients with fungating disease. The current optimal therapy would appear to be globe-sparing, macroscopic tumour debulking (without bone mobilisation) followed with early post-operative high-dose radiotherapy (~55 Gy) to the "at-risk" areas—namely, the orbital walls and cavernous sinus [61, 62]. Systemic chemotherapy, either cisplatin and doxorubicin [63] or cisplatin and 5-fluorouracil [64], appears to significantly reduce tumour burden and can be used as a pre-operative chemo-reduction, and/or a post-operative regime in addition to radiotherapy. Although not widely used, intra-arterial chemotherapy prior to exenteration has shown encouraging results in about a half of patients in whom it can be achieved [63].

Lacrimal gland ACC is histologically similar to that of breast and salivary gland, but has a worse prognosis that may be related to different profiles in molecular control [54–60], to a predominance of the basaloid variant [16, 38, 65], and to the staging of disease [66]. The prognosis for ACC is possibly better in childhood [67]. Whilst local control of disease has improved the prognosis over recent decades [61, 62], lacrimal gland ACC still has a propensity to systemic recurrence—although such recurrence appears to be delayed by the use of systemic chemotherapy [63, 64]. With a view to possible molecular therapy for ACC, expression of programmed cell death-L1 (PD-L1) protein was examined in a small cohort, but was not found to be of value [68].

4.1.3 Other Lacrimal Gland Malignancies

The lacrimal gland may be affected, either primarily or secondarily, by various rare malignancies: these include (in decreasing incidence) mucoepidermoid carcinoma, adenocarcinoma, squamous cell carcinoma, ductal adenocarcinoma, sebaceous carcinoma, acinic cell carcinoma, myoepithelial carcinoma, epithelial–myoepithelial carcinoma, carcinosarcoma, polymorphous low-grade adenocarcinoma, basal-cell carcinoma, cystadenocarcinoma, and primary undifferentiated large-cell carcinoma. If a totally undifferentiated carcinoma is revealed on biopsy, the clinician should investigate for a primary tumour elsewhere (especially gut), as *de novo* lacrimal gland adenocarcinoma is extremely rare—the latter arising more commonly within a pleomorphic adenoma. Due to the rarity of these malignancies, their optimum therapy is largely undefined.

Various benign masses have also been described within the lacrimal gland fossa, and include infantile haemangioma, solitary fibrous tumour, orbital cavernous venous malformations (cavernous haemangiomas), Kimura disease and amyloidosis.

4.2 Practical Management of Lacrimal Gland Swelling

Lacrimal gland swelling will generally fall into one of three main categories: (I) lesions with acute or subacute onset, and an imaging appearance suggesting infiltration or a diffuse lesion moulding around the globe and extraocular muscles; (II) lesions having similar imaging, but with a chronic course; and (III) well-circumscribed lesions with any duration of symptoms.

Group I lesions are predominantly inflammatory or lymphoproliferative, although they may rarely be due to a malignant epithelial tumour—particularly if the "Wedge sign" is present [53]. If there is a short history, particularly with a viral-like illness, then treatment with non-steroidal anti-inflammatories will provide symptomatic relief in many cases. If symptoms persist for more than a week, rarer causes of dacryoadenitis should be considered and imaging arranged (if not already performed): such imaging may show changes suggestive of malignancy (such as bone erosion or flecked calcification), a deep dermoid with chronic inflammation, or an unrecognised foreign body (with a remote history of trauma). Where symptoms persist, exploration through an upper eyelid skin-crease incision is appropriate—with resection of an underlying dermoid or removal of foreign body, or open biopsy of the gland where malignancy or inflammation is suspected. Whilst fine-needle biopsy has been advocated for lacrimal gland diagnosis, including pleomorphic adenoma [50], both FNAB and open biopsy should be avoided where imaging suggests the possibility of pleomorphic adenoma (PA)—namely, where an inhomogeneous, moderately-enhancing ovoid lesion causes globe compression and expansion of the lacrimal gland fossa, with intact cortical bone [51].

Group II lesions include most malignant epithelial tumours and chronic sclerosing inflammation of the lacrimal gland: In such cases, the diagnosis should be established by open biopsy or, if readily feasible, intact excision of the abnormal mass. In many chronic inflammatory masses, removal of the bulk of the lesion can very effectively relieve chronic pain, and arrest the inflammatory process. Because of the risk of malignancy in a chronically-enlarged lacrimal gland, it is imperative to avoid opening the bone, as this is likely to encourage "seeding" of malignant cells into the cancellous bone of the zygoma or calvarium [59].

Well-defined ovoid masses in the orbital lobe of the gland (especially if associated with bone scalloping or flattening of the globe) are likely to be PA and, therefore, mandate intact excision without prior incisional biopsy. With modern, high-resolution imaging of these Group III lesions, misguided incisional biopsy of PAs almost never occurs and—in contradistinction—the rate for intact excision of lesions that prove <u>not</u> to be PA is almost nil; the one exception to this latter case is, generally, where histology shows malignant transformation in a prior PA (carcinoma ex-pleomorphic adenoma).

The contemporary surgical approach for lacrimal gland lesions is through an incision based in the lateral two-thirds of the upper lid skin-crease, with or without lateral osteotomy; the incision can be extended laterally by another 10–12 mm if needed—this being especially so if osteotomy is required. Osteotomy is required only rarely to resect most lacrimal gland masses [49], and should be strenuously avoided where there is a possibility of lacrimal gland malignancy.

References

1. Bonavolontà G, Strianese D, Grassi P, et al. An analysis of 2,480 space-occupying lesions of the orbit from 1976 to 2011. Ophthal Plast Reconstr Surg. 2013;29:79–86.
2. Shields JA, Shields CL, Scartozzi R. Survey of 1264 patients with orbital tumors and simulating lesions: the 2002 Montgomery Lecture, part 1. Ophthalmology. 2004;111:997–1008.
3. Reese AB. The treatment of expanding lesions of the orbit with particular regard to those arising in the lacrimal gland; the seventh Arthur J Bedell lecture. Am J Ophthalmol. 1956;41:3–11.
4. Stewart WB, Krohel GB, Wright JE. Lacrimal gland and fossa lesions: an approach to diagnosis and management. Ophthalmology. 1979;86:886–95.
5. Shields CL, Shields JA, Eagle RC, et al. Clinicopathologic review of 142 cases of lacrimal gland lesions. Ophthalmology. 1989;96:431–5.
6. Andrew NH, McNab AA, Selva D. Review of 268 lacrimal gland biopsies in an Australian cohort. Clin Exp Ophthalmol. 2015;43:5–11.
7. Lacrimal Gland Tumor Study Group. An epidemiological survey of lacrimal fossa lesions in Japan: number of patients and their sex ratio by pathological diagnosis. Jpn J Ophthalmol. 2005;49:343–8.
8. Eldesouky MA, Elbakary MA, Sabik S, et al. Lacrimal fossa lesions: a review of 146 cases in Egypt. Clin Ophthalmol. 2014;8:1603–9.
9. Mafee MF, Edward DP, Koeller KK, et al. Lacrimal gland tumors and simulating lesions: Clinicopathologic and MR imaging features. Radiol Clin N Am. 1999;37:219–39.
10. Hughes GK, Miszkiel KA. Imaging of the lacrimal gland. Semin ultra-sound CT MR. 2006;27:476–91.
11. Won SJ, Kook JA, Mi RP, et al. The radiological spectrum of orbital pathologies that involve the lacrimal gland and the lacrimal fossa. Korean J Radiol. 2007;8:336–42.
12. Russo C, Strianese D, Perrotta M, et al. Multiparametric magnetic resonance imaging characterization of orbital lesions: a triple blind study. Semin Ophthalmol. 2020;35:95–102.
13. Vagefi MR, Hong JE, Zwick OM, et al. Atypical presentations of pleomorphic adenoma of the lacrimal gland. Ophthal Plast Reconstr Surg. 2007;23:272–4.
14. Strianese D, Elefante A, Matarazzo F, et al. Orbital lymphoma mimicking lacrimal gland pleomorphic adenoma. Case Rep Ophthalmol. 2013;4:109–13.
15. Prabhakaran VC, Cannon PS, McNab A, et al. Lesions mimicking lacrimal gland pleomorphic adenoma. Br J Ophthalmol. 2010;94:1509–12.
16. Wright JE, Rose GE, Garner A. Primary malignant neoplasms of the lacrimal gland. Br J Ophthalmol. 1992;76:401–7.
17. Tang SX, Lim RP, Al-Dahmash S, et al. Bilateral lacrimal gland disease: clinical features of 97 cases. Ophthalmology. 2014;121:2040–6.
18. Vahdani K, Rose GE. Presentation and treatment of deep orbital dermoid cysts. Ophthalmology. 2020;127:1276–8.
19. Vahdani K, Godfrey KJ, Patel P, Rose GE. Subconjunctival lipid leakage from deep orbital dermoid cysts. Ophthal Plast Reconstr Surg. 2020;36:e110–2.
20. Goold LA, Madge SN, Au A, et al. Acute suppurative bacterial dacryoadenitis: a case series. Br J Ophthalmol. 2013;97:735–8.
21. Tan LT, Davagnanam I, Isa H, et al. Clinical and imaging features of lacrimal gland involvement in granulomatosis with polyangiitis. Ophthalmology. 2015;122:2125–9.
22. Soheilian M, Bagheri A, Aletaha M. Dacryoadenitis as the earliest presenting manifestation of systemic Wegener's granulomatosis. Eur J Ophthalmol. 2002;12:241–3.
23. Kiratli H, Sekeroglu MA, Soylemezoglu F. Unilateral dacryoadenitis as the sole presenting sign of Wegener's granulomatosis. Orbit. 2008;27:157–60.
24. Ostri C, Heegaard S, Prause JU. Sclerosing Wegener's granulomatosis in the orbit. Acta Ophthalmol. 2008;86:917–20.
25. McNab AA. Orbital inflammation in Churg-Strauss syndrome. Orbit. 1998;17:203–5.
26. Berry-Brincat A, Rose GE. Idiopathic orbital inflammation: a new dimension with the discovery of immunoglobulin G4-related disease. Curr Opin Ophthalmol. 2012;23:415–9.
27. Detiger SE, Karim AF, Verdijk RM, van Hagen PM, van Laar JAM, Paridaens D. The treatment outcomes in IgG4-related orbital disease: a systematic review of the literature. Acta Ophthalmol. 2019;97:451–9.
28. Mombaerts I, Rose GE, Garrity JA. Orbital inflammation: Biopsy first. Survey Ophthalmol. 2016;61:664–9.
29. Moslehi R, Schymura MJ, Nayak S, Coles FB. Ocular adnexal non-Hodgkin's lymphoma: a review of epidemiology and risk factors. Expert Rev Ophthalmol. 2011;6:181–93.
30. Ferreri AJM, Govi S, Pasini E, et al. Chlamydophila psittaci eradication with doxycycline as first-line targeted therapy for ocular adnexae lymphoma: final results of an international phase II trial. J Clin Oncol. 2012;30:2988–94.
31. Jakobiec FA. Ocular adnexal lymphoid tumours: progress in need of clarification. Am J Ophthalmol. 2008;145:941–50.
32. Strianese D, Tranfa F, Finelli M, et al. Hepatitis C virus infection in ocular adnexal lymphomas. Arch Ophthalmol. 2010;128:1295–9.
33. Tranfa F, Di Matteo G, Strianese D, Forte R, Bonavolontà G. Primary orbital lymphoma. Orbit. 2001;20:119–24.

34. Ferry JA, Fung CY, Zukerberg L, et al. Lymphoma of the ocular adnexa: a study of 353 cases. Am J Surg Pathol. 2007;31:170–84.
35. De Cicco L, Cella L, Liuzzi R, et al. Radiation therapy in primary orbital lymphoma: a single institution retrospective analysis. Radiat Oncol. 2009;4:60–8.
36. Savino G, Battendieri R, Balia L, et al. Evaluation of intraorbital injection of rituximab for treatment of primary ocular adnexal lymphoma: a pilot study. Cancer Sci. 2011;102:1565–7.
37. Zeng J, Shi J, Li B, et al. Epithelial tumours of the lacrimal gland in the Chinese: a clinicopathologic study of 298 patients. Graefes Arch Clin Exp Ophthalmol. 2010;248:1345–9.
38. Weis E, Rootman J, Joly TJ, et al. Epithelial lacrimal gland tumours. Arch Ophthalmol. 2009;127:1016–28.
39. Ni C, Kuo PK, Dryja TP. Histopathological classification of 272 primary epithelial tumors of the lacrimal gland. Chin Med J. 1992;105:481–5.
40. Font RL, Gamel J. Epithelial tumours of the lacrimal gland: analysis of 265 cases. In: Jakobiec F, editor. Ocular and adnexal tumours. Birmingham, AL: Aesculapius; 1978. p. 787–805.
41. Von Holstein SL, Coupland SE, Briscoe D, Le Tourneau C, Heegaard S. Epithelial tumours of the lacrimal gland: a clinical, histopathological, surgical and oncological survey. Acta Ophthalmol. 2013;91:195–206.
42. Rose GE, Wright JE. Pleomorphic adenoma of the lacrimal gland. Br J Ophthalmol. 1992;76:395–400.
43. Vahdani K, Rose GE. Palpebral pleomorphic adenomas of the lacrimal gland. Ophthal Plast Reconstr Surg. 2021;37:125–8.
44. Rose GE, Vahdani K. Orbital lobe and palpebral adenomas of the lacrimal gland behave as distinct entities. Ophthal Plast Reconstr Surg. 2021;37:129–32.
45. Vahdani K, Luthert PJ, Verity DH, Rose GE. Extensive sclerosis ('mummification') in lacrimal gland pleomorphic adenoma may indicate neighbouring malignant transformation. Ophthal Plast Reconstr Surg. 2022;38:e13–7.
46. Andreasen S, von Holstein SL, Homøe P, Heegaard S. Recurrent rearrangements of the PLAG1 and HMGA2 genes in lacrimal gland pleomorphic adenoma and carcinoma ex pleomorphic adenoma. Acta Ophthalmol. 2018;96:e768–71.
47. Asahina M, Saito T, Hayashi T, Fukumura Y, Mitani K, Yao T. Clinicopathological effect of PLAG1 fusion genes in pleomorphic adenoma and carcinoma ex pleomorphic adenoma with special emphasis on histological features. Histopathology. 2019;74:514–25.
48. Currie ZI, Rose GE. Long-term risk of recurrence after intact excision of pleomorphic adenomas of the lacrimal gland. Arch Ophthalmol. 2007;125:1643–6.
49. Parker RT, Vahdani K, Rose GE. Intact removal of orbital lobe tumors of the lacrimal gland, with or without lateral wall osteotomy. Ophthal Plast Reconstr Surg. 2022;38:300–3.
50. Lai T, Prabhakaran VC, Malhotra R, et al. Pleomorphic adenoma of the lacrimal gland: is there a role for biopsy? Eye (Lond). 2009;23:2–6.
51. Rose GE. To crash or not to crash? Probability in the management of benign lacrimal gland tumours. Eye (Lond). 2009;23:1625–8.
52. Rose GE, Vahdani K, Lewis J, Rose AM. Risk and lagtime for development of lacrimal gland carcinoma expleomorphic adenoma: Observations and conjectural study. Ophthal Plast Reconstr Surg. 2022;38:563–6.
53. Lorenzano D, Rose GE. The "Wedge Sign": An imaging sign for aggressive lacrimal gland disease. Ophthalmology. 2017;124:1081–3.
54. Strianese D, Baldi G, Staibano S, et al. Expression of apoptosis-related markers in malignant epithelial tumours of the lacrimal gland and their relation to clinical outcome. Br J Ophthalmol. 2007;91:1239–43.
55. Liao Y, Zeng H, Wang X, et al. Expression patterns and prognostic significance of inhibitor of apoptosis proteins in adenoid cystic carcinoma and pleomorphic adenoma of lachrymal gland. Exp Eye Res. 2009;88:4–11.
56. Von Holstein SL, Fehr A, Persson M, et al. Adenoid cystic carcinoma of the lacrimal gland: MYB gene activation, genomic imbalances, and clinical characteristics. Ophthalmology. 2013;120:2130–8.
57. Chen TY, Keeney MG, Chintakuntlawar AV, et al. Adenoid cystic carcinoma of the lacrimal gland is frequently characterized by MYB rearrangement. Eye (Lond). 2017;31:720–5.
58. Sant DW, Tao W, Field MG, et al. Whole exome sequencing of lacrimal gland adenoid cystic carcinoma. Invest Ophthalmol Vis Sci. 2017;58:240–6.
59. Andreasen S, Tan Q, Agander TK, et al. Adenoid cystic carcinomas of the salivary gland, lacrimal gland, and breast are morphologically and genetically similar but have distinct microRNA expression profiles. Mod Pathol. 2018;31:1211–25.
60. Jiang M, Liu X, Zhang C, et al. Bioinformatics identification of the candidate microRNAs and construction of a competing endogenous RNA regulatory network in lacrimal gland adenoid cystic carcinoma high-grade transformation. Oncol Lett. 2021;21:360.
61. Rose GE, Gore SK, Plowman NP. Cranio-orbital resection does not appear to improve survival of patients with lacrimal gland carcinoma. Ophthal Plast Reconstr Surg. 2019;35:77–84.
62. Woo KI, Sagiv O, Han J, Frank SJ, Kim Y-D, Esmaeli B. Eye-preserving surgery followed by adjuvant radiotherapy for lacrimal gland carcinoma: Outcomes in 37 patients. Ophthal Plast Reconstr Surg. 2018;34:570–4.

63. Tse DT, Kossler AL, Feuer WJ, Benedetto PQ. Long-term outcomes of neoadjuvant intra-arterial cytoreductive chemotherapy for lacrimal gland adenoid cystic carcinoma. Ophthalmology. 2013;120:1313–23.
64. Manjandavida FP, Honavar SG, Murthy R, et al. Does multimodal treatment improve eye and life salvage in adenoid cystic carcinoma of the lacrimal gland? Ophthal Plast Reconstr Surg. 2022;38:348–54.
65. Gamel JW, Font RL. Adenoid cystic carcinoma of the lacrimal gland: the clinical significance of a basaloid histologic pattern. Hum Pathol. 1982;13:219–25.
66. Ahmad SM, Esmaeli B, Williams M, et al. American Joint Committee on Cancer classification predicts outcome of patients with lacrimal gland adenoid cystic carcinoma. Ophthalmology. 2009;116:1210–5.
67. Tellado MV, McLean IW, Specht CS, et al. Adenoid cystic carcinomas of the lacrimal gland in childhood and adolescence. Ophthalmology. 1997;104:1622–5.
68. Al Semari MA, Strianese D, Abu Safieh L, Al Hussain H, Abedalthagafi M, Edward DP. Expression of Programmed Cell Death-L1 (PD-L1) protein and mismatch repair mutations in orbital tumours—a pilot study. Eur J Ophthalmol. 2022;32:3097–102.

Orbital Vascular Anomalies and Vascular Tumours

Santiago Ortiz-Pérez, Francesco M. Quaranta Leoni, and David H. Verity

Key Messages

- The classification of vascular diseases of the orbit is complex and subject to frequent change and refinement.
- Broadly, vascular lesions can be divided into haemangiomas, vascular malformations, rare vascular tumours, and diseases which affect ectatic (ageing) vessels.
- Haemangiomas include capillary haemangiomas and intraosseous haemangioma.
- Vascular *malformations* include:
  - Venous-lymphatic malformations (VLM, also which include venous vascular malformations and solitary encapsulated venous-lymphatic malformations (SEVLM)).
  - Abnormal arteriovenous communications (which include high and low flow arteriovenous *fistulas*, which are usually acquired), and arteriovenous *malformations* (which are usually congenital)
- Rare vascular tumours include Kaposi's sarcoma, and Kaposiform haemangioendothelioma.
- Ectatic (ageing) vessels can be a cause for spontaneous orbital haemorrhage in the elderly. Risk factors include hypertension and diabetes.
- Orbital haemorrhage is more likely to occur in the context of low-flow than high-flow lesions.
- Low flow vascular shunts usually resolve spontaneously, whilst high flow shunts and AV malformations typically require endovascular embolisation.
- Acute orbital haemorrhage can cause a precipitous rise in orbital pressure, lead to acute loss of vision, and requires urgent intervention to prevent blindness.

1 Introduction

Classification of vascular anomalies is complex, and represents a broad spectrum of common and rare disorders. Broadly, these encompass vascular tumours, which possess a proliferative endothelium, and vascular malformations. Since 1996, the classification for these conditions has been assumed by the International Society for the Study of

S. Ortiz-Pérez (✉)
Department of Ophthalmology, Hospital Universitario Virgen de las Nieves, Granada, Spain

Department of Surgery, University of Granada - Instituto de Investigación Biosanitaria ibs.GRANADA, Granada, Spain
e-mail: santiagoortiz@ugr.es

F. M. Quaranta Leoni
Oftalmoplastica Roma, Rome, Italy

D. H. Verity
Adnexal Service, Moorfields Eye Hospital, London, UK

St John of Jerusalem Eye Hospital Group, London, UK

F. M. Quaranta Leoni et al. (eds.), *Oculoplastic, Lacrimal and Orbital Surgery*,
https://doi.org/10.1007/978-3-031-39638-0_22

Vascular Anomalies (ISSVA). The most recent classification at the time of writing was in 2018, and the reader is referred both to this Group and to a valuable review in 2022 on the ISSVA classification as it pertains to orbital disease by Tawfik and Dutton [1].

2 Haemangiomas

2.1 Capillary Haemangiomas

Infantile (capillary) haemangioma is a common periorbital benign tumour in children, affecting up to 5% of newborns. It is more frequent in females (3:1) and in premature infants. Although capillary haemangiomas often appear as solitary masses, they can be associated with other systemic conditions such as Kasabach-Merrit syndrome (thrombocytopenia, haemolytic anaemia, coagulopathy, and haemangiomas), microangiopathic haemolytic anaemia (MAHA), PHACES syndrome (**P**osterior fossa malformations, **H**aemangiomas, **A**rterial anomalies, **C**ardiac defects, **E**ye abnormalities, **S**ternal cleft, and supraumbilical raphe syndrome), Maffucci syndrome (associated with enchondromas), or associated with haemangiomas in other locations, usually in the upper respiratory tract [2–4]. The presence of four or more superficial lesions should raise suspicion of visceral involvement [2].

2.1.1 Clinical Presentation and Diagnosis

Infantile haemangiomas present during the first months of life, with up to one-third presenting at birth. Signs and symptoms may vary depending on the location of the tumour. Periorbital capillary haemangiomas are more frequently located in the upper eyelid and superomedial orbital quadrant, and can be superficial, subcutaneous, or deep. The cutaneous type presents as a typical bright red raised mass, is soft, may change in colour and size with crying, and can be blanched with pressure [3, 4].

The signs depend on the location and volume of the lesion. If located in the upper lid and brow, mechanical upper lid ptosis and astigmatism may ensue. If the tumour extends into the orbit, it can cause exophthalmos and ocular dystopia [1–4].

The natural history of these tumours includes a first phase of growth, usually during the first year of age, followed by a spontaneous regression, although during this time the lesion, as measured by ultrasonography, typically demonstrates a waxing and waning pattern [1]. Approximately 75% of lesions regress by the age of 3–7 years [4], but in some patients a fibrovascular residuum may still be demonstrable many years later [1].

The diagnosis is a clinical one for more superficial lesions, but imaging usually plays a role in defining the nature and extent of the lesion. Ultrasound can be used to evaluate the extent of periorbital involvement, with Doppler techniques confirming the vascular nature of the tumour. If deeper orbital involvement is suspected, magnetic resonance imaging (MRI) should be performed. This identifies hypointensity in the T1 sequences (which enhances significantly after contrast administration) and a hyperintense signal in the T2 sequences. Diffusion-weighted images (DWI) show increasing diffusion of water molecules, in contrast with malignant tumours which demonstrate diffusion restriction due to hypercellularity [2–4] (Fig. 1).

2.1.2 Histology

Capillary haemangiomas are hamartomas. They are more cellular during the proliferative phase and consist of anastomosing vascular channels lined by endothelial cells and pericytes. As the disease evolves, the channels enlarge, and the proportion of cells decreases. The involuting lesions are characterised by fibrosis and hyalinization of the capillary walls with luminal occlusion [2–5].

2.1.3 Management

The management of infantile haemangiomas depends on the location and whether the tumour is causing any visual impairment. Most of the cases only need follow-up as they regress with time. Indications for treatment include the risk of inducing mechanical ptosis and amblyopia, a

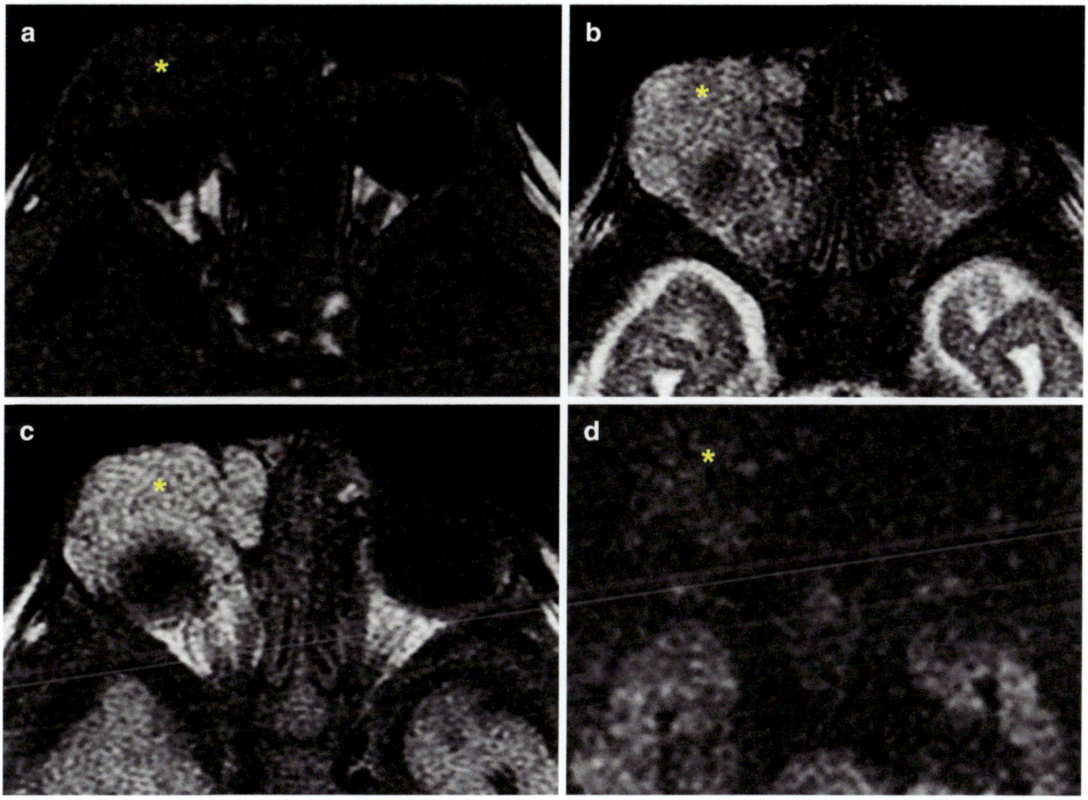

Fig. 1 MR imaging of infantile haemangioma. (**a**) T1 sequence shows a hypointense lesion affecting the inferior orbit and extending anteriorly to the lower eyelid. (**b**) T1 post-contrast image showed significant enhancement of the lesion due to its high vascular supply. (**c**) The tumour is hyperintense in T2-weighted images. (**d**) DWI-MRI at b1000 shows no restriction of diffusion, suggesting the benign nature of this tumour

severe cosmetic defect in the absence of spontaneous resolution, optic nerve compression, exposure keratopathy, infection, and necrosis [2–5].

Beta-blockers are the first-line treatment; they act suppressing vascular endothelial growth factors (VEGF) and fibroblast growth factors (FGF), both implicated in tissue proliferation [1].

Topical Timolol (0.5% gel) can be used for superficial lesions. Oral propranolol (started at the low dosage of 0.16 mg/kg/day and gradually increased to 2 mg/kg/day in three doses) is effective in deep and mixed lesions (Fig. 2). Oral beta-blocker treatment should be started under the guidance of a paediatrician or paediatric cardiologist, to monitor patients for possible systemic adverse effects, such as hypotension, bradycardia, hypoglycemia, bronchospasm, diarrhoea, hyperkalemia, and sleep disturbances.

The second-line treatment for cases with poor response to beta-blockers consists of corticosteroids; they can be used topically, injected into the lesion or given orally, depending on the size and location of the tumour. Steroids are effective only in the proliferative phase and are associated with well-known side effects.

Other treatments have been suggested, including laser photocoagulation, radiotherapy, embolization by interventional radiology, as well as other immunosuppressive drugs. Surgical resection is reserved for cases where the medical treatment fails, and there is a significant cosmetic and/or functional impairment, or for small lesions located under the skin surface [6–12].

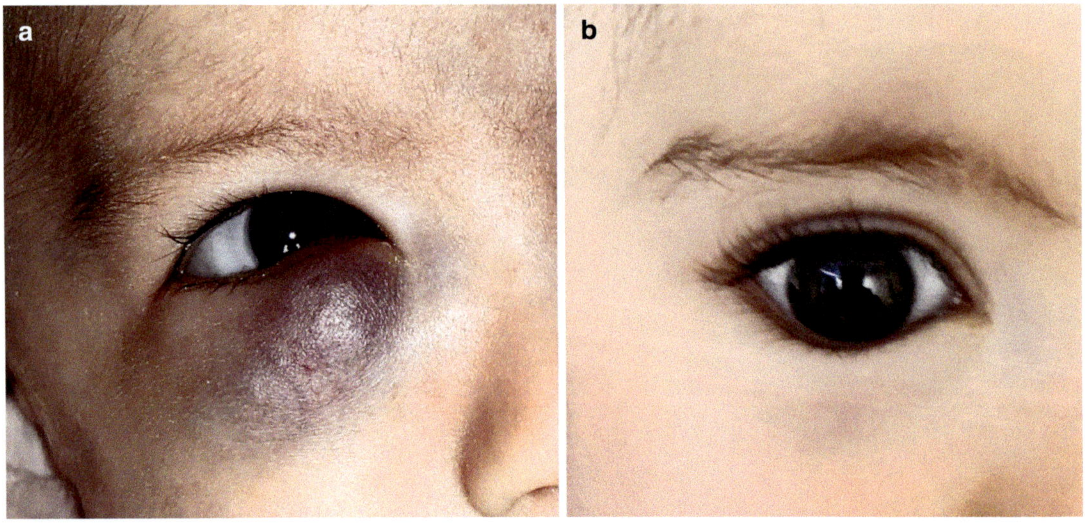

Fig. 2 Clinical picture of a patient presenting an infantile haemangioma (as per case shown in Fig. 1). (**a**) This 2-month-old patient presents with superficial and deep infantile haemangioma affecting the lower lid and the inferior orbit, causing hyperglobus, the blue mass is easily visible and palpable under the skin. (**b**) 5 months after treatment with oral propranolol showing complete resolution of the tumour

2.2 Intraosseous Haemangiomas

Intraosseous haemangiomas (IOH) are exceedingly rare benign neoplasms, accounting for 0.5–1% of all osseous neoplasms, and presenting most often in female patients in the fourth or fifth decade of life. The spine and skull are most commonly involved, with the frontal and parietal bones being preferentially affected. However, involvement of the facial skeleton, and in particular the bony orbit, is extremely rare [13–16].

2.2.1 Clinical Presentation and Diagnosis

The clinical manifestations include swelling, discomfort, or slowly growing fix to bone mass [14–16]. Although often radio*lucent* on plain film X-ray, CT imaging identifies changes similar to fibrous dysplasia. Features include an expansile, lytic lesion, usually with sclerotic changes, and a characteristic "honeycomb" or "sunburst" pattern, with fine radiating reticulated lines or trabeculae (Fig. 3).

Given the neuroimaging appearance, and the rarity of the lesion, the differential diagnosis includes fibrous dysplasia, multiple myeloma, meningioma, vascular malformation, metastatic carcinoma, eosinophilic granuloma, and haemangioma [15, 16]. Histology identifies a hamartoma consisting of anomalous proliferations of endothelial lined channels within the normal diploic space which typically erode the outer table of bone [16].

2.2.2 Management

Although en bloc excision has been advocated, partial resection has been shown to be effective in achieving good cosmetic results with no evidence of recurrence. However, biopsy or curettage can lead to severe haemorrhage, and pre-operative imaging is therefore desirable, as is pre-operative embolisation to reduce the risk of haemorrhage. Finally, post-operative radiotherapy is avoided because of the risk of malignant transformation.

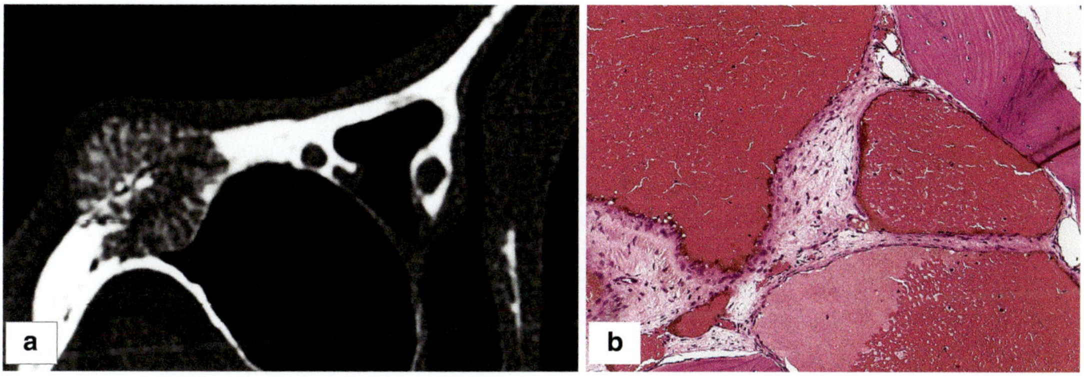

Fig. 3 Intraosseous haemangioma (IOH). (**a**) CT imaging identifies an expansile lesion a with a characteristic "honeycomb" or "sunburst" pattern, and fine radiating reticulated lines or trabeculae. (**b**) Histology shows characteristic vascular spaces between bony trabeculae, lined by a flat layer of cytologically bland endothelial cells and surrounded by loose fibrous tissue

3 Vascular Malformations

The nomenclature describing vascular malformations is complex and follows the classification of the *International Society for the Study of Vascular Anomalies* (ISSVA), itself not complete and certain to undergo further change in future. The *Orbital Society* has classified orbital vascular malformations based on their internal flow into type 1 lesions (no flow), type 2 (venous flow), and type 3 lesions (arterial flow) [17, 18].

3.1 Venous-lymphatic Malformations

The venous-lymphatic malformation, VLM, or lymphatic-venous malformation, consists of abnormal vascular spaces lined by endothelial cells. Venous or lymphatic components can be varied, accounting for venous-dominant, lymphatic-dominant, and purely lymphatic malformations. Pure lymphatic malformations (previously named lymphangiomas) are low-flow lesions, whilst combined venous-lymphatic malformations (VLM) have some degree of internal venous flow [19].

3.1.1 Clinical Presentation and Diagnosis

These benign lesions are congenital, and although can present at birth, usually become manifest during the first years of life. It has been reported that VLM is reported to comprise up to 3% of all orbital lesions, and its frequency is slightly higher in females [18–20].

VLM occur in the orbit, conjunctiva, eyelids, oropharynx, and sinuses. Associated symptoms reflect their location, size, and acute changes such as spontaneous intralesional haemorrhage (leading to the so-called *chocolate cyst*) and inflammatory changes. Proptosis, ptosis, restriction of eye movement, and swelling are among the most common clinical findings. Orbital VLM tend to insinuate within the intra- and extraconal spaces, often described radiologically as 'serpiginous'. Non-contiguous intracranial vascular malformations have been reported to occur in up to 25% of patients, including intracranial developmental venous anomalies, dural arteriovenous malformations, occlusion, or absence of dural sinuses and jugular veins, cerebral cavernous malformation, and pial arteriovenous malformations [20–22].

Diagnosis is based on clinical presentation with supportive neuroimaging. VLM can be subclassified as macrocystic (containing cysts of 2 cm or more in diameter), microcystic (less than 2 cm in diameter), or mixed, all of which may also have solid stromal components. Purely or dominant lymphatic malformations are non-distensible with the Valsalva manoeuvre, but they *can* enlarge during upper respiratory tract infections. Venous dominant malformations may show distensibility with Valsalva manoeuvres (see below) and can be decompressed [20–22].

MRI is considered the best technique for evaluating VLM. However, computed CT imaging can be also helpful, and given the complexity of managing these malformations, it may be desirable to use both MRI and CT to characterise the nature and extension of these lesions before planning treatment. CT may identify bone remodelling (being indicative of a chronic lesion), and, with a rapid acquisition time, any expansion with the Valsalva manoeuvre. MRI better characterises the nature of the lesion, the size, and the content of the cysts. The latter are characteristic in dominant lymphatic macro cystic malformations, these having a pathognomonic appearance with multiple grape-like cysts, often with a horizontal fluid level. Ultrasonography also plays a surveillance role. Finally, dynamic assessments (doppler ultrasound with and without Valsalva, CT-angiography, contrast MRI) are all crucial to determining the internal flow and the risk of bleeding during hypothetical surgical excision, and inadvertent intravenous drug delivery with proposed sclerotherapy procedures [20, 22].

3.1.2 Histology

The histologic spectrum of these lesions includes, in addition to lymphatic channels, blood vessels with venous characteristics, smooth muscle fibres, lymphocytic tissue, and blood or blood products [18, 19].

3.1.3 Management

The natural history of VLM is variable: some progress very slowly, whilst others can infiltrate the orbit and cause functional impairment due to repeated intra-lesional haemorrhages [22].

The treatment of VLM is complex and controversial. Surgical removal is a reasonable approach in cases of small or medium-sized and well-delineated malformations, but larger and diffusely infiltrative lesions can be extremely difficult to excise completely, and surgery is not without complication [23]. Surgical treatment can be performed with or without ultrasound guidance. Thus, a conservative approach is frequently the wisest for stable disease, and where expansion does not pose a risk of amblyopia.

The combination of intralesional sclerosing substances and surgical debulking may be successful in some cases, and sclerosants such as bleomycin, morrhuate sodium, polidocanol, OK-432, thrombosing agents (fibrin glue), and embolizing agents (such as cyanoacrylate glues and ethylene-vinyl alcohol copolymer) have all been proposed. Other approaches that may rarely be indicated include ultrasound-guided blood aspiration, canthotomy and cantholysis to relive the 'acute' orbit in cases of haemorrhage, orbital decompression, and even orbital exenteration in severe and disfiguring cases [24, 25].

Intralesional sclerotherapy with bleomycin—an antineoplastic antibiotic that causes marked fibrosis when injected intralesional—was previously reserved for non-resectable or treatment-resistant VLM, but has recently emerged as a primary treatment of choice for VLM (Fig. 4). However, this strategy can be challenging as the vascular spaces make up a relatively small proportion of the malformation. Although some lesions have an internal vascular network, accessible from a single point, in most cases flow is low, and a single-puncture position is unlikely to fill all vascular spaces. A long infusion time or multiple puncture sites may be an alternative approach, and usually, multiple sessions are required over time. Fluoroscopy is useful for precise targeting of lesion components in real-time, as the distribution of medication throughout the lesion can be assessed directly. Moreover, higher flow regions can be identified and avoided, reducing the risk of endovascular downstream collateral damage related to unintended sclerosis [26].

The combination of bleomycin and bevacizumab—a recombinant humanised monoclonal

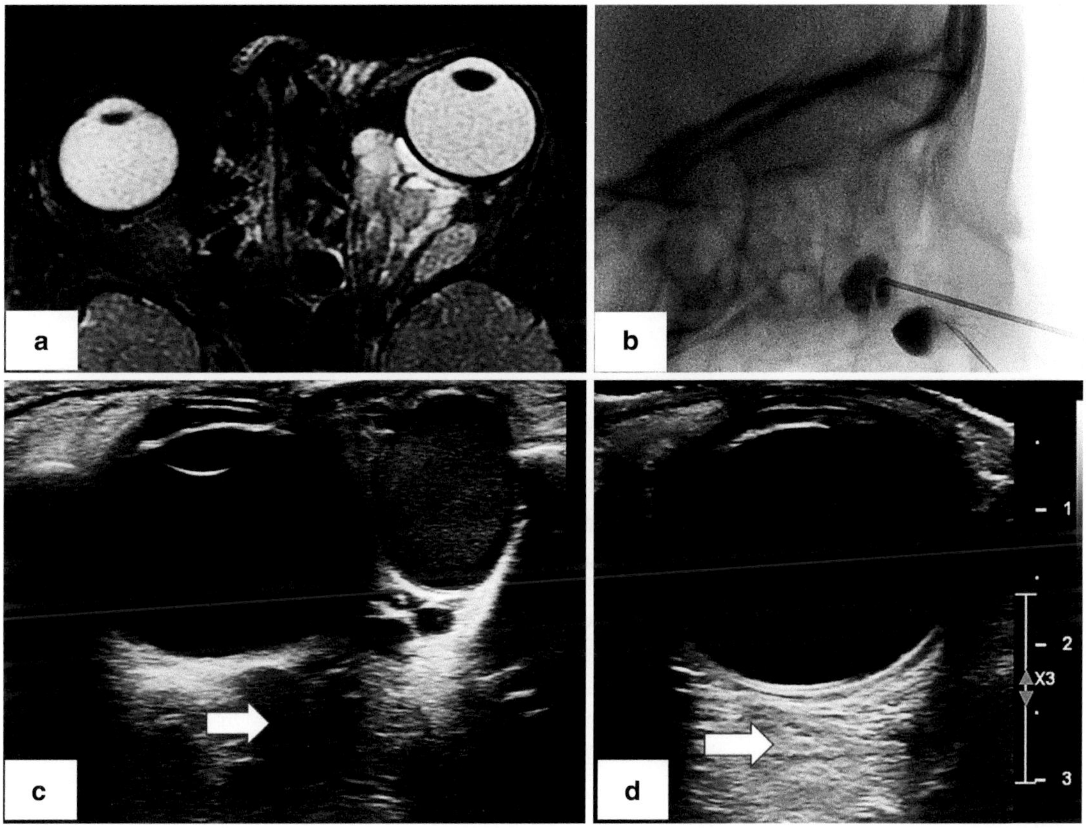

Fig. 4 4-year old child presenting with an exophthalmos and spontaneous blue discoloration around the *left* eye due to venous lymphatic malformation (VLM). (**a**) Axial T2 fat-saturated images of the MRI show an intraorbital multilocular cystic mass with fluid-fluid levels on the *left side*, suggestive of a venous lymphatic malformation (VLM). (**b**) Fluoroscopy images after ultrasound guided puncture of the cystic lesions. After confirmation of the needle position with contrast, 2500 IU bleomycin was injected. (**c**) On ultrasound during the bleomycin injection the cystic lesions are identified, note the retrobulbar *microcystic* component of the LM (*arrow*). (**d**) Follow-up ultrasound 20 months post-injection of bleomycin. The cystic lesions are significantly decreased in size and the retrobulbar component is completely resolved (*arrow*) (Source: Dr. Pieter-Jan van Doormaal (interventional radiologist) & Dr. Dion Paridaens)

antibody that blocks angiogenesis by inhibiting vascular endothelial growth factor A—has shown promising results in local treatment of recalcitrant microcystic and combined lymphatic malformations in the orbit [27, 28].

Due to the significant challenges in treating these lesions, a solely systemic approach for management would be ideal, avoiding the risk of surgical complication [26]. Recently sirolimus has emerged as a new medical treatment option for VLM. Sirolimus is a macrolide compound that has an effect on lymphatic malformation maintenance and growth by inhibiting the mechanistic target of rapamycin (mTOR) pathway that may play a role in lymphatic malformation pathogenesis [29].

Other studies have shown that sirolimus inhibits lymphangiogenesis by decreasing synthesis and promoting the degradation of vascular endothelial growth factor receptors [30]. Although further studies are needed, sirolimus appears to be a safe and effective treatment for orbital VLM, especially microcystic malformations [31]. A combination of sirolimus, and rivaroxaban, an anticoagulant medication (factor Xa inhibitor) was used successfully and kept symptoms in remission for more than 2 years in a single case [23, 32–36].

3.2 Venous Vascular Malformations (VVMs)

As described previously, venous-lymphatic malformations exhibit varying degrees of venous flow and distensibility, and are appropriately termed 'distensible venous malformations'. When located exclusively within the orbit, these lesions are termed *orbital varices* [17, 18, 24].

3.2.1 Clinical Presentation and Diagnosis

Superficial lesions, with or without a deeper component, are readily diagnosed by their clinical features, these including a soft, blood-filled lesion that expands with the Valsalva manoeuvre (Fig. 5). Deep orbital malformations are more difficult to diagnose: the symptoms can be intermittent, consisting of posture or exercise-induced pain or discomfort, proptosis, or episodes of orbital haemorrhage. Some patients may have mild enophthalmos at rest, with ophthalmic examination otherwise being normal [20, 25].

Some venous malformations, showing no evidence of distensibility, are termed 'non-distensible venous vascular malformations', this due to a relatively small communication with the systemic venous system. This group blends into the spectrum of venous–lymphatic malformation characterised by lack of, or minimal communication with, the venous outflow system [19, 20, 25]. Although haemorrhage can happen in all types of vascular malformation, this occurs less commonly in the non-distensible venous malformations [20].

Neuroimaging and management overlap with that described in the previous section (venous-lymphatic malformation). However, although these lesions have communication with the venous system, and endovascular treatment via interventional radiology can be considered, this is usually impractical. Such malformations consist of, or drain through, multiple thin-walled channels, as demonstrated by venographic studies, and this presents hazards for anterograde or retrograde catheterisation [24, 25].

3.3 Solitary Encapsulated Venous-lymphatic Malformations (SEVLM)

The SEVLM is the most frequent primary orbital mass in adults. They too are subject to on-going discussions with regard to nomenclature, in common with all other orbital vascular malformations [17]. SEVLM was previously known as cavernous haemangioma, but this term should be abandoned in preference for SEVLM.

3.3.1 Clinical Presentation and Diagnosis

SEVLM are non-distensible, low-flow vascular lesions. They present in adults, more frequently in women (60%) in the fourth and fifth decades [17, 18].

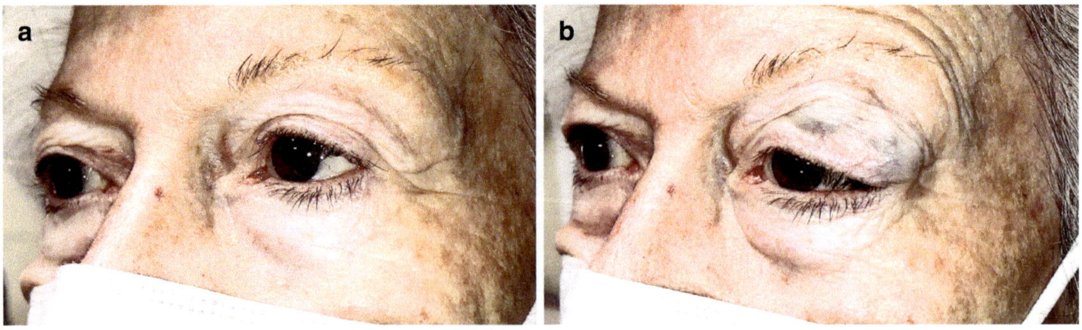

Fig. 5 Clinical image of a patient with a left orbital varix. (**a**) At rest, an orbital varix may not be clinically apparent. (**b**) After the Valsalva manoeuvre, the lesion increases in size, and the signs and symptoms become evident. In this case, the lesion affects the superolateral orbital quadrant: the superficial parts of the varix are manifest under the skin with the typical soft blue mass

The clinical manifestations depend on the location and size of the lesion. The natural history usually includes slow progression, causing a progressive painless proptosis (with a visible and palpable mass with anterior lesions), ocular dystopia, chorioretinal folds, hyperopia, optic nerve compression, increased IOP, and strabismus (Fig. 6). Circulating oestrogen and progesterone levels may play a role in clinical progression, with growth often accelerating during pregnancy. Haemorrhage within SEVLM rarely occurs, if ever [37, 38].

Clinical examination and review of previous images, when available, alerts the clinician to a slowly progressive space-occupying orbital lesion, with neuroimaging determining lesion size and location with respect to the orbital soft tissues, and its possible nature—accepting that such lesions can behave in a similar fashion to benign nerve sheath tumour (schwannoma) and solitary fibrous tumour (SFT). Not infrequently, SEVLM are encountered coincidentally when neuroimaging is performed for other reasons, such as migraine, or after a head injury [37, 38].

CT imaging identifies a well-circumscribed round or ovoid mass in the intra- or extraconal space. The rest of the orbital structures can be distorted and displaced, as compared to lymphoma which typically moulds *around* structures. CT shows homogeneous soft tissue density and may show small calcifications or phleboliths. Bony orbital walls may be remodelled in chronic cases [38–40].

MRI shows an isointense lesion on T1 weighted images and a very bright lesion on T2 imaging. Fine dark lines are due to internal septations, and hypointense pseudocapsule can be present. There is typically heterogeneous and progressive nodular enhancement on early post-contrast images, and progressive accumulation of contrast on delayed post-contrast images. However, these features can be similar to those seen in other benign tumours such as schwannoma—one of the main differential diagnoses. Diffusion techniques will show no restriction, in contrast to lymphatic tumours. Angiographic techniques are not contributory as they cannot identify the very fine feeding vessels [38–40] (Fig. 6).

3.3.2 Management

Intact excision of SEVLM is indicated for large and progressive lesions with documented change in visual functions, and the surgical approach depends on the position of the lesion relative to the optic nerve. Excision can be aided with the help of a cryoprobe, compressing the lesion against the orbital wall to reduce its volume, and passing a stabilising traction suture through the mass. Endonasal endoscopic surgery can play a role in the treatment of medial and apical SEVLM, whilst an anterior approach

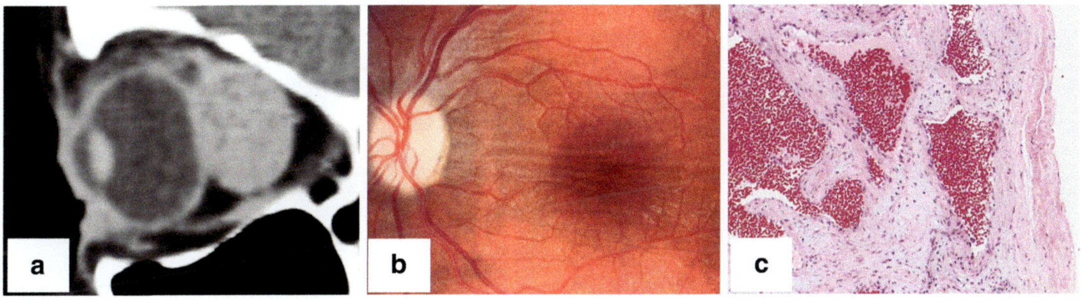

Fig. 6 Solitary encapsulated venous-lymphatic malformation (SEVLM). (**a**) CT identifies a homogenous encapsulated lesion in the intraconal space with radiological evidence for globe compression. (**b**) Fundus photograph demonstrating choroidal folds induced by the SEVLM. (**c**) Histology identifies an encapsulated lesion formed of cavernous vascular spaces separated by connective tissue stroma. The vascular spaces are lined by smooth muscle cells, are filled with blood, and are lined by flattened endothelial cell

is indicated for the great majority of lesions. This includes an upper lid skin crease approach for lesions superior to the optic nerve, a 'swinging lower lid' conjunctival approach for those inferior to the optic nerve, or a medial retrocaruncular approach for those in the medial orbit. For sizable lesions in the lateral orbit, and those extending to the lateral apex, a lateral orbitotomy approach can be preferable. Pupillary abnormalities, due to injury or ischemia to the ciliary ganglion or short ciliary nerves, occur in up to a quarter of patients undergoing surgery for intraconal SEVLM located inferotemporally or inferiorly, and in about a half of patients with apical lesions. Although most improve spontaneously, up to a third may have a persistent tonic pupil [37, 38] (Figs. 7 and 8).

Surgical management for deep SEVLM wedged in the orbital apex poses a particular challenge, and in these cases the increased risk of surgical complications, including vision loss, should be discussed carefully with the patient [26, 38]. Small apical lesions are often observed, since the natural history of such lesions is not predictable, and in rare cases, they may even regress spontaneously. Nevertheless, where there is documented evidence for progressive visual decline, such apical lesions can either be excised (with a lateral bone-swinging approach for lateral lesions), or managed with medial orbital decompression to relieve compression on the optic nerve, or fractionated stereotactic radiotherapy to reduce the size of the lesion [39].

Patients with minimal symptoms, or who are asymptomatic, can be managed conservatively and followed up with serial imaging and perimetry. Where there is any suggestion of an emerging optic neuropathy, intervention should be considered [26, 38].

3.4 Arteriovenous Malformations (AVM)

The current classification of vascular anomalies by the *International Society for the Study of Vascular Anomalies* (ISSVA) describes two categories of malformations with arterial flow

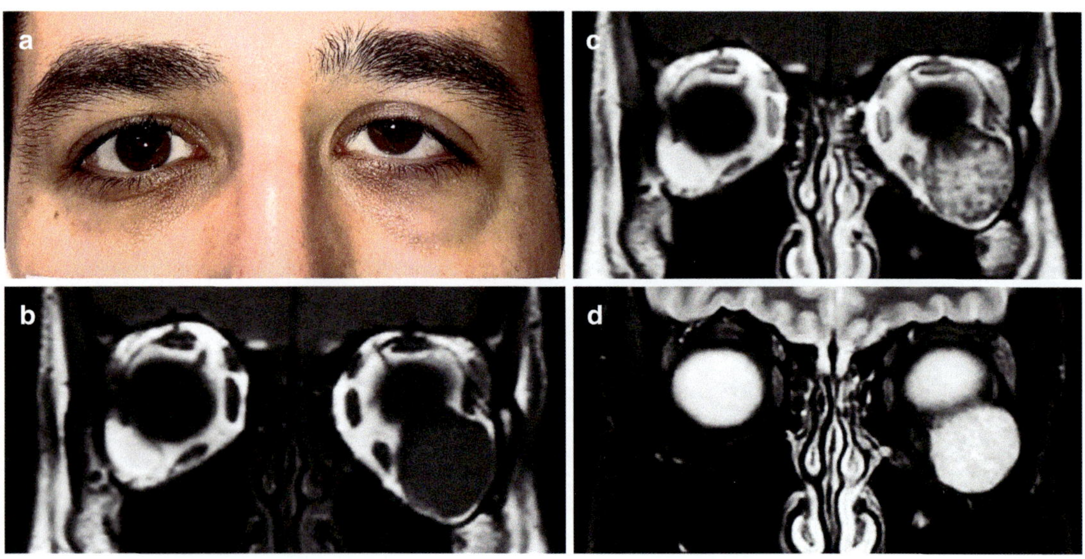

Fig. 7 Clinico-radiological correlation in a case of solitary encapsulated venous-lymphatic malformation (SEVLM). (**a**) Clinical picture of a young patient presenting with a slow-growing mass in his left inferolateral orbit, causing hyperglobus and diplopia. (**b**) T1 MRI shows an isointense and well-defined mass that causes inferior displacement of the orbital floor. (**c**) Contrast T1 sequence shows heterogeneous enhancement. (**d**) The image is hyperintense in T2 suggesting a high percentage of water within the lesion

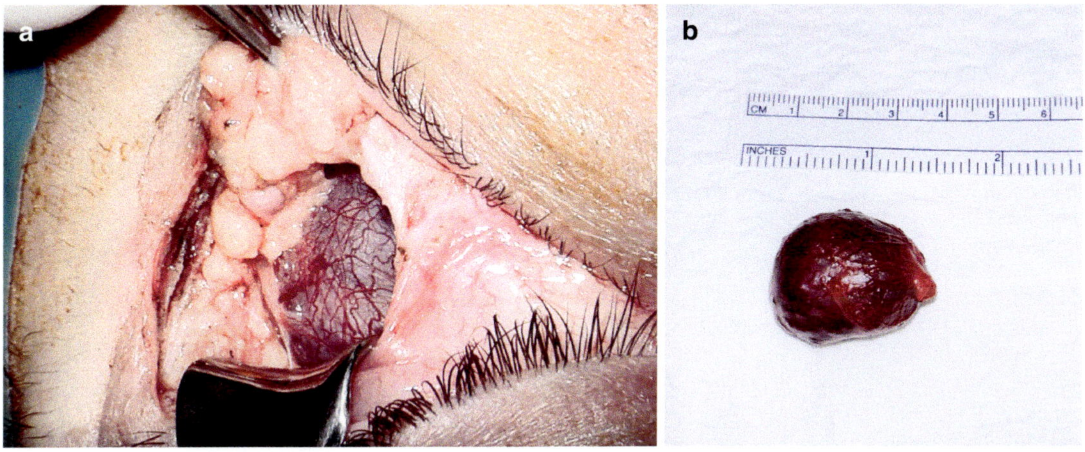

Fig. 8 Surgical images from the patient identified in Fig. 7. (**a**) Large intraconal masses are accessible via transconjunctival approaches. Typical appearance of the cavernous venous malformation with its dark *red-blueish* colour and superficial vessels, surrounded by a fine clear pseudocapsule. (**b**) Excision of an intact ovoid

arteriovenous malformation (AVM) and arterio-venous fistula [17].

3.4.1 Clinical Presentation and Diagnosis

AVM are hamartomas, where high-pressure arterial blood flows through the lesion into the venous system, without a normal capillary network. These are congenital lesions that usually remain asymptomatic and present in early adulthood and then enlarge progressively [18].

Purely *orbital* AVM are extremely rare, and more often appear in the context of head and neck AVM with involvement of the orbital vasculature. Not uncommonly such lesions have contributing arterial supplies from both the external and internal carotid systems. Clinical manifestations include the presence of a vascular mass and proptosis, with secondary signs and symptoms that vary depending on the size of the lesion and the branches implicated. Presenting ophthalmic features include dilated episcleral and conjunctival vessels, a secondary increase in intraocular pressure, ocular motility restriction with diplopia, chemosis and periorbital swelling. Variable pain or discomfort, increasing with exercise or Valsalva manoeuvre, can also occur. Pulsatility and bruit are also features of these lesions [18, 26, 41].

Diagnosis is confirmed by non-invasive cross-sectional imaging and catheter angiography [26].

3.4.2 Management

Treatment is aimed at obliteration of the abnormal arterio-venous communication, and is usually performed via an endovascular approach using liquid embolic agents to thrombose the fistula nidus. Current best practice for symptomatic or progressive AVMS is embolization of arterial feeding vessels to the lesion nidus followed by surgical debulking within a few weeks. However, complete embolization is not always possible if the lesion is supplied by feeder vessels from both the external and internal carotid systems. Current embolic agents include PHIL®, Glubran, and Onyx[1]; these agents are used for endovascular

[1]Liquid embolic agents are routinely used to close intracranial and adnexal arteriovenous fistula. These include **Glubran** (50% histoacryl/Lipiodol), **Onyx** (ethylene vinyl alcohol copolymer dissolved in dimethyl sulfoxide and suspended micronized tantalum powder to provide contrast for visualisation under fluoroscopy), and, more recently, **PHIL** (Precipitating Hydrophilic Injectable Liquid, in which the iodine component is covalently

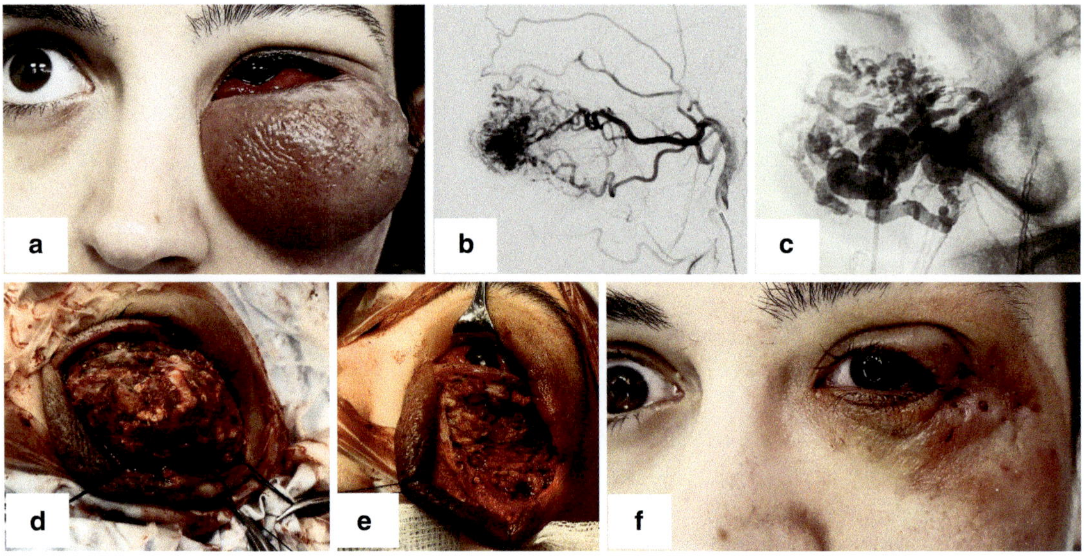

Fig. 9 (**a**) A 25 year old patient presented with a lower lid lesion that had been present for most of her life, but which had enlarged over the previous few years. (**b**) Pre-embolisation angiography demonstrates the AVM nidus with arterial tributaries from the external carotid artery. (**c**) Post-embolisation cast formed by PHIL®. (**d**) Surgical excision 1 week later via a subciliary incision. (**e**) Image showing tissue bed after removal of the AVM. (**f**) Post-operative photograph several weeks later

embolization of *cerebral* arteriovenous malformation [41] and have also been employed in the management of orbital and adnexal AVM (Fig. 9). Finally, the use of antiangiogenic drugs, especially bevacizumab, has also emerged as a promising systemic therapy [42].

3.5 Arteriovenous Fistula (Shunt)

Arteriovenous fistula (or 'shunt') is formed of an anomalous communication between arterial and venous circulations without a normal intervening capillary bed. They usually occur after injury or due to degenerative changes, but are rarely congenital [17, 18, 43–45].

3.5.1 Low-flow ("Dural") Intracranial AV Fistula (Shunt)

Dural (indirect) AV shunts are characterised by communication of meningeal branches of the internal and/or external carotid artery with the cavernous sinus, and usually occur in elderly patients with chronic arterial hypertension or other vascular disease [43–46]. These changes lead to increased pressure within the cavernous sinus which is normally a low-pressure vascular bed. The arterial contributions arise from meningeal branches of the internal and external carotid arteries: the most common supply from the *external* carotid artery is from the terminal meningeal branches of the internal maxillary artery. The most frequent source from the *internal* carotid artery is the meningo-hypophyseal trunk, and contributions from the *contralateral* dural vessels can also occur. The fistula is usually located posteriorly in the cavernous sinus.

Indirect (low flow) AV fistulas typically have a slow and insidious onset, and the diagnosis is commonly delayed or overlooked, the signs being misinterpreted for ocular surface inflammation, infection, or even thyroid-associated orbitopathy (TAO). Clinical features, which may be subtle, are due congestion within the cavernous sinus [43, 46]. These include discomfort or mild pain, with ocular redness chemosis, 'corkscrew' episcleral and conjunctival vascular engorgement, propto-

bonded to the co-polymer, giving better homogeneity of radio-opacity)

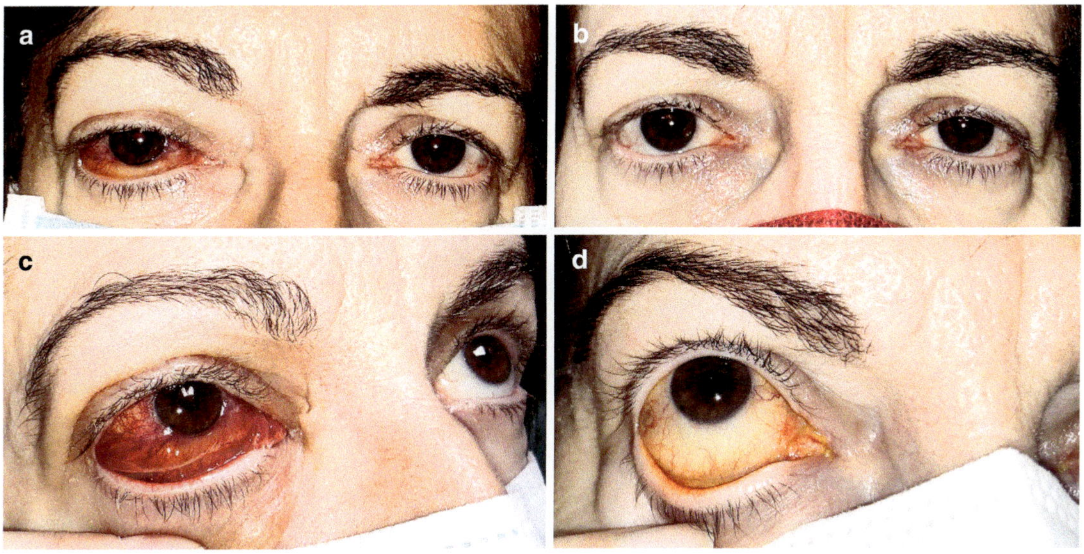

Fig. 10 Clinical pictures in a case of indirect arteriovenous fistula. (**a**) Female patient presented with right proptosis and signs of orbital congestion. (**b**) More detailed image showing dilated conjunctival vessels and chemosis. (**c**, **d**) The same patient after successful endovascular interventional treatment. Notice the significant improvement in the sign

sis, ocular motility impairment with diplopia, retinal vascular dilation, and raised intraocular pressure (Figs. 10 and 12). Rarely, subtle pulsatility of the hemicircular Goldman mires is observed through the slit lamp during contact tonometry.

3.5.2 High-flow Intracranial AV Shunt (Carotid Cavernous Fistula, CCF)

High-flow (direct) AV fistulas are usually due to cranial injury, be it accidental, or following neurosurgical or neuroradiological intervention [41]. A rupture of a branch of the internal carotid artery within the cavernous sinus (carotid-cavernous fistulas—CCF), results in a sudden and marked increase in hydrostatic pressure, accounting for the more acute and severe clinical picture than seen in an indirect AV shunt. Thus, orbital congestion can be severe, and is associated with pulsatile proptosis, conjunctival chemosis, raised intraocular pressure (with blood in Schlemm's channel), choroidal effusion, intraocular inflammation, and partial or complete ophthalmoplegia. The latter is due to extraocular muscles congestion and/or cranial nerve compression into the cavernous sinus).

Colour Doppler ultrasonography is diagnostic in both indirect and direct fistulae, identifying both arterialised and reversal of flow in a (dilated) superior ophthalmic vein with a typical Doppler waveform (Fig. 11). Neuroimaging identifies indirect signs (including superior ophthalmic vein enlargement, orbital venous filling in the early arterial phases, and cavernous sinus changes), but the gold-standard imaging remains catheter cerebral angiography, this delineating the anomalous vascular anatomy within the sinus, and whether the fistula drains posteriorly, this being relevant when planning treatment (Fig. 12). Note, posterior drainage is particularly dangerous when into the deep cerebral veins where it can cause venous hypertension and haemorrhage.

3.5.3 Intraorbital Arteriovenous Fistulas

Intraorbital arteriovenous fistulas (AVFs) are rare vascular malformations which can mimic carotid-cavernous fistulas (CCFs). These involve a fistula from the ophthalmic or facial arteries (from either or both the external and internal carotid circulations) artery to a corresponding draining vein, and can occur either spontaneously or following injury [47].

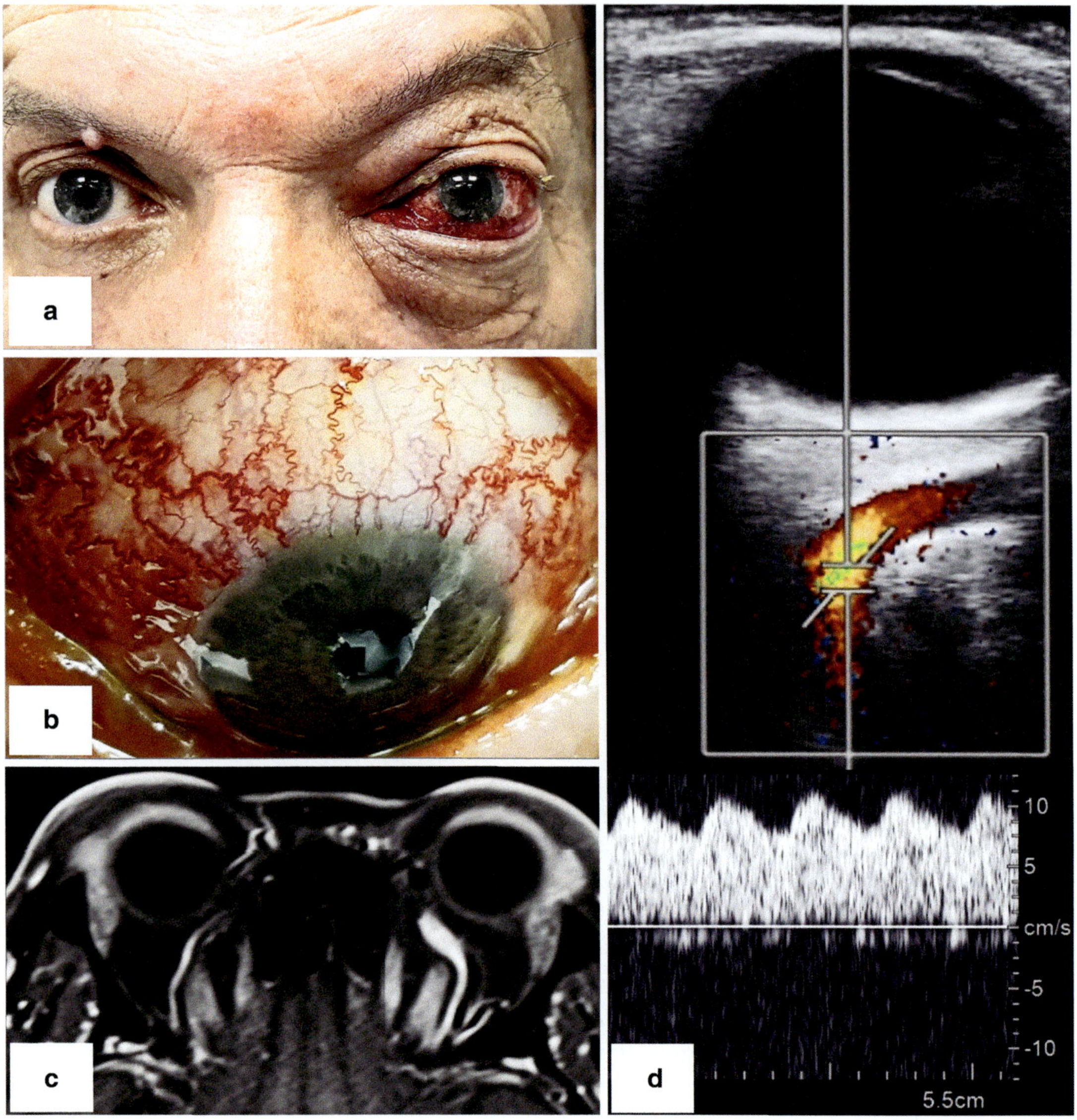

Fig. 11 Dural (low flow) carotid cavernous sinus fistula. (**a**) A patient presents with a 'red eye', proptosis, and congestion. (**b**) Slit lamp examination reveals 'snakey' or 'corkscrew' episcleral vessels. (**c**) MR imaging identifies a dilated superior ophthalmic vein (SOV). (**d**) Colour Doppler echo image (*top*) identifies arterialised flow within the vein with reversal of direction of flow. Colour Doppler energy, CDE, renders colour intensity as a function of blood flow, with red signifying flow *towards* the probe, and blue being flow *away* from the probe. Spectral Doppler examination (*bottom*) identifies a real-time velocity of blood flow within the SOV of 12 cm/s

As described above, the clinical spectrum of AV fistulas is broad; while small *indirect* fistulas typically close spontaneously (but not in all cases), larger indirect or direct fistulas usually require therapeutic intervention, with an untreated risk to the eye from exposure, vascular ischaemia, and intraocular hypertension, and a risk of intracranial haemorrhage where there is *retrograde* flow into the cerebral veins. AV fistulas are therefore co-managed by ophthalmologists, neuro-ophthalmologists, neuro-radiologists and interventional radiologists. In selected cases, embolization of the shunt can be achieved by direct exposure and canalisation of the superior ophthalmic vein via an orbital approach [43–54].

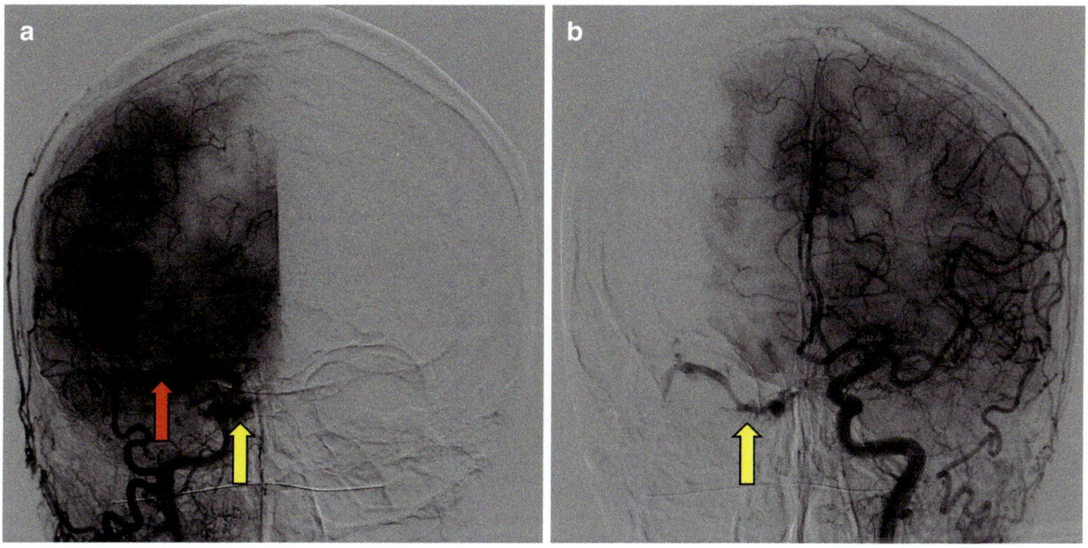

Fig. 12 Digital subtraction brain angiography of the same patient showed in Fig. 10. (**a**) Right internal carotid artery (ICA) angiogram. Note the early filling of the right cavernous sinus (*yellow arrow*) and the right superior ophthalmic vein (*red arrow*). (**b**) Left ICA angiogram. The *yellow arrow* shows the filling of the *right* superior ophthalmic vein during the early (arterial) phases of the test

3.6 Sinus Pericranii

Sinus pericranii (SP) is a rare trans-osseous venous communication between the extracranial and intracranial venous systems, usually occurring in the midline or frontal region [55]. SP is either congenital (and can be associated with venous malformations, Blue Rubber Bleb Nevus Syndrome, Von Hippel Lindau Syndrome, and craniosynostosis) or acquired following injury. It is typically asymptomatic, and presents in childhood with a nonpulsatile reducible soft tissue mass that increases in size with increased venous pressure. Although most SPs occur as solitary lesions, up to a fifth of patients have associated venous malformations elsewhere.

Evaluation requires thorough neurovascular imaging, with investigations including colour Doppler ultrasonography. Digital subtraction angiography (DSA) remains the gold-standard investigation because it clearly defines the lesional anatomy and the extent of cerebral venous sinus involvement.

There is no consensus on the optimal management for SP. 'Dominant' forms, where the anomaly forms *the major outflow for intracranial venous drainage*, is best observed, with life-time surveillance for cerebral venous hypertension or haemorrhage. 'Accessory' forms of SP care amenable to endovascular or percutaneous image-guided embolization techniques or with open surgical ligation [55, 56].

4 Other Vascular Lesions

4.1 Kaposi Sarcoma

Kaposi sarcoma (KS) is a low-grade, neoplastic disorder of vascular origin that may occur in four different forms; classic, endemic, epidemic (associated with Acquired Immune Deficiency Syndrome (AIDS)), and post-transplant [57, 58]. All four types have the same histological features and are often associated with human herpesvirus type 8 (HHV-8) infection [59]. With an increase in the world-wide incidence of immunodeficiency virus infection (HIV), the incidence of KS has increased likewise.

4.1.1 Clinical Presentation and Diagnosis

Treatment for early AIDS-related KS in previously untreated patients should start with the control of HIV with antiretrovirals, which frequently results in KS regression. KS of the eye and adnexa is thus extremely rare in patients with sero*negative* HIV infection; it is usually unilateral, although bilateral cases have been reported.

Ocular KS as the initial manifestation of HIV/AIDS is rare with only a few reported cases [58, 60, 61], and conjunctival and adnexal KS lesions have become relatively uncommon in the era of antiretroviral therapy.

KS of the eye usually occurs with the appearance of a mucocutaneous reddish brown elevated nodal lesion with conjunctival involvement [62], and can be misdiagnosed as angiosarcoma, haemangioma or pyogenic granuloma. *Orbital* KS is exceptionally rare [63], although simultaneous involvement of the lacrimal gland and the conjunctiva has been reported [64].

4.1.2 Histology

KS is composed of a spongy network of endothelial cells that form slit-like vascular spaces surrounded by spindle-shaped mesenchymal cells and collagen.

4.1.3 Management

Common therapeutic options include immune reconstitution with antiretroviral therapy in patients with HIV, surgical excision, cryotherapy, intralesional injections of chemotherapeutic agents, radiation, systemic chemotherapy, interferon, radiotherapy, and laser therapy [51]. Radical surgery can be curative. Antiretroviral therapy (HAART) combined with docetaxel, chemotherapy with INN-doxorubicin, and intralesional bleomycin have been proposed as effective treatments [58, 65–67].

4.2 Kaposiform Haemangioendothelioma

Kaposiform haemangioendothelioma (KH) is a rare, locally aggressive vascular tumour found in infants and children. It usually occurs on the trunk, extremities, and retroperitoneal regions but it may rarely primarily involve the orbit [68].

4.2.1 Clinical Presentation and Diagnosis

KH usually presents as a poorly defined purpuric mass. It can present in the orbit as a large heterogeneous hyperintense mass at T1-weighted magnetic resonance imaging with fat suppression and gadolinium enhancement, with vascular flow voids and osteolytic changes to the surrounding orbital walls [68].

Although considered a benign vascular tumour, KH may be locally aggressive, without distant metastasis. The differential diagnosis includes capillary haemangioma, dermoid cysts, rhabdomyosarcoma, neuroblastoma and fibrosarcoma [69].

The prognosis depends on tumour size. KH can be associated with Kasabach-Merrit syndrome, a coagulopathy associated with thrombocytopenia, with a mortality rate of up to 24% [68, 70].

4.2.2 Histology

KH is composed of spindle-shaped endothelial cells with hyalinized stroma with infiltrating nodules growing in an infiltrative pattern. Immunohistochemical stains are CD31 and CD34 positive with lack of immunoreactivity to GLUT1, as opposed to capillary haemangioma, which shows immunoreactivity to CD31, CD34 and GLUT1 [68].

4.2.3 Management

Treatment options include resection, embolization, laser therapy, sclerotherapy or medical treatment, including propranolol, oral corticosteroids, interferon, and cytostatic chemotherapy [68, 71–73].

Sirolimus appears to be ideal for proliferative vascular tumours through the control of tissue overgrowth disorders as an antiproliferative agent. Treatment with sirolimus can decrease pain and the fullness of vascular malformations, improve coagulation levels, and slow the growth of abnormal lymphatic vessels. Treatment of KH with sirolimus is tolerated well, and only mild reversible leukopenia was observed as a side effect [73].

5 Acute Orbital Haemorrhage

Orbital vascular disease can present with acute symptoms, and, if untreated, may lead to raised orbital pressure, reduced arterial perfusion, and consequent loss of vision. In most cases, the likely aetiology can be deduced from the clinical history and examination, and in some cases a similar such is history, with imaging, is available. High pressure at the orbital apex can result in ischaemic optic neuropathy and prompt intervention is necessary where optic nerve perfusion is threatened by excessive pressure, or where there is loss of vision [74, 75].

The classic features of an acute orbital vascular event include a sudden onset of proptosis, preceded by periocular bruising with anterior haemorrhages (note, for deeper lesions periocular ecchymosis is not immediately apparent and may even present days later). Rapid expansion of the intraorbital volume and sudden stretching of the extraocular muscles causes severe pain, nausea, and vomiting. The latter is mediated via the oculocardiac vagal reflex and is particularly troublesome in children in whom the symptoms can be incorrectly attributed to an intracranial injury.

Acute extravascular haemorrhage can embarrass the posteriorly directed venous drainage at the orbital apex and presents with episcleral venous congestion and a secondary rise in intraocular pressure. When there is significant arteriovenous shunting, the intraocular pressure may show an abnormally high variation during the cardiac cycle. A *secondary* effect of such vascular congestion and fluid egress from the intravascular compartment is increased *intracellular* fluid volume, resulting in oedematous extraocular muscles, a reduction in eye movements, and caruncular or subconjunctival oedema. Rarely, haemorrhage can occur from the orbit, and sometimes patients can be aware of a sudden onset of a pulsation within their head [75].

Spontaneous orbital haemorrhage from a normal healthy orbital vessel is rare. It may occur during an extreme rise in orbital venous pressure due to a marked Valsalva manoeuvre (delivery, exertional sports such as weightlifting), extreme venous congestion (severe vomiting or strangulation), and an orbital fracture if the small vessels which perforate the orbital walls are sheared. The site of blow can be outside the orbit (i.e. frontal fracture) and this should be considered where there is loss of vision in the absence of direct injury.

In contrast, haemorrhage from fragile vessels in the elderly patient is relatively common, and the most common cause of *all* orbital haemorrhages. Associated risk factors are antiplatelet medications, anticoagulants, uncontrolled long-standing hypertension, and chronic diabetes. In these patients, a precipitating event can result in a rapid onset of unilateral proptosis, usually with minimal reduction of vision or eye movements. Imaging typically identifies such spontaneous haemorrhages in the posterior half of the infero-temporal quadrant of the orbit.

Perhaps paradoxically, in both congenital and acquired orbital vascular lesions haemorrhage tends to occur in *low-pressure* venous or venous-lymphatic anomalies, and rarely with *high-flow* lesions. Spontaneous haemorrhage from lymphangiomas usually occur in the first decade or two of life, and become less frequent with age, thought to be due to fibrosis within the anomaly with repeated haemorrhage [75–78].

Rarely, a haemorrhage can occur spontaneously from the superior ophthalmic vein in the absence of a venous-lymphatic lesion, this presumed to be due to rupture from a susceptible past of the venous wall [79]. Radiology identifies a 'pseudoaneurysm', and the clinical features typically improve spontaneously over several months (Fig. 13).

Finally, orbital haemorrhage is also associated with necrotic orbital tumours, and long-standing silicon orbital floor implants where bleeding can occur into the enveloping fibrous sheath. These patients present with acute proptosis, and often

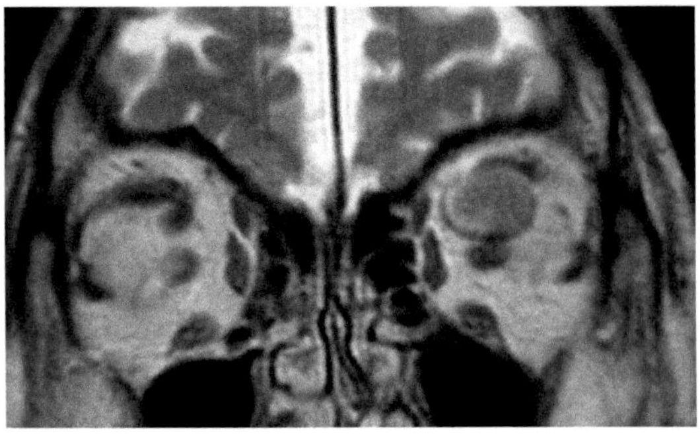

Fig. 13 Superior ophthalmic vein rupture

with hyperglobus, the appearance of periocular bruising being delayed for up to a week [80].

5.1 Management

The hydrostatic pressure generated by arterial haemorrhage is sufficient to arrest vascular perfusion at the orbital apex or in the peripapillary area, with the risk of a precipitous decline in vision. In the presence of dramatic proptosis, marked loss of eye movements and increased resistance to retropulsion, immediate treatment is mandatory to save visual function. Globe rupture must be excluded, then an intermittent firm pressure should be applied to tamponade the orbit until the bleeding subsides (due to vasospasm, platelet action and coagulation). The firm tamponade should be released at regular intervals to permit optic nerve perfusion, the haemorrhage must be drained as soon as possible and the intraorbital pressure reduced by disrupting the orbital septum [75, 81–83].

In the case of an acute *post-operative* haemorrhage, the incision should be widely reopened and, with blunt dissection, the tissues spread to permit the release of the haematoma; orbital fat prolapse results in further lowering of the orbital pressure.

Where the site of haemorrhage is known, direct drainage of the collection can readily be achieved by means of a long horizontal incision placed in the corresponding upper or lower lid skin-crease: deeper tissues are reached by blunt dissection and orbital fat pads are gently spread apart with malleable retractors to release blood and tissue fluid (Fig. 14). Care should be taken to ensure that all blood is aspirated (noting that there may be lacunae of located haemorrhage), and actively bleeding vessels are cauterised. A surgical drain should be placed.

Where the site of haemorrhage is *not* evident, the intraorbital pressure can be released by performing a lateral canthotomy and a wide lateral cantholysis, adequately opening the orbital septum to lower the intraorbital pressure (Fig. 15). The orbital septum must be divided by at least 1–2 cm both upwards and downwards around the rim. Alternatively, a full-thickness perpendicular incision of about 1 cm can be performed through the lateral ends of both eyelids; these incisions are left open (in the event that further haemorrhage occurs), and typically heal well with minimal scarring and no need for surgical revision [75, 84].

Acute intervention is usually not required with a spontaneous vasculopathic haemorrhage, as most will spontaneously reabsorb, albeit over a few months. These patients should be carefully monitored, and orbital drainage reserved for those patients who deteriorate or where there is a decline in vision. Despite the arrest of the haemorrhage, proptosis may increase slightly over the first few weeks due to the hyperosmotic effect of blood breakdown products. Cessation of antiplatelet agents and anticoagulants (having assessed the associated cardiovascular risks) reduces the risk of further haemorrhage [75, 81, 82, 85].

Orbital haemorrhages from venous-lymphatic malformations usually reabsorb over several months. Organising 'cysts' can cause optic neuropathy, globe displacement, and diplopia, and in children can threaten amblyopia. In such cases, consideration should be given to orbital exploration and drainage. Although blood cysts are readily exposed and drained, the risk of further bleeding can be reduced by excising the membrane around the haemorrhage. In the case of persistent lymphatic malformations, sclerotherapy provides a useful alternative treatment and residual lesions can often be removed intact [75].

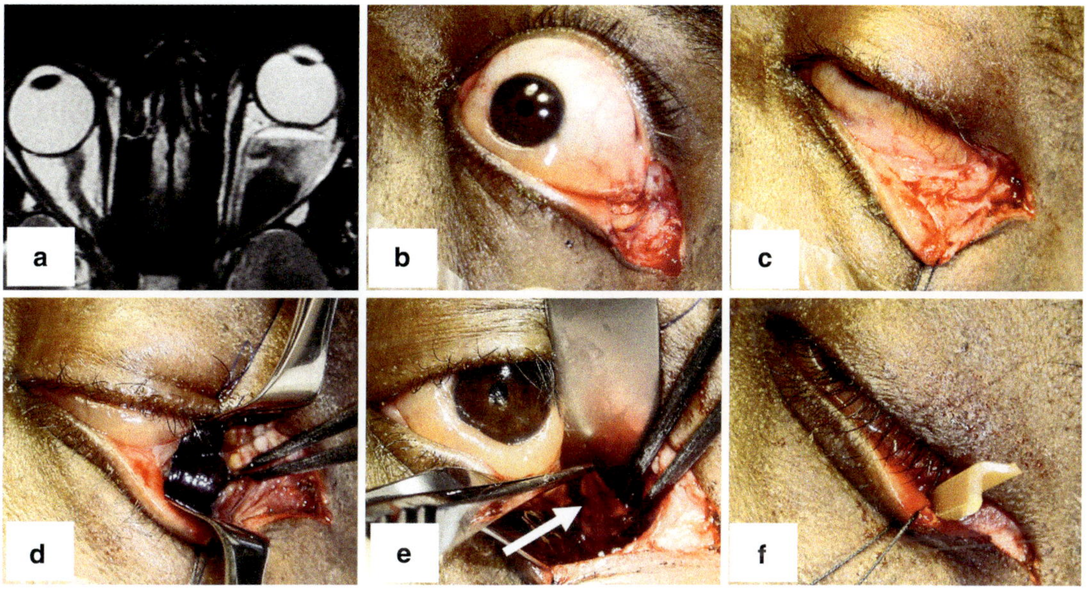

Fig. 14 A patient presented with acute orbital congestion, and reduction of vision (**a**) MR identifies layering of fresh haemorrhage within a presumed vascular anomaly. (**b–f**) The orbit is explored via a lower lid swinging flap, identifying a dilated vascular lesion containing blood, which is evacuated. Histology identifies the wall of the lesion (**e**) as part of a vascular anomaly. (**f**) A corrugated drain is placed for 24 h. Note, the patient represented 3 years later with a further orbital haemorrhage which required further drainage. No further haemorrhage occurred in the 10 years that followed

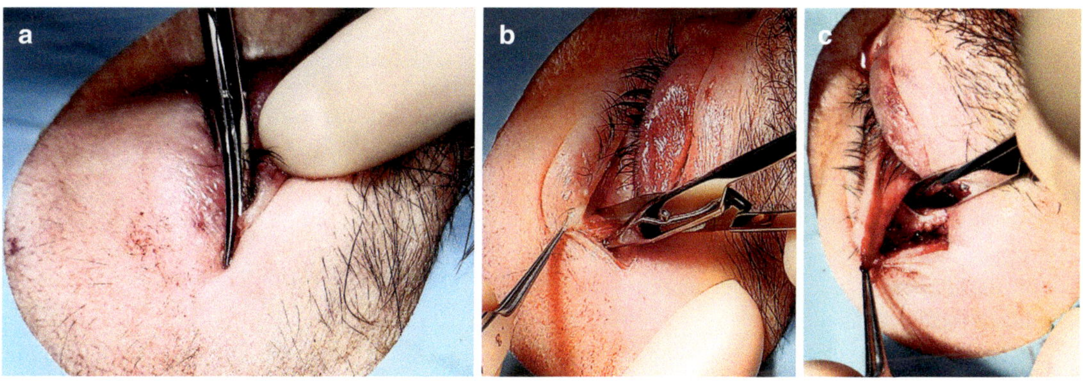

Fig. 15 Lateral canthotomy and cantholysis in case of an acute orbital haemorrhage. (**a**) Lateral canthotomy using tenotomy scissors. (**b**) Cantholysis. (**c**) Wide opening of the orbital septum is probably the most important surgical step to achieve a decrease in intraorbital pressure. Blunt scissors must be open within the orbital fat in the area of the haemorrhage (if known), or in the inferotemporal orbital quadrant (if unknown or in cases of diffuse orbital bleeding)

6 Orbital Vascular Occlusion

Acute occlusion of the orbital venous or arterial vasculature is rare and may occur in the context of underlying vascular anomaly, injury, or infection.

In patients with orbital venous anomalies, acute symptoms can be due to an intralesional haemorrhage or thrombosis, with secondary orbital congestion compromising the vision and even the eye. Surgery for these lesions carries a significant risk to normal structures and sight itself, and the benefits of surgery should always be weighed against potential risks [75].

Superior ophthalmic vein thrombosis is rare, can be uni- or bilateral, and can potentially lead to visual loss in the affected eye(s) [86]. Presenting features are similar to those described above, and the causes are broadly divided into infective, and non infective. The former include bacterial cellulitis, paranasal sinusitis, and septic cavernous sinus thrombosis. Non-infective causes include carotid-cavernous fistula, hypercoagulable states, orbital neoplasm, and idiopathic orbital inflammatory syndromes, including Tolosa-Hunt syndrome. CT venography (CTV) and MR venography (MRV) identify a linear filling defect that dilates the vein and, if originating in the vein, can extend into the ipsilateral cavernous sinus.

One of the most aggressive forms of orbital vascular occlusion occurs in rhino-orbito-cerebral mucormycosis, where invasive mucormycosis causes tissue necrosis due to fungal angioinvasion and thrombosis. This life-threatening infection causes cerebral vasculitis and infection and requires urgent treatment with the advice and support of infectious disease and intensive care physicians, head-and-neck surgeons, and neurosurgeons. Mucormycosis is usually confined to patients with altered host immune systems amongst which diabetes is considered the strongest risk factor. It is the most common opportunistic fungal infection encountered after COVID-19 infection, which causes dysregulation and alteration of the immune response, predisposing to invasive fungal infections [86]. Corticosteroid treatment greatly increases the risk of Mucormycosis. Management typically involves endoscopic sinus surgery, debridement of infected or necrotic tissues, orbital exenteration, high-dose systemic antifungal therapy (amphotericin-B, posaconazole, and isavuconazole) and can also include anticoagulation [75, 87].

Occlusion of the orbital arterial circulation is a rare event, and it is usually due to prolonged external pressure leading to closure of the arterial circulation with impaired eye movements and pupil reactions, ischaemic anterior uveitis, and loss of vision. It may occur during neurosurgical procedures in which the patient is placed in a prone position without guarding the orbit, or in an unconscious individual after a prolonged period of inadvertent pressure on the globe and the orbit [75].

References

1. Tawfik HA, Dutton JJ. Orbital vascular anomalies: A Nomenclatorial, Etiological, and Nosologic Conundrum. Ophthalmic Plast Reconstr Surg. 2022;38:108–21.
2. Verity DH, Restorie M, Rose GE. The natural history of blood velocity and lesion size in infantile orbital capillary haemangiomata. Eye. 2006;20:1228–37.
3. Stass-Isern M. Periorbital and orbital infantile hemangiomas. Int Ophthalmol Clin. 2014;54:73–82.
4. Haik BG, Karcioglu ZA, Gordon RA, Pechous BP. Capillary hemangioma (infantile periocular hemangioma). Surv Ophthalmol. 1994;38:399–426.
5. Kowalska M, Dębek W, Matuszczak E. Infantile hemangiomas: an update on pathogenesis and treatment. J Clin Med. 2021;10:4631.
6. Sebaratnam DF, Rodríguez Bandera A, l., Wong LCF, Wargon O. Infantile hemangioma. Part 2: management. J Am Acad Dermatol. 2021;85:1395–404.
7. Albanese G, Mohandas P, Wells L, Ravenscroft J, Srinivasan J, Thomas S, et al. Orbital infantile haemangioma: radiological features and treatment—case series and literature review. Orbit. 2019;38:67–71.
8. Al-Haddad C, El Salloukh NA, El Moussawi Z. β-Blockers in the treatment of periocular infantile hemangioma. Curr Opin Ophthalmol. 2019;30:319–25.
9. Xu S, Jia R, Ge S, Lin M, Fan X. Treatment of periorbital infantile haemangiomas: a systematic literature review on propranolol or steroids. J Paediatr Child Health. 2014;50:271–9.
10. Fridman G, Grieser E, Hill R, Khuddus N, Bersani T, Slonim C. Propranolol for the treatment of orbital

infantile hemangiomas. Ophthal Plast Reconstr Surg. 2011;27:190–4.
11. Men CJ, Ediriwickrema LS, Paik JS, Murdock J, Yen MT, Ng JD, et al. Surgical intervention of periocular infantile hemangiomas in the era of β-blockers. Ophthal Plast Reconstr Surg. 2020;36:70–3.
12. Hadrawi M, Alghamdi A, Alageel N, Abudawood G, Alshareef F, Abuauf M. Early vascular embolization of large orbital and periorbital infantile capillary hemangiomas; A case report. Am J Ophthalmol Case Rep. 2022;25:101377.
13. Gupta T, Rose GE, Manisali M, Minhas P, Uddin JM, Verity DH. Cranio-orbital intraosseous cavernous haemangioma. Eye (Lond). 2013;27:1320–3.
14. Choi JS, Bae YC, Bin KG, Choi KU. Intraosseous hemangioma of the orbit. Arch Craniofac Surg. 2018;19:68–71.
15. Grob SR, Wolkow N, Jakobiec FA, Lefebvre DR. Osseous cavernous hemangioma of the superior orbital rim. Orbit. 2019;38:259.
16. Hwang K. Intraosseous hemangioma of the orbit. J Craniofac Surg. 2000;11:386–7.
17. ISSVA classification for vascular anomalies© [Internet]. 2014. Available from: https://www.issva.org/UserFiles/file/ISSVA-Classification-2018.pdf.
18. Tawfik HA, Dutton JJ. Orbital vascular anomalies: a nomenclatorial, etiological, and nosologic conundrum. Ophthal Plast Reconstr Surg. 2022;38:108–21.
19. Nassiri N, Rootman J, Rootman DB, Goldberg RA. Orbital lymphaticovenous malformations: current and future treatments. Surv Ophthalmol. 2015;60:383–405.
20. Wiegand S, Eivazi B, Bloch LM, Zimmermann AP, Sesterhenn AM, Schulze S, et al. Lymphatic malformations of the orbit. Clin Exp Otorhinolaryngol. 2013;6:30–5.
21. Bisdorff A, Mulliken JB, Carrico J, Robertson RL, Burrows PE. Intracranial vascular anomalies in patients with periorbital lymphatic and lymphaticovenous malformations. AJNR Am J Neuroradiol. 2007;28:335.
22. Bilaniuk LT. Vascular lesions of the orbit in children. Neuroimaging Clin N Am. 2005;15:107–20.
23. Prat D, Gomel N, Zloto O, Anne M, Bensaid A, Bhattacharjee K, et al. Low-dose bleomycin injections for orbital lymphatic and lymphatic-venous malformations: a multicentric case series study. Ophthal Plast Reconstr Surg. 2021;37:361–5.
24. Lacey B, Rootman J, Marotta TR. Distensible venous malformations of the orbit: clinical and hemodynamic features and a new technique of management. Ophthalmology. 1999;106:1197–209.
25. Cohen LM, Grob SR, Krantz KB, Feldman KA, Rootman DB. Combined endonasal and orbital approach for resection of orbital apical tumors. Ophthal Plast Reconstr Surg. 2022;38:393–400.
26. Rootman DB, Diniz SB, Cohen LM. Clinical assessment and lesion-specific management of orbital vascular malformations. J Neurol Surg B Skull Base. 2021;82:116–28.
27. Abdelaziz O, Hassan F, Elessawy K, Emad-Eldin S, El ER. Image-guided percutaneous bleomycin and bevacizumab sclerotherapy of orbital lymphatic malformations in children. Cardiovasc Intervent Radiol. 2019;42:433–40.
28. Mustak H, Ugradar S, Goldberg R, Rootman D. Bevacizumab and bleomycin combination for treatment of orbital lymphatico-venous malformation recalcitrant to sclerosing therapy alone. Clin Experiment Ophthalmol. 2018;46:815–6.
29. Shimano KA, Eng W, Adams DM. How we approach the use of sirolimus and new agents: medical therapy to treat vascular anomalies. Pediatr Blood Cancer. 2022;69:e29603.
30. Luo Y, Liu L, Rogers D, Su W, Odaka Y, Zhou H, et al. Rapamycin inhibits lymphatic endothelial cell tube formation by downregulating vascular endothelial growth factor receptor 3 protein expression. Neoplasia. 2012;14:228–37.
31. Shoji MK, Shishido S, Freitag SK. The use of sirolimus for treatment of orbital lymphatic malformations: a systematic review. Ophthal Plast Reconstr Surg. 2020;36:215–21.
32. Purt B, Rana HS, Whitescarver TD, Chou E. Novel treatment of recurrent orbital venolymphatic malformation with sirolimus and rivaroxaban. Orbit. 2022;41:771–8.
33. Lam SC, Yuen HKL. Medical and sclerosing agents in the treatment of orbital lymphatic malformations: what's new? Curr Opin Ophthalmol. 2019;30:380–5.
34. Patel SR, Rosenberg JB, Barmettler A. Interventions for orbital lymphangioma. Cochrane Database Syst Rev. 2019;5:CD013000.
35. Sheth T, Rene C. Severe orbital inflammation and hemorrhage complicating bleomycin sclerotherapy for orbital lymphaticovenous malformation. Orbit. 2023;42:316–22.
36. Faiz K, Finitsis S, Linton J, Shankar JJS. Bleomycin for orbital and peri-orbital veno-lymphatic malformations—A systematic review. Interv Neuroradiol. 2021;27:291–7.
37. Strianese D, Bonavolontà G, Iuliano A, Mariniello G, Elefante A, Liuzzi R. Risks and benefits of surgical excision of orbital cavernous venous malformations (so-called cavernous hemangioma): factors influencing the outcome. Ophthal Plast Reconstr Surg. 2021;37:248–54.
38. Vahdani K, Rose GE. Pupillary abnormalities after excision of orbital cavernous venous malformations. Ophthalmic Plast Reconstr Surg. 2023;39:40–3.
39. Maaijwee K, Nowak PJ, van den Bosch WA, Paridaens D. Fractionated stereotactic radiotherapy for cavernous haemangioma of the orbital apex. Acta Ophthalmol. 2012;90:e655–7.
40. Rootman J, Heran MKS, Graeb DA. Vascular malformations of the orbit: classification and the role of imaging in diagnosis and treatment strategies. Ophthal Plast Reconstr Surg. 2014;30:91–104.
41. Cheung EYH, Ng RYT, Yu SCH, Zhuang JTF, Wong GKC. PHIL and squid embolization of cerebral arte-

riovenous malformation: a retrospective case series of 23 patients. Neurointervention. 2022;17:174–82.
42. Al-Samkari H, Kasthuri RS, Parambil JG, Albitar HA, Almodallal YA, Vázquez C, et al. An international, multicenter study of intravenous bevacizumab for bleeding in hereditary hemorrhagic telangiectasia: The InHIBIT-Bleed study. Haematologica. 2021;106:2161–9.
43. Kim MS, Han DH, Kwon OK, Oh CW, Han MH. Clinical characteristics of dural arteriovenous fistula. J Clin Neurosci. 2002;9:147–55.
44. De Keizer RJW. Carotid-cavernous and orbital arteriovenous fistulas: ocular features, diagnostic and hemodynamic considerations in relation to visual impairment and morbidity. Orbit. 2003;22:121–42.
45. Miller NR. Dural carotid-cavernous fistulas: epidemiology, clinical presentation, and management. Neurosurg Clin N Am. 2012;23:179–92.
46. Lacorzana J, Rocha-de-Lossada C, Ortiz-Perez S. A tricky case of unilateral orbital inflammation: carotid cavernous fistula in Graves-Basedow disease. Rom J Ophthalmol. 2021;65:201–3.
47. Naqvi J, Laitt R, Leatherbarrow B, Herwadkar A. A case of a spontaneous intraorbital arteriovenous fistula: clinico-radiological findings and treatment by transvenous embolisation via the superior ophthalmic vein. Orbit. 2013;32:124–6.
48. Sharpless M, Mahady K, Sullivan TJ. Conservative management of spontaneous intraorbital arteriovenous fistulas. Clin Experiment Ophthalmol. 2020;48:121–3.
49. Ghorbani M, Hejazian SE, Dastmalchi A, Chavoshinejad M, Asaadi S. Orbital compartment syndrome secondary to direct carotid cavernous fistula after carotid cavernous aneurysm rupture: case report and review of literature. World Neurosurg. 2020;133:409–12.
50. Tan B, Rootman J, Seah LL. Combined radiological intervention and surgical excision of a periorbital arteriovenous fistula. Orbit. 2013;32:181–3.
51. Gemmete JJ, Ansari SA, Gandhi DM. Endovascular techniques for treatment of carotid-cavernous fistula. J Neuroophthalmol. 2009;29:62–71.
52. Tjoumakaris SI, Jabbour PM, Rosenwasser RH. Neuroendovascular management of carotid cavernous fistulae. Neurosurg Clin N Am. 2009;20:447–52.
53. Williamson RW, Ducruet AF, Crowley RW, McDougall CG, Albuquerque FC. Transvenous coil embolization of an intraorbital arteriovenous fistula: case report and review of the literature. Neurosurgery. 2013;72:E130–4.
54. Akamatsu Y, Kubo Y, Chida K, Matsumoto Y, Ogasawara K. Combined surgical and endovascular treatment of an intraorbital arteriovenous fistula drained into a basal vein of Rosenthal: a technical case report. World Neurosurg. 2020;141:15–9.
55. Jones TL. Sinus pericranii. Radiol Technol. 2012;83:349–64.
56. Kang S, Hamed-Azzam S, Robertson F, Davagnanam I, Verity DH. Pulsating lid: a rare presentation of sinus pericranii. Can J Ophthalmol. 2020;55:e100–4.
57. Antman K, Chang Y. Kaposi's sarcoma. N Engl J Med. 2000;342:1027–38.
58. Fossataro F, Iuliano A, Uccello G, Lanni V, D'Andrea L, Mascolo M, et al. A rare case of bilateral conjunctival Kaposi's sarcoma in a HIV-negative patient. Am J Ophthalmol Case Rep. 2021;21:101024.
59. Viejo-Borbolla A, Schulz TF. Kaposi's sarcoma-associated herpesvirus (KSHV/HHV8): key aspects of epidemiology and pathogenesis. AIDS Rev. 2003;5:222–9.
60. Donovan C, Patel H, Shetty S, Bierman L, Lustbader JM, Oboh-Weilke AM. Aggressive conjunctival Kaposi sarcoma as the initial manifestation of acquired immunodeficiency syndrome. Am J Ophthalmol Case Rep. 2020;19:100832.
61. Coblentz J, Park JY, Discepola G, Arthurs B, Burnier M. Conjunctival Kaposi's sarcoma with orbital extension in an HIV-negative man. Can J Ophthalmol. 2018;53:e111–3.
62. Yang J, Yin XF, Li YP, Zhou SY. Case report of ocular Kaposi's sarcoma. BMC Ophthalmol. 2017;17:143.
63. Souhail H, Albouzidi A, Laktaoui A, Kriet M, Channa H, Benomar S, Terhzaz A, Alioia Z. Orbital location of Kaposi's sarcoma. J Fr Ophtalmol. 2003;26:1071–4. [Article in French].
64. Scheschonka A, Mösch M, Krieglsteiner S, Turowski B, Zanella FE. Pre- and posttreatment MR imaging in AIDS-related Kaposi sarcoma of the conjunctiva and lacrimal gland. AJNR Am J Neuroradiol. 2003;24:1327–9.
65. Ulloa-Padilla JP, Ghassibi MP, Dubovy SR, Kerr DA. Clinicopathologic correlation of Kaposi sarcoma involving the ocular adnexa: immunophenotyping of diagnostic and therapeutic targets. Ophthal Plast Reconstr Surg. 2020;36:185–90.
66. Meyer D, Gooding C. Intralesional bleomycin as an adjunct therapeutic modality in eyelid and extraocular malignancies and tumors. Middle East Afr J Ophthalmol. 2015;22:410–4.
67. Jin C, Minhas H, Kaur A, Kodali S, Gotlieb V. A case of ocular Kaposi's sarcoma successfully treated with highly active antiretroviral therapy (HAART) combined with docetaxel. Am J Case Rep. 2018;19:1074–7.
68. Gelston CD, Said S, Durairaj VD. Orbital kaposiform hemangioendothelioma. J Pediatr Ophthalmol Strabismus. 2012;49:e1–4.
69. North PE. Pediatric vascular tumors and malformations. Surg Pathol Clin. 2010;3:455–94.
70. Zukerberg LR, Nickoloff BJ, Weiss SW. Kaposiform hemangioendothelioma of infancy and childhood. An aggressive neoplasm associated with Kasabach-Merritt syndrome and lymphangiomatosis. Am J Surg Pathol. 1993;17:321–8.
71. Triana P, Dore M, Cerezo VN, Cervantes M, Sánchez AV, Ferrero MM, et al. Sirolimus in the treat-

ment of vascular anomalies. Eur J Pediatr Surg. 2017;27:086–90.
72. Lackner H, Karastaneva A, Schwinger W, Benesch M, Sovinz P, Seidel M, et al. Sirolimus for the treatment of children with various complicated vascular anomalies. Eur J Pediatr. 2015;174:1579–84.
73. Lee BB. Sirolimus in the treatment of vascular anomalies. J Vasc Surg. 2020;71:328.
74. Wright JE, Sullivan TJ, Garner A, Wulc AE, Moseley IF. Orbital venous anomalies. Ophthalmology. 1997;104:905–13.
75. Rose GE, Verity DH. Acute presentation of vascular disease within the orbit—A descriptive synopsis of mechanisms. Eye (Lond). 2013;27:299–307.
76. Sullivan TJ, Wright JE. Non-traumatic orbital haemorrhage. Clin Experiment Ophthalmol. 2000;28:26–31.
77. Atalla ML, McNab AA, Sullivan TJ, Sloan B. Nontraumatic subperiosteal orbital hemorrhage. Ophthalmology. 2001;108:183–9.
78. Moin M, Kersten RC, Bernardini F, Kulwin D, Biddinger PW, Ernst RJ, et al. Spontaneous hemorrhage in an intraorbital arteriovenous malformation. Ophthalmology. 2000;107:2215–9.
79. Vahdani K, Rose GE. Acute spontaneous rupture of the superior ophthalmic vein. Ophthalmic Plast Reconstr Surg. 2020;36:545–8.
80. Gilhotra JS, McNab AA, McKelvie P, O'Donnell BA. Late orbital haemorrhage around alloplastic orbital floor implants: a case series and review. Clin Experiment Ophthalmol. 2002;30:352–5.
81. Winterton JV, Patel K, Mizen KD. Review of management options for a retrobulbar hemorrhage. J Oral Maxillofac Surg. 2007;65:296–9.
82. Zimmerer R, Schattmann K, Essig H, Jehn P, Metzger M, Kokemüller H, et al. Efficacy of transcutaneous transseptal orbital decompression in treating acute retrobulbar hemorrhage and a literature review. Craniomaxillofac Trauma Reconstr. 2014;7:17–26.
83. Burkat CN, Lemke BN. Retrobulbar hemorrhage: inferolateral anterior orbitotomy for emergent management. Arch Ophthalmol. 2005;123:1260–2.
84. Ballard SR, Enzenauer RW, O'Donnell T, Fleming JC, Risk G, Waite AN. Emergency lateral canthotomy and cantholysis: a simple procedure to preserve vision from sight threatening orbital haemorrhage. J Spec Oper Med. 2009;9:26–32.
85. Chou BW, Rivera QN, Francis CE. Spontaneous retrobulbar haemorrhage in the setting of warfarin therapy and latent scurvy diagnosis. Orbit. 2022;41:127–9.
86. Sotoudeh H, Shafaat O, Aboueldahab N, Vaphiades M, Sotoudeh E, Bernstock J. Superior ophthalmic vein thrombosis: what radiologist and clinician must know? Eur J Radiol Open. 2019;6:258–64.
87. Naurka S, Rana N, Singh N, Kishore A, Nagpal K. COVID-19 associated rhino-orbital-cerebral mucormycosis—an institutional series. Ear Nose Throat J. 2022:1455613221077882.

Neurogenic Tumours

Peerooz Saeed and Michael Schittkowski

Key Messages

- Diagnosis and treatment of orbital neurogenic tumours remain a challenge as uncertainty persists over the aetiology, pathogenesis, and natural history of these lesions. Both optic nerve and orbital peripheral nerve sheath tumours may be associated with neurofibromatosis.
- Optic nerve sheath meningiomas arise from a proliferation of meningothelial cells within the nerve sheath of the orbital or intracanalicular portion of the optic nerve. Primary radiation therapy may improve or stabilise visual acuity.
- Secondary orbital meningiomas can invade the bone and, by hyperostosis, involve the postero-lateral orbit and push laterally into the temporal fossa. Lesser sphenoid wing meningiomas may gain access to the orbit through the superior orbital fissure, or by invasion through the bone at the orbital apex.
- Optic pathway gliomas are the most common tumours of the optic nerve and are difficult to treat due to the risk of visual loss. Observation is recommended for newly diagnosed gliomas, and resection for progressive intraorbital tumours associated with blindness, cosmetic deformity or discomfort. Radiotherapy is preferred for progressive chiasmatic tumours in older children; chemotherapy for children younger than 5 years with progressive disease.
- Peripheral nerve tumours consist primarily of neurofibromas and schwannomas (neurilemmomas). Neurofibromas may occur in a plexiform, diffuse, and solitary pattern.
- Malignant peripheral nerve sheath tumours are rare and aggressive. Combined exenteration and craniotomy may be required for tumours with an intracranial component, followed by adjuvant radiotherapy.

1 Orbital Neurogenic Tumours

Primary and secondary neurogenic tumours are common in the orbit, probably because of the many nerves supplying this region. Diagnosis and treatment remain a challenge, as uncertainty persists over the aetiology, pathogenesis, and natural history of these lesions.

This chapter reviews the most common neurogenic tumours of the orbit, including optic nerve

P. Saeed (✉)
Orbital Centre, Department of Ophthalmology, Amsterdam University Medical Center, Amsterdam, The Netherlands
e-mail: P.Saeed@amsterdamumc.nl

M. Schittkowski
Section for Strabismus and Neuroophthalmology, Department of Ophthalmology, University Medicine Goettingen, Goettingen, Germany

F. M. Quaranta Leoni et al. (eds.), *Oculoplastic, Lacrimal and Orbital Surgery*,
https://doi.org/10.1007/978-3-031-39638-0_23

sheath meningiomas, optic pathway gliomas and peripheral nerve tumours.

1.1 Anatomy

All cranial nerves are peripheral nerves, with the exception of the optic nerve, which is a tract of diencephalon (posterior portion of the forebrain). As such, the optic nerve is ensheathed in all three meningeal layers (dura mater, arachnoid, and pia mater) rather than the epineurium, perineurium, and endoneurium found in peripheral nerves [1–3]. The fibres of the optic nerve are covered with myelin produced by oligodendrocytes, rather than Schwann cells of the peripheral nervous system [3, 4].

Primary orbital meningiomas occur within the optic nerve arachnoid space or in ectopic orbital sites, while optic nerve gliomas arise from glial cells of the optic nerve [3]. Cranial nerve ganglia originate in the central nervous system.

The main peripheral nerve sheath tumours are characterised by neoplastic proliferations with Schwann cell differentiation. For instance, the Schwann cell represents the primary neoplastic cell component of neurofibroma characterised cytologically by wavy nuclear contours and S-100 protein expression. Neurofibromas also incorporate a mixture of non-neoplastic peripheral nerve components, including axons, perineurial cells, fibroblasts, and variable inflammatory elements, such as mast cells and lymphocytes [2, 5].

2 Neurofibromatoses (NF-1 and NF-2)

Both optic nerve and orbital peripheral nerve sheath tumours may be associated with one of the neurofibromatoses. These syndromes are caused by specific gene mutations and are characterised by various cutaneous pigmentary disorders, and peripheral or central nervous system benign and malignant tumours.

NF1 (von Recklinghausen's disease) is an autosomal dominant genetic disorder occurring in 1 in 3000 births and is due to a mutation in the NF1 gene at chromosome 17q11. It represents the classic peripheral neurofibromatosis with cutaneous lesions including multiple cafe-au-lait macules, axillary freckles, iris Lisch nodules and neurofibromas. In most cases, the NF-1 diagnosis is based on the minimal criterion of at least six café-au-lait spots measuring at least 15 mm in diameter. Sphenoid wing bone anomalies and optic pathway gliomas (occurring in 15% of NF1 patients) appear by the age of 3 years. Malignant transformation of tumours may occur in late adolescence or adulthood.

NF2 is a much rarer autosomal dominant genetic disorder caused by abnormalities in the NF2 gene on chromosome 22 [3]; this gene produces *merlin*, a tumour suppressor protein, and affected individuals are predisposed to various nervous system neoplasia including bilateral vestibular schwannomas, intracranial and optic nerve sheath meningiomas, and spine tumours [4]. It represents the classic central neurofibromatosis; Lisch nodules are never seen and café-au-lait macules are present in only in 50% of the cases.

The original diagnostic proposals for NF2 emphasised the necessity of a family history of the disease or bilateral vestibular schwannomas. The current diagnostic criteria take into account that peripheral nerve schwannomas, spinal tumours, cranial meningiomas and ocular abnormalities often develop before vestibular schwannomas, and that half of affected individuals do not have a family history of NF2. NF2 mosaicism manifests as mild generalised disease or as clinical features localised to one area of the nervous system, most commonly ipsilateral vestibular schwannomas and meningiomas [1, 2, 4, 6].

3 Optic Nerve Sheath Meningiomas

3.1 Pathogenesis

Optic nerve sheath meningiomas (ONSMs) arise from a proliferation of meningothelial cells within the nerve sheath of the orbital or intracanalicular portion of the optic nerve. Independent of the primary site of origin, ONSMs usually spread around the optic nerve, through the subdural and subarachnoid spaces, following pathways of least resistance such as vessels and the dural septa (Fig. 1). As they spread, they compromise nerve function by impairing blood supply to the nerve and by interfering

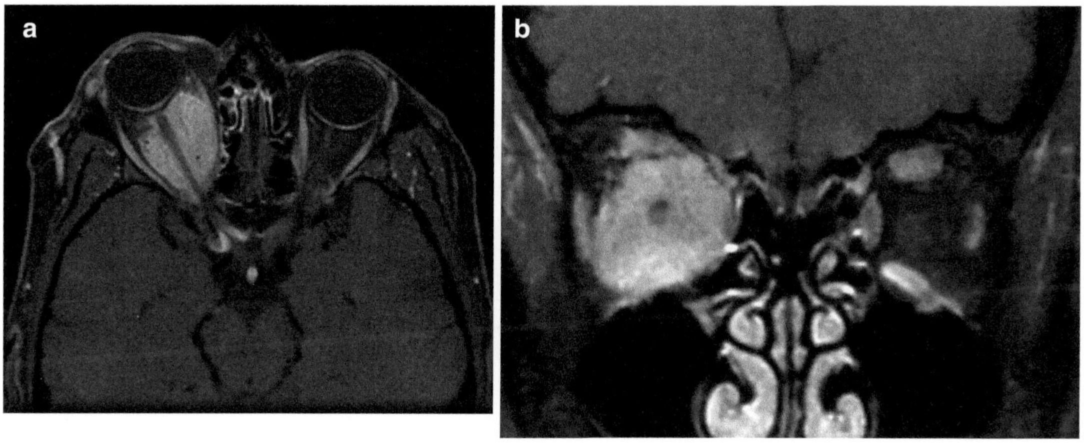

Fig. 1 Fat-suppressed T1 axial (**a**) coronal (**b**) MRI, with gadolinium showing globular configuration of optic nerve sheath meningioma with tram track sign on axial image

with axonal transport. Thus, the tumours are interposed between the nerve substance and its extradurally derived blood supply, making their resection difficult [7, 8]. Some ONSMs remain localised to a small segment of the optic nerve, whereas others spread to surround the entire length of the orbital and canalicular portions of the nerve. In rare cases, the tumour spreads through dura to infiltrate adjacent orbital structures, including fat, extraocular muscles, and bone [7, 8].

3.2 Epidemiology

Meningiomas typically arise in adults in their fourth to sixth decades of life and are rare in children. They are more common in African-Americans and in females, with a 2:1 female to male ratio in intracranial meningiomas; in Africans there seems to be a gender-equal distribution [7].

ONSMs occur more commonly in middle-aged women, but reports of the female: male distribution vary widely in the literature; ratios as high as a 5:1 female predilection have been cited [7–10].

Approximately 4–7% of ONSMs occur in childhood. Unlike those in adults, childhood ONSMs display no gender predilection, and they are often associated with NF-2. The prognosis for childhood orbital meningioma is poor compared with that in older patients. In addition to producing visual impairment, the tumour may extend to adjacent areas, such as the cavernous sinus, sella turcica, annulus of Zinn, pterygomaxillary fossa, and medial sphenoid wing [7–10].

3.3 Clinical Features

The most common symptom of the ONSMs is visual deterioration (80%). Proptosis is observed in 30% of patients and is generally small, with mean exophthalmometry of 3.2 (range, 0–13) mm. Optic disc changes are observed in 97%: disc swelling is the most frequent change, followed by atrophy and optociliary shunts. Although visual loss, optic atrophy, and optociliary shunt vessels are characteristic signs of ONSM, this triad may be seen in as few as 25% of patients. Presenting visual acuity is a broad prognostic factor: patients with better than 20/50 visual acuity tend to retain good acuity for some time [7].

3.4 Imaging

Magnetic resonance imaging (MRI) is the technique of choice for evaluating optic nerve tumours, including ONSM. CT scanning, however, is more sensitive for recognizing calcification and with contrast highlights these very vascular tumours. On T1-weighted images, ONSMs are typically isointense or slightly hypointense to brain and optic nerve tissue. T1-weighted images with gadolinium enhancement and fat suppression typically provide recognition and good definition of meningiomas, both intracranially and within the orbit and optic canal [7–10].

The diagnosis of ONSM relies heavily on radiographic growth patterns that can be described in four imaging categories:

1. Tubular with diffuse expansion growth patterns, apical expansion toward the orbital apex, or anterior nerve expansion toward the globe.
2. Globular growth pattern caused by exophytic expansion outside the nerve sheath.
3. Spindle-shaped fusiform patterns with tapers at the proximal and distal ends.
4. Focal exophytic lesions (only occasionally observed).

Calcification is observed in 31% of ONSM. The presence of dense calcification indicates slow tumour growth [7].

A radiographic study on ONSM found that among the 8% of cases confined to the optic canal, bilaterality was higher (38%) than in intraorbital ONSMs. Half the patients with bilateral ONSMs had tumours along the planum sphenoidale, continuous with the lesions in both optic canals. Thus, it appears that some cases of apparently bilateral ONSMs were truly bilateral, whereas others represent either the spread of a planum sphenoidale meningioma to both optic canals or a unilateral ONSM across the planum to the contralateral optic canal [7].

Imaging may not always definitively distinguish ONSM from other optic nerve pathology. Accurate diagnosis is aided by the clinical pattern and occasionally surgical biopsy. However, biopsies are associated with a high risk of visual loss and the spread of the tumour within the orbit, particularly in the case of ONSMs. Thus, a less invasive diagnostic procedure is desirable [11].

In vitro and *in vivo* studies have demonstrated that meningiomas have a dense, homogeneous distribution of somatostatin receptors (SSRs) and that somatostatin receptor scintigraphy (SSRS) can be used *in vivo* to identify SSR-positive tumours (Fig. 2). However, several other neoplasms, such as neuroendocrine tumours and non-Hodgkin lymphoma, also show increased

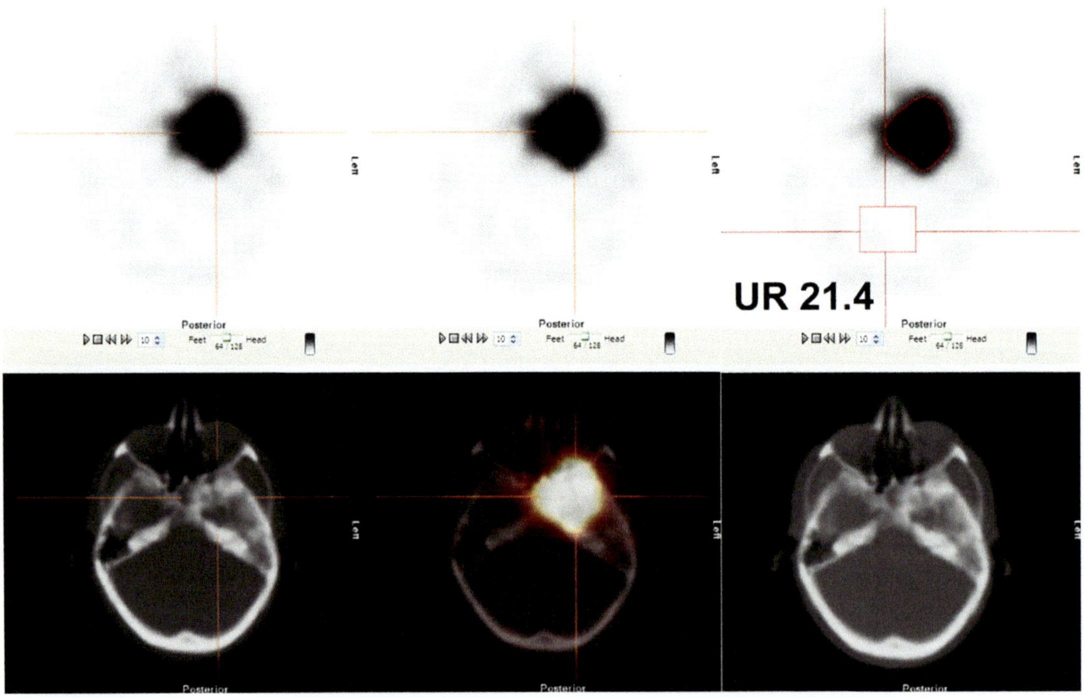

Fig. 2 Somatostatin receptor scintigraphy of an orbital meningioma with a somatostatin uptake of 21.4

somatostatin receptor expression. SSR uptake ratio in meningiomas is significantly higher than in other orbital tumour subgroups, with the exception of adenocarcinoma. Using a threshold uptake ratio of 5.9, the sensitivity of SSRS for ONSM is as high as 100%, and the specificity up to 97.2%. SSRS can be used for the differential diagnosis of ONSM, vascular lesions, non-Hodgkin lymphomas (NHLs), optic nerve gliomas, idiopathic orbital inflammation, and sarcoid, and the procedure potentially reduces the need for an intraorbital biopsy. However, SSRS cannot completely replace histopathological diagnosis because, despite the risks, atypical cases may still require biopsy [11].

Ga68-DOTATOC, a method which combines PET and MRI with Gallium-labelled octreotide, was shown to have high sensitivity in detecting ONSM and might be helpful in unclear cases to avoid risks of surgical biopsy [12].

3.5 Management

Treatment of ONSM has changed substantially over recent decades. Twenty years ago, most clinicians considered optic nerve meningioma to be untreatable. Patients were followed clinically and with imaging, and surgical resection of the nerve was only offered when the tumour threatened the optic chiasm [7, 8].

Primary radiation therapy, however, has the potential to improve or stabilise visual acuity in many patients with progressive ONSM. In one series, only 9% showed progressive visual deterioration after radiation treatment. The adverse effects of newer radiotherapy machines and fractionated stereotactic delivery methods are transient or minor [13, 14]. Recent studies recommend radiotherapy even before vision deterioration occurs [15].

3.6 Role of Surgery

Surgical excision of ONSM is technically difficult and associated with post-operative blindness; thus, in some regions it has been replaced by radiation therapy. However, surgery continues to be used for biopsies in atypical cases and in cases where visual preservation is not possible. Surgery may be indicated for orbitocranial lesions that extend to the prechiasmal and parachiasmal regions, particularly with a large intracranial component, or in cases where the planum sphenoidale is involved. Presently, vision-sparing, microsurgical dissection for primary ONSM is not feasible because of the involvement of the pial blood supply to the nerve via the meningioma [7–10].

4 Ectopic Orbital Meningiomas

Nineteen cases of orbital meningiomas with no connection to the optic nerve sheath or intracranial meninges have been reported and are known as “ectopic” or “extradural” meningiomas. Patients ranged in age from 7 to 71 years. With the exception of one 9-year-old girl, all patients were male, in contrast to most meningioma series. The tumours were located either at the orbital rim or in the medial orbital wall, with adhesion to the periosteum; in one intraconal case, the lesion was located inferomedial to the optic nerve.

Several theories have been offered to explain the origin of ectopic meningiomas. Although no arachnoidal cells have been found outside the dural sheath of the optic nerve in the orbit, Cushing found arachnoidal cells accompanying certain cranial nerves at their sites of exit through the skull foramina. Others have suggested the presence of similar cells in the arterial sheaths where vessels pierce the skull or in the periosteum. These arachnoidal cells could explain the origin of the ectopic meningiomas [13, 14, 16–19].

Additional sources for orbital ectopic meningiomas have been proposed: (1) from occasional arachnoid “nests” in the orbit, (2) from the optic nerve sheath with separation prior to clinical evaluation, and (3) from smaller nerves endowed with arachnoid cells. It has also been proposed that almost all ectopic meningiomas originate from the same location in the superomedial part of the orbit. This location suggests that ectopic orbital meningiomas could originate from an orbital meningocele or from meningeal tissue that had been trapped outside the central nervous system [13, 14, 16–19].

5 Secondary Meningiomas of the Orbit

Thirty to forty percent of all meningiomas arise from the base of the anterior or middle fossa with the potential to involve the orbit secondarily [14, 20]. Spheno-orbital meningiomas (SOMs) account for half of these tumours, while olfactory groove (OGM) and tuberculum sellae meningiomas (TSM) account for most of the remainder. Extensions of these tumours may enter the orbits, paranasal sinuses, cavernous sinus, sella, infratemporal fossa, and posterior fossa [21–31]. Visual loss is common, occurring in over 95% of patients with TSM and in over 50% of patients with OGM. Meningiomas of the medial third of the sphenoid wing (anterior clinoid meningiomas, ACM) also typically present with ipsilateral visual loss, although contralateral vision is affected in one-third of patients. The original description of the Foster Kennedy syndrome in 1911 included the triad of optic disc pallor in one eye, optic disc oedema in the fellow eye, and anosmia or hyposmia in association with anterior cranial fossa mass lesions, especially OGM and TSM. Other symptoms and signs associated with these meningiomas include headache, and mental or personality changes [4], the latter two of which are most commonly associated with OGM [20, 32–36].

Secondary orbital meningiomas that are large and longstanding show considerable overlap in signs and symptomatology. These meningiomas invade the orbit by one of two routes. They can invade the bone and, by hyperostosis, involve the postero-lateral orbit and push laterally into the temporal fossa. The other pattern of growth is seen in lesser sphenoid wing meningiomas, TSM, and OGM. Here, the tumour gains access to the orbital cavity through the superior orbital fissure, along the optic canal, or by invasion through the bone at the orbital apex [19–22, 24–29, 35–38].

6 Optic Pathway Gliomas

6.1 Pathogenesis and Aetiology

Optic pathway gliomas (OPG) are the most common tumours of the optic nerve. They are difficult to treat due to the high risk of visual loss from intervention. OPG comprise about 1% of all intracranial tumours and are of two different types: juvenile benign pilocytic astrocytoma and adult malignant glioblastoma [4, 23, 30, 31, 39, 40].

6.2 Epidemiology

The mean age of diagnosis of OPG is 8.8 years, although they may occur as late as 79 years old. Additionally, patients with OPGs that invade the hypothalamus typically present at a younger age (often by 1 year of age with diencephalic syndrome}. The female-to-male ratio is roughly equal, although there are some data that suggest that OPGs limited to the optic nerves are more common in girls [30, 40].

OPG are considered benign tumours when diagnosed in paediatric patients. Reports have shown varying levels of incidence of NF-1 among patients of OPG ranging from 10 to 70%, whereas the incidence of OPG in patients with NF-1 varies from 8 to 31%. Optic pathway gliomas that are seen in patients with NF-1 are generally felt to have a better prognosis than those found in isolation.

The true incidence of NF-1 may be considerably higher because most studies fail to mention the presence or absence of this disease in their patients [4, 23, 31, 39].

6.3 Clinical Features

Patients with OPG may be asymptomatic or may develop symptoms based on location. For example, patients with a tumour of the nerve within the orbit may present with proptosis, strabismus, or visual loss, whereas patients with intracranial

OPG can present with visual loss, endocrine/hypothalamic disturbances, spasmus nutans, and obstructive hydrocephalus.

Proptosis is usually gradual and painless; however, on rare occasions, a patient may present with acute loss of vision resulting from haemorrhage into the tumour. Optic disc swelling or pallor, visual acuity loss, visual field loss, and relative afferent pupillary defects may be seen due to the compressive effects of the tumour. The tumour eventually causes optic nerve atrophy because of pressure effects on the nerve fibres as well as the nutrient arteries. Primary and secondary strabismus is seen, along with restriction of extraocular muscle motility. Additionally, dissociated vertical nystagmus may be observed in suprasellar extending lesions.

Bilateral visual loss is associated with chiasmal involvement causing bitemporal field defects. Proptosis is more frequent in patients with NF-1 (21.5%) than in those without (5.5%), whereas patients without NF-1 are more likely to present with nystagmus and hydrocephalus [30, 40].

6.4 Imaging

CT imaging of optic nerve gliomas reveals a well-demarcated enlargement of the nerve, often with a tortuous or kinked appearance. Tumours of the chiasm exhibit various appearances, from enlargement of the chiasm to a suprasellar mass that may calcify. The tumour is usually isodense to the brain, and contrast enhancement is variable. Although OPGs may be readily apparent on CT, MRI is the preferred method. Typical MR imaging findings include an iso- to hypointense lesion on T1-weighted images, with hyperintensity seen on T2-weighted sequences and homogeneous enhancement with gadolinium administration (Fig. 3a, b). Some reports have described detailed MR imaging findings in patients with NF-1, including bilateral tumours with circumferential growth and downward kinking of the intraorbital segment of the optic nerve. Additionally, the double intensity or pseudo-CSF signal is characteristic in NF-1. This consists of a hyperintense core on T1-weighted images

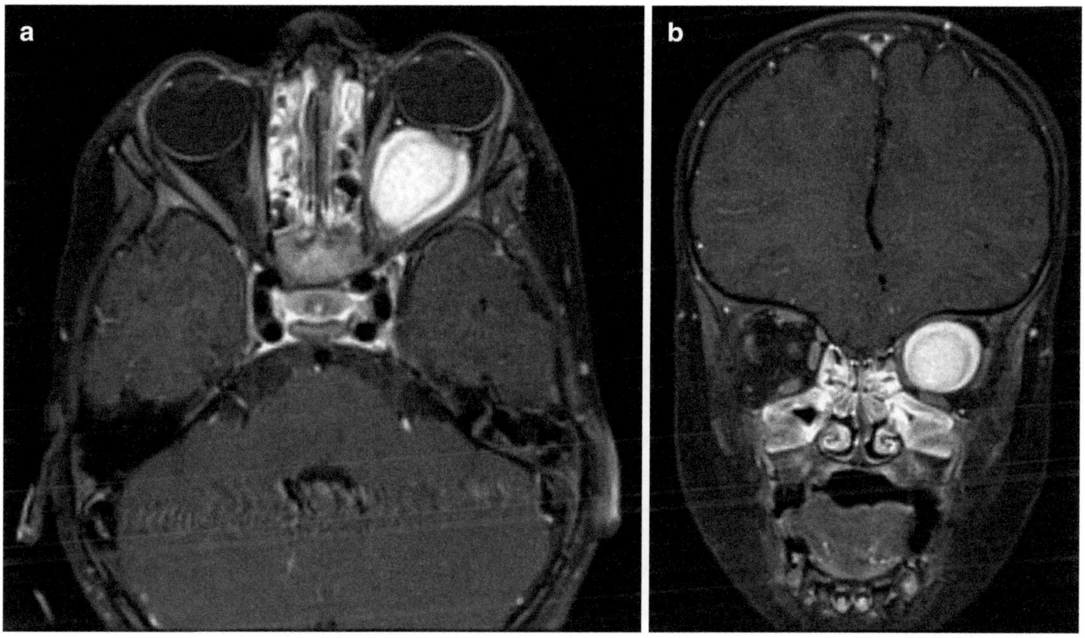

Fig. 3 Fat-suppressed T1 axial (**a**) and coronal (**b**) MRI, with gadolinium showing bulbous enlargement of the right optic nerve, consistent with an optic nerve glioma

surrounded by lower signal intensity. The inverse is seen on T2-weighted images [40–42].

Patients with NF-1 are more likely to demonstrate glioma extension along the optic tracts into the lateral geniculate ganglia and temporal lobes as well as infiltrating lesions. Positron emission tomography technology has also been shown to be useful for monitoring progression and treatment response in OPGs and may reveal changes earlier than MRI.

6.5 Histopathology

Histologically, OPGs in childhood are typically low-grade gliomas and are divided into pilocytic and fibrillary subtypes based on appearance. Pilocytic astrocytomas are more common and classically have a biphasic pattern with characteristic Rosenthal fibres and eosinophilic granular bodies. In contrast, a relatively new subgroup of OPGs has been defined: so-called pilomyxoid astrocytomas. These tumours are characterised by piloid cells in a loose fibrillary and myxoid background, are asymptomatic, and tend to be smaller. They lack Rosenthal fibres and have only rare eosinophilic granular bodies. Pilomyxoid astrocytomas were once classified with pilocytic astrocytomas, but they constitute a distinct entity with more aggressive behaviour [30, 40].

6.6 Management

The natural history of childhood OPG is almost always benign; most tumours grow slowly in a self-limited manner, and some even regress spontaneously. Some long-term studies indicate that patients who are not treated may retain stable visual function. It has been recommended that most patients with unilateral optic nerve gliomas, particularly those with NF-1, be followed at regular intervals both clinically and with neuroimaging, without intervention unless there is documented visual deterioration. Once significant visual deterioration occurs or cosmesis or discomfort becomes troubling, treatment may be considered [43].

6.7 Radiotherapy

Historically, radiation therapy was the treatment of choice for OPGs, but this has fallen out of favour in young children because of possible cognitive and endocrine disturbances, as well as radiation-induced complications such as secondary tumours and occlusive vascular disease. Currently, despite the lack of randomised trials comparing radiation therapy with other treatment modalities, radiation therapy is reserved for the treatment of progressive OPG in children older than 5–7 years of age [40, 44].

6.8 Chemotherapy

Although no single chemotherapeutic agent has been identified as a primary treatment, chemotherapy is considered first-line therapy for OPGs that cause visual loss or pituitary or hypothalamic dysfunction. It can treat tumours that have gone beyond the observation stage, even in young children, without the long-term cognitive and neuroendocrine sequelae seen with surgery and radiation therapy. Because of this, chemotherapy is now the primary treatment modality in children younger than 3 years of age with progressive or symptomatic disease. Agents including carboplatin, cisplatin, vincristine, vinblastine, actinomycin D, lomustine, thioguanine, procarbazine, etoposide, tamoxifen, and temozolomide have been used as first-line therapies. However, the most widely used regimen is a combination of carboplatin and vincristine in a 10-week induction phase, followed by 48 weeks of maintenance carboplatin/vincristine [43–45].

In summary, observation is recommended for newly diagnosed OPG and resection for progressive, large intraorbital tumours associated with blindness, cosmetic deformity or discomfort. Surgery may also be indicated in some exophytic chiasmatic tumours. Radiotherapy is preferred for progressive chiasmatic tumours in older children, and chemotherapy for those in children younger than 5 years with progressive disease [43–47].

6.9 Natural History and Clinical Course

Overall, OPGs tend to be low-grade and slow growing with long patient survival. Additionally, the presence of NF-1 and an anterior location are associated with a more favourable prognosis, whereas younger age at presentation is associated with a poorer prognosis; progression has been documented in 15–30% of OPG cases and leads to visual impairment in 30%. Worsening vision or involvement of the contralateral field has been attributed to an increase in the pressure of a pre-existing lesion on nearby axons, rather than evidence of 'true' extension into previously uninvolved tissue [42, 44, 46].

Chiasm involvement and hypothalamic involvement are associated with a decreased rate of survival, although survival is still greater than 90% for treated and untreated tumours. Even patients with progressive disease have good survival rates [42, 44]. Dutton found that 40% of patients with OPGs of the anterior visual pathway experienced progression or recurrence. 21% of patients presented with 20/40 or better vision, and 45% presented with 20/200 or better vision. 21% of patients experienced progressive visual loss, and some patients improved. Of patients with tumours confined to the optic nerve who were observed without treatment, 21% showed progression, 5% died of tumour-related causes, and 91% maintained stable vision. Patients with chiasmatic gliomas evaluated in this review demonstrated a 42% rate of progression, a 29% rate of tumour-related mortality, and a 77% rate of stable visual acuity. Treatment did not seem to change these percentages. Patients who presented with hypothalamic or third ventricle involvement fared much worse than other patients, especially if hydrocephalus was present. The tumour-related mortality rate in this group was 43%, with a 51% rate of recurrence/progression, although the prognosis for vision was similar to that of the chiasmatic tumour group, with 71% exhibiting stable vision. The subgroup of patients with pilomyxoid astrocytoma typically demonstrates a higher rate of local tumour recurrence (75% vs. 50%) and CSF dissemination [40].

Thirteen cases worldwide from 12 institutions over a 20-year period are well-documented to have shown spontaneous neuroradiological regression of OPGs. However, "spontaneous regression" can be quite misleading, because most of the individuals had significant vision loss and other neurological sequelae, such as hydrocephalus, hemiparesis, and endocrine dysfunction, despite radiological "regression." Equally important, eight of the children received no therapy, presumably being cared for prior to the era of chemotherapy. In the same retrospective review cited earlier, 32% of subjects treated with carboplatin showed improvement in visual acuity at the end of therapy. Thus, spontaneous neuroradiological regression, a rare event, is often associated with substantial and potentially preventable morbidity [41, 42, 44, 48].

7 Adult Malignant Optic Pathway Gliomas

7.1 Epidemiology

Malignant astrocytomas of the optic pathway have a rapid clinical course characterised by progressive visual loss, neurological deficits, and ultimately death. The age of presentation varies from the second to the eighth decade, and there is no specific sex predilection [47, 49–52].

7.2 Clinical Features

Patients with tumours in the proximal part of the optic nerve present with unilateral visual deterioration. Hypothalamic dysfunction, hemiparesis, and other neurological deficits develop in the later stages of the disease and death usually occurs in less than 1 year [47, 49, 50].

7.3 Investigations

Because of the acute visual loss, malignant OPG may be confused with optic neuritis or anterior ischemic optic neuropathy. In contrast to ischemic disease, however, marked enhancement of the optic nerve is seen on MRI. In the early stages of the disease, MRI with gadolinium demonstrates slight enlargement of the anterior optic pathway on post-contrast imaging, simulating optic neuritis and sarcoidosis.

The histopathology of this tumour is distinctly different from that of the paediatric optic nerve glioma, as it is characterised by extreme cellular pleomorphism, nuclear hyperchromaticity, and scattered mitoses [47, 50–52].

7.4 Management

There is currently no effective management protocol for this tumour, and radiation is only palliative. Short-term successes have been seen with a combination of chemotherapy and radiation [47, 50–52].

8 Orbital Peripheral Nerve Tumours

8.1 Aetiology and Pathogenesis

Approximately 4% of all orbital neoplasms are peripheral nerve tumours that consist primarily of neurofibromas and schwannomas (neurilemmomas). Of these, 2% of lesions are plexiform neurofibromas, 1% are isolated neurofibromas, and 1% are schwannomas. Malignant peripheral nerve tumours (malignant schwannomas, neurofibrosarcomas) do arise in the orbit but are extremely rare [53–55].

8.2 Clinical Features

Sensory nerves appear to give rise to peripheral nerve tumours with greater frequency than do motor nerves, because many patients complain of pain but retain ocular motility. As with most space-occupying lesions of the orbit, patients present with slowly progressive proptosis or displacement of the globe and may not develop diplopia until the lesion is large enough to limit ocular excursion. Visual acuity is often not affected unless the tumour compresses the optic nerve, which can occur earlier in lesions arising in the orbital apex.

Patients with benign orbital neurofibromas and schwannomas generally have a long history of progressive symptoms, although the duration of symptoms in neurofibromas is significantly longer. The similar duration of symptoms in schwannomas and malignant nerve sheath tumours would suggest that such malignant tumours are arising *de novo* and not through a malignant transformation with a preceding benign tumour.

Disturbance of trigeminal nerve function is uncommon with benign tumours and appears to occur more frequently with malignancy. Clinical and radiological signs for nerve sheath tumours, benign or malignant, are typically those of a slowly expanding orbital mass, and only a few signs, such as trigeminal sensory loss or destruction of bone, tend to favour malignancy.

Benign nerve sheath tumours occur more often in the superior orbit. This is probably a manifestation of the greater number of sensory nerves traversing this region [54–56].

8.3 Histopathology

Benign peripheral nerve sheath tumours comprise a variable proliferation and mixture of axons, Schwann cells, supporting endoneural cells, and vascular elements.

Schwannomas are generally well defined. They are often eccentric from the nerve of origin and show a predominance of spindle-shaped Schwann cells; these latter cells often display a palisading of nuclei (Antoni A pattern) or a less organised pattern (Antoni B). Axons are infrequent within, and often pass eccentrically through, the main mass of a schwannoma.

Neurofibromas more commonly arise within nerves and display more endoneural proliferation, thus expanding and forming an intimate relationship with the nerve. When there are multiple involvements with adjacent nerve branches, the effect is to produce a composite mass of thickened nerve bundles and, as such, the tumours are usually referred to as 'plexiform.'

Neurofibromas and, to a lesser degree, schwannomas can undergo degeneration, manifesting as myxoid or cystic changes and haemorrhage. Inflammatory cell infiltration may also occur with this degeneration [54, 57].

8.4 Neurofibromas

Neurofibromas may occur in several patterns: (1) plexiform, (2) diffuse, and (3) solitary.

8.4.1 Plexiform

Plexiform neurofibroma of the eyelid infiltrates the full-thickness of eyelid, causing blepharoptosis, usually greatest laterally. Skeletal changes resulting in varying degrees of aplasia of the sphenoid wing and leading to the enlargement of the superior orbital fissure, temporal lobe herniation, and pulsating exophthalmos, might accompany the disease.

The tumour tends to localise to the lateral third of the eyelid and consists of cords and nodules resulting in the classic "S-shaped" deformity and giving rise to a "bag of worms" on palpation. During adolescence, the tumour often extends to the forehead, temple, and superior orbit, leading to downward displacement of the globe. This displacement may be difficult to evaluate in the presence of extensive hypertrophy of the eyelid (Fig. 4).

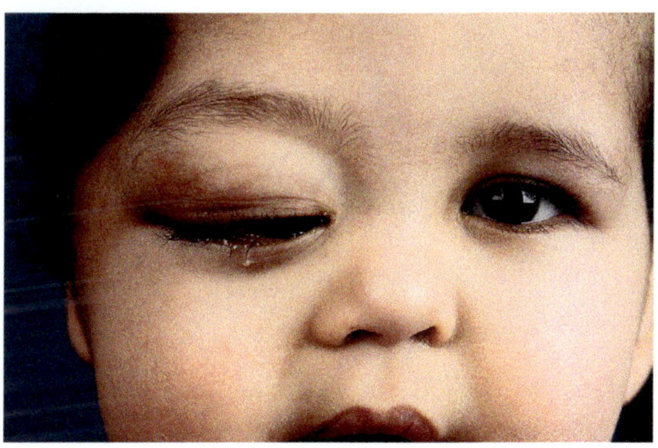

Fig. 4 3-year boy with plexiform neurofibroma of the right eyelid

Histologically, plexiform neurofibromas are unencapsulated and have an organoid appearance with proliferating units surrounded by perineurium enclosing axons, Schwann cells, and endoneurial fibroblasts. They are highly vascular, reflected by marked contrast enhancement on CT and MR imaging scans, a finding that is virtually pathognomonic for NF-1.

The treatment of plexiform neurofibromas is challenging and often disappointing. These lesions are vascular and diffusely infiltrative, often involving normal structures, such as extraocular muscles. Thus, complete removal is unachievable. The plexiform neurofibroma also has a high rate of recurrence, often requiring multiple surgeries to attain an acceptable result.

There is a fundamental difference in the management of children and adults with orbitotemporal neurofibromas. Rapid growth of neurofibromas typically occurs in children and adolescents, who therefore require close observation. Radical surgery is best delayed until disease progression has slowed. In adults, a more aggressive surgical approach can be adopted to achieve a definitive result. It is also easier to plan the time course of staged surgical procedures to correct the deformities over many months or years. However, if ptosis is threatening vision, surgery should be performed to prevent progression of amblyopia in children; conservative, staged approach is recommended [56, 58–60].

8.4.2 Diffuse

Diffuse neurofibromas appear similar to plexiform neurofibromas with infiltration of orbital fat and extraocular muscles. However, these lesions are less likely to be associated with NF-1 [57, 61, 62].

8.4.3 Solitary

Solitary neurofibroma often presents as a slow-growing tumour that exerts a mass effect, with displacement of the globe in the direction opposite to that of the tumour. The tumour may occur along any sensory nerve but is more common in the superior quadrants. When these lesions arise near the lacrimal gland, they have the clinical appearance of primary lacrimal gland tumours.

Visual acuity is often unaffected, and pain is uncommon. These lesions are most commonly seen in the third to fifth decades of life and often manifest a pseudocapsule, but a true perineurium is not seen. They are composed of wavy bundles of peripheral nerve sheath cells with comma-shaped nuclei and hyaluronic acid and collagen in the stroma [57, 61, 62].

Solitary neurofibromas and schwannomas have a similar clinical and radiological appearance. Both tumours are readily amenable to surgical excision, either through an anterolateral orbitotomy or cranio-orbitotomy when located in the posterior orbit. Surgical excision is relatively bloodless, and most can be removed intact. The primary reason to distinguish neurofibromas from schwannomas is that the former are more likely to undergo malignant transformation, although still rare [55, 60, 63–65].

8.5 Schwannomas

The vestibulo-cochlear nerve and the trigeminal nerves are the most common sites of origin for orbital schwannomas. These lesions are diagnosed most often during the second to fifth decades, with mean age of 50 years [66–69].

The schwannoma typically arises from the first division of the trigeminal nerve (supratrochlear or supraorbital branch), located in the superior orbit. Clinical features include proptosis, decreased vision diplopia, and a trigeminal distribution of numbness or pain. Globe indentation with induced hyperopia and direct optic nerve compression are causes of decreased vision. The tumour begins focally in the nerve and enlarges in a nodular fashion to become an encapsulated mass [69–71].

8.5.1 Imaging

Although there are no diagnostic neuroradiological features, orbital CT scanning frequently reveals a smooth, elongated, circumscribed intraconal or extraconal mass. Expansion of the superior orbital fissure may also be seen. Cyst formation is not uncommon. In cases of cystic degeneration within the schwannoma, heterogeneity of the lesion is a characteristic feature.

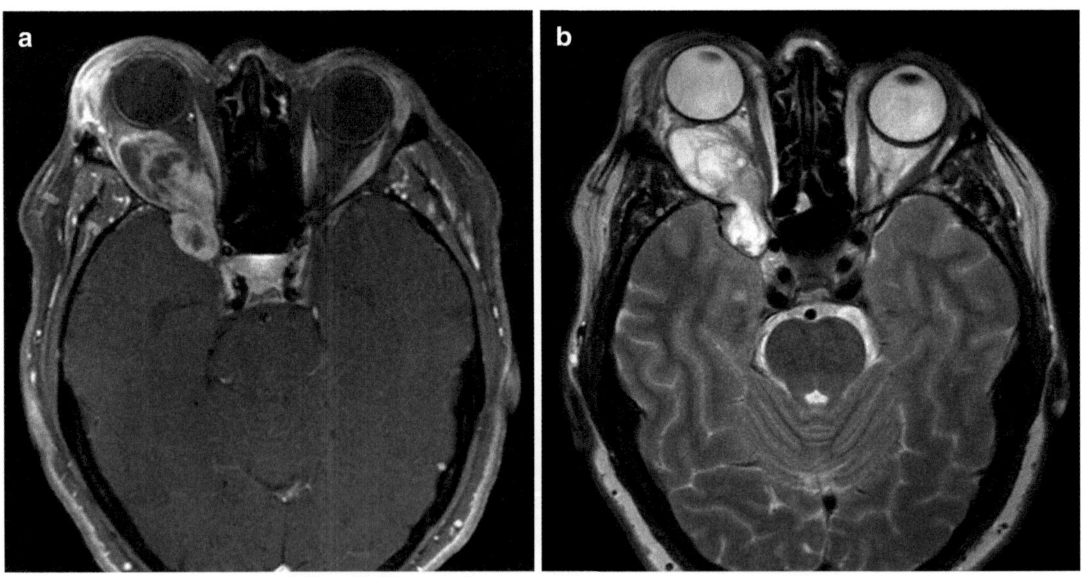

Fig. 5 Cystic schwannoma with involvement of left orbit and intracranial extension on T1 weighted axial (**a**), axial T2-weighted (**b**) and contrast enhancement. Patient underwent a combined lateral orbitotomy and pterional craniotomy. The intraorbital part was completely removed and the intracranial lesion showed no progression in 6 years. Visual acuity post-operatively remained 20/20; double vision disappeared following two strabismus surgeries

Schwannomas give low signal intensities on T1 and higher intensity signals on T2 images in non-contrast MRI (Fig. 5a, b). Recently, a study regarding dynamic contrast MRI has described the features that can differentiate between well-defined ovoid, intraconal masses. *Progressive enhancement* on the contrast imaging of later images favours the diagnosis of cavernous venous lesion rather than a schwannoma. Intramuscular schwannoma is rare and has been reported in the medial and lateral rectus muscles, inferior oblique muscle, and from the superior oblique tendon [69–74].

8.5.2 Management

Surgical removal of the tumour is the treatment of choice, and prognosis is good when complete excision is achieved. Rarely, schwannoma can recur, particularly in cases where there has been incomplete removal [6, 66, 67, 69].

9 Malignant Peripheral Nerve Sheath Tumours

9.1 Pathogenesis and Aetiology

Malignant peripheral nerve sheath tumours (MPNST) are very rare and aggressive neoplasms. MPNST is a non-specific term referring to any malignant tumour that arises from or differentiates to cells of the peripheral nerve sheath, including malignant schwannoma and neurofibrosarcoma. It is often difficult to ascertain the true cell of origin. The tumour may arise *de novo* or as a consequence of malignant transformation of a neurofibroma. MPNST accounts for approximately 10% of all soft-tissue sarcomas in the body [6, 75–85].

These tumours usually arise from ophthalmic or maxillary sensory branches of the trigeminal nerve, especially the supraorbital branch [6, 76, 77].

9.2 Epidemiology

MPNST is predominantly an adult disease, with most tumours occurring in patients between 20 and 50 years of age. Cases arising in individuals with NF-1 have an earlier age of onset, with some reported even in early infancy. In sporadic cases of MPNST, there is no gender predilection, but male patients predominate when the tumour arises in patients with NF-1 [6, 75–85].

9.3 Clinical Features

Typically, patients develop orbital pain and swelling over several months. These lesions may appear deceptively benign on clinical examination. Hypesthesia or anaesthesia may be present in the distribution of the involved nerve, with neuroparalytic keratitis reported in cases of trigeminal nerve involvement [6, 75–85].

9.4 Imaging

MRI of MPNSTs usually shows a well-defined mass lesion with mixed components. Cystic components are sometimes present within the tumour, and perineural invasion can be observed by enlargement of the nerve or neural enhancement in contrast-enhanced images. Because these lesions grow inside the nerve sheath, they adopt a spindle or globular well-circumscribed appearance. They usually do not have a true capsule but rather a pseudocapsule.

9.5 Histopathology

MPNST is composed of highly cellular, spindle-shaped cells that resemble soft-tissue sarcoma, but with differentiation toward elements of the nerve sheath, Schwann cell, and perineural cell. Numerous variations exist, including a biphasic spindle and epithelioid cell pattern, or including necrotic and myxoid areas. The diagnosis of malignancy is based on the presence of cells with irregular size and shape, nuclear enlargement, and hyperchromatism.

Immunohistochemical staining typically provides the best markers for MPNSTs. HMB-45 is usually negative, and cytokeratin focal S-100 protein positivity is seen in 70% of tumour cells. MPNSTs may also show reactivity for CD56 or myelin basic protein.

9.6 Management

MPNST is highly aggressive; thorough surgical excision of MPNST is justified because of its tendency to recur at the site of the initial tumour, regardless of its location. Because of the tendency of MPNST to grow toward intracranial structures, orbital exenteration is probably the best currently available treatment option. Where feasible, a combined exenteration and craniotomy would be required for orbital MPNST with an intracranial component. Adjuvant irradiation at a dose of >60 Gy may improve local control of disease [6, 75–85].

References

1. Levin LA, Jakobiec FA. Peripheral nerve sheath tumors of the orbit. In: Albert D, Miller J, Azar D, Young LH, editors. Albert and Jakobiec's principles and practice of ophthalmology. WB Saunders; 1994. p. 1978–2327.
2. Powers CJ, Friedman AH. A brief history of surgery for peripheral nerve sheath tumors. Neurosurg Focus. 2007;22:E1.
3. Selhorst JB, Chen Y. The optic nerve. Semin Neurol. 2009;29:29–35.
4. Ferner RE. Neurofibromatosis 1 and neurofibromatosis 2: a twenty first century perspective. Lancet Neurol. 2007;6:340–51.
5. Turbin RE, Pokorny K. Diagnosis and treatment of orbital optic nerve sheath meningioma. Cancer Control. 2004;11:334–41.
6. Fay A, Dolman PJ. Neurogenic tumors of the orbit. Diseases and disorders of the orbit and ocular adnexa: In, Elsevier; 2016.
7. Saeed P, Rootman J, Nugent RA, White VA, Mackenzie IR, Koornneef L. Optic nerve sheath meningiomas. Ophthalmology. 2003;110:2019–30.
8. Dutton JJ. Optic nerve sheath meningiomas. Surv Ophthalmol. 1992;37:167–83.
9. Kennerdell JS, Maroon JC, Malton M, Warren FA. The management of optic nerve sheath meningiomas. Am J Ophthalmol. 1988;106:450–7.
10. Eddleman CS, Liu JK. Optic nerve sheath meningioma: current diagnosis and treatment. Neurosurg Focus. 2007;23:E4.
11. Saeed P, Tanck MWT, Freling N, Baldeschi L, Mourits MP, Bennink RJ. Somatostatin receptor scintigraphy for optic nerve sheath meningiomas. Ophthalmology. 2009;116:1581–6.
12. Graef J, Furth C, Kluge AK, Acker G, Kord M, Zimmermann Z, et al. 68Ga-DOTATOC-PET/MRI-A secure one-stop shop imaging tool for robotic radiosurgery treatment planning in patients with optic nerve sheath meningioma. Cancers (Basel). 2021;13:3305.
13. Johnson TE, Weatherhead RG, Nasr AM, Siqueira EB. Ectopic (extradural) meningioma of the orbit: a report of two cases in children. J Pediatr Ophthalmol Strabismus. 1993;30:43–7.
14. Craig WMK, Gogela LJ. Intraorbital meningiomas; a clinicopathologic study. Am J Ophthalmol. 1949;32:1663–80.
15. Pintea B, Boström A, Katsigiannis S, Gousias K, Pintea R, Baumert B, et al. Prognostic factors for functional outcome of patients with optic nerve sheath meningiomas treated with stereotactic radiotherapy-evaluation of own and meta-analysis of published data. Cancers (Basel). 2021;13:1–8.
16. Farah SE, Konrad H, Huang DT, Geist CE. Ectopic orbital meningioma: a case report and review. Ophthal Plast Reconstr Surg. 1999;15:463–6.
17. Wolter JR, Benz SC. Ectopic meningioma of the superior orbital rim. Arch Ophthalmol. 1976;94:1920–2.
18. Tan KK, Lim ASM. Primary extradural intra-orbital meningioma in a Chinese girl. Br J Ophthalmol. 1965;49:377–80.
19. Decock CE, Kataria S, Breusegem CM, Van Den Broecke CM, Claerhout IJ. Ectopic meningioma anterior to the lacrimal gland fossa. Ophthal Plast Reconstr Surg. 2009;25:57–9.
20. Bondy M, Lee LB. Epidemiology and etiology of intracranial meningiomas: a review. J Neurooncol. 1996;29:197–205.
21. Dreyer N, Loughlin J, Rothman K. Cause-specific mortality in cellular telephone users. JAMA. 1999;282:1814–6.
22. El Gindi S. Olfactory groove meningioma: surgical techniques and pitfalls. Surg Neurol. 2000;54:415–7.
23. North KN, Riccardi V, Samango-Sprouse C, Ferner R, Moore B, Legius E, et al. Cognitive function and academic performance in neurofibromatosis. 1: consensus statement from the NF1 Cognitive Disorders Task Force. Neurology. 1997;48:1121–7.
24. Foote K, Friedman W, Buatti J, Bova F, Meeks S. Linear accelerator radiosurgery in brain tumor management. Neurosurg Clin N Am. 1999;10:203–42.
25. Goel A, Muzumdar D, Desai KI. Tuberculum sellae meningioma: a report on management on the basis of a surgical experience with 70 patients. Neurosurgery. 2002;51:1358–63.
26. Gökalp HZ, Arasil E, Kanpolat Y, Balim T. Meningiomas of the tuberculum sella. Neurosurg Rev. 1993;16:111–4.

27. Hentschel SJ, DeMonte F. Olfactory groove meningiomas. Neurosurg Focus. 2003;14:6.
28. Saeed P, Van Furth WR, Tanck M, Kooremans F, Freling N, Streekstra GI, et al. Natural history of spheno-orbital meningiomas. Acta Neurochir. 2011;153:395–401.
29. Saeed P, Van Furth WR, Tanck M, Freling N, Van Der Sprenkel JWB, Stalpers LJA, et al. Surgical treatment of sphenoorbital meningiomas. Br J Ophthalmol. 2011;95:996–1000.
30. Avery RA, Fisher MJ, Liu GT. Optic pathway gliomas. J Neuroophthalmol. 2011;31:269–78.
31. Listernick R, Ferner RE, Liu GT, Gutmann DH. Optic pathway gliomas in neurofibromatosis-1: controversies and recommendations. Ann Neurol. 2007;61:189–98.
32. Al-Mefty O. Operative atlas of meningiomas. Philadelphia: Lippincott Williams & Wilkins; 1998.
33. Babu R, Barton A, Kasoff SS. Resection of olfactory groove meningiomas: technical note revisited. Surg Neurol. 1995;44:567–71.
34. Black PM. Meningiomas. Neurosurgery. 1993;32:643–57.
35. Bonnal J, Thibaut A, Brotchi J, Born J. Invading meningiomas of the sphenoid ridge. J Neurosurg. 1980;53:587–99.
36. Boulos PT, Dumont AS, Mandell JW, Jane JA. Meningiomas of the orbit: contemporary considerations. Neurosurg Focus 2001;10:E5.
37. Chou SP, Miles J. The pathology of meningiomas. In: Almefty O, editor. Meningiomas. New York: Raven; 1991. p. 37–57.
38. De Jesús O, Toledo MM. Surgical management of meningioma en plaque of the sphenoid ridge. Surg Neurol. 2001;55:265–9.
39. Fisher MJ, Loguidice M, Gutmann DH, Listernick R, Ferner RE, Ullrich NJ, et al. Visual outcomes in children with neurofibromatosis type 1-associated optic pathway glioma following chemotherapy: a multicenter retrospective analysis. Neuro Oncol. 2012;14:790–7.
40. Dutton JJ. Gliomas of the anterior visual pathway. Surv Ophthalmol. 1994;38:427–52.
41. Parsa CF, Hoyt CS, Lesser RL, Weinstein JM, Strother CM, Muci-Mendoza R, et al. Spontaneous regression of optic gliomas: thirteen cases documented by serial neuroimaging. Arch Ophthalmol. 2001;119:516–29.
42. Astrup J. Natural history and clinical management of optic pathway glioma. Br J Neurosurg. 2003;17:327–35.
43. Nicolin G, Parkin P, Mabbott D, Hargrave D, Bartels U, Tabori U, et al. Natural history and outcome of optic pathway gliomas in children. Pediatr Blood Cancer. 2009;53:1231–7.
44. Binning MJ, Liu JK, Kestle JRW, Brockmeyer DL, Walker ML. Optic pathway gliomas: a review. Neurosurg Focus. 2007;23:1–8.
45. Listernick R, Ferner RE, Piersall L, Sharif S, Gutmann DH, Charrow J. Late-onset optic pathway tumors in children with neurofibromatosis 1. Neurology. 2004;63:1944–6.
46. Opocher E, Kremer LCM, Da Dalt L, van de Wetering MD, Viscardi E, Caron HN, et al. Prognostic factors for progression of childhood optic pathway glioma: a systematic review. Eur J Cancer. 2006;42:1807–16.
47. Miyamoto J, Sasajima H, Owada K, Mineura K. Surgical decision for adult optic glioma based on [18F]fluorodeoxyglucose positron emission tomography study. Neurol Med Chir (Tokyo). 2006;46:500–3.
48. Liu GT, Lessell S. Spontaneous visual improvement in chiasmal gliomas. Am J Ophthalmol. 1992;114:193–201.
49. Dinh TT, Wang YY, Rosenfeld JV, Cherny M. Glioblastoma of the optic chiasm. J Clin Neurosci. 2007;14:502–5.
50. Wabbels B, Demmler A, Seitz J, Woenckhaus M, Bloß HG, Lorenz B. Unilateral adult malignant optic nerve glioma. Graefes Arch Clin Exp Ophthalmol. 2004;242:741–8.
51. Hoyt WF, Meshel LG, Lessell S, Schatz NJ, Suckling RD. Malignant optic glioma of adulthood. Brain. 1973;96:121–32.
52. Raikar SS, Halloran DR, Elliot M, McHugh M, Patel S, Gauvain KM. Outcomes of pediatric low-grade gliomas treated with radiation therapy: a single-institution study. J Pediatr Hematol Oncol. 2014;36:e366–70.
53. Grabb WC, Dingman RO, Oneal RM, Dempsey PD. Facial hamartomas in children: neurofibroma, lymphangioma, and hemangioma. Plast Reconstr Surg. 1980;66:509–27.
54. Adekeye EO, Abiose A, Ord RA. Neurofibromatosis of the head and neck: clinical presentation and treatment. J Maxillofac Surg. 1984;12:78–85.
55. Jackson IT, Laws ER, Martin RD. The surgical management of orbital neurofibromatosis. Plast Reconstr Surg. 1983;71:751–8.
56. Marchac D, Britto JA. Remodelling the upper eyelid in the management of orbitopalpebral neurofibromatosis. Br J Plast Surg. 2005;58:944–56.
57. Harkin JC. Pathology of nerve sheath tumors. Ann N Y Acad Sci. 1986;486:147–54.
58. Lee V, Ragge NK, Collin JRO. Orbitotemporal neurofibromatosis. Clinical features and surgical management. Ophthalmology. 2004;111:382–8.
59. Van Der Meulen JC, Moscona AR, Vandrachen M, Hirshowitz B. The management of orbitofacial neurofibromatosis. Ann Plast Surg. 1982;8:213–20.
60. Madill KE, Brammar R, Leatherbarrow B. A novel approach to the management of severe facial disfigurement in neurofibromatosis type 1. Ophthal Plast Reconstr Surg. 2007;23:227–8.
61. North K. Neurofibromatosis type 1 in childhood. London: MacKeith Press; 1997. p. 31–3.
62. Bloem JJAM, var der Meulen JC. Neurofibromatosis in plastic surgery. Br J Plast Surg. 1978;31:50–3.
63. Adkins J, Ravitch M. The operative management of von Recklinghausen's neurofibromatosis in children, with special reference to lesions of the head and neck. Surgery. 1977;82:342–8.

64. Morax S, Herdan ML, Hurbli T. The surgical management of orbitopalpebral neurofibromatosis. Ophthal Plast Reconstr Surg. 1988;4:203–13.
65. Carroll GS, Haik BG, Fleming JC, Weiss RA, Mafee MF. Peripheral nerve tumors of the orbit. Radiol Clin North Am. 1999;37:195–202.
66. Levin LA, Jakobiec FA. Peripheral nerve sheath tumors of the orbit. In: Albert and Jakobiec's principles and practice of ophthalmology. WB Saunders; 1994. p. 1978–2327.
67. Pollock S. Tumors of cranial and peripheral nerves. In: Miller NR, Newman NJ, editors. Walsh and Hoyt's clinical neuro-ophthalmology. Baltimore: Williams & Wilkins; 1998. p. 2297–327.
68. Schatz H. Benign orbital neurilemoma. Sarcomatous transformation in von Recklinghausen's disease. Arch Ophthalmol. 1971;86:268–73.
69. Rootman J, Goldberg C, Robertson W. Primary orbital schwannomas. Br J Ophthalmol. 1982;66:194–204.
70. Abe T, Kawamura N, Homma H, Sasaki K, Izumiyama H, Matsumoto K. MRI of orbital schwannomas. Neuroradiology. 2000;42:466–8.
71. Wang Y, Xiao LH. Orbital schwannomas: findings from magnetic resonance imaging in 62 cases. Eye (Lond). 2008;22:1034–9.
72. Dehaene I, Marchau M, Vanhooren G. Schwannoma of the optic sheath. J Clin Neuroophthalmol. 1987;7:219–22.
73. Tanaka A, Mihara F, Yoshiura T, Togao O, Kuwabara Y, Natori Y, et al. Differentiation of cavernous hemangioma from schwannoma of the orbit: a dynamic MRI study. AJR Am J Roentgenol. 2004;183:1799–804.
74. Mafee MF, Putterman AM, Valvassori G, Campos M, Capek V. Orbital space-occupying lesions: role of computed tomography and magnetic resonance imaging. An analysis of 145 cases. Radiol Clin North Am. 1987;25:529–59.
75. Wong WW, Hirose T, Scheithauer BW, Schild SE, Gunderson LL. Malignant peripheral nerve sheath tumor: analysis of treatment outcome. Int J Radiat Oncol Biol Phys. 1998;42:351–60.
76. Jakobiec FA, Font R, Zimmerman L. Malignant peripheral nerve sheath tumors of the orbit: a clinicopathologic study of eight cases. Trans Am Ophthalmol Soc. 1985;83:332–66.
77. Briscoe D, Mahmood S, O'Donovan D, Bonshek R, Leatherbarrow B, Eyden B. Malignant peripheral nerve sheath tumor in the orbit of a child with acute proptosis. Arch Ophthalmol. 2002;120:653–5.
78. Stark AM, Buhl R, Hugo HH, Mehdorn HM. Malignant peripheral nerve sheath tumours—report of 8 cases and review of the literature. Acta Neurochir. 2001;143:357–64.
79. Hrehorovich PA, Franke HR, Maximin S, Caracta P. Malignant peripheral nerve sheath tumor. Radiographics. 2003;23:790–4.
80. Schmidt RF, Yick F, Boghani Z, Eloy JA, Liu JK. Malignant peripheral nerve sheath tumors of the trigeminal nerve: a systematic review of 36 cases. Neurosurg Focus. 2013;34:E5.
81. Martinez-Devesa P, Mitchell T, Scott I, Moffat D. Malignant peripheral nerve sheath tumors of the head and neck: two cases and a review of the literature. Ear Nose Throat J. 2006;85:392–6.
82. Ducatman B, Scheithauer B, Piepgras D, Reiman H, Ilstrup D. Malignant peripheral nerve sheath tumors. A clinicopathologic study of 120 cases. Cancer. 1986;57:2006–21.
83. Cheng SF, Chen YI, Chang CY, Peng Y, Liao SL. Malignant peripheral nerve sheath tumor of the orbit: malignant transformation from neurofibroma without neurofibromatosis. Ophthal Plast Reconstr Surg. 2008;24:413–5.
84. Williams Z, Coumans J-V, Bredella MA, Torriani M, Hornicek F, Ouellette H, et al. Role of positron emission tomography imaging in the surgical management of peripheral nerve sheath tumors in patients with neurofibromatosis type 1. Neurosurgery. 2007;61:202.
85. Lyons CJ, McNab AA, Garner A, Wright JE. Orbital malignant peripheral nerve sheath tumours. Br J Ophthalmol. 1989;73:731–8.

Mesenchymal Tumours of the Orbit

Kaveh Vahdani, David H. Verity, and Geoffrey E. Rose

Key Messages

- Mesenchymal tumours are benign and malignant neoplasms that account for 5–9% of all orbital tumours.
- They originate from mesodermal-derived precursor cells that develop into different connective tissues in the orbit. Mesenchymal tumours arising in the adjacent sino-nasal cavities and skull base, as well as metastatic tumours, can also affect the orbit.
- Rhabdomyosarcoma in childhood and solitary fibrous tumours in adults are two of the most common entities.
- Benign mesenchymal tumours commonly cause mass effect and varying degrees of functional impairment, and some lesions, such as solitary fibrous tumours, may develop recurrent disease or malignant transformation. The main treatment modality for these lesions is surgery with complete excision.
- Malignant mesenchymal tumours tend to be aggressive, with propensity for both local and distant invasion. A multidisciplinary approach is required, with surgery (wide local resection or orbital exenteration) being the mainstay of treatment, however radiation and/or chemotherapy may also be used depending on the histology and stage of the tumour.

1 Introduction

Mesenchymal tumours are benign and malignant neoplasms that account for 5–9% of all orbital tumours [1, 2]. They originate from mesodermal-derived precursor cells that develop into different connective tissues in the orbit, including striated extraocular muscles, fibroblasts of connective tissue septa, orbital adipocytes, the trochlear cartilage, vascular wall smooth muscle, and Müller's muscle. The orbit may also be affected by mesenchymal tumours originating in the surrounding sino-nasal cavities and skull base, as well as by metastatic tumours [1–3]. The commonest orbital mesenchymal tumours are classified in this chapter according to their cellular differentiation: fibrocytic, myogenic, adipocytic, cartilaginous, osseous and miscellaneous (Table 1). Tumours of vascular origin are described in chapter "Orbital Vascular Anomalies and Vascular Tumours".

K. Vahdani (✉) · G. E. Rose
Adnexal Service, Moorfields Eye Hospital, London, UK
e-mail: kaveh.vahdani@nhs.net

D. H. Verity
Adnexal Service, Moorfields Eye Hospital, London, UK

St John of Jerusalem Eye Hospital Group, London, UK

F. M. Quaranta Leoni et al. (eds.), *Oculoplastic, Lacrimal and Orbital Surgery*,
https://doi.org/10.1007/978-3-031-39638-0_24

Table 1 Classification for mesenchymal tumours of the orbit

Tumour sub-group	Benign	Malignant
Fibrocytic	Solitary fibrous tumour Nodular fasciitis Myofibroma Myofibromatosis	Fibrosarcoma
Myogenic—striated muscle	Rhabdomyoma	Rhabdomyosarcoma
Myogenic—smooth muscle	Leiomyoma	Leiomyosarcoma
Adipocytic	Lipoma	Liposarcoma
Chondrogenic	Chondroma	Chondrosarcoma
Osseous and fibro-osseous	Osteoma Fibrous dysplasia Ossifying fibroma	Osteogenic sarcoma
Other	Myxoma	Alveolar soft part sarcoma Synovial sarcoma

2 Fibrocytic Tumours

2.1 Solitary Fibrous Tumours

Originally described in the pleura, solitary fibrous tumours (SFTs) are an uncommon spindle-cell tumour that can also affect extraserosal tissues, including the orbit. Immunohistochemistry, cytogenetics, and molecular studies have revealed that "SFT' 'is the correct group terminology for a spectrum of morphologically-similar mesenchymal fibroblastic neoplasms that include haemangiopericytoma, giant cell angiofibroma, and fibrous histiocytoma [1–4]. SFTs can arise anywhere in the orbit, conjunctiva, eyelids, or lacrimal drainage system. They usually have a benign clinical course, but recurrent tumours can be locally-aggressive or display malignant features with extraorbital extension [1–4].

2.1.1 Clinical Presentation

Presentation is usually during fourth to sixth decades, but it can affect all ages, with no gender predilection. Depending on the size and anatomical position of the tumour, most patients report a slowly-progressive painless proptosis and globe displacement (Fig. 1a, b), that may be accompanied with impaired visual function, reduced ocular motility, blepharoptosis, or an anteriorly palpable mass. The lacrimal outflow system may become involved, resulting in medial canthal mass, epiphora, or dacryocystitis [1–3].

2.1.2 Imaging

CT usually shows as well-defined homogenous and strongly-enhancing soft-tissue mass, that may be located in any part of the orbit and associated with displacement of normal orbital structures or bone remodelling. Bone destruction or infiltration may be seen in recurrent disease or malignant transformation. On MRI, the lesion appears isointense on T1-weighted images, and heterogenous isointense to hyperintense on T2-weighted images, with avid post-gadolinium enhancement (Fig. 1c, d) and quite frequently vascular flow-voids within the tumour [4]. Perfusion-weighted MRI may aid in distinguishing SFT from other lesions with similar morphology, such as orbital cavernous venous malformations and neurilemmoma.

2.1.3 Histology

SFTs are composed of haphazardly arranged bland spindle-shaped cells within a variably collagenous stroma, mixed with staghorn-pattern of branching thin-walled sinusoidal-like (haemangiopericytomatous) blood vessels. Immunohistochemistry usually shows positive staining for vimentin, CD34, bcl-2 and CD99 (Fig. 1f–h), and negative staining for S100, cytokeratin, desmin, factor VIII-related antigen and smooth muscle actin. Immunostaining for the protein STAT6 is a sensitive and specific surrogate marker for the NAB2-STAT6 gene fusions that are pathognomonic for SFT [1, 2, 5].

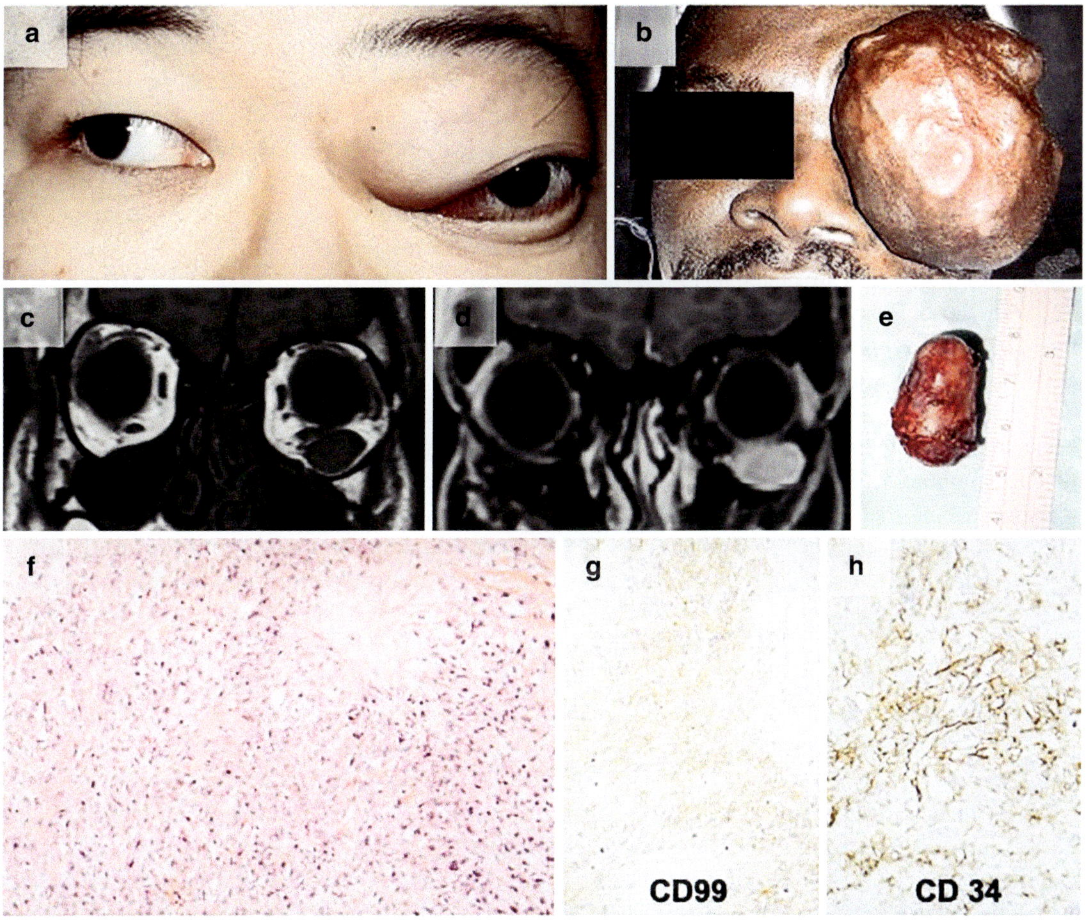

Fig. 1 Solitary fibrous tumour (SFT): (**a**) East-Asian female presenting with left superonasal quadrant mass, proptosis, infero-lateral globe displacement and mild chemosis having undergone sub-brow incisional biopsy. (**b**) African male with giant left SFT and prominent tumour vascularity. (**c**) T1-weighted MRI showing a left well-circumscribed, isointense, avidly-enhancing ovoid mass in the inferior orbit, causing hyperglobus (**d**). (**e**) The mass was excised intact with histology confirming SFT. (**f**) Histopathology of SFT showing bland arrangement of spindle-shaped cells within a collagenous stroma with positive immunohistochemistry for CD99 (**g**) and CD34 (**h**)

2.1.4 Management and Prognosis

Intact excision is the treatment of choice and usually curative (Fig. 1e). Although some patients with residual benign disease can remain stable for many years after piecemeal excision, the latter procedure may increase the risk of recurrence—often with a higher mitotic index and a propensity for locally-aggressive disease—or risk of malignant transformation. All patients should have long-term clinico-radiological surveillance, since late asymptomatic recurrence can occur even in those who had intact tumour excision [1, 2]. The role of radiotherapy is controversial, is mainly reserved for recurrent disease, malignant transformation or metastasis, and orbital exenteration may rarely be required for extensive incurable tumours [2, 6].

2.2 Nodular Fasciitis

Originally termed as "subcutaneous pseudosarcomatous fibromatosis", nodular fasciitis is a reactive benign proliferation of fibroblasts and myofibroblasts that generally affects the superficial fascia. Orbital involvement is rare, accounting for 15% of all fibrocytic lesions and for <1% of all orbital masses [3]. Presentation is usually in children and young adults with fairly rapid onset of well-circumscribed superficial palpable mass at the orbital rim or in epibulbar tissues, with occasional pain or inflammatory features, and rarely proptosis due to a more posteriorly-located mass.

Histologically they are characterised by a proliferation of plump and immature-appearing fibroblasts or myofibroblasts with more eosinophilic cytoplasm than resting fibroblasts. The tumour can easily be misdiagnosed as sarcoma because of its hypercellularity and high mitotic index. Immunohistochemistry shows positive staining for smooth muscle actin (SMA) and vimentin, but not desmin [2]. Local excision is the recommended treatment and recurrence is rare.

2.3 Myofibroma and Myofibromatosis

Myofibromas are benign non-encapsulated fibrous tumours with contractile myoid elements, and may present as solitary or generalised lesions. Although both forms can affect all ages, the generalised form (myofibromatosis) is often seen in infants with multiple nodules in the skin, muscles, viscera and bones, and potentially lethal due to respiratory or gastrointestinal complications.

Orbital involvement is uncommon, with most lesions being solitary myofibromas that present with well-circumscribed eyelid or anterior orbital painless hard masses (Fig. 2a), although deeper lesions originating from the bone may cause proptosis. Radiologically, most lesions are fairly well-circumscribed and isodense on CT.

Histologically, it is nodular or multinodular, commonly displaying a biphasic or zonal appearance, composed of nodular fascicles of spindle cells surrounding cellular zones of undifferentiated cells in a background of a collagenous matrix. Mitotic activity is uncommon and, on immunohistochemistry, the myofibroblasts positively stain for vimentin and smooth muscle actin (SMA), but not S100, keratin, desmin or epithelial membrane antigen (EMA).

Complete surgical excision is usually curative, although lesions may also regress spontaneously after incomplete removal.

2.4 Fibrosarcoma

Fibrosarcomas (FSs) usually affect the limbs, and are malignant tumours originating from mesenchymal cells with fibroblastic or myofibroblastic differentiation. FS can develop as a primary orbital tumour, secondary to prior orbital radiotherapy (after hereditary retinoblastoma) or secondary to a primary sinonasal tumour invading the orbit. Juvenile and adult variants are described, the former having a better prognosis despite histological similarity.

Depending on the tumour location, patients may present with progressive proptosis, eyelid swelling, blepharoptosis, with or without orbital pain (Fig. 2b). Imaging studies usually show grossly-circumscribed homogeneous lesions in the anterior orbit that are isodense on CT and have low-intermediate signal intensity on T1 and T2-weighted images, with moderate contrast enhancement. Lytic lesions within the bone may also be present. Histological examination shows spindle-shaped cells arranged in a collagen matrix to form fascicles which interdigitate in a characteristic chevron-like pattern; the presence of spindle cells and a high amount of collagen distinguishes this lesion from rhabdomyosarcoma.

Local recurrence occurs in up to 50% of cases, particularly in those with radiation-induced or secondary tumours with a poor prognosis. Wide local excision or exenteration with adjuvant radiotherapy (50–60 Gy) and or chemotherapy is the mainstay of treatment [1, 2].

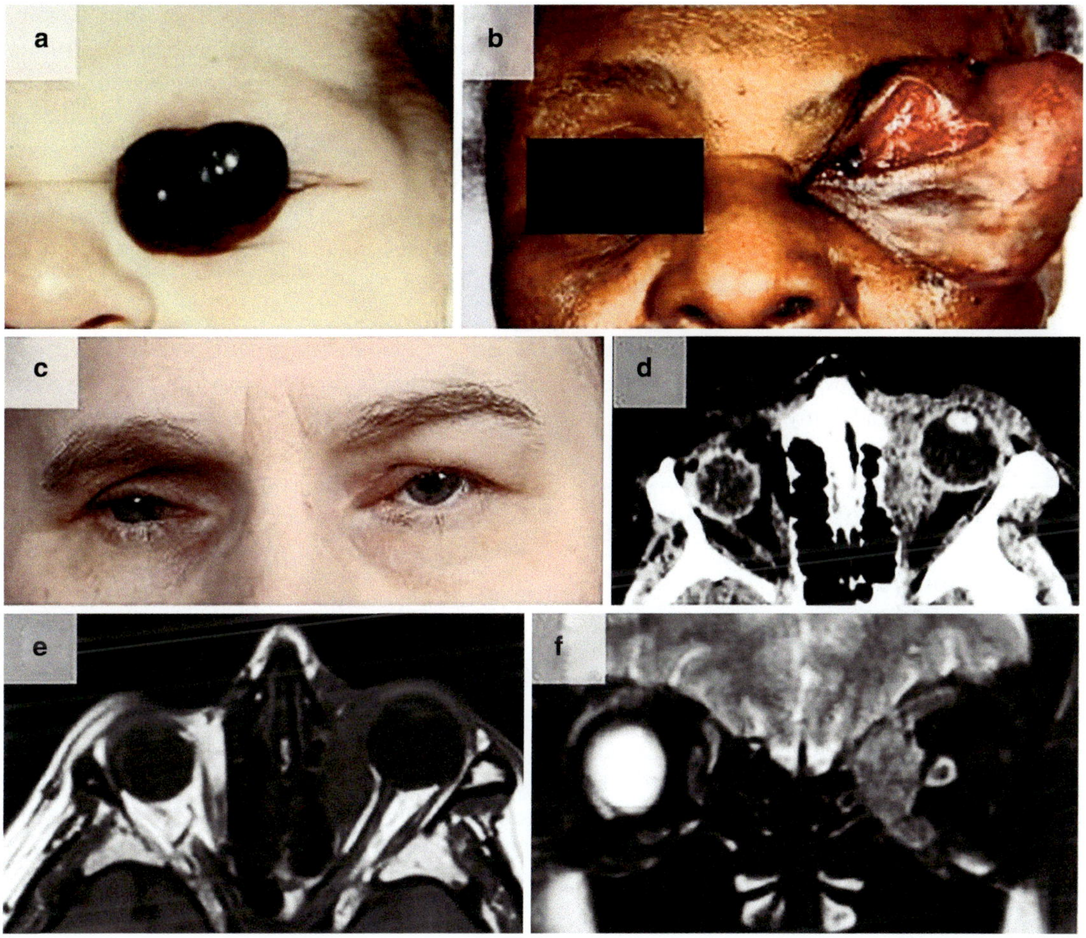

Fig. 2 (**a**) Infant with left medial canthal spontaneously infarcted myofibroma. (**b**) Left locally advanced fibrosarcoma. (**c**) Leiomyosarcoma following radiotherapy in infancy for retinoblastoma presenting with left superonasal palpable mass. (**d**) CT shows a heterogenous medial orbital lesion contiguous with medial rectus and associated with adjacent bone remodelling. The lesion appears isointense on T1-weighted MRI (**e**), with moderate heterogenous post-gadolinium enhancement (**f**)

3 Tumours of Striated Muscle

3.1 Rhabdomyoma

Rhabdomyoma is a benign soft tissue neoplasm with skeletal muscle differentiation, accounting for ~2% of all striated muscle tumours in children. Most tumours arise in the head and neck (oral and retroauricular area), with orbital involvement rarely reported in the first three decades. Foetal rhabdomyoma may be associated with basal cell naevus syndrome, which is caused by mutations in the tumour suppressor gene PTCH1.

Presentation is usually with slowly-progressive proptosis. On MRI, the mass is well-circumscribed, isointense, and exhibits homogenous enhancement with no surrounding infiltration, necrosis, haemorrhage, or bone destruction (although bone remodelling may be seen). Histology shows a circumscribed, but unencapsulated, mass displaying bland primitive spindle cells associated with foetal myotubules in a myxoid stroma. Immunohistochemistry shows skeletal muscle differentiation with positive staining for myoglobin, desmin, and muscle-specific actin. The tumour can be adequately managed by a local excision [2].

3.2 Rhabdomyosarcoma

Rhabdomyosarcoma is the commonest childhood soft tissue mesenchymal tumour and orbital malignancy. The clinical presentation and management of rhabdomyosarcomas are described in chapter “Orbital Rhabdomyosarcomas”.

4 Tumours of Smooth Muscle

4.1 Leiomyoma

Leiomyoma is a rare benign tumour of the smooth muscle, that can arise from Müller's muscle, lower eyelid retractors, vascular walls, or muscular elements within orbital septa. Most tumours arise in children or young adults, with a male predilection.

Anteriorly-located tumours may be painful and present with eyelid swelling or palpable mass, whilst intraconal lesions tend to cause proptosis. Visual impairment and reduced ocular motility are uncommon. Imaging generally shows a well-circumscribed non-enhancing mass with no specific features to differentiate from other orbital lesions. Histology shows fascicles of elongated spindle cells with no mitotic activity, and immunohistochemistry is positive for vimentin, smooth muscle actin, and desmin. Intact local excision is the treatment of choice, although it may be difficult due to profound adherence between the tumour capsule and surrounding orbital tissues.

4.2 Leiomyosarcoma

Leiomyosarcoma is a malignant smooth muscle neoplasm, accounting for 5–10% of soft tissue sarcomas. Primary orbital involvement is very uncommon, with lesions arising from smooth muscle in blood vessels, Müller's muscle, orbital fascial septa or *de novo* from smooth muscle precursors. It usually affects the older or middle-aged women, although it has also been observed in children and young individuals with prior orbital or periorbital radiation. Midface or metastatic lesions may also cause secondary orbital involvement [1, 2].

4.2.1 Clinical Presentation

Patients usually present with rapidly progressive proptosis and variable impairment of vision or motility, due to tumour infiltration (Fig. 2c). Congestive or compressive features—including conjunctival hyperaemia, disc swelling, retinal venous engorgement, or choroidal folds—may also be present.

4.2.2 Imaging

CT usually shows a dense, heterogeneous, round mass with moderate post-contrast enhancement, sometimes associated with bone remodelling or destruction (Fig. 2d). The lesions are isointense on T1-weighted MRI and hypointense on T2-weighting, with occasional post-gadolinium peripheral enhancement [2] (Fig. 2e, f). Occasionally, extraorbital extension may be present.

4.2.3 Histopathology

Microscopy shows solid proliferation of spindle cells with abundant mitotic activity and numerous parallel myofibrils along the cells that stain deep-red with Masson trichrome. There is a prominent vascular component and smooth muscle actin, desmin and h-caldesmon are positive in most tumours.

4.2.4 Management

Intact excision of small encapsulated tumours should be performed but, due to their infiltrative nature, this is often difficult and wide local resection—including surrounding bone—or orbital exenteration is often necessary. Adjuvant radiotherapy is commonly used and chemotherapy is indicated for systemic disease.

5 Adipocytic Tumours

5.1 Lipoma

Lipomas are the most frequent adipose-derived mesenchymal tumours, commonly arising in the subcutaneous tissues, but rarely found in the orbit—where spindle cell lipoma, angiolipoma, pleomorphic lipoma, and myolipoma have been reported. Clinical presentation of lipomas, particularly pleomorphic subtype, may be similar to prolapsed orbital fat, with eyelid swelling or palpable mass. Diagnosis can be overlooked as many patients elect not to undergo surgery, and because the adipose tissue is usually discarded after surgery.

Imaging reveals a well-circumscribed non-enhancing mass that is radiolucent on CT and isointense on MRI and moulded around the orbital structures (Fig. 3a, b). Histologically, the tumour is composed of mature adipocytes and may be differentiated from normal orbital fat by thicker fibrous septa between fat lobules, greater vascularity, a more variegated appearance to the diameters of the univacuolar adipocytes, and occasionally dispersed spindle cells and smooth muscle cells. Lipomas are readily treated by surgical excision without any significant complication (Fig. 3c, d).

5.2 Liposarcoma

Liposarcomas (LSS) arise from primitive mesenchymal lipoblasts, and are the most common soft tissue sarcoma—accounting for ~20% of all sarcomas. Primary orbital involvement is rare, occurs mostly in middle age, and is often initially overlooked due to its inconspicuous resemblance to prolapsed orbital fat or lipoma. Orbital metastatic LS can rarely arise from primary tumours of the extremities or retroperitoneum [1, 2, 7].

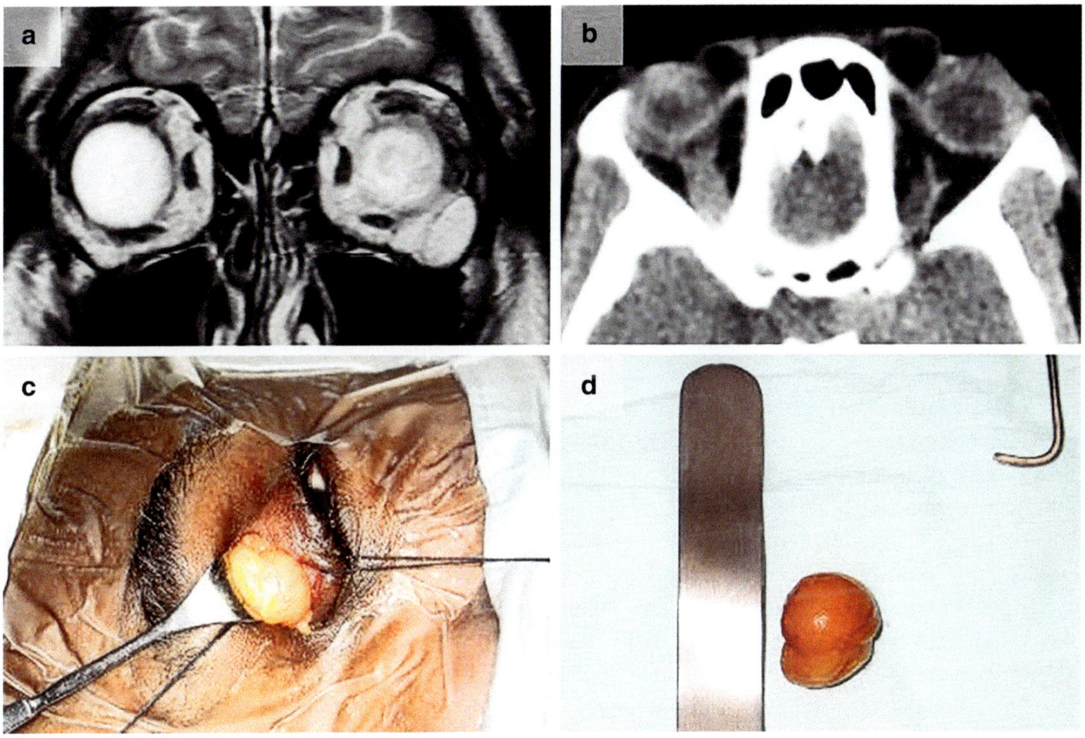

Fig. 3 Orbital lipomas: (**a**) T-2 weighted MRI shows a well-circumscribed fat-intensity infero-temporal quadrant ovoid mass. (**b**) CT shows bilateral round superonasal quadrant hypodense lesions intimately related to superior oblique tendons. (**c**) Operative appearance of the left superonasal quadrant lipoma and (**d**) the same lesion being excised intact

5.2.1 Clinical Presentation

Presenting features include slowly progressive painless proptosis, globe displacement, reduced visual function or ocular motility, and a palpable rubbery mass when anteriorly-located.

5.2.2 Imaging

The tumour is often located in the superior, lateral and retrobulbar areas. On CT, it is usually a well-defined, lobulated, fat-attenuation mass with dense intralesional septa and moderate-to-marked heterogenous post-contrast enhancement. MRI shows iso- or hyperintense mass on T1-weighted and hypointense on T2-sequences, with septa appearing as low-intensity lines, and variable enhancement that is greater in the periphery.

5.2.3 Histopathology

The tumour is composed of round, stellate or spindle-shaped lipoblasts in a myxoid or mucopolysaccharide-rich stroma, with a complex vascular network. Well-differentiated, myxoid, round-cell, dedifferentiated, and pleomorphic are the five subtypes that have been identified, with myxoid and well-differentiated lesions being the commonest orbital variants.

5.2.4 Management and Prognosis

With primary orbital lesions, smaller tumour size and well-differentiated subtypes have a better prognosis, and metastasis is rare. Complete excision is difficult due to the infiltrative nature, and therefore wide local resection is recommended for local control. Even after extensive surgery, recurrence is common, and partial resection has a greater risk of recurrence and de-differentiation into more aggressive phenotypes.

The role of adjuvant radiotherapy is controversial and mainly reserved for recurrences. When local excision and adjunctive radiotherapy fail, exenteration should be offered to prevent extra-orbital spread. Most tumours are chemo-resistant, and cytotoxic agents are reserved for palliative treatment.

6 Chondrogenic Tumours

6.1 Chondroma

Chondroma is a benign tumour composed of well-differentiated, mature hyaline cartilage and primary orbital lesions are exceedingly rare, with two types described: the "true chondroma," considered to develop from the trochlea, and the "cartilaginous hamartoma," thought to arise from primitive mesenchymal cells. Primary skull base or paranasal sinus chondromas may also affect the orbit.

'Cartilaginous hamartomas' typically present as circumscribed orbital masses in children, while 'true chondromas' are more typically present in adults with a slowly progressive well-defined mass located in the superonasal quadrant of the orbit, with features of Brown's syndrome. The prognosis is generally good, although malignant transformation into chondrosarcoma can rarely occur. Intact surgical excision is the main treatment for symptomatic or progressive lesions.

6.2 Chondrosarcoma

Chondrosarcoma is a malignant cartilaginous tumour mostly arising in the extremities, pelvis and ribs, with orbital involvement usually being secondary to extension from sinonasal tumours (Fig. 4) [8]. Various associations, such as trauma, previous irradiation or Paget's disease, have been reported and genomic studies suggest a possible genetic propensity. Low-grade periorbital chondrosarcoma can also occur in multiple enchondromatosis (Ollier's disease).

6.2.1 Clinical Presentation

Commonly occurring in young adults, the tumour may present with ocular displacement, diplopia, visual impairment, palpable inferior or medial orbital mass, with or without pain, or with sino-nasal symptoms.

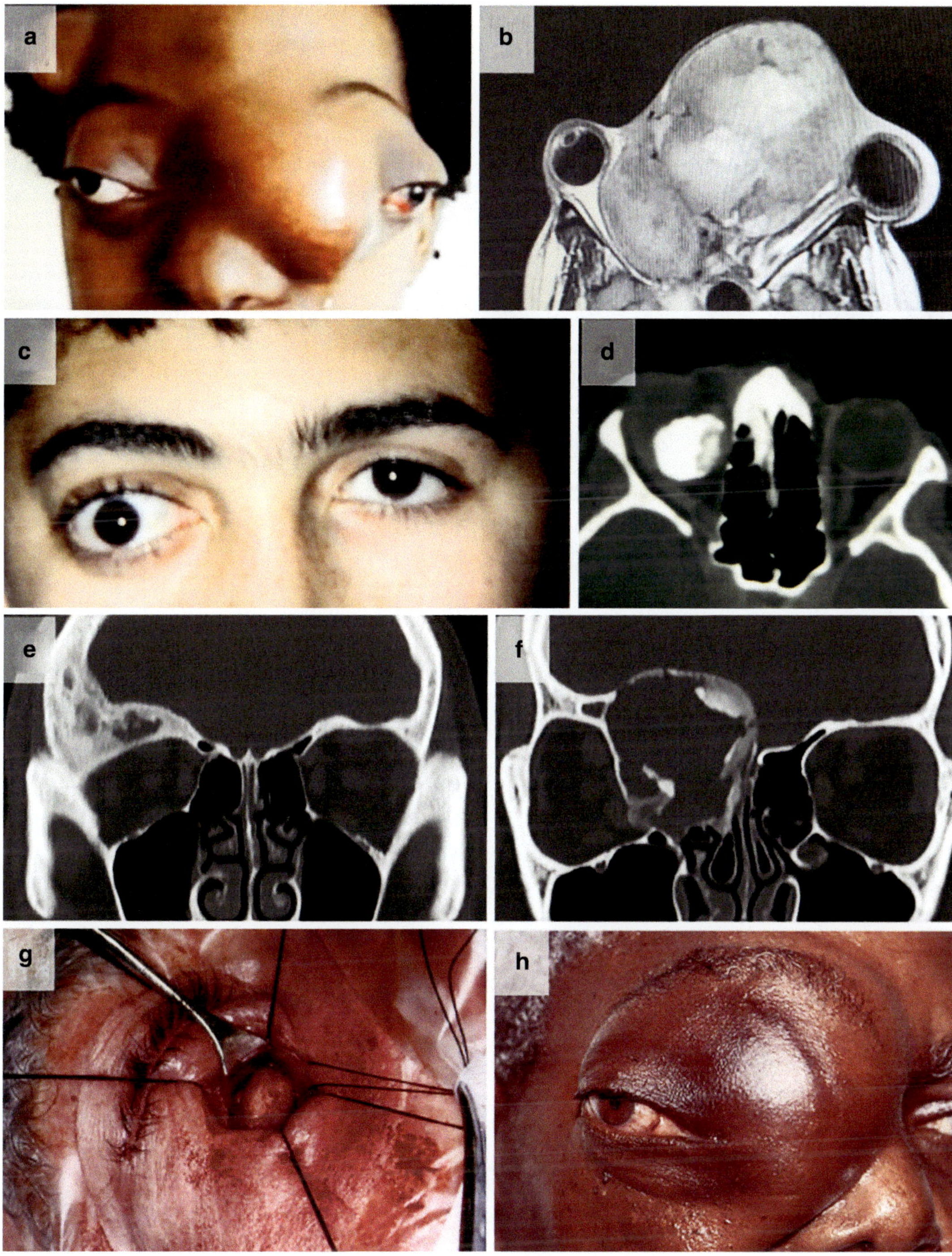

Fig. 4 (**a**) Bilateral advanced chondrosarcoma. (**b**) Axial T-1 weighted MRI of large well-delineated sinonasal chondrosarcoma invading both orbits. (**c**) Right infero-temporal globe displacement due to fronto-ethmoid ivory osteoma (**d**). (**e**) Fibrous dysplasia involving the right orbital roof, with ground glass appearance of the medullary bone and cystic changes. (**f**) Right ossifying fibroma involving the orbit, frontal and ethmoidal sinuses, and the skull base. (**g**) Intra-operative appearance of right ossifying fibroma involving the orbital floor/maxillary bone. (**h**) Osteosarcoma with large expansile mass and lateral globe displacement

6.2.2 Imaging

The tumour is fairly well-defined on CT, with radiolucent matrix and areas of sclerosis, may have a sclerotic rim, and have variable contrast enhancement. Erosion of the orbital plate around the base of the tumour and intracranial extension may be seen. The lesion appears hyperintense on T1-weighted MRI, and isointense to hyperintense on T2-weighted images.

6.2.3 Histology

Histologically, the lesions appear as irregularly-shaped lobules with atypical chondrocytes separated by fibrous bands or bony trabeculae. Based on level of differentiation they are graded into: Grade I tumours—well differentiated, resembling a chondroma; Grade II tumours—moderately differentiated, showing maturation with multiple cells in lacunae with a greater degree of nuclear atypia; and Grade III—poorly differentiated tumours showing atypia with frequent mitoses, anaplastic stroma, and sometimes with foci of osteoid formation. Histological variants include clear cell, myxoid, mesenchymal and dedifferentiated chondrosarcomas, the latter two having the worst prognosis. Mesenchymal chondrosarcoma is the most common variant of primary chondrosarcoma in the orbit.

6.2.4 Management and Prognosis

Complete surgical resection can be challenging due to infiltrative borders of the tumour, usually requiring a multidisciplinary approach. Adjuvant radiotherapy may have some effect in slowing progression of non-resectable tumours and the role of chemotherapy is unclear. Long-term surveillance is needed as local recurrence may occur in 65% of the cases within 5 years, and it is the main cause of death.

7 Osseous and Fibro-osseous Tumours

7.1 Osteoma

With possible aetiologies including trauma and chronic sinusitis, osteomas are the most frequent benign bone tumours of paranasal sinuses, especially the frontal and ethmoidal sinuses. Most orbital osteomas are intrusions by sino-nasal lesions, and usually discovered incidentally. However, they are rarely part of Gardner's syndrome, which comprises soft-tissue tumours, intestinal polyposis, secondary bowel cancer, and retinal pigmentary changes. Ivory (compact), cancellous, and fibrous (spongiosa) are three variants of osteoma [1, 2, 9].

7.1.1 Clinical Presentation

Osteomas are more common in males, with a peak incidence in the fourth decade. The tumour can be asymptomatic, or may cause globe displacement (Fig. 4c), pain, headache or palpable hard mass—typically in the superonasal quadrant of the orbit. Chronic sinusitis or secondary mucocele may arise if the bony mass obstructs sinus drainage.

7.1.2 Imaging

Typically, a hyperdense, ovoid, or multilobular superior or superonasal mass, encroaching into the orbit, is seen on CT (Fig. 4d). The ivory type shows bone density, whereas the fibrous variant is less dense and resembles fibrous dysplasia.

7.1.3 Histopathology

The ivory osteoma has minimal fibrous stroma, while the less mature cancellous variant may have more visible interconnecting fibrous pathways and osteoblastic activity. Fibrous osteomas have a significant fibrous stroma with scant bone spiculation, and may be part of the spectrum comprising fibrous dysplasia and ossifying fibroma.

7.1.4 Management

Surgical excision is indicated for larger and symptomatic osteomas or those causing aesthetic deformities. The lesions can be removed through external, endoscopic or combined approaches. Recurrence is uncommon, even after incomplete excision.

7.2 Fibrous Dysplasia

Fibrous dysplasia (FD, characterised by expansion and replacement of medullary bone by fibro-osseous tissue, is a non-inherited bone disease that can affect a single bone (monostotic) or multiple bones (polyostotic). Polyostotic FD can occur in isolation or as part of endocrinopathies and abnormalities of cutaneous pigmentation in McCune-Albright syndrome, as well as with intramuscular myxomas in Mazabraud syndrome. Most lesions are monostotic and 20% involve craniofacial bone—the frontal, sphenoid, and ethmoid bones being most affected [1–3, 9].

7.2.1 Clinical Presentation

Presentation is usually in childhood or adolescence, but the monostotic form may remain asymptomatic until adulthood. Typical features include facial asymmetry, proptosis and hypoglobus due to commonly involved frontal bone. Facial pain, strabismus, epiphora and visual loss—due to encasement of the optic canal, spontaneous bleeding, formation of sinus mucocoele or aneurysmal bone cyst—may also occur. Progression is usually slow and it may stop in middle age. Although almost invariably benign, FD can undergo transformation into osteosarcoma, fibrosarcoma, or other malignancies, especially following irradiation.

7.2.2 Imaging

Classically the lesions have a "ground glass" appearance with medullary expansion and thinning of the cortical bone (Fig. 4e). Depending on the stage of development of the lesion, the radiological characteristics of FD range from radiolucent areas in the early stages to extensive sclerotic changes with ill-defined borders in later stages. MRI usually shows areas of low-to-intermediate signal intensity equal to that of muscle, with moderate to marked post-contrast enhancement.

7.2.3 Histopathology

FD is characterised by fibrous tissue with randomly oriented bony trabeculae composed of immature woven bone that are not lined by osteoblasts, although focal osteoblastic rimming may be seen. Trabeculae have a variety of forms, ranging from solid, circular islands to short, irregular, curved, or serpiginous shapes, giving them the "Chinese character" or "alphabet soup" appearance.

7.2.4 Management

Before puberty management is generally conservative. Bisphosphonates and monoclonal antibodies, such as tocilizumab or denosumab, have been utilised for controlling severe persistent bone pain in polyostotic disease.

Surgery is indicated for functional orbital impairment, progressive deformity, chronic pain, intralesional cysts near orbital apex, or when malignant transformation is suspected. Conservative surgical excision is preferred, as complete resection is usually impractical, and neurosurgical decompression may occasionally be required if the optic canal is compromised. Radiotherapy is contraindicated due to risk of malignant transformation. These and other management guidelines are detailed in chapter "Neuro-Orbital Diseases".

7.3 Ossifying Fibroma

Ossifying fibroma (OF) is a slow-growing benign tumour composed of highly-cellular fibrous tissue with varying amounts of osseous or cement-like tissue. The lesion typically develops in young adults, with a predilection for mandible or maxilla, and orbital involvement is usually secondary to paranasal sinus lesions. OF tends to have a more aggressive clinical behaviour than FD, starting with a gradually expansile lesion that may eventually involve the contralateral orbit, or extend intracranially [1–3, 9].

7.3.1 Clinical Presentation

Depending on the size and location of the lesion, there is progressive proptosis and lateral or upward globe displacement, which in some cases is accompanied with pain or compressive optic neuropathy.

7.3.2 Imaging

CT reveals a well-circumscribed ovoid mass in the affected bone, with an inhomogeneous matrix and thin sclerotic margin (Fig. 4f). Internal septations and foci of calcification may be noted. MRI shows a heterogeneous signal, with intermediate intensity on T1-weighted images and hypointense T2-weighted images, and marked post-contrast enhancement of the sclerotic rim.

7.3.3 Histopathology

OF consists of benign spindle cells in a vascular fibrous stroma, with scattered bony ossicles surrounded by a narrow ring of osteoblasts, a feature that distinguishes OF from FD.

7.3.4 Management

Wide local resection (Fig. 4g) is the mainstay of treatment, often requiring a combined orbital, skull base, and neurosurgical approach, together with skull base reconstruction using bone grafts or alloplastic materials. Recurrence can occur after incomplete excision, and long-term clinico-radiological observation is advised.

7.4 Osteosarcoma

Usually affecting the extremities, osteosarcoma (or osteogenic sarcoma) is the commonest primary malignant bone tumour and primary orbital involvement is rare—with most lesions arising from neighbouring paranasal sinuses. The tumours may also develop after irradiation for hereditary retinoblastoma, and malignant transformation of fibrous dysplasia or Paget's disease [1–3, 9].

Orbital osteosarcomas commonly present in the fourth to fifth decades, with rapidly-progressive globe displacement, deep orbital pain, a palpable mass and/or reduced vision (Fig. 4h). Imaging generally shows an irregular, lytic bony lesion with foci of calcification, associated with soft tissue component infiltrating the adjacent structures, which is best visible on MRI.

Histologically, osteosarcoma is a highly anaplastic and pleomorphic tumour composed of spindle, epithelioid, plasmacytoid, fusiform, ovoid, small round cells, clear cells and giant cells. Osteoid and neoplastic bone formation is present, with the tumour matrix often containing varying amounts of chondroid or fibrous tissues.

In most cases, extensive local resection or exenteration is necessary, along with adjuvant chemotherapy or radiation. Orbital osteosarcoma has a poor prognosis, with a 5-year survival of less than 50%.

8 Other Mesenchymal Tumours

8.1 Myxoma

Myxoma is a rare benign mesenchymal tumour that affects the skeletal muscles of the limbs, the skin, the heart, and the genitourinary system. Deriving from fibroblast-like cells, myxomas generate a lot of glycosaminoglycans, especially hyaluronic acid, and very little collagen. Carney syndrome, Mazabraud syndrome, and McCune–Albright syndrome are known associations, but orbital involvement is extremely rare.

Orbital myxomas generally present with painless proptosis, and imaging usually shows a mass located in the mid or posterior orbit (Fig. 5a, b). Histologically they are composed of stellate cells and delicate fibrillary reticulin, within a loose mucoid stroma containing sparse blood vessels. Although myxomas are benign, wide local resection is recommended as incomplete excision may result in local recurrence. Presumed non-progressive asymptomatic lesions may be observed.

8.2 Alveolar Soft-part Sarcoma

Representing <1% of all sarcomas, alveolar soft-part sarcoma (ASPS) is an extremely rare malignant mesenchymal tumour and most commonly arises in the head and neck. It has an uncertain line of differentiation and is thought to be a muscle-derived tumour [10].

Orbital ASPS is very rare and patients generally present in young adulthood with a painless slowly-growing mass, eyelid swelling or propto-

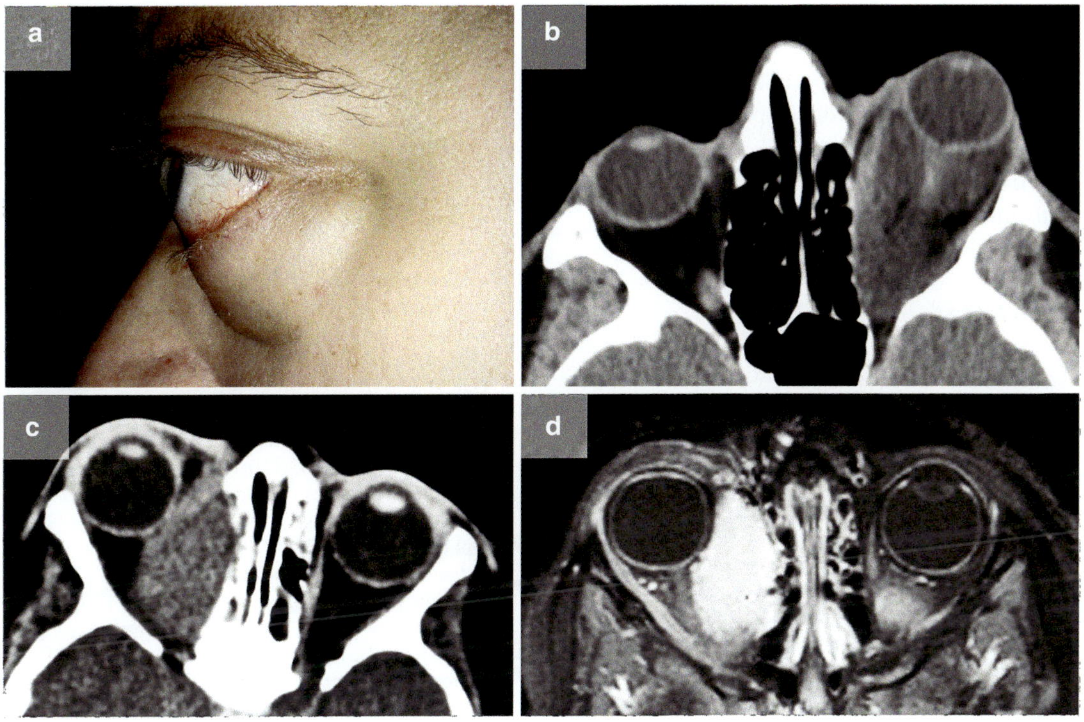

Fig. 5 (**a**) Left orbital myxoma presenting with severe proptosis. (**b**) Axial CT of left orbital myxoma appearing as diffuse infiltrative mass throughout the orbit. (**c**) CT imaging of alveolar soft part sarcoma showing right medial orbital soft-tissue mass with adjacent bone remodelling and marked contrast enhancement on MRI (**d**)

sis. Imaging shows a homogeneous soft-tissue mass with marked contrast enhancement on both CT and MRI (Fig. 5c, d). The tumour is composed of large epithelioid cells arranged in a distinct organoid or "nesting" pattern, surrounded by thin fibrovascular septa; the nests develop a "pseudo-alveolar" pattern due to loss of cellular cohesion and a central necrosis.

ASPS have a variable biological behaviour, but most have a relatively indolent clinical course, and orbital tumours are reported to be smaller and have a better prognosis compared to other locations. Complete surgical excision is the established treatment for ASPS, with adjuvant radiotherapy reported to reduce the risk of local recurrence.

8.3 Synovial Sarcoma

Accounting for 10% of all soft-tissue sarcomas, synovial sarcoma (SS) is the second most common soft-tissue sarcoma in children, and most affect the extremities or head and neck, with a only few reported orbital cases; it affects mainly young adults and has a female preponderance. SS arises from primitive mesenchymal stem cells and is associated with a unique DNA translocation, resulting in an SYT-SSX fusion gene [11].

Clinical features include, periorbital pain, eyelid swelling, ophthalmoplegia or palpable mass. Radiologically the tumours appear in continuity with extraocular muscles, most commonly medial rectus, and sometimes displays prominent calcification within the tumour—a relatively uncommon feature in other soft-tissue sarcomas.

Orbital SS is a poorly-differentiated sarcoma composed of primitive round or spindle cells, while classic SS shows a biphasic population of spindle and epithelial cells. Detecting the unique (X;18) translocation, or the resultant SYT–SSX fusion gene product, helps confirm the diagnosis and distinguish this entity from other primitive soft-tissue cancers that are more frequent in the orbit.

Five-year survival for all SS is 80% and about a half of patients will develop metastases. Most of the reported orbital SS underwent local resection without margin control, and some had adjuvant chemotherapy or radiotherapy.

References

1. Garrity JA, Henderson JW, Cameron JD. Henderson's tumors of primitive mesoderm, striated muscle, adipose tissue and smooth muscle. In: Garrity JA, Henderson JW, Cameron JD, editors. Henderson's orbital tumors. 4th ed. Philadelphia: Lippincott Williams & Wilkins; 2007. p. 123–41.
2. Lane KA, Nilyk JR, Jakobiec FA. Mesenchymal, fibroosseous, and cartilaginous orbital tumors. In: Albert DM, Miller JW, Azar DT, editors. Albert & Jakobiec's principles and practice of ophthalmology. 3rd ed. Philadelphia: Saunders/Elsevier; 2008. p. 3159–201.
3. Shields JA, Shields CL, Scartozzi R. Survey of 1264 patients with orbital tumors and simulating lesions: The 2002 Montgomery Lecture, Part 1. Ophthalmology. 2004;111:997–1008.
4. Furusato E, Valenzuela IA, Fanburg-Smith JC, et al. Orbital solitary fibrous tumor: encompassing terminology for hemangiopericytoma, giant cell angiofibroma, and fibrous histiocytoma of the orbit: reappraisal of 41 cases. Hum Pathol. 2011;42:120–8.
5. Blessing NW, Bermudez-Magner JA, Fernandez MP, Rosenberg AE, Dubovy SR, Johnson TE. Solitary fibrous tumor of the orbit: a case series with clinicopathologic correlation and evaluation of STAT6 as a diagnostic marker. Ophthalmic Plast Reconstr Surg. 2020;36:164–71.
6. Thompson LDR, Liou SS, Feldman KA. Orbit solitary fibrous tumor: a proposed risk prediction model based on a case series and comprehensive literature review. Head Neck Pathol. 2021;15:138–52.
7. Daniel CS, Beaconsfield M, Rose GE, Luthert PJ, Heathcote JG, Clark BJ. Pleomorphic lipoma of the orbit: a case series and review of literature. Ophthalmology. 2003;110:101–5.
8. Kiratli H, Dikmetas O, Tarlan B, et al. Orbital chondrosarcoma arising from paranasal sinuses. Int Ophthalmol. 2013;33:403–7.
9. Selva D, White VA, O'Connell JX, Rootman J. Primary bone tumors of the orbit. Surv Ophthalmol. 2004;49:328–42.
10. Hei Y, Kang L, Yang X, et al. Orbital alveolar soft part sarcoma: A report of 8 cases and review of the literature. Oncol Lett. 2018;15:304–14.
11. Stagner AM, Jakobiec FA, Fay A. Primary orbital synovial sarcoma: A clinicopathologic review with a differential diagnosis and discussion of molecular genetics. Surv Ophthalmol. 2017;62:227–36.

Secondary Orbital Tumours and Orbital Metastases

Diego Strianese, Adriana Iuliano, and Francesco M. Quaranta Leoni

Key Messages

- Secondary orbital tumours are lesions that originate from contiguous structures. Basal cell eyelid carcinoma and squamous cell conjunctival carcinoma are the two most frequent tumours which can lead to a secondary orbital invasion.
- Basal cell carcinomas invading the orbit have been successfully treated in recent years with medications that target the sonic hedgehog pathway.
- Immune checkpoint inhibitors and epidermal growth-factor receptor inhibitors are effective for treatment of patients with locally advanced or metastatic squamous cell carcinoma of the head and neck. Exenteration may be considered in patients with orbital involvement and poor residual visual acuity.
- Most orbital metastases are carcinomas; sarcomas and melanomas are considerably less common. Breast is the most common primary site of metastatic orbital lesions, followed by lung and prostate.
- Treatment of orbital metastatic lesions aim to control the growth of the tumour, preserve visual function, and improve patient comfort. There is no standard treatment: surgery, radiotherapy or neoadjuvant therapy may have favourable responses, although the prognosis usually remains poor.

1 Secondary Orbital Tumours

Secondary orbital tumours are lesions that originate from contiguous structures such as the eyelids, conjunctiva, eye, paranasal sinuses, nasopharynx, and that grow large enough to invade the orbit. Metastatic orbital tumours are those that spread to the orbit by blood from distant foci. The classification of the distribution of secondary orbital tumours is shown in Table 1 [1, 2].

Eyelid basal cell carcinoma and eyelid and conjunctival squamous cell carcinoma are the two most frequent tumours which can lead to a secondary orbital invasion. Early diagnosis and proper treatment of eyelid carcinomas have

D. Strianese · A. Iuliano
Orbital Unit, University of Naples Federico II, Naples, Italy

F. M. Quaranta Leoni (✉)
Oftalmoplastica Roma, Rome, Italy
e-mail: fquarantaleoni@gmail.com

F. M. Quaranta Leoni et al. (eds.), *Oculoplastic, Lacrimal and Orbital Surgery*,
https://doi.org/10.1007/978-3-031-39638-0_25

Table 1 Classification of secondary orbital tumours

Lesion
Eyelid
Basal cell carcinoma
Squamous cell carcinoma
Sebaceous gland carcinoma
Merkel cell carcinoma
Malignant melanoma
Intraocular
Retinoblastoma
Uveal melanoma
Conjunctiva
Squamous cell carcinoma
Malignant melanoma
Mucoepidermoid carcinoma
Nasopharynx
Carcinoma
Angiofibroma
Sinus carcinoma
Intracranial meningioma
Chordoma

reduced the incidence of secondary orbital invasion in recent years. However, as the COVID-19 outbreak has led to a limited access to healthcare for patients worldwide, a new wave of orbital secondary invasion from the aforementioned carcinomas has been observed [3].

1.1 Eyelid Basal Cell Carcinoma

Basal cell carcinoma (BCC) is, overall, the most frequently occurring malignant lesion of the eyelid. BCC is a slowly growing tumour with the tendency to invade surrounding tissues particularly when located in the medial canthal area [4]. Due to a relatively greater amount of sun exposure of the lower eyelid, BCC has a predilection for this region (Fig. 1), followed by the medial canthus (Fig. 2). Metastases are diminishingly rare [4].

1.1.1 Physical Examination

Careful examination of an eyelid lesion is essential when BCC is suspected, and macroscopic features of the lesion are useful in differential diagnosis and in the decision-making process. When a large lesion is encountered, evaluation of ocular motility and proptosis are essential in excluding orbital extension (Fig. 3), and impairment of an extraocular muscle in the region of a suspected BCC can represent an early sign of orbital invasion [4]. Medial canthal lesions are critical and require computed tomography (CT) or magnetic resonance imaging (MRI) to rule out possible orbital invasion.

Examination of the lesion includes assessment for:

- General appearance and extent of the lesion and periocular skin
- Distortion of eyelid architecture or eyelid malposition
- Presence of skin ulceration
- Madarosis
- Telangiectasias
- Blood clot due to bleeding of the lesion
- Pigmentation and skin colour changes—useful for differential diagnosis and BCC variants

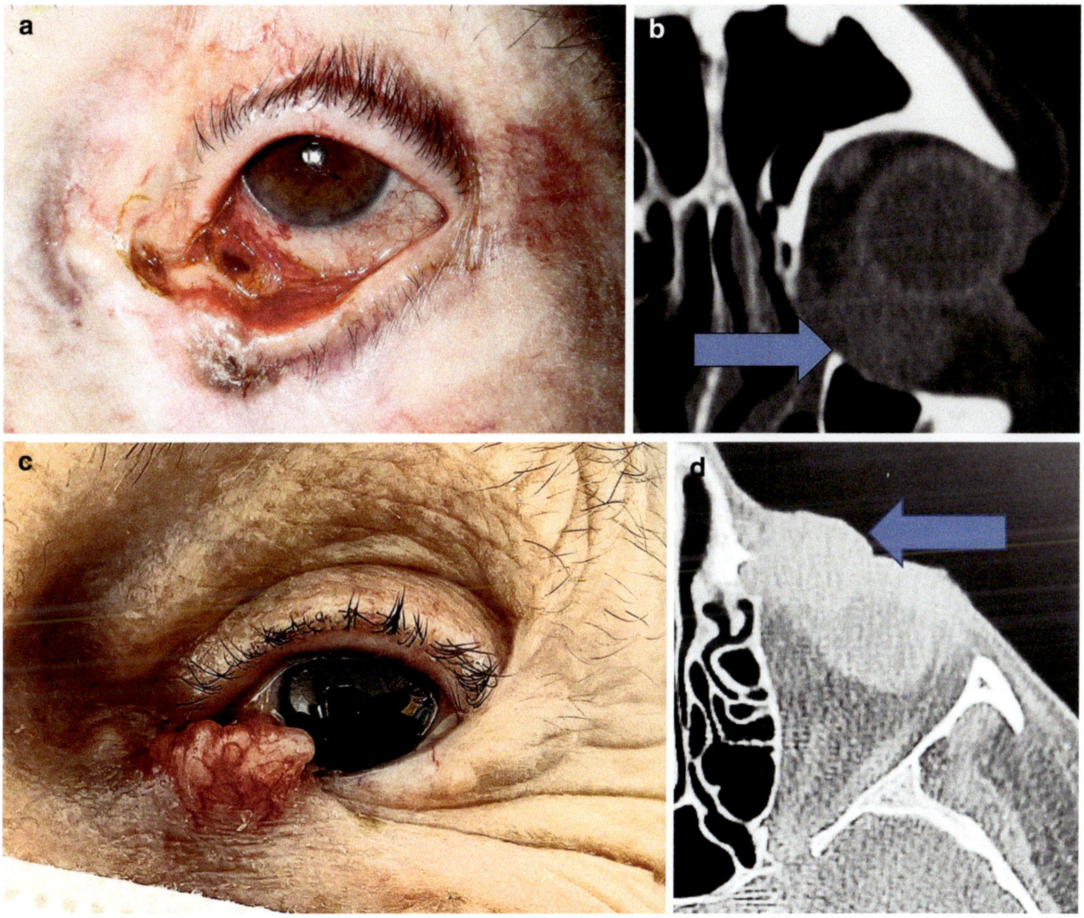

Fig. 1 (**a**, **c**) Recurrent basal cell carcinomas of the left lower eyelid in two separate patients, with respective CT imaging (**b**, **d**) identifying orbital invasion in each case (Courtesy of F. Quaranta Leoni)

BCC may be indolent (and thus neglected by the patient), or present as an ulcerated and non-healing lesion with recurrent bleeding and crusting of the skin. Eyelash loss (madarosis), distortion of normal eyelid margin sclerodermic growth may also be observed (see chapter "Periocular Skin Lesions and Eyelid Tumours").

1.1.2 Management

Treatment aims to a complete surgical excision with clear margin. Margin control is performed with good results either with frozen sections or Mohs' technique (see chapter "Eyelid Tumour Excision: Frozen Section Versus Mohs Surgery").

Globe-sparing surgery for locally advanced BCCs—with the intention of preserving visual function—can still result in visual impairment or loss due to ocular misalignment and surface disorders. Surgery can be complicated by late recurrence that develops rapidly, despite silent neuroimaging for years. These patients require lifelong surveillance as morbidity and chance of recurrence are not well elucidated [5].

Pervasive BCCs—invading vital structures or surgically unresectable due to the general condition of the patient—have been successfully treated in recent years with medication that targets the sonic hedgehog pathway, such as vismo-

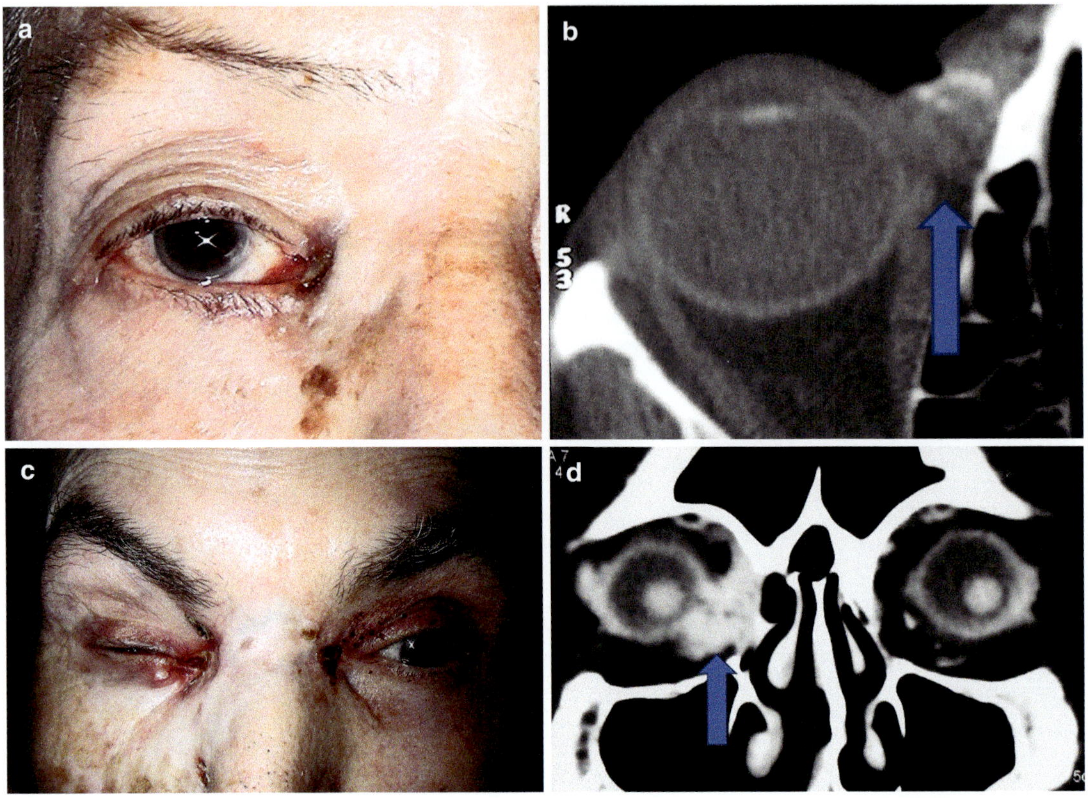

Fig. 2 (**a**, **c**) Recurrent basal cell carcinomas of the right medial canthus in two separate patients, with respective CT imaging (**b**, **d**) identifying orbital invasion in each case (Courtesy of F. Quaranta Leoni)

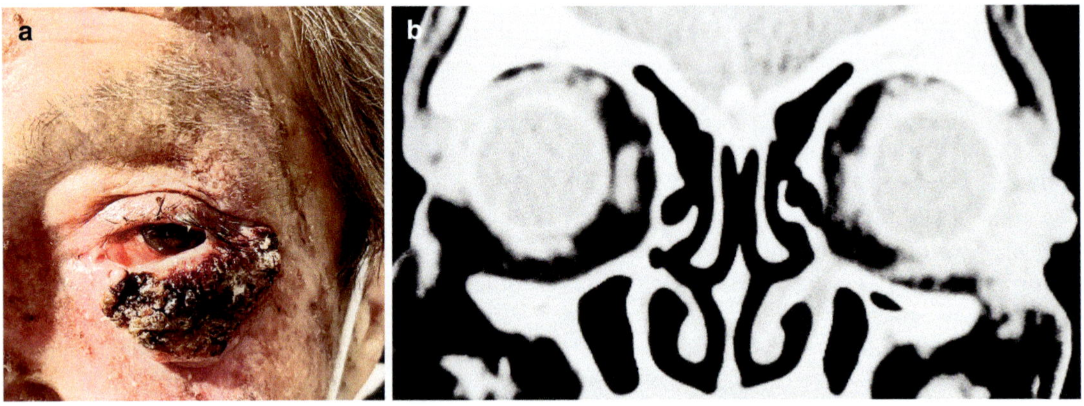

Fig. 3 (**a**) Recurrent basosquamous carcinoma of left lower lid and lateral canthus. These tumours may be difficult to differentiate from squamous cell carcinomas and should be treated as such. (**b**) Coronal CT scan shows orbital invasion (Courtesy of F. Quaranta Leoni)

degib (Fig. 4) and sonidegib (see chapter "Management of Locally Invasive and Metastatic Eyelid Tumours") [6].

Sonic hedgehog inhibitors are effective in preserving essential ocular structures and visual acuity in patients with advanced BCC [7], decreasing the need for orbital exenteration that results in a significant reduction in the quality of life.

Brachytherapy has been used for locally advanced eyelid BCC and squamous cell carci-

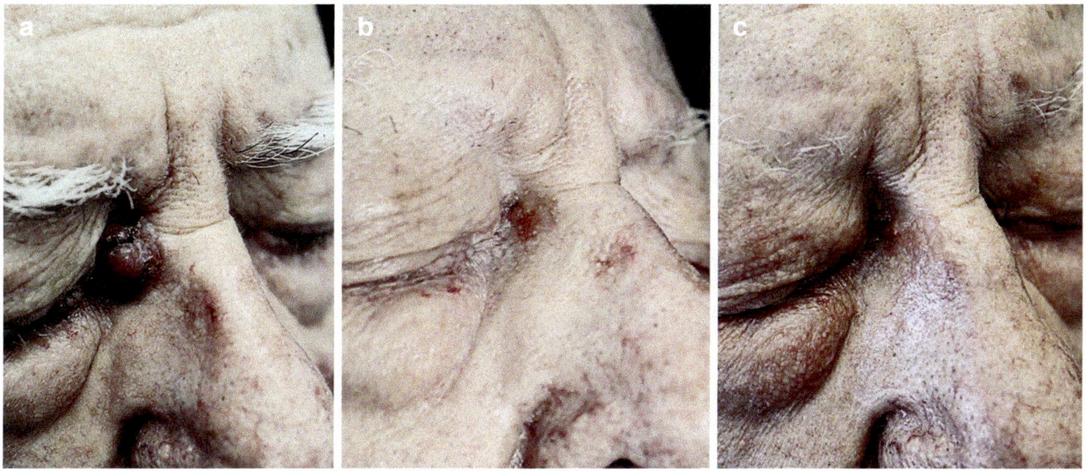

Fig. 4 (**a**) 84 year-old man with recurrent invasive basal cell carcinoma of the right medial canthus, after cryotherapy and surgical excision with no clear margins. (**b**) After 4 months of treatment with vismodegib. (**c**) After 8 months of treatment with vismodegib there is good response with regression of the tumour (Courtesy of G. Savino, P. Sollena, A. Di Stefani)

noma (SCC) as independent treatment or as adjuvant treatment after surgery in case of patients that had undergone surgery and suffered relapse of the disease. The advantage of interstitial brachytherapy is the possibility of placing applicators inside the target, which makes it possible to administer a high dose within the clinical target volume (CTV). The rapid decrease in the dose with the growing distance from the applicator allows for the protection of adjacent structures for a significant dose reduction within the most sensitive structures. In a recent series, none of the patients treated experienced optic neuropathy, retinopathy, or visual impairment, and no relapse or metastasis were observed after a median follow-up time of 51 months [8].

1.2 Eyelid Squamous Cell Carcinoma

Eyelid SCC is less frequent than BCC, but has a more aggressive course with a higher propensity for orbital invasion. SCC is the second most common malignant eyelid tumour and accounts for 5% of malignancies of the eyelid [9]. It may develop *de novo* but often may arise from preexisting lesions such as actinic keratosis, squamous cell carcinoma in situ (Bowen's disease), xeroderma pigmentosum, or following radiotherapy. The most frequent periocular sites are lower eyelid and medial canthus, followed by upper eyelid and lateral canthus.

Orbital invasion has been reported to occur in up to 5.9% of all non-melanoma malignant eyelid carcinomas. Reported rates of metastasis for eyelid SCC vary from 1 to 21% [10].

1.2.1 Physical Examination

SCC lesions usually present as a raised nodule or plaque with overlying keratinization, scaling, or ulceration typically in the elderly.

A thorough ophthalmic examination, with reference to ocular motility, exophthalmometry, and periocular sensation is essential, and may identify early evidence for orbital invasion. Presence of a mass adherent to the bone, globe displacement, impaired ocular motility, and periocular paraesthesia or anaesthesia are highly suggestive of orbital involvement.

Palpation of regional lymph nodes, preauricular, sublingual, submandibular, and cervical is also essential, with regional lymph node metastasis reported as many as 24% of patients, common

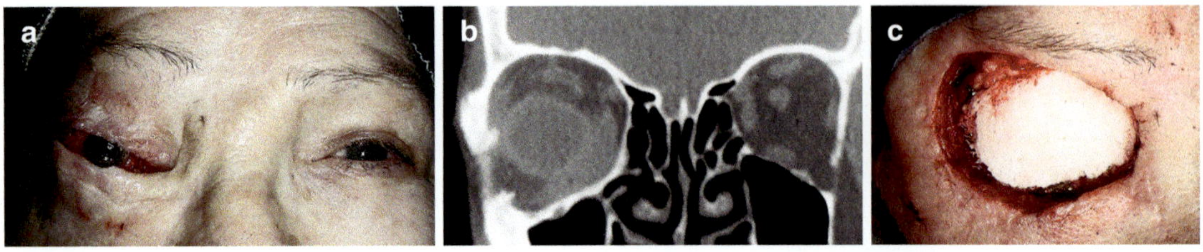

Fig. 5 (**a**) Recurrent squamous cell carcinoma invading the right orbit, after several operations. (**b**) CT scan showing orbital invasion and absence of bone of the lateral wall. Bone removal should not be performed. (**c**) The patient after palliative exenteration due to intractable pain (Courtesy of F. Quaranta Leoni)

sites being the preauricular, parotid, and submandibular lymph nodes [10].

Examination includes:

- The general appearance of the lesion and periocular skin
- Presence of skin ulceration
- Distortion of eyelid architecture or eyelid malposition
- Madarosis
- Telangiectasias

1.2.2 Management

Surgical excision is the treatment of choice. To achieve clearance, Mohs' micrographic surgery or excision with frozen-section control are frequently employed [11, 12]. Globe-sparing excisional surgery can be considered in selected cases with anterior orbital invasion, to avoid cosmetic disfigurement and loss of vision due to orbital exenteration [11], but lifelong clinical and imaging surveillance are necessary to detect possible recurrences.

Exenteration can be considered in patients with orbital involvement and poor residual visual acuity (Fig. 5), the goal of treatment being to obtain tumour free-surgical margins in order to prevent distance metastases or intracranial invasion [12].

Patients with large and extensive lesions or recurrent lesions should undergo sentinel lymph node biopsy, and the possibility of lymphatic invasion should be considered in all patients with a diagnosis of SCC. Non-invasive techniques such as echo-colour Doppler, neck MRI or CT scan with contrast enhancement all play a role in the evaluation of local lymph nodes. Radical dissection of neck lymph nodes is only indicated in cases where there is documented invasion and advanced disease, but no distant metastasis. In case of metastasis, a combination of chemotherapy and radiotherapy is recommended [12].

If orbital invasion is diagnosed, collaboration with a multidisciplinary team (oncologists, radiotherapists) helps in planning management.

Cemiplimab—a monoclonal antibody that targets the cellular pathway known as PD-1 acting as a checkpoint inhibitor—is indicated for the treatment of patients with metastatic cutaneous SCC or locally advanced SCC who are not candidates for curative surgery or curative radiotherapy (Fig. 6) [13].

Epidermal growth-factor receptor (EGFR) inhibitors are effective in the management of locally advanced or metastatic SCC of the head and neck (see chapter "Management of Locally Invasive and Metastatic Eyelid Tumours").

1.2.3 Follow Up and Prognosis

Where eyelid SCC is detected early and cleared with free margins, the prognosis is good [13]. The frequency and overall duration of follow up varies, and are based on the individual case.

Any recurrence should be treated aggressively. Unfavourable prognostic factors include: poorly differentiated tumours, perineural spread, orbital invasion, and immunosuppression. Perineural invasion with associated cranial neuropathies (trigeminal and facial nerve most commonly) occurs in 3–14% of SCC and is correlated with a worse prognosis [13].

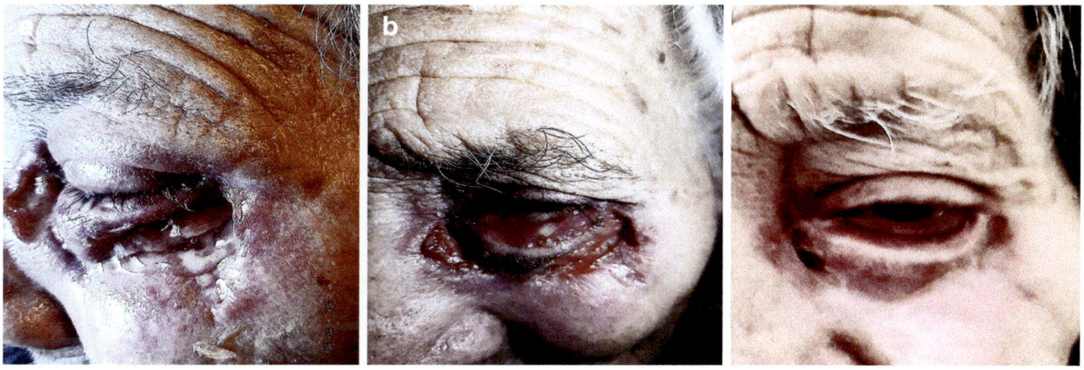

Fig. 6 (**a**) Recurrent squamous cell carcinoma invading the left orbit. (**b**) Same patient after 1 month of treatment with cemiplimab. (**c**) After 3 months of treatment with cemiplimab there is a good clinical response (Courtesy of D. Strianese and A. Iuliano)

1.3 Eyelid Sebaceous Gland Cell Carcinoma

Sebaceous gland cell carcinoma (SGC) is a rare, highly malignant, and potentially lethal tumour of the skin, which most commonly occurs in the eyelid. The neoplasm arises from sebaceous glands, such as those of the meibomian glands in the tarsus, the Zeis glands of the eyelashes, the caruncle, and the skin of the eyebrow. The lesion occurs more often in the upper eyelid, most likely due to the presence of a greater number of meibomian glands (see chapter "Periocular Skin Lesions and Eyelid Tumours").

1.3.1 Physical Examination

SGC is yellow in appearance due to intracellular lipid content. It arises from sebaceous glands, usually at the lid margin, and can extend to the palpebral conjunctiva.

SGC is one of the great masqueraders, as can mimic other lesions such as chronic unilateral blepharitis, BCC, SCC, superior limbic keratoconjunctivitis, chronic ocular surface disease, ocular cicatricial pemphigoid, and chalazia.

1.3.2 Diagnostic Procedures

One of the hallmark features of SGC is pagetoid spread in which malignant cells spread into epithelium discontinuous with the main tumour mass. The mainstay of treatment is surgical. It is important to obtain a full thickness biopsy specimen, in addition to mapping biopsies of the tarsal and bulbar conjunctiva. Mohs' micrographic surgery is an effective treatment for SGC, although invasive or widespread ocular surface disease may require orbital exenteration. This is especially true for large, deeply invasive lesions, or significant bulbar conjunctival involvement. Staging is assessed using the TNM definitions as provided by the American Joint Committee on Cancer recommendations. Sentinel lymph node biopsies can be obtained. According to the AJCC it seems reasonable to recommend sentinel lymph node biopsy or at least strict regional lymph node surveillance for patients with SGC of the eyelid who have T category of T2b or worse, or tumours of 10 mm or more in greatest dimension [14]. A combination of cisplatin/5-fluorouracil or cisplatin/paclitaxel as neoadjuvant systemic chemotherapy can downstage the tumour, and allows less aggressive and organ-sparing surgeries [15].

1.3.3 Follow Up and Prognosis

Despite previously reported associations with poorer outcomes, there is no consensus in the definition for discrete microinvasive or clinical disease presentations in periocular SGC. It has been suggested that multicentric disease (foci of microinvasive tumour with basement membrane disruption) should be differentiated from multifocal disease (clinically evident nodules involving both the upper and lower eyelids): this may improve risk stratification and help to identify patients who require more aggressive management and surveillance. Discrete microinvasion is associated with high rates of misdiagnosis, simultaneous involvement of both upper and lower eyelids, pagetoid spread, multinodular growth, local tumour spread, and local recurrence. Eyelid multifocality is associated with more advanced disease including orbital extension and regional invasion [16].

SGC can recur in up to 33% of the cases. The category of T2b or worse is correlated with regional lymph nodes metastases; [14] metastasis can occur in about 25% of cases [16]. T category of T3a or worse is correlated with distant metastases and death. In the AJCC's study of 50 consecutive patients with sebaceous carcinoma, 5 (10%) died. No tumours <12 mm were associated with distant metastases or death [14].

1.4 Eyelid Merkel Cell Carcinoma

Merkel cell carcinoma (MCC) is a rare but highly aggressive cutaneous malignancy with neuroendocrine features that has 33–46% mortality (see chapter "Periocular Skin Lesions and Eyelid Tumours"). The clinical features of MCC are summarised in the acronym AEIOU—Asymptomatic, Expanding rapidly, Immune suppression, Older than 50, ultraviolet (UV)-exposed site on a person with fair skin. The most common primary sites of MCC are head and neck (45%), and eyelid tumours represent only 2.5% of cases [17].

1.4.1 Management

Wide excision of the tumour in combination with adjuvant radiation therapy to the primary site is the first-line strategy. Chemotherapy and immunotherapy can be used to treat metastatic or unresectable MCC [17, 18].

Avelumab, an anti-PDL1 inhibitor was approved by FDA/EMA in 2017 for treatment of metastatic Merkel cell carcinoma. Studies have shown some responses continuing at up to 2 years when compared to standard chemotherapy, with improved health-related quality of life [18].

Pembrolizumab and nivolumab have also demonstrated efficacy in the treatment of advanced MCC, though there are no reported cases assessing their use for advanced periocular lesions [18].

As tumour angiogenesis is one of the features of MCC, the inhibition of vascular endothelial growth factor (VEGF) signalling pathway can represent a possible therapy. Apatinib—an inhibitor of VEGFR-2 tyrosine kinase activity targeting the intracellular ATP binding site of the receptor—has shown a favourable effect with great durability in a case of locally advanced periocular MCC, with adverse events including hypertension, proteinuria, and hand–foot syndrome [19].

1.5 Eyelid Malignant Melanoma

Cutaneous malignant melanoma of the eyelid skin arises from the malignant proliferation of melanocytes. It can arise de novo or from a preexisting nevus (see chapter "Periocular Skin Lesions and Eyelid Tumours") [17–22].

1.5.1 Epidemiology

Primary melanomas of the eyelid skin are rare. They account for <1% of all cutaneous malignant melanomas. The most common location of eyelid melanomas is the lower eyelid, where it is approximately 2.6 times more likely to occur than the upper eyelid [23]. Malignant melanoma accounts for 5–20% of metastatic and secondary orbital malignancies (Fig. 7a–c), but only a small proportion of primary orbital neoplasia [17–22], with only about 50 cases reported to date.

1.5.2 Risk Factors

As with cutaneous melanomas of other sites, eyelid melanomas are usually a result of DNA damage from exposure to UV light, particularly UVB (290–320 nm). In addition to UV exposure, other common risk factors include fair skin, the presence of dysplastic or congenital naevi, family history of melanoma, and older age [23].

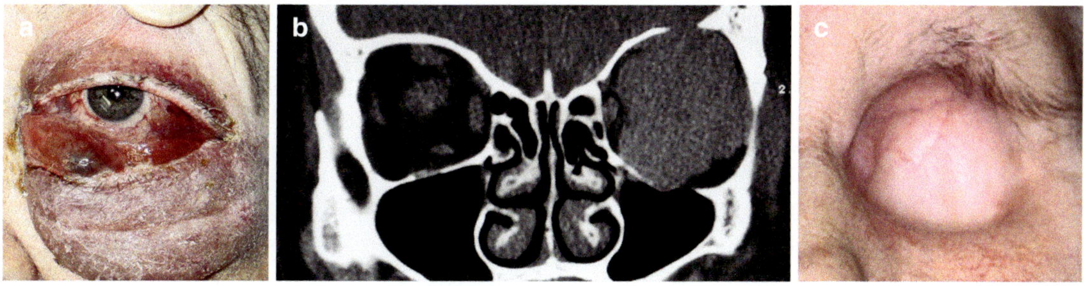

Fig. 7 (**a**) Malignant melanoma accounts for 5–20% of metastatic and secondary orbital malignancies. This image shows left orbital invasion by an untreated choroidal melanoma. (**b**) Coronal orbital CT showing a mass occupying the left orbit. (**c**) Following left exenteration (Courtesy of F. Quaranta Leoni)

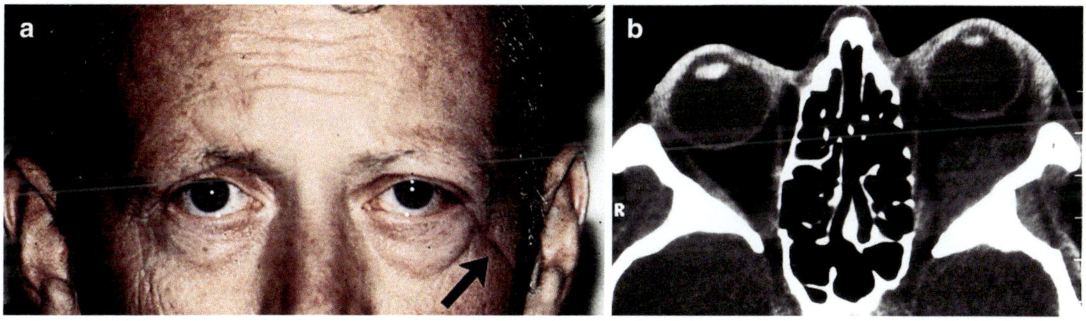

Fig. 8 (**a**) 48 year-old man with left sided recent onset proptosis and previous history of excision of a cutaneous melanoma from his left temporal cheek (arrow). (**b**) Coronal orbital CT depicting a mass in the inferolateral orbit. Histological examination of the biopsy specimen showed findings suggestive of melanoma with neurotropic spread. The tumour had probably spread along the zygomatico-facial or zygomatico-temporal nerve into the orbit (Courtesy of D. Paridaens)

1.5.3 Clinical Examination

The diagnosis of cutaneous malignant melanoma of the eyelid is suspected clinically and confirmed histologically.

Suspicious lesions can be identified using the classic "ABCD" method of evaluation (Asymmetry, Border irregularity, Colour variation, Diameter). Examination should also include palpation for regional lymphadenopathy.

Suspicious lesions can present with a spectrum ranging from flat tan macules, with irregular borders, to nodular or elevated lesions varying in colour with lesions being tan, black, grey, pink, blue, and even white [23, 24].

1.5.4 Management

Eyelid malignant melanoma management has been discussed in chapters "Periocular Skin Lesions and Eyelid Tumours" and "Management of Locally Invasive and Metastatic Eyelid Tumours". Where orbital invasion is suspected and imaging shows orbital disease, an incisional biopsy must be performed without mobilisation of bone.

Secondary orbital melanoma usually forms a well-defined mass at the time of presentation (Fig. 8) and, in such cases, the mass can be excised intact through a bone-sparing anterior orbitotomy. Where macroscopically intact excision is not possible, the lesion should be meticulously isolated from the neighbouring tissues, and surgical debulking can be performed.

Palliative orbital exenteration can be considered if orbital disease is causing major disfigurement (Fig. 7); local radiotherapy can be used as adjuvant therapy when there are no distant metastases [20]. Chemotherapy plays a role when there is systemic metastatic disease at orbital presentation. Treatment options are changing rapidly with the advent of targeted therapy for periocular melanoma (see chapter "Management of Locally Invasive and Metastatic Eyelid Tumours"). Immunotherapy for metastatic cutaneous melanoma markedly improves survival, with the most dramatic being ipilimumab and nivolumab combination therapy [25].

1.5.5 Prognosis

Providing an accurate prognosis to patients with orbital melanoma remains problematic due to the highly variable survival curves, likely due to genetic variation in tumour biology between patients, as well as location of origin. The development of new immunotherapeutic agents, including BRAF-inhibitors, offer hope of a better outcome, if not (yet) a cure.

1.6 Conjunctival Squamous Cell Carcinoma

1.6.1 Epidemiology

Squamous cell carcinoma (SCC) of the conjunctiva is a rare malignancy that is part of the spectrum of ocular surface squamous neoplasia (OSSN). It is reported to be the most common malignant tumour of the ocular surface. Its incidence varies between 0.02 and 3.5/100.000 [26, 27].

1.6.2 Aetiology and Risk factors

In SCC of the conjunctiva, abnormal cells extend through the basement membrane into the conjunctival stroma, whereas in *intraepithelial* neoplasia (CIN) the malignant cells are confined to the surface epithelium.

The aetiology of SSC appears to be multifactorial, and likely involves a variety of environmental factors in a susceptible host [26–28].

Orbital extension of OSSN is overall rare. Outdoor occupation, HIV infection, larger and thicker tumours in the inferior quadrant with forniceal and/or tarsal conjunctival involvement with nodular or nodulo-ulcerative morphology, poor tumour differentiation, SSC, spindle cell and mucoepidermoid variants on histopathology are at increased risk for orbital tumour extension [28].

SCC has the potential to penetrate the corneoscleral lamella into the anterior chamber of the eye, as well as breach the orbital septum to invade the soft tissues of the orbit, sinuses, and the brain; lymphatic and haematogenous metastasis can also occur. Thus, due to their potentially aggressive behaviour, conjunctival SCCs are considered to be sight and life threatening [26, 27].

1.6.3 Clinical Examination

The clinical presentation of OSSN is variable, making diagnosis sometimes difficult. Typically, patients present with a gelatinous or plaque-like interpalpebral conjunctival grey or white lesion. Approximately 95% of CIN lesions occur at the limbus, where the most actively mitotic cells reside [26, 27].

1.6.4 Management

Selected cases can be treated with IFN α-2b, mitomycin C, or 5-fluorouracil [29]. CIN and SCC lesions involving the limbus should be excised with wide tumour-free conjunctival margins, using a no-touch technique. Where complete tumour excision is not feasible due to the site or the size of the lesion, adjuvant chemotherapy with topical interferon (IFN) α-2b is suggested [30].

Sentinel node biopsy may be appropriate to stage the disease [31]. Radiation therapy can be considered as adjunctive therapy in cases that have not responded to other treatments. Gamma knife stereotactic radiosurgery is a potential alternative to orbital exenteration surgery for conjunctival SCC extending into the anterior orbit in patients refusing orbital exenteration or with a second blind eye [32]. However, the disease is more likely to recur than with exenteration surgery, hence lifelong monitoring and low threshold for surgical intervention or retreatment is advisable.

1.6.5 Follow Up and Prognosis

Recurrence of OSSN after surgical excision can occur in over half of cases. The rate of recurrence is substantially higher in the setting of positive surgical margins. Even if the surgical margins are negative, up to one third of patients may experience a recurrence within 10 years [33].

Patients should be placed on a strict follow-up program with clinical visits every 3–6 months. Although recurrences can occur many years after primary surgery, most recurrences are noted during the first year of follow-up [33].

1.7 Conjunctival Malignant Melanoma

Conjunctival melanomas most commonly arise from PAM, as well as naevi, and can also occur *de novo:* 71% of conjunctival melanomas are reported to arise from PAM with atypia, and 17% from a naevus. When conjunctival melanoma arises from a naevus, or *de novo,* it appears as a solitary pigmented or amelanotic smooth vascular nodule, commonly in the limbal area.

Increased vascularity and adherence to the underlying sclera may be present. Melanomas are more frequently observed in Caucasians and exhibit a nodular or diffuse growth. Suspicious lesions need to be completely excised and submitted for histopathological investigation. Once the diagnosis is confirmed, systemic work-up is required [34].

1.7.1 Management

The primary treatment of conjunctival melanoma is excision of the entire tumour with wide surgical margins [34]. If there is scleral involvement then sclero-conjunctivectomy should be considered [35]. A "dry" technique (throw the BSS of the surgical field) should be employed so that cells are not spread to other areas of conjunctiva. A "no touch" technique should also be used taking care not to touch any cancerous cells with surgical instruments which could also spread cells. Most surgeons will also add an adjuvant therapy to primary excision including cryotherapy in a double freeze thaw fashion to the base and edges. If a wide excision is performed, a membrane graft will be needed in the form of either amniotic membrane available off the shelf or a mucous membrane graft from the oral mucosa. Sentinel lymph node biopsy should be considered for lesions thicker than 2 mm [36].

Early secondary exenteration (after a number of local recurrences less than or equal to 4) may reduce the occurrence of metastases and improve patient survival in conjunctival melanoma. Thus, secondary exenteration might be a curative surgery in some patients with recurrent disease [37]. This is in contrast with a previous study that stated that conjunctival melanomas thicker than 1.0 mm were associated with a mortality varying between 33 and 50%, independent of whether exenteration was performed as primary or secondary treatment [38].

Although the current data are limited to case reports and small case series, there is evidence for the role of immunotherapy for patients with locally advanced, recurrent, or metastatic conjunctival melanoma [36].

1.7.2 Prognosis and Follow-up

Patients with conjunctival melanoma should be periodically followed up and investigated for local recurrence. Systemic work-up is also mandatory as the mortality is about 25%.

Conjunctival melanomas have a risk of local recurrence in 20–50% of cases. Melanoma-related mortality at 10 years ranges from 13 to 38%. Lesions that involve the fornix or the palpebral conjunctiva have a higher risk for metastasis and locally aggressive disease than bulbar lesions [38]. Caruncular disease has the worst outcome, may infiltrate the orbit, and is associated with 50% mortality at 3 years. Melanomas arising de novo seem to carry a higher risk of metastasis and death compared with those cases arising from PAM or nevus. Conjunctival melanomas with orbital invasion show a higher frequency of prior eyelid incisional biopsy [39]. Melanomas with orbital invasion at presentation demonstrate larger, more extensive tumours involving the fornix or tarsus, with greater rate of metastasis and death [39].

1.8 Conjunctival Mucoepidermoid Carcinoma

Mucoepidermoid carcinoma is an aggressive variation of the conjunctival invasive squamous cell carcinoma, accounting for less than 5% of these tumours. It commonly arises from the salivary glands in the head and neck region. Ocular and ocular adnexa involvement is rare, and the primary site of origin is usually from the conjunctiva, lacrimal gland, or lacrimal sac [40].

1.8.1 Clinical Features

Mucoepidermoid carcinoma is more frequent in elderly men (>70 years old). It can originate from the bulbar conjunctiva but can also be present in the caruncle. It can have a yellow, globular and cystic appearance. This tumour tends to invade the globe, the orbit, the paranasal sinuses, and orbital metastases typically cause mass effect and bony involvement [21]. Extraocular movement restriction may be out of proportion to proptosis. In the intraocular space, the mucoepidermoid can produce a mucinous cyst in the suprauveal space. The mucin production is more frequent in the intraocular space than in the bulbar conjunctiva [40].

Wolfish *et al.* reported a case series of 19 cases of a sinonasal tract of mucoepidermoid: the majority presented with a mass within the nasal cavity or paranasal sinus [41]. Ophthalmologic features included diplopia, proptosis, and visual field changes.

1.8.2 Treatment

Orbital exenteration may be needed to eradicate a high grade and invasive carcinoma. Radiotherapy should be considered for cases with high risk of recurrence and poor prognosis [41].

1.8.3 Prognosis and Follow Up

Prognosis for orbital metastases is generally poor even if the local orbital tumour can be controlled, and two-year survival rate is 27% [42]. The most significant prognostic factors are the patient's age and treatment method. Patients aged 56 and older have a poorer prognosis. Patients who are treated with surgery and radiation have better prognosis [43].

1.9 Sinonasal: Nasopharyngeal Carcinoma

Due to the close anatomical relationship of the eyes with the nose and the sinuses, the orbit is secondarily involved in numerous sinonasal and nasopharyngeal pathologies. A significant portion of the orbital bony architecture is related to the paranasal sinuses: the roof is the floor of frontal sinus, the medial wall the lateral wall of the ethmoid labyrinth, the inferior wall the roof of the maxillary sinus, and the posteromedial wall the anterolateral wall of the sphenoid sinus [44]. Ocular involvement from sinonasal diseases occur due to direct spread to orbit, venous spread due to valveless nature of veins, cranial nerve involvement, nasolacrimal apparatus involvement and intracranial spread [45, 46].

Sinonasal disease with secondary orbital involvement can present with proptosis, preseptal cellulitis, epiphora, diplopia, ophthalmoplegia, blurring of vision, enophthalmos, ptosis, orbital cellulitis, and loss of vision [45]. Proptosis is a common sign in clinical presentation of neoplastic lesions of nose and paranasal sinuses [47].

1.10 Intracranial Meningiomas

Meningiomas are typically slow growing, benign neoplasms. Secondary orbital meningiomas arise from adjacent structures and extend into the orbit via the optic canal or the superior orbital fissure: sphenoid wing (SOM), anterior clinoid, cavernous sinus, tuberculum sellae, and olfactory groove. These tumours are treated in detail in chapters "Neurogenic Tumours" and "Neuro-orbital Diseases".

2 Orbital Metastasis

Metastatic orbital lesions have been estimated to account for 1–13% of all orbital tumours [21, 48, 49]. The mean age at time of presentation is 60 years [42, 50]. However, the incidence of reported orbital metastases has increased [21]. This may be due to improved treatment leading to an increase in the median survival. Other considerations include advances in the diagnosis and widespread use of imaging techniques which has led to a more accurate detection of these lesions [51].

Two to 5% of patients with systemic cancer are reported to have an orbital metastasis, due to haematogenous spread of the primary tumour [52].

Most orbital metastases are carcinomas; sarcomas and melanomas are considerably less common [48, 53]. Breast consistently ranks the most common primary site, with 29 to 53% [54–56], of metastatic orbital lesions [57], followed by lung (11%), and prostate (8%, Fig. 9) [54, 58]. Other sites include kidney, thyroid, stomach, melanoma, and pancreas [59]. The frequency at each of the sites can differ depending on the demographics and the country of origin of the study [48, 50, 51].

In 19–25% of cases patients may have no history of systemic cancer when presenting with ophthalmic symptoms [21]. Prognosis is generally poor.

2.1 Orbital Metastases from Breast Cancer

Orbital metastases due to breast cancer can be the result of a cellular tropism caused by estrogens produced by periorbital fat, which correlates with the majority of cases secondary to hormone-sensitive tumours (Fig. 10). Oestrogen receptor positivity has been found in conjunctiva, tear glands and tarsal conjunctiva, which could explain the affinity to these sites [60].

Orbital metastases may be the first sign of an undiagnosed primary tumour, mostly invasive lobular breast cancer, as the orbit represents a rich in fat niche which may attract disseminated invasive lobular breast cancer cells (Fig. 11). On the other hand, invasive ductal breast cancer expresses E-cadherin, which limits cell dispersion and rarely brings to orbital metastases [60].

The average age at diagnosis is 61 years [54]. The time from diagnosis of breast cancer to the onset of orbital metastases is usually prolonged, with an average of 2–8.5 years, [60] although there are reports up to 28 years [61]. Orbital activity is presented as the first manifestation of breast cancer in 30% of cases. There is no more frequent laterality and it is bilateral in less than 10% [62].

Although extraocular muscles are rarely infiltrated by metastatic tumours from distant sites, orbital metastases of breast carcinoma have a tendency to spread to the extraocular muscles and to orbital fat [21]. The rarity of extraocular muscle involvement by metastases has been attributed to the constant movement of these muscles, which prevents lodging of neoplastic cells, and to their unfavourable chemical environment for neoplastic growth [63]. As treatment for primary breast cancer has improved and the life expectancy has increased, the incidence of orbital metastases is expected to rise [21, 64].

Diplopia and ocular motility disorders in a patient with neoplastic disease should raise suspicion of tumour involvement of the extraocular muscles; however, broad differential diagnosis is

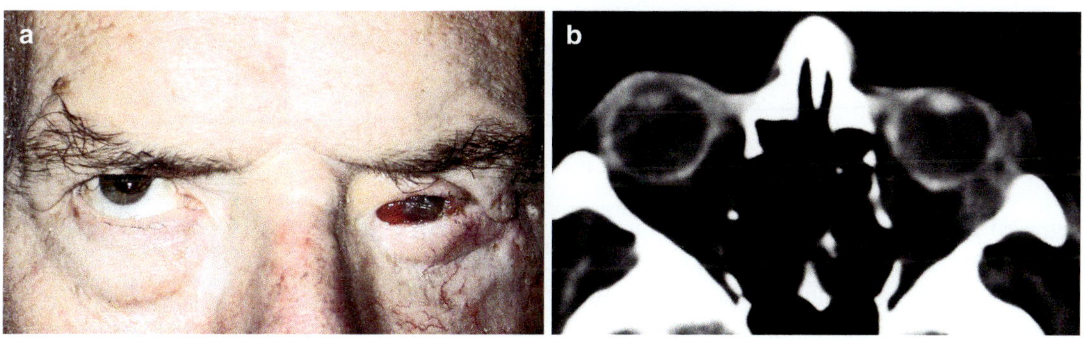

Fig. 9 (**a**) 71 year-old man with left sided rapidly progressive proptosis and eye deterioration and previous surgery for prostate cancer. (**b**) Axial CT scan identifies a mass in the lacrimal gland fossa adherent to the globe. Histological examination of the biopsy specimens identified an infiltrating tumour indicative of a metastasis of earlier diagnosed prostate carcinoma (Courtesy of F. Quaranta Leoni)

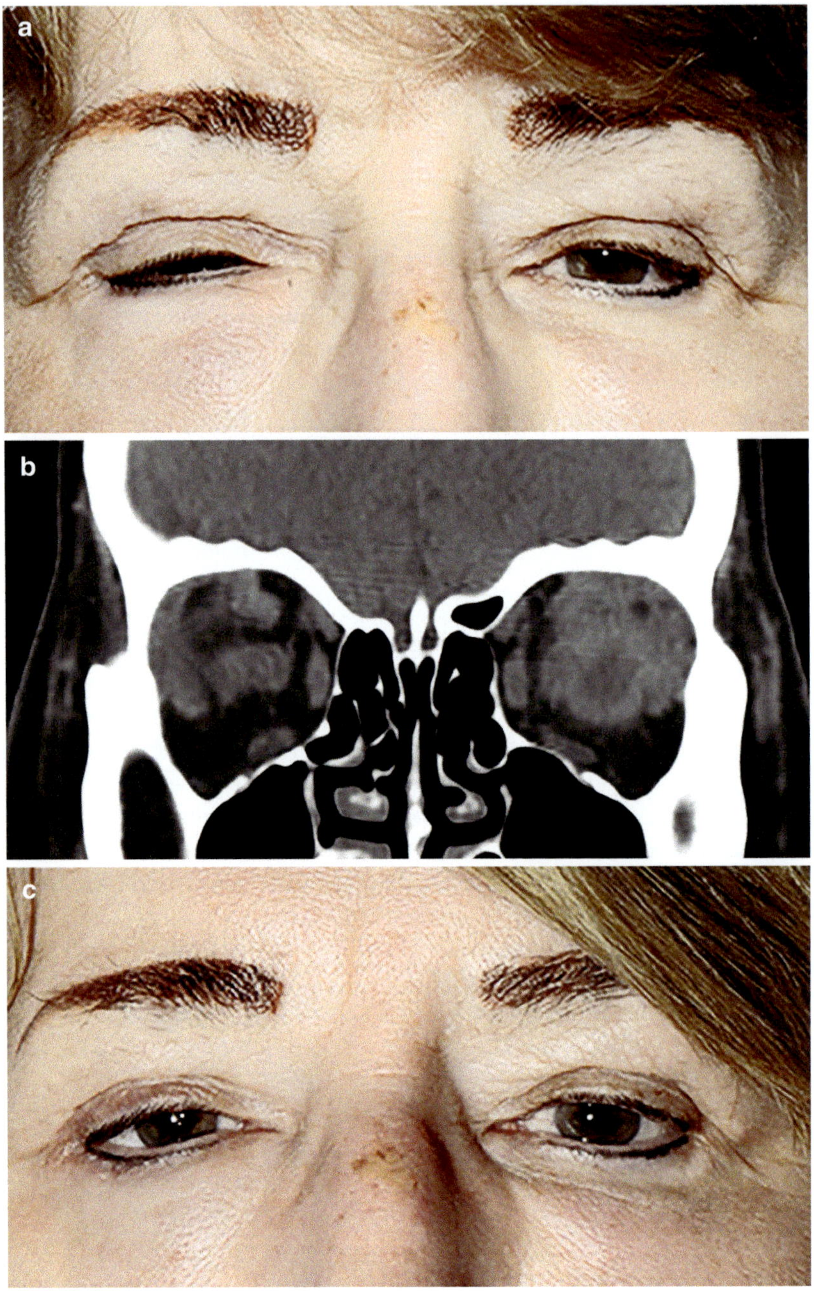

Fig. 10 (**a**) 47 year-old lady with a history of breast carcinoma presented with a 5-month history of periocular swelling. (**b**) Coronal CT scan identifies diffuse changes in each orbit. Histological examination of the biopsy specimens confirmed a diffusely infiltrating tumour suggestive of metastasis of earlier diagnosed ductal breast carcinoma. (**c**) The patient showed some degree of improvement after 2 months of treatment with aromatase inhibitors (Courtesy of W.A. van den Bosch and D. Paridaens)

required to determine the cause and to institute appropriate treatment. CT scan and MRI are helpful in demonstrating extraocular muscle enlargement and determining the extent of orbital involvement. Laboratory studies should be carried out to exclude other conditions that may cause extraocular muscle enlargement like vasculitis, endocrine and immunologic diseases.

Biopsy of the involved tissue is necessary for the diagnosis. In breast carcinoma cases, discordance of ER, PR and HER2/neu status between the primary tumour and subsequent metastases is well recognized [65]. Several studies have reported hormone receptor discordance rates between 30 and 40% between primary breast carcinoma and metastatic disease [66, 67].

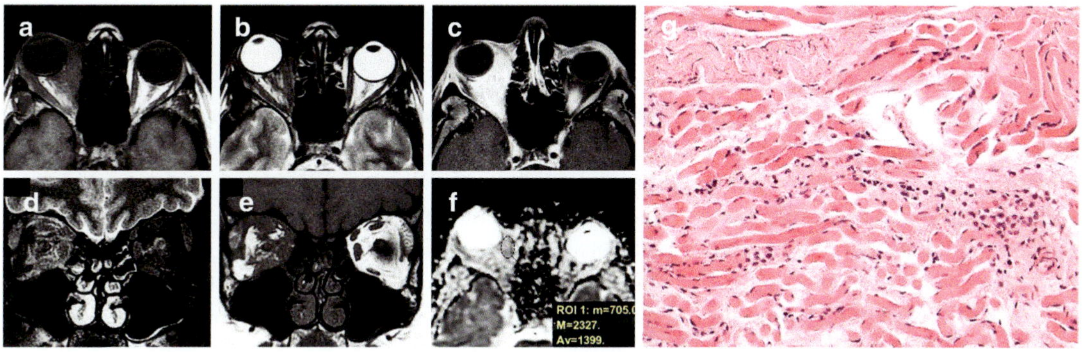

Fig. 11 Imaging and pathology of an infiltrating breast lobular carcinoma metastasized to the right orbit. The lesion is hypointense on MRI T1w (**a**, **d**), and iso-hyperintense on T2w images (**b**, **e**); contrast enhancement (**c**) is diffuse and homogeneous. On apparent diffusion coefficient (ADC) maps (**f**) average value in the region of interest (ROI) is 705 × 10–6 mm2/s. (**g**) Pathology shows small to medium-sized tumour cells that grow in single files (Indian files) between striated muscle fibres ER+, PR+, Ki67+ (Courtesy of G. Savino)

The treatment of orbital metastatic lesions may help to control the growth of the tumour, to preserve visual function, and to improve patient comfort. There is no standard treatment; surgery, radiotherapy or systemic treatment (chemotherapy, hormone therapy) may have favourable responses, although the prognosis is usually poor, with an average survival of 2–34 months. External-beam radiotherapy to the orbital metastatic lesion is the mainstay treatment [21].

2.2 Clinical Features

Proptosis is the main clinical sign at diagnosis (49%) and is often associated with diplopia (48%), pain (19%), visual impairment (16%), ptosis (10%) and presence of a palpable mass [21]. Scirrhous breast carcinoma may present with enophthalmos (see Fig. 21, chapter "Orbital Imaging"). Henderson has emphasised the clinical syndrome of the scirrhous types of metastatic carcinoma [68]. While the initial orbit symptoms are similar to those of other adenocarcinomas, a diffusely infiltrating tumour may lead to a progressively immobilised globe with enophthalmos rather than exophthalmos.

Orbital neoplastic infiltration alone does not explain the phenomenon of enophthalmos. In general, three mechanisms alone or in combination can lead to enophthalmos: structural abnormality (orbital asymmetry, maxillary hypoplasia, microphthalmos, destruction of the orbital bones, trauma), fat atrophy (orbital varix, scleroderma, following irradiation, following orbital haemorrhage, lipodystrophy), and traction (following surgical shortening of an extraocular muscle). The normal orbital fat is replaced by a tumour that has a relatively smaller volume; the maturation of the collagen matrix is associated with contracture similar to that seen in maturing scar tissue [60].

The mean time of presentation of an orbital metastasis after the diagnosis of primary cancer has been found to be 52 months; however, orbital metastasis can occur at any time after initial cancer diagnosis, with one case presenting after 35 years [69].

2.3 Evaluation of the Suspected Orbital Metastasis

When an orbital mass occurs in a patient with a cancer history, history, ocular and systemic evaluation and imaging usually help to determine if the mass is likely to be a metastasis. Some metastases are relatively slow growing and may mimic a benign lesion; however, orbital metastases very rarely present as a slowly progressive mass [48].

Although any space occupying mass may result in axial displacement of the globe, most metastases will produce a motility deficit, pain, or decrease in vision [21]. Metastatic lesions are more commonly found in the anterior orbit [53]. Well-encapsulated, discrete, and focal intraconal masses are unlikely to be metastases, while masses which involve the extraocular muscles and bone are much more likely to be metastases. No area of the orbit is immune to a metastasis, with case reports of metastases to every anatomic structure of the orbit, including the subperiosteal space [70]. Tumour pattern can vary from diffuse infiltrative to a focal mass. Metastases from carcinoid, renal cell carcinoma, and melanoma tend to be circumscribed. Imaging features are not specific: CT commonly shows a solid enhancing mass located often within the orbital fat, and bone erosion can be present. Orbital metastases from breast cancer present diffuse and irregular infiltration, often growing along rectus muscles and fascial planes. Standardised B- and A-scan echography can be useful in case of muscle involvement or more superficial lesions. MRI provides an accurate resolution of the mass, and most orbital metastases show some enhancement on MRI with contrast [71].

It is critical to review all of the patient's imaging. Oncologic patients usually have previous brain imaging, that includes the orbit. Detection of a mass that was not present in previous imaging is highly suggestive of a metastasis, while a lesion that was present on previous imaging and looks unchanged is less likely to be a metastasis.

The definitive diagnosis of orbital metastasis is made by biopsy and histopathological examination.

2.4 When and How to Biopsy a Suspected Orbital Metastasis

Incisional biopsy of the orbital mass suspected to be a metastasis should be performed where requested by the oncologist. In patients with widespread disease and a new orbital mass, biopsy rarely needs to be performed to confirm metastasis. A biopsy may be necessary in presence of a solitary metastasis to the orbit with no other metastatic disease, or when decreasing tumour burden may result in more effective chemotherapy or radiation therapy. In addition, biopsy of the orbit may present less risk than other sites, when additional material may be needed for staging or therapeutic decisions. This is especially true if targeted therapy depends on the molecular analysis of the tumour, or when the metastasis is behaving in a different manner as compared to the primary tumour. An anterior orbital location of the metastasis has been reported in 66% of cases, allowing easy surgical access [48]. In those cases, which only need a confirming biopsy, fine needle aspiration biopsy (FNAB) can be an alternative [72], and is usually suggested when the mass is located deep within the orbit and the patient is at risk for surgery [73].

Availability of previous pathology enables the cytopathologist to determine if the FNAB specimen has the same characteristics of the primary tumour [72, 73].

2.5 Management

Management of the orbital metastasis depends on the primary tumour and staging of the systemic disease. Surgical removal or debulking can be associated with orbital irradiation, and treatment of systemic malignancy with chemotherapy or hormone therapy. If the tumour is well circumscribed, an excisional biopsy can be performed. Radiotherapy and/or chemotherapy are designed on the basis of the specific protocol therapy [74].

Potential threat to visual function and general health condition of the patient should be carefully considered. In patients with progressive worsening of vision due to mass compression, either surgical removal or debulking of the lesion can be suggested. Orbital exenteration should only be used for palliation if other types of treatments fail, or if massive orbital infiltration is present. Observation is reserved to patients who refuse further treatment.

2.6 Outcome

Orbital metastases are associated with poor prognosis. The median survival of patients with orbital metastasis was reported to be 15.6 months [75], and few cases with longer survival have been described [76].

References

1. Shields JA, Bakewell B, Augsburger JJ, Donoso LA, Bernardino V. Space-occupying orbital masses in children. A review of 250 consecutive biopsies. Ophthalmology. 1986;93:379–84.
2. Shinder R, Al-Zubidi N, Esmaeli B. Survey of orbital tumors at a comprehensive cancer center in the United States. Head Neck. 2011;33:610–4.
3. Lanni V, Iuliano A, Laezza MP, Uccello G, Tranfa F, Strianese D. Oculoplastic management of patients in the Covid-19 era: experience from an Italian tertiary referral center. Orbit. 2020;39:391–3.
4. Iuliano A, Strianese D, Uccello G, Diplomatico A, Tebaldi S, Bonavolontà G. Risk factors for orbital exenteration in periocular basal cell carcinoma. Am J Ophthalmol. 2012;153:238–41.
5. Tong JY, Martin PA, Tumuluri K, Selva D. Recurrence following globe sparing excision for basal cell carcinoma with anterior orbital invasion. Ophthalmic Plast Reconstr Surg. 2023;39:374–80.
6. Gill HS, Moscato EE, Chang AL, Soon S, Silkiss RZ. Vismodegib for periocular and orbital basal cell carcinoma. JAMA Ophthalmol. 2013;131:1591–4.
7. Kahana A, Unsworth SP, Andrews CA, et al. Vismodegib for preservation of visual function in patients with advanced periocular basal cell carcinoma: The VISORB Trial. Oncologist. 2021;26:e1240–9.
8. Cisek P, Kieszko D, Bilski M, Dębicki R, Grywalska E, Hrynkiewicz R, Bębnowska D, Kordzińska-Cisek I, Rolińska A, Niedźwiedzka-Rystwej P, Grzybowska-Szatkowska L. Interstitial HDR brachytherapy in the treatment of non-melanocytic skin cancers around the eye. Cancers (Basel). 2021;13:1425.
9. Font RL. Eyelids and lacrimal drainage system. In: Spencer WH, editor. Ophthalmic pathology. an atlas and textbook. 3rd ed. Philadelphia: WB Saunders; 1996. p. 2229–32.
10. Loeffler M, Hornblass A. Characteristics and behavior of eyelid carcinoma. Ophthalmic Surg. 1990;21:513–8.
11. Bergmann MJ, de Keizer ROB, Paridaens D. Globe-sparing surgical treatment for periocular malignancies with anterior orbital invasion: a consecutive case series. Orbit. 2023:1–9. Epub ahead of print
12. Mehta VJ, Ling J, Sobel RK. Review of targeted therapies for periocular tumors. Int Ophthalmol Clin. 2017;57:153–68.
13. Dhillon J, Li DQ, Burnier M, Shenouda G, Arthurs BP, El-Hadad C. Cemiplimab for metastatic squamous cell carcinoma of the orbit, periocular adnexa, and thigh. Orbit. 2022:1–7.
14. Bita E, et al. American Joint Committee on Cancer T category for eyelid sebaceous carcinoma correlates with nodal metastasis and survival. Ophthalmology. 2012;119:1078–82.
15. Verma S, Kumar N, Meel R, Sen S, Kashyap S, Sharma S, Pushker N, Pushpam D, Bakhshi S. Neoadjuvant systemic chemotherapy in sebaceous gland carcinoma of the eyelid: a retrospective study. Ocul Oncol Pathol. 2021;7:251–6.
16. Magazin M, Dalvin LA, Salomao DR, Castner NB, Halbach C, Tooley AA. Sebaceous carcinoma of the eyelid: proposed nomenclature for multifocal and multicentric disease. Ophthalmic Plast Reconstr Surg. 2023;39:117–22.
17. Garcia GA, Kossler AL. Avelumab as an emerging therapy for eyelid and periocular Merkel cell carcinoma. Int Ophthalmol Clin. 2020 Spring;60:91–102.
18. Cowey CL, Liu FX, Kim R, Boyd M, Fulcher N, Krulewicz S, Kasturi V, Bhanegaonkar A. Real-world clinical outcomes with first-line avelumab in locally advanced/metastatic Merkel cell carcinoma in the USA: SPEAR-Merkel. Future Oncol. 2021;17:2339–50.
19. Feng Y, Song X, Jia R. Case report: favorable response to the tyrosine kinase inhibitor Apatinib in recurrent Merkel cell carcinoma. Front Oncol. 2021;11:625360.
20. Zografos L, Ducrey N, Beati D, Schalenbourg A, Spahn B, Balmer A, et al. Metastatic melanoma in the eye and orbit. Ophthalmology. 2003;110:2245–56.
21. Ahmad SM, Esmaeli B. Metastatic tumours of the orbit and ocular adnexa. Curr Opin Ophthalmol. 2007;18:405–13.
22. Rose AM, Luthert PJ, Jayasena CN, Verity DH, Rose GE. Primary orbital melanoma: presentation, treatment, and long-term outcomes for 13 patients. Front Oncol. 2017;7:316.
23. Boulos PR, Rubin PA. Cutaneous melanomas of the eyelid. Semin Ophthalmol. 2006;21:195–206.
24. Odashiro AN, Arthurs B, Pereira PR, Filho JP, Belfort E, Burnier MN Jr. Primary orbital melanoma associated with a blue nevus. Ophthal Plast Reconstr Surg. 2005;21:247–8.
25. Larkin J, Chiarion-Sileni V, Gonzalez R, Grob JJ, Cowey CL, Lao CD, et al. Combined Nivolumab and Ipilimumab or monotherapy in untreated melanoma. N Engl J Med. 2015;373:23–34.
26. Shields CL, Shields JA. Tumors of the conjunctiva and cornea. Surv Ophthalmol. 2004;49:3–24. [PubMed]
27. Yeoh CHY, Lee JJR, Lim BXH, Sundar G, Mehta JS, Chan ASY, Lim DKA, Watson SL, Honavar SG, Manotosh R, Lim CHL. The management of ocular surface squamous neoplasia (OSSN). Int J Mol Sci. 2022;24:713.
28. Kaliki S, Wagh RD, Vempuluru VS, Kapoor AG, Jakati S, Mishra DK, Mohamed A. Ocular surface squamous neoplasia with orbital tumour extension: risk factors and outcomes. Eye (Lond). 2023;37:446–52.

29. Sepulveda R, Pe'er J, Midena E, Seregard S, Dua HS, Singh AD, et al. Topical chemotherapy for ocular surface squamous neoplasia: current status. Br J Ophthalmol. 2010;94:532–5.
30. Shields CL, Shields JA. Tumors of the conjunctiva and cornea. Indian J Ophthalmol. 2019;67:1930–48.
31. Krachmer JH, Mannis MJ, Holland EJ. Cornea: fundamentals, diagnosis and management. Philadelphia: Elsevier Mosby; 2005.
32. Schechter BA, Koreishi AF, Karp CL, Feuer W. Long-term follow-up of conjunctival and corneal intraepithelial neoplasia treated with topical interferon alfa-2b. Ophthalmology. 2008;115:1291–6, 1296.e1
33. Bata BM, Radatz MWR, Salvi SM. Gamma knife stereotactic radiosurgery for conjunctival squamous cell carcinoma invading the anterior orbit: a case series. Ocul Oncol Pathol. 2021;7:206–14.
34. Damato B, Coupland SE. Management of conjunctival melanoma. Expert Rev Anticancer Ther. 2009;9:1227–39.
35. Grossniklaus HE, Margo CE, Solomon AR. Indeterminate melanocytic proliferations of the conjunctiva. Trans Am Ophthalmol Soc. 1999;97:157–70.
36. Sa HS, Daniel C, Esmaeli B. Update on immune checkpoint inhibitors for conjunctival melanoma. J Ophthalmic Vis Res. 2022;17:405–12.
37. Lemaître S, Lévy-Gabriel C, Dendale R, Vincent-Salomon A, Lumbroso-Le Rouic L, Cassoux N, Couturaud B, Desjardins L. Secondary orbital exenteration for conjunctival melanoma: a study of 25 cases. J Fr Ophtalmol. 2021;44:415–9.
38. Paridaens AD, McCartney AC, Minassian DC, Hungerford JL. Orbital exenteration in 95 cases of primary conjunctival malignant melanoma. Br J Ophthalmol. 1994;78:520–8.
39. Shields JA, Shields CL. Conjunctival melanoma in 430 cases: comparative analysis of the impact of orbital invasion on tumor recurrence, metastasis, and death. Ophthal Plast Reconstr Surg. 2023;39:49–57.
40. Dithmar S, Wojno TH, Washington C, Grossniklaus HE. Mucoepidermoid carcinoma of an accessory lacrimal gland with orbital invasion. Ophthal Plast Reconstr Surg. 2000;16:162–6.
41. Wolfish EB, Nelson BL, Thompson LD. Sinonasal tract mucoepidermoid carcinoma: a clinicopathologic and immunophenotypic study of 19 cases combined with a comprehensive review of the literature. Head Neck Pathol. 2012;6:191–207.
42. Char DH, Miller T, Kroll S. Orbital metastases: diagnosis and course. Br J Ophthalmol. 1997;81:386–90.
43. Ozawa H, Tomita T, Sakamoto K, Tagawa T, Fujii R, Kanzaki S, et al. Mucoepidermoid carcinoma of the head and neck: clinical analysis of 43 patients. Jpn J Clin Oncol. 2008;38:414–8.
44. Sayed YE. Orbital involvement in sinonasal disease. Saudi J Ophthalmol. 1995;9:29–37.
45. Sikarwari V, Bishti RS, Kumari D, Shukla RK. Ophthalmic manifestations in ENT diseases and surgical procedures. IOSR J Dent Med Sci. 2013;11:87–92.
46. Williamson Noble FA. Diseases of the orbit and its contents, secondary to pathological conditions of the nose and paranasal sinuses. Ann R Coll Surg Engl. 1954;15:46–64.
47. Sinha V, Bharadwaj D, George A, Memon RA. Proptosis through eyes of ENT surgeon. Indian J Otolaryngol Head Neck Surg. 2005;57:207–9.
48. Magliozzi P, Strianese D, Bonavolontà P, Ferrara M, Ruggiero P, Carandente R, et al. Orbital metastases in Italy. Int J Ophthalmol. 2015;8:1018–23.
49. Bonavolontà G, Strianese D, Grassi P, et al. An analysis of 2,480 space-occupying lesions of the orbit from 1976 to 2011. Ophthalmic Plast Reconstr Surg. 2013;29:79–86.
50. Günalp I, Gündüz K. Metastatic orbital tumors. Jpn J Ophthalmol. 1995;39:65–70.
51. Eldesouky MA, Elbakary MA. Clinical and imaging characteristics of orbital metastatic lesions among Egyptian patients. Clin Ophthalmol. 2015;9:1683–7.
52. Matlach J, Nowak J, Göbel W. Papilledema of unknown cause. Ophthalmologe. 2013;110:543–5.
53. Shields JA, Shields CL, Brotman HK, Carvalho C, Perez N, Eagle RC Jr. Cancer metastatic to the orbit: the 2000 Robert M. Curts Lecture. Ophthalmic Plast Reconstr Surg. 2001;17:54.
54. Shields JA, Shields CL, Scartozzi R. Survey of 1264 patients with orbital tumors and simulating lesions: the 2002 Montgomery Lecture, Part 1. Ophthalmology. 2004;111:997–1008.
55. Henderson JW, Farrow GM. Metastatic carcinomas. 3rd ed. New York: Raven Press; 1994.
56. Weigelt B, Reis-Filho S. Histological and molecular types of breast cancer: is there a unifying taxonomy? Nat Rev Clin Oncol. 2009;6:718–30.
57. Meltzer DE, Chang AH, Shatzkes DR. Case 152: orbital metastatic disease from breast carcinoma. Radiology. 2009;253:893–6.
58. Civit T, Colnat-Coulbois S, Freppel S. Orbital metastasis. Neurochirurgie. 2010;56:148–5.
59. Fahmy P, Heegaard S, Jensen OA, Prause JU. Metastases in the ophthalmic region in Denmark 1969-98. A histopathological study. Acta Ophthalmol Scand. 2003;81:47–50.
60. Pierson T, Tebit E, Sayed AE, Smolkin M, Dillon P. Orbital metastases from breast cancer: retrospective analysis at an Academic Cancer Center. Breast J. 2016;22:447–50.
61. Milman T, Pliner L, Langer PD. Breast carcinoma metastatic to the orbit: an unusually late presentation. Ophthalmic Plast Reconstr Surg. 2008;24:480–2.
62. Rossi L, Zancla S, Civitelli L, Ranieri E. An unusual orbital metastasis of breast cancer. Breast Dis. 2014;34:173–6.
63. Ashton N, Morgan G. Discrete carcinomatous metastases in the extraocular muscles. Br J Ophthalmol. 1974;58:112–7.
64. Fenton S, Kemp EG, Harnett AN. Screening for ophthalmic involvement in asymptomatic patients with metastatic breast carcinoma. Eye (Lond). 2004;18:38–40.

65. Aurilio G, Disalvatore D, Pruneri G, Bagnardi V, Viale G, Curigliano G, Adamoli L, Munzone E, Sciandivasci A, De Vita F, Goldhirsch A, Nolè F. A metaanalysis of oestrogen receptor, progesterone receptor and human epidermal growth factor receptor 2 discordance between primary breast cancer and metastases. Eur J Cancer. 2014;50:277–89.
66. Lower EE, Glass EL, Bradley DA, Blau R, Heffelfinger S. Impact of metastatic estrogen receptor and progesterone receptor status on survival. Breast Cancer Res Treat. 2005;90:65–70.
67. Li MH, Hou CL, Wang C, Sun AJ. HER-2, ER, PR status concordance in primary breast cancer and corresponding metastatic lesion in lymph nodes in Chinese women. Pathol Res Pract. 2016;212:252–7.
68. Henderson JW. Orbital tumors. Philadelphia: WB Saunders; 1973. p. 479.
69. Spraker MB, Francis CE, Korde L, Kim J, Halasz L. Solitary orbital metastasis 35 years after a diagnosis of lobular carcinoma *in situ*. Cureus. 2017;9:e1404.
70. Nash S, Bartels H, Pemberton J. Metastatic cervical adenocarcinoma to the orbital subperiosteal space. Can J Ophthalmol. 2017;52:e60–2.
71. Khan SN, Sepahdari AR. Orbital masses: CT and MRI of common vascular lesions, benign tumors, and malignancies. Saudi J Ophthalmol. 2012;26:373–83.
72. Dresner SC, Kennerdell JS, Dekker A. Fine needle aspiration of metastatic orbital tumors. Surv Ophthalmol. 1983;27:397–8.
73. Bagchi K, Giri A, Sarkar R, Das S, Nag S. Fine needle aspiration biopsy in the diagnosis of intraocular and extra-ocular mass lesions. J Indian Med Assoc. 2010;108:457–9.
74. Marwaha G, Macklis R, Singh AD. Radiation therapy: orbital tumors. Dev Ophthalmol. 2013;52:94–101.
75. Ferry AP, Font RL. Carcinoma metastatic to the eye and orbit II. A clinicopathological study of 26 patients with carcinoma metastatic to the anterior segment of the eye. Arch Ophthalmol. 1975;93:472–82.
76. Chong VF. The orbits in cancer imaging. Cancer Imaging. 2006;6:S27–31.

Neuro-Orbital Disease

Michelle Khan, Stijn van der Meeren, and David H. Verity

Key Messages

- Diseases which straddle the orbito-cranial junction require multi-specialty management.
- The oculoplastic specialist should be competent at examining the cranial nerves as they relate to the orbit and facial structures, with a knowledge of their anatomy.
- Sphenoid wing meningioma (SWM) is a benign condition in the great majority of cases with no current medical or surgical cure. Radiotherapy for SWM plays a role, but the indications and timing remain uncertain in some cases. Surgery can cause more morbidity than the disease itself, including irreversible sight loss and blindness. Dotatate CT/MR imaging and somatostatin receptor PET/CT (SSTR PET) imaging can be diagnostic in suspected cases of atypical or recurrent SWM.
- Fibrous dysplasia (FD) is a rare bone disease that can lead to facial deformities and fractures, although can also be an asymptomatic, coincidental finding. Imaging (CT or MR) identifies 'woven' bone within a fibrous stroma - described as 'ground glass' in appearance. Activity is determined with 18F-NaF PET/CT in concert with serum alkaline phosphatase levels. Treatment is symptomatic, and Bisphosphonates, which induce osteoclast apoptosis, may be effective.
- 50% of all patients presenting with presumed *solitary* EMP in the orbit are found to have occult multiple myeloma (MM) within 6 months of an orbital biopsy; such patients should be carefully screened for systemic disease.
- Orbital apex syndrome (OAS), superior orbital fissure syndrome(SOFS) and cavernous sinus syndrome (CSS) present with distinct clinical features, but share similar aetiologies. The optic nerve is affected in OAS and CSS, but not SOFS. In CSS sympathetic fibres and the maxillary branch of the trigeminal nerve (V2) are also involved.

1 Introduction

This chapter examines a selection of pathologies which straddle the orbit-cranial junction and which can present with orbital or neurological symptoms, or both. Management of these conditions frequently requires close collaboration with both neurosurgeons and neuro-ophthalmology

M. Khan
Department of Ophthalmology and Vision Sciences, University of Toronto, Toronto, ON, Canada

S. van der Meeren
Department of Ophthalmology, Leiden University Medical Center, Leiden, The Netherlands

D. H. Verity (✉)
Adnexal Service, Moorfields Eye Hospital, London, UK

St John of Jerusalem Eye Hospital Group, London, UK
e-mail: david.verity@nhs.net

F. M. Quaranta Leoni et al. (eds.), *Oculoplastic, Lacrimal and Orbital Surgery*, https://doi.org/10.1007/978-3-031-39638-0_26

colleagues. Such diseases can present with orbital mass effect, axial and non axial displacement of the globe, pain, vascular congestion, cranial neuropathies, and vision loss.

Diagnosis requires a careful history, examination with particular attention to the function of the cranial nerves (II, III, IV, V, VI, and VII), and appropriate imaging. CT is preferred for solely orbital disease, but MRI is used to investigate optic nerve, cavernous sinus, and intracranial pathology.

Vascular malformations, idiopathic orbital inflammatory and histiocytic lesions, primary optic nerve disorders, and sino-orbital diseases are discussed elsewhere.

2 Sphenoid Wing Meningioma

Meningiomas are the most common primary intracranial tumours in adults [1]. Arising from arachnoid cap cells, approximately 18% of all meningiomas are located near the sphenoid wing, with about half of these in the medial portion of the wing [2]. Sphenoid wing meningiomas (SWM) have two main growth patterns, the nodular or *en-masse* pattern, or the more diffuse *en-plaque* pattern, which can be distinguished radiologically. They are classified according to their site of origin along the sphenoid ridge: lateral, middle or clinoidal. Tumours affecting the clinoid process can be further subdivided into three different types, according to their relationship to the optic nerves, chiasm and carotid cistern as well as the presence or absence of interfacing arachnoid membranes between the tumour and cerebral vessels [3].

Presenting symptoms of SWM vary depending on the location of the primary tumour. The tumour can extend from the intracranial space into the orbit through bone, the superior orbital fissure or the cavernous sinus. They can present with progressive symptoms of an orbital or temporal fossa mass, including temporal fullness, orbital mass effect, ptosis, and impaired extraocular motility (Figs. 1 and 7, Table 1). Tumours near the sella or optic nerve can cause visual field defects, optic disc oedema and atrophy [2, 4]. The orbital mass effect of SWM includes eyelid oedema, chemosis, proptosis, inferomedial globe displacement, limitation of extraocular muscles, globe distortion, and compressive optic neuropathy; hyperostosis of the optic canal, intracranial disease, and refractive changes and keratopathy can also reduce vision (Figs. 2 and 3, Table 2).

2.1 Radiological Features

Both computed tomography (CT) and magnetic resonance imaging (MRI) play a role in monitoring and managing patients with SWM. MRI identifies soft tissue disease, whilst CT better defines the associated hyperostosis, and is particularly valuable in determining the likely contribution of hyperostosis of the optic canal to visual loss. Imaging of sphenoid wing meningiomas demonstrate a thick homogeneous tumour bed with relative sparing of anatomic structures. The tumours

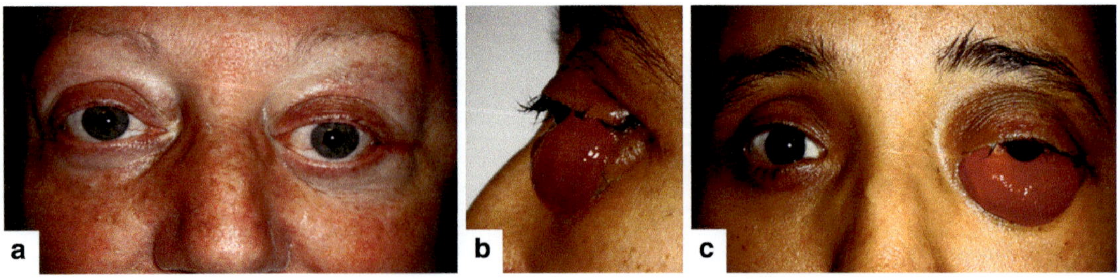

Fig. 1 Presenting features of SWM: Patient with SWM presenting with inferior globe displacement and proptosis (**a**). Chronic inferior conjunctival chemosis due to orbital congestion (**b, c**)

Table 1 Presenting symptoms of sphenoid wing and spheno-orbital meningiomas [4]

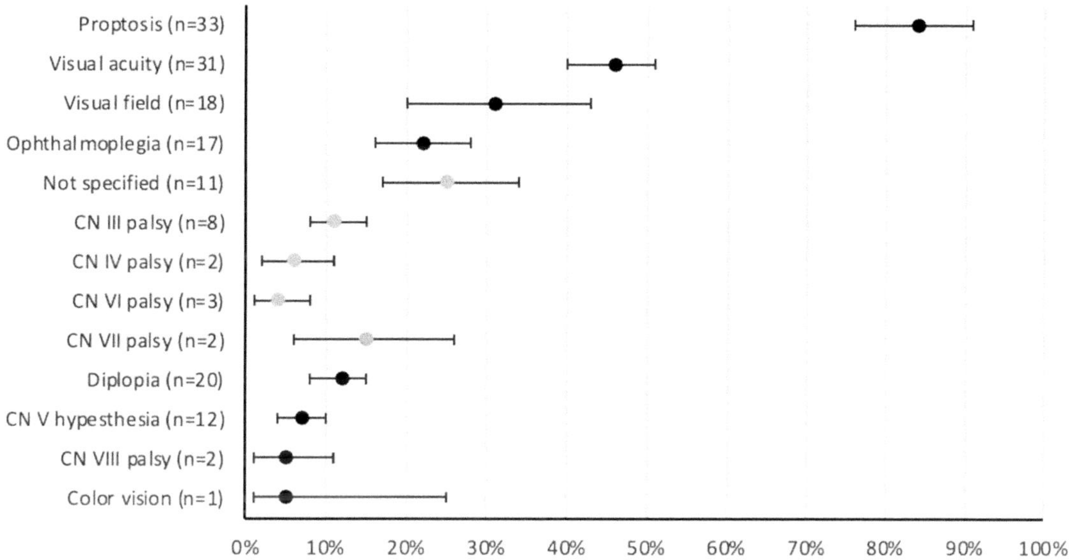

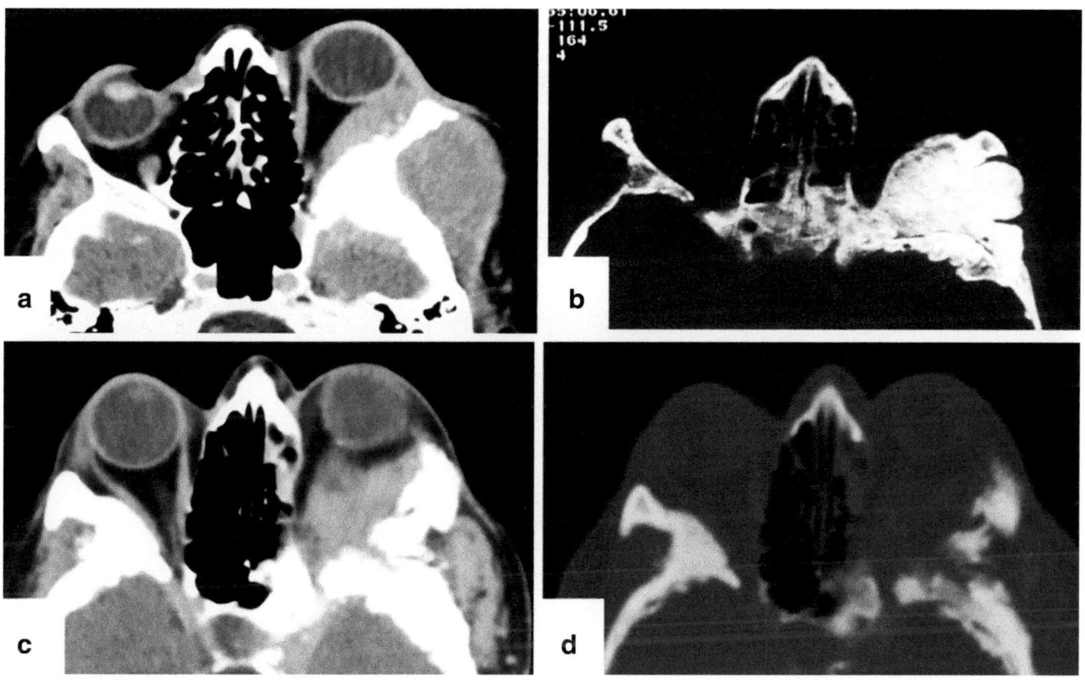

Fig. 2 CT identifying intra- and extra-orbital soft tissue disease (**a**), in addition to massive bony involvement (**b**). Bilateral disease, with tumour extending into the orbital apex and through the orbital fissures. Soft tissue is also seen in the left temporalis fossa and the middle cranial fossa (**c**, **d**)

are slow growing and have a tendency to conform around structures and cause compression rather than tissue invasion. The average annual growth rate of meningiomas is 1–3 mm per year [5].

On CT, meningiomas are iso- to slightly hyper-attenuating and exhibit homogenous and intense enhancement after injection of iodinated contrast. On MRI they appear as well circumscribed dural

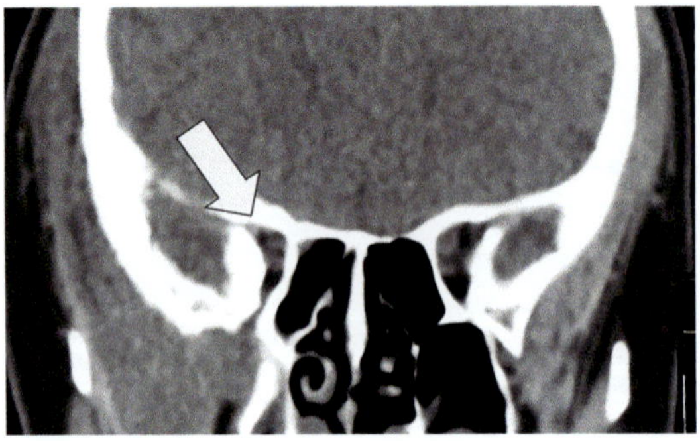

Fig. 3 Compression of the optic canal causing optic neuropathy

Table 2 Orbital features of sphenoid wing meningioma

Mass effect
• Gradual globe displacement with proptosis and/or inferior displacement
• Reduced globe movement & squint
• Globe distortion leading to refractive changes
• Incomplete blink cycle
Vascular congestion
• Diurnal oedema of the eyelid and cheek
• Chronic conjunctival chemosis
• Chronically dilated episcleral vessels
Visual impairment
• Exposure keratopathy
• Intra-orbital compressive optic neuropathy
• Retro orbital ischemic optic neuropathy
• Compression of the cavernous sinus

masses, with variable T1 and T2 signal characteristics. T2 is typically iso or hyperintense, and a dural tail is not uncommon in almost 75% of cases. An indication of vascularity may be present on routine imaging, and there may or may not be vasogenic oedema. Up to 50% of tumours have some vasogenic oedema, but this does not correlate with tumour size. They also tend to exhibit hyperostosis and calcifications in up to 20%, which can be seen on either CT or MRI.

Meningiomas express somatostatin receptors which bind to 68-Gallium dotatate. In dotatate CT/MR imaging, and somatostatin receptor PET/CT (SSTR PET) imaging, radio-labelled gallium avidly attaches to the receptor (Fig. 4). SST PET is valuable where there is diagnostic uncertainty, or where subtle recurrence is suspected.

2.2 Tumour Grading

The pathological and clinical classification of meningiomas is based upon the WHO classification system for brain tumours [6, 7].

- WHO Grade I (benign): includes secretory, microcystic,clearcell,lymphoplasmocyte-rich,

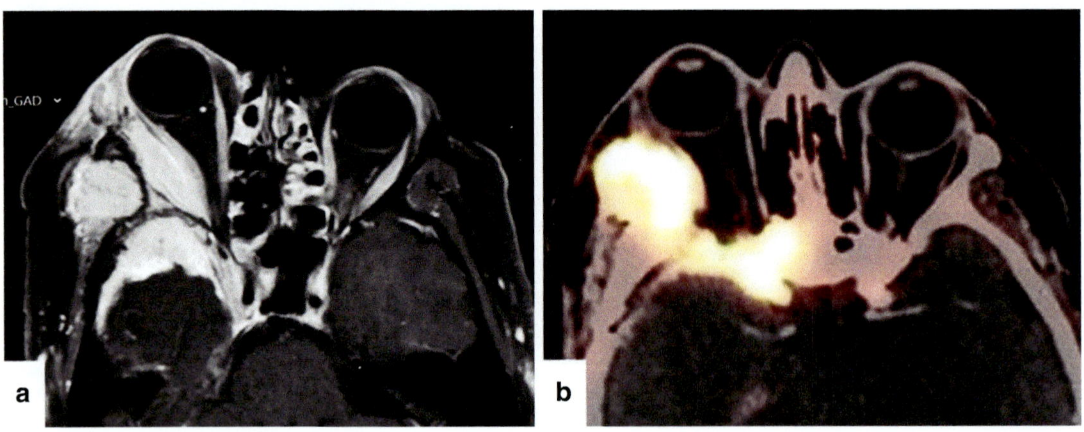

Fig. 4 Meningiomas express somatostatin receptors which bind to 68-Gallium dotatate. In dotatate CT/MR imaging, and somatostatin receptor PET/CT (SSTR PET) imaging, radio-labelled gallium avidly attaches to the receptor. SST PET is valuable where there is diagnostic uncertainty, or where subtle recurrence is suspected (**a**, **b**)

and chordoid variants. Despite invasion of the adjacent bony structures, grade I meningiomas do not invade the brain parenchyma. WHO Grade I accounts for approximately 80% of all cases.
- WHO Grade II (atypical): includes atypical variant. This type of meningioma shows frequent mitosis and an increased nuclear-cytoplasmic ratio. WHO Grade II accounts for approximately 18% of all cases.
- WHO Grade III/IV (malignant): include rhabdoid and anaplastic variants. This type of meningioma shows even greater mitosis, necrosis, and invasion of brain parenchyma. These constitute less than 1% of all meningiomas.

Because meningiomas are heterogeneous in terms of prognosis, even within a WHO grade, it is recommended to assess a DNA methylation profile for better characterization of the tumour [8]. More recently, a classification system was suggested that combines several DNA/RNA genetic profiles to predict clinical outcomes more accurately [9].

2.3 Management

Treatment of SWM is based on symptoms, signs, and rate of progression, and as such varies between patients. Both surgery and radiation may be indicated where there is symptomatic and progressive disease.

2.3.1 Radiotherapy

Radiotherapy for SWM includes stereotactic radiosurgery, fractionated stereotactic radiotherapy (FSRT), intensity modulated radiotherapy (IMRT), and particle radiotherapy (also known as "proton beam"), and the indications are broadly based on WHO tumour grade (Table 3).

In stereotactic radiosurgery, radiation is pulsed at the tumour in one fraction, while in FSRT and IMRT, the dose is given in multiple fractions over time. The main difference between FSRT and IMRT is that IMRT can accommodate more complex shapes and larger tumours because it improves the ability of the radiation to conform to the tumour edge and minimise damage to important normal structures [10]. Clinically, radiosurgery is a safe alternative to skull-base meningioma resection in patients who are not good surgical candidates; however, limitations exist for tumours in close proximity to critical and radiosensitive structures. FSRT and IMRT are generally used when the tumour is around radiosensitive structures such as the optic nerve or chiasm. For radiation therapy as a whole, local control rates of 92–100% have been reported. Rates of permanent neurological deficits range from 1.6% to 9.8% [11]. After radiation therapy, tumour volume decreases in approximately 33% of cases at 2 years and 36% at 3 years [10, 12].

Table 3 Radiation treatment recommendations based on WHO tumour grade in sphenoid wing meningioma patients

Tumour grade	Treatment recommendation
Grade I	No urgency to irradiate but consider radiotherapy for inoperable tumours, particularly if they are progressing, sub totally resected, or the patient is symptomatic.
Grade II	Radiotherapy indicated, significant recurrence risk (between 40 to 60%) 5–10 years following surgical resection.
Grade III	Radiotherapy is indicated even after complete surgical resection.

2.3.2 Surgical Management

Surgical resection has long been considered the primary and definitive treatment for meningioma patients [12]. Surgical resection of SWM is difficult because of the complicated intracranial, intraosseous and intraorbital growth patterns, with tumour frequently in close proximity to neurovascular structures and the cavernous sinus. Although, in principle, surgery entails maximal tumour removal, including both soft tissue and bony hyperostosis, in practice this requires major expertise [13], carries a risk to vision, and is never curative. Nonetheless, when indicated, surgery can result in rapid reduction of an intracranial mass effect, confirmation of the pathology and grade, and relief of both proptosis, and visual pathway compression.

Treatment options for SWM with *periorbital* invasion depend on the surgeon's personal training, experience and surgical preference [14]. Ringel et al. reported that prognosis is good even if a remnant of disease is present without radical resection, and that the surgical aim should be symptom relief rather than radical resection [15]. On the other hand, Mariniello et al. reported that recurrence rate of the tumour depends on the extent of resection [16]. A recent large meta analysis found surgery to be both safe and effective: there is improvement of visual acuity in 91%, visual fields in 87% and proptosis in 96% [4]. There is yet no consensus on the surgical methods of radical and safe resections of SWM based on the presence of periorbital invasion [17].

Surgery is typically performed using multistage procedures with different techniques (e.g. endoscopic endonasal surgery for anterior skull base lesions, pterional craniotomy for advanced inner ridge tumours with large hyperostosis and orbital surgery for orbital mass lesions). Endoscopic techniques may reduce morbidity rates associated with resection through craniotomy [11, 18]. Rates of gross total resection are approximately 50%, complete removal of large lesions is hardly ever possible. Surgical complications range from 1–18%, much less compared to intracranial surgery where there is a 20–40% complication rate. The 5-year recurrence free survival for WHO Grade I meningiomas is 88%. For patients with periorbital invasion, gross total resection of tumour has been associated with lower recurrence rates compared to subtotal resection [19].

Orbital decompression is useful in cases of compressive optic neuropathy or where there is significant proptosis e.g. when a large intraorbital mass is present or the hyperostosis affects the orbital apex (Fig. 5.) *Medial* orbital decompression via a retro-caruncular route affords an 'open sky' view of the medial wall of the orbit, permitting decompression of the orbital apex, and removal of the posterior orbital floor and the ethmoid-maxillary 'strut', these two latter areas of decompression resulting in significantly greater reduction of apical orbital pressure (Figs. 6 and 7). *Lateral* orbital wall decompres-

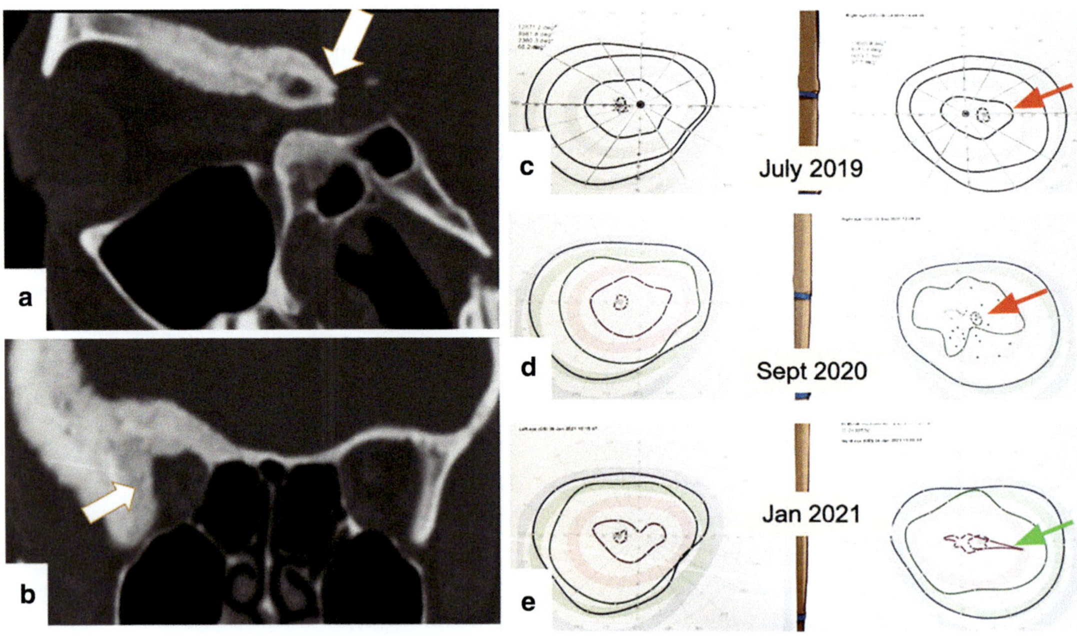

Fig. 5 SWM case study 1. Radiology identifying SWM with bony involvement of the optic canal (white arrows, **a**, **b**)). Reduction of the right visual field due to SWM with apical crowding and bony optic canal involvement. Red arrows identify contracture of the inner isoptre (**c**, **d**). Following medial wall decompression, the inner isoptre has enlarged (green arrow, **e**). However, decompression of the canal *per se* may still be necessary if the disease progresses (as, indeed, it subsequently did in this patient)

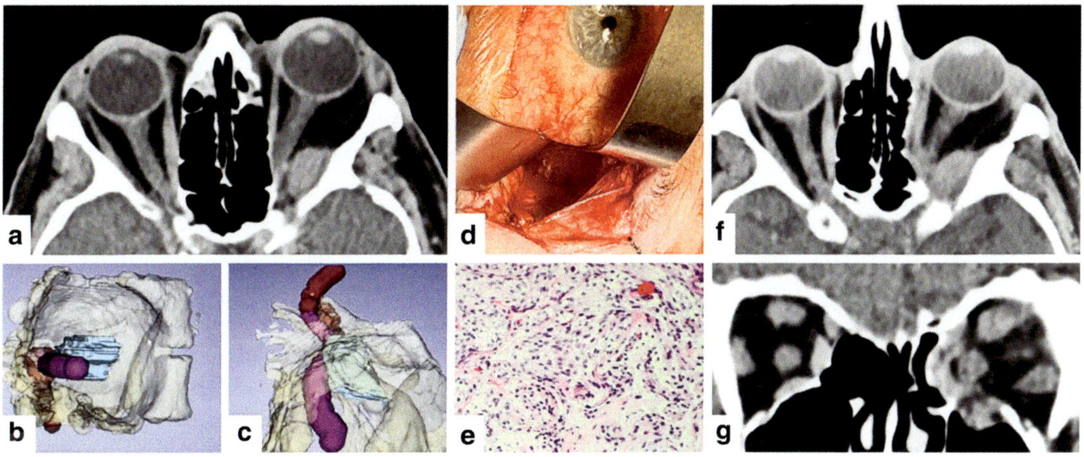

Fig. 6 SWM case study 2. CT of a 70 year old patient presenting with reduced visual acuity and proptosis over the previous 4 month. Imaging identified a soft tissue lesion at the orbital apex displacing the optic nerve medially (**a**). Colour-coded CT 3-D reconstruction showing compression of the optic nerve by the lesion (**b**, **c**). Biopsy via a lateral canthotomy (**d**) approach revealed a meningioma (figure e showing whorls of meningothelial cells). Medial decompression (**f**, **g**) proved inadequate in relieving the optic nerve compression due to the bony spur of the wall of the posterior ethmoid air cell. Further decompression via the endonasal approach proved more successful

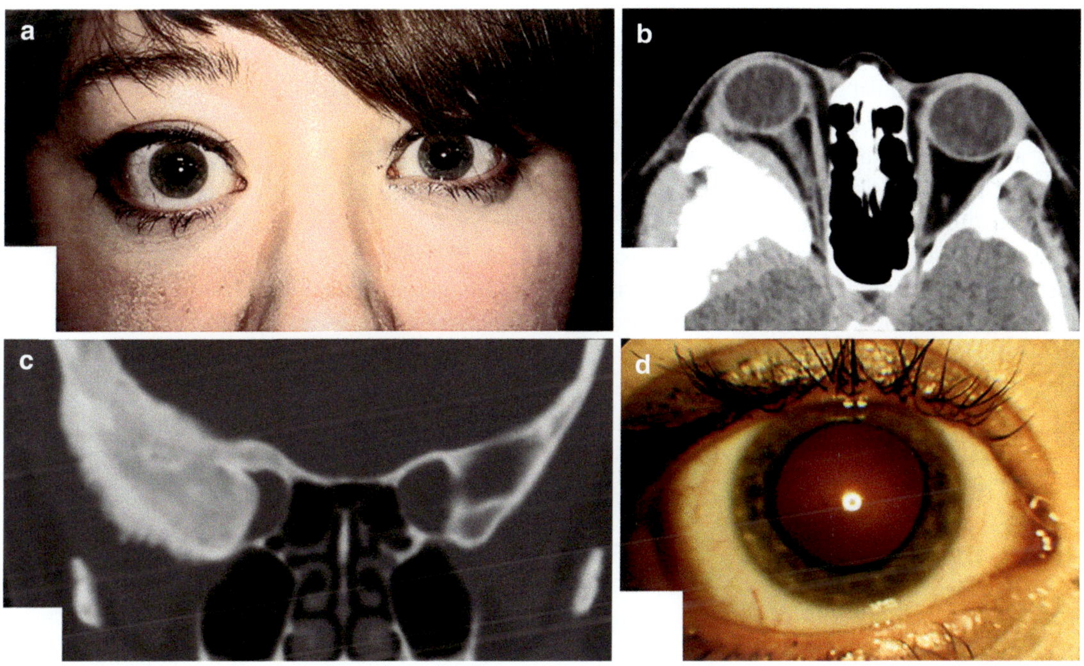

Fig. 7 SWM case study 3. A 30 year old female presented with gradual onset proptosis (**a**) due to sphenoid wing meningioma involving the lateral orbital wall, temporalis fossa and middle cranial fossa (**b**, **c**). Medial wall decompression was performed to reduce proptosis. Towards the end of surgery, a dramatic mydriasis occurred (**d**), presumed due to compression of the ciliary nerves against the medially-bowed lateral wall. However, vision was preserved, and the mydriasis resolved over several months

Table 4 The complex challenge of sphenoid wing meningioma: Keypoints

- Meningiomas are largely benign
- Treatment *per se* can cause significant morbidity, including blindness
- Management is conservative in the absence of visual symptoms
- Consider orbital decompression for proptosis or intra-orbital nerve compression
- Where visual pathway compression is posterior to the orbital apex, consider endoscopic decompression of the optic canal, or cranial decompression
- Avoid hormone replacement treatment (progesterone)
- Radiotherapy plays a role in slowing down disease progression

sion - including the rim in advanced cases - debulks both the hyperostotic bone along the lateral orbital wall and roof, and overlying soft tissue tumour. The latter is removed most effectively with a radiofrequency loop electrode. In such patients with progressive congestion and/or optic neuropathy, adjunctive radiotherapy is often indicated to slow or halt progression of the disease.

In summary, the management of SWM is complex, and whilst surgical intervention can reduce the mass effect on the optic pathways, it is also associated with visual loss, particularly in cases of hyperostotic apical or optic canal compression. Radiotherapy is indicated in WHO grade 2 tumours and above, but may also be indicated in grade 1 tumours where there is progression with mass effect that cannot be addressed surgically. Finally, in all cases progesterone supplements must be avoided (Table 4).

3 Fibrous Dysplasia

3.1 Overview

Fibrous dysplasia (FD) is a rare bone disease with an estimated incidence of 1 in 10.000 people. It is a genetic but non-inheritable disease, caused by a missense mutation in chromosome 20q13, changing the GNAS protein [20]. Changes in this protein cause osteoclast activity (abnormal high resorption of normal bone), abnormal proliferation and differentiation of osteoblasts (leading to abnormal high bone formation) and proliferation of fibroblasts. As a result, normal bone is replaced by fibro-osseous lesions of poor quality and with mineralization defects. These bony lesions can be painful or lead to deformities or fractures.

Because of the somatic mosaicism, clinical manifestations of the disease vary widely.

If only one bone is affected it is called monostotic whereas multiple bones are affected it is called polyostotic disease. McCune Albright Syndrome (MAS) is the combination of polyostotic FD, pubertas praecox and 'café au lait' skin lesions. Mazabraud's syndrome is the combination of FD with intramuscular myxoma. Monostotic disease can be asymptomatic whereas MAS patients can be severely affected [21].

Because of the asymptomatic subset of patients, the prevalence remains unknown. In symptomatic patients pain and impaired mobility are common, as well as susceptibility to fractures or deformity.

Prevalence of craniofacial fibrous dysplasia (CFD) within the FD/MAS population is reported to be as high as 56% in patients with monostotic FD and craniofacial bones are also affected in nearly half of the patients with polyostotic FD. The orbital bones are the second most prevalent parts of the skull that are affected in patients with FD/MAS [22].

Imaging (CT or MR, Figs. 8, 9 and 10) show lesions of non-cortical, specular aspects of woven bone within a fibrous stroma, called 'ground glass' appearance, that can be compact, lytic or mixed. The radiographic density depends on the amount of woven bone and its mineralization. Note, it is not unusual for this disease to be an incidental finding since it is often asymptomatic [23].

Biopsy with histological evaluation of suspected bone disease is often not necessary. If the diagnosis is questionable or if malignancy is considered, the tissue should be processed fresh (frozen) in order to enable genetic testing for GNAS mutation. Among the differential diagnosis of CFD are intraosseous venous malformation, hyperostosis caused by meningioma (en plaque) and juvenile psammomatoid osseous fibroma.

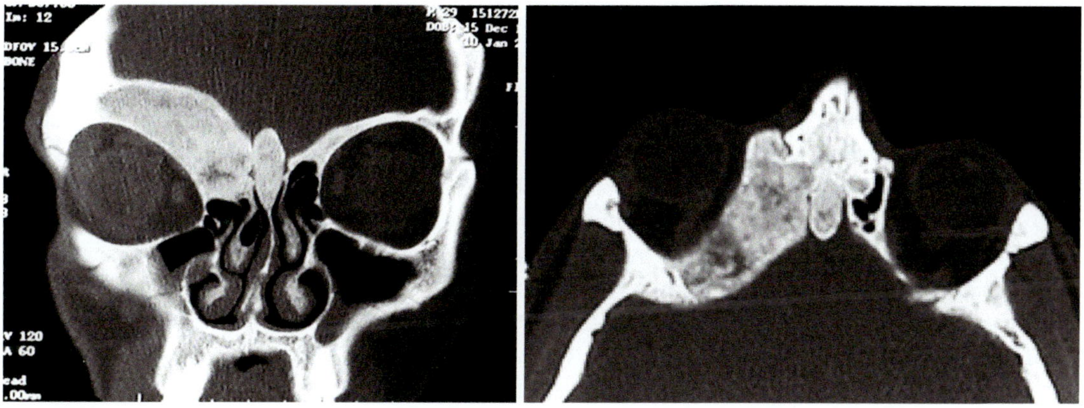

Fig. 8 Fibrous dysplasia of the right frontal bone (CT with bone windows)

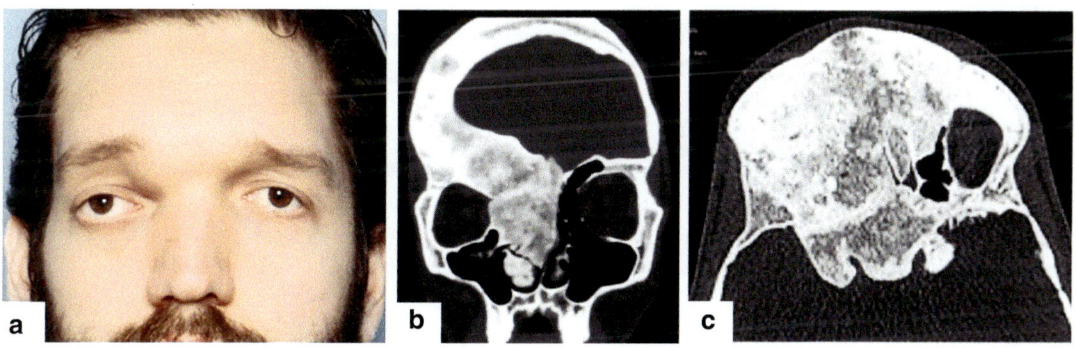

Fig. 9 Image showing a 27 year old male with craniofacial fibrous dysplasia, previously treated with bisphosphonates but not surgery. The disease had been stable for over 7 years with visual acuity of OD 1/300 and OS 0.2 Snellen (**a**). CT, coronal plane (**b**). CT, axial plane (**c**)

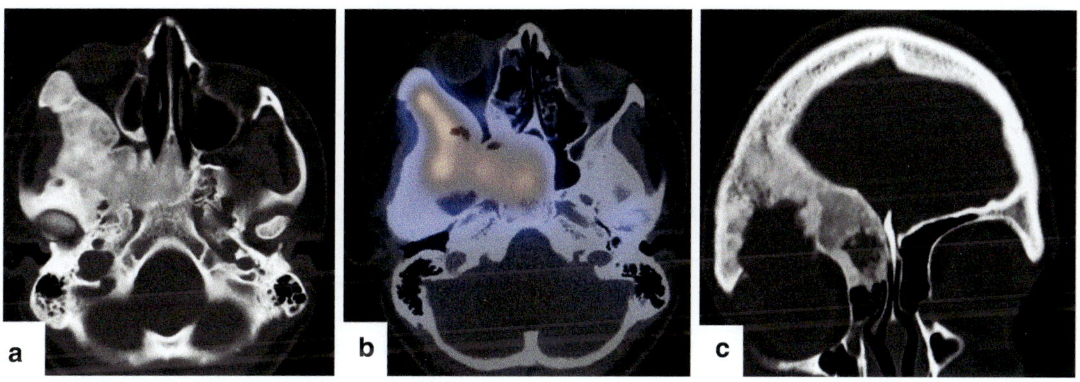

Fig. 10 Fibrous dysplasia in a 21 year old male, untreated, and without visual signs or symptoms (**a**). CT axial plane (**b**). CT axial plane combined with NAF-PET showing bone turnover activity (**c**)

If the diagnosis is made or suspected, FD/MAS needs to be staged in order to assess the extent of the disease. This includes physical examination of the skeletal system, bone related laboratory testing and whole body imaging.

Activity of the lesions can be shown with 18F-NaF PET/CT, combined with serum bone turnover markers such as serum alkaline phosphatase levels [24]. (Fig. 10) The extent, distribution and impact of the craniofacial FD should be defined using CT imaging. If nerve impairment or functional impairment is suspected, treatment in a multidisciplinary team including endocrinologist, maxillofacial surgeon, neurosurgeon and/or ENT/audiology is needed.

Patients can suffer from pain, facial deformity and impairment of vision, hearing or jaw movement. The majority of CFD lesions are reported to be detected by the age of 3 years. Patients with CFD have been known to have impaired quality of life and are affected by the disease differently compared to patients without craniofacial localizations [25].

The optic canal is frequently involved in CFD, and narrowing of the canal can cause optic neuropathy (Fig. 10). Until skeletal growth is complete, patients are at risk of optic canal narrowing but also the formation of aneurysmal bone cysts (ABC., Fig. 10)). A cyst, especially located near the orbital apex or optic canal, can cause a sudden compressive optic neuropathy, needing urgent surgical treatment. Extensive skull involvement has been reported to cause intracranial hypertension, and can be associated with optic disc oedema and visual field loss [26].

Facial deformity is not uncommon but diplopia in the absence of cranial nerve paralysis is very rare. Pain is frequently reported and very difficult to treat. Bone deformities can cause abnormal mechanical forces but also the undermineralization of the affected bone is thought to contribute to pain: the bone is less rigid and more dynamic, potentially causing the periosteum to 'slide' over the bone, resembling the pain that is also seen in bone fractures [27]. Other possible explanations for pain include the mechanisms comparable with bone metastases and neuropathic involvement [28–30].

3.2 Monitoring and Treatment

Management guidelines have been established by the FD/MAS international consortium to address the various diagnostic and therapeutic challenges in fibrous dysplasia [31]. These include a care pathway for diagnosis, staging principles (to establish disease extent), and monitoring and treatment guidelines. The latter encompass pharmacological therapy and surgical principles based on expert opinion and published studies.

In all cases, an endocrinologist should be involved and disease staging will reveal which other subspecialties should be consulted. Since there is no cure for FD, treatment is symptomatic and aims to alter functional impairment, to relieve pain and/or to reduce bone turnover [32].

If the optic canal is involved and stable disease has not been determined, it is recommended to monitor patients for compressive optic neuropathy. Periodic visual field examination, colour vision testing and/or VEP can aid in diagnosing optic neuropathy. CT imaging is regularly needed to rule out the presence of aneurysmal bone cyst. If needed, surgery should be performed to decompress the optic nerve in order to maintain or preserve normal visual function. Surgery should be performed by a surgical team with fibrous dysplasia experience because the lesions vary in tissue density. Surgery should be avoided in the absence of functional deficits.

It is unknown whether bone activity returns to normal when skeletal growth is completed. Adult patients with active lesions can still be at risk of narrowing of the optic canal, although this risk seems to be higher in children. Nevertheless, adult patients should also be monitored until disease stability is confirmed [31].

Bisphosphonates induce osteoclast apoptosis and are often prescribed with the aim of decreasing bone resorption and bone turnover [33]. They also appear to ameliorate pain in certain patients. More recently, Denosumab, an anti-RANK ligand antibody, has emerged as a potential new treatment. Denosumab decreases bone resorption by inhibiting the differentiation of osteoclasts, but its safety profile, particularly in children (in whom adequate phosphate levels are essential for normal growth), awaits further trials [34]. Furthermore, other endocrinopathies known to be associated with FD (including FGF-23 mediated hypophosphatemia, growth hormone excess, and thyroid abnormalities), should be identified and treated before such treatment is considered.

Finally, although frontal lesions often affect globe position, diplopia rarely occurs, but surgery may be indicated in patients with stable disease and with severe facial asymmetry or extreme proptosis.

4 Solitary Extramedullary Plasmacytomas and Multiple Myeloma (SEMP)

Plasma cells develop from activated B cells, and with malignant proliferation lead to multiple myeloma (MM) , either confined to the bone marrow compartment, or identified as solitary extramedullary lesion(s) (solitary extramedullary plasmacytoma, SEMP). Most SEMPs arise in the head and neck, especially along the upper respiratory/sinonasal tract [35].

Periocular SEMPs are rare, as periocular plasmacytomas occur mainly as part of MM [36]. Most patients present with proptosis, periorbital swelling, altered vision and pain. Usually there is globe displacement and reduced ocular motility. Around 60% presents with a palpable mass. The lesions are most often located in the superolateral anterior orbit with a soft tissue mass "exploding" from the frontal bone or the greater wing of the sphenoid [37] (Fig. 11).

Radiological features of SEMPs may vary, and not all lesions are contiguous with bone. Lesions that *are* contiguous with bone are usually larger, hypointense to isointense on T1-weighted images, and isointense to hyperintense on T2-weighted images. Lesions non-contiguous with bone are more often hypointense on T2-weighted images [38].

Suspected lesions can be biopsied with or without tumour debulking. Since there is no histological difference between SEMPs and MM, the diagnosis of SEMP is made in the *absence* of clinical, radiological or histological evidence of systemic disease [39]. Thus, all patients should be referred to a haematologist for a full systemic review and staging.

In approximately 10–30% of patients SEMPs progress to MM [40]. In one study, of all patients presenting with periocular disease, approximately half already had known systemic disease, and of the other half, a further 50% were found to have occult MM within 6 months of orbital biopsy [37]. However, of the remaining 50% (a quarter of the cohort), none developed MM over an average follow-up of more than 9 years.

Treatment of SEMP is local radiotherapy with curative intent. Chemotherapy can be considered in multifocal, persistent or recurrent disease. The estimated 5-year survival for periocular SEMP is around 50%, however, more than 50% develop MM in 2 years after treatment [37, 41]. MM is a haematological malignancy, treated by chemo-

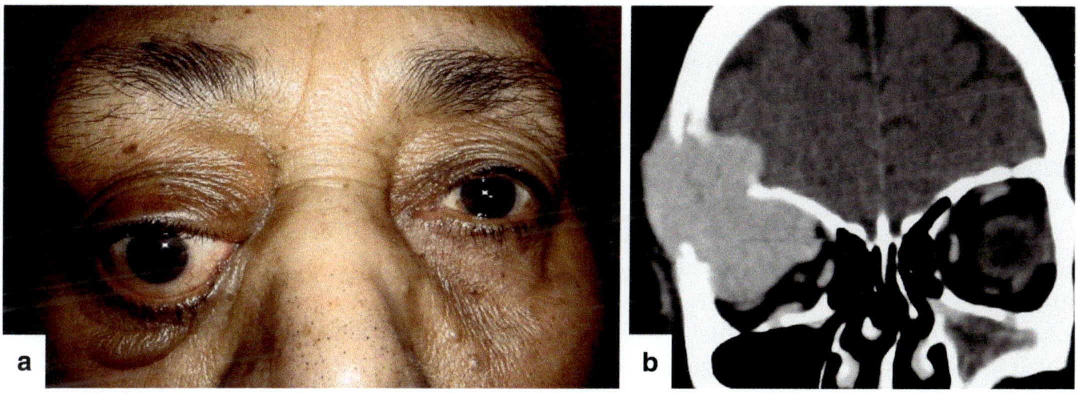

Fig. 11 Orbito-cranial plasmacytoma deposit presenting with severe axial and non-axial proptosis (**a**). CT identifies a bone-lytic soft tissue lesion (**b**)

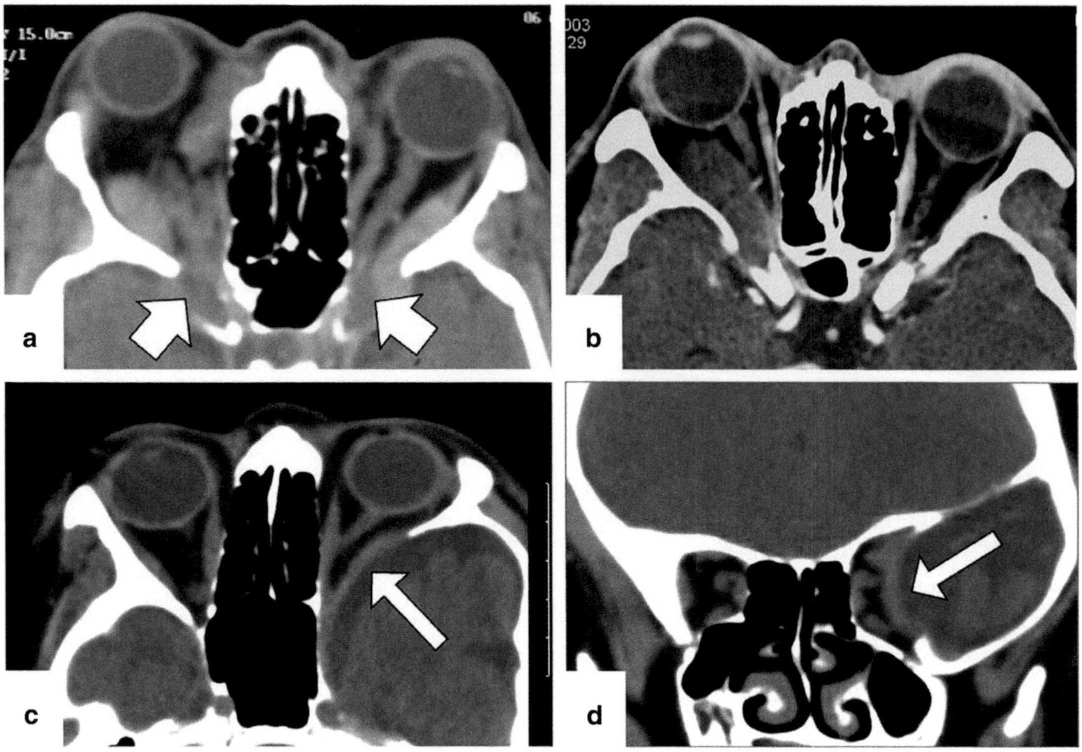

Fig. 12 CT identifying bilateral lateral neurofibromata with expansion of the superior ophthalmic fissures (short arrows, (**a**)). Superolateral neurofibroma extending to cavernous sinus and superior orbital fissure (**b**). Sphenoid wing dysplasia (long arrow), with expansion of the left middle cranial fossa and a consequent reduction in the volume of the bony orbit (**c**, **d**)

therapy, usually combined with autologous hematopoietic stem cell transplantation followed by maintenance medical treatment. The median progression-free survival of MM is around 40 months [42].

5 Orbital Neurofibromatosis

Neurofibromatosis (NF-1 and NF-2) is discussed in Chapter "Neurogenic Tumours". NF1 can involve the orbit with plexiform neurofibromas of the intra-orbital cranial nerves, optic nerve sheath and sclera, and dysplasia of the sphenoid wing. The latter presents with pulsating exophthalmos, and accounts for the so-called '**bare orbit sign'**, a radiological reference which refers to an absent **'innominate line'** (a projection of the greater wing of the sphenoid), and which can also be associated with an antero-posterior enlargement of the middle cranial fossa (Fig. 12).

6 Orbital Apex, Superior Orbital Fissure, and Cavernous Sinus Syndromes

Orbital apex syndrome (OAS), superior orbital fissure syndrome(SOFS), and cavernous sinus syndrome (CSS) each present with distinct clinical features, but share similar aetiologies.

6.1 Anatomy of the Orbital Apex

Anatomically, the orbital apex is the posterior part of the orbit where the four orbital walls converge; it has the shape of a pyramid, with the apex directed posteriorly. It includes the optic canal and the superior and inferior orbital fissures (Fig. 13). The cavernous sinus is located posteriorly from the orbital apex and is contiguous with the orbital apex and superior orbital fissure [43]. The optic canal contains the optic nerve (surrounded by meninges), the ophthalmic artery (lateral to the optic nerve) and the postganglionic sympathetic nerves that arise from the carotid plexus. The superior orbital fissure (SOF) is located within the sphenoid bone, inferolateral to the optic canal. Within the orbital apex, a tendinous ring of the thickened periorbita, the annulus of Zinn, divides the SOF into a superolateral, central and inferior part. The superolateral part transmits the lacrimal (CNV1), frontal (CNV1) and trochlear (CNIV) nerves, the superior ophthalmic vein and recurrent meningeal artery. The middle part transmits the superior and inferior branches of the oculomotor nerve (CNIII), the nasociliary nerve (CN V1), and the abducens nerve (CNVI). The inferior part transmits the inferior branch of the ophthalmic vein [44]. The contents of the optic canal and the central portion of the SOF run through the annulus of Zinn.

6.2 Clinical Signs

OAS involves cranial neuropathies in association with optic nerve dysfunction. The most common presenting manifestation of OAS is visual loss and ophthalmoplegia involving multiple cranial nerves, including the oculomotor, trochlear, and abducens nerves, and the ophthalmic branch of the trigeminal nerve (V1) (Table 5). Radiological signs include subtle reduction or loss of the apical fat plane (Fig. 14).

OAS is a distinct clinical presentation and differs from superior orbital fissure syndrome (SOFS) in which the optic nerve is *not* involved [45]. In cavernous sinus syndrome (CSS), the clinical features reflect a combination of OAS and the involvement of sympathetic fibres and the maxillary branch of the trigeminal nerve (V2). Patients who have features of SOFS may subsequently develop OAS and CSS [46].

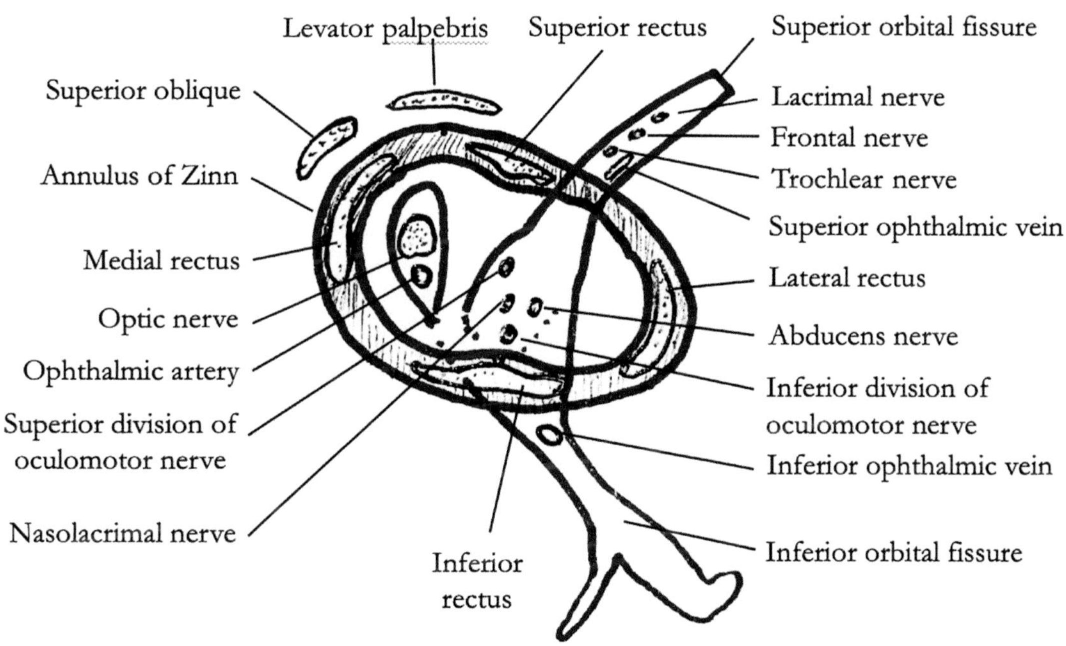

Fig. 13 Structures at the orbital apex

Table 5 Presenting features of orbital apex syndrome

- Mass effect
  - Proptosis with or without orbital congestion
  - Chemosis
  - Choroidal folds
- CN II
  - Visual loss
  - Optic disc oedema
  - Afferent pupillary defect (RAPD)
  - Optic disc atrophy (which may develop within weeks to months)
- CNIII, IV, VI
  - Efferent pupillary abnormalities
  - Ophthalmoplegia with variable diplopia, mydriasis, and ptosis
  - Reduced corneal sensation and corneal reflex
  - Periorbital/facial pain and hypo-esthesia of the forehead

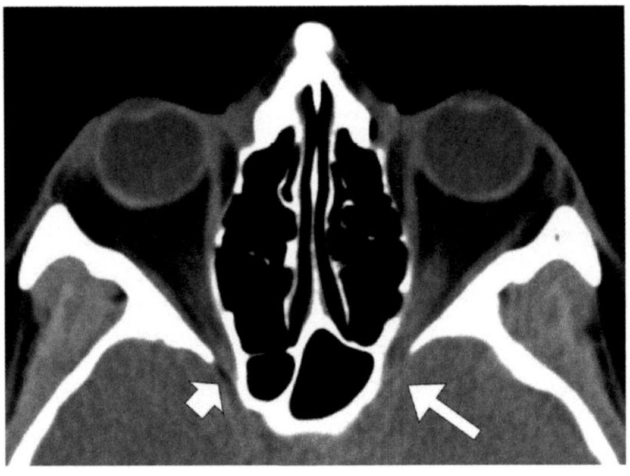

Fig. 14 Loss of the fat plane at the left orbital apex due to (presumed) orbital sarcoid. The short arrow shows the fat plane at the normal orbital apex on the right, with loss of the fat plane on the left (long arrow)

6.3 Causes

A wide variety of pathologies can lead to orbital apex syndrome, including the following:

6.3.1 Inflammatory

Churg-Strauss syndrome, giant cell arteritis, granulomatosis with polyangiitis, idiopathic orbital inflammation, IgG4 related orbital disease, sarcoidosis (Figs. 14, 15, and 16), systemic lupus erythematosus (SLE), thyroid-associated orbitopathy, Tolosa Hunt Syndrome.

6.3.2 Infectious

Post-septal bacterial orbital cellulitis or invasive fungal sinusitis; aggressive bacterial sinusitis can cause OAS with virtually absent cellulitis [47]. Specific infectious agents include fungi (aspergillosis, Mucormycosis), bacteria (streptococcus, staphylococcus, actinomyces, gram-negative bacilli, anaerobes, mycobacterium tuberculosis), spirochetes (treponema pallidum), and viruses (Herpes Zoster).

6.3.3 Neoplastic

Primary orbital tumours such as adenoid cystic carcinoma.

Head and neck tumours e.g. nasopharyngeal carcinoma with extension into the orbit.

Neural tumours such as neurofibroma, meningioma, glioma, ciliary neurinoma, schwannoma.

Metastatic lesions among which originate from lung, breast, renal cell, melanoma.

Hematological neoplasms such as Burkitt lymphoma, non-Hodgkin lymphoma, leukaemia.

Cutaneous squamous cell carcinoma is also known to cause apical lesions by perineural invasion.

6.3.4 Injury (Traumatic/Iatrogenic)

Direct injury, usually as a result of displacement of bony fragments or a hematoma that causes compression of the apical nerves and vessels.

Indirect injuries result from shearing forces to the anatomic structures of the superior orbital fissure and/or optic nerve from high impact forces.

Iatrogenic causes include sinonasal/skull base surgery, orbital surgery and facial surgery.

6.3.5 Vascular

Carotid cavernous aneurysm, carotid cavernous fistula, cavernous sinus thrombosis.

6.3.6 Other

Fibrous dysplasia (aneurysmal bone cyst), mucocele, neurofibromatosis.

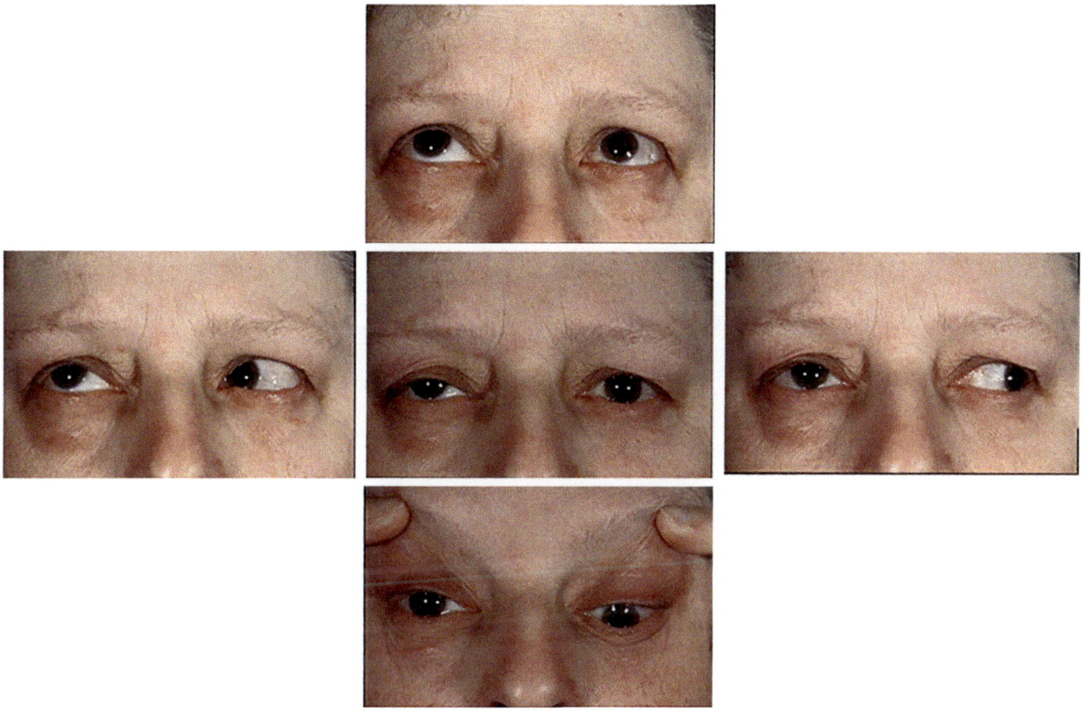

Fig. 15 This patient, with known systemic sarcoidosis, presented with reduced right abduction and depression (oculomotor nerve paresis), and failure of right abduction (abducens nerve paresis)

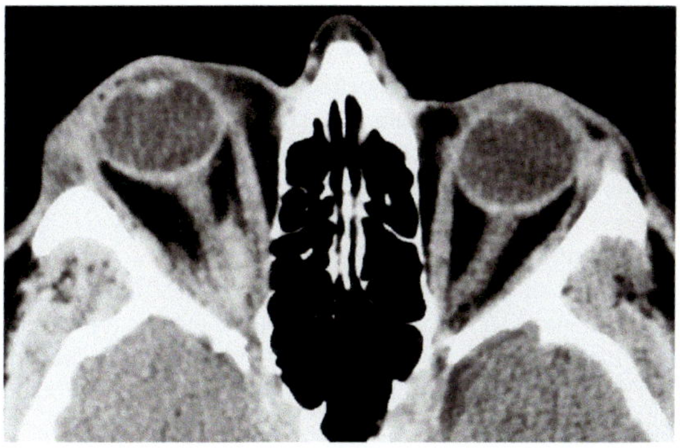

Fig. 16 CT imaging of patient shown in Fig. 15 identifying a mass at the orbital apex and loss of the fat plane. The physical signs promptly resolved on systemic corticosteroid treatment. The patient relapsed several years later with an anterior orbital lesion, biopsy of which confirmed granulomatous inflammation compatible with a diagnosis of sarcoidosis

6.4 Management

6.4.1 Inflammatory

Both corticosteroids and steroid-sparing agents can be used to treat inflammatory disease, depending on the underlying cause and clinical presentation. Usually a diagnostic biopsy is needed [48]. In some cases radiotherapy can be considered to reduce inflammation. Surgical decompression of the apex has proven to be beneficial e.g. in dysthyroid optic neuropathy [49].

6.4.2 Infectious

Antibiotic therapy will be needed in cases of bacterial cellulitis whereas antifungal and antiviral medication will benefit patients with fungal or viral disease. Acute OAS caused by orbital abscess or subperiosteal empyema will benefit from surgical intervention using an endoscopic, transcaruncular or direct approach [50].

6.4.3 Neoplastic

Radiological features do not often reduce the need for a diagnostic biopsy. Treatment of neoplasms causing OAS depends on the exact aetiology and clinical features and can include surgery, radiotherapy or chemotherapy.

6.4.4 Injury (Traumatic/Iatrogenic)

A CT-scan will be able to show orbital (comminuted) fractures. Some patients may benefit from high dose corticosteroids in case of optic nerve compression. In case of orbital compartment syndrome, urgent intervention is needed to prevent optic nerve damage and permanent loss of vision. Lateral canthotomy and cantholysis may decrease compression of the orbita but some cases require corticosteroids and/or decompressive surgery [51].

6.4.5 Vascular

Imaging using both CT and MRI are often required to allow for adequate diagnosis. In general, carotid cavernous fistula and aneurysms can be managed conservatively but in cases with cranial nerve dysfunction, management includes surgical or endovascular intervention [52, 53]. Cavernous sinus thrombosis requires anticoagulation, possible adjunctive corticosteroid therapy, and aggressive broad-spectrum antibiotic therapy if septic [54].

References

1. Low JT, Ostrom QT, Cioffi G, Neff C, Waite KA, Kruchko C, et al. Primary brain and other central nervous system tumors in the United States (2014-2018): a summary of the CBTRUS statistical report for clinicians. Neurooncol Pract. 2022;9:165–82.
2. Korn BS. 2021–2022 Basic and clinical science course, section 07: oculofacial plastic and orbital... Surgery. San Francisco, CA: American Academy of Ophthalmology; 2021.
3. Al-Mefty O. Clinoidal meningiomas. J Neurosurg. 1990;73:840–9.
4. Fisher FL, Zamanipoor Najafabadi AH, Schoones JW, Genders SW, van Furth WR. Surgery as a safe and effective treatment option for spheno-orbital meningioma: a systematic review and meta-analysis of surgical techniques and outcomes. Acta Ophthalmol. 2021;99:26–36.
5. Sherman WJ, Raizer JJ. Chemotherapy: what is its role in meningioma? Expert Rev Neurother. 2012;12:1189–95. quiz 96.
6. Louis DN, Ohgaki H, Wiestler OD, Cavenee WK, Burger PC, Jouvet A, et al. The 2007 WHO classification of tumours of the central nervous system. Acta Neuropathol. 2007;114:97–109.
7. Louis DN, Perry A, Wesseling P, Brat DJ, Cree IA, Figarella-Branger D, et al. The 2021 WHO classification of tumors of the central nervous system: a summary. Neuro-Oncology. 2021;23:1231–51.
8. Sahm F, Schrimpf D, Stichel D, Jones DTW, Hielscher T, Schefzyk S, et al. DNA methylation-based classification and grading system for meningioma: a multicentre, retrospective analysis. Lancet Oncol. 2017;18:682–94.
9. Nassiri F, Liu J, Patil V, Mamatjan Y, Wang JZ, Hugh-White R, et al. A clinically applicable integrative molecular classification of meningiomas. Nature. 2021;597:119–25.
10. Combs SE, Ganswindt U, Foote RL, Kondziolka D, Tonn JC. State-of-the-art treatment alternatives for base of skull meningiomas: complementing and controversial indications for neurosurgery, stereotactic and robotic based radiosurgery or modern fractionated radiation techniques. Radiat Oncol. 2012;7:226.
11. Oostra A, van Furth W, Georgalas C. Extended endoscopic endonasal skull base surgery: from the Sella to the anterior and posterior cranial fossa. ANZ J Surg. 2012;82:122–30.
12. Pechlivanis I, Wawrzyniak S, Engelhardt M, Schmieder K. Evidence level in the treatment of meningioma with focus on the comparison between surgery versus radiotherapy. A review. J Neurosurg Sci. 2011;55:319–28.
13. Park GO, Park HH, Yoo J, Hong CK, Oh J. Surgical outcomes of sphenoid wing meningioma with periorbital invasion. J Korean Neurosurg Soc. 2022;65:449–56.
14. Elborady MA, Nazim WM. Spheno-orbital meningiomas: surgical techniques and results. Egypt J Neurol Psychiatry Neurosurg. 2021;57:18.
15. Ringel F, Cedzich C, Schramm J. Microsurgical technique and results of a series of 63 spheno-orbital meningiomas. Neurosurgery. 2007;60:214–21. discussion 21–2.
16. Mariniello G, Maiuri F, Strianese D, Donzelli R, Iuliano A, Tranfa F, et al. Spheno-orbital meningiomas: surgical approaches and outcome according to the intraorbital tumor extent. Zentralbl Neurochir. 2008;69:175–81.
17. Kiyofuji S, Casabella AM, Graffeo CS, Perry A, Garrity JA, Link MJ. Sphenoorbital meningioma: a unique skull base tumor. Surgical technique and results. J Neurosurg. 2019:1–8.
18. Kim W, Ghodrati F, Mozaffari K, Samarage HM, Zhang AB, Pradhan A, et al. Endoscopic endonasal approach for resection of a recurrent spheno-orbital meningioma resulting in complete resolution of visual symptoms: a case report and review of literature. J Neuro-Oncol. 2022;160:545–53.
19. Komotar RJ, Starke RM, Raper DM, Anand VK, Schwartz TH. Endoscopic endonasal versus open transcranial resection of anterior midline skull base meningiomas. World Neurosurg. 2012;77:713–24.

20. Robinson C, Collins MT, Boyce AM. Fibrous dysplasia/McCune-Albright syndrome: clinical and translational perspectives. Curr Osteoporos Rep. 2016;14:178–86.
21. Chapurlat RD, Orcel P. Fibrous dysplasia of bone and McCune-Albright syndrome. Best Pract Res Clin Rheumatol. 2008;22:55–69.
22. Yang L, Wu H, Lu J, Teng L. Prevalence of different forms and involved bones of craniofacial fibrous dysplasia. J Craniofac Surg. 2017;28:21–5.
23. Thomsen MD, Rejnmark L. Clinical and radiological observations in a case series of 26 patients with fibrous dysplasia. Calcif Tissue Int. 2014;94:384–95.
24. Papadakis GZ, Manikis GC, Karantanas AH, Florenzano P, Bagci U, Marias K, et al. (18) F-NaF PET/CT imaging in fibrous dysplasia of bone. J Bone Miner Res. 2019;34:1619–31.
25. Hagelstein-Rotman M, Genders SW, Andela CD, Dijkstra S, Majoor BCJ, Notting IC, et al. Patients with isolated craniofacial dysplasia report better quality of life compared with those with craniofacial dysplasia and extracranial involvement. Ophthalmic Plast Reconstr Surg. 2020;36:292–7.
26. Jaulent P, Vignot E, Chapurlat R. Fibrous dysplasia of occipital bone revealed by acute intracranial hypertension. Osteoporos Int. 2019;30:691–3.
27. Riminucci M, Robey PG, Bianco P. The pathology of fibrous dysplasia and the McCune-Albright syndrome. Pediatr Endocrinol Rev. 2007;4:401–11.
28. Chapurlat RD, Gensburger D, Jimenez-Andrade JM, Ghilardi JR, Kelly M, Mantyh P. Pathophysiology and medical treatment of pain in fibrous dysplasia of bone. Orphanet J Rare Dis. 2012;7:S3.
29. Jimenez-Andrade JM, Mantyh WG, Bloom AP, Xu H, Ferng AS, Dussor G, et al. A phenotypically restricted set of primary afferent nerve fibers innervate the bone versus skin: therapeutic opportunity for treating skeletal pain. Bone. 2010;46:306–13.
30. Mundy GR. Metastasis to bone: causes, consequences and therapeutic opportunities. Nat Rev Cancer. 2002;2:584–93.
31. Javaid MK, Boyce A, Appelman-Dijkstra N, Ong J, Defabianis P, Offiah A, et al. Best practice management guidelines for fibrous dysplasia/McCune-Albright syndrome: a consensus statement from the FD/MAS international consortium. Orphanet J Rare Dis. 2019;14:139.
32. Rotman M, Hamdy NAT, Appelman-Dijkstra NM. Clinical and translational pharmacological aspects of the management of fibrous dysplasia of bone. Br J Clin Pharmacol. 2019;85:1169–79.
33. Luckman SP, Hughes DE, Coxon FP, Graham R, Russell G, Rogers MJ. Nitrogen-containing bisphosphonates inhibit the mevalonate pathway and prevent post-translational prenylation of GTP-binding proteins, including Ras. J Bone Miner Res. 1998;13:581–9.
34. Raborn LN, Burke AB, Ebb DH, Collins MT, Kaban LB, Boyce AM. Denosumab for craniofacial fibrous dysplasia: duration of efficacy and post-treatment effects. Osteoporos Int. 2021;32:1889–93.
35. Bachar G, Goldstein D, Brown D, Tsang R, Lockwood G, Perez-Ordonez B, et al. Solitary extramedullary plasmacytoma of the head and neck--long-term outcome analysis of 68 cases. Head Neck. 2008;30:1012–9.
36. Shields JA, Shields CL, Scartozzi R. Survey of 1264 patients with orbital tumors and simulating lesions: the 2002 Montgomery lecture, part 1. Ophthalmology. 2004;111:997–1008.
37. Zloto O, Vahdani K, Stack R, Verity DH, Rose GE. Periocular presentation of solitary Plasmacytomas and multiple myeloma. Ophthalmic Plast Reconstr Surg. 2022;38:180–4.
38. Tirumani SH, Shinagare AB, Jagannathan JP, Krajewski KM, Munshi NC, Ramaiya NH. MRI features of extramedullary myeloma. AJR Am J Roentgenol. 2014;202:803–10.
39. Soutar R, Lucraft H, Jackson G, Reece A, Bird J, Low E, et al. Guidelines on the diagnosis and management of solitary plasmacytoma of bone and solitary extramedullary plasmacytoma. Br J Haematol. 2004;124:717–26.
40. de Waal EG, Leene M, Veeger N, Vos HJ, Ong F, Smit WG, et al. Progression of a solitary plasmacytoma to multiple myeloma. A population-based registry of the Northern Netherlands. Br J Haematol. 2016;175:661–7.
41. Caers J, Garderet L, Kortum KM, O'Dwyer ME, van de Donk N, Binder M, et al. European myeloma network recommendations on tools for the diagnosis and monitoring of multiple myeloma: what to use and when. Haematologica. 2018;103:1772–84.
42. Cowan AJ, Green DJ, Kwok M, Lee S, Coffey DG, Holmberg LA, et al. Diagnosis and management of multiple myeloma: a review. JAMA. 2022;327:464–77.
43. Engin Ö, Adriaensen G, Hoefnagels FWA, Saeed P. A systematic review of the surgical anatomy of the orbital apex. Surg Radiol Anat. 2021;43:169–78.
44. Badakere A, Patil-Chhablani P. Orbital apex syndrome: a review. Eye Brain. 2019;11:63–72.
45. Kline LB. The Tolosa-hunt syndrome. Surv Ophthalmol. 1982;27:79–95.
46. Yeh S, Foroozan R. Orbital apex syndrome. Curr Opin Ophthalmol. 2004;15:490–8.
47. Pfeiffer ML, Merritt HA, Bailey LA, Richani K, Phillips ME. Orbital apex syndrome from bacterial sinusitis without orbital cellulitis. Am J Ophthalmol Case Rep. 2018;10:84–6.
48. Mombaerts I, Rose GE, Garrity JA. Orbital inflammation: biopsy first. Surv Ophthalmol. 2016;61:664–9.

49. Saeed P, Tavakoli Rad S, Bisschop P. Dysthyroid optic neuropathy. Ophthalmic Plast Reconstr Surg. 2018;34:S60–7.
50. Smith JM, Bratton EM, DeWitt P, Davies BW, Hink EM, Durairaj VD. Predicting the need for surgical intervention in pediatric orbital cellulitis. Am J Ophthalmol. 2014;158:387–94 e1.
51. Warner N, Eggenberger E. Traumatic optic neuropathy: a review of the current literature. Curr Opin Ophthalmol. 2010;21:459–62.
52. Eddleman CS, Hurley MC, Bendok BR, Batjer HH. Cavernous carotid aneurysms: to treat or not to treat? Neurosurg Focus. 2009;26:E4.
53. Ellis JA, Goldstein H, Connolly ES Jr, Meyers PM. Carotid-cavernous fistulas. Neurosurg Focus. 2012;32:E9.
54. Coutinho JM, Stam J. How to treat cerebral venous and sinus thrombosis. J Thromb Haemost. 2010;8:877–83.

Surgical Approaches to the Orbit

Kaveh Vahdani, Dion Paridaens,
and Geoffrey E. Rose

Key Messages

- It is generally possible to deal with all solely orbital disease using six basic orbital approaches, all of which respect periocular aesthetics.
- These key approaches include (1) upper lid skin crease, (2) swinging lower eyelid flap (with "high" and "low" variants), (3) lateral canthotomy, (4) lateral orbitotomy with bone mobilisation, (5) transconjunctival retrocaruncular approach, and (6) transconjunctival peritomy.
- A multidisciplinary approach including neurosurgeons, maxillo-facial or head-and-neck surgeons is recommended when the disease extends beyond the orbit into the adjacent structures.
- The risk of functional impairment following orbital surgery varies significantly depending on the depth of the orbit, with variability within each zone.
- Due to the crowding of the neurovascular structures in the orbital apex, operating in the posterior third of the orbit carries a high risk of complication, many being serious or permanent.

1 Introduction

Historically performed by neurosurgeons [1], orbital surgery is now an ophthalmic speciality that employs more refined and aesthetic approaches with less morbidity than transcranial methods. However, where the disease spreads outside the orbit into the cranium, paranasal sinuses, or pterygopalatine fossa, a multidisciplinary approach with neurosurgeons, maxillo-facial or head-and-neck surgeons is advisable. This chapter covers six key approaches that provide good access to all areas of the orbit, as well as pre-operative, intra-operative and post-operative considerations (Table 1). With these six fundamental techniques, all of which respect periocular aesthetics, it is generally possible to address all solely orbital pathology, with little or no contemporary indication for other approaches—such as a lid-split orbitotomy, "lazy-S" incision (Stallard-Wright), or bicoronal flap—in such cases.

The authors have no conflict of interest to declare.

K. Vahdani (✉) · G. E. Rose
Adnexal Service, Moorfields Eye Hospital, London, UK
e-mail: kaveh.vahdani@nhs.net

D. Paridaens
Department of Oculoplastic, Orbital and Lacrimal Surgery, The Rotterdam Eye Hospital and Erasmus Medical Center, Rotterdam, The Netherlands

F. M. Quaranta Leoni et al. (eds.), *Oculoplastic, Lacrimal and Orbital Surgery*,
https://doi.org/10.1007/978-3-031-39638-0_27

Table 1 Approaches to the orbit

Six key approaches for solely orbital disease	• Upper eyelid skin-crease approach • Swinging lower eyelid approach (two variants) • Lateral canthotomy approach • Bone-swinging lateral orbitotomy • Transconjunctival retrocaruncular approach • Conjunctival peritomy approach
Orbital and sino-nasal/midfacial disease	• Trans-antral endoscopic approach • Lateral rhinotomy approach • Trans-oral midfacial degloving approach • Midfacial resection via bicoronal flap • frontal osteoplastic flap
Orbital and intracranial disease	• Frontal osteotomy via bicoronal approach • Superotemporal panoramic orbitotomy • Frontal ridge osteotomy • Intervention radiology

Table 2 Risks and complications of orbital surgery

Intra-operative	
	• Haemorrhage • Vasospasm at the orbital apex (due to tissue manipulation or thermal injury) • Ocular ischaemia (due to sustained pressure on the globe) • Mydriasis (prolonged compression of globe or ciliary ganglion) • Ocular surface exposure • CSF leak (due to injury of ethmoidal roof or superolateral bony orbit)
Post-operative	
General risks	• Visual loss (low) • Haemorrhage • Infection (rare)
Orbital roof	• Sensory changes (frontal nerve and supratrochlear nerve territories) • Diplopia (injury to trochlea or superior oblique tendon) • CSF leak
Medial orbit	• Watery eye (injury to lacrimal outflow system) • Medial wall fracture • Ipsilateral sensory loss on nasal ala (nasociliary nerve)
Orbital floor	• Sensory changes (infraorbital nerve) • Orbital floor fracture
Lateral orbit	• Dry eye (lacrimal gland damage/removal) • Loss of reflex tearing (lacrimal nerve transection) • Mydriasis (ciliary ganglion damage)
Posterior orbit	• Irreversible visual loss (complete or partial) • Ophthalmoplegia • Blepharoptosis • Periocular sensory loss

2 The Surgical 'Conoid of View'

The orbit is a tetrahedral soft-tissue structure surrounded by bone, and unless the bony wall(s) are displaced or removed, all surgical approaches to the orbit are restricted by the anterior orbital aperture (generally less than 3 cm) and the extent to which the globe can be displaced. Therefore, with an orbital apex lesion, the surgeon's maximum theoretical binocular 'conoid of view' is around 50° by 30°, although practically it is narrower since soft tissues restrict the operative field even more, with the operative view becoming monocular in the depths of the surgical field. The conoid of view can be enhanced by either shifting the incision closer to the location of the lesion, in order to shorten the conoid "depth" (for example, lateral canthotomy approach to lateral masses), or displacing an orbital wall outwards (as performed in bone-swinging lateral orbitotomy).

3 The Risks of Orbital Surgery

The risk of orbital function impairment varies significantly at different depths within the orbit, with variations within each zone (Table 2). Surgery for lesions alongside the globe in the anterior one-third of the orbit is associated with a significantly lower risk of collateral injury than surgery in the posterior third of the orbit, where the conoid of view is restricted and structures are viewed more obliquely.

The most serious risk whilst operating in the middle third of the orbit is (relatively rare) visual loss due to ischaemia of the optic nerve, but the ciliary ganglion is probably the most vulnerable structure in this region, with persistent mydriasis a relatively common complication after the removal of retrobulbar tumors.

Due to the crowding of the neurovascular structures in the orbital apex, operating in the posterior third of the orbit carries a high risk of complication, many being serious or permanent. Complete visual loss—due to vasospasm at the orbital apex—is quite common with removal of "peanut" tumours wedged in the apex, especially with tumours located below the optic nerve, alongside the ophthalmic artery [2]. Complete ophthalmoplegia is common after operating near the superior orbital fissure, this ophthalmoplegia often improving markedly at about 3 months after surgery, but occasionally leaving a selective neuropraxia.

The appropriate risks of surgery should be explained to the patient, as well as the risks of choosing to not having surgery, and any alternatives to surgery. In contrast to suspected malignancy, where the benefit of surgery outweighs the risks, it is recommended to wait for evidence of progressive visual impairment before considering intervention for well-defined "benign" looking apical lesions that may carry a significant risk of major complication with surgery.

4 Perioperative Considerations

Pre-operative considerations include the type of anaesthesia, general medical status, the use of anticoagulant and antiplatelet medications, and the need for early post-operative hospitalisation.

Orbital surgery, particularly for more anterior procedures (for example, lacrimal gland biopsy), can be performed with local anaesthesia or regional blocks under sedation. However, unless the risks are deemed unacceptable, general anaesthesia is preferable as it allows for better intra-operative control of systemic blood pressure. Medical conditions such as hypertension, diabetes, or dysthyroid state should be well controlled in all patients undergoing routine orbital surgery, and a pre-operative assessment by an anaesthetist is indicated where hypotensive general anaesthesia is required. General anaesthesia with controlled hypotension, improves the operative field by reducing arterial and venous bleeding, can be efficiently achieved with total intravenous anaesthesia (TIVA) using Propofol and Remifentanyl, or a mixture of volatile inhalational agents (such as isofluorane) with titrated small doses of a beta-blocker to avoid compensatory tachycardia.

To avoid the risks of haemorrhage, antiplatelet agents such as aspirin and clopidogrel should be stopped (if safe to do so) for at least 2 weeks before surgery and direct oral anticoagulants (dabigatran, rivaroxaban, apixaban, edoxaban) for 2 days. In patients on warfarin, the INR should be <1.5, and low molecular weight heparin should be considered where anticoagulation cannot be discontinued (for example, with metallic heart valves). All herbal remedies, garlic, ginger, ginseng and ginkgo should also be avoided completely for a few weeks before surgery.

Per-operative measures that help to reduce the risk bleeding include positioning of the patient during surgery, with a 15° head-up, reverse Trendelenburg, position to reduce the venous return, an intravenous antifibrinolytic agent such as tranexamic acid, and control of perioperative pain with regional infiltration using a long-acting local anaesthetic, such as bupivacaine.

5 The Six Principal Approaches to the Orbit

All regions of the orbit can be accessed through one of 6 principal orbitotomies (Table 1), although occasionally a combination of two such routes might be required for large or diffuse masses, extensive trauma, or decompression of multiple walls.

The choice of surgical approach is largely dependent on the location and depth of the required access. When incisional biopsy is indicated, a trans-lid approach (through the upper lid skin crease or inferior conjunctiva) is usually adequate. In contrast, for intact excision of a deeper lesion, a lower lid swinging flap or bone-swinging lateral orbitotomy may be necessary to increase the surgeon's conoid of view, and allow greater access to the posterior orbit.

5.1 Anterior Orbitotomy: Upper Eyelid Skin-Crease Approach

The upper two-thirds of the orbit are accessible via the upper eyelid approach (Fig. 1), this healing with no visible scar and allowing access right back to the superior orbital fissure and orbital apex. It is ideal for incisional or excisional biopsies, with the skin incision biased medially for supero-nasal masses and laterally for lacrimal gland masses and those alongside the lateral orbital wall.

After making the skin incision, the orbicularis muscle is divided along the length of the incision, and the skin/muscle flaps are put on traction (usually with a 2/0 silk suture), followed by an upward, preseptal dissection to avoid damage to the underlying levator muscle aponeurosis.

For non-lacrimal masses, the orbital septum is entered a few millimetres below the arcus marginalis, then divided medially and/or laterally, according to the quadrant in which orbital exploration is needed (Fig. 1b). Masses along the orbital roof are best reached by downward displacement of the preaponeurotic fat pad, and masses involving the superior rectus or levator muscles reached by passage in the plane below the fat pad. The intraconal space is reached by

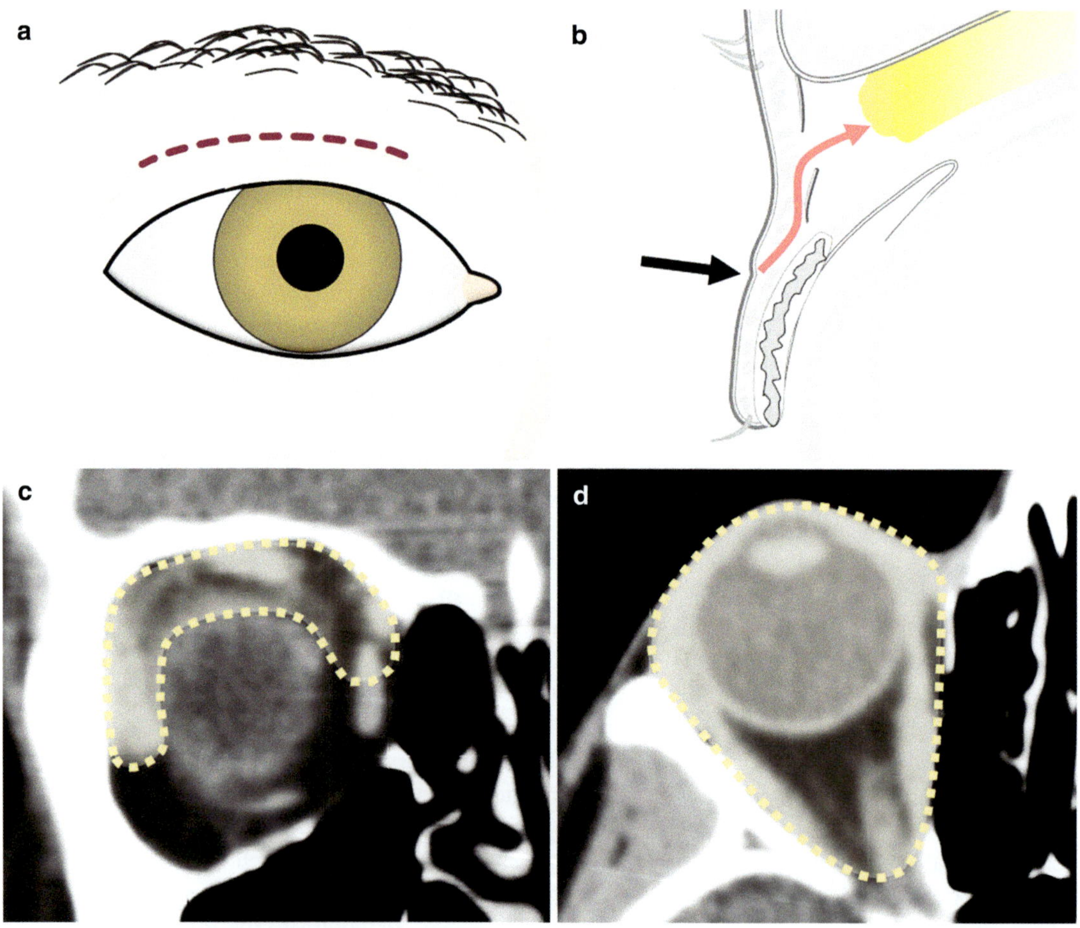

Fig. 1 Upper lid skin crease approach. (**a**) Skin crease incision (dashed line), the position of which can be biased medially or laterally. (**b**) Schematic route to superior extraconal and intraconal spaces—sub-orbicularis dissection and opening the septum below the arcus marginalis. (**c** and **d**) Regions of the orbit accessible through this approach

either lateral or medial displacement of the superior rectus/levator complex and blunt dissection through to the intraconal fat.

A closed pair of blunt-ended scissors is directed towards the mass, through the fat, and then opened widely, with 13–16 mm retractors on either side of the scissors to maintain the plane and depth of exploration. The orbital mass is typically revealed after repeating this manoeuvre several times, with the assistant gently retracting the surrounding tissues to maintain a good view of the targeted area. If intact excision of a well-defined mass is intended, it should be carefully separated from surrounding tissues with gentle diathermy and the division of any bridging vascular pedicles, whereas incisional biopsy of ill-defined masses is a preferably achieved with a *single* grip of the tissues specimen so as to reduce crush artefacts. After obtaining haemostasis, a vacuum drain should be placed where there has been surgery within the deep orbit, to reduce the serum collection and pressure rise at the apex, thereby minimising the risk of optic nerve ischaemia and visual loss; the drain trocar may be passed through the eyebrow to avoid a visible scar.

For lacrimal gland biopsy, the preseptal plane is followed to the supero-lateral orbital rim, the arcus marginalis divided for 2 cm above the lateral canthal tubercle, to mobilise the orbital lobe of the gland inferomedially and a good-sized specimen of abnormal tissue taken for biopsy; biopsies of the *orbital* lobe are much preferred to transconjunctival biopsies of the palpebral lobe, as many lacrimal gland diseases tend to spare the latter and its biopsy carries a major risk of dry eye.

After adequate haemostasis, the orbicularis and skin are closed with a running 6/0 nylon suture that can be removed between 1–2 weeks after surgery or, where an absorbable suture is required (as in a child, or with no follow-up) 8/0 polyglactan, and a firm eye pad applied. The eyepad and drain can usually be removed within 12–24 h following surgery, or earlier if there is any element of severe or increasing orbital pain (when vision should be checked).

5.2 Anterior Orbitotomy: Lower Lid Swinging Flaps

The lower two-thirds of the orbit can be reached through several routes, of which the "tear-trough" skin incision is effectively obsolete, due to the risks of visible lower lid scar, fistula formation, lower eyelid retraction or adhesions to the underlying bone. Similarly, the subciliary blepharoplasty incision, whilst useful for removal of redundant skin, tends to be unnecessarily vascular, thereby hindering orbital exploration, and may cause scarring.

The modern approach for inferior orbitotomy is the lower lid swinging flap, of which there are two variants (Fig. 2). The first is the "high" flap (Fig. 2c), with conjunctival incision 1 mm below the lower border or the tarsus, which allows access, via the *preseptal* plane, to the inferior orbital rim, from which excellent access to the orbital floor and medial wall is achieved. The "low" flap (Fig. 2d), with the conjunctival incision located in the depths of the lower fornix, exposes the *postseptal* extraconal fat pad and, from here, all of the orbit, except the supero-medial part of both the intraconal and extraconal space, can be accessed. Understanding the fundamental difference between the two types of lower lid swinging flaps, which were not highlighted in the original description for this approach [3, 4], allows a rational application of these extremely valuable techniques.

5.2.1 The "High" Variant of Lower Lid Swinging Flap

The lower lid is disinserted by a slightly downward-directed lateral canthotomy and cantholysis, and the conjunctiva then opened along its horizontal extent at 1 mm below the lower tarsal border (Fig. 2c), with care taken to avoid inadvertent canalicular damage. The cornea can be protected by anchoring the cut edge of the lower conjunctiva to the upper lid margin with a 4/0 nylon suture on a bow. After dissection in the preseptal plane down to the orbital rim, the periosteum is incised along the orbital rim to expose the extraperiosteal space as widely as required;

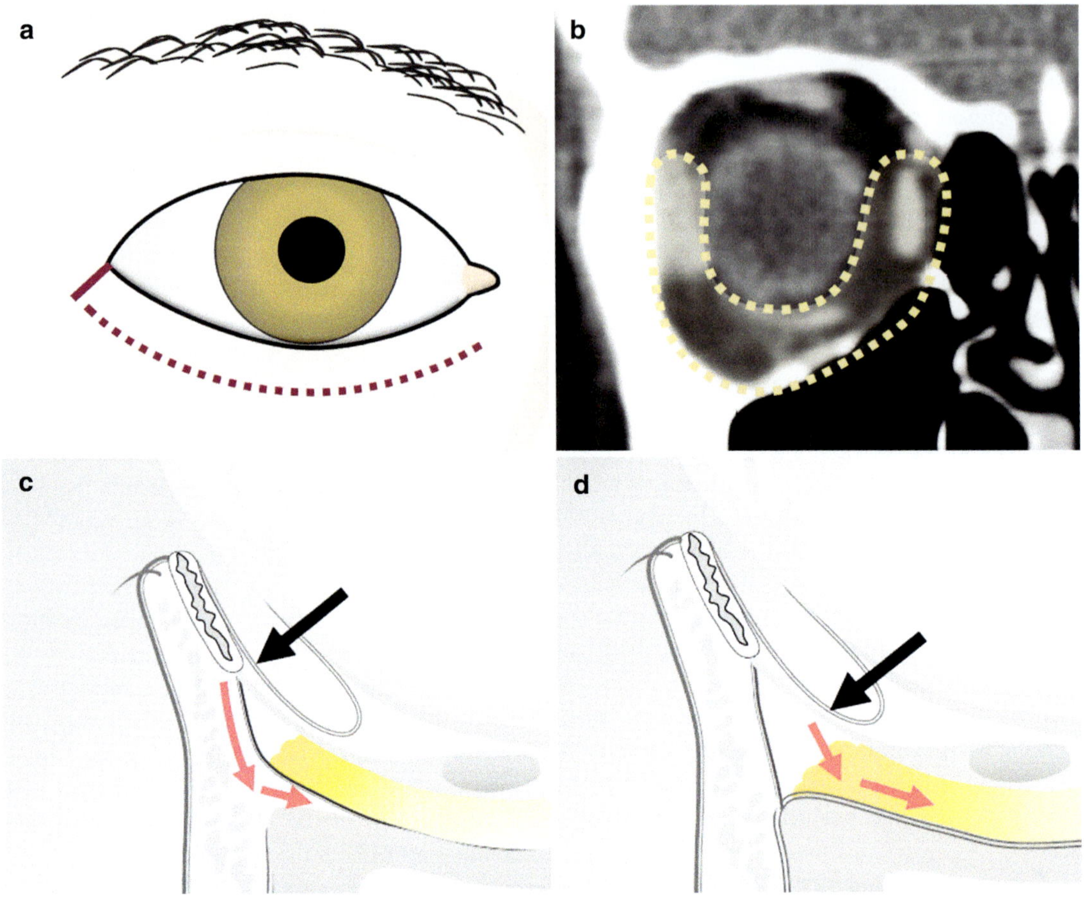

Fig. 2 Swinging lower eyelid flap. (**a**) Lateral canthotomy with division of the lower limb of the canthal tendon, followed by conjunctival incision (marked by dotted line) and (**b**) the areas of the orbit accessible through this approach. (**c**) The "high variant" used for extraperiosteal approaches to the orbital floor and medial orbit, and (**d**) "low variant" used for intraperiosteal exploration of the extraconal or intraconal orbital spaces

for periosteal elevation across the whole floor, it is necessary to cauterise and divide the artery crossing from the infraorbital canal to the orbit. Where extensive access to the medial wall as well as the floor is required, the incision can be extended superomedially into a retrocaruncular incision with temporary division of the origin of the inferior oblique muscle. The anterior and posterior ethmoidal neurovascular bundles, which are generally visible during surgery, limit upward extraperiosteal dissection. Such an approach is typically used for repair of orbital fractures or when three-wall decompression is required in cases of extreme proptosis.

The swinging flaps are repaired in a layered fashion, by closing the lateral end of the conjunctival incision with a 6/0 polyglactan suture, followed by lateral canthal repair with grey-line and lash-line alignment sutures, suturing the cut end of the lower tarsus and the upper limb of the lateral canthal tendon, and finally closing the skin incision.

5.2.2 The "Low" Variant of the Lower Lid Swinging Flap

Following an inferolateral canthotomy and cantholysis similar to "high" variant, the conjunctiva is opened along the lowest point in the inferior fornix (Fig. 2d) and its length varies according to the required field of view; This post-septal route allows excellent access to the lateral, inferior and, if needed, medial extraconal space and may be used to biopsy or resect large inflammatory masses, tumours, and vascular anomalies in these areas. Masses overlying an expanded inferior orbital fissure may also be debulked right back and into the pterygo-palatine fossa. Intraconal masses, such as cavernous venous malformations, can be removed by entering the intraconal fat-space between the inferior and lateral recti, these muscles being the most widely spaced. This is also a versatile approach for biopsy or resection of the optic nerve lesions; for example, for removal of the entire intraorbital portion of the optic nerve in cases of solely orbital optic nerve tumour with painful, blind severe proptosis. Likewise, the less oblique approach to the inferior rectus, as opposed to a conjunctival route, facilitates representative biopsy of the muscle belly.

5.3 Anterior Orbitotomy: Lateral Canthotomy Approach

The lateral half of the orbit can be reached through a horizontal lateral canthotomy, without division of the upper or lower limbs of the lateral canthal tendon (Fig. 3); this has the advantages of rapid access and closure, short operative time, no loss of eyelid stability and a completely hidden scar [5].

This approach is particularly useful where a diffuse process, such as inflammation or lymphoma, involves multiple tissues and biopsy is required from muscle, fat and lacrimal gland.

The outer canthus is divided 1–1.5 cm horizontally (to the bone) with a pair of scissors and a traction suture placed through the lateral end of the upper and lower eyelid, this creating a rhomboid-

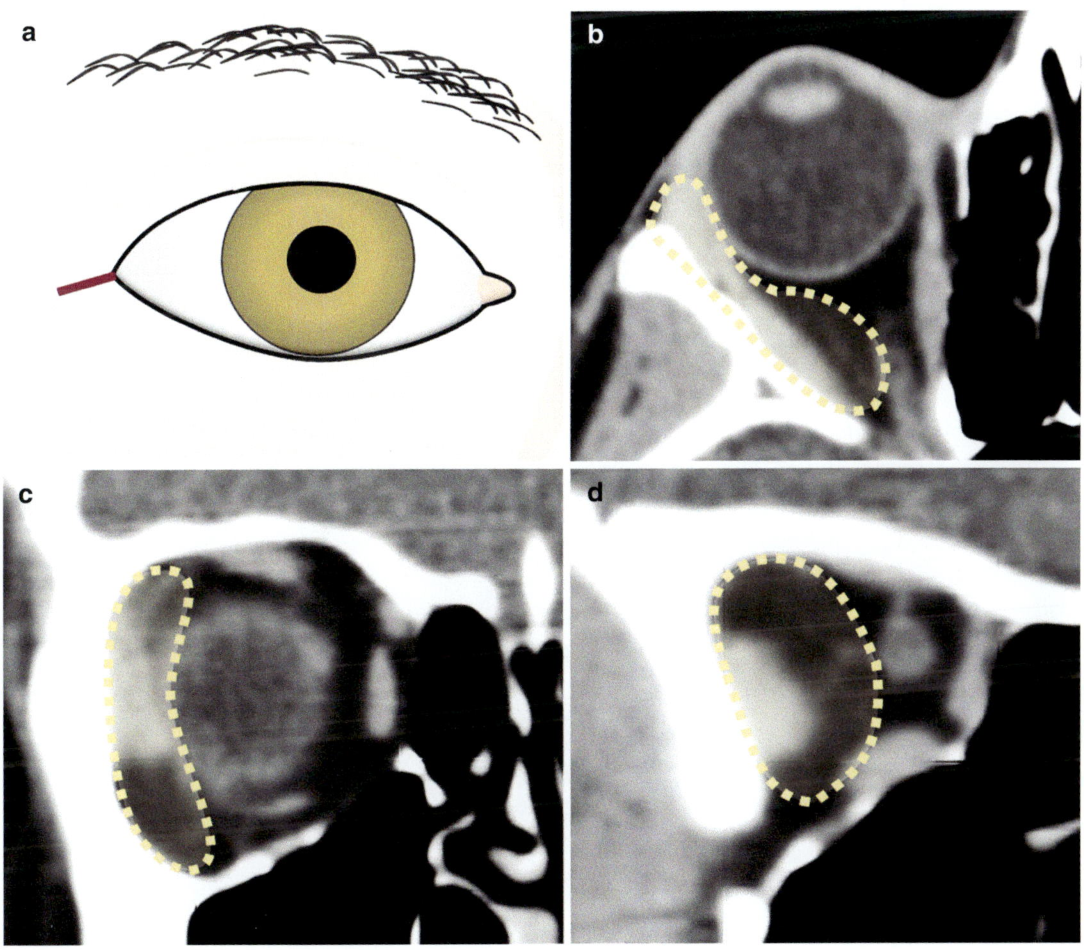

Fig. 3 Lateral canthotomy approach and the accessible parts of the orbit through this route (**a–d**)

shaped access. The tissues are then spread and retracted to expose the lateral extraconal and intraconal space; if greater access is required, the lower canthal tendon can be divided to convert it to a 'low' lower lid swinging flap. Canthotomy closure is readily accomplished by alignment of the lid margins with a 6/0 absorbable suture, then apposition of the upper and lower limbs of the tendon and skin closure.

5.4 Lateral Orbitotomy with Bone Mobilisation

Moving the lateral orbital wall outwards during surgery (lateral osteotomy) provides improved access to the orbital apex, and markedly increases the "conoid of view" by both widening the entrance incision and also shortening the path length [6, 7]. With the increased use of the 'low' variant of the lower lid swinging flap, the need for bone-swinging lateral orbitotomy is considerably reduced, although it is still valuable for the intact removal of very large lacrimal gland lesions and for removing "peanut lesions" wedged into the orbital apex.

Contemporary techniques utilise an extended upper eyelid skin-crease incision (Fig. 4), rather than the unsightly extended brow incision, and avoid removal (and devitalisation) of the bone flap by just hinging it laterally on the temporalis muscle.

A skin-crease incision in the lateral half of the upper lid is extended for about 1–1.5 cm into the

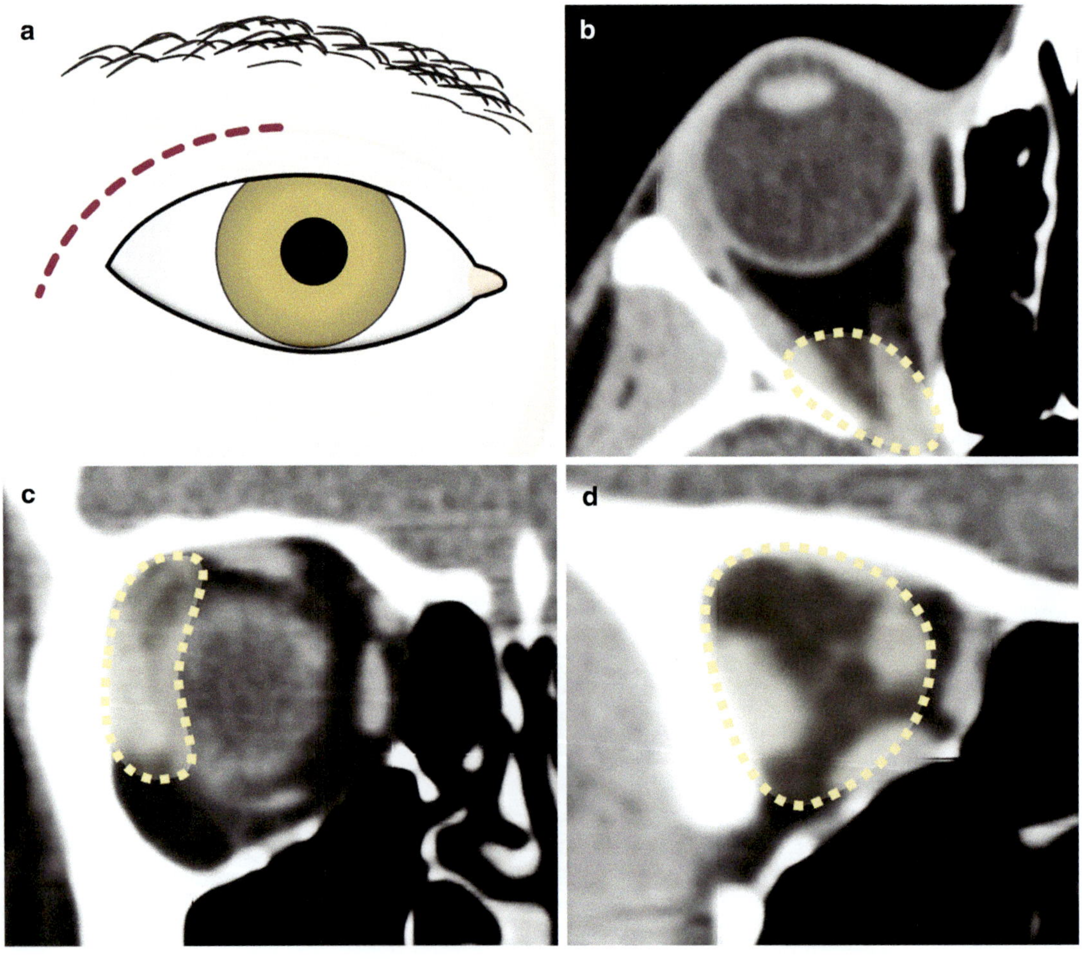

Fig. 4 Lateral orbitotomy with bone mobilisation via a laterally-extended upper lid skin crease incision, and the corresponding surgical fields that may be reached (**a**–**d**)

infero-lateral rhytid, and the orbital rim is exposed. The periosteum is incised widely at about 6–7 mm outside the rim, and the periosteal leaf raised anteriorly, over the orbital rim, and then posteriorly across the lateral orbital wall, taking care to divide any perforating vessels. Two parallel anteroposterior cuts are made through the lateral wall with a high-frequency oscillating saw, the upper cut being at the level of the superficial temporal line and the lower cut just above the level of the zygomatic arch; the temporalis muscle is then incised for 1 cm lateral to these two cuts to provide a "muscle hinge" on which the bone can later be mobilised. A pair of 2 mm drill holes are made into the rim on either side of the osteotomies (to allow later suture fixation of the flap), and the internal face of the lateral wall can also be weakened by "scoring" the bone about 1 cm behind the rim. Whilst protecting the orbital contents with a large retractor, the bone is out-fractured and the remaining jagged posterior edges is trimmed with bone rongeurs, especially backwards to enhance access to the orbital apex; bone wax is applied to the sphenoidal marrow space if there is significant bleeding. The orbital contents can then be accessed by opening the periosteum just behind the arcus marginalis (which is seen as an inflexion in the periosteum) and incising posteriorly towards the orbital apex.

Following surgery, the bone flap is repositioned and held in place with 4/0 absorbable sutures passed through the drill holes, the external leaf of periosteum closed with the same suture, and the skin incision closed with a running 6/0 nylon suture.

5.5 Transconjunctival Retrocaruncular Approach

The retrocaruncular (often inappropriately referred to as 'transcaruncular') approach [8, 9], provides excellent access to the medial orbital wall, ethmoid sinuses, the medial half of the orbital floor, and to masses located medially within the orbit (Fig. 5). This approach is quick, avoids the lacrimal sac, and leaves no visible scar—rendering it far superior to the previously popular Lynch incision. The retrocaruncular approach is particularly valuable where decompression is required for compressive thyroid optic neuropathy.

The medial eyelids are retracted with 2/0 silk sutures, gentle conjunctival diathermy applied to the back edge of the caruncle and continued in an arc about 5 mm superiorly and inferiorly along the fornices, caution being taken to avoid damage to the canaliculi. The conjunctiva is opened along this line (Fig. 5a), and closed scissors are directed 45° postero-medially, behind the posterior lacrimal fascia, to reach the posterior lacrimal crest, with the lacrimal sac protected by an 11 mm malleable retractor and orbital soft tissues gently displaced laterally with a 16 mm malleable retractor. The dissection plane remains intraperiosteal for reaching lesions in the medial orbit while, for access to the medial wall (e.g. medial wall decompression or fracture repair), the extraperiosteal space is entered immediately behind the posterior lacrimal crest (Fig. 5b) and the medial periosteum reflected laterally with a 16 mm malleable retractor to gain access to the orbital apex. The anterior and posterior ethmoidal neurovascular bundles demarcate the upper limit for peeling periosteum from the underlying bone, while the lower limit can be extended to the infraorbital nerve canal. The conjunctival incision is closed with 7/0 absorbable sutures placed at the upper and lower edges of the caruncle.

5.6 Transconjunctival Peritomy Approach

Although conjunctival peritomy has a simple incision and closure, as compared to the larger incision of eyelid approaches it provides only a limited and oblique view of deep orbital structures—often predisposing to inadequately-sized, crushed or non-representative biopsy samples. This approach can still be useful for exploration of masses along-

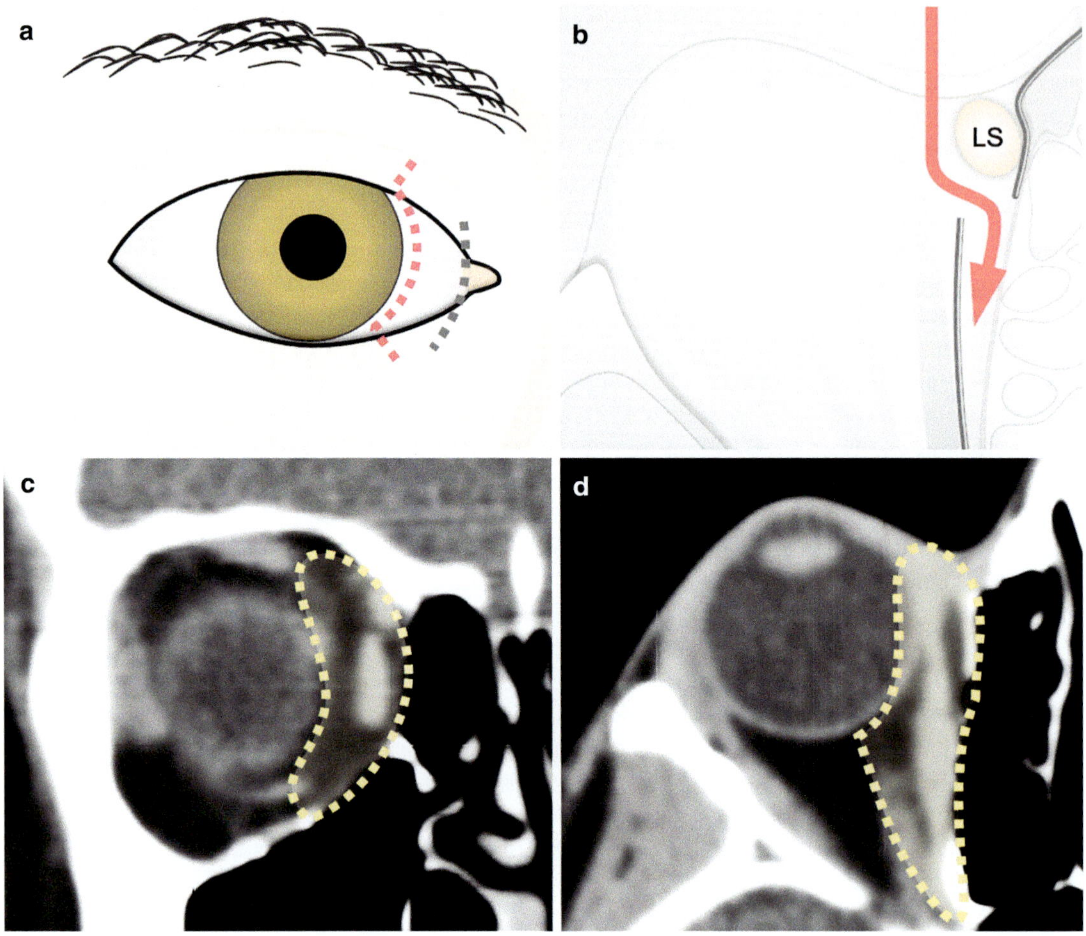

Fig. 5 Transconjunctival retrocaruncular (grey line) and peritomy (pink line) approaches (**a**). (**b**) Retrocaruncular approach to the medial orbital wall, to reach the extraperiosteal space and the ethmoid sinuses, with orbital periosteum opened immediately behind the crest. "LS" denotes lacrimal sac. (**c** and **d**) The regions of the orbit, ethmoidal sinus and maxillary sinus that may be accessed through a retrocaruncular approach

side the globe, with the parabulbar space being reached through a 120–180° conjunctival peritomy with radial relieving incisions (Fig. 5a), and the retrobulbar intraconal space accessed by appropriate fenestration of the posterior Tenon's fascia. Conjunctival closure is achieved with 8/0 absorbable sutures at the limbus.

6 Post-operative Care

After surgery, accumulation of fluid and inflammatory mediators can be reduced by placement of a vacuum drain (typically for 12 h), by padding the operated orbit moderately firmly (for 12–24 h), and by nursing the patient in a semi-recumbent position to reduce orbital venous pressure. Early post-operative instructions should emphasize the importance of seeking medical attention if there is severe and increasing pain, as this may indicate intraorbital arterial haemorrhage; urgent release of any sutured closure and drainage of haemorrhage should be considered where a "rock-hard" proptosis has developed, with mechanical restriction of eye movements and signs of optic neuropathy.

When surgery is performed in the mid-orbit or apex, intra-operative parenteral corticosteroids should be administered (to reduce exudation of inflammatory mediators and provide neuroprotection), followed by a tapering course of oral steroids over 10–14 days to minimize post-operative inflammation. Antibiotics should be given in cases of prolonged surgery, disruption of the paranasal sinuses, or placement of an orbital implant.

Patients are informed that eyelid swelling, ptosis, and diplopia are common after deep orbital surgery and might last for weeks or months. Normal gentle activities can be resumed the day after surgery, but heavy lifting, strenuous activity, and intensive sports should be avoided for 3 weeks. Nose-blowing and flying should be avoided for at least 2 weeks after fracture repairs or decompression of the medial orbital wall or floor.

References

1. Dandy W. Results following the transcranial attack of orbital tumours. Arch Ophthalmol. 1941;25:191–6.
2. Rose GE. The "devil's touch"; visual loss and orbital surgery. A synopsis of the Mustardé lecture, 2006. Orbit. 2007;26:147–58.
3. De Riu G, Meloni SM, Gobbi R, et al. Subciliary versus swinging eyelid approach to the orbital floor. J Craniomaxillofac Surg. 2008;36:439–42.
4. McCord CD Jr, Moses JL. Exposure of the inferior orbit with fornix incision and lateral canthotomy. Ophthalmic Surg. 1979;10:53–63.
5. Hamed-Azzam S, Verity DH, Rose GE. Lateral canthotomy orbitotomy: a rapid approach to the orbit. Eye (Lond). 2018;32:333–7.
6. McNab AA, Wright JE. Lateral orbitotomy–a review. Aust N Z J Ophthalmol. 1990;18:281–6.
7. Harris GJ, Logani SC. Eyelid crease incision for lateral orbitotomy. Ophthal Plast Reconstr Surg. 1999;15:9–16.
8. Shorr N, Bayliss HI, Goldberg RA, et al. Transcaruncular approach to the medial orbit and orbital apex. Ophthalmol. 2000;107:1459–63.
9. Garcia GH, Goldberg RA, Shorr N. The transcaruncular approach in repair of orbital fractures: a retrospective study. J Craniomaxillofac Trauma. 1998;4:7–12.

Fine Needle Aspiration Biopsy in Orbital Disease

Eva Dafgård Kopp and Lelio Baldeschi

Key Messages

- FNAB is a rapid and minimally invasive procedure done during an office visit without anaesthesia and can be used as an initial diagnostic technique.
- When cytology is integrated with clinical and radiographic findings, FNAB can reliably differ neoplastic from non-neoplastic conditions.
- Orbitotomies may be avoided in nonresectable lesions that can be managed with medical therapies or radiotherapy.
- FNAB is particularly helpful to diagnose an orbital recurrence or metastasis diagnose which can be obtained without any surgical intervention.
- Nondiagnostic aspirates may sometimes be obtained, and an inconclusive FNAB should not be ignored if not sufficient information is given, a second FNAB should be considered or an incisional open biopsy.

Orbital masses are multifaceted in nature. Epidemiology, clinical presentation and findings and radiological picture guide the diagnosis by narrowing the case scenario of possible differential diagnosis. Often a biopsy is needed to support or confirm the possible diagnosis.

An open sky biopsy is diagnostically conclusive in 98–99% [1] but the harvesting of the necessary sample requires surgery which, in a delicate context such as the orbital one, can be connected with an elevated degree of morbidity, additionally local anaesthesia is not always an option and many cases need narcosis.

Fine needle aspiration biopsy (FNAB) also named fine needle aspiration cytology (FNAC) being an in-office procedure, which does not require anaesthesia, is a rapid and minimally invasive diagnostic technique, which represent a valid alternative to open sky biopsy in adult patients.

When properly used in well-indicated patients, FNAB of orbital and periorbital lesions is a very useful and convenient adjunct diagnostic technique, but requires close cooperation between the ophthalmologist/orbitologist and cytopathologist and sometimes a radiologist.

E. Dafgård Kopp (✉)
Department of Oculoplastic, Lacrimal and Orbital Surgery, St. Erik Eye Hospital, Karolinska Institutet, Stockholm, Sweden
e-mail: Eva.dafgard-kopp@regionstockholm.se

L. Baldeschi
Department of Ophthalmology, Catholic University of Louvain, Academic Hospital Saint Luc, Brussels, Belgium

F. M. Quaranta Leoni et al. (eds.), *Oculoplastic, Lacrimal and Orbital Surgery*,
https://doi.org/10.1007/978-3-031-39638-0_28

1 Historical Notes

The importance of diagnostic cytology in modern clinical oncology was first introduced by Papanicolau in the late twenties and later further popularised by the same authors in the early "40 of last century". His contributions on exfoliative cytology applied to gynaecological cancerology however are closely linked to observations of around one century before when the peculiar characteristics of tumoural cells were described [2].

Needle biopsy was first proposed by Kun in 1847 [3], applied to breast tumours by Paget and Erichsen around 1850 [4], to the lung in 1882 [5] further developed first by Graig and Gray on lymph nodes at the beginning of last century [6]. In the twenties and thirties of last century FNA was developed to full at Memorial Cancer Center of New York and at the Karolinska Institute of Stockholm, where the possibilities of FNA cytology as well as FNA histology performed with an 18-gauge needle were underscored [4]. Finally, the greatest contribution to modern FNAB was given by Godwin who, in 1964, described most of the cytologic characteristics of the commonest types of cancers [7]. For orbital tumours the technique was first demonstrated by Schyberg in 1975 [8].

FNAB applied to the orbit has its major contribution in a recent study on 225 cases co-authored by one of the authors of the present chapter in which FNAB resulted in effective and exceedingly safe [9].

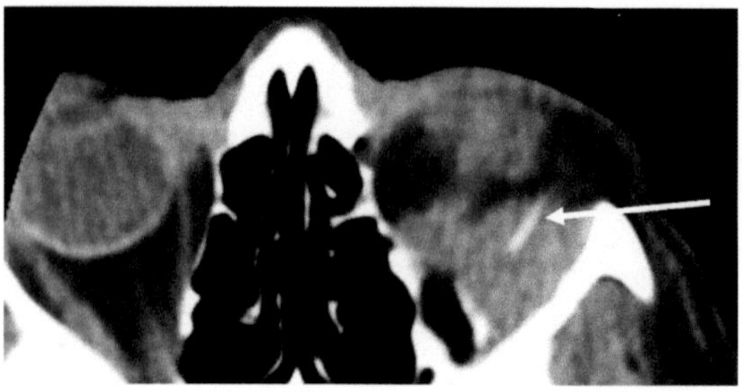

Fig. 1 A CT scan of an 85-year-old patient affected by a Non-Hodgkin's lymphoma of the left orbit: the tumour and the needle used for a FNAB are indicated by the arrow

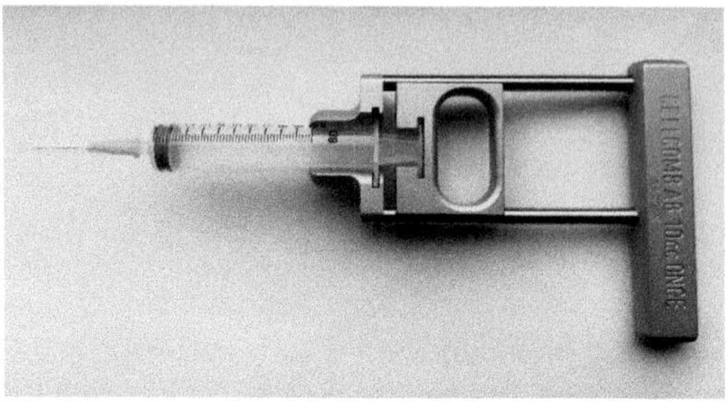

Fig. 2 A Syringe equipped with a needle mounted in a holder pistol. (Courtesy of Edneia Tani, MD)

2 Technique

In adults it is an outpatient procedure and no local anaesthesia or sedation is required. FNAB on superficial and palpable lesions are performed by an ophthalmologist or a cytopathologist while non-palpable more posterior tumours can be better punctured under guided by ultrasounds [10–12] or computerised tomography (CT) imaging together with a radiologist (Fig. 1). Anticoagulant therapy is to be discontinued before the FNAB, the same applies to antiaggregant therapy particularly when dealing with lesions deeply located within the orbit.

Typically a 23-gauge needle (22- to 27-gauge) is attached to a 10 cc syringe mounted in a one-hand grip pistol holder (Fig. 2). The needle is passed into the orbital lesion and the piston is withdrawn, creating a negative pressure within the lumen of the needle. The needle is then moved up and forward in different directions within the tumour. Aspirate pressure is released before the needle is removed. This manoeuvre brings tumour cells and tumour fragments within the needle or occasionally within the syringe. The syringe is detached from the needle and a new syringe loaded with air is connected to the needle to propel possible harvested material onto a glass slide, after this a smear is created for morphological examination following staining with May-Grünwald-Giemsa and immediately examined by the cytopathologist. The remaining material within the needle or the syringe used for the harvesting can be rinsed in phosphate-buffered saline to a cell suspension for additional techniques such as flow cytometry, immunostaining on cytospin preparations and cytogenetic analysis. When the cytology performed on spot fails to detect a sufficient cell sample or when the harvested material is not evaluated to be representative for the suspect lesion FNAB is repeated.

3 Non Conclusive Aspirates

FNAB does not always provide a sufficient number of cells, or the morphology of the harvested cells may be insufficiently preserved to provide adequate material for subsequent examination. Papers published between 1990 and 2016 report that up to 29% of aspirates were inadequate for cytological evaluation. Common reasons are difficult accessibility, as in tumours of the orbital apex [13], or that the cells in the sample resemble normally occurring cells in the orbit, such as in vascular malformations and benign nerve tumours [14, 15]. However, the most common reason is that the sample yields sparse cells, such as in chronic inflammation with fibrosis, and reactive lesions where the aspirates are poorly cellular [9, 10, 13, 15–18].

Depending on the degree of suspicion, when a negative aspirate is obtained (being 'inconclusive', or describing 'normal findings'), a second or even third FNAB can be done. Following the second or third cytologically inconclusive FNAB, and incisional 'opensky' biopsy should be considered if immunocytochemistry and cytometry are also inconclusive [16, 19].

4 Diagnostic Accuracy

The use of immunocytochemistry, flow cytometry, and cytogenetic testing have markedly improved diagnostic accuracy. Earlier studies report a correct diagnosis as low as 70% of orbital FNAB, though more recent data showed a diagnostic certainty of up to 100% [10, 20, 21] if smears are followed by more sophisticated testing procedures.

The outcome of FNAB appears to be dependent on operators and on the harvesting techniques employed. Liu et al. [22] showed that surgeons with experience of performing more than 25 orbital FNAB had a harvesting accuracy ranging from 75 to 100%, whereas surgeons with experience less than 15 FNAB had a range of 0 to 100% success rate. Performing the aspirations with guidance of ultrasound or CT have also increased the diagnostic accuracy [15]. When dealing with orbital neoplasms the success of FNAB is higher with palpable masses (90% success) than with non palpable lesions (75%) and with masses located behind the eyeball the success of FNAB is lower (71%) as compared with more superficially located orbital lesions (87%) [9]. The same study did not show any correlation between success of FNAB and size, quadrant of location, or radiological appearance (diffuse or focal) of orbital lesions.

With FNAB, false negative and false positive smears may rarely occur. Cytologic diagnosis of inflammation have later resulted in histologically proven lymphoma, metastatic breast cancer, mucoepidermoid carcinoma and rhabdomyosarcoma [9, 13, 15, 23].

Conversely, conventional incisional biopsies can also lead to false positive histological diagnoses, with lymphoma and lacrimal gland neoplasia diagnosed in the presence of inflammation alone [9, 16, 24].

These pitfalls stress the importance of a careful interpretation of the aspirates by an experienced pathologist.

5 Clinical Indications

5.1 Lacrimal Gland Lesions

Lacrimal gland tumours can be difficult to diagnose by clinical and radiological features alone. The most common epithelial tumour in the lacrimal gland is pleomorphic adenoma (LGPA). LGPA can present atypically and various other lesions have been reported as mimicking LGPA based on only clinical and radiological criteria [25]. In general, persistent lacrimal gland masses are investigated by incisional biopsy [26]. However, LGPA has typical radiological features, and where these are present, or where there is doubt, complete *intact* excision of the mass should be performed to avoid the risk of seeding adenomatous cells throughout the orbit, each with a risk of subsequent neoplastic transformation [27].

5.2 Lymphoproliferative Lesions

Lymphoproliferative lesions are the most common primary orbital tumours in older adults. They may be secondary or arise primarily in the orbit. Benign reactive lymphoid hyperplasia and low grade malignant lymphoproliferative disorders in the orbit and ocular adnexa are clinically and radiologically indistinguishable from each other.

The presence of a monomorphic population of lymphoid cells generally suggests a lymphoma. The majority of lymphomas are low-grade small cell lymphomas with extranodal marginal zone lymphoma of the mucosa associated lymphoid tissue (MALT) subtype being the most common subtype.

An incisional biopsy has traditionally been the gold standard for the diagnosis for lymphoma, with the use of FNAB for initial diagnosis being controversial. However, the development of sensitive flow cytometry and molecular genetic testing has made it possible to assess clonality in small samples with a diagnostic accuracy of more than 90% [16, 18, 28, 29]. Subclassification rates according to WHO (2008) is reported between 40–60% [30, 31]. Unclassified cases have been diagnosed in two main categories, B cell lymphoma of large cell morphology and small B cell lymphoma.

In recent years, the importance of a biopsy in diagnosing orbital inflammation has been highlighted. FNAB is not recommended in cases of a suspicious orbital inflammation, particularly in sub acute or chronic cases where fibrosis is expected, and for this reason the diagnostic yield from FNAB is low and a histopathological evaluation is to be preferred.

5.3 Cysts

Cystic lesions in the orbit are benign and usually have a typical radiological appearance. In cases where the diagnosis cannot be confirmed on clinical and radiological grounds, a FNAB can be performed, with reasonable possibilities to reach a correct diagnosis.

5.4 Metastases

Of all tumours of the orbit, up to 13% are metastases. In the paediatric population neuroblastoma is the most common orbital metastasis. Ewing sarcomas are the most frequent orbital metastases in adolescents, while in adults breast cancer is the most common type, followed by lung and prostatic cancer. In most patients, the primary cancer is known, but a metastasis to the orbit may be the first sign of a disseminated cancer. Radiologically, the typical finding is a change involving extraocular muscles and bones, but a diffuse growth pattern may also occur. FNAB is particularly helpful in diagnosing an orbital metastasis because a definitive diagnosis can be obtained without additional surgical intervention. Many primary tumours show characteristic immunoreactivity for antigens and the same profile is usually repeated for metastases and further use of a panel of monoclonal antibodies may suggest the origin of an unknown primary tumour (Fig. 3).

A pitfall may be encountered with scirrhous metastatic breast cancer which can be highly fibrotic with scarce if any cellularity, and FNAB can yield results similar to chronic inflammation [9].

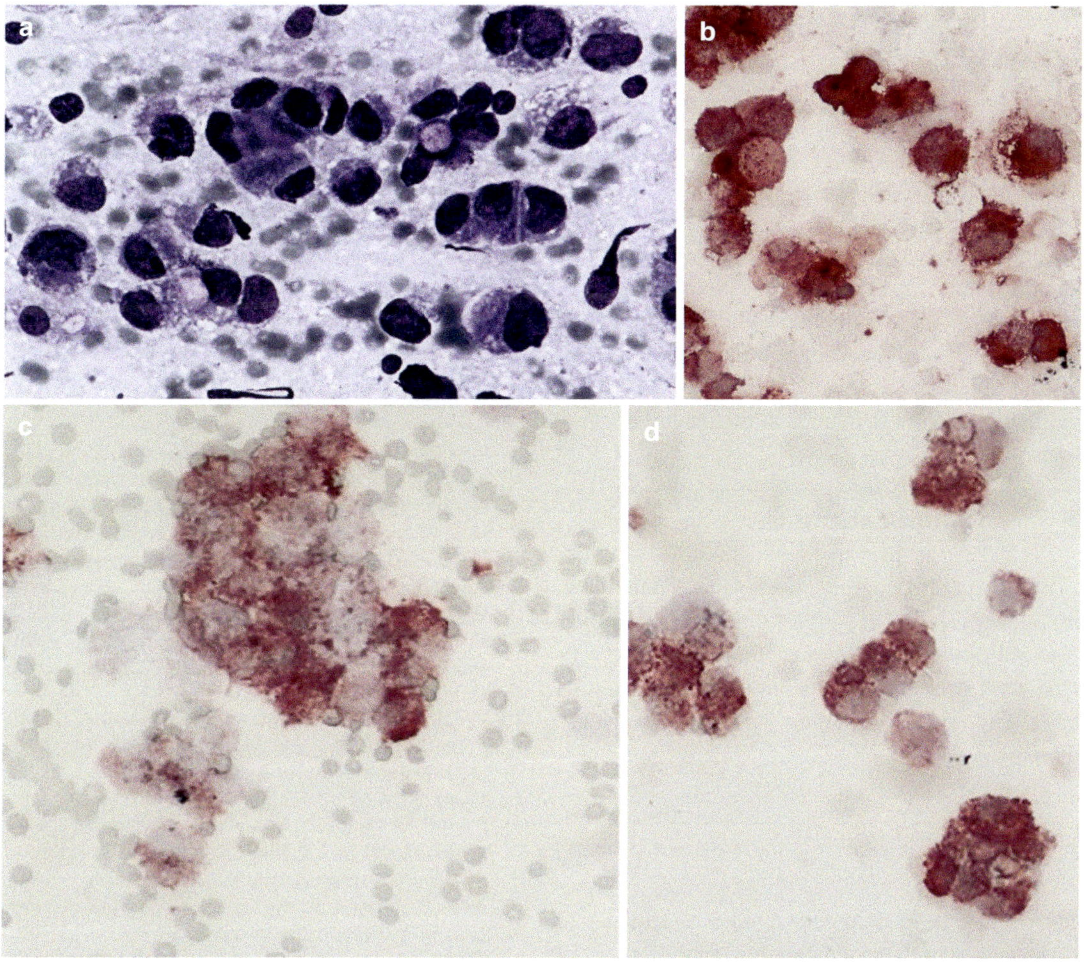

Fig. 3 (**a**–**d**) Smears from an orbital tumour. (**a**) FNAB smear shows loose clusters of tumour cells with eccentric nuclei and some with large cytoplasmic vacuoles (May-Grünwald-Giemsa stain). The tumour cells from FNAB material stained positive for (**b**) CEA, (**c**) cytokeratin 7 and (**d**) cytokeratin 20. This profile is consistent with gastric cancer cells (alkaline phosphatase immunostaining). (Courtesy of Edneia Tani, MD)

5.5 Other Primary Malignant Neoplasms

Cytological examinations are relatively reliable in distinguishing benign from malignant lesions [15]. There are many reports on the usefulness of FNAB in the diagnosis of malignant orbital neoplasms and, in addition to the orbital lesions described above, FNAB may be appropriate as a first diagnostic step in suspecting a primary malignant orbital tumour such as sarcoma and carcinoma, as well as retinoblastoma, melanoma, and leukaemia [32, 33]. However, no radical procedure such as exenteration or tumour excision with large surgical margins should be planned on the basis of FNAB, and an incisional biopsy is required in these cases to confirm the diagnosis.

6 Lesions Not Suitable for FNAB

Some tumours are less suited for FNAB, especially those which consist chiefly of cells that normally appear in the orbit. One of these is cavernous hemangioma, consisting of endothelial cells, fibroblasts, and erythrocytes which could mimic a haemorrhage. Furthermore, a FNAB of a lymphatic or a venous-lymphatic malformation may cause an orbital haemorrhage. Deep posterior lesions should be avoided due to the risk of damaging the delicate structures at the orbital apex.

7 Complications

In earlier reports, complications such as damage to the globe, motility disturbance, ptosis, and infection are described. However, these are now very rare, with small hematomas in the aspiration area or eyelid rarely resulting in any permanent damage.

8 Summary

FNAB can be considered a valid alternative to open biopsy in the evaluation and management of orbital lesions. It requires close cooperation between the ophthalmologist and an experienced cytopathologist. FNAB is a reliable and safe diagnostic technique and is performed as an outpatient procedure. It is of specific value in the diagnosis of lacrimal gland tumours (with the express exception of pleomorphic adenoma), metastases, recurrences, identifying differences between malignant and benign tumours, in deep lymphoproliferative lesions, and granulomatous inflammations. When a non-diagnostic smear is obtained or when the clinical suspicion is in disagreement with the cytological findings, a re-FNAB or an incisional biopsy for histopathological examination should be performed. Finally, FNAB is less useful for apical tumours, vascular malformations, optic nerve tumours, inflammations, and reactive lesions.

References

1. Ting DSJ, Perez-Lopez M, Chew NJ, Clarke L, Dickinson AJ, Neoh C. A 10-year review of orbital biopsy: the newcastle eye Centre study. Eye. 2015;29:1162–6.
2. Grunze SA. History of clinical cytology: a selection of documents. Darmstadt: Viernheim G Verlag Ernst Giebeler; 1980.
3. Kun M. A new instrument for the diagnosis of tumors. Mon J Med Sci. 1847;7:853.
4. Webb AJ. Through a glass darkly (the development oF FNAB). Bristol Med Chir J. 1974;89:59–68.
5. Leyden O. Uber infectiose Pneumonie. Dtsch Med Wochenschr. 1883;9:52–4, Berliner medicinische Gesellschaft.
6. Grieg E, Gray A. Note on lymphatic glands in sleeping sickness. Br Med J. 1904;1:1252.
7. Godwin J. Cytologic diagnosis of aspiration biopsies of solid or cystic tumors. Acta Cytol. 1964;8:206–15.
8. Schyberg E. Fine needle biopsy of orbital tumours. Acta Ophthalmol Suppl. 1975;125:11.
9. Wiktorin ACH, Dafgård Kopp EME, Tani E, Söderén B, Allen RC. Fine-needle aspiration biopsy in orbital lesions: a retrospective study of 225 cases. Am J Ophthalmol. 2016;166:37–42.
10. Pagni F, Jaconi M, Smith AJ, Brenna A, Valente MG, Leoni S, Leni D, Vacirca F, Sozzi D. The role of fine needle aspiration of orbital lesions: a case series. Acta Cytol. 2016;60:31–8.
11. Gupta N, Kaur J, Rajwanshi A, Nijhawan R, Srinivasan R, Dey P, Singh U, Gupta P. Spectrum of orbital and ocular adnexal lesions: an analysis of 389 cases diagnosed by fine needle aspiration cytology. Diagn Cytopathol. 2012;40:582–5.
12. Timmis A, Touska P, Uddin J, Pilcher J. The role of ultrasound-guided tissue sampling techniques in the management of extra-ocular orbital lesions. Ultrasound. 2018;26:145–52.
13. Zeppa P, Tranfa F, Errico ME, Troncone G, Fulciniti F, Vetrani A, Bonavolontà G, Palombini L. Fine needle aspiration (FNA) biopsy of orbital masses: a critical review of 51 cases. Cytopathology. 1997;8:366–72.
14. Agrawal P, Dey P, Saikia UN, Gupta N, Radhika S, Nijhawan R, Rajwanshi A. Fine-needle aspiration cytology of orbital meningiomas. Diagn Cytopathol. 2012;40:967–9.
15. Amoli FA, Tarri AS, Doost KH, Kamalian N, Tabriz HM. Comparison of the results of fine needle aspiration biopsy specimens and permanent histopathologic preparation in orbital mass lesion. Iran J Pathol. 2011;6:124–32.
16. Tani E, Seregard S, Rupp G, Söderlund V, Skoog L. Fine-needle aspiration cytology and immunocytochemistry of orbital masses. Diagn Cytopathol. 2006;34:1–5.

17. Khan L, Malukani K, Malaiya S, Yeshwante P, Ishrat S, Nandedkar SS. Role of fine needle aspiration cytology as a diagnostic tool in orbital and adnexal lesions. J Ophthalmic Vis Res. 2016;11:287–95.
18. Nassar DL, Raab SS, Silverman JF, Kennerdell JS, Sturgis CD. Fine-needle aspiration for the diagnosis of orbital hematolymphoid lesions. Diagn Cytopathol. 2000;23:314–7.
19. Tijl JW, Koornneef L. Fine needle aspiration biopsy in orbital tumours. Br J Ophthalmol. 1991;75:491–2.
20. Rastogi A, Jain S. Fine needle aspiration biopsy in orbital lesions. Orbit. 2001;20:11–23.
21. Solo S, Siddaraju N, Srinivasan R. Use of fine needle cytology in the diagnosis of orbital and eyelid mass lesions. Acta Cytol. 2009;53:41–52.
22. Liu D. Complications of fine needle aspiration biopsy of the orbit. Ophthalmology. 1985;92:1768–71.
23. Char DH, Cole TB, Miller TR. False negative orbital fine needle biopsy. Orbit. 2012;31:194–6.
24. Nair LK, Sankar S. Role of fine needle aspiration cytology in the diagnosis of orbital masses: a study of 41 cases. J Cytol. 2014;31:87–90.
25. Prabhakaran VC, Cannon PS, McNab A, Davis G, O'Donnell B, Dolman PJ, Ghabrial R, Selva D. Lesions mimicking lacrimal gland pleomorphic adenoma. Br J Ophthalmol. 2010;94:1509–12.
26. Lai T, Prabhakaran VC, Malhotra R, Selva D. Pleomorphic adenoma of the lacrimal gland: is there a role for biopsy? Eye. 2009;23:2–6.
27. Kopp ED, Sahlin S, Tani E, Skoog L, Seregard S. Fine-needle aspiration biopsy in lacrimal gland pleomorphic adenoma. Eye. 2010;24:386.
28. Agrawal P, Dey P, Lal A. Fine-needle aspiration cytology of orbital and eyelid lesions. Diagn Cytopathol. 2013;41:1000–11.
29. Stephen N, Manivannan P, Gochhait D, Sreerekha J, Ramasubramanian N, Srinivas BH, Kar R, Kasturi N, Basu D, Siddaraju N. The utility of fine needle aspiration cytology in orbital haematolymphoid neoplasms. Cytopathology. 2021;32:217–26.
30. Jelloul FZ, Navarro M, Navale P, Hagan T, Cocker RS, Das K, Rosen L, Zhang X, Sheikh-Fayyaz S. Diagnosis of lymphoma using fine-needle aspiration biopsy and core-needle biopsy: a single-institution experience. Acta Cytol. 2019;63:198–205.
31. Norin C, Dafgård KE. Fine-needle aspiration biopsy in orbital lymphoma. Abstract ESOPRS Annual Meeting; 2017. p. 314.
32. Kapatia G, Rajasekaran S, Rohilla M, Gupta P, Gupta N, Srinivasan R, Rajwanshi A, Saikia UN, Dey P. Fine-needle aspiration cytology of extra-salivary adenoid cystic carcinoma. Cytopathology. 2020;31:215–22.
33. Siddaraju N, Solo S, Soundararaghavan J, Srinivasan R. Fine needle aspiration biopsy of pleomorphic adenoma and adenoid cystic carcinoma of the lacrimal gland. Acta Cytol. 2008;52:515–7.

Endoscopic Orbital Surgery

Benjamin S. Bleier and Suzanne K. Freitag

Key Messages

- Endoscopic orbital surgery is a rapidly advancing field created from a multidisciplinary collaboration between skilled rhinologic and orbital surgeons that provides a minimally invasive route to management of orbital tumours and other pathology.
- Staging systems have been created to allow for standardised discussion and reporting of orbital tumours with regard to endonasal accessibility and expanding clinical experience has led to a growing body of literature on the topic.
- This broadening experience is likely to translate into safer surgical options with less patient morbidity in the management of orbital tumours.
- Possible complications of endoscopic orbital surgery include standard complications of transnasal endoscopic surgery and orbital surgery. Careful medial rectus retraction is important to reduce the risk of diplopia. However, some patients with pre-operative diplopia due to the orbital mass may experience resolution after surgery.

B. S. Bleier
Department of Otolaryngology, Massachusetts Eye and Ear, Harvard Medical School, Boston, MA, USA

S. K. Freitag (✉)
Ophthalmic Plastic Surgery Service, Department of Ophthalmology, Massachusetts Eye and Ear, Harvard Medical School, Boston, MA, USA
e-mail: Suzanne_Freitag@meei.harvard.edu

1 Introduction

Surgical approaches to the orbit traditionally have included a variety of options depending on the goals of surgery, suspected pathologic diagnosis, size and location of lesion, and surgeon experience and preference. These include transcutaneous, transcaruncular, or transconjunctival orbitotomy, frontotemporal craniotomy with orbito-zygomatic osteotomy, or combinations thereof. Lesions located in the orbital apex have historically posed a particular challenge to surgeons due to the need for deep dissection through the confined space within the bony walls of the orbit, limited illumination, difficulty manoeuvring through orbital fat, the need for meticulous hemostasis, and avoidance of damage to the globe and complex neurovasculature of the orbit.

Endoscopic sinus surgery was developed in the 1980’s, and in the years to follow, advances in technology and technical skill in addition to collaboration with oculoplastic surgeons have allowed for expansion of the field to manage pathology within the orbit. The earliest of these procedures involved endoscopic dacryocystorhinostomy, followed by orbital decompression with removal of bones of the medial wall and orbital floor for relief of compressive optic neuropathy from thyroid-associated orbitopathy (TAO) or expansile lesions within the orbit. The endonasal management of sinonasal tumours with orbital extension led to a proliferation of techniques that has resulted in the use of this approach for purely orbital pathology. Initially this was reserved for medial

F. M. Quaranta Leoni et al. (eds.), *Oculoplastic, Lacrimal and Orbital Surgery*,
https://doi.org/10.1007/978-3-031-39638-0_29

extraconal orbital tumours and foreign bodies, but with expanding experience, much of the extra- and intraconal portions of the orbit may be reached from an endonasal approach with or without transorbital assistance. Stereotactic image guidance systems, which are commonplace in endoscopic sinus surgery, are often utilised in these cases.

The advantages conferred via a transnasal endoscopic approach over traditional orbitotomy routes include higher magnification and brighter illumination of the surgical field, and avoidance of the need for globe retraction and cutaneous incisions. The transnasal endoscopic approach is often the most direct route to pathology within the orbit, primarily traversing the air-filled sinuses rather than the complex intracranial or intraorbital space. Hence, the multidisciplinary collaboration of skilled rhinologic and orbital surgeons has advanced the field to offer minimally invasive surgical options for the management of orbital neoplasms, foreign bodies, and other pathology requiring access to this compact but intricate anatomic area.

2 Anatomy

The orbit is bounded medially and inferiorly by the bones of the sinonasal labyrinth which must be selectively resected to provide endoscopic access to the medial orbital structures. These include the ethmoid bone and its associated ethmoid air cells and lamina papyracea along the medial wall, the maxillary bone forming the orbital floor inferiorly, and the orbital process of the palatine bone which contributes to the posteromedial floor. Each of these bones articulates with the sphenoid bone either through direct suture lines or contiguous soft tissue compartments. The sphenoid bone and its foramina form the posterior and medial boundaries of the orbital apex and optic canal.

The medial extraconal space is defined as the space between the lamina papyracea and the medial rectus muscle. The intraconal compartment is defined as the conical space within the musculofascial cone formed by the extraocular muscles. These muscles insert within the tendinous ring called the annulus of Zinn at the orbital apex. The intraconal space contains the ophthalmic artery, cranial nerves II, III, V1 branches and VI as well as orbital fat. The extraconal space contains the lacrimal gland and sac, a portion of the superior ophthalmic vein, the lacrimal and frontal branches of cranial nerve V1, cranial nerve IV as well as fat. The superior rectus and levator muscles are innervated by the superior division of CN III (oculomotor nerve). The inferior rectus, medial rectus, and inferior oblique muscles are innervated by the inferior division of CN III. The lateral rectus is innervated by CN VI (abducens nerve), while CN IV innervates the superior oblique muscle. The cranial nerves to the rectus muscles enter the orbit posteriorly through the superior orbital fissure.

The medial rectus muscle functions as the doorway to the intraconal space from an endoscopic perspective [1, 2]. Variability of the neurovascular supply to the medial rectus muscle is the rule. A mean of 1.5 arterial branches derived from the inferomedial muscular trunk of the ophthalmic artery insert on the lateral aspect of the muscle at a mean of 8.8 mm from the sphenoid face. The oculomotor nerve segment to the medial rectus contains a large proximal trunk 5.5 ± 1.1 mm in length which then arborizes 13.2 ± 2.7 mm from the sphenoid face to diffusely innervate the muscle. The most anterior neurovascular pedicle extends anteriorly 17 mm (nerve) and 15 mm (artery), respectively. These general branching patterns of the inferior division of the oculomotor nerve and inferomedial muscular trunk of the ophthalmic artery enable a conceptualization of the medial intraconal space into two broad compartments, one anterior to the inferomedial muscular trunk takeoff and one posterior to this. Within the posterior compartment, all of the neurovascular structures critical to proper visual function coalesce within millimetres of one another making this space the most challenging to work within [1].

3 Staging Systems

This compartmental approach has recently led to the iteration of several endoscopic orbital tumour staging systems which have been designed to enable standardised, prospective, outcome reporting across institutions. The original CHEER (Cavernous Hemangioma Exclusively Endoscopic Resection) staging system [2, 3] has recently been revised to a more comprehensive ORBIT (Orbital Resection by Intranasal Technique) system which incorporates outcomes for all primary tumours of the orbit and permits both exclusively endoscopic and combined transorbital-transnasal resection. The stages of the ORBIT system are as follows: I—Extraconal; II- Intraconal and anterior to the inferomedial muscular trunk of the ophthalmic artery; III—Intraconal and posterior to the inferomedial muscular trunk of the ophthalmic artery with/without extension into the optic canal; IV-Any lesion with extra-orbital extension into the pterygopalatine/infratemporal fossa; and V—Any lesion with extra-orbital extension into the intracranial space (Fig. 1).

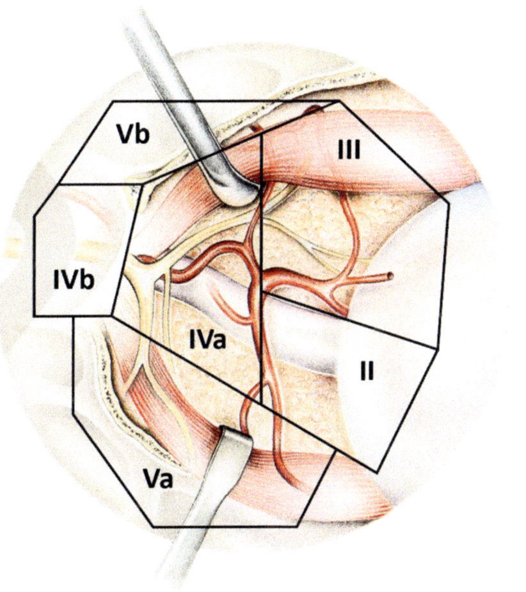

Fig. 1 Schematic of compartments associated with the CHEER staging system. Stage I (e.g. extraconal) lesions are not depicted

4 Indications

A variety of orbital conditions are amenable to an endonasal surgical approach. Neoplasms located in the ORBIT classification regions I to V are suitable for endoscopic diagnostic incisional biopsy or subtotal or total excision. Careful review of pre-operative imaging allow surgeons to determine the most likely aetiology of orbital lesions, in order to avoid unintentional incision of a vascular or lymphatic malformation, optic nerve associated neoplasm, or other pathology which could lead to uncontrolled haemorrhage or visual loss. Cavernous hemangiomas, now sometimes referred to as low-flow venous malformations, are the most common primary orbital neoplasm and are usually minimally adherent to surrounding structures. Surgeons new to this approach may therefore wish to consider attempting removal of cavernous hemangiomas during the steep, early learning-curve of this technique. Common medial orbital lesions that are slightly more adherent include solitary fibrous tumours. Orbital schwannomas are often much more adherent and when tumours such as this are suspected pre-operatively, preparation should be made for a possible combined transorbital approach to assist dissection from the lateral side.

Non-organic foreign bodies of the orbit are often observed, however if it is determined that foreign body removal is required, this may be performed endoscopically in the same areas as are suitable for neoplasms. This situation may arise if a patient requires magnetic resonance imaging for another medical condition or if the presence of the foreign body is affecting the vision by causing gaze-evoked amaurosis or optic neuropathy.

This endonasal approach may also be used for orbital decompression to relieve compressive optic neuropathy due to TAO or a neoplasm exerting pressure on the optic nerve. This is reserved for neoplasms known to be benign, as opening the orbit to allow spillage of malignant cells into the sinus cavity is contraindicated.

5 Patient Selection

All patients presenting with an orbital tumour potentially amenable for endoscopic resection require evaluation by a multidisciplinary team including an oculoplastic surgeon, otolaryngologist, and if necessary, a neurosurgeon. The multidisciplinary team should have experience working together and discuss preferred approach, goals of surgery, anticipated outcomes, and potential for complications. All patients should obtain a complete ophthalmological examination including formal visual field testing and exophthalmometry measurements. Neurosurgical consultation should be obtained when there is concern for intracranial extension or the potential need for a transcranial superior approach.

A high resolution, non-contrast, computed tomography (CT) scan should be performed to assess the bony anatomy while neurovascular structures and lesion flow and enhancement characteristics should be assessed with magnetic resonance imaging (MRI). If the inter-relationship of the optic nerve and tumour remains unclear on tri-planar imaging, three dimensional (3D) reconstruction can be very helpful while providing an estimate of the tumour volume and morphology. 3D reconstruction may also help to determine the "plane of resectability" which predicts the tumour volume lateral, yet inferior, to the optic nerve that may still be resectable by a primary endoscopic approach via the contralateral trajectory afforded by a binarial approach (Fig. 2a, b).

Angiography may be considered in vascular lesions or if an ophthalmic artery aneurysm is suspected, however it is generally not universally required.

In patients with lesions extending anterior to the meridian of the globe or above the plane of resectability, an exclusively endoscopic approach is contraindicated and alternative primary or combination approaches should be considered.

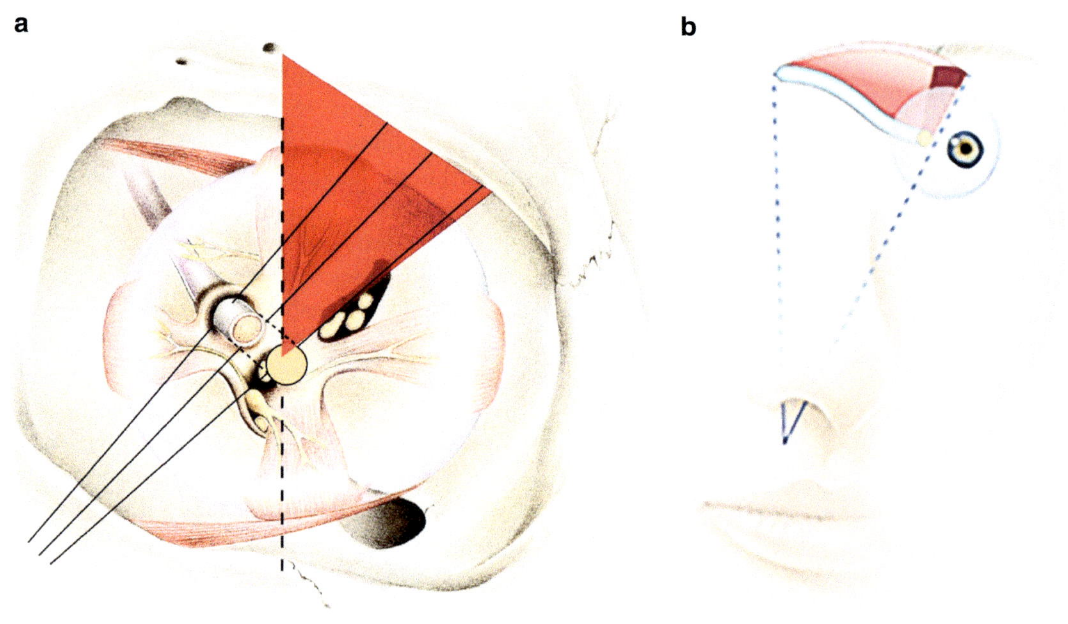

Fig. 2 (**a**) Coronal illustration of the orbit with the three solid lines demonstrating the plane of resectability (POR). Lesions superior and lateral to this plane cannot be resected using an exclusively endoscopic approach. (**b**) Facial view demonstrating the concept of the POR where the orbital approach from the contralateral nare enables dissection within the inferolateral orbit without requiring direct optic nerve retraction

6 Surgical Technique

6.1 Sinus Surgery

The first step in an endoscopic orbital approach is endoscopic sinus surgery to gain access to the medial and/or inferior orbit and optic canal. Optimization of hemostasis is critical and includes head elevation and topicalization using 1:1000 fluorescein labelled epinephrine soaked neuro-patties. Local anaesthetic may also be injected to target the anterior ethmoid vascular bed. The initial surgery may be performed with a 0° endoscope. The uncinate process is resected at its insertion on the maxillary line. Unlike in traditional endoscopic sinus surgery, the superior insertion of the uncinate process is left in place to protect the frontal recess from secondary obstruction by orbital fat.

The maxillary sinus should be opened in all cases to prevent iatrogenic maxillary obstruction. The ethmoid bulla, vertical basal lamella, and posterior ethmoid cells are removed completely. It is important to extend the dissection to the entire skull base. A wide opening of the sphenoid sinus and a partial resection of the superior turbinate should be performed to identify the lateral sphenoid wall structures including the optic canal, carotid protuberance, and optico-carotid recess. A concurrent septoplasty may be performed as needed. Middle turbinate resection should only be performed when necessary as removal carries the risk of olfactory disruption, frontal sinus obstruction, and post-operative epistaxis.

6.2 Medial Orbital Decompression

The mucosa may be stripped from the lamina papyracea to the lateral skull base to avoid post-operative mucocele formation. The resection of the lamina papyracea may be performed by creating a fracture and then removing the thin bony fragments with a blakesley forceps or a ball tipped probe. The sphenoid suture line may be identified as the transition of the thinner lamina papyracea to the thicker sphenoid bone. Care should be taken not to injure the anterior and posterior ethmoid arteries as the laminectomy is carried superiorly to the skull base.

6.3 Orbital Process Palatine Bone

The orbital process of the palatine bone restricts inferomedial orbital access and inferolateral retraction. When this access is required, the orbital process may be isolated and resected. The superior maxillary sinus mucosa should be reflected laterally before bone resection and may be redraped afterwards [4]. The thick process may be thinned under direct visualisation using a high-speed drill. Down-fracturing of the residual bone in an anterior-inferior vector enables resection while avoiding injury to the sphenopalatine neurovascular bundle and infraorbital nerve [5].

6.4 Management of the Septum

Employment of a 4-handed approach requires binarial access which, in turn, necessitates the creation of transeptal access. For lesions of the posterior orbit this may be achieved through a simple posterior septectomy. For lesions in the mid to anterior orbit, a transeptal approach is favoured. This approach begins with a hemi-transfixion incision on the side contralateral to the lesion. The mucosa is then elevated in a submucoperichondrial plane and the quandrangular cartilage is resected while preserving at least a 1 cm caudal and dorsal strut. The contralateral mucosa may then either be opened using a horizontal incision or fully removed in the form of a vascularized nasoseptal flap which can be stored in the nasopharynx and used to reconstruct the medial orbital wall. At the conclusion of the surgery, the hemi-transfixion incision can be closed thereby avoiding the development of a septal perforation (Fig. 3).

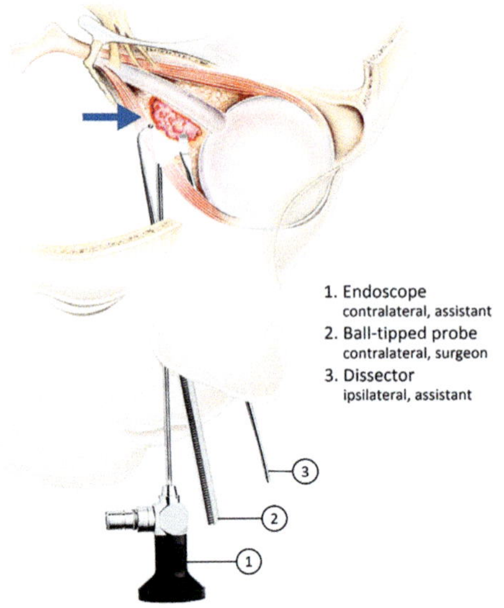

Fig. 3 Illustration of instrument and endoscope placement during a binarial approach to a left intraconal lesion

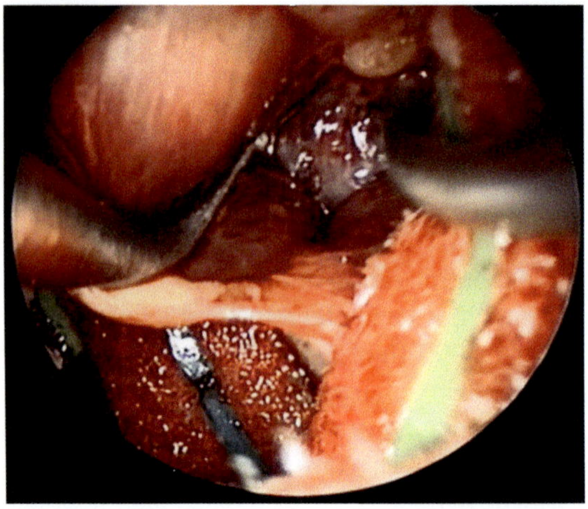

Fig. 4 Endoscopic view demonstrating a three handed approach to a left CHEER Stage IVa lesion where a ball-tipped probe is used to retract the medial rectus while a Penfield dissector over a saline soaked neuropattie is used to expose the tumor capsule

7 Medial Rectus Retraction

The medial rectus muscle is the principal structure restricting endoscopic access to the intraconal space, and must be meticulously preserved in a functional manner. Several retraction techniques have been described in the literature. These include retraction at the globe insertion point using a vessel loop, static trans-septal and retro-choanal retraction, and dynamic four-handed trans-septal retraction using an instrument such as a ball tipped probe or penfield dissector [6–9]. The four-handed transseptal approach with medial rectus muscle retraction allows for greatest intraconal space exposure while ensuring protection of the neuromuscular inputs to the medial rectus [8]. Depending on the location of the tumour, retraction may be carried out inferiorly or superiorly. Prolonged medial rectus retraction should be avoided in order to prevent neurovascular traction injury and allow perfusion of the muscle [9].

8 Dissection Technique

Dissection of the intra-or extraconal tumour may be performed using blunt instruments such as the ball-tipped probe and angled penfield dissector. The capsule of the tumour should be identified and carefully followed. The suction may be used as a second dissecting instrument and is applied over a saline-soaked neuro-pattie. The great advantage of this technique is the simultaneous dissection and optimization of vision due to control of blood pooling. The four-handed approach enables bimanual dissection while providing good visualisation with the endoscope. Depending on the location of the tumour, 0° or angled scopes may be used. An angled scope may be more useful for more anterior and lateral lesions (Fig. 4).

For tumours that are minimally adherent, such as cavernous hemangiomas, it may be possible to free the majority of the tumour from surrounding structures from a purely endonasal approach. When this has been accomplished, the tumour can be grasped with a Blakesley or cupped forceps and gentle tractional force is exerted to deliver the mass into the ethmoid sinus and then out through the naris. When the mass has poorly defined borders, is adherent to surrounding structures, or extends superior to the frontoethmoidal suture line or anterior to the insertion of the optic nerve on the globe, it is prudent to consider a combined transorbital approach. This is often accomplished via a minimally invasive transcaruncular incision. A Westcott scissors is used to incise along the pos-

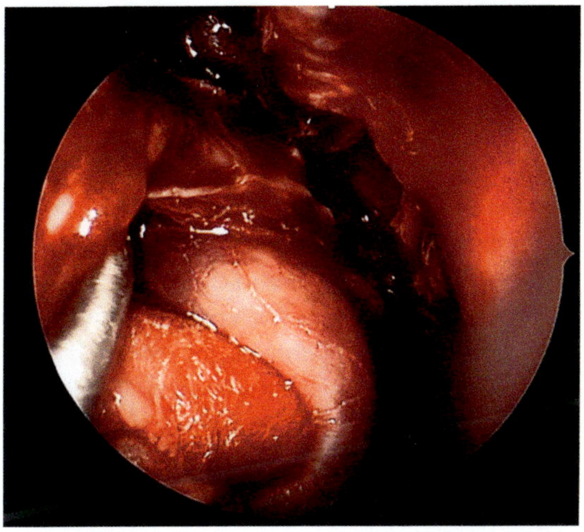

Fig. 5 Endoscopic view of a combined transnasal/transcaruncular approach to a right orbital schwannoma. In this image, the anterior edge of the schwannoma is being delivered into the nose via the transcaruncular approach using a cotton-tipped applicator

terior aspect of the caruncle. A Stevens scissors carefully identifies the posterior lacrimal crest which delineates the anterior border of dissection along the medial wall of the orbit. The tumour is visually identified via this approach and dissection can be carried out along its lateral aspect. The opening in the medial orbital wall created endonasally allows for medial displacement of the tumour, creating additional intraorbital space for dissection and manipulation of the lateral aspect of the tumour. At this point, both surgeons working simultaneously through the nose and orbit can develop a strategy to complete dissection of the tumour and deliver it (Fig. 5).

9 Orbital Fat Management

One of the most challenging aspects of orbital surgery is manoeuvring through the orbital fat. Fat obstructs visualisation and when retracted often slips into a new position necessitating a different angle of retraction, creating a continuous need for creative manipulation. This is particularly challenging from an endoscopic approach, because the orbital fat prolapses into the sinus, obstructing endoscopic visualisation. Orbital fat should not be excised in these cases, nor should it be cauterised for shrinkage, as this further decreases the volume of the orbital contents, and risks damage to delicate surrounding structures. Orbital fat may be retracted endonasally with saline-soaked neuropatties, which both maintain a dissection plane and absorb blood. Suctioning through the neuropatties can provide an effective barrier to orbital fat becoming incarcerated in the suction tip.

10 Haemostasis

Hemostasis represents a particular challenge within the orbit for a variety of reasons. The proximity of the optic nerve and other critical neurovascular structures limits use of cautery to judicious use of bipolar on low settings. Similarly, vasoconstrictive agents are contraindicated following opening of the periorbita for fear of inducing ophthalmic arterial vasospasm and retinal ischemia. Finally, absorbable hemostatic materials carry the concern of intraconal scarring and extraocular muscle dysfunction. As a result of these limitations, hemostasis should be maintained by adequate head elevation, anaesthetic regulation of cardiac output, and cool saline irrigation, as well as pre-operative avoidance of anticoagulants. Fortunately, the surgical communication of the orbit to the intranasal cavity provides a pathway for blood egress thereby limiting the risk of retrobulbar hematoma and orbital compartment syndrome. For this reason, non-absorbable nasal packing should be avoided following any orbital procedure and, if necessary, should never place direct pressure on the medial orbital wall.

11 Management of Medial Orbital Wall

Endoscopic approaches to the orbit necessarily violate the medial orbital wall, expose intraorbital fat, induce muscular oedema, bleeding, and fluid transudation. Furthermore, these approaches result in a significant reduction in orbital volume following tumour removal. As a result, patients are at risk of enophthalmos with its attendant risks of diplopia and poor cosmetic outcome. Consequently, immediate medial and inferior orbital reconstruction is advocated, particularly for intraconal tumours at the mid and anterior orbit. A nasoseptal flap, pedicled on the posterior septal artery, has been shown to be capable of providing complete coverage of the entire medial and inferior orbit [10, 11]. The flap may be raised using a needle-tipped Bovie and Cottle elevator, may be carried out as far anteriorly as needed, and can be incorporated into the trans-septal approach [12]. This technique has the advantage of providing a "delayed" or soft reconstruction as the flap contracts around the orbitotomy. This provides for immediate blood egress and resolution of oedema while avoiding the development of an orbital compartment syndrome which could occur with immediate rigid reconstruction. Gelfoam or tissue glues may be considered on the nasal surface of the flap to provide support and minimise the risk of flap migration during healing. Delayed reconstruction of the orbital walls may also be undertaken if needed to improve globe malposition utilising a variety of rigid materials commonly used for orbital fracture repair, including porous polyethylene sheets or titanium mesh.

12 Orbital Decompression

Decompression of the medial orbital wall and floor may also be performed endonasally. The patient is placed under general anaesthesia and supine in a reverse Trendelenburg position. The entire surgery may be performed with a 0° endoscope however angled scopes are useful in the setting of inferomedial strut preservation and assessing completeness of the lateral floor resection. Septoplasty or middle turbinate resection may be performed as needed. Middle turbinate resection should only be performed when it limits the decompression as it may confer an increased risk of olfactory disruption, remnant lateralization with frontal sinus obstruction and post-operative epistaxis.

A standard sphenoid-ethmoidectomy should be performed first. It is crucial to dissect the entire skull base to ensure maximal space for decompression. The mucosa along the lamina and lateral skull base may be stripped to avoid possible mucocele formation. For medial orbital decompression, the lamina papyracea should be cleaned of all adjacent ethmoid air cells. A curette may be used to fracture the lamina medially. The posterior limit of the lamina is the sphenoid bone. This suture line can be easily identified as the bone becomes much thicker. Early uncontrolled penetration of the periorbita should be avoided at first as herniated orbital fat may obscure visualisation of the surgical field.

The orbital floor may also be removed for additional inferior decompression. A maxillary antrostomy with bone removal from the natural ostium to the posterior maxillary wall should be performed with a 0° endoscope. The superior maxillary sinus mucosa may be reflected laterally prior to bone removal to assist in post-operative re-mucosalisation. The floor may then be down-fractured by using a spoon curette which generally travels laterally to the level of the infraorbital canal in a single fragment. Preserving the inferomedial strut has been described a successful and safe procedure in patients without prior diplopia to minimise post-operative double vision [13–16]. In this case, a 4-mm high-speed tapered 70° diamond burr is used to thin the bone from the lateral edge of the inferomedial strut to the medial border of the infraorbital canal. A double ball probe can be used to fracture the thinned bone away from the periorbita. Further bone may be removed using a frontal sinus through-biting punches.

The next step in decompression is performing the periorbital incision. Depending on the desired degree of decompression, the extent of the periorbital incision can vary. To limit diplopia rates, a strip of periorbita may be left over the medial rectus muscle [17]. After incision of the periorbita, the fat will typically decompress into the nasal cavity. However, multiple fascial bands will often remain and the fat should be feathered medially with a blunt instrument, under gentle tonic pressure on the globe. After sufficient decompression, the preserved maxillary sinus mucosa should be laid back gently.

13 Post-operative Considerations

Placement of an eye patch at the end of any surgery involving the orbit is not recommended, as prompt identification of orbital haemorrhage by the patient noticing visual changes or an observer identifying significant eyelid oedema and ecchymosis is critical to allow for rapid intervention to avoid permanent visual loss. If an orbital haemorrhage occurs, the instinct to hold pressure on the orbit should be avoided, as this will allow for a dangerous elevation of intraorbital pressure which can lead to central retinal artery occlusion and irreversible blindness. Instead, the orbit should be opened via the previous incisions to allow for egress of blood. Consideration should also be given to performing lateral canthotomy and inferior cantholysis to allow for decompression.

Upon awakening in the recovery room, patients should be examined including assessment of visual acuity, colour vision, pupillary size and reaction, extraocular motility, and intraocular pressure. The orbit should be palpated and visually evaluated for evidence of elevated pressure or retrobulbar haemorrhage and the nose evaluated for epistaxis. Consideration should be given to prescribing oral antibiotics for 5 to 7 days. Oral corticosteroid can help to reduce orbital oedema and is recommended in a tapered dosing for 1 to 2 weeks post-operatively. Patients should be instructed to avoid nose blowing to decrease the risk of forcing air into the orbit via the sinuses.

14 Outcomes

Surgical outcomes for both purely endonasal procedures and procedures combined with orbitotomy assistance have demonstrated very good results with regard to effectiveness of achieving surgical goals as well as safety and minimising complications. Cavernous hemangiomas, because of their usual lack of adhesion to surrounding structures, can be expected to be amenable to complete excision in the majority of cases. A systematic review of 39 articles describing this endoscopic technique by Dubal et al. reported that complete tumour resection was possible in 73 to 100% of intraconal cases and in almost all extraconal cases [18]. More adherent tumours that are inseparable from the extraocular muscles and deep orbital neurovasculature may be less amenable to complete excision, and pre-operative examination and review of imaging as well as intra-operative judgement should dictate when subtotal excision should be considered. Bleier et al. reported that intraconal lesions are more likely to be incompletely resected and have a higher incidence of post-operative enophthalmos and diplopia compared with extraconal lesions [19]. This is likely a result of the larger medial wall exposure and increased surgical time and manipulation of the medial rectus required in such cases.

15 Complications

Possible complications of these procedures include standard complications of transnasal endoscopic surgery and orbital surgery, including: epistaxis, cerebrospinal fluid leak, obstructive sinusitis, trigeminal hypesthesia, orbital haemorrhage, damage to optic nerve or globe, enophthalmos, and diplopia. Diplopia may be transient or permanent, and is often very debilitating. Attention to careful medial rectus retraction is important to reduce the risk of this complication. However, some patients with pre-operative diplopia due to mass effect from an orbital lesion may experience resolution of diplopia after surgery.

References

1. Bleier BS, Healy DYJ, Chhabra N, Freitag S. Compartmental endoscopic surgical anatomy of the medial intraconal orbital space. Int Forum Allergy Rhinol. 2014;4:587–91.
2. Jafari A, von Sneidern M, Lehmann AE, Shen SA, Shishido S, Freitag SK, Bleier BS. Exclusively endo-

scopic endonasal resection of benign orbital tumors: a systematic review and meta-analysis. Int Forum Allergy Rhinol. 2021;11:924–34.
3. El Rassi E, Adappa ND, Battaglia P, Castelnuovo P, Dallan I, Freitag SK, Gardner PA, Lenzi R, Lubbe D, Metson R, Moe KS, Muscatello L, Mustak H, Nogueira JF, Palmer JN, Prepageran N, Ramakirshnan VR, Sacks R, Snyderman CH, Stefko ST, Turri-Zanoni M, Wang EW, Zhou B, Bleier BS. Development of the international orbital Cavernous Hemangioma Exclusively Endonasal Resection (CHEER) staging system. Int Forum Allergy Rhinol. 2019;9:804–12.
4. Palmer N, Chiu A. Atlas of endoscopic sinus and skull base surgery. 1st ed. Philadelphia, PA: Elsevier; 2013. p. 255.
5. Mueller S, Freitag S, Bleier B. Morphometric analysis of the orbital process of the palatine bone and its relationship to endoscopic orbital apex surgery. Ophthal Plast Reconstr Surg. 2018;34:254.
6. Lenzi R, Bleier B, Felisati G, Muscatello L. Purely endoscopic trans-nasal management of orbital intraconal cavernous haemangiomas: a systematic review of the literature. Eur Arch Otorhinolaryngol. 2016;273:2319–22.
7. Yao W, Bleier B. Endoscopic management of orbital tumors. Curr Opin Otolaryngol Head Neck Surg. 2016;24:57–62.
8. Lin G, Freitag S, Kocharyan A, Yoon M, Lefebvre D, Bleier B. Comparative techniques of medial rectus muscle retraction for endoscopic exposure of the medial intraconal space. Am J Rhinol Allergy. 2016;30:226–9.
9. Shafi F, Zaidi S, Mehta P, Ahluwalia H, Ahmed S. Endoscopic medial rectus sling: a window into the intraconal orbital apex. Ophthal Plast Reconstr Surg. 2016;32:233–6.
10. Chhabra N, Healy D, Freitag S, Bleier B. The nasoseptal flap for reconstruction of the medial and inferior orbit. Int Forum Allergy Rhinol. 2014;4:763–6.
11. Healy DJ, Lee N, Freitag S, Bleier B. Endoscopic bimanual approach to an intraconal cavernous hemangioma of the orbital apex with vascularized flap reconstruction. Ophthal Plast Reconstr Surg. 2014;30:e104–6.
12. Hadad G, Bassagasteguy L, Carrau R, Mataza J, Kassam A, Snyderman C, et al. A novel reconstructive technique after endoscopic expanded endonasal approaches: vascular pedicle nasoseptal flap. Laryngoscope. 2006;116:1882–6.
13. Bleier B, Lefebvre D, Freitag S. Endoscopic orbital floor decompression with preservation of the inferomedial strut. Int Forum Allergy Rhinol. 2014;4:82–4.
14. Goldberg R, Shorr N, Cohen M. The medial orbital strut in the prevention of post decompression dystopia in dysthyroid ophthalmopathy. Ophthal Plast Reconstr Surg. 1992;8:32–4.
15. Wright ED, Davidson J, Codere F, Desrosiers M. Endoscopic orbital decompression with preservation of an inferomedial bony strut: minimization of postoperative diplopia. J Otolayrngol. 1999;28:252–6.
16. Finn A, Bleier B, Cestari D, Kazlas M, Dagi L, Lefebvre D, Yoon M, Freitag S. A retrospective review of orbital decompression for thyroid orbitopathy with endoscopic preservation of the interfomedial orbital strut. Ophthal Plast Reconstr Surg. 2017;33:334–9.
17. Metson R, Samaha M. Reduction of diplopia following endoscopic orbital decompression: the orbital sling technique. Laryngoscope. 2002;112:1753–7.
18. Dubal PM, Svider PF, Denis D, Folbe AJ, Eljoy JA. Short-term outcomes of purley endoscopic endonasal resection of orbital tumors: a systematic review. Int Forum Allergy Rhinol. 2014;4:1008–15.
19. Bleier B, Castelnuovo P, Battaglia P, Turri-Zanoni M, Dallan I, Metson R, et al. Endoscopic endonasal orbital cavernous hemangioma resection: global experience in techniques and outcomes. Int Forum Allergy Rhinol. 2016;6:156–61.

Navigation in Orbital Surgery

Cornelia Caron, Maarten Koudstaal,
Dion Paridaens, and Eppo Wolvius

Key Messages

- Navigation enables real-time localization of instruments during surgery, which is of great importance when operating in the orbital apex and close proximity to the optic nerve.
- Regardless of the indication, use of navigation reduces the risk for trauma to surrounding structures and reduces the risk for perioperative morbidity, which leads to a reduction in the number of revision procedures.
- Accurate target location by correct pre-operative planning in combination with navigation makes it possible to operate through cosmetically acceptable incisions and define the most ideal surgical approach. This leads to more impressive and individualised surgery with better outcomes.

C. Caron · M. Koudstaal · E. Wolvius
Orbital Center, Department of Maxillofacial Surgery, Erasmus MC, Rotterdam, The Netherlands

D. Paridaens (✉)
Department of Oculoplastic, Orbital and Lacrimal Surgery, The Rotterdam Eye Hospital and Erasmus Medical Center, Rotterdam, The Netherlands
e-mail: a.paridaens@erasmusmc.nl; d.paridaens@oogziekenhuis.nl

1 History

Navigation finds its basis in stereotactic surgery, a technique dating back to the early 1900s, and was initially used for neurosurgical and psychiatric procedures in the late 1940s and early 1950s [1–5]. It was designed accurately to insert a wire or cannula into a desired anatomical area in the skull with minimal injury to surrounding structures [4]. This conventional stereotactic system required a rigid, localization frame to be secured to the skull to provide reference points for targeting via an X, Y, Z-axes coordinate system. Development of technologies such as Computed Tomography (CT) and Magnetic Resonance Imaging (MRI), and increasing capabilities of computer technologies enlarged the anatomical field in which the technique could be used and with that also enlarged the field of indications.

Frame-based stereotaxy was the standard method for accurately localising small intracranial lesions until the end of the 1980s, later these systems were replaced by frameless systems. Frameless and computer-aided navigation systems enable real time visualisation of the position of an instrument in the corresponding images. This can be achieved without the need for a stereotactic localization frame and is very useful when performing a procedure where one cannot see the tip of the instrument. One of the first frameless navigation systems used a pointer emitting ultrasound sources [6]. Later, magnetic sources and infrared light-emitting diodes (LED) were described [7, 8].

F. M. Quaranta Leoni et al. (eds.), *Oculoplastic, Lacrimal and Orbital Surgery*,
https://doi.org/10.1007/978-3-031-39638-0_30

The accuracy of today's navigation systems is approximately 2 mm, but is highly dependent on setup and the quality of imaging.

Frameless navigation systems allow for more flexibility for the surgeon, increasing the indications beyond the borders of neurosurgery. With its aesthetic importance, tightly enclosed muscular and neurovascular structures, and thin walls, the orbit can be a challenging operation site and it was thought that orbital surgeons might benefit from navigation. Use of navigation in surgical procedures of the orbit was firstly described in 2001 by Camara et al. [9], whilst the use of frameless navigation in orbital surgery was first described in 2006 by N. Hejazi [10].

2 Frameless Navigation

Frameless navigation can be categorized into four types.

2.1 Articulated Arm Systems

Articulated arm systems are a descendant of the early tethered arm systems and the first widely used navigation tool. An articulated arm with position sensors in several joints is clamped to the operating table. The position of each joint is known, allowing the computer to calculate the arm configuration and thus the tip location in space relative to its base. The arm tip is then used to mark certain points on the patient's head. In addition, the same points are selected on the preoperative images displayed on the computer screen allowing for the computer to determine the 3D head position and the anatomical points to that region. This way of localising positions in 3D-space has proven to be accurate, but limits the degrees of freedom for surgeons [11–13].

2.2 Acoustical Systems

Acoustical systems use ultrasound emitting electrodes and microphones as detectors to localise a pointer or microscope by repeatedly measuring the transit times of ultrasonic sounds travelling between the electrodes on the microscope or instrument and microphones attached to a reference frame. Use of at least three ultrasound emitting electrodes and three microphones enables unique determination of the position of the microscope or instrument. Use of the system is influenced by air temperature, humidity and turbulence, but also by ultrasonic noise and echoes in the operating room. All these factors together and the need for an unobstructed field between the emitter and receiver make it an inaccurate, and therewith, a suboptimal system to use in a clinical setting [14–18].

2.3 Optical Systems

Optical systems use a camera-array to localise the position of an instrument with either infrared light-emitting diodes (LEDs) or infrared light reflecting spheres attached (Fig. 1). The use of

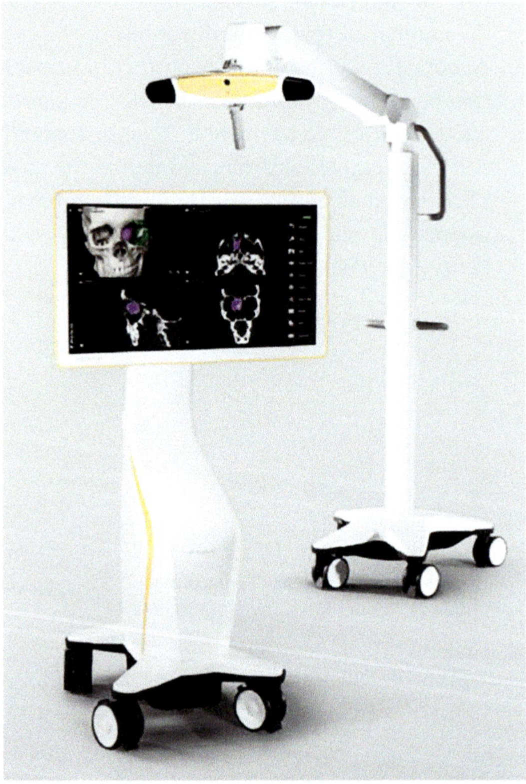

Fig. 1 Curve® Navigation allows users to plan, review, document and stream surgery from anywhere in the operating room. (Source: Brainlab)

two cameras leads to 'stereoscopic' information, better known as optical triangulation. Like the acoustic systems, the line-of-sight between the device cameras, the probe or the microscope should not be obstructed. However, the system is easy to use and allows for no limitation of degrees of freedom for surgeons. It is therefore a popular system that is routinely used, regardless of the surgical environment [8, 14, 19, 20]. For orbital surgery, optical systems are mainly used to allow for the greatest range of motion for the surgeon.

2.4 Electromagnetic Systems

The electromagnetic system uses a reference source generating a low-frequency electromagnetic field within which the orientation and position of a magnetic field sensor could be determined (Fig. 2). The accuracy of this system is within the 2-mm-range and there are no limitations of degrees of freedom for the surgeon, no need for an articulated arm, and no line-of-sight problems. However, the magnetic receiver, and thus the accuracy of the system, can be disturbed by metallic objects in the surgical field [7, 14, 21].

3 Practical Applications

There are several applications for navigation in orbital surgery, namely planning, performing, and evaluating the outcome of surgeries. In addition, navigation can be used for research purposes, however this lies beyond the scope of this chapter and will therefore not be further discussed.

This chapter will discuss the most common applications of navigation in orbital surgery, varying from orbital reconstruction and orbital decompression to surgery on the lacrimal drainage system and tumour resection.

3.1 Orbital Reconstruction

The largest number of studies describing navigation in orbital surgery are related to reconstruction of the orbit following facial trauma. In maxillofacial traumatology, fractures of the orbito-zygomatic complex are among the most commonly diagnosed fractures, and treatment is often dependent on the degree of displacement of the bony structures. Unfortunately, revision sur-

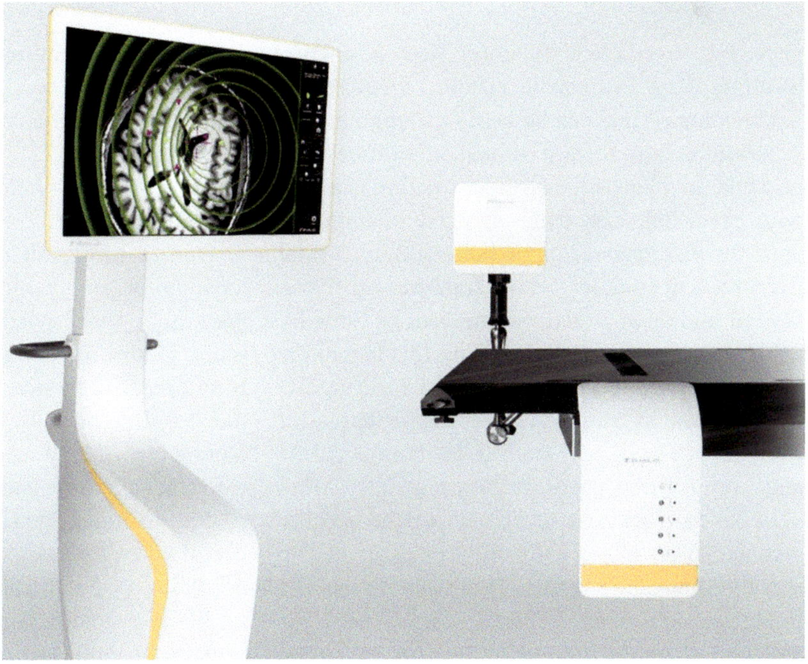

Fig. 2 Electromagnetic (EM) tracking allows users to perform pinless procedures and eliminate line-of-sight issues for neurosurgical procedures. (Source: Brainlab)

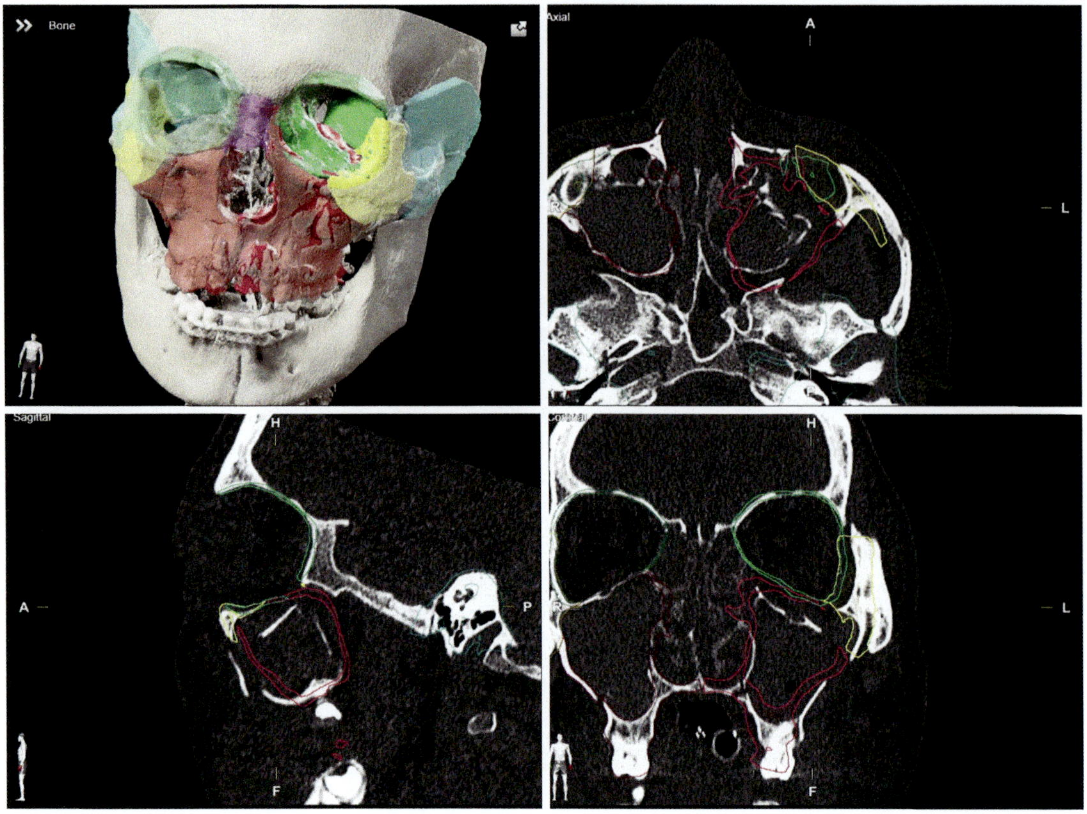

Fig. 3 Unilateral defects allow for the utilisation of templates from the healthy side. Choose segmented objects with Elements Object Manipulation and mirror them to the affected side. Mirrored structures can be easily manipulated and positioned according to existing anatomical structures of the affected side. (Source: Brainlab)

gery for insufficient function and aesthetics resulting from inadequate primary treatment is not uncommon and can be very challenging.

With the introduction of navigation it became possible to plan orbital reconstruction surgery with precision. Computer assisted planning is used for planning repair of both solitary orbital fractures and complex orbital fractures involving several midfacial structures, and can be done by using a mirroring technique. With this technique it is possible to reposition bones in a virtual 3D environment by mirroring the unaffected orbit over the affected orbit leading to more accurate and symmetric post-operative results. This 3D-plan can be used to create patient specific reconstruction plates (implants) or estimate the size for a standard implant. These patient specific implants could more precisely restore the original contouring and volume of the orbit. Accurate pre-operative planning by mirroring the unaffected side over the affected side could improve the outcome of surgery, and decrease the need for revision surgery [22]. However, further research is needed to scientifically substantiate this theory (Fig. 3).

During surgery it is possible to confirm the location of an instrument, which might be of great importance when operating in close proximity to the orbital apex and the optic nerve. Intra-operatively, it is also possible to evaluate the position of bony structures and plates by combining the images of the pre-operative CT-scan with the images of the surgical planning. According to some surgeons this is especially useful when the posterior ledge is absent. When normal bony landmarks are present, there seems to be less tendency to have patient specific implants manufactured. Navigation in these cases

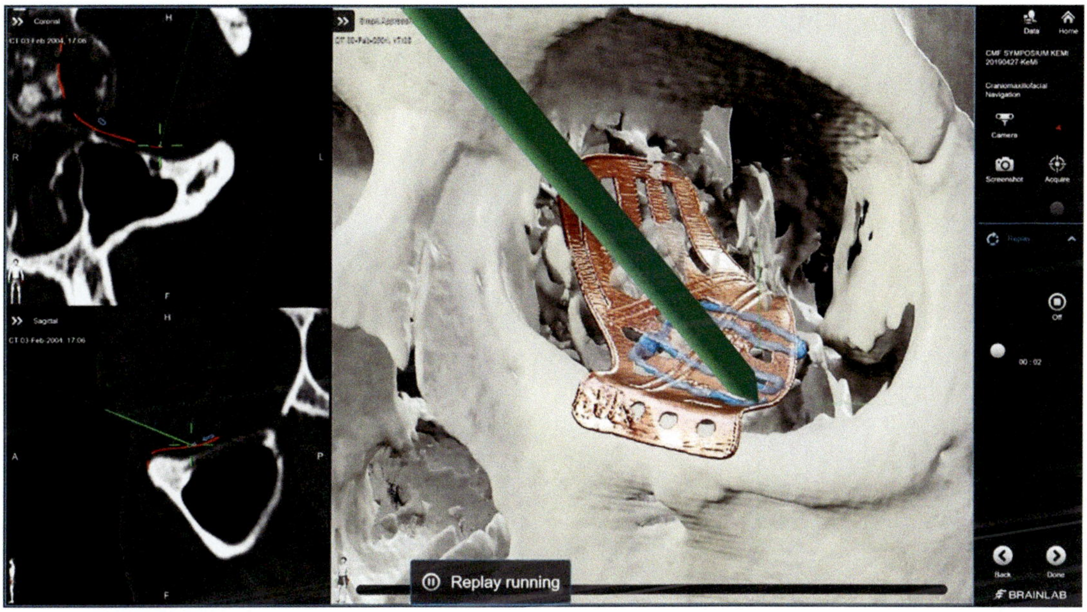

Fig. 4 Quality control with intra-operative navigation offers real-time information about the position of implants. (Source: Brainlab)

is then mainly used to guide the surgeon with regards to instrument positioning. Image guidance in orbital reconstruction is becoming increasingly routine [22–25]. According to Cai et al., post-operative complications and the need for repeat procedures decreased when using navigation for orbital reconstruction in trauma patients [26]. The use of image-guided navigation during orbital reconstruction has been shown to reduce post-operative complications, including diplopia, infraorbital hypesthesia, ophthalmoplegia, and exophthalmos [26, 27] (Fig. 4).

3.2 Surgery on the Lacrimal Drainage System

The use of navigation during surgery on the lacrimal drainage system is described in both dacryocystectomy and dacryocystorhinostomy. Some authors find navigation or CT-guidance during these procedures only helpful in challenging cases or in case of secondary acquired nasolacrimal duct obstruction. Invading tumours of the lacrimal sac or severe distortion of the anatomy after previous surgery, e.g., hemimaxillectomy, rhinectomy, post trauma or post reconstruction following sinonasal tumours, can make surgery of the lacrimal drainage system challenging. The use of navigation in these cases could be useful as injuries to surrounding structures could be avoided [28–30].

According to Reichel et al. the use of navigation can also be useful in patients undergoing routine procedures to the lacrimal drainage system, such as endoscopic DCR [31]. The use of navigation enhances both comfort for the surgeon and safety for the patient. With the help of image guidance, the location of the lacrimal sac could be determined with an accuracy of 1 mm, despite variations in anatomy of the nasal cavity, turbinates and nasal septum. In addition, image guidance made adequate opening of the bony nasolacrimal canal and adequate removal of the medial wall of the lacrimal sac possible, resulting in a significant increase in preservation of nasal mucosa and minimal exposure of bone, and with that a higher success rate [31, 32]. So far, there is no information available on the influence of the obstruction site on the success rate of endoscopic DCR with navigation.

3.3 Orbital Decompression

Orbital decompression involves the removal of one or more orbital walls to treat (thyroid-disease associated) exophthalmos. In some cases, a variable degree of periorbital fat removal is also needed. Orbital decompression is technically challenging, as the goal of reducing proptosis competes with aesthetic requests and post-operative complications, such as diplopia, ophthalmoplegia, infra-orbital hypesthesia, and insufficient reduction of the proptosis [33, 34].

To optimise the surgical outcome and reduce the risk for post-operative complications, several techniques for orbital decompression have been developed and described, for example inferomedial orbital decompression with retention of the inferomedial strut, balanced orbital decompression with decompression of both the medial and lateral wall, and lateral wall decompression. However, the combination of anatomical variations, the presence of important neurovascular structures and the proximity to the brain can make every used technique for maximal orbital decompression a challenge. To ensure an appropriate level of decompression with minimal iatrogenic damage precise surgical planning and execution is key [33, 34].

Therefore, the use of navigation during orbital decompression has gained greater attention over the last couple of years. With the right pre-operative planning, navigation can be very useful in identifying the exact bony landmarks and other anatomical structures, it enables measurement of the thickness of the orbital walls, and it makes it possible to determine the endpoint of decompression [33–38].

Several studies showed a greater reduction in proptosis and/or strabismus rates when using navigation. This could be the result of more aggressive bone removal laterally to enhance proptosis reduction, while enabling more nuanced bone removal medially at the level of the belly of the medial rectus muscle [35, 36]. According to Millar et al., navigation is especially useful in decompression of the (deep) lateral wall, as the surgical limits in this area vary and are not universally agreed. To their experience, it is difficult to intra-operatively define the posterior limits of the deep lateral wall, and it is difficult to standardise these surgical limits. Visualising the exact location of instruments during surgery leads to more impressive and individualised orbital decompressions with better outcomes and enhances safety [33]. Surgical navigation provides objective control in removing bone that would otherwise would have been left in place, and it is thought that navigation is an absolute surplus value in cases where maximal decompression is desired [33, 34, 37, 38]. Interestingly, use of surgical navigation in orbital decompressions also leads to a significant reduction in operating time as more cases are performed, it reduces surgical stress, makes it possible to operate through small cosmetically acceptable incisions, and reduces the number of revision procedures [33, 37, 38].

3.4 Intraorbital Foreign Body

Orbital foreign bodies are not uncommon and typically the result of facial injury. Intraorbital foreign objects can lead to infection, pain, vision problems, blindness, and can reduce the function of extraocular muscles. Therefore, removal of foreign bodies is often necessary [39, 40].

The main difficulty in removing intraorbital foreign bodies is the localization and determining its relation to vital orbital structures when using conventional pre-operative radiography. Even if the foreign body is visible on conventional radiography, it can be difficult to determine its exact position in the orbit. With the arrival of 3D imaging localising foreign bodies and their relation to surrounding tissues became easier. Using 3D imaging in combination with pre-operative planning and intra-operative navigation build the fundament for the best surgical outcome [39–41]. It should be taken into account that metallic foreign bodies may cause beam hardening and photon starvation artefacts. Artefact reduction algorithms have been developed to reduce this effect and make high-quality detailed 3D reconstruction models possible, but it should always be taken into account when planning for surgery [41].

Traditionally, open approaches were used to remove intraorbital foreign bodies. Detecting a foreign body in a deep, narrow area with poor visibility increases the risk of iatrogenic damage. Image-guided navigated removal of foreign bodies has proven to be an effective treatment modality improving surgical outcome, especially when combined with (transnasal) endoscopic surgery [40].

Minimally invasive surgery has the advantage that it gives direct access without the risk of further scarring. In addition, endoscopic guidance with good illumination and image magnification helps visualise the orbital structures. When combined with navigation it is possible to directly correlate the endoscopy images with the pre-operative 3D-images reducing the risk for trauma to surrounding structures. It allows for safer manipulation of instruments and easier location of the foreign object. This is especially valuable in situations where the normal anatomy is distorted, e.g., trauma, fibrous wrapping of the foreign body, previous attempts removing the foreign body [39–41]. The complication rates, including bleeding, iatrogenic trauma, and infection rates, are lower in patients when navigation is used. Routine use of navigation (with minimally invasive surgical techniques) in removal of intraorbital foreign bodies is therefore recommended [39, 42, 43].

3.5 Intraorbital Tumours

Resection of orbital or complex orbitofacial tumours is often the most promising and effective therapy with regards to recurrence rate and preservation of visual function. Furthermore, resection allows histological diagnosis and decompression of at-risk anatomical structures. However, removal of orbital or complex orbitofacial tumours can be challenging and is associated with increased perioperative morbidity because of limited space and the proximity to sensitive structures. Surgery on apical orbital masses is particularly fraught with difficulty. Visual loss, and damage to either cranial nerves or extraocular muscles as a consequence of surgery are frequently reported [44, 45].

Navigation is helpful in accurate target localization, determination of the optimum trajectory for biopsy, defining the most ideal surgical approach, establishing tumour margins for resection, and is helpful in avoiding damage to surrounding tissues. Use of additional CT angiographic guidance helps to avoid vascular injuries during tumour removal. Furthermore, use of colour-coding software allows marking of the tumour, optic nerve, vessels and other important structures [9, 44–49] (Fig. 5).

For soft tissue tumours it should be remembered that surgical manipulation moves the structures within the orbit, therefore pre-operative scans may be of limited value during surgery *per se*. However, in surgeries involving osseous structures navigation undoubtedly reduces perioperative morbidity and improves resection grades [22].

Further decrease of perioperative morbidity and more aggressive tumour resection can be achieved with additional intra-operative CT or MRI imaging. These intra-operative images are directly uploaded to the navigation system. This allows for control of resection and updating of pre-operative data. Use of this technique could lead to more aggressive yet safe tumour removal, without additional perioperative morbidity, and thus a better outcome. This effect was seen in specific cases, e.g., patients with complex tumours, distorted anatomy due to tumour growth or previous operations, and it is therefore not yet recommended to use intra-operative imaging as a standard procedure for all tumour resections [45].

3.6 Navigation-Guided Optic Canal Decompression in Traumatic Optic Neuropathy

Inaccurate intra-operative localization of the bony fragments that impinge on the optic nerve is one of the many causes of failure of surgical optic

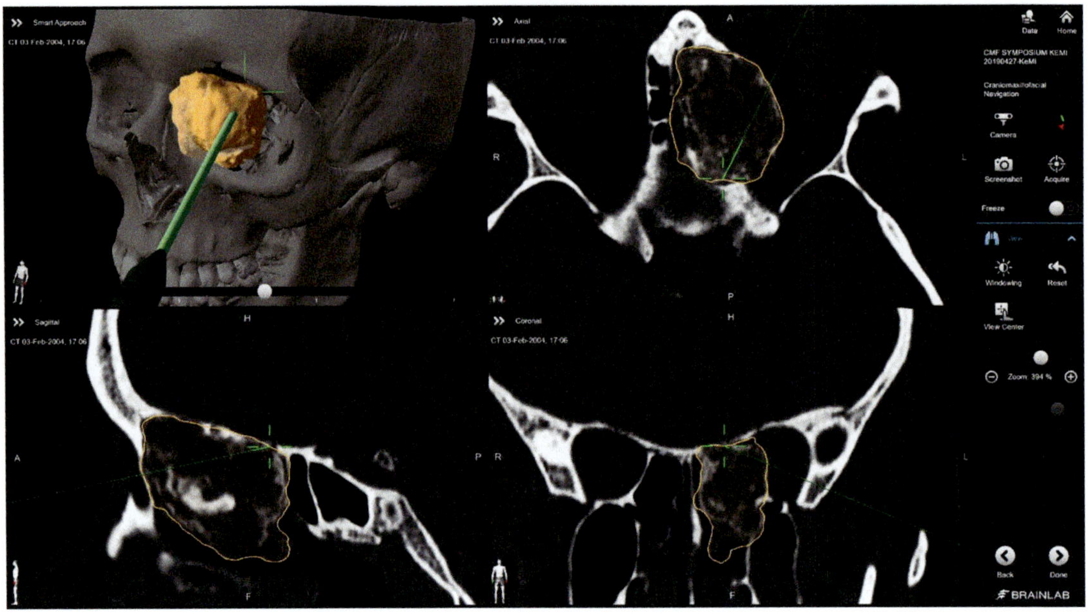

Fig. 5 Surgical navigation is used for precision guidance during craniomaxillofacial tumour surgery. (Source: Brainlab)

canal decompression. Moreover, it may even leads to inadvertent damage to the optic nerve. Navigation allows for more precision and safety. Additionally, high-resolution imaging gives important information on possible further contributors to optic nerve injury, e.g., optic nerve oedema, retrobulbar haemorrhage, intraorbital emphysema, and optic canal fracture. In combination with an angiogram, information can be obtained regarding the exact localization of blood vessels in the surgical area [22, 23, 50, 51].

4 Advantages of Navigation in Orbital Surgery

4.1 Improved Accuracy

Regardless the indication, pre-operative planning allows for proper navigation and makes intra-operative accurate localization of pathology possible. In a complex anatomical structure such as the orbit conventional imaging and approaches were not always sufficient, leading to a less predictable outcome of surgery. With the use of navigation less revision procedures are needed [22–24, 45].

4.2 Safety

The conical shape of the orbit makes direct visualisation of structures and exact localization of instruments during surgery difficult, especially at the apex of the orbit. Real-time localization of instruments in relation to the anatomic structures is possible with navigation leading to a reduction in surgical stress. This allows safer and more controlled surgery, less perioperative morbidity, and reduced frequency of revision procedures [33, 34].

4.3 Effectiveness and Reduction in Operating Time

Navigation makes it possible to operate through smaller cosmetically acceptable incisions. Furthermore, knowing where one is with real-time localization of instruments leads to more effective surgical movements, and with that reduction in operating time. As there is a learning curve, this effect is specifically notable after several cases have been performed with navigation [33–35, 37].

4.4 Educational Purposes

Navigation plays a significant role in the education and training of trainee surgeons. It can familiarise them with the complex anatomy of the orbit, give them more self-esteem, and reduce the surgical learning curve [36, 52].

5 Disadvantages of Navigation in Orbital Surgery

5.1 Longer Operating Time

In the beginning, both the pre-operative planning and setting up the system before surgery take time. It is thought that surgical time initially is increased by approximately 40 min. However, once one becomes familiar with the system, there is a reduction in operating time when compared to cases were navigation is not used. This decrease in operating time will likely be less evident in surgeries performed by junior surgeons given their relative inexperience [35, 36].

5.2 Costs

The required equipment is expensive, and the technology is upgraded continuously, adding extra costs to maintain the hardware and software. The costs vary widely, and some health insurances do not pay for technology when used. This makes it difficult to convince certain hospitals to invest in navigation, and it seems likely that purchasing a navigational system is only interesting for clinics performing orbital surgery in a considerable number of patients or in clinics where use of a navigation system can be shared between multiple disciplines, e.g., craniomaxillofacial surgery, ENT, neurosurgery and orthopaedics [33, 34].

5.3 False Sense of Safety

Navigation can never replace anatomical mastery and surgical experience and should always be seen as a tool. Sufficient knowledge of the orbital anatomy always remains important as one should be able to determine the position of an instrument and its relation to surrounding structures, even when CT-angiograms or colour-coding of intraorbital structures are used [38].

6 Case Report

A 76-year-old male with a medical history of previous excision of myositis ossificans of the right orbital roof in 2006 presented with severe swelling and ptosis of the right upper eyelid. The right globe was difficult to examine because of compression due to swelling. His vision was severely diminished to light perception in the right eye. In addition, there was ophthalmoplegia. A biopsy of the swelling identified a solitary fibrous tumour and resection was planned with the help of navigation.

Following disinfection, positioning, and fixation of the reference system, an upper lid crease incision over the swelling of the eyelid was made. To remove the tumour in total, we performed a lateral orbitotomy. The tumour was dissected, adhesion of the tumour was seen dorsally and cranially to scar tissue of the previous (neurosurgical) operation. Cranially the tumour was

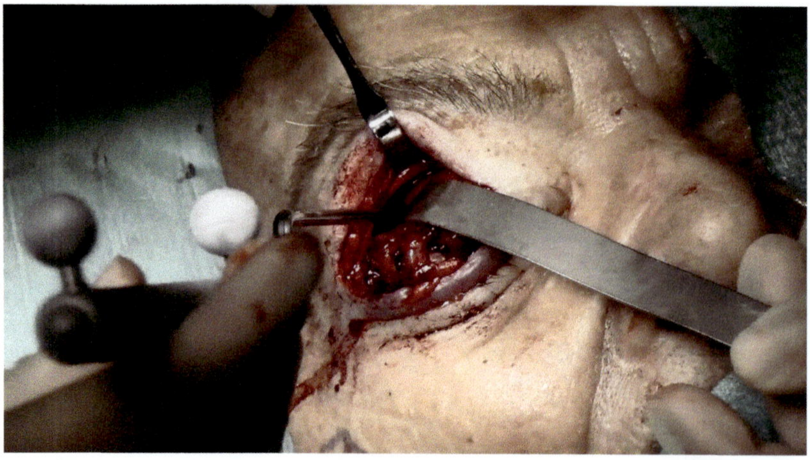

Fig. 6 Identification of the meninges with the help of navigation (surgeons: Dion Paridaens and Elske Strabbing)

adhered to the meninges. Navigation was used to identify the meninges (Fig. 6). Once the tumour was removed, the lateral orbital rim was replaced and fixated with screws.

7 Future Perspectives

The use of navigation has become more common practice in the operating room in recent years and has significantly improved surgical outcome and patient safety. However, technical development and advancement in healthcare are an ongoing process. With conventional navigation, surgeons still have to switch their attention between the surgical area and the display. Mixed and augmented reality resolve this issue by integrating the information of the navigational system into the surgical field-of-view (Fig. 7). Thus far, this technique has not been routinely used in orbital surgery and is still under research and development, both technically and clinically [53].

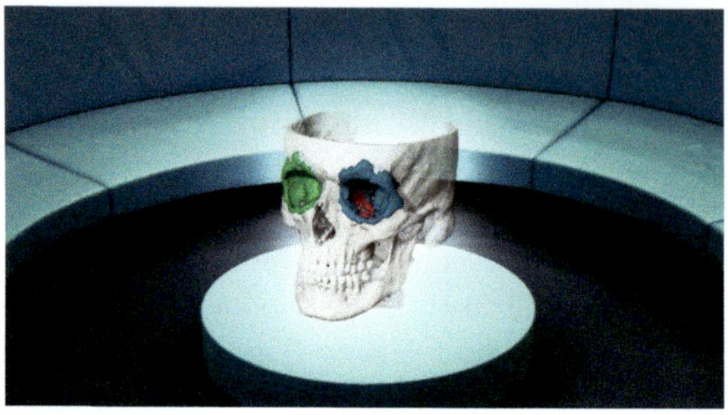

Fig. 7 Navigation and Mixed Reality helps users view spatial relationships between bone, tumour, and implant in 3D for craniomaxillofacial trauma fractures and tumour cases. (Source: Brainlab)

References

1. Leksell L. A stereotactic apparatus for intracranial surgery. Acta Chir Scand. 1949;99:229.
2. Riechert T, Wolff M. [A new directive apparatus for the coagulation of the ganglion gasseri and other intracerebral procedures]. Ein neues Zielgerat fur die Koagulation des ganglion Gasseri und andere intracerebrale Eingriffe. Acta Neurochir. 1952;2:405–7.
3. Spiegel EA, Wycis HT, Freed H. Stereoencephalotomy in thalamotomy and related procedures. J Am Med Assoc. 1952;148:446.
4. Spiegel EA, Wycis HT, Marks M, Lee AJ. Stereotaxic apparatus for operations on the human brain. Science. 1947;106:349–50.
5. Talairach DJ. Recherches sur la coagulation therapeutique des structures sous-corticales chez l'homme. Rev Neurol. 1949;81:4.
6. Reinhardt H, Meyer H, Amrein E. A computer-assisted device for the intraoperative CT-correlated localization of brain tumours. Eur Surg Res. 1988;20:51–8.
7. Kato A, Yoshimine T, Hayakawa T, Tomita Y, Ikeda T, Mitomo M, Harada K, Mogami H. A frameless, armless navigational system for computer-assisted neurosurgery. Technical note. J Neurosurg. 1991;74:845–9.
8. Zamorano LJ, Nolte L, Kadi AM, Jiang Z. Interactive intraoperative localization using an infrared-based system. Neurol Res. 1993;15:290–8.
9. Camara JG, Nguyen LT, Fernandez-Suntay JP, Nardin GF, Sua AS. The use of a computer-assisted image-guided system (InstaTrak) in orbital surgery. Ophthalmic Plast Reconstr Surg. 2001;17:447–51.
10. Hejazi N. Frameless image-guided neuronavigation in orbital surgery: practical applications. Neurosurg Rev. 2006;29:118–22.
11. Dorward NL. Neuronavigation—the surgeon's sextant. Br J Neurosurg. 1997;11:101–3.
12. Wirtz CR, Tronnier VM, Bonsanto MM, Hassfeld S, Knauth M, Kunze S. [Neuronavigation. Methods and prospects] Neuronavigation. Methoden und Ausblick. Nervenarzt. 1998;69:1029.
13. Benardete EA, Leonard MA, Weiner HL. Comparison of frameless stereotactic systems: accuracy, precision, and applications. Neurosurgery. 2001;49:1409–16.
14. Willems PW, van der Sprenkel JW, Tulleken CA, Viergever MA, Taphoorn MJ. Neuronavigation and surgery of intracerebral tumours. J Neurol. 2006;253:1123–36.
15. Ivanov M, Ciurea AV. Neuronavigation. Principles surgical technique. J Med Life. 2009;2:29–35.
16. Reinhardt HF, Zweifel HJ. Interactive sonar-operated device for stereotactic and open surgery. Stereotact Funct Neurosurg. 1990;54-55:393–7.
17. Horstmann GA, Reinhardt HF. Ranging accuracy test of the sonic microstereometric system. Neurosurgery. 1994;34:754–5.
18. Roberts DW, Strohbehn JW, Hatch JF, Murray W, Kettenberger H. A frameless stereotaxic integration of computerised tomographic imaging and the operating microscope. J Neurosurg. 1986;65:545–9.
19. Gumprecht HK, Widenka DC, Lumenta CB. BrainLab VectorVision Neuronavigation system: technology and clinical experiences in 131 cases. Neurosurgery. 1999;44:97–104.
20. Germano IM, Villalobos H, Silvers A, Post KD. Clinical use of the optical digitizer for intracranial neuronavigation. Neurosurgery. 1999;45:261–9.
21. Tan KK, Grzeszczuk R, Levin DN, Pelizzari CA, Chen GT, Erickson RK, Johnson D, Dohrmann GJ. A frameless stereotactic approach to neurosurgical planning based on retrospective patient-image registration. Technical note. J Neurosurg. 1993;79:296–303.
22. Udhay P, Bhattacharjee K, Ananthnarayanan P, Sundar G. Computer-assisted navigation in orbitofacial surgery. Indian J Ophthalmol. 2019;67:995.
23. DeLong MR, Gandolfi BM, Barr ML, Datta N, Willson TD, Jarrahy R. Intraoperative image-guided navigation in craniofacial surgery: review and grading of the current literature. J Craniofac Surg. 2019;30:465–72.
24. Moe KS, Murr AH, Wester ST. Orbital Fractures. Facial Plast Surg Clin North Am. 2018;26:237–51.
25. Sukegawa S, Kanno T, Furuki Y. Application of computer-assisted navigation systems in oral and maxillofacial surgery. Jpn Dent Sci Rev. 2018;54:139–49.
26. Cai EZ, Koh YP, Hing EC, Low JR, Shen JY, Wong HC, Sundar G, Lim TC. Computer-assisted navigational surgery improves outcomes in orbital reconstructive surgery. J Craniofac Surg. 2012;23:1567–73.
27. Zavattero E, Ramieri G, Roccia F, Gerbino G. Comparison of the outcomes of complex orbital fracture repair with and without a surgical navigation system: a prospective cohort study with historical controls. Plast Reconstr Surg. 2017;139:957–65.
28. Ali MJ, Naik MN. Image-guided dacryolocalization (IGDL) in traumatic secondary acquired lacrimal drainage obstructions (SALDO). Ophthalmic Plast Reconstr Surg. 2015;31:406–9.
29. Day S, Hwang TN, Pletcher SD, Bhatki A, McCulley TJ. Interactive image-guided endoscopic dacryocystorhinostomy. Ophthalmic Plast Reconstr Surg. 2008;24:338–40.
30. Kent JS, Allen LH, Rotenberg BW. Image-guided transnasal endoscopic techniques in the management of orbital disease. Orbit. 2010;29:328–33.
31. Reichel O, Taxeidis M. Use of an image-guided navigation system for routine endonasal endoscopic dacryocystorhinostomy. J Laryngol Otol. 2019;133:685–90.
32. Leong SC, Macewen CJ, White PS. A systematic review of outcomes after dacryocystorhinostomy in adults. Am J Rhinol Allergy. 2010;24:81–90.
33. Millar MJ, Maloof AJ. The application of stereotactic navigation surgery to orbital decompression for thyroid-associated orbitopathy. Eye (Lond). 2009;23:1565–71.
34. Patel BC. Stereotactic navigation for lateral orbital wall decompression. Eye (Lond). 2009;23:1493–5.

35. Heisel CJ, Tuohy MM, Riddering AL, Sha C, Kahana A. Stereotactic navigation improves outcomes of orbital decompression surgery for thyroid associated orbitopathy. Ophthalmic Plast Reconstr Surg. 2020;36:553–6.
36. Prevost A, Dekeister C, Caron P, Imbert P, Cavallier Z, Lauwers F, Boutault F. Outcomes of orbital decompression using surgical navigation in thyroid-associated ophthalmopathy. Int J Oral Maxillofac Surg. 2020;49:1279–85.
37. Servat JJ, Elia MD, Gong D, Manes RP, Black EH, Levin F. Electromagnetic image-guided orbital decompression: technique, principles, and preliminary experience with 6 consecutive cases. Orbit. 2014;33:433–6.
38. Wu CY, Kahana A. Stereotactic navigation with a registration mask in orbital decompression surgery: preliminary results. Ophthalmic Plast Reconstr Surg. 2015;31:440–4.
39. Gui H, Yang H, Shen SG, Xu B, Zhang S, Bautista JS. Image-guided surgical navigation for removal of foreign bodies in the deep maxillofacial region. J Oral Maxillofac Surg. 2013;71:1563–71.
40. Koo Ng NK, Jaberoo MC, Pulido M, Olver JM, Saleh HA. Image guidance removal of a foreign body in the orbital apex. Orbit. 2009;28:404–7.
41. Zhao Y, Li Y, Li Z, Deng Y. Removal of orbital metallic foreign bodies with image-guided surgical navigation. Ophthalmic Plast Reconstr Surg. 2020;36:305–10.
42. Ewers R, Schicho K, Undt G, Wanschitz F, Truppe M, Seemann R, Wagner A. Basic research and 12 years of clinical experience in computer-assisted navigation technology: a review. Int J Oral Maxillofac Surg. 2005;34:1–8.
43. Grobe A, Klatt J, Heiland M, Schmelzle R, Pohlenz P. Diagnostic and therapeutic aspects in the treatment of gunshot wounds of the viscerocranium. Eur J Trauma Emerg Surg. 2011;37:41–7.
44. Berger M, Char DH. Interactive image guidance for surgical localization of orbital apical tumors. Orbit. 2002;21:199–203.
45. Terpolilli NA, Rachinger W, Kunz M, Thon N, Flatz WH, Tonn JC, Schichor C. Orbit-associated tumors: navigation and control of resection using intraoperative computed tomography. J Neurosurg. 2016;124:1319–27.
46. Enchev Y, Tzekov C, Ferdinandov D, Cekov A, Spiriev T. Neuronavigation in cranio orbital neurosurgery—do we really need it? Turk Neurosurg. 2011;21:119.
47. Karcioglu ZA, Mascott CR. Computer-assisted image-guided orbit surgery. Eur J Ophthalmol. 2006;16:446–52.
48. Lee KY, Ang BT, Ng I, Looi A. Stereotaxy for surgical navigation in orbital surgery. Ophthalmic Plast Reconstr Surg. 2009;25:300–2.
49. Marcus H, Schwindack C, Santarius T, Mannion R, Kirollos R. Image-guided resection of spheno-orbital skull-base meningiomas with predominant intraosseous component. Acta Neurochir. 2013;155:981–8.
50. Bhattacharjee K, Serasiya S, Kapoor D, Bhattacharjee H. Navigation-guided optic canal decompression for traumatic optic neuropathy: two case reports. Indian J Ophthalmol. 2018;66:879–82.
51. Yan W, Chen Y, Qian Z, Selva D, Pelaez D, Tu Y, Wu W. Incidence of optic canal fracture in the traumatic optic neuropathy and its effect on the visual outcome. Br J Ophthalmol. 2017;101:261.
52. Seyler TM, Lai LP, Sprinkle DI, Ward WG, Jinnah RH. Does computer-assisted surgery improve accuracy and decrease the learning curve in hip resurfacing? A radiographic analysis. J Bone Joint Surg Am. 2008;90:71–80.
53. Benmahdjoub M, van Walsum T, van Twisk P, Wolvius EB. Augmented reality in craniomaxillofacial surgery: added value and proposed recommendations through a systematic review of the literature. Int J Oral Maxillofac Surg. 2021;50:969–78.

Orbital Injury – Anatomical Based Reconstruction

Paola Bonavolontà, Santiago Ortiz Pérez,
Cornelia Caron, Maarten Koudstaal,
and Simon Holmes

Key Messages

- Orbital fractures are common and evidence based treatment planning is essential to avoid increased risk of poor long term functional and aesthetic outcomes.
- Pure orbital fractures are limited to the orbital walls without fracturing the orbital rim; impure orbital fractures involve the orbital rim and are often seen as part of larger fracture patterns involving adjacent bony structures.
- Indications for treatment of orbital floor fractures are entrapment of the medial or inferior rectus muscles, or persistent changes in the orbital volume. Entrapment requires immediate surgical intervention. Changes in the orbital volume can be the result of lack of support for the orbital contents, leading to hypophthalmos, enophthalmos and/or diplopia.
- Fracture patterns in children are related to the characteristic developmental anatomy of the craniofacial skeleton at the time of injury. Entrapment of the inferior rectus muscle in young children is rare, but possible. The presentation of these fractures is known as a 'white eye blow out' and may present with nausea, vomiting and bradycardia. Delay to surgery is possibly linked to long term functional outcomes.
- Computer assisted surgery is useful to obtain a virtual pre-operative planning of the desired reconstruction using pre-operative CT scans and adequate software. Computer-aided-design (CAD) implants and computer-aided-manufacturing (CAM) implants may support the orbital reconstruction procedure, providing a customised implant for reconstruction directly on the patient's anatomy.

P. Bonavolontà
Maxillofacial Unit, University of Naples Federico II, Naples, Italy

S. O. Pérez
Department of Ophthalmology, Hospital Universitario Virgen de las Nieves., Granada, Spain

Department of Surgery, University of Granada - Instituto de Investigación Biosanitaria ibs. GRANADA , Granada, Spain

C. Caron · M. Koudstaal
Orbital Center, Department of Maxillofacial Surgery, Erasmus MC, Rotterdam, The Netherlands

S. Holmes (✉)
Department of Oral and Maxillofacial Surgery, Barts Health NHS Trust, London, UK
e-mail: s.holmes@qmul.ac.uk

F. M. Quaranta Leoni et al. (eds.), *Oculoplastic, Lacrimal and Orbital Surgery*,
https://doi.org/10.1007/978-3-031-39638-0_31

1 Introduction

Orbital fractures are common and present to different specialties according to local referral pathways. The presentation is stereotypical and prescient diagnosis and evidence based treatment planning is essential to avoid increased risk of poor long term functional and aesthetic outcomes.

2 Epidemiology of Orbital Trauma

Orbital floor and medial wall fracture is a common sequelae following moderate to severe energy transfer. The fracture pattern may be described as 'pure' should the orbital rim remain intact and 'impure' if this is violated. Impure fractures are a heterogenous group and orbital involvement is common in other facial fractures including those of the inferior orbital margin, zygoma, maxilla at Le Fort 2 and 3 level, naso -orbito- ethmoid, and craniofacial patterns.

There are many papers concerning the aetiology of facial injuries [1–3] and a common theme around mechanisms including interpersonal violence, falls, motor vehicle accidents, sporting and industrial accidents, and of course conflict. In most studies there is an acceptance that male sex is heavily represented with typical age distribution focussed in the second and third decades. Whilst there are regional differences in aetiologies [4], the global burden of facial trauma was articulated in a recent paper [5] as approximately 7.5 million cases giving an incidence of 98/100,000. There is however no detail on orbital trauma per se.

In a recent study [6] of 582 patients with orbital trauma treated over a 5 year period, 82% were male, with a peak incidence in 20–29 years of age. Whilst assault was most common (55%) falls (20%) and motor vehicle accidents (12%) were also often observed.

3 Orbital Fracture Patterns

With a prevalence of up to 55%, facial fractures involving the orbits are not uncommon in the adult population [7, 8]. The underlying insult is largely predictive for the type of fracture that arises and several fracture patterns can be distinguished [9, 10]. This paragraph discusses the different orbital fracture patterns with a main focus on 'pure' and 'impure' orbital fractures.

3.1 Pure and Impure Fractures of the Orbit

A variety of classifications has been proposed to assess orbital fractures, however the most frequently used classification for orbital fractures was proposed in the 1960s, categorising orbital fractures in two separate groups, i.e. 'pure' and 'impure' orbital fractures [11, 12].

3.1.1 Pure Orbital Fractures

Pure orbital fractures are limited to the orbital walls without fracturing the orbital rim. It is thought these fractures are often the result of the application of a nonpenetrating, blunt force over the orbital contents leading to posterior displacement of the orbital contents into a smaller portion of the orbit. This process leads to increased intraorbital pressure resulting in a fracture of one or more orbital walls, mostly at its weakest point(s) [13]. However, different mechanisms are also possible and are discussed below when applicable. Four to sixteen percent of facial skeletal injuries are isolated orbital fractures [10]. There are four general types of pure orbital fractures:

Orbital Roof Fractures

These make up 1 to 9% of all orbital fractures. The orbital roof belongs to the anterior skull base, and separates the orbit from the anterior cranial fossa. Usually these fractures are related to adjacent trauma to the orbital rim, however intracranial injuries caused by occipital trauma, e.g. contrecoup injuries and frontal contusions, can also lead to orbital roof fractures [14, 15].

Lateral Orbital Wall Fractures

Isolated lateral orbital wall fractures are rare and are the result of an isolated trauma to the lateral orbital wall. When compared to the other orbital walls, higher energy is necessary to fracture this firm structure. Treatment is only needed in case of severe displacement. Lateral orbital wall fractures are mainly associated with fractures of the zygomatic maxillary complex and/or more severe facial traumas such as cranial base injuries [14, 15].

Medial Orbital Wall Fractures

According to the literature, isolated medial wall fractures are diagnosed in 0 to 55% of the cases of facial injury [15]. Isolated medial fractures are easily missed, especially initially when acute clinical symptoms mask deformity. Treatment is needed in case of entrapment or in case of clinically evident hypophthalmos. For isolated medial wall fractures it is hard to predict who will develop late hypophthalmos or enophthalmos, and who will not [14, 15].

Orbital Floor Fractures

There are two main theories on how orbital floor fractures can occur. As described above, the first theory describes the transfer of hydraulic forces through the orbital contents onto the weakest point of the orbit, often blowing out the orbital floor. Interestingly, the lamina papyracea is thinner than the orbital floor. However, this bony structure is buttressed by the ethmoid partitions possibly making it more resistant to a sudden rise in intraorbital pressure, which could explain the higher incidence of orbital floor fractures. The second theory states that traumatic forces on the orbital rim can lead to buckling of the orbital floor, resulting in it to fracture at its weakest point [13, 15–17].

Indications for treatment of orbital floor fractures are entrapment of the medial or inferior rectus muscles, or persistent, aesthetically disturbing changes in the orbital volume. Entrapment always requires immediate surgical intervention. True entrapment of the muscle itself can compromise the vascular supply of the entrapped muscle, leading to necrosis, fibrosis and ultimately scarring. This can result in motility disorders. However, motility disorders can also be the result of fat entrapment, without involvement of a muscle. Of note, entrapment is rare in the adult population. Changes in the orbital volume can be the result of lack of support for the orbital contents, leading to hypophthalmos, enophthalmos and/or diplopia. However, the degree of floor loss requiring surgical intervention is strongly debated. Several authors suggest as a general rule, >50% involvement of the floor or > 2 mm of hypophthalmos will necessitate surgical repair [14]. Whilst this is a strong guide, clinical correlation is mandatory and influenced by persistent diplopia after the swelling has subsided or a clinically obvious enophthalmos or hypoglobus which the patient can identify.

3.1.2 Impure Orbital Fractures

These fractures involve the orbital rim and are often seen as part of larger fracture patterns involving adjacent bony structures, i.e. fractures of the zygomatic maxillary complex, the naso-orbitoethmoid complex or Le Fort II/III fractures. Orbital fractures in combination with the zygomatic maxillary complex or the naso-orbitoethmoid complex account for 30 to 55% of the facial skeletal injuries [9, 10, 14, 15].

3.2 Fracture Patterns in Children

Fracture patterns in children differ from adult fracture patterns as they are related to a child's activities and the characteristic developmental anatomy of the craniofacial skeleton at the time of injury. Several factors of development play a role. The first factor is related to the presence of a higher proportion of cancellous bone and cartilage in the growing sutures in children. These characteristics make paediatric bone more elastic and allow it to absorb more energy without resulting in a fracture. The second factor playing an essential role are the different stages of sinus development [18, 19].

The maxillary sinuses are the first to develop. This occurs biphasic and it is not until the age of 12 years that the maxillary sinus expands, which is related to eruption of the permanent dentition. It is thought that the presence of unerupted maxillary dentition protects the orbital floor from fracturing in young children. The maxillary sinus reaches adult size at the age of 16 years [19].

The ethmoid sinuses are usually not seen on radiographs until the age of 1 year old and gradually reach adult size by the age of 12 years.

During ethmoid sinus development the medial orbital wall becomes progressively thin, making it more susceptible to fracture [19].

Ossification of the frontal bone starts around age 2, whereas pneumatization of the frontal sinus starts around the age of 7 years. Development completes during adulthood. Frontal bone and orbital roof fractures are more common in children than in adults. This is the result of incomplete pneumatization and the high cranium-to-face ratio. Furthermore, the frontal bone and supraorbital rim are more prominent in the paediatric skull, and therewith receive the initial impact of a trauma [19].

Previous studies showed that until the age of 7 years, orbital roof fractures are the most common orbital fractures to occur in childhood. From the age of 7, fractures of the orbital floor become more common, which is the result of maxillary sinus development [20, 21]. Even though certain fractures are more likely to occur at a certain age than others, one should always bear in mind that due to anatomical and developmental differences between patients even the *unexpected can happen*. For example, entrapment of the inferior rectus muscle in a 3-year old is rare, but possible. Decent knowledge of the clinical features is therefore essential. The presentation of these fractures is known as a 'white eye blow out' and is commonly missed [22], and may present with nausea, vomiting, and bradycardia to the paediatric surgeons following an incidental finding [23]. Delay to surgery is possibly linked to long term functional outcomes [24] and emphasises a need for a high index of suspicion.

4 Clinical Features

Periocular trauma has a variety of presentations depending on the degree of hard and soft tissue involvement.

Orbital trauma might be considered according to three main principles which guide our diagnostic protocol and subsequent treatment plan [25–27].

- Penetrating trauma including intraocular foreign body.
- Orbital haemorrhage—potentially sight threatening.
- Orbital fractures.

The main clinical signs and symptoms are stereotypical and should be sought in every patient with orbital trauma.

4.1 External Appearance

1. Periorbital ecchymosis and subconjunctival haemorrhage. These are the most frequent signs of presentation, but its absence does not rule out a fracture, particularly in the paediatric population.
2. Emphysema. The presence of air within the soft tissues is a common sign in orbital fractures that communicate the orbital cavity with a paranasal sinus, especially the ethmoid. The emphysema might also be visible under the conjunctiva (chemosis).
3. Globe malposition. Typically, enophthalmos is due to the increase in the orbital volume, but it is also possible to see exophthalmos in cases of severe orbital haemorrhage, hypoglobus, or even globe dislocation into the maxillary sinus. The hypoglobus is a sign of wide floor fractures (Fig. 1a–c).
4. Periorbital deformity, such as orbital asymmetry, telecanthus, superior sulcus deepening, and upper lid ptosis. The telecanthus might denote medial fractures with medial canthal tendon disinsertion, frequent in Naso-Orbito-Ethmoid Fractures [15].
5. Orbital tension and difficulties in opening the eye are suggestive of compartment syndrome [25–28]. Rapid diagnosis and management with a lateral cantholysis is mandatory and should be expected with the following findings.
   (a) Severe orbital pain.
   (b) Ophthalmoplegia.
   (c) Loss of pupillary reflex.
   (d) Diminished acuity.

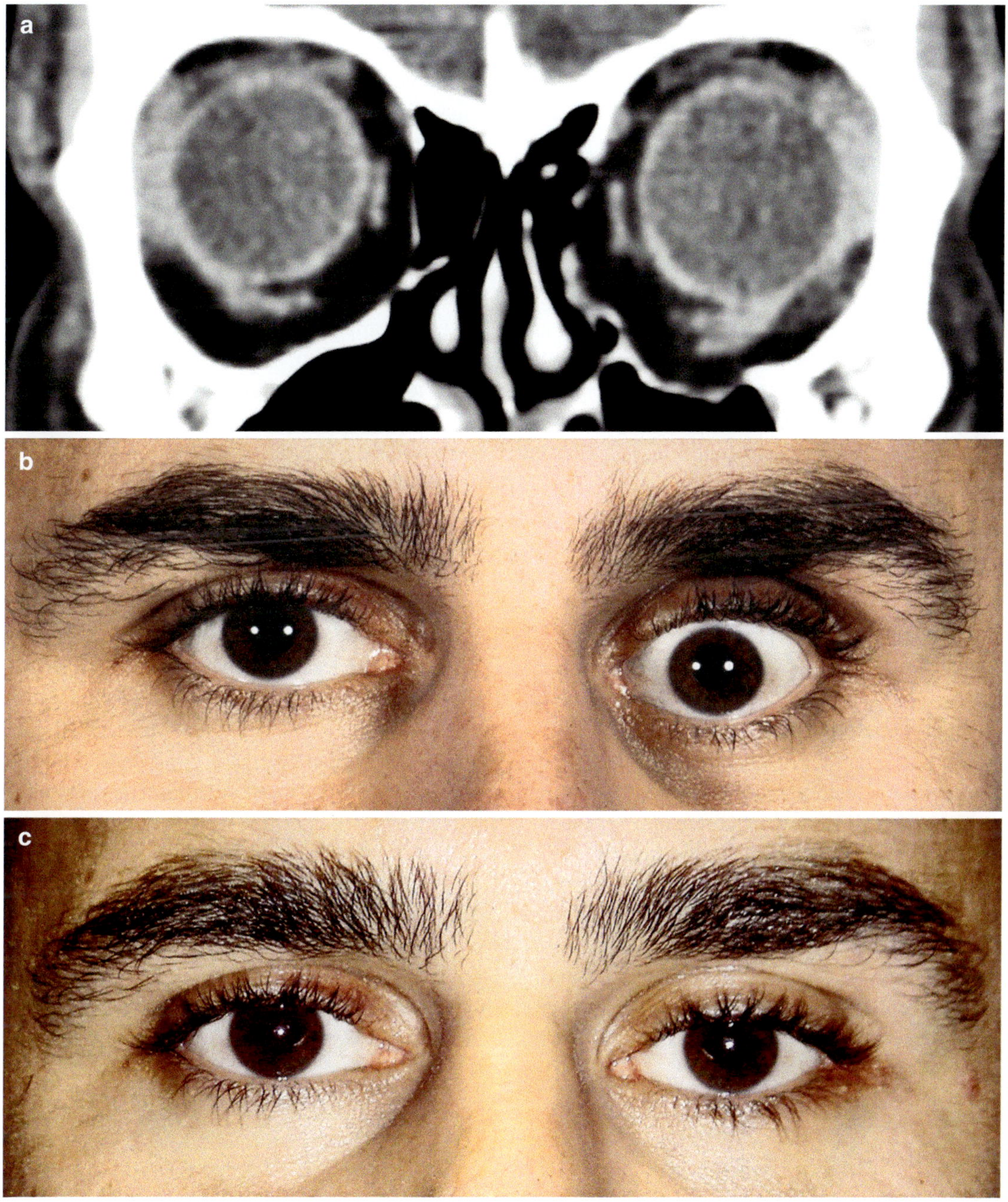

Fig. 1 (**a**) CT identifying a large left orbital floor and medial wall fracture following blunt injury. (**b**) The patient presented with diplopia, left enophthalmos and hypoglobus. (**c**) Post left orbital floor and medial wall implants placed via a swinging lower eyelid transconjunctival approach Orbital Injury – Anatomical Based Reconstruction (images courtesy of Mr David H. Verity)

(e) Proptosis.
(f) Loss of red colour perception.

4.2 Patient Symptoms

1. Neurosensorial impairment. The lower eyelid and cheek hypoesthesia (infraorbital nerve territory) are frequent in cases of floor fractures that affect the infraorbital nerve.
2. Diplopia. This is a frequent symptom and very useful for a clinical diagnosis, although it may be masked by pain or swelling. Should diplopia be present it is highly suggestive of an orbital fracture and functional assessment by an orthoptist is mandatory.
3. Visual disturbances. Ocular pathology is common following orbital trauma [29] with sequelae of minimal blurring to blindness, depending on other injuries affecting the eye and the optic nerve [25–28].

4.3 Ocular Motility

Diplopia and ocular motility impairment might be related to different mechanisms: soft tissue/muscle entrapment, soft tissue/muscle hematoma and oedema, muscle ischemia, motor nerve palsy, and central nervous system (brainstem) injury [15].

General motility restriction may be a sign of increasing orbital tension (compartment syndrome) or fractures affecting the orbital apex [27].

Restriction in one or two gaze positions is most frequent, it is usually due to one or two-wall fractures, but it may also be present in nerve palsy, or rarely due to an intra-orbital foreign body.

Muscle entrapment is more frequent affecting the medial wall and floor, and usually in the equator of the orbit. Generally, if the trap is in the equator or more anterior, the motility limitation is on the contrary gaze (i.e. if the inferior rectus is trapped anteriorly, there will be a limitation in up-gaze), if the entrapment is more posterior, the restriction occurs in the same gaze (i.e. if the inferior rectus is trapped posteriorly, there will be a limitation in down-gaze) [25].

Systemic signs and symptoms, such as bradycardia, nausea, dizziness, severe pain, etc., during eye movements, especially if motility restriction is significant, are indicative of muscle entrapment. This situation is described typically in "white-eye" or linear trapdoor fractures, seen in the paediatric population, where the muscle (usually the inferior) is trapped within the fracture line, with very few external signs of trauma (Fig. 2a–c). It has been described that up to 43% of orbital floor fractures in children present without external signs [28].

4.4 Systemic Signs and Symptoms

These include headache, nausea and vomiting, and bradycardia. These symptoms might be due to the oculo-cardiac reflex, and are more frequent if there is muscle entrapment [25–27].

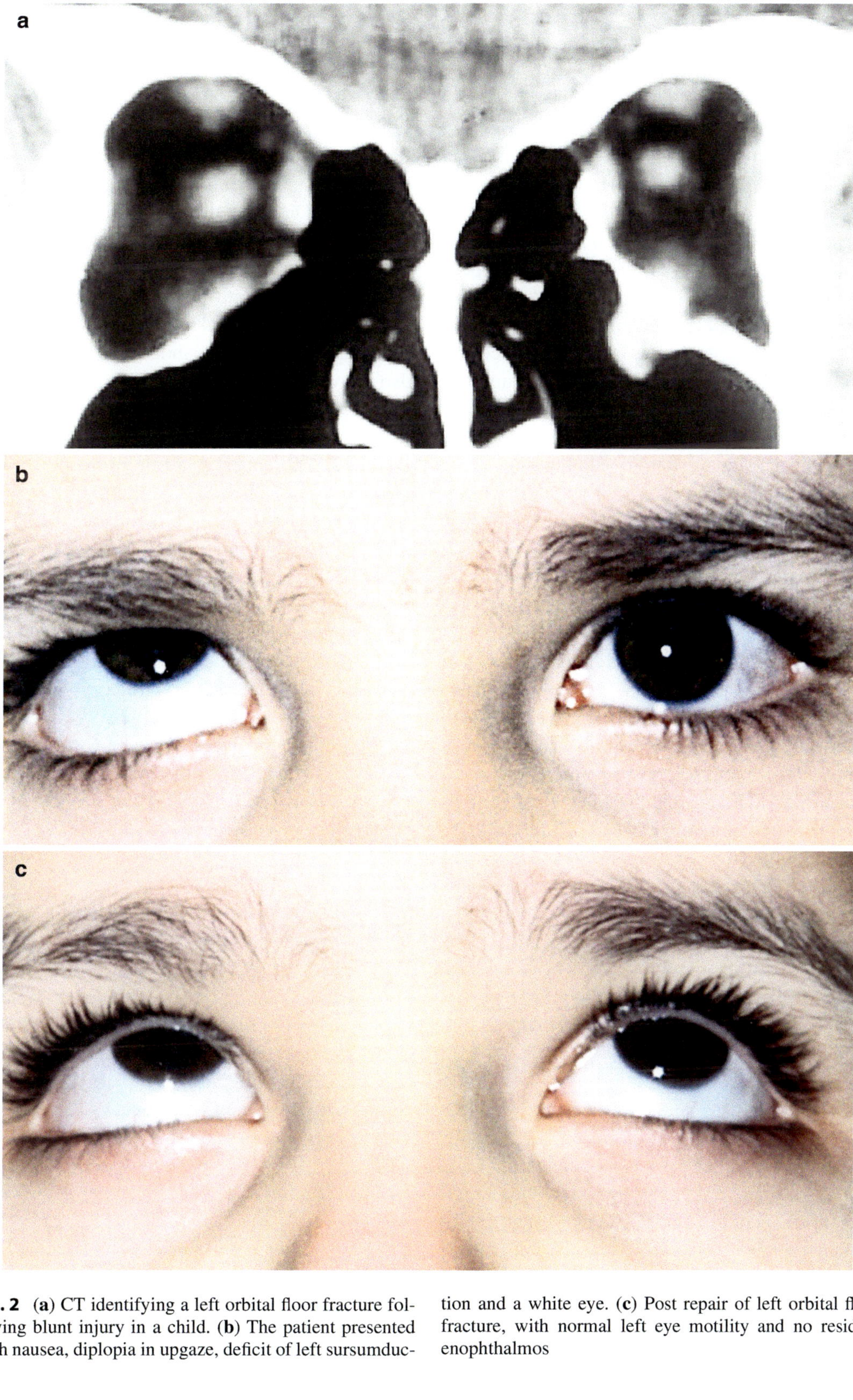

Fig. 2 (**a**) CT identifying a left orbital floor fracture following blunt injury in a child. (**b**) The patient presented with nausea, diplopia in upgaze, deficit of left sursumduction and a white eye. (**c**) Post repair of left orbital floor fracture, with normal left eye motility and no residual enophthalmos

5 Complications

5.1 Compartment Syndrome

The orbit is a cavity with rigid walls (either bone or the fibrous periorbita). If there is an acute rise in the orbital pressure, the venous flow can be altered, and this severe complication establishes. The aetiology is either an orbital haemorrhage or emphysema or even an abscess that may appear days after the trauma. It can be suspected if there is orbital and eyelid tension on palpation, proptosis, signs of optic nerve impairment (colour vision impairment, relative afferent pupillary defect—RAPD, visual decrease), global ocular motility restriction, ocular hypertension, and retinal hypoperfusion in fundus examination. This syndrome is an emergency that should be managed urgently [25–27].

5.2 Traumatic Optic Neuropathy

This is a rare but severe complication; it has been described to occur in up to 10% of patients with craniofacial fractures. It can be secondary to direct (foreign bodies, nerve avulsion, bone fragments, etc.) or indirect nerve injury. The main symptom is a visual impairment, which can be variable depending on the degree of the damage; also, colour vision impairment, and RAPD, are signs that should make clinicians presume this complication [27, 30].

6 Diagnostic Principles: Role of Orthoptics: Treatment Planning

Managing orbital trauma follows a systematic approach, prioritising life-threatening injuries first, the eye and orbital vision-threatening injuries second, preserving the eye and orbital anatomy third, and, finally, aesthetic concerns. To remember this, a simple mnemotechnic rule is used—"LIVES": [25, 26].

- LI: life
- V: vision
- E: eye and orbit
- S: aesthetic

6.1 History

The mechanism of injury may indicate the type of fracture. Direct eye trauma with a blunt object, sometimes of relatively minor energy, may lead to a blow-out fracture of the medial wall and/or the orbital floor, with lateral wall (zygomatico-maxillary) and orbital roof fractures usually requiring a high-energy shock [25, 26, 31]. It is also relevant to ask about past ophthalmic history that may influence the examination (i.e., previous visual problems, strabismus surgery, orbital surgery, etc.). Moreover, as a rule in medicine, it is important to ask about allergies and medications, especially those that may affect the blood coagulation and could increase the risk of orbital haemorrhage.

In cases of severe trauma, where a patient presents with loss of consciousness, it is not possible to obtain a full medical and surgical history. In these cases a collateral history should be sought from witnesses or emergency services. On occasion it may be necessary to perform diagnostic or even therapeutic measures without knowing a full history in potential life or vision threatening injuries.

6.2 External and Ophthalmic Examination

The external examination gives useful information in cases of periocular trauma. Specific signs may guide diagnosis. Palpation may demonstrate "step-offs" in orbital rim fractures, or the presence of emphysema in medial/floor fractures [15, 27].

A comprehensive ophthalmic examination is very important and must always be done during the initial phase, and should include:

- Visual acuity and visual field (confrontation)
- Colour vision
- Slit-lamp examination
- Intraocular pressure
- Ocular fundus

- Pupillary responses
- Ocular motility (see below)

6.3 Ocular Motility and Orthoptics

Orbital trauma commonly affects ocular motility and can be dependent on soft tissue oedema and haemorrhage, soft tissue/muscle entrapment into the fracture lines, and be associated with motor nerve palsits and brain injuries.

Although a full orthoptic examination is also desirable, it is usually difficult in the acute phase and often deferred until resolution of swelling.

On admission, if the patient cooperates, ocular motility in all gazes should be examined, paying attention to any restriction. Clinical photographs may be of help to study the ocular motility in these cases.

A forced duction test may be performed to exclude muscle entrapment. It should be done under anaesthesia, either under topical or as a prelude to operative intervention.

Full orthoptic evaluation, including the Hess-Lancaster test or video-oculography, is important in the follow-up of these patients, as motility impairment and diplopia are reported in up to 82%. Independent of the aetiology, the strabismus is likely to change post operatively, and sequential orthoptic measurements are frequently needed during the first 6 months after injury [32].

6.4 Neuroimaging

Neuroimaging plays a central role both in the initial diagnosis and in the treatment plan for these patients.

- CT scan is the test of choice in orbital trauma: it allows excellent visualisation of the bony structures and gives information about the anatomical integrity of soft tissues.
- X-ray (Water, Caldwell, Rhesse, and lateral) may be useful in specific cases, floor fractures or intra-orbital foreign bodies can be diagnosed with these techniques, but they are indicated only if a CT-scan is not available.
- MRI is not usually needed in most cases of orbital trauma. It may be useful to study some structures in-depth and investigate complications concerning the optic nerve, extraocular muscles, etc. MRI is contraindicated if a metallic foreign body is suspected.

The modern techniques of virtual surgical planning and navigation might be useful in complex cases; they allow pre-operative planning and a very accurate orbital navigation during surgery. However, they are expensive and only available in tertiary referral centres [15, 25–28].

7 Surgical Approach

The orbital contents can be approached via the skin or conjunctiva. Whilst the final choice comes down to surgeon preference there is evidence of better outcome with the latter approach [33].

Surgery entails an extraperiosteal approach to the fracture site and elevation of all the soft tissue from the defect, this described in detail by Evans [34].

7.1 Evolution of Materials Used in Fracture Repair

The goal of orbital repair is to free incarcerated soft tissue by bridging the defect(s) with autologous, allogenic, or alloplastic materials, and to restore orbital volume [35]. A wide variety of materials have been used for this purpose, each with its own advantages and disadvantages. However, there is still no consensus on which material is the most effective. An ideal material should be biocompatible, dimensionally stable, resistant to infection, radio-opaque, non-carcinogenic, and easy to manipulate and maintain in position. Ideally it would be readily affordable.

Whilst there is no internationally accepted universal evidence based operating procedure, most surgeons recommend using materials that restore anatomical shape and reliably partition the orbit from adjacent anatomical structures. A variety of autologous materials have been used including naso-septal and auricular cartilage, maxillary and mandibular bone, iliac crest, rib and internal and external calvaria. All these materials share certain problems associated with the morbidity of the donor site and exhibit variable degrees of resorption.

Alloplastic materials avoid donor site morbidity and reduce operating time and can be subdivided into non-resorbable and resorbable materials. A variety of resorbable materials have been used e.g. poly L lactide, polyglactin-910, and polydioxanone sulphate (PDS) [36, 37]. Non-resorbable alloplastic implants are permanent foreign bodies, and late complications, such as infection, extrusion, implant migration, recurrent haemorrhage or residual diplopia, may occur [38], requiring subsequent implant removal, sometimes many years post-operatively. Despite documented failures, silastic was the mainstream material used for many years [39].

In relation to large defects, titanium has been shown to be superior to bone [40], and subsequent refinements in implant shape have followed. Pre-formed anatomical implants based on studies of orbital shape [41] can help restore the complex internal orbital anatomy [42]. The use of more advanced techniques such as computer-aided-design (CAD) and computer-aided-manufacturing (CAM) implants (see below) may prove invaluable in the large orbital defects including those with secondary changes seen in previously operated or delayed cases (Figs. 3, 4) [43].

The choice of implant is largely surgeon-derived within certain fracture types and there is no scientific evidence to support the ideal choice. However, with the aid of modern imaging analysis we will be able to quantitatively assess the surgical results and stability over time of the different materials used, providing important information for future clinical practice.

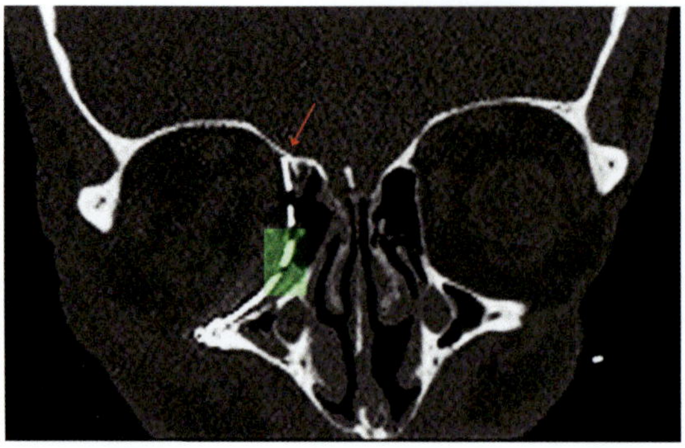

Fig. 3 Coronal CT demonstrating CAD CAM plate in situ. The green box illustrates the junctional zone, and the articulation of the skull base is identified by the red arrow

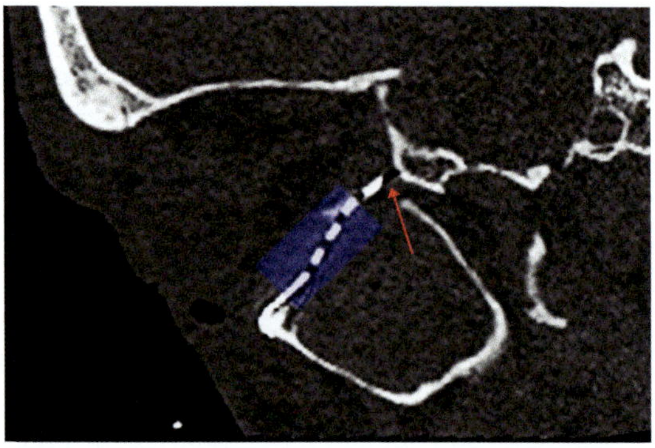

Fig. 4 Sagittal CT showing the posterior articulation—in this case the orbital process of the palatine bone was involved in the fracture (red arrow), the S shaped curvature is also demonstrated (blue box)

7.2 Computer Assisted Surgery: Virtual Planning and Use of Navigation

Computer assisted surgery can be an important tool during the treatment of complex orbital fractures. It is expedient to obtain a virtual pre-operative planning of the desired reconstruction using pre-operative CT scans and adequate software.

Several studies have highlighted how CAD and CAM technologies may support the orbital reconstruction procedure, providing a customised implant for reconstruction directly on the patient's anatomy. The CAD-CAM systems available on the market allow reconstruction work with preformed plates, laser synthesising customised plates, or hand-crafting plates on a stereolithographic model [43, 44].

The main indications for orbital navigation are complex orbital fractures, especially those involving more than one wall and approaching the orbital apex or orbital roof, for example, Jaquiery IV and V patterns [45]. The goals of the surgery are to restore the orbital frame and volume, prevent enophthalmos, avoid extraocular muscle restriction and visual disturbance, and finally to obtain an adequate aesthetic result.

Jaquiery Category	
I	Isolated defect of orbital floor or medial wall, 1–2 cm^2 within anterior two thirds
II	Defect of orbital floor and/or medial wall >2 cm^2 within anterior two thirds with preservation of medial ledge
III	Defect of orbital floor and/or medial wall >2 cm^2 within anterior two thirds with missing medial ledge
IV	Defect of entire orbital floor and medial wall extending into posterior third with missing bone ledge medially
V	Defect of entire orbital floor and medial wall extending into posterior third with missing bone ledge medially and defect extends into orbital roof

Pre-surgical Planning: The first step is to obtain a computer tomography (CT) scan of high-resolution with a 0.5 mm slice and multiplanar views consisting of axial, coronal, sagittal and 3D-reconstruction. Fiducial markers can be fixed to dental splints or titanium bone screws (at least 3–5 screws) can be inserted into the skull prior to CT scanning. Skin fiducials or laser surface scanning are applicable only if the soft tissue is intact.

Various types of software have been developed for imaging management and manipulation for surgical navigation (one of the most commonly used is iPlan Cranial Brainlab, Munich, Germany). Digital Imaging and Communications in Medicine (DICOM) of the CT scan is used to perform the correct orbital orientation and obtain the orbital auto segmentation of the unaffected side. In the case of a unilateral fracture, it is possible to perform the mirroring using the DICOM data of the specular contralateral orbit as a reference for the reconstruction of the bone defect. During this phase a virtual insertion of an anatomically preformed titanium mesh can be performed. The implant can be pre-modeled on a stereolithographic 3 D model, pre-printed by exporting the patient's Standard Triangulation Language (STL) files of the skull. The skull model can be the exact reproduction of the patient's anatomy or can be printed using the mirroring of the unaffected orbital side. The stereolithographic model can easily be printed by means of a modern 3D printer, also in-house [46] The model facilitates surgery during the phase of mesh modelling (Fig. 5a–c), which will be implanted during the surgery. Alternatively, if preformed meshes are used, the adequacy of the reconstruction can be verified with the virtual insertion of the mesh, this tool allowing a pre-operative selection of the correct implant size. The virtual orbital reconstruction facilitates a correct 3-dimensional positioning of the virtual implant.

Intra-operative navigation: The first stage of surgery involves the recording phase of the patient; a tracking of the patient's head is obtained

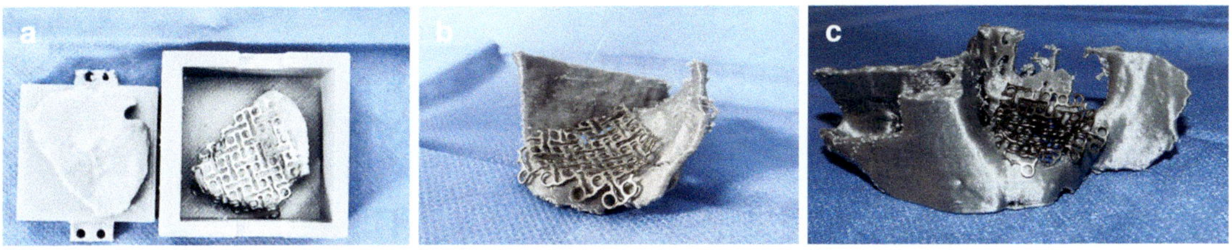

Fig. 5 (**a**) Shaping of the titanium mesh and its accurate fitting to the orbital floor printed model. (**b**) Mirrored orbit model. (**c**) Involved orbit model

with a dynamic reference frame (DRF) attached to the Mayfield clamp, or the patient's parietal bone. The CT data need to be imported into the Surgical Navigator and it is necessary to match the patients within the surgical area. For intra-operative recording, a star-shaped tool is needed, which is fixed directly onto the skull.

Localization: The optical references consist of reflective spheres that the navigator identifies through infrared video cameras. Landmarks, which were defined during the planning stage, are identified.

The surgical steps are no different from those adopted during traditional surgery. However, navigation allows the surgeon to check instantaneously the position of the surgical instrument on the CT images and to verify, during the surgery, if the reconstruction has been performed properly according to the pre-surgical planning (Fig. 6a–c).

After the operation it is possible to confirm the adequacy of the procedure by performing a CT scan. Thanks to the common software used, the analysis of the pre-operative and post-operative images is conducted by means of merging the pre-operative and post-operative images and comparing the reduction and/or reconstruction quality (Fig. 7).

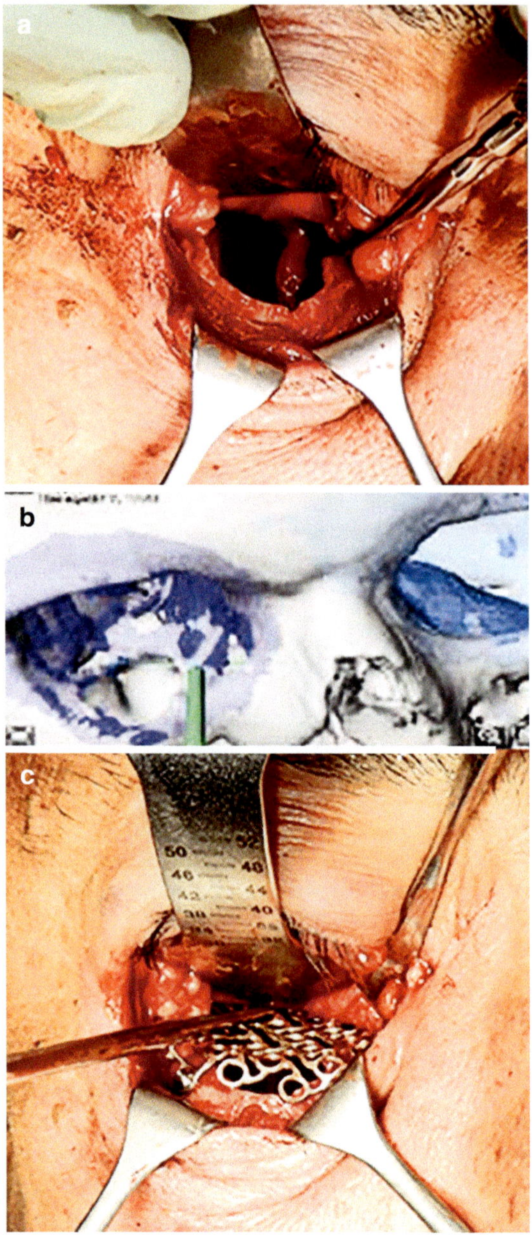

Fig. 6 (**a**) Right orbital floor defect. (**b**) Checking under navigator control. (**c**) Patient-specific mesh placement

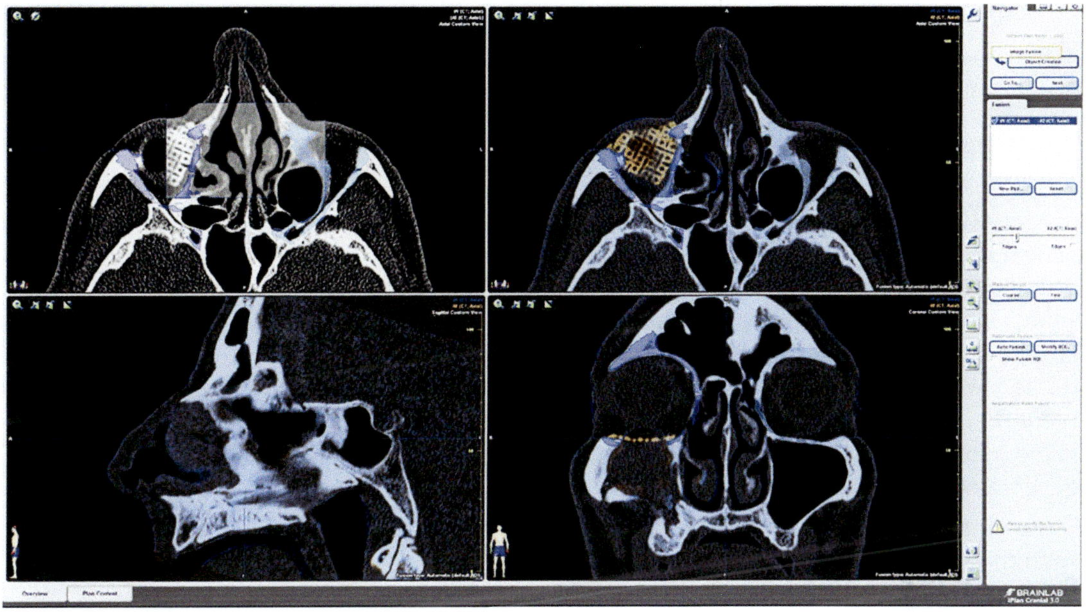

Fig. 7 Point-to-point discrepancy measurement on the overlap analysis in iPlan Cranial 3.0

8 Aftercare

The diagnosis and pre-and post-operative care of orbital injuries requires a multidisciplinary approach for optimal results.

The multidisciplinary team includes the orbital surgeon, ophthalmologist, and the orthoptist, and the injury pattern and collateral damage is carefully assessed and documented.

Following emergency management, patients are seen in the first weeks by both the orbital surgeon, the ophthalmologist and at least twice by the orthoptist for objective measurements to be recorded.

If, after the initial swelling has subsided, diplopia or an aesthetically disturbing enophthalmos is not present, the patient is seen at 6, 12, 26, and 52 weeks after trauma by either the orbital surgeon or ophthalmologist. Orthoptic reassessment is indicated to manage post-operative diplopia and referral to a strabismus surgeon as required. During these follow up consultations, subjective and objective diplopia, globe position, skin sensation, and Hertel measurements are checked and noted in the charts. Clinical photographs are taken at timepoints 6 and 52 weeks.

In cases where the initial swelling has subsided, but diplopia and/or aesthetically disturbing enophthalmos is present, surgical options are discussed with the patient.

In surgical cases the patient is ideally operated within 1–2 weeks, with one post-operative night stay for eye observations and pain control. Hourly vision checks are performed until 6 hours after the procedure, as this is the time window where most post-operative haemorrhage occurs. Thereafter, vision checks may continue every 2 hours until the next day, being the day of discharge. Depending on the implant used antibiotics and analgesics are prescribed and the patient is advised not to blow the nose or sneeze with a closed nose for 3 weeks. The patient is seen at 1 week, 3 weeks, 6, 12, 26 and 52 weeks after surgery by the orbital surgeon, and by the ophthalmologist, should there be evidence of ocular dysfunction. The orthoptist is consulted at 3 weeks and as indicated according to diplopia progression. Clinical photographs are taken at timepoints 6 and 52 weeks [47, 48].

9 Post-operative Imaging

The discussions around indications are unnecessarily controversial and articulated well by Paul Manson [49] with respect to zygomatic—orbital fractures. Whilst there is a degree of tolerance for a poorly positioned orbital plate, the anatomical complexity of the repair and proximity to vital structures together with functional compromise with impingement of ocular muscles demands radiological surveillance. In cases of bioresorbable membranes which are difficult to identify on post-operative scans there is less of an indication. One of the advantages of navigation, particularly with screen capture is the avoidance of a post-operative scan, provided there is no ocular dysmotility.

References

1. Ruslin M, Brucoli M, Boffano P, Benech A, Dediol E, Uglesic V, et al. Motor vehicle accidents-related maxillofacial injuries: a multicentre and prospective study. Oral Surg Oral Med Oral Pathol Oral Radiol. 2019;128:199–204.
2. Brucoli M, Boffano P, Broccardo E, Benech A, Corre P, Bertin H, et al. The “European zygomatic fracture” research project: the epidemiological results from a multicenter European collaboration. J Craniomaxillofac Surg. 2019;47:616–21.
3. Boffano P, Roccia F, Zavattero E, Dediol E, Uglesic V, Kovacic Z, et al. European maxillofacial trauma (EURMAT) project: a multicentre and prospective study. J Craniomaxillofac Surg. 2015;43:62–70.
4. Boffano P, Kommers SC, Karagozoglu KH, Forouzanfar T. Aetiology of maxillofacial fractures: a review of published studies during the last 30 years. Br J Oral Maxillofac Surg. 2014;52:901–6.
5. Lalloo R, Lucchesi LR, Bisignano C, Castle CD, Dingels ZV, Fox JT, et al. Epidemiology of facial fractures: incidence, prevalence and years lived with disability estimates from the global burden of disease 2017 study. Inj Prev. 2020;26:i27–35.
6. Moffatt J, Hughes D, Bhatti N, Holmes S. Orbital bone fractures in a Central London trauma center: a retrospective study of 582 patients. J Craniofac Surg. 2021;32:1334; Publish Ahead of Print.
7. Catherine Z, Courvoisier DS, Scolozzi P. Is the pure and impure distinction of orbital fractures clinically relevant with respect to ocular and periocular injuries? A retrospective study of 473 patients. J Craniomaxillofac Surg. 2019;47:1935–42.
8. Shere JLBJ, Holtel M, Amorosa PJ. An analysis of 3599 midfacial and 1141 orbital blowout fractures among 4426 United States Army soldiers 1980-2. Otolaryngol Head Neck Surg. 2004;130:164–70.
9. Louis M, Agrawal N, Kaufman M, Truong TA. Midface fractures I. Semin Plast Surg. 2017;31:85–93.
10. Manana W, Odhiambo WA, Chindia ML, Koech K. The pattern of orbital fractures managed at two referral centers in Nairobi, Kenya. J Craniofac Surg. 2017;28:e338–e42.
11. Converse JMSB, Obear MF, Woos-Smith D. Orbital blowout fractures: a ten-year survey. Plast Reconstr Surg. 1967;39:20–36.
12. Cramer LM, Tooze FM, Lerman S. Blowout fractures of the orbit. Br J Plast Surg. 1965;18:171–9.
13. Pfeiffer R. Traumatic enophthalmos. Arch Ophthamol. 1943;30:293–304.
14. Kunz C, Audige L, Cornelius CP, Buitrago-Tellez CH, Rudderman R, Prein J. The comprehensive AOCMF classification system: orbital fractures—level 3 tutorial. Craniomaxillofac Trauma Reconstr. 2014;7:S092–102.
15. Lozada KN, Cleveland PW, Smith JE. Orbital trauma. Semin Plast Surg. 2019;33:106–13.
16. Kunz C, Audige L, Cornelius CP, Buitrago-Tellez CH, Frodel J, Rudderman R, et al. The comprehensive AOCMF classification system: midface fractures—level 2 tutorial. Craniomaxillofac Trauma Reconstr. 2014;7:S059–67.
17. Tessier P. The classic reprint. Experimental study of fractures of the upper jaw. I and II. Rene Le Fort, M.D. Plast Reconstr Surg. 1972;50:497–506; contd.
18. Hink EM, Wei LA, Durairaj VD. Clinical features and treatment of pediatric orbit fractures. Ophthalmic Plast Reconstr Surg. 2014;30:124–31.

19. Oppenheimer AJ, Monson LA, Buchman SR. Pediatric orbital fractures. Craniomaxillofac Trauma Reconstr. 2013;6:9–20.
20. Fortunato MA, Fielding AF, Guernsey LH. Facial bone fractures in children. Oral Surg Oral Med Oral Pathol. 1982;53:225–30.
21. Koltai PJ, Amjad I, Meyer D, Feustel PJ. Orbital fractures in children. Arch Otolaryngol Head Neck Surg. 1995;121:1375–9.
22. Holmes SBCJ, Metafa A. Lesson of the week—blunt orbital trauma. BMJ. 2000;321:750–1.
23. Cobb A, Murthy R, Manisali M, Uddin J, Toma A. Oculovagal reflex in paediatric orbital floor fractures mimicking head injury. Emerg Med J. 2009;26:351–3.
24. Gerber B, Kiwanuka P, Dhariwal D. Orbital fractures in children: a review of outcomes. Br J Oral Maxillofac Surg. 2013;51:789–93.
25. Ophthalmology TAao. Basic and clinical science course:orbit, eyelids and lacrimal. System. 2020;1:139–49.
26. Manolidis SWB, Kirby M, Scarlett M, Hollier L. Classification and surgical management of orbital fractures_experience with 111 orbital reconstructions. J Craniofac Surg. 2002;13:726–37.
27. Dolman PRJ. Orbital trauma. Orbital surgery: a conceptual approach. 2nd ed. Philadelphia, PA: Wolters Kluwer Health; 2013.
28. Roth FS, Koshy JC, Goldberg JS, Soparkar CN. Pearls of orbital trauma management. Semin Plast Surg. 2010;24:398–410.
29. Al-Qurainy IASL, Dutton GN, Moos KF, El-Attar. The characteristics of midfacial fractures and the association with ocular injury: a prospective study. Br J Oral Maxillofac Surg. 1991;29:291–301.
30. Karimi S, Arabi A, Ansari I, Shahraki T, Safi S. A systematic literature review on traumatic optic neuropathy. J Ophthalmol. 2021;2021:5553885–10.
31. Cruz AEG. Epidemiology and management of orbital fractures. Curr Opin Ophthalmol. 2004;15:416–21.
32. Braaksma-Besselink Y, Jellema HM. Orthoptic evaluation and treatment in orbital fractures. Atlas Oral Maxillofac Surg Clin North Am. 2021;29:41–50.
33. De Riu G, Meloni SM, Gobbi R, Soma D, Baj A, Tullio A. Subciliary versus swinging eyelid approach to the orbital floor. J Craniomaxillofac Surg. 2008;36:439–42.
34. Evans BT, Webb AA. Post-traumatic orbital reconstruction: anatomical landmarks and the concept of the deep orbit. Br J Oral Maxillofac Surg. 2007;45:183–9.
35. Bite UJI, Forbes GS, Gehring DG. Orbital volume measurements in enophthalmos using three-dimensional CT imaging. Plast Reconstr Surg. 1985;74:502–7.
36. Tuncer SYR, Kandal S, Demir YH, Ozmen S, Latifoglu O, Atabay K. Reconstruction of traumatic orbital floor fractures with resorbable mesh plate. J Craniofac Surg. 2007;18:598–605.
37. Buchel P, Rahal A, Seto I, Iizuka T. Reconstruction of orbital floor fracture with polyglactin 910/polydioxanon patch (ethisorb): a retrospective study. J Oral Maxillofac Surg. 2005;63:646–50.
38. Morrison ADSC, Moos KF. The use of silastic as an orbital implant for reconstruction of orbital wall defect. J Oral Maxillofac Surg. 1995;53:412–7.
39. Courtney DJ, Thomas S, Whitfield PH. Isolated orbital blowout fractures: survey and review. Br J Oral Maxillofac Surg. 2000;38:496–504.
40. Ellis E 3rd, Tan Y. Assessment of internal orbital reconstructions for pure blowout fractures: cranial bone grafts versus titanium mesh. J Oral Maxillofac Surg. 2003;61:442–53.
41. Metzger MC, Schon R, Tetzlaf R, Weyer N, Rafii A, Gellrich NC, et al. Topographical CT-data analysis of the human orbital floor. Int J Oral Maxillofac Surg. 2007;36:45–53.
42. Scolozzi P, Momjian A, Heuberger J, Andersen E, Broome M, Terzic A, et al. Accuracy and predictability in use of AO three-dimensionally preformed titanium mesh plates for posttraumatic orbital reconstruction: a pilot study. J Craniofac Surg. 2009;20:1108–13.
43. Bhatti N, Kanzaria A, Huxham-Owen N, Bridle C, Holmes S. Management of complex orbital fractures. Br J Oral Maxillofac Surg. 2016;54:719–23.
44. Mustafa SF, Evans PL, Bocca A, Patton DW, Sugar AW, Baxter PW. Customized titanium reconstruction of post-traumatic orbital wall defects: a review of 22 cases. Int J Oral Maxillofac Surg. 2011;40:1357–62.
45. Jaquiery C, Aeppli C, Cornelius P, Palmowsky A, Kunz C, Hammer B. Reconstruction of orbital wall defects: critical review of 72 patients. Int J Oral Maxillofac Surg. 2007;36:193–9.
46. Maglitto F, Dell'Aversana Orabona G, Committeri U, Salzano G, De Fazio GR, Vaira LA, et al. Virtual surgical planning and the "in-house" rapid prototyping technique in maxillofacial surgery: the current situation and future perspectives. Appl Sci. 2021; 11:1.
47. Holmes S, Perry M, McQuillan J, White S. Orbital fractures. In: Atlas of operative maxillofacial trauma surgery. London: Springer; 2014. p. 359–439.
48. Holmes S, Bhatti N. Secondary management of the orbit. In: Atlas of operative maxillofacial trauma surgery—post traumatic deformity. London: Springer; 2020.
49. Manson PN. Commentary on: the role of postoperative imaging after orbital floor repair. Craniomaxillofac Trauma Reconstr. 2018;11:102–3.

Part III

Thyroid-Associated Orbitopathy

Clinical Manifestations of Thyroid-Associated Orbitopathy

Onur Konuk, Segun Awotesu, and Raghavan Sampath

Key Messages

- Thyroid-associated orbitopathy (TAO) is an autoimmune mediated disease that typically affects middle-aged females. It has been described as having a biphasic curve characterised by inflammation, stabilisation, and regression. Clinical features include signs of inflammation, lid retraction, lid lag, proptosis and extraocular motility problems.
- TAO is typically seen in the context of Graves hyperthyroidism but may also occur in euthyroid and hypothyroid patients as well. Diagnosis is clinically based but may also be aided by laboratory studies and imaging of the orbit. Imaging may show two broad groups; one in which muscle enlargement predominates and a second group with marked orbital fat enlargement.
- Disease activity refers to the presence of inflammatory features more prominent in the early stages of the condition, whilst severity describes the disease burden on the patient.
- Different evaluation protocols have been described to guide when intervention is indicated such as the clinical activity scale.
- Disease severity ranges from mild, which is amenable to conservative measures, to severe disease, this needing prompt medical and or surgical intervention.
- Severe sequelae include exposure keratopathy and optic neuropathy, these manifesting with visual disturbance and a range of clinical signs.

1 Introduction

Graves' orbitopathy (GO), or thyroid-associated orbitopathy (TAO), is a major extrathyroidal manifestation of Graves' disease. The pathophysiological pathway of this autoimmune disorder is still obscure, but the most common theory is that TAO is triggered by an immune reaction against one or more antigens shared by the thyroid and orbit. The thyrotropin (TSH) receptor and insulin-like growth factor-1 (IGF-1) receptor are the most popular targets, and their relationship with the occurrence of orbital disease and related treatment protocols are still under investigation [1, 2]. The estimated incidence of TAO is 0.54–0.9 cases/100,000/year in men, 2.67–3.3 cases/100,000/year in women [3, 4]. A recent study from the European Group on Graves' Orbitopathy (EUGOGO) reported the approximate prevalence of TAO of all degrees in Europe between 90 and 155/100,000 population [5].

O. Konuk (✉)
Department of Ophthalmology, Oculoplastic and Orbital Unit, Gazi University Medical School, Ankara, Turkey
e-mail: dronurkonuk@yahoo.com

S. Awotesu
Ophthalmology Department, Leicester Royal Infirmary, Leicester, UK

R. Sampath
Department of Ophthalmology, University Hospitals of Leicester NHS Trust, Leicester Royal Infirmary, Leicester, UK

F. M. Quaranta Leoni et al. (eds.), *Oculoplastic, Lacrimal and Orbital Surgery*,
https://doi.org/10.1007/978-3-031-39638-0_32

TAO develops in up to 45% of patients with thyroid disease [6]. Of these, 3–5% develop more severe features such as soft tissue congestion, impaired motility, or compressive optic neuropathy [7, 8]. Tanda et al. [9] reported less than 3% progression to moderate-to-severe TAO in a series of 346 recent onset and untreated Graves' patients. In another study 196 Graves' patients were evaluated and 81 (41%) developed TAO [10].

The natural course of TAO was described by Rundle and Wilson [11], modelled in two stages for evaluating the clinical findings and predicting the therapeutic results. It is proposed that the clinical features of TAO are initially inflammatory in nature (the active phase), including oedema, redness, and pain in the periorbital area. This phase is usually seen within 18 months before or after the onset of thyroid disease. The inflammatory findings stabilise and subside within 18–24 months with resultant sequelae of TAO (inactive phase) [12, 13].

2 Diagnosis

Early diagnosis of TAO is important to prevent progression to more severe stages. A careful examination by an endocrinologist, internist, or ophthalmologist plays a vital role in the detection of early clinical findings and determining the activity and severity of TAO. Combined thyroid eye clinics which include an endocrinologist and an ophthalmologist have a critical role in optimising the strategy for evaluation and treatment [14].

The diagnosis of TAO is usually based on clinical and laboratory criteria. Exophthalmos, periorbital soft tissue inflammation, eyelid retraction and strabismus in a patient with known Graves' thyrotoxicosis is usually sufficient for the diagnosis of TAO. However, euthyroid and unilateral or asymmetric orbital involvement may require additional clinical and radiological examination to elucidate the diagnosis.

3 Symptoms and Clinical Features

In clinical practice, most patients have no or mild ocular signs. These changes are usually recognized by friends, family relatives, or detected in photographs. In more severe forms of the disease, patients usually present with soft tissue inflammatory signs of TAO such as excessive tearing, ocular irritation, grittiness, photophobia, ocular redness, eyelid swelling, and pain. In some cases diplopia and blurred vision with a decrease in visual acuity may occur with the progression of orbital inflammation. These symptoms usually correspond to the clinical findings of eyelid retraction, redness of the eyelids and conjunctiva, and swelling of the eyelids, caruncle, and conjunctiva (chemosis) [7]. Other symptoms including proptosis, limitation of eye movements, superficial punctate keratitis or ulceration, and decrease in visual acuity due to optic nerve involvement usually demonstrate progression in the severity of ophthalmic involvement [15].

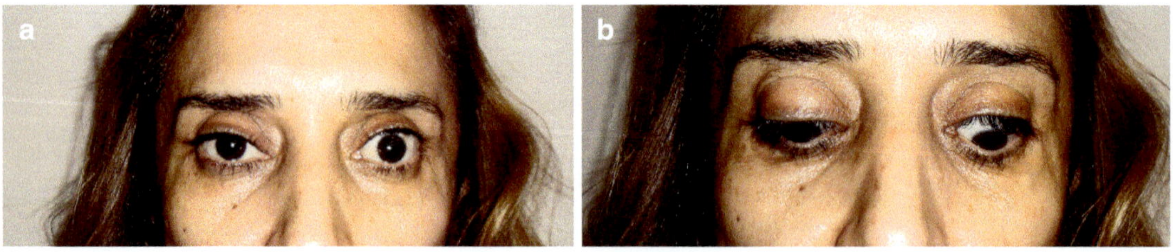

Fig. 1 (**a**, **b**) Upper eyelid retraction is the most common clinical feature of thyroid-associated orbitopathy. It is characterized by *lid lag* in down gaze

3.1 Upper Eyelid Retraction

Upper eyelid retraction (see Chapter "Management of Eyelid Retraction") can lead to the classic "thyroid stare" which can change with fixation or emotion (Dalrymple's sign), and which is usually associated with *lid lag* during down gaze (Von Graefe's sign), or spasmodic eyelid overaction on up gaze (Kocher's sign) (Fig. 1). The exact cause of upper eyelid retraction is not understood. There are three proposed mechanisms. First, increased muscle activity of levator palpebralis superior muscle (which may be isolated or secondary to inferior rectus restriction), and increased hyperreactivity of Muller's muscle to sympathomimetic stimulus that is supposed to be due to adrenergic activity of increased thyroid hormones. Second, the inflammation of the levator-Müller muscle complex ends up with fibrosis and causes shortening of the upper eyelid retractors. And third, extreme proptosis may rarely cause upper eyelid retraction in which the eyelid settles on the equator of the globe rather than the cornea [16].

3.2 Adnexal Inflammation and Congestion

Symptoms of adnexal inflammation are periorbital pain, eyelid oedema and redness, conjunctival redness, caruncular oedema and chemosis [7] (Fig. 2). Diurnal variation with worsening of the symptoms in the morning is more evident in the early active stages of the disease. All these symptoms and findings are subjective and may change during the daytime. Additionally, their interpretation depends on the examiners' experience. It is very important to distinguish between pain due to inflammation of the adnexal and orbital tissues, and pain due to corneal exposure. Similarly, conjunctival redness can be a sign of inflammation or exposure of the ocular surface and dry eye. Periorbital oedema can easily be confused with orbital fat prolapse. More importantly, it may be difficult to differentiate inflammatory findings from orbital congestion [17]. Both pathophysiological mechanisms give the same clinical findings but may need different management strategies. The predictability of these assessments may be improved by repeated examinations and by using a reference atlas of standardised photos of the patient [15].

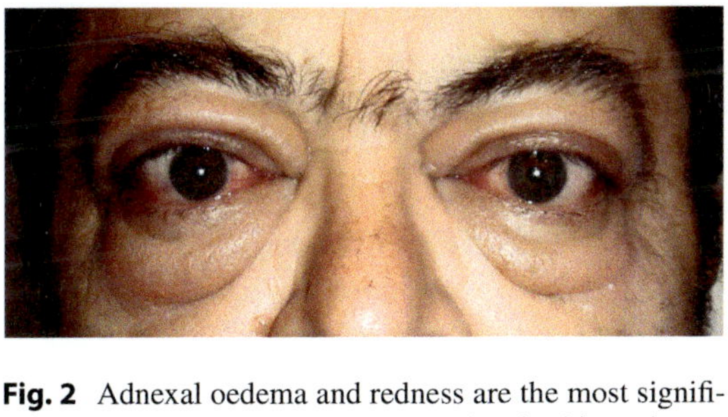

Fig. 2 Adnexal oedema and redness are the most significant findings for active thyroid-associated orbitopathy

3.3 Proptosis

Proptosis (exophthalmos) is one of the most common symptoms of TAO that usually needs surgical correction for both functional and cosmetic reasons (Fig. 3). Orbital inflammation causes an increase of extraocular muscles and orbital fibroadipose tissue volume in combination with the possible role of orbital vascular congestion in the restricted area of bony orbit is the primary cause of prominent globes. The degree of proptosis is measured between the apex of the cornea and the anterior surface of the bony lateral orbital rim in millimetres with an exopthalmometer. The values show a wide range in healthy individuals depending on the race and gender [18–20]. An asymmetry more than 2 mm between the two eyes suggests proptosis, as well as values more than

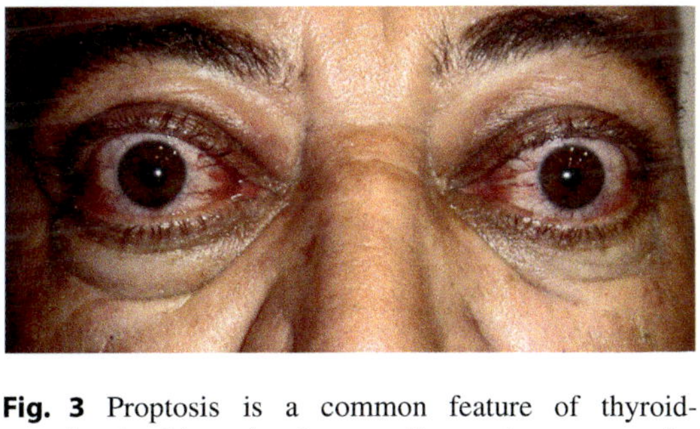

Fig. 3 Proptosis is a common feature of thyroid-associated orbitopathy that usually requires surgery for both functional and cosmetic reasons

16–18 mm for Asians, 18–20 mm for Caucasians, and 20–22 mm for patients of African ancestry may be diagnosed as proptosis [21, 22]. Hertel exophthalmometry is the most popular instrument for evaluating proptosis, however it requires the patient to have intact lateral orbital rims. In cases with disturbed lateral rim due to previous decompression or tumour surgery, a Naugle exophthalmometer can be used as its fixation points are slightly above and below the superior and inferior orbital rims.

3.4 Strabismus

The effect of thyroid disease on the extraocular muscles occurs in two phases. The first stage is the inflammatory phase which is characterised by lymphocytic infiltration of the extraocular muscles and orbital tissues. The second shows fibrosis of the tissues with a decrease of inflammation. The inferior and medial recti muscles are mostly involved, resulting in hypotropia and esotropia (Fig. 4). Although the oblique muscles are rarely involved, any of the rectus muscles can be involved, leading to any type of strabismus [23] (see chapter "Strabismus in Thyroid-Associated Orbitopathy").

3.5 Exposure Keratopathy

Corneal involvement is usually seen in moderate to severe cases of TAO due to severe proptosis or upper eyelid retraction. In early cases, foreign body sensation and mild hyperemia of the conjunctiva is the main symptom that can be easily treated with ocular lubrication. In more severe forms of corneal exposure, ulceration, keratitis, and corneal perforation can be encountered. In these cases, frequent lubrication of the ocular surface, temporary tarsorrhaphy, recession of upper eyelid retractors, and orbital decompression should be performed [24].

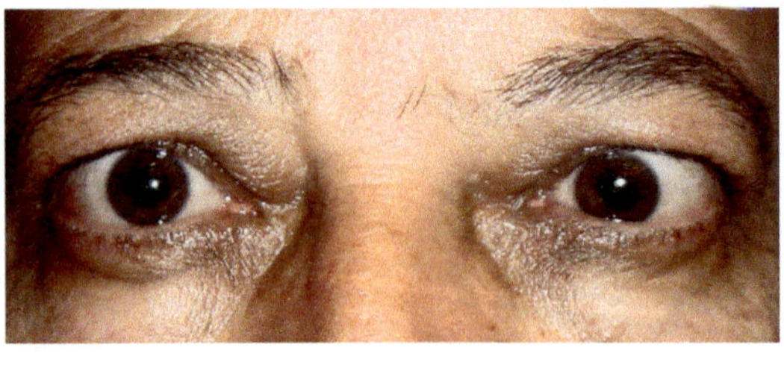

Fig. 4 Involvement of inferior and medial recti muscles is typical for thyroid-associated orbitopathy, presenting with hypotropia and esotropia

3.6 Dysthyroid Optic Neuropathy

The clinical features of dysthyroid optic neuropathy (DON) are decrease of visual acuity, loss of contrast sensitivity and visual field, relative afferent pupillary defect and optic disc oedema. A patient with DON may have a normal appearing disc, but the presence of disc swelling, if present, is a very specific indicator of DON. Proptosis if present is not correlated with DON. It is important to be aware that patients with minimal or no proptosis may develop DON [25] (Fig. 5). The proposed causes of optic nerve dysfunction were reported as increased retrobulbar pressure and mechanical compression on the optic nerve at the orbital apex by enlarged extraocular muscles. The optimum management strategy for DON is controversial. Systemic corticosteroids are the treatment of choice as a first line treatment in most cases, but orbital decompression by removal of one or more orbital walls may provide an improvement in visual functions if steroid therapy fails (see chapter "Dysthyroid Optic Neuropathy") [24–29].

4 Laboratory and Radiological Findings

TAO is mainly based on clinical findings. Laboratory tests and radiology investigations can be used to confirm the TAO when clinical features are equivocal or atypical. Elevated serum levels of serum thyroxine or triiodothyronine and decreased TSH levels and the absence of thyroid radioiodine uptake suppression after administration of triiodothyronine of thyroid is suggestive of thyroid dysfunction [4].

The presence of TSH receptor antibodies (TrAb), thyroid peroxidase antibodies and thyroid stimulating immunoglobulins e.g. anti-

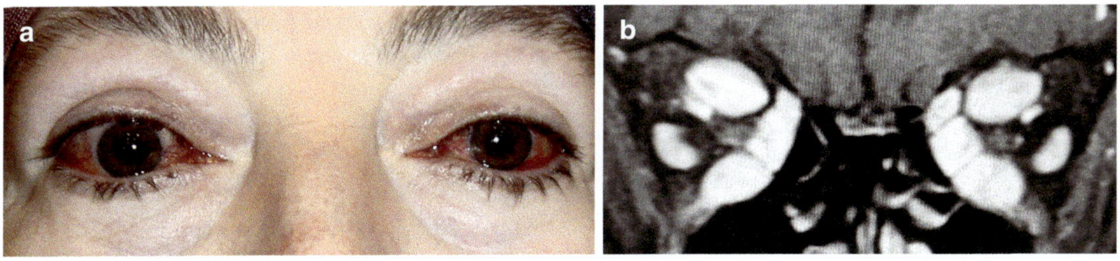

Fig. 5 A case of dysthyroid ophthalmopathy (**a**) showing enlarged extraocular muscles in MRI (**b**). Note that proptosis may not be encountered in some cases

thyroglobulin can also be tested. There is positive correlation with the levels of TrAb values and severity of TAO, and this antibody can therefore be a marker for the management protocols and follow up period [1].

Ultrasonography (USG) can be used to visualise the orbital structures and to determine recti muscle enlargement in TAO, and USG findings may correlate with CAS [30–32]. Advantages of this modality is its low cost, lack of ionising radiation and relatively short examination time. The role of orbital USG is limited by intra and inter observer variability and the inability to image the orbital apex and bony structures [30]. Several studies evaluated orbital doppler imaging of the superior ophthalmic vein (SOV) velocity with disease severity. Monteiro et al. [33] showed significantly reduced SOV flow in patients with active congestive orbitopathy or myogenic fibrotic TAO. Similar studies have also shown that a decrease in flow velocity in orbital veins correlates with disease severity [34, 35].

Computed tomography (CT) is often the first imaging modality of choice not only for the differential diagnosis of TAO, but also for surgical planning for orbital decompression. CT evaluates the bony orbit and sinus walls due to its ability to demonstrate both bony and soft tissue pathology. Several studies have evaluated the success of CT in assessing disease activity [36, 37]. CT findings can be used to predict the presence of optic neuropathy in patients with TAO. Several early studies established a quantitative relationship between DON and extraocular muscle enlargement, pointing to a compressive aetiology [38, 39].

Magnetic resonance imaging (MRI) gives detailed images of orbital softs tissues and can measure interstitial oedema especially in extraocular muscles and fat. The particular limitations are its inability to show bony details, long timing of the procedure, and its relatively high cost. Additionally, it cannot be used in patients with metallic implants, and those with electronic cardiac devices require special evaluation before imaging can be performed [40].

MRI is considered superior to CT in assessing disease activity in TAO. Several studies have found a relationship between MRI signal intensity and disease severity, emphasising that inflammatory and oedematous muscular changes are central to active disease [40–44].

5 Disease Activity and Severity

The diagnosis of TAO is quite straightforward in cases with hyperthyroidism, bilateral exophthalmos, eyelid oedema and retraction, and strabismus [7, 8]. However, it is essential to detect early cases and identify high-risk patients and evaluate the activity and severity of the disease to predict the treatment outcome with either medical or surgical interventions. In clinical practice the term *activity*, and the protocols to evaluate clinical activity, are usually used to differentiate the early inflammatory phase from chronic fibrotic phase of the disease. Patients with active inflammatory findings typically show improvement with medical anti-inflammatory treatment, whereas those in the chronic fibrotic phase are usually resistant to anti-inflammatory treatment but significantly improve with appropriate surgical treatment options [8–11]. The term *severity* refers to the extent of orbital involvement and is graded as 'disease severity'. The evaluation protocols for disease severity are used to standardise and optimise the follow up and treatment protocols as much as possible.

5.1 Evaluation of Disease Activity

5.1.1 Disease Duration

It was Rundle [11] who first attempted to explain the natural history of the TAO and developed a model known as "Rundle's curve" (Fig. 6). Rundle reported that the disease has an initial progressive phase lasting a few months, followed by a plateau phase, and then a slow progressive improving phase, which may last several years. Menconi et al. [45] again later questioned this in 2014 and agreed that peak activity is encountered between 13 and 24 months. It is shown that disease duration less than 16 months can be a predictor for positive results for immunosuppressive treatment [46]. Similarly, in patients with moderate-to-severe and active TAO, the results of immunosuppressive treatment are usually better if treatment starts within 1 year from the onset of TAO [47].

5.1.2 Clinical Activity Score

In 1989 Mourits et al. [48] created the clinical activity score based on features of acute inflammation aimed at identifying active disease. This score has been modified subsequently to include four out of five features of inflammation, namely pain, redness, swelling, and impaired function [49] (Table 1). For each item present a point is given, and the sum of these is the clinical activity score (CAS). The score has a maximum of 7 at the initial examination and 10 at subsequent visits. Clinically "active" TAO is defined as a score of 3/7 initially or 4/10 at follow-up examination. Chemosis, caruncle swelling, increase in proptosis, decrease in motility and visual acuity, although present only in a small minority of patients, were all highly specific for disease activity and therapeutic outcome [49]. The CAS score of 4 or higher has been shown to have an 80% positive predictive value and a 64% negative predictive value in predicting response to corticosteroid therapy [48].

One criticism of the CAS scoring model is that it is a binary response assessment, and it scores each finding equally as 1 point. This raises a potential problem as less serious signs like eye-

Table 1 The clinical activity score (CAS)

Pain	Spontaneous orbital pain	+1
	Gaze evoked orbital pain	+1
Redness	Conjunctival redness	+1
	Eyelid erythema	+1
Swelling	Eyelid swelling	+1
	Chemosis	+1
	Caruncle/Plica swelling	+1
	Increase of >2 mm in proptosis	+1
Impaired function	**Decrease in uniocular excursion >8 degrees**	+1
	Decrease of 1 line Snellen Acuity	+1
Total	**Active: >3/7—at initial exam**	
	Active: >4/10 at successive exam	

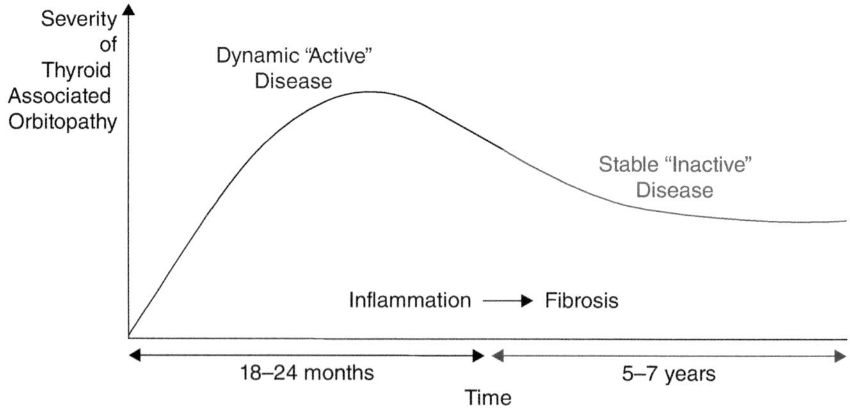

Fig. 6 Rundle's curve

lid redness have the same score with the more serious signs such as drop in one line of Snellen Visual Acuity which may be a finding for DON. Additionally, patients with high CAS scores may have long-standing congestive changes that are unresponsive to any immunotherapy. Additionally, severe disease complications such as DON, eyelid retraction, or proptosis may develop despite low CAS scores [50].

5.2 Disease Severity

There have been many classification methods used to grade TAO. Each of these methods have their own advantages and limitations.

The NOSPECS was first developed in 1969 and has six grades; Grade 0 (N) being no signs or symptoms, Grade I (O) is only limited signs such as *lid lag* or retraction, Grade II (S) is involvement of soft tissues, Grade III (P) is the presence of proptosis, and Grade IV (E) is the extraocular muscle involvement, Grade V (C) represents corneal involvement, and Grade VI (S) shows the optic nerve involvement and sight loss [51]. This classification is practical with its mnemonic and useful for determining disease severity but does not make a distinction between inflammatory progressive disease from stable non inflammatory disease [52].

The current grading methods used for the assessment of TAO are European Group of Graves' Orbitopathy (EUGOGO) Classification [24], and the VISA Classification (vision, inflammation strabismus, and appearance) [53] (Table 2). VISA is more commonly used in North America and Canada, while EUGOGO is in Europe. These protocols are not interchangeable, and a single method should be used to follow up each patient.

Table 2 Evaluation of activity in VISA classification

VISA inflammatory score	Total 0-8
Clinical finding	Score
Orbital pain (none, at rest, with gaze)	0-2
Chemosis	0-2
Eyelid oedema	0-2
Conjunctival injection	0-1
Eyelid injection	0-1

The EUGOGO classification assesses disease activity based on the CAS. The system allows comparison of disease parameters with a standardised image atlas [15].

The EUGOGO severity assessment classifies TAO as:

Mild TAO

Patients whose features of TAO have only a minor impact on daily life insufficient to justify immunomodulation or surgical treatment. They usually have one or more of the following:

- minor eyelid retraction (<2 mm)
- mild soft-tissue involvement
- exophthalmos
- <3 mm above normal for race and gender
- no or intermittent diplopia and corneal exposure responsive to lubricants

Moderate-to-severe TAO

Patients without sight-threatening TAO whose eye disease has sufficient impact on daily life to justify the risks of immunosuppression (if active) or surgical intervention (if inactive). They usually have two or more of the following:

- eyelid retraction ≥2 mm
- moderate or severe soft-tissue involvement
- exophthalmos ≥3 mm above normal for race and gender
- inconstant or constant diplopia

Sight-threatening (very severe) TAO

Patients with dysthyroid optic neuropathy and/or significant corneal exposure

The VISA system was developed by Dolman and Rootman [53] and evaluates both TAO activity and severity considering subjective and objective indicators of vision, inflammatory changes, strabismus/motility problems and appearance/exposure. The sequence of the sections reflects the order in which the problems should be managed, with vision being the number one priority. Vision is evaluated by best-corrected visual acuity, pupillary light reflexes, colour vision testing and optic nerve assessment. The primary goal of this section is to rule out TAO optic neuropathy. Inflammation is graded based on symptoms such as orbital pain at rest, and signs including degree of conjunctival chemosis and redness, and eyelid oedema.

The authors modified the CAS and omitted caruncular oedema as a separate sign and graded pain, chemosis and eyelid oedema with a 0–2 scale. They recommend immunosuppressive treatment or RT if the inflammatory grade is 5 or more. Strabismus is assessed by eliciting a history of diplopia from no diplopia, diplopia with horizontal or vertical gaze, intermittent diplopia in straight gaze, and constant diplopia in straight gaze as well as by assessing ocular ductions and prism cover testing using Hirshberg principle and graded from 0° to 45° in four directions. Appearance is assessed subjectively regarding eyelid retraction, proptosis, foreign body sensation or tearing and objectively by measuring levator function, eyelid retraction, Hertel exophthalmometry, and intraocular pressure. All the findings are subjectively graded as the same, better or worse.

References

1. Nicolì F, Lanzolla G, Mantuano M, Ionni I, Mazzi B, Leo M, et al. Correlation between serum anti-TSH receptor autoantibodies (TRAbs) and the clinical feature of Graves' orbitopathy. J Endocrinol Invest. 2021;44:581–5.
2. Smith TJ, Kahaly GJ, Ezra DG, Fleming JC, Dailey RA, Tang RA, et al. Teprotumumab for thyroid-associated ophthalmopathy. N Engl J Med. 2017;376:1748–61.
3. Perros P, Zarkovic M, Azzolini C, Ayvaz G, Baldeschi L, Bartalena L, et al. PREGO (presentation of Graves' orbitopathy) study: changes in referral patterns to European Group on Graves' orbitopathy (EUGOGO) centers over the period from 2000 to 2012. Br J Ophthalmol. 2015;99:1531–5.
4. Bartalena L, Piantanida E, Gallo D, Lai A, Tanda ML. Epidemiology, natural history, risk factors, and prevention of Graves' orbitopathy. Front Endocrinol (Lausanne). 2020;30:615993.
5. Perros P, Hegedus L, Bartalena L, Marcocci C, Kahaly GJ, Baldeschi L, et al. Graves' orbitopathy as a rare disease in Europe: a European Group on Graves' Orbitopathy (EUGOGO) position statement. Orphanet J Rare Dis. 2017;12:72.
6. Chin YH, Ng CH, Lee MH, et al. Prevalence of thyroid eye disease in Graves' disease: A meta-analysis and systematic review. Clin Endocrinol (Oxf). 2020; 93: 363–374.
7. Kendall-Taylor P, Perros P. Clinical presentation of thyroid associated orbitopathy. Thyroid. 1998;8:427–8.
8. Perros P, Kendall-Taylor P. Natural history of thyroid eye disease. Thyroid. 1998;8:423–5.
9. Tanda ML, Piantanida E, Liparulo L, Veronesi G, Lai A, Sassi L, et al. Prevalence and natural history of Graves' orbitopathy in a large series of patients with newly diagnosed Graves' hyperthyroidism seen at a single center. J Clin Endocrinol Metab. 2013;98:1443–9.
10. Noth D, Gebauer M, Muller B, Burgi U, Diem P. Graves' ophthalmopathy: natural history and treatment outcomes. Swiss Med Wkly. 2001;131:603–9.
11. Rundle FF, Wilson CW. Development and course of exophthalmos and ophthalmoplegia in Graves' disease with special reference to the effect of thyroidectomy. Clin Sci. 1945;5:177–94.
12. Marcocci C, Bartalena L, Bogazzi F, Panicucci M, Pinchera A. Studies on the occurrence of ophthalmopathy in Graves' disease. Acta Endocrinol. 1989;120:473–8.
13. Wiersinga WM, Bartalena L. Epidemiology and prevention of Graves'ophthalmopathy. Thyroid. 2002;12:855–60.
14. Toruner FB, Konuk O, Ayvaz G. Combined eye clinics. In: Wiersinga M, Kahaly GJ, editors. Graves' orbitopathy: a multidisciplinary approach—questions and answers. Basel: Karger; 2017. p. 113–8.
15. Dickinson AJ, Perros P. Controversies in the clinical evaluation of active thyroid-associated orbitopathy: use of a detailed protocol with comparative photographs for objective assessment. Clin Endocrinol (Oxf). 2001;55:283–303.
16. Cruz AA, Ribeiro SF, Garcia DM, Akaishi PM, Pinto CT. Graves upper eyelid retraction. Surv Ophthalmol. 2013;58:63–76.
17. Uddin JM, Rubinstein T, Hamed-Azzam S. Phenotypes of thyroid eye disease. Ophthalmic Plast Reconstr Surg. 2018;34:S28–33.
18. Mourits MP, Lombardo SH, van der Sluijs FA, Fenton S. Reliability of exophthalmos measurement and exophthalmometry value distribution in a healthy Dutch population and in Graves' patients: an exploratory study. Orbit. 2004 Sep;23:161–8.
19. Kashkouli MB, Nojomi M, Parvaresh MM, Sanjari MS, Modarres M, Noorani MM. Normal values of Hertel exophthalmometry in children, teenagers, and adults from Tehran, Iran. Optom Vis Sci. 2008;85:1012–7.

20. Beden U, Ozarslan Y, Oztürk HE, Sönmez B, Erkan D, Oge I. Exophthalmometry values of Turkish adult population and the effect of age, sex, refractive status, and Hertel base values on Hertel readings. Eur J Ophthalmol. 2008;18:165–71.
21. Migliori ME, Gladstone GJ. Determination of the normal range of exophthalmometric values for black and white adults. Am J Ophthalmol. 1984;98:438–42.
22. Amino N, Yuasa T, Yabu Y, Miyai K, Kumahara Y. Exophthalmos in autoimmune thyroid disease. J Clin Endocrinol Metab. 1980;51:1232–4.
23. Buckley EG. Restrictive strabismus. In: Plager DA, editor. Strabismus surgery: basic and advanced strategies. Oxford: Oxford University Press; 2004.
24. Bartalena L, Kahaly GJ, Baldeschi L, Dayan CM, Eckstein A, Marcocci C, et al. The 2021 European Group on Graves' orbitopathy (EUGOGO) clinical practice guidelines for the medical management of Graves' orbitopathy. Eur J Endocrinol. 2021;185:G43–67.
25. McKeag D, Lane C, Lazarus JH, Baldeschi L, Boboridis K, Dickinson AJ, et al. Clinical features of dysthyroid optic neuropathy: a European Group on Graves' Orbitopathy (EUGOGO) survey. Br J Ophthalmol. 2007;91:455–8.
26. Garip Kuebler A, Wiecha C, Reznicek L, Klingenstein A, Halfter K, Priglinger S, et al. Evaluation of medical and surgical decompression in patients with dysthyroid optic neuropathy. Eye (Lond). 2020;34:1702–9.
27. Mourits MP, Bijl H, Altea MA, Baldeschi L, Boboridis K, Currò N, et al. Outcome of orbital decompression for disfiguring proptosis in patients with Graves' orbitopathy using various surgical procedures. European Group on Graves' Orbitopathy (EUGOGO). Br J Ophthalmol. 2009;93:1518–23.
28. Korkmaz S, Konuk O. Surgical treatment of dysthyroid optic neuropathy: long-term visual outcomes with comparison of 2-wall versus 3-wall orbital decompression. Curr Eye Res. 2016;41:159–64.
29. Reich SS, Null RC, Timoney PJ, Sokol JA. Trends in orbital decompression techniques of surveyed ASOPRS members. Ophthalmic Plast Reconstr Surg. 2016;32:434–7.
30. Demer JL, Kerman BM. Comparison of standardized echography with magnetic resonance imaging to measure extraocular muscle size. Am J Ophthalmol. 1994;118:351–61.
31. Yamamoto K, Itoh K, Yoshida S, Saito K, Sakamoto Y, Matsuda A, et al. A quantitative analysis of orbital soft tissue in Graves' disease based on B-mode ultrasonography. Endocrinol Jpn. 1979;26:255–6.
32. Gerding MN, Prummel MF, Wiersinga WM. Assessment of disease activity in Graves' ophthalmopathy by orbital ultrasonography and clinical parameters. Clin Endocrinol (Oxf). 2000;52:641–6.
33. Monteiro MLR, Angotti-Neto H, Benabou JE, Betinjane AJ. Color Doppler imaging of the superior ophthalmic vein in different clinical forms of Graves' orbitopathy. Jpn J Ophthalmol. 2008;52:483–8.
34. Yanik B, Conkbayir I, Acaroglu G, Hekimoglu B. Graves' ophthalmopathy: comparison of the Doppler sonography parameters with the clinical activity score. J Clin Ultrasound. 2005;33:375–80.
35. Konuk O, Onaran Z, Ozhan Oktar S, Yucel C, Unal M. Intraocular pressure and superior ophthalmic vein blood flow velocity in Graves' orbitopathy: relation with the clinical features. Graefes Arch Clin Exp Ophthalmol. 2009;247:1555–9.
36. Le Moli R, Pluchino A, Muscia V, Regalbuto C, Luciani B, Squatrito S, et al. Graves' orbitopathy: extraocular muscle/total orbit area ratio is positively related to the clinical activity score. Eur J Ophthalmol. 2012;22:301–8.
37. Byun JS, Moon NJ, Lee JK. Quantitative analysis of orbital soft tissues on computed tomography to assess the activity of thyroid-associated orbitopathy. Graefes Arch Clin Exp Ophthalmol. 2017;255:413–20.
38. Gonçalves AC, Silva LN, Gebrim EM, Matayoshi S, Monteiro ML. Predicting dysthyroid optic neuropathy using computed tomography volumetric analyses of orbital structures. Clinics (Sao Paulo). 2012;67:891–6.
39. Weis E, Heran MK, Jhamb A, Chan AK, Chiu JP, Hurley MC, et al. Quantitative computed tomographic predictors of compressive optic neuropathy in patients with thyroid orbitopathy: a volumetric analysis. Ophthalmology. 2012;119:2174–8.
40. Kirsch E, von Arx G, Hammer B. Imaging in Graves' orbitopathy. Orbit. 2009;28:219–25.
41. Mayer E, Herdman G, Burnett C, Kabala J, Goddard P, Potts MJ. Serial STIR magnetic resonance imaging correlates with clinical score of activity in thyroid eye disease. Eye (Lond). 2001;15:313–8.
42. Tortora F, Cirillo M, Ferrara M, Belfiore MP, Carella C, Caranci F, et al. Disease activity in Graves' ophthalmopathy: diagnosis with orbital MR imaging and correlation with clinical score. Neuroradiol J. 2013;26:555–64.
43. Jiang H, Wang Z, Xian J, Li J, Chen Q, Ai L. Evaluation of rectus extraocular muscles using dynamic contrast-enhanced MR imaging in patients with Graves' ophthalmopathy for assessment of disease activity. Acta Radiol. 2012;53:87–94.
44. Kvetny J, Puhakka KB, Røhl L. Magnetic resonance imaging determination of extraocular eye muscle volume in patients with thyroid-associated ophthalmopathy and proptosis. Acta Ophthalmol Scand. 2006;84:419–23.
45. Menconi F, Profilo MA, Leo M, Sisti E, Altea MA, Rocchi R, et al. Spontaneous improvement of untreated mild Graves' ophthalmopathy: Rundle's curve revisited. Thyroid. 2014;24:60–6.
46. Terwee CB, Prummel MF, Gerding MN, Kahaly GJ, Dekker FW, Wiersinga WM. Measuring disease activity to predict therapeutic outcome in Graves' ophthalmopathy. Clin Endocrinol (Oxf). 2005;62:145–55.
47. Kahaly GJ. Management of moderately severe Graves orbitopathy. In: Wiersinga WM, Kahaly GJ, editors. Graves' orbitopathy: a multidisciplinary

approach—questions and answers. Basel: Karger; 2017. p. 140–71.

48. Mourits MP, Koornneef L, Wiersinga WM, Prummel MF, Berghout A, van der Gaag R. Clinical criteria for the assessment of disease activity in Graves' ophthalmopathy: a novel approach. Br J Ophthalmol. 1989;73:639–44.
49. Mourits MP, Prummel MF, Wiersinga WM, Koornneef L. Clinical activity score as a guide in the management of patients with Graves' ophthalmopathy. Clin Endocrinol (Oxf). 1997;47:9–14.
50. Barrio-Barrio J, Sabater AL, Bonet-Farriol E, Velázquez-Villoria Á, Galofré JC. Graves' ophthalmopathy: VISA versus EUGOGO classification, assessment, and management. J Ophthalmol. 2015;2015:249125.
51. Werner SC. Modification of the classification of the eye changes of Graves' disease: recommendations of the Ad Hoc Committee of the American Thyroid Association. J Clin Endocrinol Metab. 1977;44:203–4.
52. Frueh BR. Why the NOSPECS classification of Graves' eye disease should be abandoned, with suggestions for the characterization of this disease. Thyroid. 1992;2:85–8.
53. Dolman PJ, Rootman J. VISA classification for Graves orbitopathy. Ophthalmic Plast Reconstr Surg. 2006;22:319–24.

Different Phenotypes and Ocular Surface Changes in Thyroid-Associated Orbitopathy

Jimmy M. Uddin and Shirin Hamed Azzam

Key Messages

- Thyroid-associated orbitopathy (TAO) is an autoimmune disease which is heterogenous.
- Multiple drivers affect the disease in its clinical, radiological, and biochemical appearance.
- Phenotype is a consequence of the interaction of the tissues and how the disease processes its response.
- There are six different phenotypes of TAO: (1) Congestive phenotype, (2) White eye expansion, (3) White eye apex, (4) Hydraulic apex, (5) Cicatricial active and (6) Cicatricial passive. The clinical manifestations of those phenotypes and their response to the treatment modalities are different.
- Classifying TAO patients according to this suggested phenotype classification is the key to choosing the best treatment options and providing a best tailored treatment.
- There are numerous factors for the pathogenesis of dry eye in TAO such as changes in tear volume, tear film osmolarity and instability, corneal sensitivity, and meibomian gland loss.

J. M. Uddin (✉)
Adnexal Service, Moorfields Eye Hospital, London, UK
e-mail: jmuddin@aol.com

S. H. Azzam
Baruch Padeh Medical Center, Poriya, Israel

1 Thyroid-Associated Orbitopathy is Heterogenous

Why do patients with Thyroid-Associated Orbitopathy (TAO) have different clinical manifestations, natural histories and different responses to treatment?

TAO is heterogenous and not driven by a single pathophysiology. There are multiple drivers of disease which will manifest differently in their clinical, radiological and biochemical appearance, also called phenotypes (Fig. 1).

There are problems with current classifications of TAO leading to confounding and misleading clinical assumptions and conclusions of disease activity and severity, including ocular surface changes such conjunctival chemosis, injection or redness.

These also have contributed to problems in inclusion criteria and outcomes in studies, which may make conclusions less reliable.

Severity does *not* always follow as with "NOSPECS" where there is progression from signs to soft-tissue changes and then proptosis; followed by motility, corneal and eventually sight-loss manifestations.

There is often an *inverse* correlation with proptosis and optic neuropathy, with patients less proptosed having higher risk of developing optic neuropathy due to crowding of the orbital apex and increased intraorbital tension.

F. M. Quaranta Leoni et al. (eds.), *Oculoplastic, Lacrimal and Orbital Surgery*,
https://doi.org/10.1007/978-3-031-39638-0_33

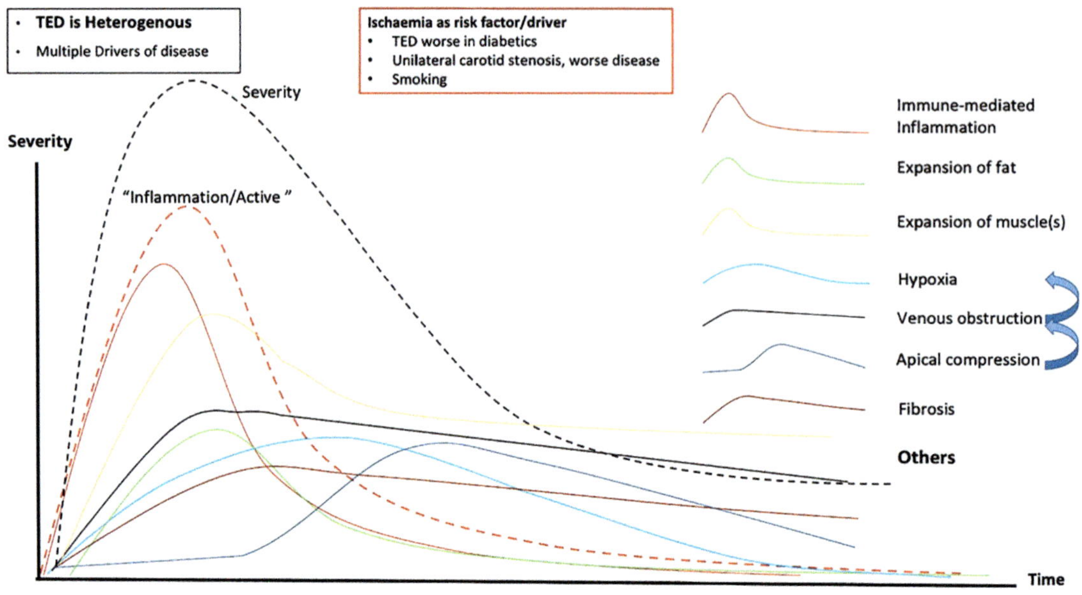

Fig. 1 Drivers and manifestations of thyroid-associated orbitopathy

There are predominantly single parameter manifestations of TAO, where there is no or little progression from one parameter to another, and these are not dependent or always sequential. Some patients have severe disease with optic neuropathy, but very little chemosis and redness. Others have persistent chemosis and redness but are not in the active inflammatory phase. There are subtypes who have progressive motility changes late in disease but are unlikely to be active inflammatory.

2 Drivers for Thyroid-Associated Orbitopathy

TAO is initially an autoimmune disease and the main extrathyroidal manifestation of Graves' disease that accounts for 80% of bilateral exophthalmos [1–3]. It primarily produces expansion of the extraocular muscles and fat in the orbit. The pathogenesis can be summarised by four main phenomena: (1) Inflammation of the periorbital soft tissues; (2) Overproduction of glycosaminoglycans by orbital fibroblasts; (3) Hyperplasia of adipose tissue and (4) Other poorly defined mechanical and vascular factors [4–6].

In addition, autoantibodies to the TSH receptor (TSH-R Ab) may have an independent drive in TAO. There are also fatty and fibrotic changes in the extraocular muscles (EOM) which have continued longer term effects, even in the "late/inactive" phase of TAO. These may be amenable to specific current or future treatments.

The natural history of TAO has been described for many years according to Rundle's curve [7–11]: which only plotted prominence of the eye (proptosis against time). The initial phase is the active phase where there is usually worsening of signs and symptoms that lasts for 6–18 months, and then there is an improvement to a plateau phase which is inactive inflammatory disease, without resolving into a normal condition [7–12]. It is essential to differentiate between activity and severity as the curve of the activity often precedes the severity peak by a few months [9–11] and the treatment modality is different during the different phases.

Initial and continual inflammation should respond to anti-inflammatory modalities, including immunosuppression drug interventions and radiotherapy.

Mechanical factors could be modified by reducing the orbital "tension" by reducing orbital swelling, EOM and fat expansion: or by expanding the orbital space to accommodate more room by bony decompression surgery. This will be dependent on where the orbital tension is most prominent, which in certain phenotypes is the posterior apical orbit.

The vascular component may be mainly mechanical with reduced venous outflow in the orbit and increased vascular congestion in the orbit or associated with inflammation.

There may also be a "hypoxic" element to worsening of TAO contributed by vascular congestion as well as smoking, diabetes and other vascular disease (including ischaemia due to ipsilateral carotid artery stenosis).

Continued TSH-R mediated disease may be modifiable by specific targeted therapies to that pathway (currently teprotumumab) [13, 14].

Anti-fibrotic agents may also have a role in late disease.

All these factors and others will determine the type of TAO and which treatment modality is more likely to work, as well as why treatments fail to make a difference.

We are now also re-evaluating concepts of active (inflammatory) disease and reversibility of disease with the changes that are seen with targeted therapies, including teprotumumab.

3 Phenotypes of Thyroid Associated Orbitopathy

Nunery described two classifications for TAO [15]. Type I patients (lipogenic variant) present with symmetrical proptosis but without inflammatory signs; CT demonstrates increased volume of orbital fat. Type II (muscle variant/restrictive myopathy) patients present with symmetrical/asymmetrical proptosis and diplopia; CT shows asymmetrical enlargement of extraocular muscles [15, 16].

Phenotype refers to the observable physical properties of an organism. What an organism looks like as a consequence of the interaction of its genotype and the environment; what the disease looks like as a consequence of the interaction of the tissues and the disease process(es) its response [17]. The same principles can apply to TAO.

Phenotypes are identifiable subtypes of TAO which will have specific clinical, radiological and biochemical parameters (T4, T3, TSH-R Ab) which support a more predictable course of disease and response to treatment modalities, allowing for more personalised care.

JMU et al. published six different phenotypes of TAO and their response to different treatment modalities [18]:

1. Congestive
2. White eye expansion
3. White eye apex
4. Hydraulic apex
5. Cicatricial active
6. Cicatricial passive

The clinical manifestations of those phenotypes and their response to the treatment modalities are different. Therefore, it is crucial to classify the phenotype to each TAO patient, in order to offer them the best tailored treatment.

3.1 Congestive (Active Inflammatory) Phenotype

The patients present in the early stage of the disease (weeks to months) with eye discomfort, secondary to inflammatory pathogenesis. Physical examination includes, redness, swelling of the eyelids, conjunctival hyperaemia, mild to moderate proptosis with diplopia. Usually, they do not develop signs of optic neuropathy. Imaging demonstrates enlargement of the extraocular muscles with or without fat expansion (Figs. 2a–d and 3). They respond well to immunosuppression treatments [19] and teprotumumab.

3.2 White Eye Expansion Phenotype

The patients present due to "prominent" eyes insidiously over a few months or even years, without inflammatory symptoms of redness or pain. Their examination reveals mild to moderate proptosis with soft orbit. There is often no or mild

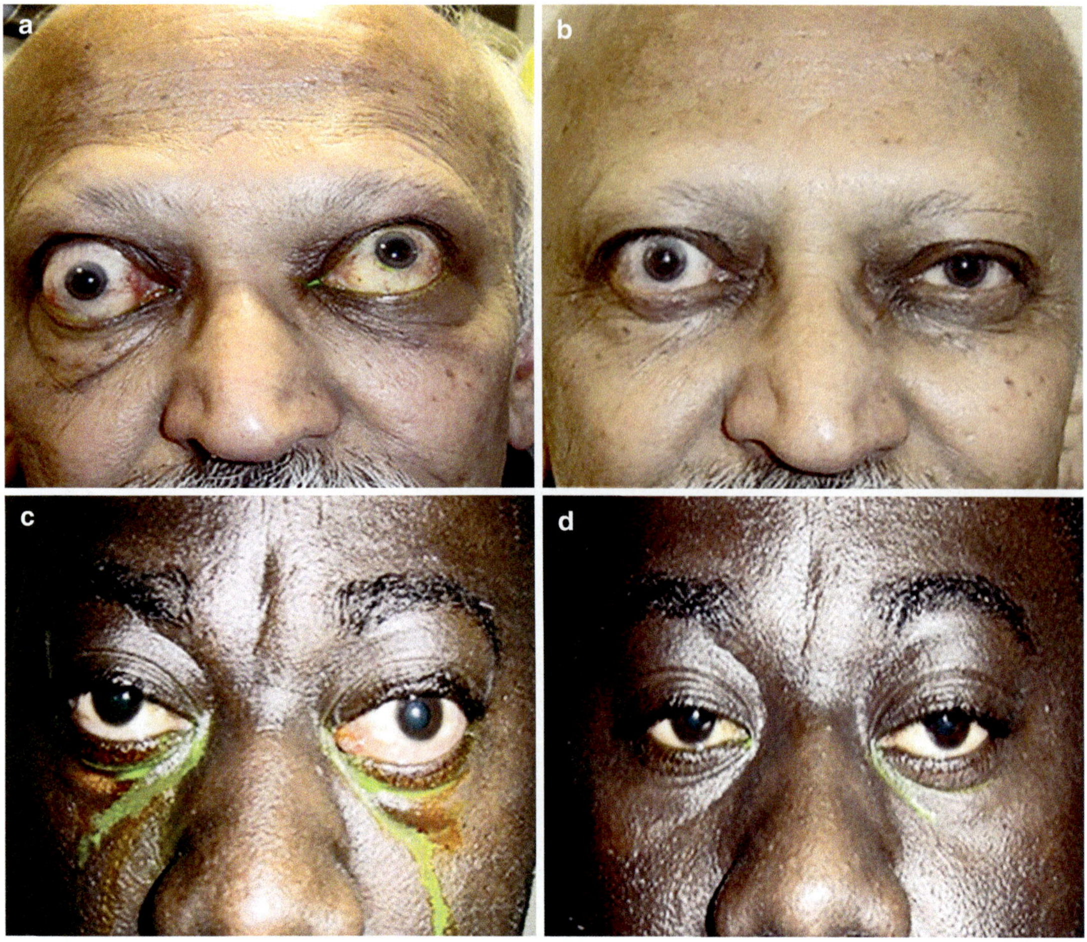

Fig. 2 Phenotype 1: Congestive (active inflammatory) TAO before (**a**, **c**) and after (**b**, **d**) immunosuppression, with a good response

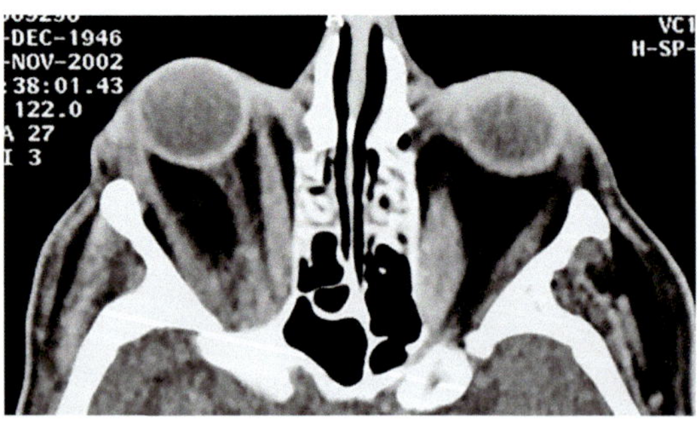

Fig. 3 Phenotype 1: Congestive (active inflammatory) TAO. Expansion of muscle and fat on CT scan

restriction of their extraocular movements without optic neuropathy. Ocular surface often is good. Imaging reveals mainly orbital fat expansion (Fig. 4a–d). This phenotype is similar to Type I by Nunery [15] and is common among paediatric TAO, and certain ethnic groups such as Indian population (Naik M, presented at International TAO Society Symposium, London, United Kingdom, 2016 [20]). Their response to immunosuppression is unknown, but likely to be poorly responsive; whereas orbital decompression surgery can be offered as rehabilitative reconstructive surgery. Teprotumumab may be less effective in these groups.

3.3 White Eye Apex Phenotype

Patients with this phenotype present with white prominent eyes over weeks to months. Most cases complain of deep pain in the orbit. Their ophthalmic examination reveals minimal conjunctival hyperaemia, mild eyelid retraction,

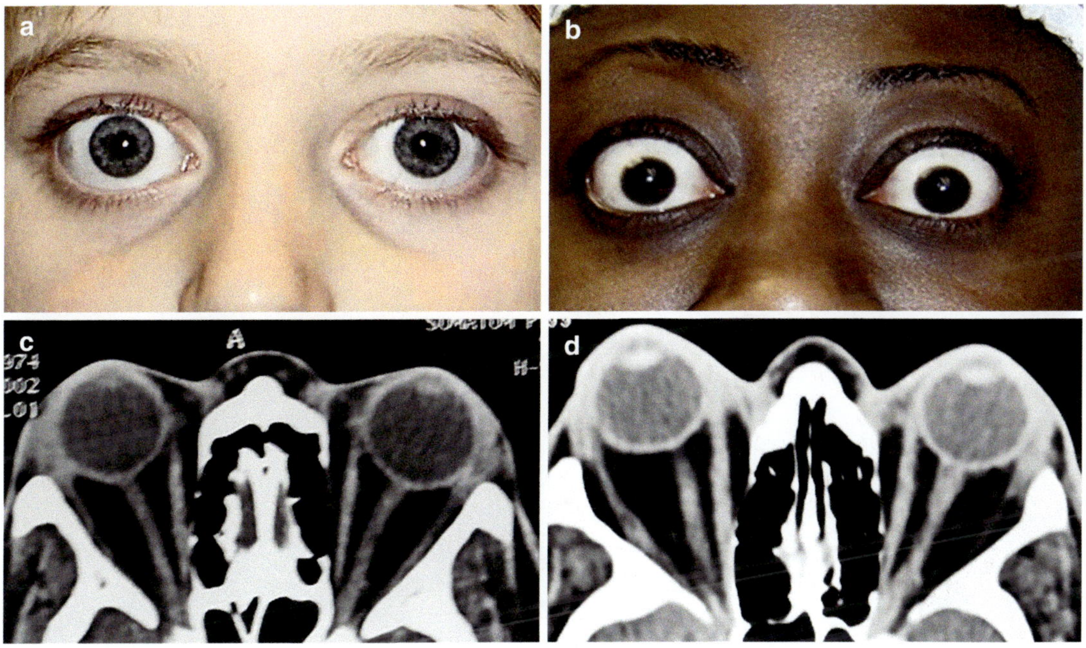

Fig. 4 Phenotype 2: White eye expansion TAO (**a**, **b**) with fat expansion on CT (**c**, **d**)

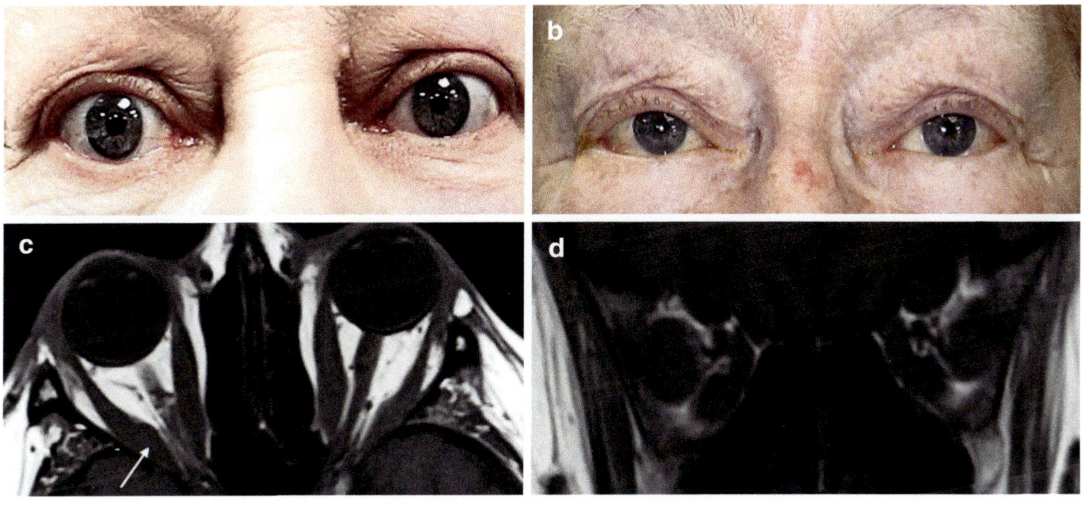

Fig. 5 Phenotype 3: White eye apex (**a**, **b**). Imaging shows posterior apical crowding (**c**, **d**)

moderate motility restriction with minimal proptosis. There is a biphasic phenomenon when pressing the orbit—it is moderate to retropulsion, and firmer when pressing deeper. The hallmark of this phenotype is optic neuropathy. Imaging reveals a crowded apex in the posterior third of the orbit (Fig. 5a–d). They respond poorly or partially to immunosuppression, but well to apical decompression surgery.

3.4 Hydraulic Apex Phenotype

Rose described this variant in 2006 [21]. Patients present late in their inflammatory disease with progressive history of discomfort and red prominent eyes. Diplopia is common due to restrictive eye movements and the orbit is moderate to firm to retropulsion. Usually there are characteristic deep, dilated conjuncti-

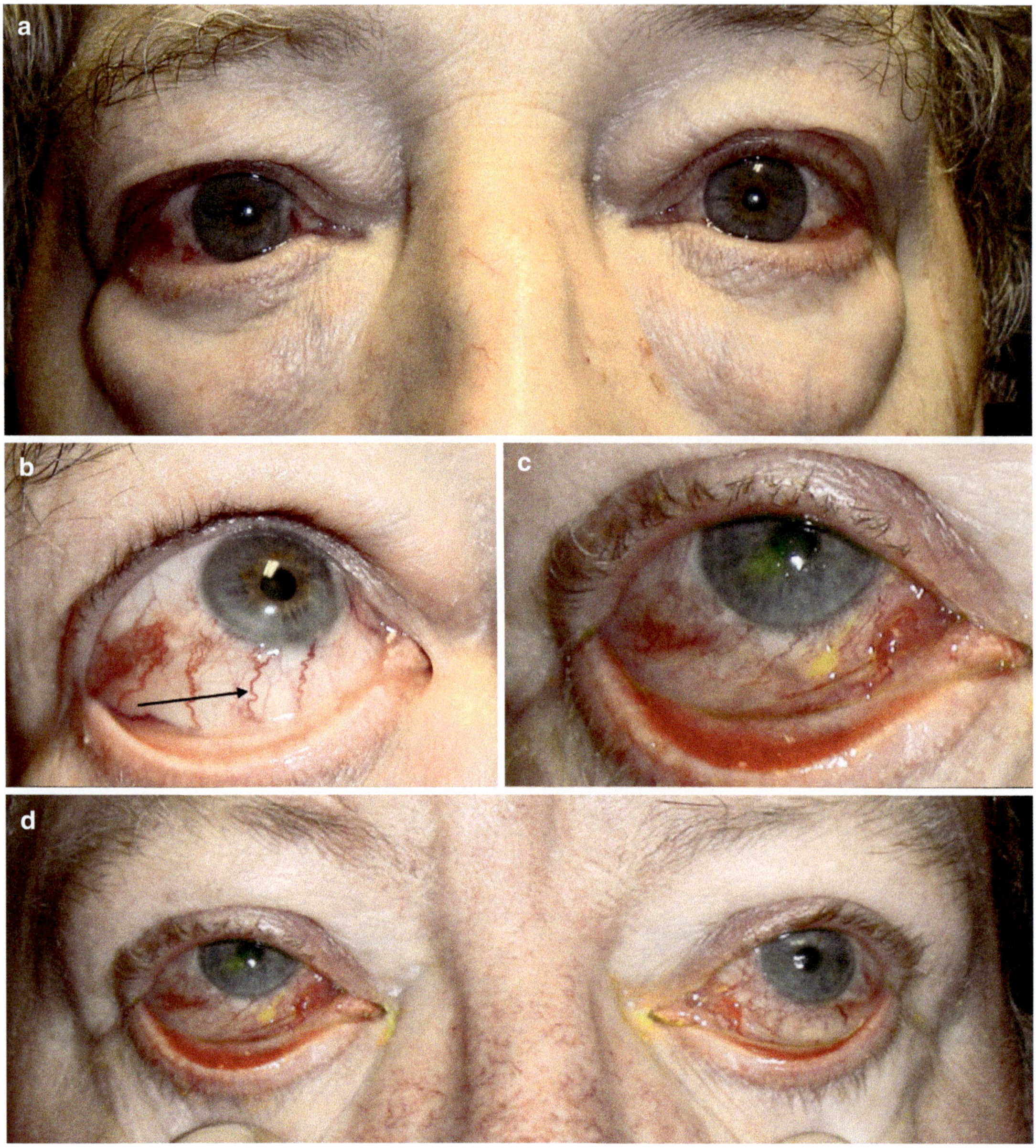

Fig. 6 Phenotype 4: Conjunctival vessel pattern is similar for a low flow fistula (**a** + **b**) and hydraulic apex TAO (**c** + **d**)

val vessels, which is similar to low-flow carotid-cavernous fistula (Fig. 6a–d). The pathogenesis is a crowded orbit, with tight septum that increases the orbital pressure and subsequent optic nerve ischemia. Orbital imaging demonstrates enlarged EOM with crowding within posterior third to half of the orbit. This phenotype does not respond to immunosuppression, whereas it responds well to orbital decompression surgery (Fig. 7a–d).

3.5 Cicatricial Active Phenotype

The patients present during the early phase of the disease with progressive strabismus or eyelid retraction with white eyes, over weeks to few months. They might complain about pain in eye movements, especially in the direction opposite to the affected muscle. Progressive strabismus is the predominant feature in this phenotype. Mild to moderate proptosis may present with soft orbit and eyelid retraction,

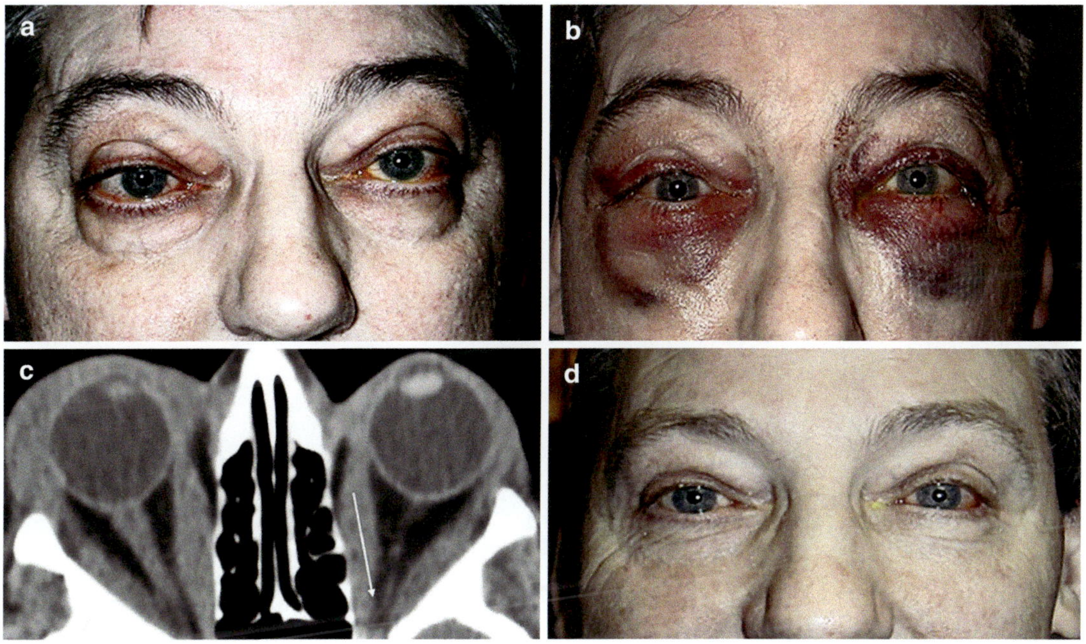

Fig. 7 Phenotype 4: Hydraulic apex (**a**) with marked muscle expansion on CT (**c**). Patient had prolonged and very high doses of IV steroids. The disease is "switched off" following decompression (**b**, **d**)

and typically there is no optic neuropathy. There is minimal conjunctival chemosis and injection, leading to a conclusion of "inactive inflammatory" disease. However, this due to the localised inflammation of the affected muscle (inferior rectus or levator muscle) being unseen clinically as its "hidden" from surface examination. Imaging reveals single predominant enlarged extraocular muscle, commonly inferior rectus or levator palpebrae superioris muscle in cases affecting the upper eyelid. MRI may be helpful in showing the inflammatory signs of the enlarged muscle as it reveals high water content in the affected muscle (Fig. 8a–e). Immunosuppression may help, but due to the asymmetric nature of the disease, may result in little manifest improvement of signs and symptoms. Local steroid injection may have a role in this variant [22].

3.6 Cicatricial Passive Phenotype

The patients present during the late phase of the disease with slowly, progressive strabismus, over months to a year. They may have mild discomfort with worsening of the diplopia. Mild to moderate proptosis may present with soft orbit. Eyelid retraction may be present. Optic neuropathy is not a feature. It is a late inactive phase of the disease, compared to the cicatricial active phenotype, that indicates fibrosis of the muscle. They are often mistaken for active progressive disease, but will have a low water content on MRI. They do not respond to immunosuppression modalities or steroid injections. Anti-fibrotic agents and teprotumumab may have a role.

In summary, not all TAO patients present with inflammatory signs during their early or late disease. For instance, 'white eye apex' phenotype, has minimal clinical activity score, despite a treatable optic neuropathy. Moreover, 'cicatricial active phenotype' has minimal active score when it is in the early inflammatory phase. Therefore, it is important to classify TAO patients according to this suggested phenotype classification, in order to understand the different behaviours of each phenotype and their response to the different treatment modalities. This is key to choosing the best treatment options and providing a personalised treatment plan.

We await future trials and studies to understand the pathogenesis of further emerging phenotypes.

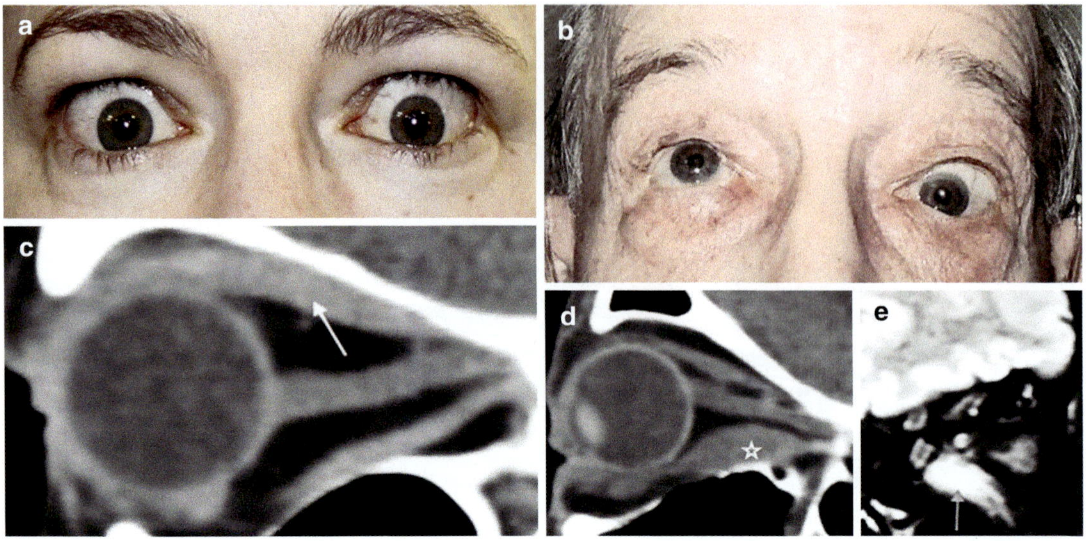

Fig. 8 Phenotype 5: Cicatricial active TAO. With upper eyelid retraction (**a**) or a "tight" inferior rectus and marked hypotropia with poor elevation (**b**). CT scan confirms enlargement of the levator in the first patient (**c**) and the inferior rectus in the second (**d**). MRI in this patient confirms activity in the inferior rectus muscle with high signal (**e**)

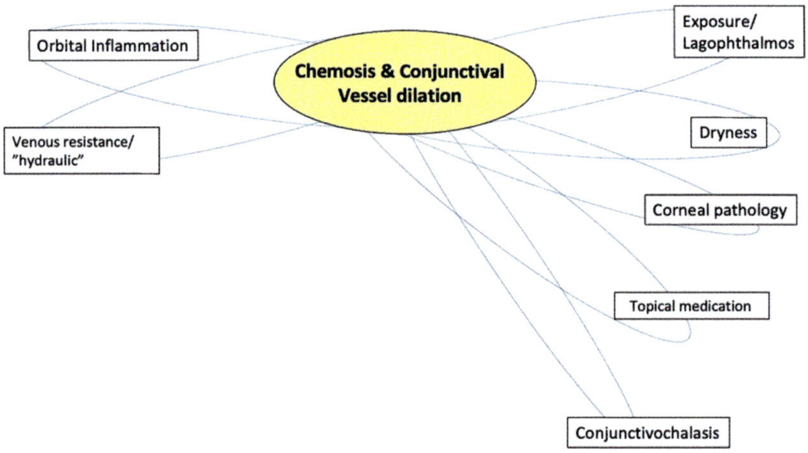

Fig. 9 Drivers for conjunctival chemosis and vessel dilation

4 Confounding Ocular Surface Signs

Confounding ocular surface factors for TAO signs and symptoms may result in inappropriate classification and misleading conclusions about the nature of TAO and possible treatment responses.

Ocular surface signs are not always indicative of clinical activity score (CAS) and disease activity. Chemosis and conjunctival vessel dilation can be caused by orbital inflammation, vascular resistance (hydraulic phenotype), lagophthalmos, dryness, corneal pathology and topical medication (Fig. 9).

Persistent redness, conjunctival injection and chemosis may be more indicative of ocular surface disease, rather than disease activity. The location of signs is important and sometimes this can be revealed by seeing the interpalpebral nature with sparing of the bulbar conjunctiva under the upper eyelid, which is demonstrated with the eye looking down and the upper eyelid being held up (Fig. 10b).

Conjunctivochalasis may be mistaken for chemosis and persistent activity (Fig. 10a–c).

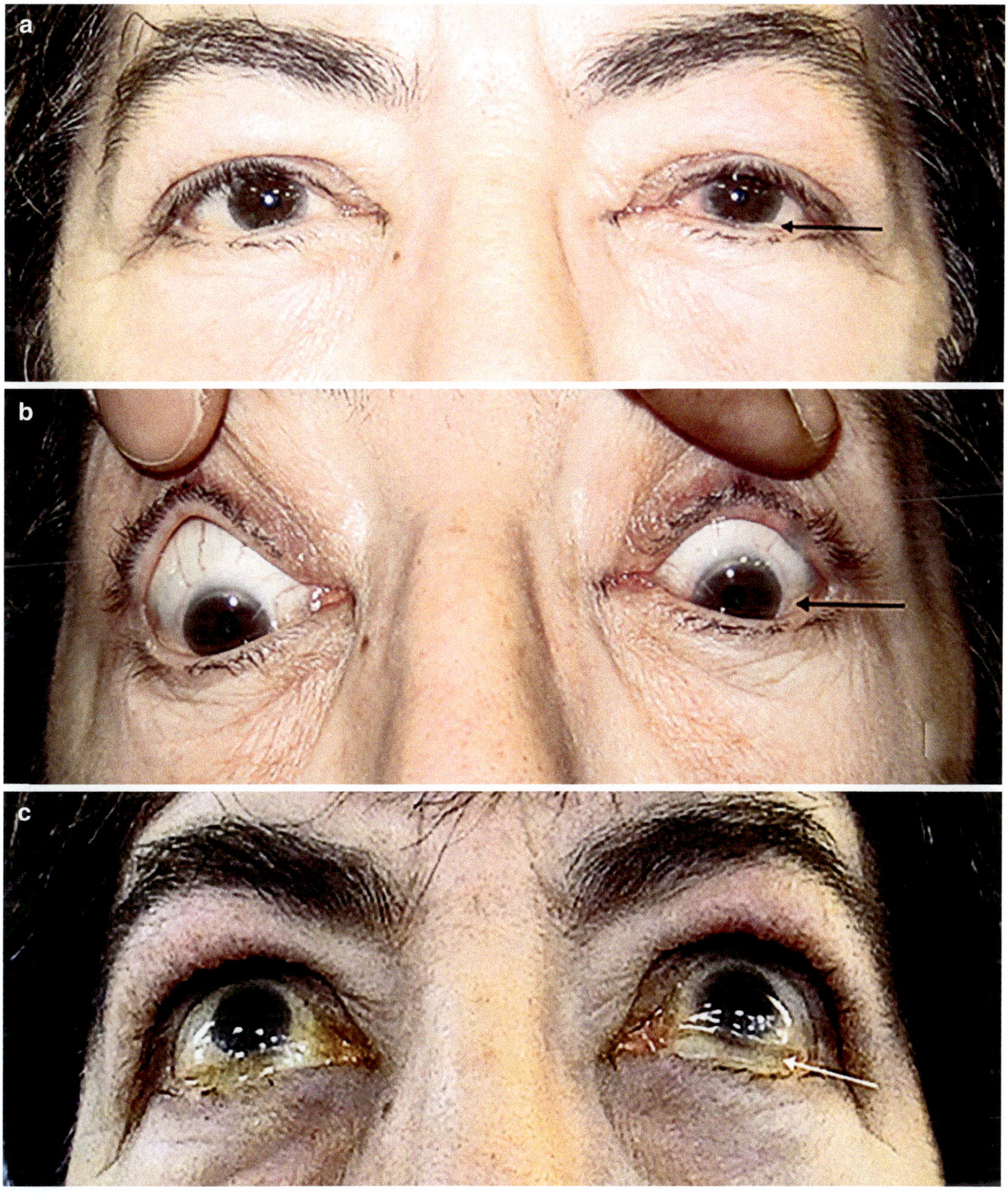

Fig. 10 Patient treated with immunosuppression for persistent "active" TAO, due to high CAS score and conjunctival chemosis and injection (**a**). Superior bulbar conjunctiva was white (**b**) and conjunctivochalasis was demonstrated (**c**). Patient improved with cessation of immunosuppression and increased topical lubrication

Different types of conjunctival injection and vessel dilation may support different pathophysiology. Superficial, intermediate and deep conjunctival vessel changes can be seen. Deep dilated vessels are seen more with hydraulic phenotype with little oedema and injection between the vessels (Fig. 11). Whereas, congestive phenotype has both deep and superficial dilated vessels with injection and oedema between deep vessels (Fig. 12).

See summary of the six different phenotypes of TAO in Fig. 13.

5 Ocular Surface Changes in Thyroid-Associated Orbitopathy

5.1 Prevalence

Dry eye disease (DED) was defined recently according to the Tear Film and Ocular Surface Society International Dry Eye Workshop II (TFOS DEWS II) definition as ocular surface symptoms presence and other signs of DED (ocular surface disease index score (OSDI) more than 13 and any 1 sign of abnormal tear break up time (TBUT) or abnormal ocular surface staining) [23]. The prevalence of DED is 20% in the United Kingdom, 39.2% in France and 14.5% in America [24]. The prevalence increases with ageing (around 25–45%) and in women is 1.74 times more than in men [25]. DED symptoms include burning, itching, blurred vision, redness, and sensitivity to light. Although dry eye symptoms are reported commonly among TAO patients (around 65–85%) [26, 27], few studies have investigated the association between DED and TAO [24, 26–34].

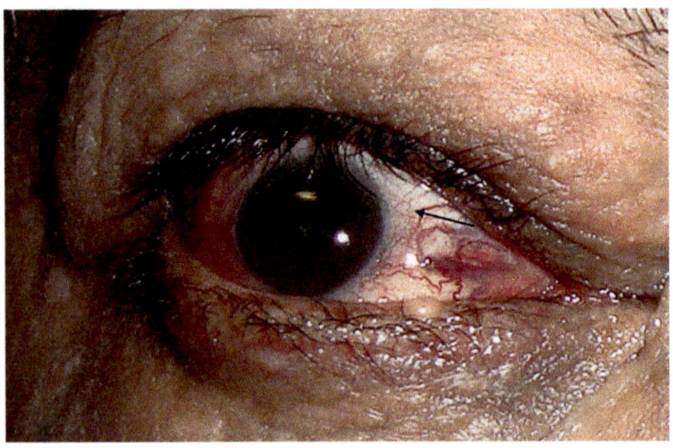

Fig. 11 Deep dilated vessels in hydraulic apex TAO

5.2 Pathogenesis

The mechanisms of DED in TAO are not fully known. It is multifactorial with synergistic effect and caused by (Table 1):

1. *Immunological changes*: T-cell mediated inflammation and TSH-receptors expression in the acinar cells of the lacrimal gland causes a decrease in the tear volume [28, 35]. In addition, previous evidence suggests that TAO patients have abnormally high tear film osmolarity [36] that stimulates pro-inflammatory cytokines and causes an activation of the mitogen-activated protein kinase (MAPK)

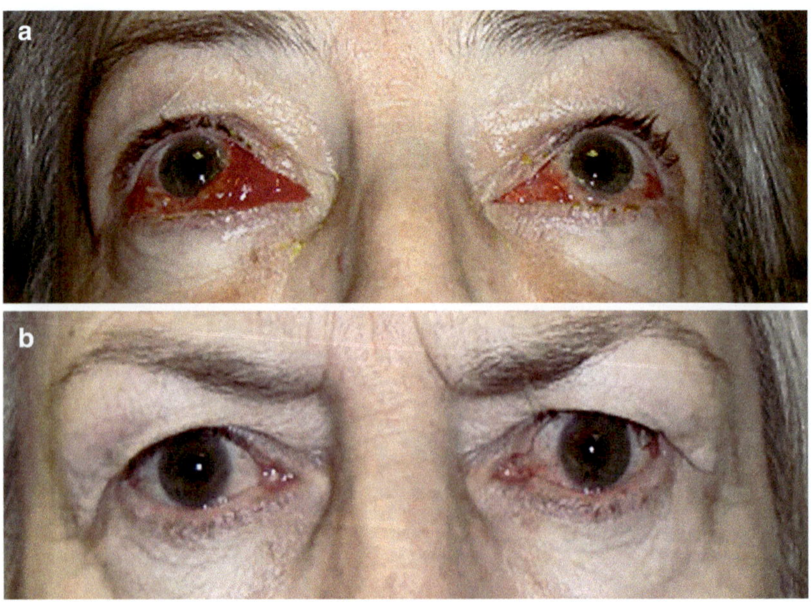

Fig. 12 Mixed vessel dilation and chemosis with congestive TAO, despite high dose of steroids (**a**). Resolves following decompression surgery (**b**)

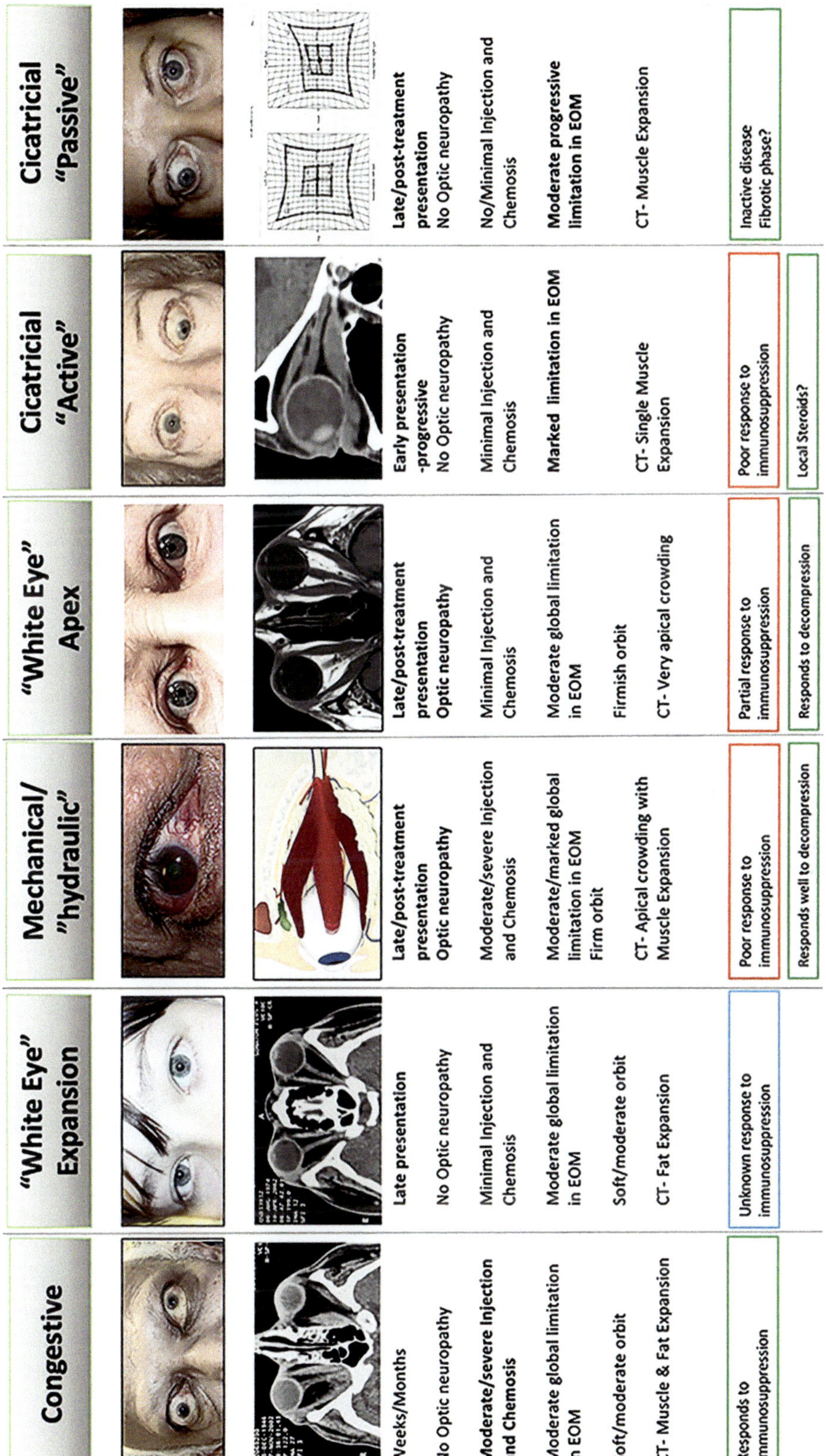

Fig. 13 Summary of thyroid-associated orbitopathy phenotypes including symptoms, signs and treatments for each phenotype

Table 1 Pathogenesis of dry eye disease in thyroid-associated orbitopathy

Factor	Change
Tear volume	↓
Tear film osmolarity	↑
Tear film instability	↑
Protein component in tear film	↑
Corneal sensitivity	↓
Palpebral aperture	↑
Incomplete blinking	↑
Meibomian gland loss	↑

cascade and further inflammatory cytokines stimulation [37]. This leads to worsening of the ocular inflammation that is important in DED pathogenesis. Moreover, Tear hyperosmolarity causes pathological changes to the corneal epithelium cells which increases the inflammatory cytokines in the tear film and DED [38]. Achtsidis et al. have revealed a significant reduction in the corneal sensitivity in TAO, showing an association with DED [26]. Furthermore, TAO patients have an abnormal proteinaceous composition of their tear film that is consistent with dysfunction in the lacrimal gland [31]. A previous study showed that 28% of TAO patients have an abnormal tear film protein profile [39].

2. *Morphological and functional changes*: proptosis and higher palpebral aperture cause incomplete blinking and increase in tear evaporation [40]. In addition, a previous study showed that there is a correlation between palpebral aperture and TBUT. Patients with a wider aperture suffer from shorter TBUT, which leads to tear film instability [41]. Moreover, secondary to the incomplete blinking, TAO patients suffer from meibomian gland dysfunction as was demonstrated by higher meibomian gland loss in meibography [42].

5.3 Clinical Diagnosis of DED

Diagnosis of DED among TAO patients is part of the clinical ophthalmic examination that includes objective and subjective evaluations.

Objective measurements- TBUT to measure the tear stability, Fluorescein and lissamine green staining to detect de-epithelized and devitalized ocular surface areas, respectively. In addition, Schirmer test to detect aqueous deficiency and meibography to evaluate meibomian gland loss.

Subjective measurements include questionnaires to assess the symptoms of ocular irritation and the environmental triggers. The Ocular Surface Disease Index (OSDI) is one of the commonly used questionnaires. It consists of 12 questions that are filled by the patient. OSDI is higher in inflammatory disease [43]. Wu et al., showed that both active and inactive TAO patients suffer from DED and their OSDI (50.00, 27.08, respectively) were significantly higher than those of healthy controls [44].

DED causes eye discomfort and influences the patients' quality of life [24]. The GO-QOL questionnaire is widely used and assesses the quality of life among TAO patients through two main scales: appearance and visual functioning [45]. Lin et al. found that the score in appearance and visual functioning had significant correlation with the activity and severity of TAO [46] (see chapter "Quality of Life in Patients with Thyroid-Associated Orbitopathy").

5.4 Treatment of DED in TAO

Lubricants and anti-inflammatory drops can be used to treat DED among TAO patients. Preservative-free lubricants through the day and overnight can be very helpful, mainly for patients with lagophthalmos [47]. A hypotonic solution can be used to decrease the elevated tear osmolarity, but it has only a transient effect [48]. Surgical treatments such as orbital decompression and eyelid surgeries can protect the ocular surface and tear film.

Anti-inflammatory drops such as steroids can improve the dry eye symptoms among TAO patients. Cyclosporine A inhibits T-cell proliferation and stops apoptosis of ocular surface cells [49]. However, there is conflicting evidence regarding the impact of cyclosporine A for DED in TAO patients [38, 50].

References

1. Iyer S, Bahn R. Immunopathogenesis of Graves' ophthalmopathy: The role of the TSH receptor. Best Pract Res Clin Endocrinol Metab. 2012;26:281–9.
2. Ludgate M, Baker G. Unlocking the immunological mechanisms and orbital inflammation in thyroid eye disease. Clin Exp Immunol. 2002;127:193–8.
3. Bartalena L, Baldeschi L, Dickinson A, et al. Consenus statement of the European Group on Graves' orbitopathy (EUGOGO) on management of GO. Eur J Endocrinol. 2008;158:273–85.
4. Bahn RS. Graves' ophthalmopathy. N Engl J Med. 2010;362:726–38.
5. Barrio-Barrio J, Sabater AL, Bonet-Farriol E, Velazquez-Villoria A, Galofre JC. Graves' ophthalmopathy: VISA versus EUGOGO classification, assessment, and management. J Ophthalmol. 2015;2015:249125.
6. Stan MN, Bahn RS. Risk factors for development or deterioration of Graves' ophthalmopathy. Thyroid. 2010;20:777–83.
7. Rundle FF, Wilson CW. Development and course of exophthalmos and ophthalmoplegia in Graves' disease with special reference to the effect of thyroidectomy. Clin Sci. 1945;5:177–94.
8. Rundle FF. Management of exophthalmos and related ocular changes in Graves; disease. Metabolism. 1957;6:36–48.
9. Bartley GB. Rundle and his curve. Arch Ophthalmol. 2011;129:356–8.
10. Wiersinga WM. Immunosuppressive treatment of Graves' ophthalmopathy. Thyroid. 1992;2:229–33.
11. Perros P, Kendall-Taylor P. Natural history of thyroid eye disease. Thyroid. 1998;8:423–5.
12. Wiersinga WM, Perros P, Kahaly GJ, et al. Clinical assessment of patients with Graves' orbitopathy: The European Group on Graves' Orbitopathy recommendations to generalists, specialists and clinical researches. Eur J Endocrinol. 2006;155:387–9.
13. Douglas R, Kahaly G, Patel A, et al. Teprotumumab for the treatment of active thyroid eye disease. N Engl J Med. 2020;382:341–52.
14. Ugradar S, Kang J, Kossler A, et al. Teprotumumab for the treatment of chronic thyroid eye disease. Eye (Lond). 2022;36:1553–9.
15. Nunery WR. Ophthalmic Graves' disease: a dual theory of pathogenesis. Ophthalmol Clin North Am. 1991;4:73–87.
16. Rubin P, Watkins L, Rumelt S, Sutula F, Dallow R. Orbital computed tomographic characteristics of globe subluxation in thyroid orbitopathy. Ophthalmology. 1998;105:2061–4.
17. Miravitlles M, Soler-Cataluna JJ, Calle M, et al. Treatment of COPD by clinical phenotypes: putting old evidence into clinical practice. Eur Respir J. 2013;41:1252–6.
18. Uddin JM, Rubinstein T, Hamed-Azzam S. Phenotypes of thyroid eye disease. Ophthal Plast Reconstr Surg. 2018;34:S28–33.
19. Mourits MP, Prummel MF, Wiersinga WM, et al. Clinical activity score as a guide in the management of patients with Graves' ophthalmopathy. Clin Endocrinol (Oxf). 1997;47:9–14.
20. Goldstein SM, Katowitz WR, Moshang T, et al. Pediatric thyroid associated orbitopathy: the Children's Hospital of Philadelphia experience and literature review. Thyroid. 2008;18:997–9.
21. Rose GE. Postural visual obscurations in patients with inactive thyroid eye disease; a variant of 'hydraulic' disease. Eye (Lond). 2006;20:1178–85.
22. Lee SJ, Rim TH, Jang SY, et al. Treatment of upper eyelid retraction related to thyroid-associated ophthalmopathy using subconjunctival triamcinolone injections. Graefes Arch Clin Exp Ophthalmol. 2013;251:261–70.
23. Craig JP, Nicholas KK, Apkek EK, Caffery B, Dua HS, Joo CK, et al. TFOS DEWS II definition and classification report. Ocul Surf. 2017;15:276–83.
24. Sun R, Zhou HF, Fan XQ. Ocular surface changes in Graves' ophthalmopathy. Int J Ophthalmol. 2021;14:616–21.
25. Stapleton F, Alves M, Bunua VY, Jalbert I, Lekhanont K, Malet F, et al. TFOS DEWS II epidemiology report. Ocul Surf. 2017;15:334–65.
26. Achtsidis V, Tentolouris N, Theodoropoulou S, Panagiotidis D, Vaikoussis E, Saldana M, et al. Dry eye in Graves ophthalmopathy: correlation with corneal hypoesthesia. Eur J Ophthalmol. 2013;23:473–9.
27. Ismailova DS, Fedorov AA, Grusha YO. Ocular surface changes in thyroid eye disease. Orbit. 2013;32:87–90.
28. Bahn RS, Dutton CM, Natt N, Joba W, Spitzweg C, Heufelder AE. Thyrotropin receptor expression in Graves' orbital adipose/connective tissues: potential autoantigen in Graves' ophthalmopathy. J Clin Endocrinol Metab. 1998;83:998–1002.
29. Gurdal C, Sarac O, Genc I, Kirimlioglu H, Takmaz T, Can I. Ocular surface and dry eye in Graves' disease. Curr Eye Res. 2011;36:8–13.
30. Eckstein AK, Finkenrath A, Heiligenhaus A, Renzing-Kohler K, Esser J, Kruger C, et al. Dry eye syndrome in thyroid-associated ophthalmopathy: lacrimal expression of TSH receptor suggests involvement of TSHR-specific autoantibodies. Acta Ophthalmol Scand. 2004;82:291–7.
31. Selter JH, Gire AI, Sikder S. The relationship between Graves' ophthalmopathy and dry eye syndrome. Clin Ophtalmol. 2014;9:57–62.
32. Rocha EM, Mnatelli F, Nominato LF, Bonini S. Hormes and dry eye syndrome: An update on what we do and don't know. Curr Opin Ophthalmol. 2013;24:348–55.
33. Villani E, Viola F, Sala R, Salvi M, Mapelli C, Curro N, et al. Corneal involvement in Graves' orbitopathy: An in vivo confocal study. Invest Ophthalmol Vis Sci. 2010;51:4574–8.

34. Inoue S, Kawashima M, Arita R, Kozaki A, Tsubota K. Investigation of meibomian gland function and dry eye disease in patients with Graves' ophthalmopathy. J Clin Med. 2020;9:2814.
35. Lehmann GM, Feldon SE, Smith TJ, Phipps RP. Immune mechanisms in thyroid eye disease. Thyroid. 2008;18:959–65.
36. Gilbard JP, Farris RL. Ocular surface drying and tear film osmolarity in thyroid eye disease. Acta Ophthalmol. 1983;61:108–16.
37. Luo L, Li D-Q, Corrales RM, Pflugfelder SC. Hyperosmolar saline is a proinflammatory stress on the mouse ocular surface. Eye Contact Lens. 2005;31:186–93.
38. Gurdal C, Genc I, Sarac O, Gonul I, Takmaz T, Can I. Topical cyclosporine in thyroid orbitopathy-related dry eye: clinical findings, conjunctival epithelial apoptosis, and MMP-9 expression. Curr Eye Res. 2010;35:771–7.
39. Khalil HA, De Keizer RJ, Kijlstra A. Analysis of tear proteins in Graves' ophthalmopathy by high performance liquid chtomatography. Am J Ophthalmol. 1988;106:186–90.
40. Iskeleli G, Karakoc Y, Abdula A. Tear film osmolarity in patients with thyroid ophthalmopathy. Jpn J Ophthalmol. 2008;52:323–6.
41. Brasil MV, Brasil OFM, Vieira RP, Vaisman M, Amaral Filho OMB. Tear film analysis and its relation with palpebral fissure height and exophthalmos in Graves' ophthalmopathy. Arq Bras Oftalmol. 2005;68:615–8.
42. Park J, Baek S. Dry eye syndrome in thyroid eye disease patients: The role of increased incomplete blinking and meibmoian gland loss. Acta Ophthalmol. 2019;97:e800–6.
43. Garcia DM, Reis de Oliveira F, Modulo CM, Faustino J, Barbosa AP, Alves M, Rocha EM. Is Sjogren's syndrome dry eye similar to dry eye caused by other etiologies? Discriminating different diseases by dry eye tests. PLoS One. 2018;13:e0208420.
44. Wu LQ, Cheng JW, Cai JP, Le QH, Ma XY, Gao LD, Wei RL. Observation of corneal Langerhans cells by in vivo confocal microscopy in thyroid-associated ophthalmopathy. Curr Eye Res. 2016;41:927–32.
45. Wiersinga WM. Quality of life in Graves' ophthalmopathy. Best Pract Res Clin Endocrinol Metab. 2012;26:359–70.
46. Lin IC, Lee CC, Liao SL. Assessing quality of life in Taiwanese patients with Graves; ophthalmopathy. J Formos Med Assoc. 2015;114:1047–54.
47. Sokol J, Foulks GN, Haider A, Nunery WR. Ocular surface effects of thyroid disease. Ocul Surf. 2010;8:29–39.
48. Holly FJ, Lamberts DW. Effect of nonisotonic solutions on tear film osmolality. Invest Ophthalmol Vis Sci. 1981;20:236–45.
49. Pflugfelder SC. Anti-inflmmatory therapy of dry eye. Ocul Surf. 2003;1:31–6.
50. Altiparmak UE, Acar DE, Ozer PA, et al. Topical cyclosporine A for the dry eye findings of thyroid orbitopathy patients. Eye. 2010;24:1044–50.

Medical Management of Thyroid-Associated Orbitopathy

Maarten P. Mourits and Pari N. Shams

Key Messages

- The management of thyroid-associated orbitopathy (TAO) is complex and the treatment should be provided as part of a multidisciplinary team, including ophthalmologist, orthoptist, endocrinologist and the family doctor.
- Thyroid dysfunction must be managed together with comorbidities, such as smoking and diabetes mellitus, and these should be addressed simultaneously.
- Treatment should be started at the time of diagnosis to decrease the final severity of the disease, as it is more effective when initiated early in the active phase of the disease.
- Both hyperthyroidism and hypothyroidism negatively influence TAO. Hypothyroidism can be corrected with oral supplementation; there are three options for treatment of hyperthyroidism: antithyroid drugs, radio-active iodine, and thyroidectomy.
- Establishing whether a patient has active or inactive TAO is important, as immunosuppression with corticosteroids or orbital radiotherapy are effective in the active stage of the disease. Surgical treatments should only be undertaken when the disease is inactive and has remained stable for at least 3–6 months.

1 Introduction

Management of thyroid-associated orbitopathy (TAO) is complex (Table 1). The treatment must be provided as part of a multidisciplinary team [1], including ophthalmologist, orthoptist, endocrinologist and the family doctor as a minimum. There is often associated thyroid dysfunction, which must be simultaneously managed, and there are medical conditions and comorbidities, such as smoking and diabetes mellitus, that have to be addressed as part of the management of TAO. Patients often require lifestyle modification and psychological support, which if not managed appropriately may have a significant negative impact on the outcome of their disease and quality of life, during an often long and difficult period of treatment. Uncontrolled thyroid function has been shown to negatively influence the natural history TAO and must be managed simultaneously and is a matter of priority [2]. The management, medical or surgical, of TAO should begin with an assessment of disease activity and severity. A true understanding of disease activity can only be made in a longitudinal fashion, following a minimum of two consultations. However, even following the initial consultation,

M. P. Mourits (✉)
Orbital Center, Department of Ophthalmology, Amsterdam University Medical Centers, Amsterdam, The Netherlands
e-mail: mpmourits@gmail.com

P. N. Shams
Adnexal Service, Moorfields Eye Hospital, London, UK

F. M. Quaranta Leoni et al. (eds.), *Oculoplastic, Lacrimal and Orbital Surgery*,
https://doi.org/10.1007/978-3-031-39638-0_34

Table 1 Flow chart for management of TAO

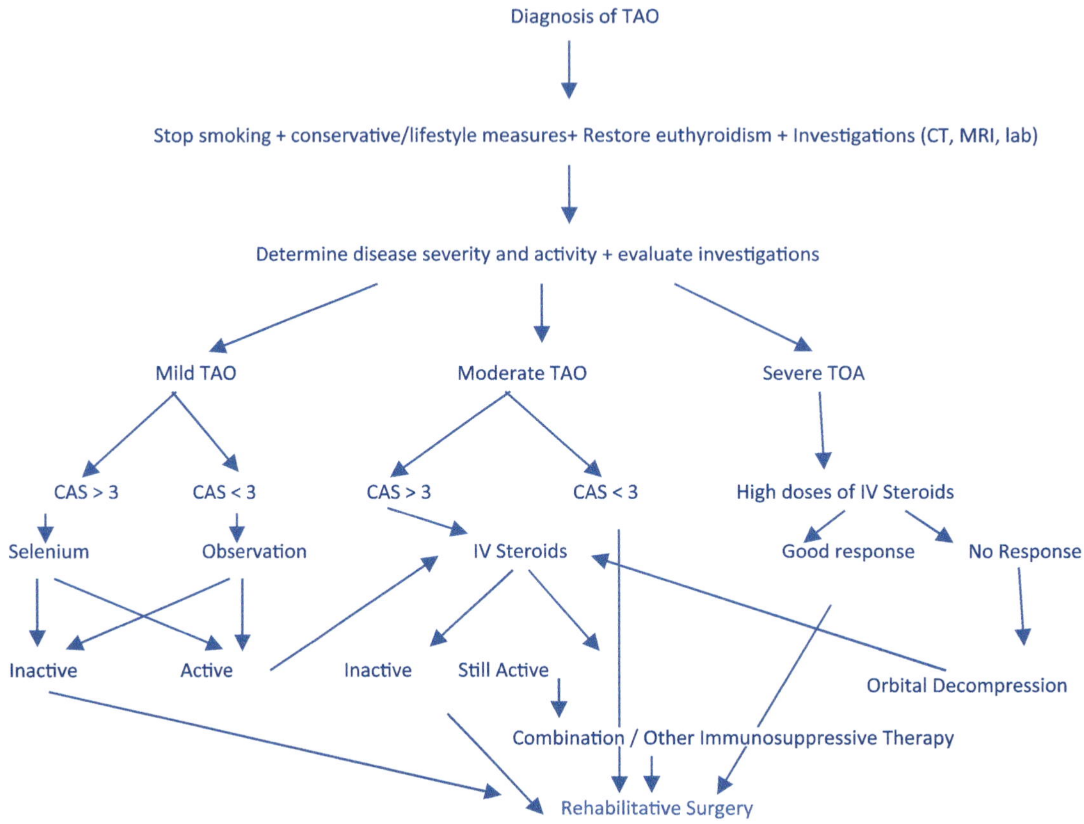

once a provisional diagnosis has been made, some (temporary) measures can be taken. Representatives of thyroid or TAO patient associations can help patients with TAO cope with their disease by offering support and information [3]. One of the first and most important goals of systemic management of patients with TAO is to achieve a stable euthyroid state, which can take 3 months or more to achieve. This period can be employed to assess whether the orbitopathy is active or quiescent. Moreover, this period can be applied to collect relevant information, such as lab-values, scans, etc. After 3 months, a definite treatment plan can be started. Exclusion should be made for patients with the most severe form of TAO, i.e. dysthyroid optic neuropathy (DON). Generally, they have to be admitted to the hospital immediately and courses of methylprednisolone pulse therapy have to be initiated as soon as possible.

It is important to initiate treatment for TAO at the time of diagnosis in order to decrease the final severity of the disease, which has been shown to be most effective when treatment is initiated early in the active phase of the disease to allow to bring inflammation and swelling under control and decrease the degree of permanent tissue scarring and functional damage (Fig. 1a, b).

2 Therapeutic Measures at the First Visit

Once a diagnosis of TAO has been made, the treatment will depend on the activity and severity of disease at presentation. The majority of patients with TAO have mild to moderate disease, and require only supportive care.

Approximately 90% of patients with TAO will have upper eyelid retraction [4] and a reduced

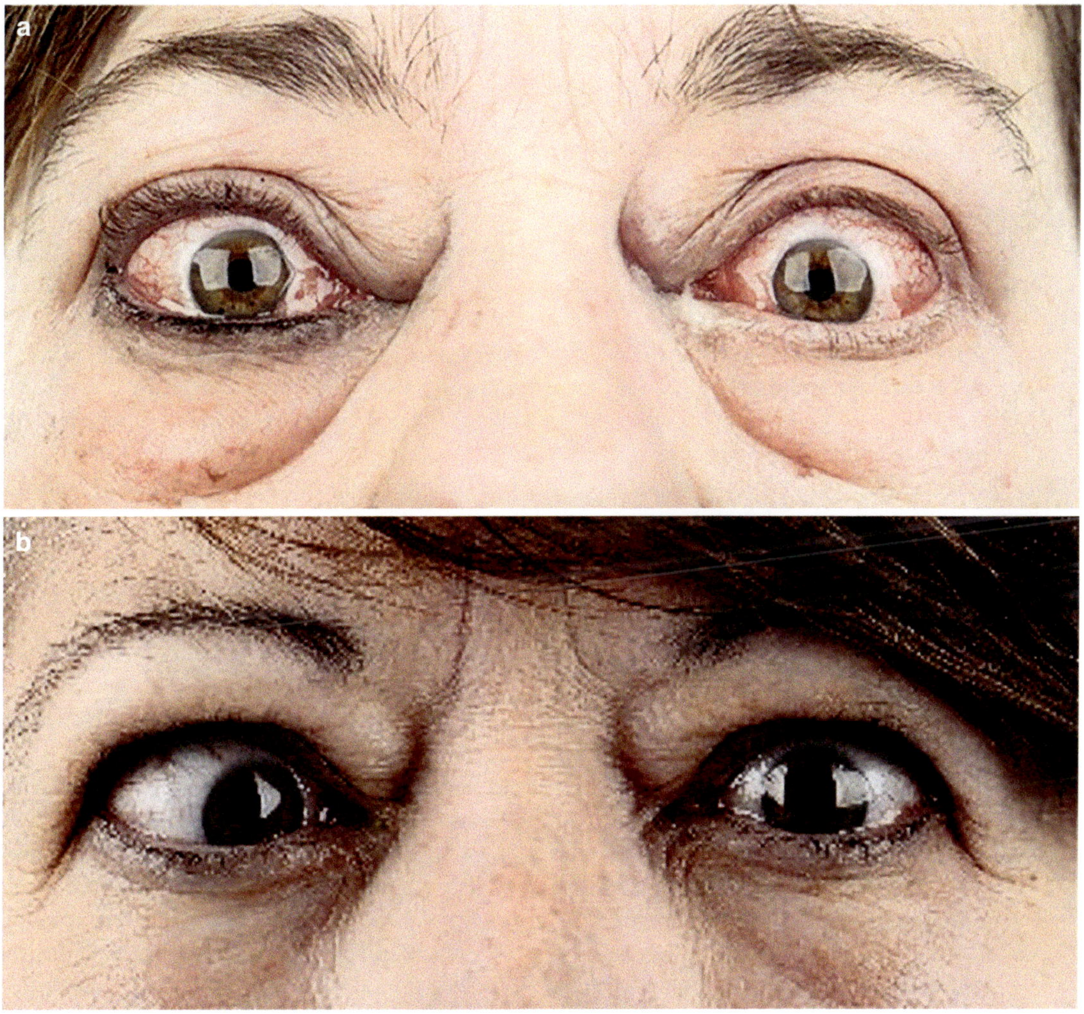

Fig. 1 Patient with active TAO (**a**) with inactive TAO (**b**)

blink rate (Stellwag's sign, 1869) resulting in dry eye symptoms due to evaporative tear loss. Lubricants, given as drops, gels and ointments for the night, will help to manage these symptoms. Photophobia and dry eye can be decreased with dark protective glasses. Approximately 40% of the patients with TAO will show some form of motility impairment [5], who may be helped by Fresnel prisms or some form of eye occlusion.

3 Lifestyle Modifications

Smoking cessation can help maintain stable thyroid hormone levels, as well as decrease the duration of the active phase of the disease. Smoking greatly increases the risk for TAO (odds ratio, 7.7; 95% confidence interval, 4.3–13.7) [6]. Smoking increases the risk of developing TAO by seven fold compared to nonsmokers, but also increases the severity of TAO, reduces the effectiveness of many treatments and negatively influences the outcome of treatment of TAO. Smoking, therefore, should be discouraged. Refraining from smoking may be extremely difficult, and smoking cessations programs often have to be deployed. Encouraging patients to maintain good general health and well-being can reduce stress and anxiety levels. Optimizing dietary habits, vitamin D and selenium levels can also be of benefit to patients. Selenium has been shown to be beneficial in patients with mild orbitopathy in

Europe where the soil is selenium deficient. Sodium restriction reduces water retention in the tissues surrounding the eyes. Sleeping with the head of the bed elevated and applying cool packs can reduce facial swelling. Oral non-steroidal anti-inflammatory drugs (NSAIDs) may relieve eye pain and eyelid swelling.

4 Restoration and Maintenance of a Euthyroid State

Both hyperthyroidism and hypothyroidism negatively influence TAO [2]. Whereas hypothyroidism can simply be corrected with levothyroxine tablets, treatment of hyperthyroidism is more complicated. There are three options for treatment of hyperthyroidism:

1. Antithyroid drugs
   (a) *Titration method*: Antithyroid drugs are given in such a dosage that euthyroidism is reached. The disadvantage of this approach is that levels of thyroid hormones may fluctuate considerably and more than several months are needed to bring the patient in a stable position.
   (b) *Block and Replacement:* Enough antithyroid drugs are given to completely block the patient's own production. At the same time, the required thyroid hormone (levothyroxine) is supplemented.

The advantages of antithyroid drug treatment are that they quickly restore euthyroidism, especially with the 'block and replace' regimen and that they can then be stopped after a period of 2 years without creating lifelong dependency. As autoimmune hyperthyroidism and TAO are self-limiting diseases, approximately 60% will stay euthyroid with 30–40% developing recurrent hyperthyroidism. For this reason it is good practice to maintain TAO-patients on antithyroid medications until the eye disease is inactive and stable for 6 months [7]. As such, in more severe cases, antithyroid drugs are often given for years, though not infinitely. If there is relapse of hyperthyroidism after discontinuation of antithyroid medications, or if the patient develops an allergic or adverse reaction to them, other treatment modalities may be considered by the patient's endocrinologist.

2. Radio-active iodine

The radioiodine I-131 is taken orally in a capsule or liquid form and is quickly absorbed into the bloodstream and concentrated by the thyroid gland, where it begins destroying the gland's thyroid cells. It can permanently treat hyperthyroidism, but radioactive iodine has a number of disadvantages:

(a) Patients not responding sufficiently need a second or even third treatment with this isotope.
(b) Euthyroidism is rarely achieved, and hypothyroidism has to be managed through lifelong levothyroxine replacement.
(c) The destruction of the thyroid cells process takes days to weeks and during this period the symptoms may worsen.
(d) Radio-active iodine elicits or worsens TAO in 15% [8]. At risk patients include recent and/or active TAO, severe hyperthyroidism, high levels of TSH-receptor antibodies and smokers. Patients with these risk factors should not be offered I^{131}-treatment or treated with caution. Worsening of TAO can be prevented using concomitant treatment with oral corticosteroids (0.3–0.4 mg/kg oral prednisone for 3 months). Patients without these risk factors can be offered I^{131}-treatment safely without steroid cover.
(e) Post I^{131}-hypothyroidism may exacerbate TAO and has to be anticipated and corrected as soon as possible.

Despite these disadvantages, radio-active iodine has a 50 year history and is a well-established treatment option for hyperthyroidism worldwide with few long-term side-effects.

3. Thyroidectomy

Subtotal or total thyroidectomy will result in hypothyroidism, which has to be anticipated and corrected with levothyroxine as it will otherwise exacerbate TAO. Accidental removal of parathyroid glands and surgical damage to the recurrent laryngeal nerve, causing a hoarse voice, are possible complications of surgery, but in experienced hands mostly avoidable. Nevertheless, thyroidectomy is a less commonly used treatment modality compared to radio-active iodine.

5 Severity and Disease Activity of TAO

When assessing patients with TAO, it is important to document both the current activity and severity of disease at each and every visit. This enables the establishment of the current degree of activity and severity, on which management decisions are based, and importantly also helps to track the course of the disease as to whether the patient is improving, deteriorating or has remained stable.

5.1 Severity of TAO

For grading the disease severity, there are several well established classification systems including the Werner's NOSPECS classification and the VISA classification [9, 10]. The EUGOGO classification has been widely adopted as the gold standard for assessment of patients with TAO [11], and classifies severity into three categories:

1. Mild TAO: 60% of all patients with TAO, with mild impact on quality of life

    - Clinical signs and symptoms insufficient to justify immunosuppression or surgical intervention and can include any of the following:
        - Mild eyelid retraction (<2 mm)
        - Mild soft tissue involvement
        - Proptosis <3 mm (correlate to race and gender)
        - Transient or no diplopia
        - Dry eye symptoms responsive to topical lubricants

2. Moderate-to-Severe TAO: 35% of all Patients with TAO

    - Non sight-threatening, but clinical signs and symptoms have sufficient impact on quality of life to justify immunosuppression or surgical intervention, and can include any of the following:
        - Eyelid retraction ≥2 mm
        - Moderate or severe soft tissue involvement
        - Proptosis >3 mm (correlate to race and gender)
        - Transient or constant diplopia

Assessment of disease activity is of utmost importance in this group, since patients are initially treated with immunosuppressive therapy and rehabilitative surgical surgery is undertaken when the disease is stable and inactive.

3. Sight-threatening or Dysthyroid Optic Neuropathy: <5% of all Patients with TAO
    - Clinical signs of optic neuropathy and/or corneal breakdown
    - Required urgent immunosuppression with or without surgical intervention

Dysthyroid Optic Neuropathy (DON) occurs due to a combination of extreme orbital soft tissue swelling and a tight orbital septum with subsequent raised intraorbital pressure [12], causing optic nerve compression and loss of vision. A tight orbital septum is believed to prevent auto-decompression, hence the degree of proptosis may not be significant [13, 14]. Patients with DON always have active TAO.

5.2 Activity of TAO

Establishing whether a patient has active or inactive TAO is important as immunosuppression with corticosteroids or orbital radiotherapy are only thought to be effective in the active stage of the disease. On the other hand, certain surgical treatments, such as strabismus surgery, should only be undertaken when the disease is inactive and has remained stable for at least 3–6 months. Patients with active moderate or severe TAO should be treated with immunosuppressive therapy, whereas patients with inactive and stable TAO can be scheduled for surgical intervention(s).

To assess the activity of TAO, the Clinical Activity Score (CAS) has been developed [15]. The CAS is based on the classic signs of inflammation, e.g. rubor (redness), dolor (pain), tumor (swelling) and functio laesa (impaired function). The fifth classic sign (calor) has not been included, because the CAS is a clinical score that should be practically applied without special instruments such as a heat detector.

The Clinical Activity Score is used to assess the activity of TAO. At the initial visit, patients are given a CAS score of 1–7, one point for each sign or symptom. If the CAS is ≥3 the disease is considered active.

1. Orbital pain in primary gaze
2. Gaze-evoked orbital pain
3. Eyelid swelling
4. Eyelid erythema
5. Conjunctival injection
6. Conjunctival Chemosis
7. Inflammation of caruncle or plica semilunaris

At the follow-up visit in addition to the above seven criteria the following are evaluated, one point each sign or symptom. If the CAS is ≥4 the disease is considered active.

8. Increase of ≥2 mm proptosis in the last 1–3 months
9. Deterioration in uniocular motility in any one direction of ≥5°
10. Decrease in visual acuity equivalent to 1 Snellen line

Patients with a CAS of three or more out of ten respond well to immunosuppressive treatment, while those with less than three points were likely not to respond [15].

The CAS has been criticized for several reasons. Firstly, each criteria is given equal weighting, and it is not clear whether this is appropriate. Secondly, the first seven criteria can be subjective. Thirdly, the scoring is binary. Often small degrees of improvement are not sufficient to alter the score of each item. Therefore, a photographic atlas of graded inflammatory signs for EUGOGO has been developed, available at https://www.eugogo.org/, to overcome some of these drawbacks [16]. Despite its disadvantages, the CAS has become widely adopted as a standardized measure of disease activity of TAO, and in particular utilized in randomized clinical trials [17–19], with inter-observer agreement in 86% of cases [20]. In a study testing the effectiveness of the CAS, it was shown that, using a cut-off point of 4 on a scale of 10, the positive predictive value of the CAS was 80%, the negative predictive value 64%, the sensitivity 55% and the specificity 86% [21]. It should be understood that response to corticosteroids or orbital radiation as a quality measure of the CAS is a derivative and does not take into account that treatments are ineffective in some individuals [22].

The intrinsic value of the CAS has been further established by its relationship with serum levels of thyroid-stimulating antibodies and thyrotropin-binding inhibitory immunoglobulins, ultrasonography and octreotide uptake on octreotide scintigraphy, all of which are considered parameters of disease activity [23–25]. Over the years there has been a tendency to use the first 7 items of the CAS only, which has the advantage that a score can be assessed on the same day during the first visit. However the 7-item CAS has never been evaluated for its predictive value. In recent studies, the 7-items CAS with a cut-off point of 3 is usually used.

Both activity and severity of TAO can also be assessed with the VISA analysis, which evaluates Vision, Inflammation, Strabismus, and Appearance and is used at the first and subsequent visits. It has the advantage of providing a detailed, standardized and comprehensive scoring system, encompassing CAS for disease activity and specific criteria to assess disease severity. This requires the observer to give an objective score, which can be used to assess disease activity and severity at the initial visit and crucially also for the longitudinal assessment of patients at subsequent visits.

6 Management of Mild TAO

Mild TAO is a self-limiting disease, and a period of observation, together with conservative measures to address any symptoms and cessation of smoking, is typically sufficient (Table 1). Patients with a CAS of 3 or more out of 7 can be offered the antioxidant 'selenium' (100 μg selenium twice daily). The trace element selenium is inexpensive and no side effects have been reported. A placebo-controlled trial demonstrated a greater improvement in TAO in the selenium group as compared to the placebo group (61% vs. 36%, $p < 0.001$), and progression of TAO from mild to severe form was significantly lower in the selenium group (7% vs. 26%) [26]. A validated quality-of-life questionnaire (GO-QoL) also supported the use of selenium. Surgical intervention in patients with mild TAO can be undertaken after a period of 3–6 months of disease stability and inactivity.

7 Management of Moderately Severe TAO

7.1 Corticosteroid Treatment

The oldest immunosuppressive treatment, corticosteroids are still the medical treatment of choice for patients with active and moderately severe TAO (Table 1). Corticosteroids have multiple mechanisms of action in TAO, leading to a reduction in periocular inflammation. They down-regulate the immune system through:

- Anti-inflammatory actions
- Interference with the function of T and B lymphocytes
- Reduction in the recruitment of neutrophils, monocytes, and macrophages
- Inhibition of the function of immunocompetent cells
- Inhibition of the release of cytokines
- Decrease glycosaminoglycans (GAGs) synthesis and secretion by orbital fibroblasts

Over the years corticosteroid treatment has had a questionable reputation, due to its moderate efficacy and many side-effects. However, this presumed moderate effectiveness was in large part due to the fact that oral prednisone had been used to treat patients with active and with *inactive* TAO. Its side-effects were predominantly due to unnecessary prolonged use. Moreover, bone and gastric protection, with bisphosphonates and proton pump-inhibitors respectively, were not routinely administered as they are today. The efficacy of prednisone in active TAO management has now been demonstrated in a number of randomized controlled clinical studies [27, 28]. Treatment with oral steroids (e.g. prednisone) is most common, typically starting with a high dose, and slowly tapering over several months. While the success rate of oral prednisone is approximately 60%, intravenous (IV) methylprednisolone administered in pulses has a success rate exceeding 80% [29, 30]. Moreover, IV methylprednisolone is better tolerated than oral prednisone [30]. Hence, methylprednisolone IV pulse therapy has become the gold standard treatment in the management of patients with active and moderately severe TAO, and is now advocated by the European Group of Graves' Orbitopathy [31]. EUGOGO recommends, based on a dose finding study [32], a regimen of 500 mg methylprednisolone IV once a week for 6 weeks, followed by 250 mg once a week for another a further 6 weeks. Such a regimen results in a total dose of 4.5 g. High-dose IV corticosteroids have a higher risk of toxicity but this decreases with lower IV doses. Infusions of methylprednisolone can be administered in an outpatient setting where the patient can be monitored for side-effects. The significant inconvenience and cost of multiple hospital visits and an attempt to improve the availability of high-dose corticosteroid treatment, particularly during the COVID-19 pandemic, has accelerated the use of oral methylprednisolone given at equivalent high doses to IV methylprednisolone. In one small study the clinical efficacy and safety of oral methylprednisolone compared with IV administration was found to be non-inferior [33].

However, many patients do not respond or only partially respond to corticosteroid treatment [22], whilst others relapse with dose reduction or discontinuation of corticosteroids. Important side effects include Cushing syndrome, weight gain, mood and sleep disturbance, increased risk of infection, steroid induced or loss of control of diabetes and hypertension and osteoporosis. A low risk of cardiac and liver toxicity [34], electrolyte disturbances, and arrhythmias exists. Frequent monitoring of electrolytes, liver function, blood glucose and blood pressure is required. Steroids, therefore, should not be used in patients with a history of recent viral hepatitis or marked reduced liver function, severe cardiovascular or psychiatric disorders and cumulative doses of 8 mg should be avoided, as well as daily doses of more than 1 g [34].

Corticosteroids have been first line therapy for TAO and are effective against the inflammatory signs of TAO and can improve ocular motility, but generally have little effect on proptosis. Yang et al. found that IV administered methylprednisolone pulses stabilize active TAO in 85% and reduces the severity of TAO in 38% [35]. When effective and tolerated they help to inactivate the disease and allow patients to undergo surgical rehabilitation. If no change in disease status is observed after 6 weeks of treatment with corticosteroids, there should be no more delay in switching the patient to an alternative immunosuppressive treatment. The response to IV pulsed methylprednisolone therapy may be increased by combining with a second line immunosuppressive agent such as mycophenolate mofetil [36]. The latter reduces proliferation of B and T cells of the immune system and also suppresses antibody formation by B cells.

7.2 Orbital Radiotherapy

External beam orbital radiotherapy has been used in the treatment of TAO for almost a century [37]. It is presumed to work by inducing terminal differentiation in progenitor fibroblasts, suppressing the downstream consequences of fibroblast activation, and by reducing the secretion of proinflammatory cytokines from activated lymphocytes. Current high-energy linear accelerators provide targeted delivery of radiation to the retrobulbar orbital tissues. Several randomized clinical trials have demonstrated the efficacy of radiotherapy for patients with moderately severe as well as mild TAO [17, 38, 39]. Orbital radiotherapy may not show benefit for several days to weeks, but its effects are longer-lasting. In some patients there may be a temporary exacerbation of TAO, which can be covered with corticosteroids. Indeed concurrent use of corticosteroids with orbital radiotherapy has been found to be more efficacious than orbital radiotherapy alone [40, 41]. Most treatment regimens administer a total of 20 Gy given at 2 Gy per day over 10 days. Orbital radiotherapy decreases inflammatory eye signs and improves ocular motility in about 60%. Orbital radiotherapy seems to shorten the duration of the disease, thus allowing earlier performance of eventual rehabilitative surgery [42]. Side-effects of radiotherapy are limited to a modest increase of retinopathy in patients with diabetes mellitus [43]. It is generally recommended that orbital radiotherapy is restricted to patients older than 35 years of age and without systemic vascular disease. The rate of compressive optic neuropathy has been shown to be significantly lower, and improvement in ocular motility greater, in patients receiving orbital radiotherapy in addition to corticosteroids [44]. Patients with active TAO appear to have an effective and sustained response to orbital radiotherapy combined with corticosteroids that is protective against disease progression and the development of compressive optic neuropathy.

7.3 Rituximab

Rituximab is a chimeric monoclonal antibody against a surface protein on B-cells called CD20. It causes depletion of these B-cells, thereby influencing the autoimmune response of TAO. The outcome of two randomized clinical trials in active, moderately severe TAO have been conflicting [45, 46]. Therefore currently, rituximab (1000 mg given twice over 2 weeks) is considered primarily in patients with insufficient response to methylprednisolone pulse therapy. Its role in the treatment of TAO requires further study.

7.4 Tumor Necrosis Factor-Alpha and Interleukin-6-Receptor Monoclonal Antibodies

At the time of writing there is insufficient evidence for a role of these treatment options in patients with active and moderately severe TAO.

7.5 Combination Treatment

Where there is insufficient response or intolerance to corticosteroid treatment, combinations of steroid sparing immunosuppressive modalities can be given. In a double blind randomized clinical trial, cyclosporine alone appeared to be ineffective in patients with active and moderately severe TAO. However, the combination of oral prednisone and cyclosporine (7.5 mg per kg body weight per day during 12 weeks) was effective in 56% of patients who had no or insufficient response to oral prednisone alone [2].

7.6 Teprotumumab

This monoclonal antibody blocking the IGF-1 receptor on orbital fibroblasts and lymphocytes appears as an exciting new drug in our armamentarium in the treatment of TAO, as it is the first drug that not only improves inflammatory signs of TAO and ocular motility, but also significantly reduces proptosis [18, 47]. It is administered at 10 mg per kg body weight initially, followed by seven infusions of 20 mg per kg once every 3 weeks over 24 weeks (see chapter "Novel Immunomodulatory Treatment Modalities in Thyroid-Associated Orbitopathy").

8 Management of Severe TAO and Dysthyroid Optic Neuropathy

Management of patients with very severe, vision-threatening TAO is well established as per the EUGOGO protocol. Patients with Dysthyroid Optic Neuropathy (DON) are treated with IV pulses of methylprednisolone 1.0 g per day for 3 consecutive days, which can be repeated after 1 week. If the response is insufficient, urgent orbital decompression should be considered. In patients with corneal ulcers corneal exposure protocols should be followed and surgical procedures to protect the cornea should be considered early on. Surgical decompression of the orbit reduces orbital congestion in TAO, but does not halt disease activity or progression of muscle enlargement, orbital volume expansion, or optic nerve compression [38]. Hence, even after successful orbital decompression, immunosuppressive treatment may be necessary and patients should be monitored closely for relapse of DON.

9 Quality of Life

It is good practice to have the outcomes of treatment judged by patients themselves. The GO-QoL questionnaire is very suitable for this (see chapter "Quality of Life in Patients with Thyroid-Associated Orbitopathy") [48].

References

1. Estcourt S, Hickey J, Perros P, Dayan C, Vaidya B. The patient experiences of services for thyroid eye disease in the United Kingdom: results of a nationwide survey. Eur J Endocrinol. 2009;161:483–7.
2. Prummel MF, Wiersinga W, Mourits M, Koornneef L, Berghout A, van der Gaag R. Amelioration of eye changes of Graves' ophthalmopathy by achieving euthyroidism. Acta Endocrinol. 1989;121:185–9.
3. Perros P, Zarkovic M, Azzolini C, Ayvaz G, Baldeschi L, Bartalena L, et al. PREGO (presentation of Graves' orbitopathy) study: changes in referral patterns to European Group on Graves' Orbitopathy (EUGOGO) centers over the period from 2000 to 2012. Br J Ophthalmol. 2015;99:1531–5.
4. Bartley GB, Fatourechi V, Kadrmas EF, Jacobsen SJ, Ilstrup DM, Garrity JA, Gorman CA. Clinical features of Graves' ophthalmopathy in an incidence cohort. Am J Ophthalmol. 1996;121:284–90.
5. Sasim IV, Berendschot TT, van Isterdael C, Mourits MP. Planning health care for patients with Graves' orbitopathy. Graefes Arch Clin Exp Ophthalmol. 2008;246:1315–21.
6. Prummel MF, Wiersinga WM. Smoking and risk of Graves' disease. JAMA. 1993;27:479–82.

7. Elbers L, Mourits M, Wiersinga W. Outcome of very long-term treatment with antithyroid drugs in Graves' hyperthyroidism associated with Graves' orbitopathy. Thyroid. 2011;21:279–83.
8. Traisk E, Tallstedt L, Abraham-Nordling M, Andersson T, Berg G, Calissendorff J, et al. Thyroid-associated ophthalmopathy after treatment for Graves' hyperthyroidism with antithyroid drugs or iodine-131. J Clin Endocrinol Metab. 2009;94:3700–7.
9. Werner SC. Modification of the classification of the eye changes of Graves' disease. Am J Ophthalmol. 1977;83:725–7.
10. Dolman PJ, Rootman J. VISA classification for Graves orbitopathy. Ophthal Plast Reconstr Surg. 2006;22:319–24.
11. European Group on Graves' Orbitopathy (EUGOGO), Wiersinga WM, Perros P, Kahaly GJ, Mourits MP, Baldeschi L, Boboridis K, Boschi A, Dickinson AJ, Kendall-Taylor P, Krassas GE, Lane CM, Lazarus JH, Marcocci C, Marino M, Nardi M, Neoh C, Orgiazzi J, Pinchera A, Pitz S, Prummel MF, Sartini MS, Stahl M, Von Arx G. Clinical assessment of patients with Graves' orbitopathy: The European Group on Graves' Orbitopathy recommendations to generalists, specialists and clinical researchers. Eur J Endocrinol. 2006;155:387–9.
12. McKeag D, Lane C, Lazarus JH, Baldeschi L, Boboridis K, Dickinson AJ, Hullo AI, Kahaly G, Krassas G, Marcocci C, Marinò M, Mourits MP, Nardi M, Neoh C, Orgiazzi J, Perros P, Pinchera A, Pitz S, Prummel MF, Sartini MS, Wiersinga WM, European Group on Graves' Orbitopathy (EUGOGO). Clinical features of dysthyroid optic neuropathy: A European Group on Graves' Orbitopathy (EUGOGO) survey. Br J Ophthalmol. 2007;91:455–8.
13. Otto AJ, Koornneef L, Mourits MP, Deen-Van LL. Retrobulbar pressures measured during surgical decompression of the orbit. Br J Ophthalmol. 1996;80:1042–5.
14. Koornneef L. Eyelid and orbital fascial attachments and their clinical significance. Eye. 1988;2:130–4.
15. Mourits MP, Koornneef L, Wiersinga WM, Prummel MF, Berghout A, Van Der Gaag R. Clinical criteria for the assessment of disease activity in Graves' ophthalmopathy: a novel approach. Br J Ophthalmol. 1989;73:639–44.
16. Dickinson AJ, Perros P. Controversies in the clinical evaluation of active thyroid-associated orbitopathy: use of a detailed protocol with comparative photographs for objective assessment. Clin Endocrinol (Oxf). 2001;55:283–303.
17. Mourits MP, Van Kempen-Harteveld ML, García MB, Koppeschaar HP, Tick L, Terwee CB. Radiotherapy for Graves' orbitopathy: randomised placebo-controlled study. Lancet. 2000;355:1505–9.
18. Douglas RS, Kahaly GJ, Patel A, Sile S, Thompson EHZ, Perdok R, Fleming JC, Fowler BT, Marcocci C, Marinò M, Antonelli A, Dailey R, Harris GJ, Eckstein A, Schiffman J, Tang R, Nelson C, Salvi M, Wester S, Sherman JW, Vescio T, Holt RJ, Smith TJ. Teprotumumab for the treatment of active thyroid eye disease. N Engl J Med. 2020;382:341–52.
19. Kahaly GJ, Riedl M, König J, Pitz S, Ponto K, Diana T, Kampmann E, Kolbe E, Eckstein A, Moeller LC, Führer D, Salvi M, Curro N, Campi I, Covelli D, Leo M, Marinò M, Menconi F, Marcocci C, Bartalena L, Perros P, Wiersinga WM, European Group on Graves' Orbitopathy (EUGOGO). Mycophenolate plus methylprednisolone versus methylprednisolone alone in active, moderate-to-severe Graves' orbitopathy (MINGO): a randomised, observer-masked, multicentre trial. Lancet Diabetes Endocrinol. 2018;6:287–98.
20. Gerding MN, Prummel MF, Kalmann R, Koornneef L, Wiersinga WM. The use of colour slides in the assessment of changes in soft-tissue involvement in Graves' ophthalmopathy. J Endocrinol Invest. 1998;21:459–62.
21. Mourits MP, Prummel MF, Wiersinga WM, Koornneef L. Clinical activity score as a guide in the management of patients with Graves' ophthalmopathy. Clin Endocrinol (Oxf). 1997;47:9–14.
22. Bartalena L, Veronesi G, Krassas GE, Wiersinga WM, Marcocci C, Marinò M, Salvi M, Daumerie C, Bournaud C, Stahl M, Sassi L, Azzolini C, Boboridis KG, Mourits MP, Soeters MR, Baldeschi L, Nardi M, Currò N, Boschi A, Bernard M, Von Arx G, Perros P, Kahaly GJ, European Group on Graves' Orbitopathy (EUGOGO). Does early response to intravenous glucocorticoids predict the final outcome in patients with moderate-to-severe and active Graves' orbitopathy? J Endocrinol Invest. 2017;40:547–53.
23. Gerding MN, Van Der Meer JW, Broenink M, Bakker O, Wiersinga WM, Prummel MF. Association of thyrotrophin receptor antibodies with the clinical features of Graves' ophthalmopathy. Clin Endocrinol (Oxf). 2000;52:267–71.
24. Gerding MN, Prummel MF, Wiersinga WM. Assessment of disease activity in Graves' ophthalmopathy by orbital ultrasonography and clinical parameters. Clin Endocrinol (Oxf). 2000;52:641–6.
25. Gerding MN, Van Der Zant FM, Van Royen EA, Koornneef L, Krenning EP, Wiersinga WM, Prummel MF. Octreotide-scintigraphy is a disease-activity parameter in Graves' ophthalmopathy. Clin Endocrinol (Oxf). 1999;50:373–9.
26. Marcocci C, Kahaly GJ, Krassas GE, Bartalena L, Prummel M, Stahl M, Altea MA, Nardi M, Pitz S, Boboridis K, Sivelli P, Von Arx G, Mourits MP, Baldeschi L, Bencivelli W, Wiersinga WM, European Group on Graves' Orbitopathy. Selenium and the course of mild Graves' orbitopathy. N Engl J Med. 2011;364:1920–31.
27. Prummel MF, Mourits MP, Berghout A, Krenning EP, van der Gaag R, Koornneef L, Wiersinga WM. Prednisone and cyclosporine in the treatment of severe Graves' ophthalmopathy. N Engl J Med. 1989;321:1353–9.
28. Marcocci C, Bartalena L, Panicucci M, Marconcini C, Cartei F, Cavallacci G, Laddaga M, Campobasso G, Baschieri L, Pinchera A. Orbital cobalt irradia-

tion combined with retrobulbar or systemic corticosteroids for Graves' ophthalmopathy: a comparative study. Clin Endocrinol (Oxf). 1987;27:33–42.
29. van Geest RJ, Sasim IV, Koppeschaar HP, Kalmann R, Stravers SN, Bijlsma WR, Mourits MP. Methylprednisolone pulse therapy for patients with moderately severe Graves' ophthalmopathy: prospective, randomized, placebo-controlled study. Eur J Endocrinol. 2008;15:229–37.
30. Kahaly GJ, Pitz S, Hommel G, Dittmar M. Randomized, single-blind trial of intravenous versus oral steroid monotherapy in Graves' orbitopathy. J Clin Endocrinol Metab. 2005;90:5234–40.
31. Bartalena L, Baldeschi L, Boboridis K, Eckstein A, Kahaly GJ, Marcocci C, Perros P, Salvi M, Wiersinga WM, European Group on Graves' Orbitopathy (EUGOGO). The 2016 European Thyroid Association/European Group on Graves' Orbitopathy Guidelines for the Management of Graves' Orbitopathy. Eur Thyroid J. 2016;5:9–26.
32. Bartalena L, Krassas GE, Wiersinga W, Marcocci C, Salvi M, Daumerie C, et al. Efficacy and safety of three different cumulative doses of intravenous methylprednisolone for moderate to severe and active Graves' orbitopathy. J Clin Endocrinol Metab. 2012;97:4454–63.
33. Shams PN. High-dose oral methylprednisolone for the management of severe active thyroid eye disease during the Coronavirus disease 2019 pandemic. Ophthalmic Plast Reconstr Surg. 2020;36:418–9.
34. Marino M, Morabito E, Brunetto MR, Bartalena L, Pinchera A, Marcocci C. Acute and severe liver damage associated with intravenous glucocorticoid pulse therapy in patients with Graves' ophthalmopathy. Thyroid. 2004;14:403–6.
35. Yang M, Wiersinga WM, Soeters MR, Mourits MP. What is the aim of immunosuppressive treatment in patients with Graves' orbitopathy? Ophthalmic Plast Reconstr Surg. 2014;30:157–61.
36. Kahaly GJ, Riedl M, König J, Pitz S, Ponto K, Diana T, Kampmann E, Kolbe E, Eckstein A, Moeller LC, Führer D, Salvi M, Curro N, Campi I, Covelli D, Leo M, Marinò M, Menconi F, Marcocci C, Bartalena L, Perros P, Wiersinga WM, European Group on Graves' Orbitopathy (EUGOGO). Mycophenolate plus methylprednisolone versus methylprednisolone alone in active, moderate-to-severe Graves' orbitopathy (MINGO): a randomized, observer-masked, multicentre trial. Lancet Diabetes Endocrinol. 2018;6:287–98.
37. Kazim M, Garrity JA. Orbital radiation therapy for thyroid eye disease. J Neuroophthalmol. 2012;32:172–6.
38. Prummel MF, Mourits MP, Blank L, Berghout A, Koornneef L, Wiersinga WM. Randomized double-blind trial of prednisone versus radiotherapy in Graves' ophthalmopathy. Lancet. 1993;342:949–54.
39. Prummel MF, Terwee CB, Gerding MN, Baldeschi L, Mourits MP, Blank L, Dekker FW, Wiersinga WM. A randomized controlled trial of orbital radiotherapy versus sham irradiation in patients with mild Graves' ophthalmopathy. J Clin Endocrinol Metab. 2004;89:15–20.
40. Zoumalan CI, Cockerham KP, Turbin RE, Volpe NJ, Kazim M, Douglas RS, Feldon SE. Efficacy of corticosteroids and external beam radiation in the management of moderate to severe thyroid eye disease. J Neuroophthalmol. 2007;27:205–14.
41. Stiebel-Kalish H, Robenshtok E, Hasanreisoglu M, Ezrachi D, Shimon I, Leibovici L. Treatment modalities for Graves' ophthalmopathy: systematic review and metaanalysis. J Clin Endocrinol Metab. 2009;94:2708–16.
42. Pitz S, Kahaly G, Rösler HP, Krummenauer F, Wagner B, Stübler M, Pfeiffer N. Retrobulbar irradiation for Graves' ophthalmopathy-long-term results. Klin Monbl Augenheilkd. 2002;219:876–82.
43. Wakelkamp IM, Tan H, Saeed P, Schlingemann RO, Verbraak FD, Blank LE, Prummel MF, Wiersinga WM. Orbital irradiation for Graves' ophthalmopathy: is it safe? A long-term follow-up study. Ophthalmology. 2004;111:1557–62.
44. Shams PN, Ma R, Pickles T, Rootman J, Dolman PJ. Reduced risk of compressive optic neuropathy using orbital radiotherapy in patients with active thyroid eye disease. Am J Ophthalmol. 2014;157:1299–305.
45. Stan MN, Garrity JA, Carranza Leon BG, Prabin T, Bradley EA, Bahn RS. Randomized controlled trial of rituximab in patients with Graves' orbitopathy. J Clin Endocrinol Metab. 2015;100:432–41.
46. Salvi M, Vannucchi G, Campi I, Curro N, Dazzi D, Simonetta S, et al. Efficacy of B-cell targeted therapy with rituximab in patients with active moderate to severe Graves' orbitopathy: a randomized controlled study. J Clin Endocrinol Metab. 2015;100:422–31.
47. Smith TJ, Kahaly GJ, Ezra DG, Fleming JC, Dailey RA, Tang RA, et al. Teprotumumab for thyroid-associated ophthalmopathy. N Engl J Med. 2017;376:1748–61.
48. Terwee CB, Dekker FW, Mourits MP, Gerding MN, Baldeschi L, Kalmann R, et al. Interpretation and validity of changes in scores on the Graves' ophthalmopathy quality of life questionnaire (GO-QoL) after different treatments. Clin Endocrinol (Oxf). 2005;54:391–8.

Dysthyroid Optic Neuropathy

Peerooz Saeed and Kaveh Vahdani

Key Messages

- Dysthyroid optic neuropathy (DON) is a serious and potentially blinding complication of thyroid-associated orbitopathy (TAO).
- The main pathogenic mechanism is direct compression of the optic nerve by enlarged extra-ocular muscles within the rigid orbital apex, causing increased apical hydrostatic pressure and restriction of the posterior optic nerve blood supply.
- Other factors such as neighbouring inflammation, metabolic changes or optic nerve stretch may also increase the susceptibility of the optic nerve to the compressive damage.
- Prompt recognition and management of DON are crucial in preventing irreversible sight loss.
- High dose intravenous methylprednisolone is the first line of treatment, followed by early surgical decompression of the posteromedial orbit, if response to medical treatment is inadequate. Post-operatively, patients should be closely monitored and supplemental treatment may be required to maximise recovery of the orbital functions.

P. Saeed (✉)
Orbital Centre, Department of Ophthalmology, Amsterdam University Medical Center, Amsterdam, The Netherlands
e-mail: P.Saeed@amsterdamumc.nl

K. Vahdani
Adnexal Service, Moorfields Eye Hospital, London, UK

1 Introduction

Dysthyroid optic neuropathy (DON) is a relatively uncommon, but serious complication of thyroid-associated orbitopathy (TAO), and requires prompt diagnosis and intervention to prevent permanent vision loss.

Although most commonly seen in the setting of orbital congestion and inflammation, atypical presentation with minimal overt inflammatory signs may delay recognition and adequate management, particularly in the presence of other causes of visual impairment [1, 2].

2 Epidemiology and Risk Factors

The reported annual adjusted incidence of TAO is 16 females and 3 males per 100,000 population, with no significant ethnic predisposition [3]. DON occurs in ≈5% of patients with TAO [4], with an estimated annual incidence of 0.75 cases per million population, according to a recent United Kingdom survey [5].

Risk factors for DON include older age, male gender, smoking, comorbidities such as diabetes, uncontrolled thyroid function, and treatments for hyperthyroidism [6–8].

The age at presentation in DON is significantly higher compared to those with TAO alone (54 years vs. 46 years), [8–10] and for every

F. M. Quaranta Leoni et al. (eds.), *Oculoplastic, Lacrimal and Orbital Surgery*,
https://doi.org/10.1007/978-3-031-39638-0_35

decade, the odds of developing DON may increase by approximately 60% [6]. DON is also more common in males, especially with advancing age [9–11].

Smoking is associated with up to eight-fold increase in risk of developing TAO, [12] greater disease severity and less favourable response to treatment. Smoking is also recognised as an independent modifiable risk factor for DON, although substantial evidence is lacking [6, 13, 14]. Diabetic microangiopathy, particularly in insulin-dependent patients, has been associated with optic nerve hypoxia, thus increasing its vulnerability to compressive optic neuropathy [7].

Dysthyroidism is strongly correlated with the development, severity and progression of TAO. The majority of DON occurs in hyperthyroid patients, although it may also develop in the setting of hypothyroidism or euthyroidism [15]. Rapid establishment and maintenance of euthyroid status following anti-hyperthyroid treatments is essential. Radio-iodine therapy, a well-known risk factor for progression of TAO [16], may also increase the risk of developing DON, although strong evidence is lacking.

3 Pathogenesis

The pathogenesis of DON is complex and involves mechanical, vascular, metabolic, and inflammatory factors. The generally accepted mechanism is optic nerve compression or restriction of its blood supply by enlarged extraocular muscles (EOM) [1, 9, 10, 17, 18].

EOM enlargement in the rigid orbital apex causes a significant increase in the apical pressure [19], this probably determining DON by a microvascular posterior optic neuropathy. Several clinical and orbital volumetric studies support the role of muscle and/or fat enlargement in DON, and certain orbital shapes, such as that of Asians, are likely to be at greater risk [10, 17, 20, 21]. The typically rapid recovery of DON following apical bone decompression also supports a reversible microvascular ischaemia in DON, and, similarly, orbital decompression leads to immediate relief of postural visual obscurations due to peripapillary vasculopathy in patients with "hydraulic" TAO (see chapter "Different Phenotypes and Ocular Surface Changes in Thyroid-Associated Orbitopathy") [2].

DON may occasionally develop in the absence of evident apical optic nerve compression; in such cases, it has been suggested that optic nerve stretch may be a contributory factor—this being caused by increased intraorbital soft tissues volumes (i.e., fat or muscle expansion) and pressure, leading to a gradual and persistent strain on the optic nerve, and consequently dysfunction of the optic nerve [22–24]. Classically, this has been described in orbits with marked proptosis, straightening of the optic nerve and tenting of the posterior globe. However, the relationship between proptosis and DON in unclear, and many patients with DON do not have significant proptosis [18, 21, 25–27].

While the optic nerve length has been observed to be significantly greater in DON, the optic nerve profile and compliance estimates have been shown to be almost identical in DON and TAO without DON, suggesting that optic nerve elongation in DON, though significant, is not extending optic nerve to its elastic limits and is, therefore, unlikely to be causing metabolic stress to the optic nerve [28]. However, it is possible that marked elongation may render the optic nerve more susceptible to pressure-induced microvascular ischaemia, optic neuritis due to neighbouring orbital inflammation, or mechanical and metabolic changes in axoplasmic flow within the optic nerve [28].

4 Clinical Presentation

DON is primarily a clinical diagnosis based on impaired visual function, supported by radiological evidence of apical crowding, with no established diagnostic "gold standard" [29]. Blurring of vision, reduced colour perception, and or new visual field defects indicate early DON [30]. As the apical pressure increases, more severe visual impairment, postural visual obscurations, relative afferent pupillary defect (RAPD) or optic disc abnormalities may develop (Fig. 1).

Although DON is commonly observed in the context of severely inflamed orbits, with a

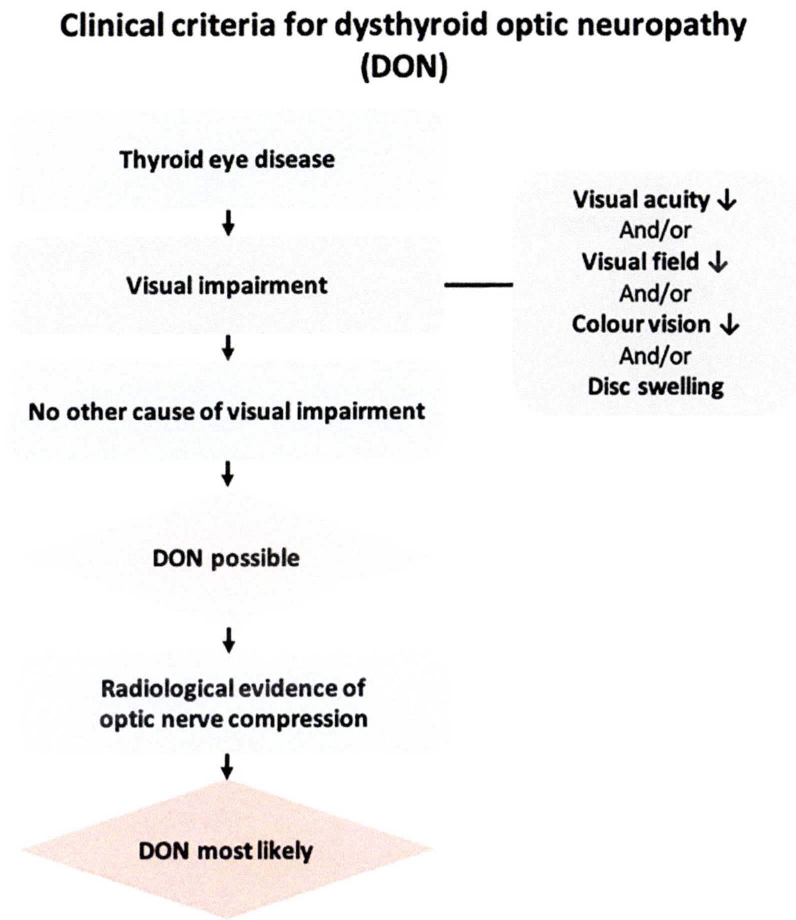

Fig. 1 Flowchart of diagnostic criteria for dysthyroid optic neuropathy (DON)

reported median clinical activity score (CAS) 4/7, it can also occur with minimal or no congestive features—25% of DON with visual acuity of ≤20/40 have a CAS score ≤3 [29]. Furthermore, signs or symptoms of DON may not always be present in subclinical or atypical forms. Good visual acuity or lack of RAPD cannot rule out the diagnosis of DON, with 50–70% of DON patients having an acuity of 20/40 or better, and absent RAPD in 50% of the cases (probably due to bilateral symmetrical involvement) [8, 29, 31]. Optic disc swelling, if present, is a very specific indicator of DON, however the optic disc appearance is normal in over half of the DON cases [29].

Marked proptosis is often absent in patients with DON and the degree of exophthalmos may not correlate with the severity of neuropathy [29, 30]. Furthermore, lack of proptosis or stable exophthalmometry should not be interpreted as normal orbital pressure, but may instead indicate containment of the orbital soft tissues by a robust orbital septum with increased hydrostatic pressure of the orbit, that can rapidly escalate and precipitate severe optic neuropathy. In such cases, the only clinical features may be a firm orbit on retropulsion, with or without optic disc oedema, and severe apical crowding on imaging [30].

5 Investigations

5.1 Visual Fields (VF)

VF testing is a sensitive tool for detecting early DON and monitoring response to treatment. Various patterns of VF deficit are found in over two-thirds of patients with DON, including central or paracentral scotoma, inferior arcuate or altitudinal defects, enlarged blind spot, nerve fibre bundle defects and generalised constriction; the inferior VF defects are more common [32].

5.2 Optical Coherence Tomography (OCT)

OCT provides reproducible qualitative and quantitative data allowing detection of retinal nerve fibre layer and macular ganglion cell complex loss in subclinical stages [33]. In addition, OCT angiography can show decreased peripapillary vascular density and attenuated perfusion in eyes with DON, which significantly correlates with the extent of visual impairment [34].

5.3 Visual Evoked Potentials (VEP)

VEP offers electrophysiological evidence for DON and it is possibly more sensitive than kinetic perimetry. VEP abnormalities, specifically prolonged P100 latency, are a sensitive indicator of diminished optic nerve conduction and may be present in three-quarters of patients [35].

5.4 Doppler Ultrasonography

Doppler ultrasound is particularly useful in assessing the flow characteristics in the superior ophthalmic vein (SOV), which is often reduced or reversed in DON; [36] dilated SOVs are also more commonly found in orbits with concomitant DON, these changes reflecting apical compression by the enlarged EOMs.

5.5 Computerised Tomography (CT) and Magnetic Resonance Imaging (MRI)

Radiological evaluation using CT and MRI is paramount in diagnosing DON [25] (Figs. 2 and 3). Both imaging modalities are useful for assessing disease activity by extra-ocular muscle (EOM) contrast enhancement on CT, and higher water content on T2-weighted and fat-suppressed images using short tau inversion recovery (STIR) MRI sequences. While MRI has a superior soft tissue definition, CT provides better imaging of the bony orbital anatomy, which is crucial for surgical planning.

Typical findings in DON are EOM volume expansion and apical crowding. The muscle index represents a means of estimating the relative EOM volume within the orbit—this being significantly greater in DON orbits than TAO alone, with two-thirds of DONs showing a muscle index of greater than 70%, while muscle indices of <50% excludes DON in most cases [17] Apical crowding, best shown on coronal sections, is a good predictor for DON and its severity can be graded based on the extent of perineural fat effacement, with almost 80% of the DON orbits having severe apical crowding compared to approximately 13% of the orbits without DON [37].

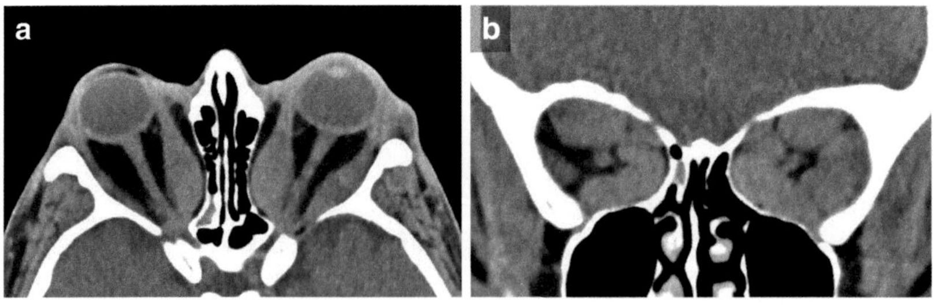

Fig. 2 Computerised tomography of a 35-year-old heavy-smoker female with hyperthyroidism, presenting with progressive bilateral optic neuropathy, non-responsive to intravenous steroids. (**a**) Axial section shows bilateral marked proptosis with enlarged medial recti and auto-decompressed medial orbital walls. (**b**) Coronal sections show severe apical crowding and effacement of the perineural fat (*left* more than *right*)

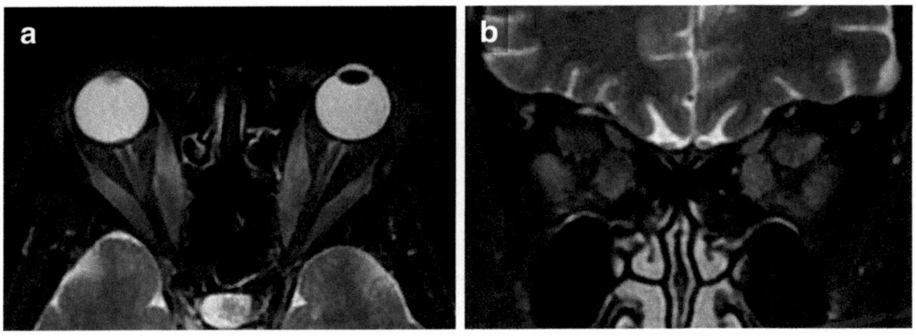

Fig. 3 MRI STIR (short-tau inversion recovery) sequences of a 75-year-old east Asian female presenting with severe bilateral asymmetrical dysthyroid optic neuropathy, bilateral swollen discs and orbital congestion, non-responsive to systemic steroids. (**a**) Axial and (**b**) Coronal section show mild bilateral proptosis, straightening of the optic nerves, enlarged oedematous recti muscles with apical crowding

The shape of the bony orbit may also be an independent predictor, with narrower orbits, such as that of Asians, being more susceptible to develop DON [21]. Other features that may be present are dilated SOV or prolapsed orbital fat through the superior orbital fissure, that are less specific for DON [29].

6 Medical Treatment

High-dose intravenous methylprednisolone (IVMP) is the first line of treatment for DON, and prompt surgical decompression is indicated for those who fail to respond. Although there is no universally accepted dosing regimen, a commonly used protocol for IVMP is 500–1000 mg daily for 3 consecutive days, repeated if necessary, after 1 week. Such regimen may lead to complete visual recovery in approximately 43% of cases and avoid surgery in up to half of these patients [38]. The cumulative dose of IVMP should not exceed 8 g to reduce the risk of acute liver failure, and patients should be closely monitored for systemic side effects [39]. Urgent orbital decompression should be performed if there is inadequate or absent response within 2 weeks (Fig. 4) [30, 39].

Low-dose radiotherapy is a useful adjunct to corticosteroids, reducing the risk of progression to DON in high-risk TAO patients, or even obviating the need for surgery in DON [40]. Commonly, a total dose of 20 Gy per orbit is administered in 10 fractions over a 2-week period. In view of the delay in treatment response, radiotherapy should not be used alone, and should only be used with great caution in patients with DM and hypertension, who have a higher risk of developing radiation retinopathy [41].

Various immunosuppressive and biologic agents have been investigated in DON and are generally used as second line therapies. Rituximab, an anti-CD20 monoclonal antibody, and tocilizumab, an anti-IL-6 monoclonal antibody, have been proposed for treating severe active TAO and/or DON refractory to steroid therapy, although strong level of evidence is lacking [39, 42–44].

Teprotumumab, an insulin-like growth factor I receptor (IGF-IR) which is overexpressed by orbital fibroblasts and B and T cells in TAO, has been shown to be superior to placebo in reducing CAS score and proptosis in patients with moderate-severe TAO [45]. However, the efficacy of teprotumumab compared to gold-standard treatment with steroids is yet to be confirmed. Early findings show that teprotumumab may be useful in patients with DON who have not yet developed significant optic atrophy, particularly those who are poor surgical candidates or have failed previous therapeutic interventions [46].

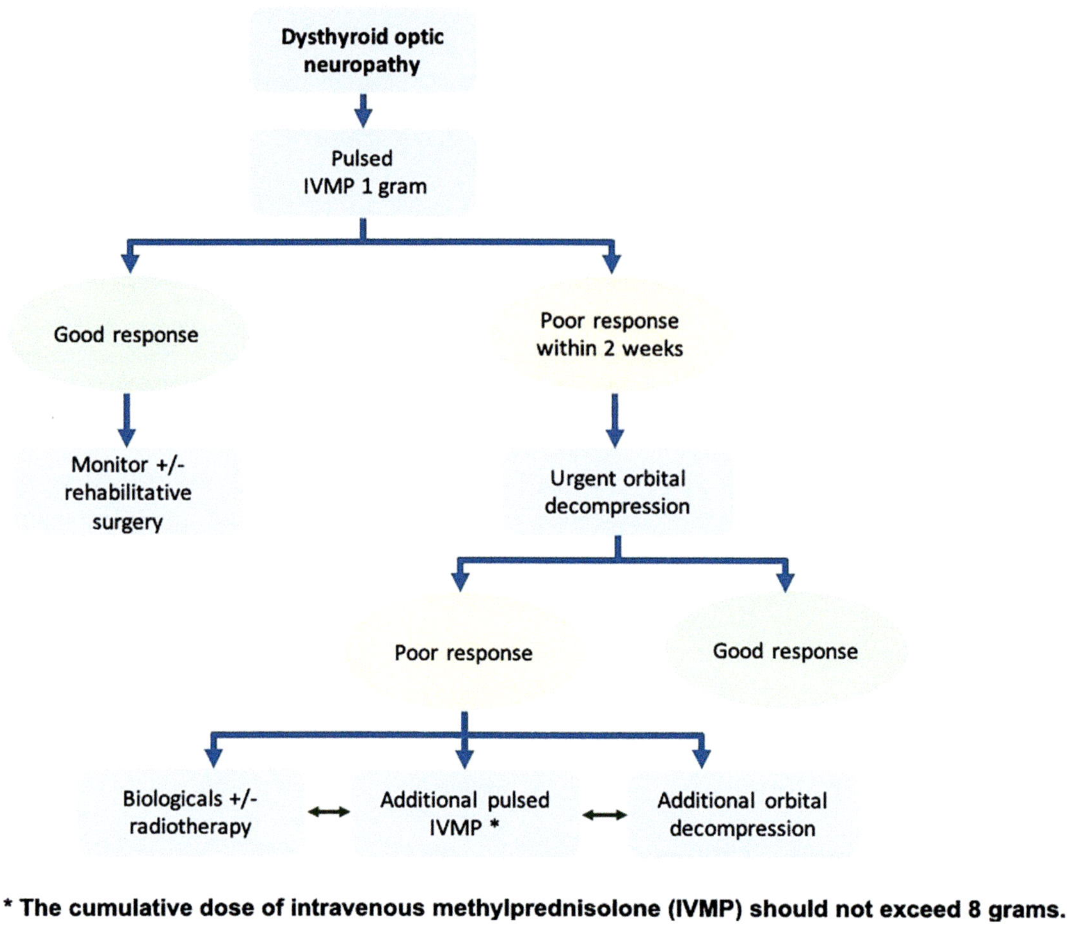

Fig. 4 Flowchart with suggested treatment protocol for dysthyroid optic neuropathy (DON)

7 Surgical Treatment

Orbital decompression is considered when response to medical therapy is not prompt and adequate [29, 30]. The goal of the surgery is to lower the hydrostatic pressure at the orbital apex, thereby reducing orbital congestion and improving optic nerve perfusion. Surgically, the bony medial wall is removed as far posteriorly as the annulus of Zinn, with posterior and mid-ethmoid air cells, and the posterior half of the maxillo-ethmoidal strut [30, 47]. Medial wall decompression is commonly performed through retrocaruncular or endoscopic approaches—both enabling a wider visualisation of the entire medial orbital wall and the maxillo-ethmoidal strut (Fig. 5a), allowing effective decompression of the orbital apex with a broad excision of the medial periosteum [30].

Removal of the deep lateral orbital bone, either alone or in combination with other techniques, is an alternative option for apical decompression [48]. Orbital fat removal may provide additional decompression, and in selected cases is performed as an isolated procedure [23].

Visual recovery following surgery depends on the duration of the DON, and return of full visual function can occur rapidly in patients having an acute history of optic neuropathy. Marked rapid improvement has also been observed in some patients with 6 months or longer period of pre-existing compressive optic neuropathy [30]. Restoration of central vision to 20/40 or better in over 85% of the cases, has been reported

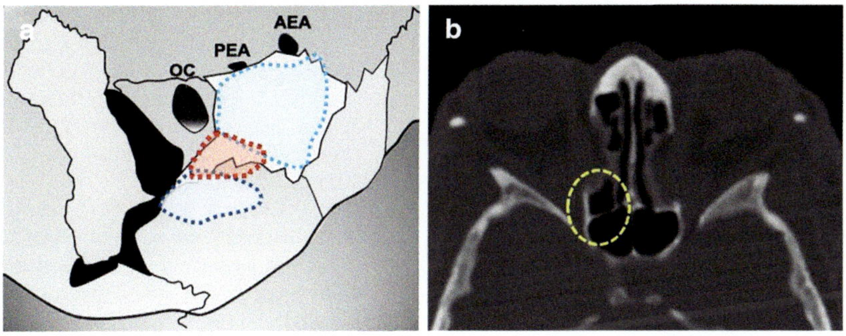

Fig. 5 (**a**) Schematic illustration of right orbit demonstrating the extent of medial wall decompression. AEA, denotes anterior ethmoidal artery, PEA, posterior ethmoidal artery, OC, optic canal. Blue dotted areas are lamina papyracea and posterior medial floor. *Red dotted area* is the posterior maxillo-ethmoidal strut. (**b**) Bony window axial CT section following bilateral endoscopic medial wall and ab-externo lateral wall decompression showing adequate left but incomplete right medial wall decompression with residual posterior lamina papyracea and ethmoidal air cell (*yellow dotted area*)

irrespective of severity of the visual loss or surgery delay [49]. Some authors reported almost 70% complete visual recovery [31].

Occasionally, absent or poor visual recovery, or even visual deterioration might be due to insufficient orbital decompression (Fig. 5b), and in such cases, a complete removal of the medial wall or further lateral wall decompression should be considered [1]. Post-operatively, 20% of the patients may require additional immunosuppressive therapy or radiation to control the ongoing inflammatory process [50].

References

1. Saeed P, Tavakoli Rad S, Bisschop P. Dysthyroid optic neuropathy. Ophthalmic Plast Reconstr Surg. 2018;34:S60–S7.
2. Rose GE. Postural visual obscurations in patients with inactive thyroid eye disease; a variant of 'hydraulic' disease. Eye (Lond). 2006;20:1178–85.
3. Bartley GB, Fatourechi V, Kadrmas EF, Jacobsen SJ, Ilstrup DM, Garrity JA, et al. The incidence of Graves' ophthalmopathy in Olmsted County, Minnesota. Am J Ophthalmol. 1995;120:511–7.
4. Bartley GB, Fatourechi V, Kadrmas EF, Jacobsen SJ, Ilstrup DM, Garrity JA, et al. Clinical features of Graves' ophthalmopathy in an incidence cohort. Am J Ophthalmol. 1996;121:284–90.
5. Wong Y, Dickinson J, Perros P, Dayan C, Veeramani P, Morris D, et al. A British Ophthalmological Surveillance Unit (BOSU) study into dysthyroid optic neuropathy in the United Kingdom. Eye (Lond). 2018;32:1555–62.
6. Khong JJ, Finch S, De Silva C, Rylander S, Craig JE, Selva D, et al. Risk factors for Graves' orbitopathy; the Australian Thyroid-Associated Orbitopathy Research (ATOR) Study. J Clin Endocrinol Metab. 2016;101:2711–20.
7. Kalmann R, Mourits MP. Diabetes mellitus: a risk factor in patients with Graves' orbitopathy. Br J Ophthalmol. 1999;83:463–5.
8. Blandford AD, Zhang D, Chundury RV, Perry JD. Dysthyroid optic neuropathy: update on pathogenesis, diagnosis, and management. Expert Rev Ophthalmol. 2017;12:111–21.
9. Trobe JD, Glaser JS, Laflamme P. Dysthyroid optic neuropathy. Clinical profile and rationale for management. Arch Ophthalmol. 1978;96:1199–209.
10. Neigel JM, Rootman J, Belkin RI, Nugent RA, Drance SM, Beattie CW, et al. Dysthyroid optic neuropathy. The crowded orbital apex syndrome. Ophthalmology. 1988;95:1515–21.
11. Perros P, Crombie AL, Matthews JN, Kendall-Taylor P. Age and gender influence the severity of thyroid-associated ophthalmopathy: a study of 101 patients attending a combined thyroid-eye clinic. Clin Endocrinol (Oxf). 1993;38:367–72.
12. Prummel MF, Wiersinga WM. Smoking and risk of Graves' disease. JAMA. 1993;269:479–82.
13. Wiersinga WM. Management of Graves' ophthalmopathy. Nat Clin Pract Endocrinol Metab. 2007;3:396–404.
14. Lee JH, Lee SY, Yoon JS. Risk factors associated with the severity of thyroid-associated orbitopathy in Korean patients. Korean J Ophthalmol. 2010;24:267–73.
15. Bartalena L, Macchia PE, Marcocci C, Salvi M, Vermiglio F. Effects of treatment modalities for Graves' hyperthyroidism on Graves' orbitopathy:

a 2015 Italian Society of Endocrinology Consensus Statement. J Endocrinol Invest. 2015;38:481–7.
16. Stan MN, Bahn RS. Risk factors for development or deterioration of Graves' ophthalmopathy. Thyroid. 2010;20:777–83.
17. Barrett L, Glatt HJ, Burde RM, Gado MH. Optic nerve dysfunction in thyroid eye disease: CT. Radiology. 1988;167:503–7.
18. Feldon SE, Muramatsu S, Weiner JM. Clinical classification of Graves' ophthalmopathy. Identification of risk factors for optic neuropathy. Arch Ophthalmol. 1984;102:1469–72.
19. Riemann CD, Foster JA, Kosmorsky GS. Direct orbital manometry in patients with thyroid-associated orbitopathy. Ophthalmology. 1999;106:1296–302.
20. Kennerdell JS, Rosenbaum AE, El-Hoshy MH. Apical optic nerve compression of dysthyroid optic neuropathy on computed tomography. Arch Ophthalmol. 1981;99:807–9.
21. Chan LL, Tan HE, Fook-Chong S, Teo TH, Lim LH, Seah LL. Graves ophthalmopathy: the bony orbit in optic neuropathy, its apical angular capacity, and impact on prediction of risk. AJNR Am J Neuroradiol. 2009;30:597–602.
22. Anderson RL, Tweeten JP, Patrinely JR, Garland PE, Thiese SM. Dysthyroid optic neuropathy without extraocular muscle involvement. Ophthalmic Surg. 1989;20:568–74.
23. Kazim M, Trokel SL, Acaroglu G, Elliott A. Reversal of dysthyroid optic neuropathy following orbital fat decompression. Br J Ophthalmol. 2000;84:600–5.
24. Soni CR, Johnson LN. Visual neuropraxia and progressive vision loss from thyroid-associated stretch optic neuropathy. Eur J Ophthalmol. 2010;20:429–36.
25. Giaconi JA, Kazim M, Rho T, Pfaff C. CT scan evidence of dysthyroid optic neuropathy. Ophthalmic Plast Reconstr Surg. 2002;18:177–82.
26. Trobe JD. Optic nerve involvement in dysthyroidism. Ophthalmology. 1981;88:488–92.
27. Nanda T, Dunbar KE, Campbell AA, Bathras RM, Kazim M. Greater proptosis is not associated with improved compressive optic neuropathy in thyroid eye disease. Ophthalmic Plast Reconstr Surg. 2018;34:S72–S4.
28. Rose GE, Vahdani K. Optic nerve stretch is unlikely to be a significant causative factor in dysthyroid optic neuropathy. Ophthalmic Plast Reconstr Surg. 2020;36:157–63.
29. McKeag D, Lane C, Lazarus JH, Baldeschi L, Boboridis K, Dickinson AJ, et al. Clinical features of dysthyroid optic neuropathy: a European Group on Graves' Orbitopathy (EUGOGO) survey. Br J Ophthalmol. 2007;91:455–8.
30. Verity DH, Rose GE. Acute thyroid eye disease (TED): principles of medical and surgical management. Eye (Lond). 2013;27:308–19.
31. Jeon C, Shin JH, Woo KI, Kim YD. Clinical profile and visual outcomes after treatment in patients with dysthyroid optic neuropathy. Korean J Ophthalmol. 2012;26:73–9.
32. Choi CJ, Oropesa S, Callahan AB, Glass LR, Teo L, Cestari DM, et al. Patterns of visual field changes in thyroid eye disease. Orbit. 2017;36:201–7.
33. Micieli JA, Newman NJ, Biousse V. The role of optical coherence tomography in the evaluation of compressive optic neuropathies. Curr Opin Neurol. 2019;32:115–23.
34. Zhang T, Xiao W, Ye H, Chen R, Mao Y, Yang H. Peripapillary and macular vessel density in dysthyroid optic neuropathy: an optical coherence tomography angiography study. Invest Ophthalmol Vis Sci. 2019;60:1863–9.
35. Iao TWU, Rong SS, Ling AN, Brelen ME, Young AL, Chong KKL. Electrophysiological studies in thyroid associated orbitopathy: a systematic review. Sci Rep. 2017;7:12108.
36. Walasik-Szemplinska D, Pauk-Domanska M, Sanocka U, Sudol-Szopinska I. Doppler imaging of orbital vessels in the assessment of the activity and severity of thyroid-associated orbitopathy. J Ultrason. 2015;15:388–97.
37. Nugent RA, Belkin RI, Neigel JM, Rootman J, Robertson WD, Spinelli J, et al. Graves orbitopathy: correlation of CT and clinical findings. Radiology. 1990;177:675–82.
38. Vannucchi G, Covelli D, Campi I, Origo D, Curro N, Cirello V, et al. The therapeutic outcome to intravenous steroid therapy for active Graves' orbitopathy is influenced by the time of response but not polymorphisms of the glucocorticoid receptor. Eur J Endocrinol. 2014;170:55–61.
39. Bartalena L, Baldeschi L, Boboridis K, Eckstein A, Kahaly GJ, Marcocci C, et al. The 2016 European Thyroid Association/European Group on Graves' Orbitopathy Guidelines for the Management of Graves' Orbitopathy. Eur Thyroid J. 2016;5:9–26.
40. Gold KG, Scofield S, Isaacson SR, Stewart MW, Kazim M. Orbital radiotherapy combined with corticosteroid treatment for thyroid eye disease-compressive optic neuropathy. Ophthalmic Plast Reconstr Surg. 2018;34:172–7.
41. Dolman PJ, Rath S. Orbital radiotherapy for thyroid eye disease. Curr Opin Ophthalmol. 2012;23:427–32.
42. Salvi M, Vannucchi G, Curro N, Campi I, Covelli D, Dazzi D, et al. Efficacy of B-cell targeted therapy with rituximab in patients with active moderate to severe Graves' orbitopathy: a randomized controlled study. J Clin Endocrinol Metab. 2015;100:422–31.
43. Khanna D, Chong KK, Afifiyan NF, Hwang CJ, Lee DK, Garneau HC, et al. Rituximab treatment of patients with severe, corticosteroid-resistant thyroid-associated ophthalmopathy. Ophthalmology. 2010;117:133–9 e2.
44. Perez-Moreiras JV, Gomez-Reino JJ, Maneiro JR, Perez-Pampin E, Romo Lopez A, Rodriguez Alvarez FM, et al. Efficacy of tocilizumab in patients with moderate-to-severe corticosteroid-resistant graves orbitopathy: a randomized clinical trial. Am J Ophthalmol. 2018;195:181–90.

45. Smith TJ, Kahaly GJ, Ezra DG, Fleming JC, Dailey RA, Tang RA, et al. Teprotumumab for thyroid-associated ophthalmopathy. N Engl J Med. 2017;376:1748–61.
46. Sears CM, Wang Y, Bailey LA, Turbin R, Subramanian PS, Douglas R, et al. Early efficacy of teprotumumab for the treatment of dysthyroid optic neuropathy: a multicenter study. Am J Ophthalmol Case Rep. 2021;23:101111.
47. Finn AP, Bleier B, Cestari DM, Kazlas MA, Dagi LR, Lefebvre DR, et al. A retrospective review of orbital decompression for thyroid orbitopathy with endoscopic preservation of the inferomedial orbital bone strut. Ophthalmic Plast Reconstr Surg. 2017;33:334–9.
48. Choe CH, Cho RI, Elner VM. Comparison of lateral and medial orbital decompression for the treatment of compressive optic neuropathy in thyroid eye disease. Ophthalmic Plast Reconstr Surg. 2011;27:4–11.
49. Dolman PJ. Dysthyroid optic neuropathy: evaluation and management. J Endocrinol Invest. 2021;44:421–9.
50. McCord CD Jr. Current trends in orbital decompression. Ophthalmology. 1985;92:21–33.

Orbital Decompression Surgery

David H. Verity, Lelio Baldeschi,
Jimmy M. Uddin, and Dion Paridaens

Key Messages

- There are three main indications for surgery: active severe thyroid-associated orbitopathy (TAO) with optic neuropathy or corneal exposure unresponsive to immunosuppression, rehabilitation after active disease, and 'congestive' orbitopathy.
- In cases of mild to moderate exophthalmos (<26 mm) lateral wall and fat decompression alone may be sufficient to restore globe position with minimal diplopia risk.
- For more severe exophthalmos and congestive TAO, a 'balanced' two-wall decompression is preferred, this involving the lateral and medial orbital walls, with or without removal of the posterior-medial floor.
- For optic neuropathy with little proptosis and "white eye apex" TAO, removal of the posterior medial wall and medial floor is effective in most cases in relieving DON.

1 Introduction

Thyroid-associated orbitopathy (TAO) is an autoimmune orbital inflammation that results in increasing orbital adipocytes and extracellular matrix [1]. The inflammatory phase of TAO mainly affects the extraocular muscles and orbital adipose tissue, with increasing accrual of tissue oedema, pro-inflammatory cytokines and lymphocytes [2]. This expansion of orbital soft tissues can compromise orbital blood flow, resulting in optic nerve ischaemia and secondary retardation of axonal flow (dysthyroid optic neuropathy; DON) and hydraulic TAO. Where the orbital septum is non-compliant, forward expansion of the soft tissues is restricted, and this increases the risk of both DON and congestive orbitopathy. TAO is manifest in about a half of patients with Graves' disease and, although DON can be challenging to treat, fortunately only 5% of all patients with TAO will develop such severe disease [3].

The typical course of TAO is one of an 'active' inflammatory phase lasting 12–24 months, followed by an 'inactive' fibrotic stage [4].

Surgical decompression during the active phase of moderate disease is an uncommon indication. Early orbital decompression should be considered in the presence of failed medical treatment of TAO with severe congestive features

D. H. Verity (✉)
Adnexal Service, Moorfields Eye Hospital, London, UK

St John of Jerusalem Eye Hospital Group, London, UK
e-mail: david.verity@nhs.net

L. Baldeschi
Department of Ophthalmology, Catholic University of Louvain, Academic Hospital Saint Luc, Brussels, Belgium

J. M. Uddin
Adnexal Service, Moorfields Eye Hospital, London, UK

D. Paridaens
Department of Oculoplastic, Orbital and Lacrimal Surgery, The Rotterdam Eye Hospital and Erasmus Medical Center, Rotterdam, The Netherlands

F. M. Quaranta Leoni et al. (eds.), *Oculoplastic, Lacrimal and Orbital Surgery*,
https://doi.org/10.1007/978-3-031-39638-0_36

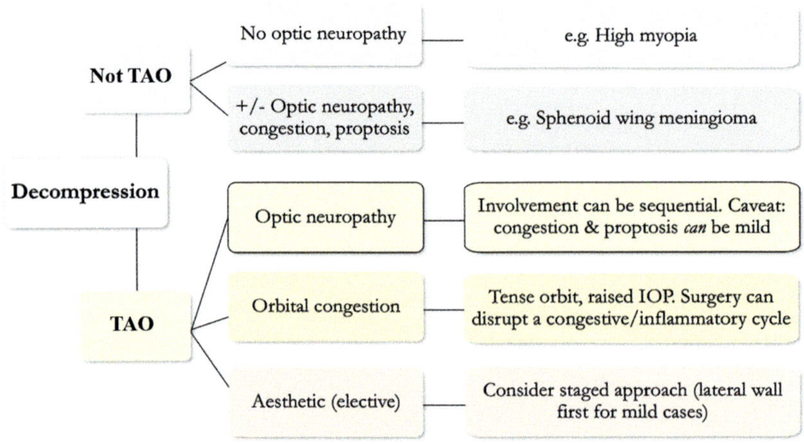

Fig. 1 Guide to indications for orbital decompression

(to limit and reverse progression of TAO), *severe* acute TAO with visual loss due to marked exposure keratopathy, 'hydraulic' features, compressive optic neuropathy and white eye apex TAO. When patients do not respond promptly (within 1–2 weeks) to high-dose corticosteroid treatment, urgent decompression of the deep medial orbital wall and postero-medial floor is indicated; this rapidly relieves congestion and restores optic nerve perfusion [5].

When the active inflammatory phase has abated, decompression can be performed for functional and aesthetic reasons. Indications include to improve: globe position, eyelid displacement ("retraction') caused by orbital tissue expansion, persistent congestion, orbital fat displacement and expansion (contributing to "puffy eyelids and lacrimal gland displacement) and strabismus contributed by limited orbital space. This is usually followed by surgery to address diplopia and upper eyelid retractors recession or lower eyelid surgery, including blepharoplasty and eyelid fat reduction [6].

Rehabilitative orbital decompression, which can also include fat removal, has been employed since the early 1980s [7], and is not exclusively reserved for patients with TAO (Fig. 1). Several approaches are described, and include removal of the medial, lateral, and inferior bony walls, thus expanding the orbital space into paranasal sinuses or temporalis fossa [8]. However, despite extensive literature on the subject, there remains no consensus on the most effective intervention: some authors advocate fat decompression alone, whilst others prefer bony decompression with a graded approach, with both external [8, 9] and internal [10] approaches described.

This chapter presents a practical approach to decompression, with reference to surgical techniques.

2 History

In the past, orbital surgery has been performed by general, ophthalmic, and neuro-surgeons. Walter Dandy, a preeminent neurosurgeon in the 1940s, wrote that "*all orbital surgery should be performed through the transcranial route*" and that "*such surgery results in less morbidity than the commonly-used orbital approach*" [11]. Nevertheless, during the second half of the twentieth century, surgical practice changed in favour of less invasive approaches to avoid the higher morbidity of the intracranial route.

In 1889 Kronlein described a lateral orbital approach which involved removal of bone for excision of a dermoid cyst [12]. This approach was also used by Dollinger in 1890 to reduce exophthalmos in TAO, but, due to the associated scar, the technique was not widely adopted. Nevertheless, this approach resulted in prolapse of the orbital contents into the temporalis fossa, and was the first description of a successful orbital decompression. In 1929 Hirsch described an approach for orbital *floor* decompression [12], and the neurosurgeon Naffziger reported an approach to decompress the orbital *roof* in 1931. In 1939 Kistner was the first to describe a *medial* wall decompression (by ethmoidectomy) [12], and in 1957 Walsh and Ogura popularised a trans-antral approach for medial wall *and* floor decompression [13]. Later, in 1990, Kennedy described an endoscopic approach to the medial wall [14]. Since then, orbital surgeons have increasingly undertaken such surgery, initially using the Ogura technique [15], and now using minimally invasive transorbital approaches, having altogether abandoned neurosurgical approaches [16].

Several techniques for lateral decompression have been described, these initially involving removal of anterior portions of the lateral orbital wall [17]. More recently described approaches remove wider areas of bone from the posterior lateral wall and basin of the inferior orbital fissure, these referred to as the 'door jamb' and the 'deep lacrimal keyhole', with both external (transcutaneous) and transconjunctival approaches employed [10, 18, 19]. Other authors advocate orbital fat removal on the basis that exophthalmos in TAO is due expansion of orbital soft tissues. This approach was first published by Olivari in 1991 and by Trokel in 1993 [20, 21].

Orbital decompression for mild to moderate degrees of exophthalmos is increasingly tending towards lateral wall surgery alone (Fig. 3), performed by orbital surgeons through minimally invasive approaches [22]. Note, indications for orbital decompression can include other compressive pathologies such as sphenoid wing meningioma and posterior vascular lesions, and high myopia (Fig. 1).

3 Practical and Anatomical Considerations

The total orbital volume, formed by a bony tetrahedral cavity with an anterior aperture, is approximately 30–32 cm [3], and is larger in males, with ethnic variation. Unless these wall(s) are displaced or removed, surgical access to the orbit is limited by the anterior orbital opening (measuring 40 mm by 35 mm) and the extent to which the globe can be displaced during surgery. Five bony areas can be decompressed including the deep and anterior lateral wall, the medial wall and the orbital floor (medial and lateral to the infraorbital canal) (Fig. 2). Orbital fat compartments may also be removed alone or in conjunction with bony decompression.

Since both extraocular muscle function and eyelid positions are dependent on the position of the globe, orbital decompression (which can alter both axial and non-axial proptosis) should precede strabismus and eyelid interventions [23], although some advocate simultaneous eyelid lowering and decompression surgery to reduce recovery time [24]. However, since eyelid lowering under general anaesthesia can have unpredictable results, a better result is achieved by undertaking eyelid surgery with local anaesthesia once all post-operative oedema has resolved.

Finally, the patient's occupation and the functional impact of post-operative diplopia is relevant in surgical planning: for example, a self-employed taxi driver with significant exophthalmos may choose lateral wall decompression

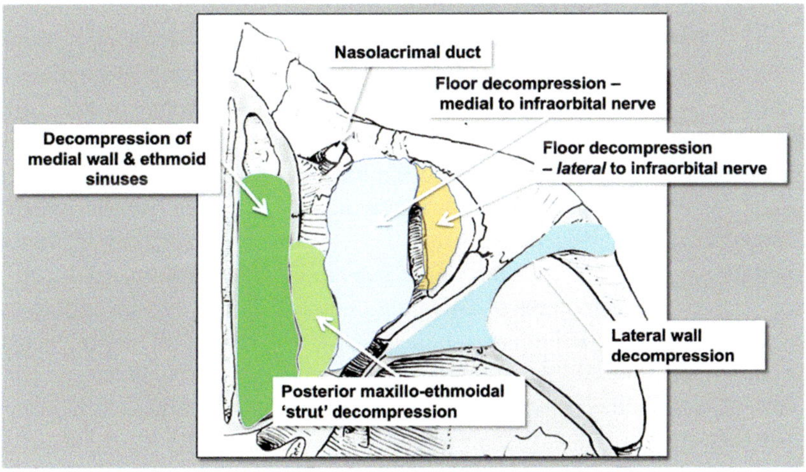

Fig. 2 Schematic showing orbital decompression 'zones'

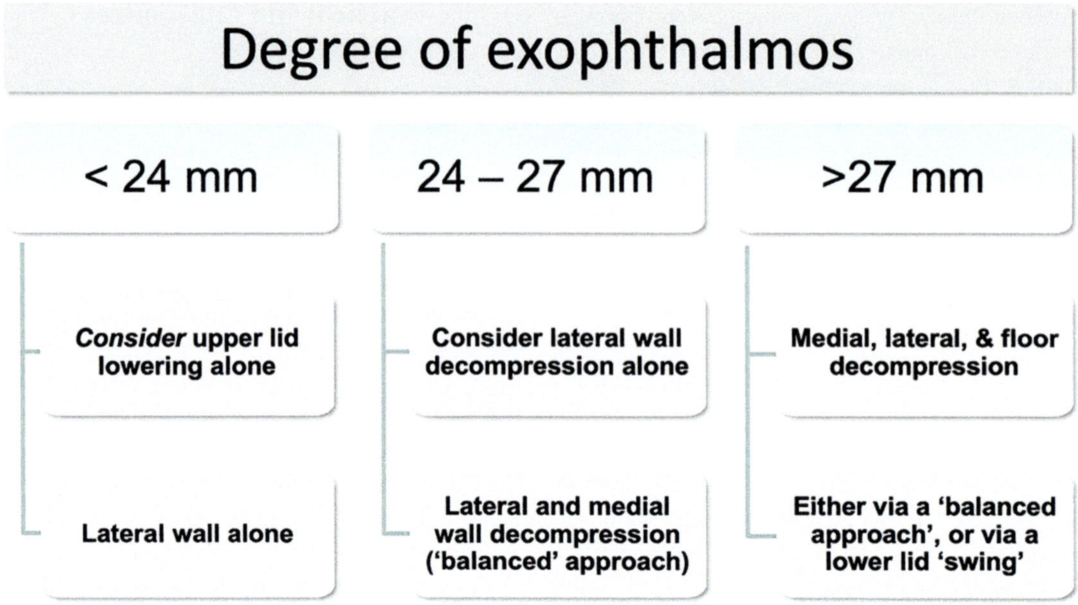

Fig. 3 An algorithmic approach for aesthetic bone decompression. Note, this serves as a *general guide*; the approach in each individual varies according to the degree of pre-morbid exophthalmos and the desired degree of decompression

(accepting a suboptimal reduction in exophthalmos, but with a low risk of post-operative diplopia) in preference to the greater risk of diplopia with medial wall decompression [25]. A broad approach to decompression, based on degree of exophthalmos, and not intended to be didactic, is given in Fig. 3.

4 A Logical Approach to Orbital Decompression for Thyroid-Associated Orbitopathy

Oculoplastic and orbital surgery is rarely necessary in the *acute* phase of TAO, and indicated for functional and aesthetic rehabilitation after the inflammatory phase has subsided, and in those with major orbital *congestion*. There are three main indications for surgery: severely active TAO with corneal exposure or optic neuropathy unresponsive to immunosuppression, rehabilitation following active disease, and congestive orbitopathy (Fig. 1).

4.1 Severe Active TAO

Orbital decompression is indicated when acute fulminant TAO fails to respond promptly and adequately to adequate immunosuppression, typically high-dose intravenous methylprednisolone. Such patients can present with a tense orbit and unilateral or bilateral dysthyroid optic neuropathy (DON). Occasionally, there are fewer outward signs of congestion, but optic neuropathy is present, as with "white eye" apex TAO. Relieving the orbital congestion disrupts the cycle of increased orbital pressure, vascular engorgement and further inflammation, and such patients rarely require prolonged steroid treatment following successful surgery.

The features of early optic neuropathy include deterioration of vision unresponsive to topical lubrication, reduced colour appreciation on *objective* testing (note, patients are often only aware of *subtle* 'greying' of objects), and early visual field defects [26]. In contrast to the patient presenting with *florid* inflammatory signs and

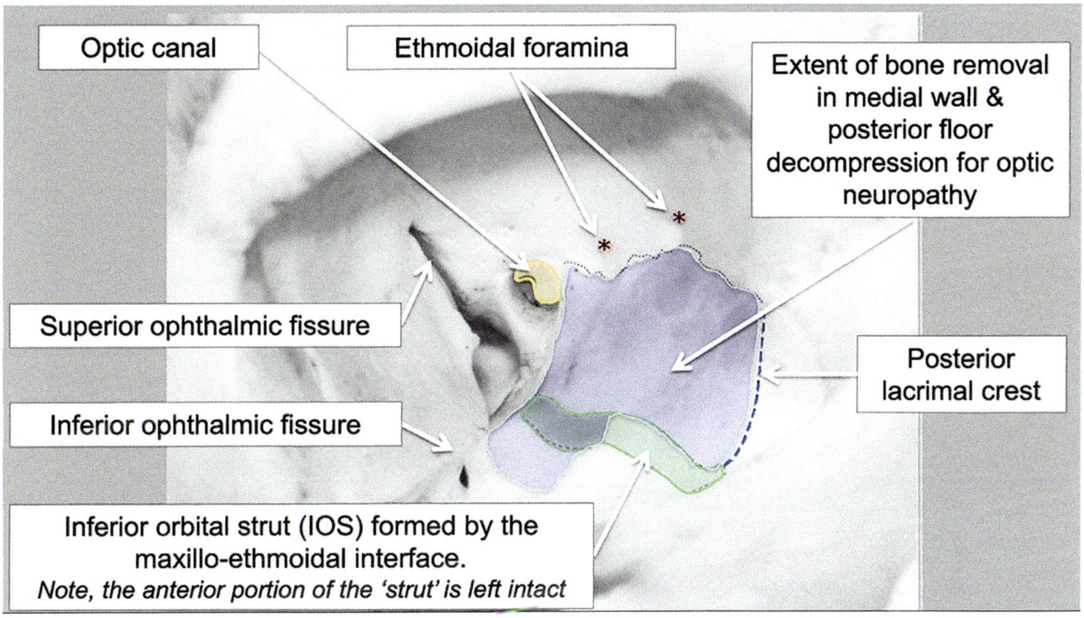

Fig. 4 Anatomical landmarks superimposed on a cadaveric specimen identifying the extent of bone removal in patients with optic neuropathy. Note, the extent to which the medial wall is decompressed anteriorly depends on the degree of associated exophthalmos, but is usually taken as far as the posterior lacrimal crest

DON, as noted above, others can present with reduced distance and colour acuity, orbital tenseness and established optic disc oedema, but *without* overt inflammatory signs. This paradoxical presentation, thought to be due to congestion at the orbital *apex*, can result in a delayed diagnosis. Indeed, in bilateral cases, where a *relative* afferent pupillary defect may be absent, quite severe visual loss can wrongly be attributed to cataract or macular disease. Despite a diagnostic delay of weeks to months, severe DON can still be reversed with medial wall and medial floor decompression, with removal of the most apical lamina papyracea being essential to relieve all apical compression [27], and visual recovery rates approaching 100% in a number of studies [28–31].

Thus, only decompression of the orbital apex can sufficiently reduce local hydrostatic pressure to allow reperfusion of the optic nerve [32]. The annulus of Zinn, origin of the four recti, is situated slightly more posteriorly at its *medial* border [33], and an effective medial decompression will therefore ensure maximum removal of bone medially and inferiorly, with removal of the posterior maxillo-ethmoidal interface (junction of the medial wall and floor), or 'infero-medial bone strut' (Fig. 4).

The medial orbital wall is reached via a medial eyelid or transconjunctival retro-caruncular approach, each affording the surgeon an 'open-sky' view of the medial orbit, the latter giving access to the orbital floor as far lateral as the infraorbital canal. Endoscopic trans-nasal approach to the medial wall, inferomedial strut and medial floor can be employed by competent endoscopic surgeons, resulting in similar bone removal.

Broadly, the technique is as follows: 2/0 silk traction sutures are placed full-thickness through the medial upper and lower eyelids, this being more practical than the use of a speculum (Fig. 5). The intended retro-caruncular conjunctival incision can be marked, and the conjunctiva widely opened to prevent subsequent tearing of the tissues. A pair of closed tissue scissors are placed into the defect, advanced towards the posterior lacrimal crest, and widely opened just posterior to the axis of the crest, thereby dividing the overlying tissues. The lacrimal apparatus is protected with a small Desmarres

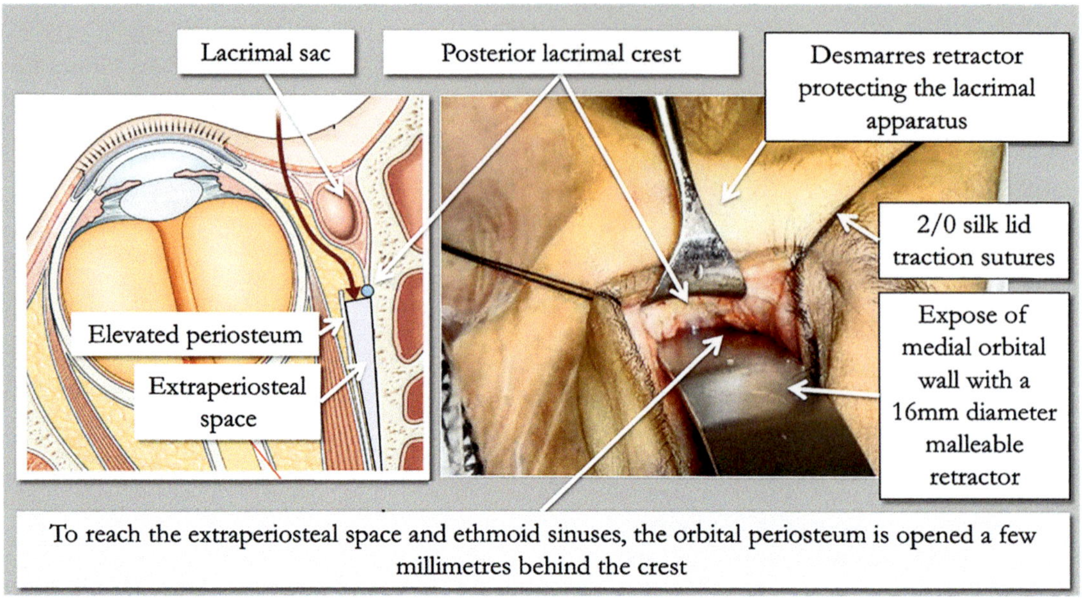

Fig. 5 Retrocaruncular approach to the medial orbital wall

retractor or an angulated 11 mm malleable retractor, and a 16 mm retractor is used to displace the orbital tissues laterally to expose the medial orbital wall. Further division of the soft tissues, either by blunt dissection or using orbital diathermy forceps, exposes the periosteum immediately behind the posterior lacrimal crest; the periosteum can then be opened with a blade or periosteal elevator. In most patients an intact periosteal opening can be achieved between the level of the ethmoidal foramina superiorly and the medial orbital floor below. The periosteal sheet (if intact) is then separated from the medial wall as far back as the annulus of Zinn (to which it is tightly bound), and infero-laterally as far across as the infra-orbital canal. Where the tissues are friable, or the lamina papyracea particularly fragile, the surgeon should begin the manoeuvre over the (firmer) maxillo-ethmoidal suture, or the medial floor itself, where both the bone and the periosteum tend to be stronger.

Once elevated, the periosteum is widely separated from the bone using a 16 mm malleable retractor angulated to about 70° and a MacDonald's elevator. This degree of angulation enables the surgeon, sitting to the side of the patient, to control any prolapse of the fat into the surgical field, and gives a clear 'open-sky' view of the entire medial wall and medial floor. Care should be taken not to work *above* the level of the anterior and posterior ethmoidal vessels, as these define the lowest level of the anterior cranial fossa.

Less experienced surgeons may prefer to decompress the medial floor prior to the medial wall, as this identifies the posterior limit of the maxillary antrum early in the procedure. This landmark lies approximately 8–10 mm in front of the annulus of Zinn, and helps in determining the *posterior* limits for the subsequent ethmoidectomy. In-fracture at the midpoint of the floor, medial to the infra-orbital canal, is performed with a large artery clip, and bone is removed anteriorly (to within 5 mm of the inferior orbital rim) with an up-cutting rongeur, and posteriorly with an *end*-cutting rongeur until there is no remaining posterior 'ledge'. Decompression of the floor can be extended as far laterally as the infraorbital nerve according to the degree of proptosis and required extent of decompression (Fig. 6). Bridging arteriolar tributaries of the distal maxillary artery, found at the medial border of the infraorbital nerve, should be cauterised because these can cause *major* haemorrhage.

Medial wall decompression is achieved by in-fracture of the lamina papyracea below the level of the anterior ethmoidal artery, and removal of the wall with extirpation of the ethmoid air cells; this is achieved anteriorly by using an up-cutting rongeur, and posteriorly with the Tilley-Henkle

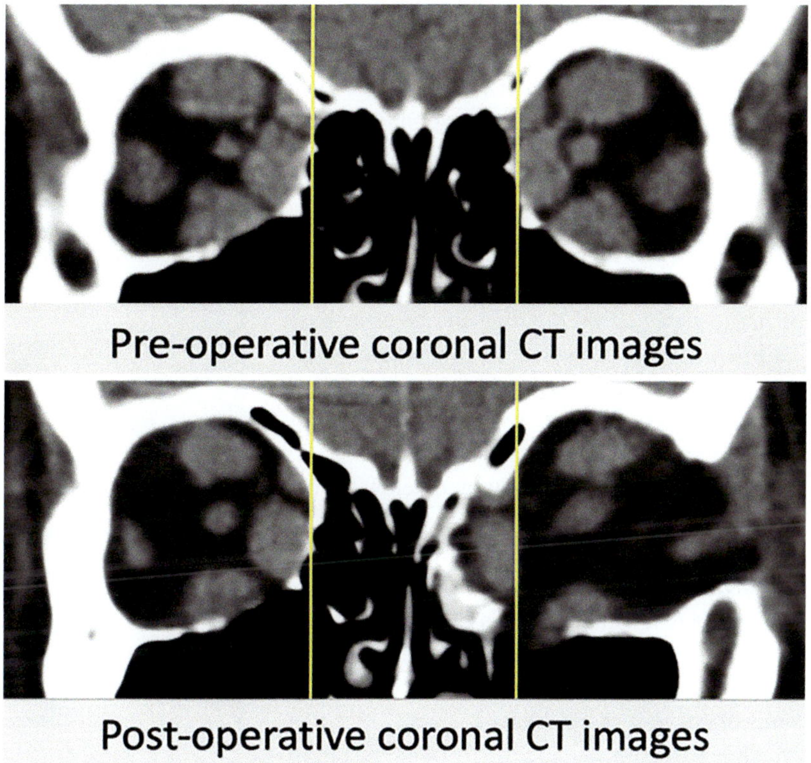

Fig. 6 Pre- and post-operative coronal CT images identifying radiological changes after left bony medial wall and medial floor decompression (*vertical yellow bars* aligning similar bony landmarks pre and post surgery)

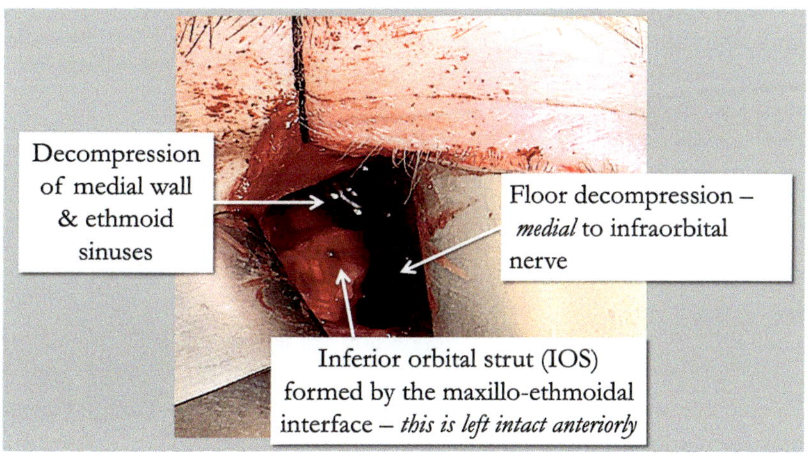

Fig. 7 Per-operative image identifying intact anterior maxillo-ethmoid 'strut' in patient undergoing medial wall and medial floor bone decompression. Collapse or complete removal of the strut compromises drainage of the maxillary sinus

ethmoidectomy forceps. The surgical field of view is increasingly restricted in the posterior orbit, often being monocular at the deepest point of the surgical bed. Measures to improve the surgical field should include cessation of all non-steroidal and antiplatelet medications for at least two weeks prior to surgery, positioning the patient in a head-up position, maintaining the systolic blood pressure at 80–85 mmHg (unless posing unacceptable anaesthetic risks), perioperative tranexamic acid, and frequent aspiration of blood. With a good view the surgeon is able to remove the most posterior ethmoid air cell(s), in-fracture the bony septum between the posterior ethmoid air cells and the sphenoid sinus, and remove the final 2–3 mm of medial wall adjacent to the annulus of Zinn. Finally, the *posterior* half of the bony maxillo-ethmoidal interface (the 'strut') is removed (maintaining integrity of the anterior half, Figs. 4, and 7) and its tri-radiate base ground down using end-cutting rongeurs. This manoeuver is essential if adequate release of *apical* pressure is to be achieved: the periosteum is opened in a tapering 'V' configuration corresponding to one linear cut opening along the skull base, and another along the lateral border of the floor defect. The incisions are brought to a "point" at the orbital apex, this tip of released periosteum being drawn anteriorly out of the orbit, and the triangle of tissue removed by dividing the anterior base. This periosteal excision leads to a prolapse of apical tissues over about a 180° arc, from the skull base superiorly to the lateral antrum below. Conjunctival closure is achieved with a 7/0 absorbable suture placed above and below the caruncle, antibiotic ointment or gel instilled into the conjunctival sac, and the patient double padded overnight in the semi-recumbent position. Nose-blowing is discouraged for ten days after surgery to reduce the risk of surgical emphysema, and the patient should avoid flying for two weeks whilst sinus drainage is re-established.

Almost irrespective of severity of DON, inferomedial decompression as described usually results in major recovery of DON within day(s) of surgery, and patients with optic neuropathy who fail to respond to the first 3 or 4 courses of Intravenous methylprednisolone (IVMP) should be considered for decompression of the posterior medial orbital wall and posteromedial floor and not be consigned to protracted course(s) of immunosuppression. Where greater volume decompression is required, the bony fenestration can be extended as far as, or lateral to, the infraorbital canal, and also combined with lateral wall decompression via a separate incision.

Sequelae of medial wall and floor decompression include esotropia (Fig. 8), late imploding antrum syndrome following excessive removal of the maxillo-ethmoidal bony 'strut' (Fig. 9) [34], and paraesthesia of the upper cheek, gums, and teeth. Very rare, but significant complications include haemorrhage, injury to the recti muscles, and visual loss. Damage to the lacrimal sac is entirely avoidable and is not generally a concern. Finally, and similarly avoidable if relevant landmarks are observed, cranial perforation along the low-lying central fovea ethmoidalis or cribriform plate has been reported—this potentially leading to catastrophic complications [35]. Dural breaks with CSF leakage can be patched with autologous tissues including temporalis fascia, fat,

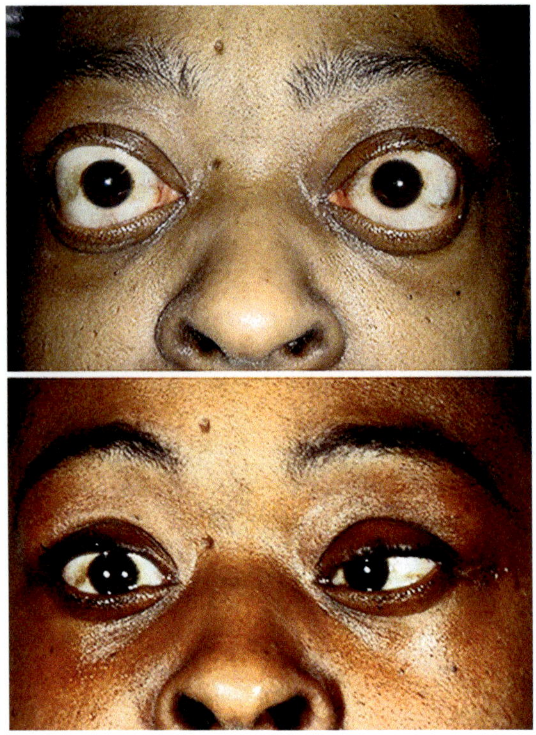

Fig. 8 Pre- and post-operative images: three wall orbital decompression (swinging eyelid) and upper eyelid lengthening for inactive TAO. Note major reduction of exophthalmos, resolution of the inferior scleral show, but, in addition, secondary esotropia

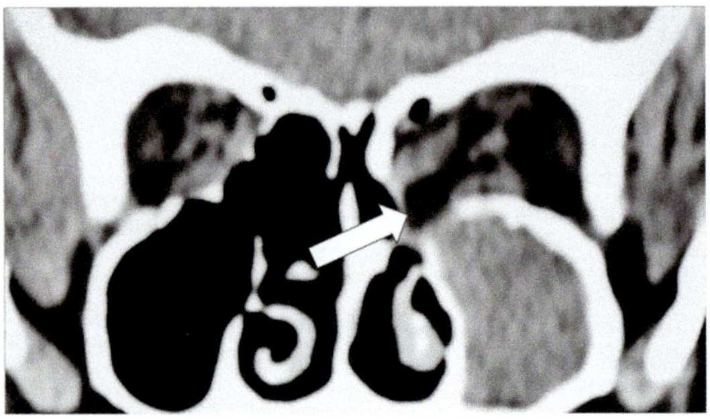

Fig. 9 Obstructed maxillary sinus drainage following medial decompression. Arrow identifies fat prolapse onto the sinus ostium following inadvertent removal of the anterior half of the maxillo-ethmoid 'strut', with complete opacification of the sinus

muscle, and acellular dermal grafts, the graft being stabilised with glue [36]. Finally, inadvertent posterior extension within the sphenoid sinus can lead to carotid artery damage [36].

Surgery can be combined with intra-operative navigation to confirm anatomical positions and landmarks.

4.2 Inactive TAO

TAO tends to be 'monophasic' with an active, inflammatory phase of 6–12 months. This phase can be more protracted in smokers and those with poor thyroid control, and can occasionally reactivate spontaneously or following surgery [37]. Once the inflammation has abated, rehabilitative measures aim to restore the globe position within the orbit, address troublesome diplopia, and re-establish a natural eyelid height, contour and volume (Fig. 10).

Where there is photographic evidence of increased and troublesome proptosis (that is, the proptosis is not 'constitutional'), and where exophthalmometry is greater than approximately 22 mm, consideration should be given to orbital decompression. For mild to moderate degrees of exophthalmos, a deep lateral wall decompression is preferred by many, this typically resulting in up to 5–7 mm reduction in exophthalmos, albeit with significant variation between patients Fig. 11). Equally, the lateral wall fenestration (especially anterior superolateral) allows the lacrimal gland to prolapse posteriorly into the lateral window, this addressing much of the 'fullness' of the eyelid sulcus which cannot be addressed by blepharoplasty alone. Many past techniques were based on an extended brow incision [38], but the lateral upper eyelid skin crease incision, lateral canthotomy or swinging eyelid approach affords excellent access, better cosmesis, and no thinning of the brow hairs [7, 10, 17, 19, 33, 39, 40]. Rarely, troublesome hollowness of the temporalis fossa posterior to the lateral bony rim can occur, in addition to masticatory oscillopsia, temple tenderness, 'clicking' sensation and gaze-evoked ocular pain [41, 42].

A trans upper-lid approach to orbital rim-sparing lateral wall decompression entails a skin-crease incision in the lateral third of the upper eyelid, extended for about a centimetre into the infero-lateral rhytid [9]. The soft tissues overlying the bony rim are opened, with a Desmarres retractor used to displace tissues either side of the incision. Using a D15 blade or sharp periosteal elevator, the periosteum is widely incised along the posterior external face of the lateral rim and raised anteriorly over the rim. A 19 mm mallea-

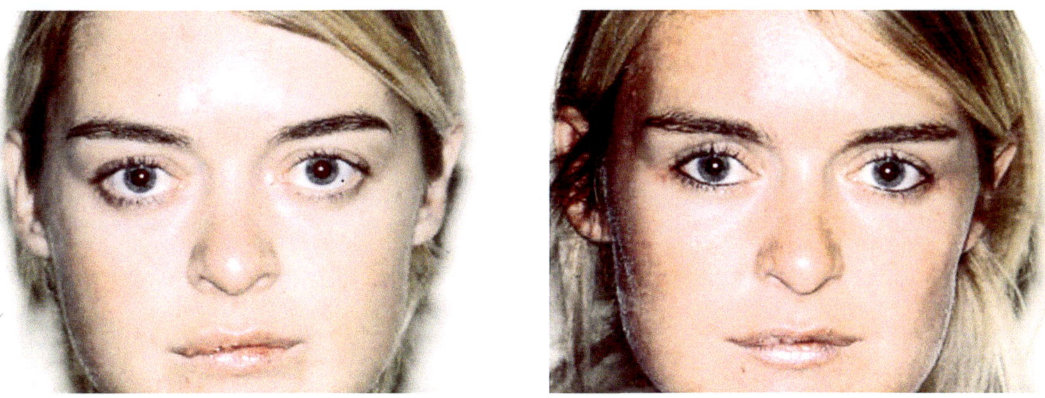

Fig. 10 Pre-operative view (*left*) of a young female patient with burnt-out TAO, presenting with mild proptosis and cosmetically disturbing lower scleral show. She expressed a reduced quality of life due to the changes in appearance. Post-operative view (*right*) 2 months after inferomedial orbital decompression. Note the reduction of the lower scleral show. No post-operative diplopia or other side-effects occurred (Courtesy of D. Paridaens)

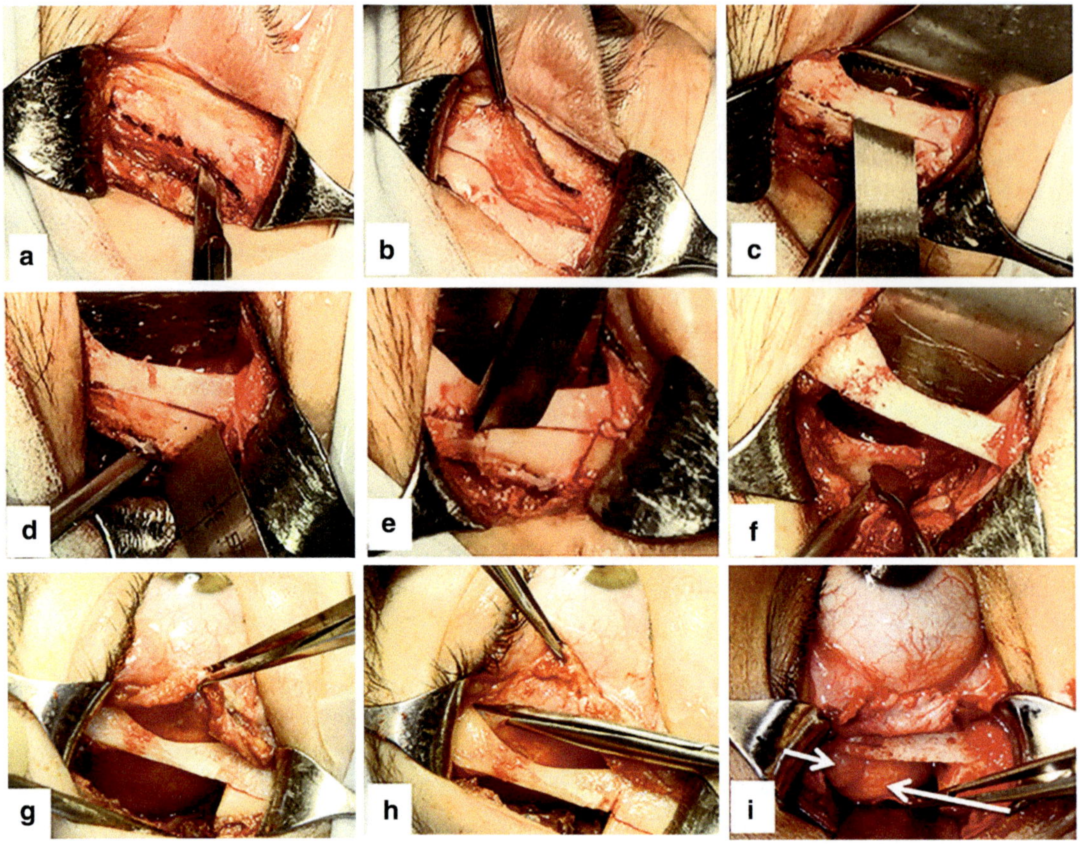

Fig. 11 Steps involved in *ab externo* lateral wall bone decompression. (**a**) A lateral upper eyelid skin crease incision is made, the orbital rim exposed, and the periosteum incised immediately anterior to the insertion of the temporalis fascia (*dotted line*). (**b**) Using a periosteal elevator, with 'back-cuts' superiorly and inferiorly, the periosteum is reflected over the lateral rim. Malleable retractors are employed, with the aid of the elevator, to continue this reflection off the internal aspect of the lateral orbital wall. (**c**) A full-thickness bone cut is made in the coronal plane with an oscillating saw approximately 5 mm posterior to the lateral orbital rim. (**d**) A second such incision is made inferiorly at approximately 70° to the first incision. (**e**) A block of lateral orbital wall is displaced posteriorly with a hammer and chisel, taking care not to fracture the bar of the anterior orbital rim. A 19 mm diameter malleable retractor protects the orbital soft tissues throughout. (**f**) The posterior extent of the initial osteotomy is identified with the periosteal elevator: this is enlarged and extended to the trigone of the sphenoid using rongeurs and/or a burr. Venous bleeding from the marrow space of the posterior lateral wall can be tamponaded with bone wax. Some authors advocate deep bone removal to expose dura. Sufficient inferolateral bone removal is essential. (**g**) Note the intact lateral periosteum beginning to bulge into the bony osteotomy. (**h**) The periosteum is opened to create an aperture wider than the bony osteotomy. An incision is made 2 mm posterior to the original arcus marginalis, continued superiorly beyond the lacrimal gland, and inferiorly. The periosteal opening is completed with several incisions running posteriorly. (**i**) Note the lacrimal gland (*short arrow, pale white/pink*)—now in the superior osteotomy—and the orbital fat (*long arrow, yellow*). Blunt wide opening of the inferolateral fat planes encourages further soft tissue prolapse

ble retractor and periosteal elevator are used to reflect the periosteal sheet medially away from the lateral orbital wall, dividing vascular bridges as necessary. Protecting the orbital soft tissues with the retractor, two full-thickness osteotomies are made using an oscillating saw. The first is made in the coronal plane, 3 mm behind the lateral rim, and the second at about 70° to the first and positioned just above the inflexion of the zygomatic arch. The thin bridge of orbital rim is preserved, and an anterior wedge of bony wall is **out**-fractured using a hammer and chisel on the external surface.

Removal of bone and access through the orbital rim can also be achieved using a cutting burr (instead of the saw). A 4–6 mm cutting burr is used to remove a window of bone anteriorly, the size of which can be limited to the surgeon's choice. Being careful to reflect and protect temporalis, a full thickness perforation can be made and extended into the temporalis fossa. Bone punches or a 4 mm cutting burr can be used to remove further lateral wall from an external or internal approach, including the trigone. Diamond burrs may be employed when close to soft tissue such as dura.

Once achieved, the lateral window is then widely enlarged superiorly (to allow the lacrimal gland to prolapse backwards), posteriorly (using an angulated 135° 'down-cutting' rongeur), and inferiorly, permitting prolapse of fat from the infero-temporal quadrant of the orbit. Posteriorly, bone excision is taken into the marrow-space of the trigone of the sphenoid, with haemostasis from the marrow space achieved with bone wax.

To enable prolapse of adipose tissue and lacrimal gland into the bone window, a linear periosteal incision is made immediately behind the arcus marginalis, enlarged with several posteriorly-directed incisions. Disruption of the fat and fibrous septae in the infero-lateral fat compartment with wide blunt dissection is necessary to allow adequate soft tissue prolapse and decompress the orbit. Inferolateral orbital fat may also be excised through this approach to enhance the decompression. The periosteum and deep tissues are then closed with a 5/0 absorbable suture and a suction drain placed into the depths of the orbit. Skin closure is achieved with a running 6/0 nylon suture, and the orbit padded for 8–10 h.

Another efficient and elegant method to perform a rim-sparing lateral wall decompression is the *ab interno* approach via a (minimal incision) *swinging eyelid* approach, which can also be used to access the orbital floor (Figs. 12, 13, and 14) [10, 43]. Under general anaesthesia, the lateral canthus and lower eyelid are infiltrated with lignocaine 2% with 1:200,000 adrenaline. A lateral extended canthotomy of about 10–15 mm parallel to the relaxed skin tension lines is made. The underlying orbicularis muscle and the inferior crus of the lateral canthal ligament is incised. While the lower eyelid is retracted downwards with Adson forceps, the lower eyelid retractors and conjunctiva are cut from the lateral canthus towards the centre of the lower eyelid. The periosteum is incised just anterior of the orbital margin. Periosteum elevators and curved retractors are used to dissect the periosteum/periorbita from the orbital margin and the area of the orbit to be decompressed, be it medial, inferior, or lateral wall (Figs. 12, 13, 14, and 15). For the lateral wall, this area is fully exposed after cauterisation and division of the zygomaticofacial and zygomaticotemporal arteries and nerves. A hammer and chisel are used to create a bony opening in the lateral wall, while the orbital contents are carefully protected with curved retractors. With rongeurs the opening is enlarged in all directions, after blunt dissection of the temporalis muscle with a Freer periosteal elevator. Thick bone is removed by chiselling or burring. With adequate retraction of the temporalis muscle laterally and the orbital contents medially, the deep lateral wall is visualised and bone can be removed up to the inner table of the greater wing of the sphenoid. Bone can be excised as far as the inferior and superior orbital fissures. Any bleeding from diploic vessels is stopped with bone wax. The lateral periorbita is opened with a bent 18 gauge needle, and after visible herniation of orbital fat, an Arthro-Lok reverse cutting blade (no 6083, Beaver) or No 15 surgical blade is used to cut the periorbita in an anteroposterior direction. This results in herniation of orbital fat, which can be augmented through blunt dissection with scissors in the spaces between the rectus muscles. Drains are left in the temporal fossa only in case of poor haemostasis. The periosteum and conjunctiva are closed with interrupted absorbable sutures. The lateral canthus is sutured with an absorbable suture (Vicryl® 5.0 or 6.0), and the skin is closed with a continuous absorbable or non-absorbable suture. In orbital decompression, the amount of

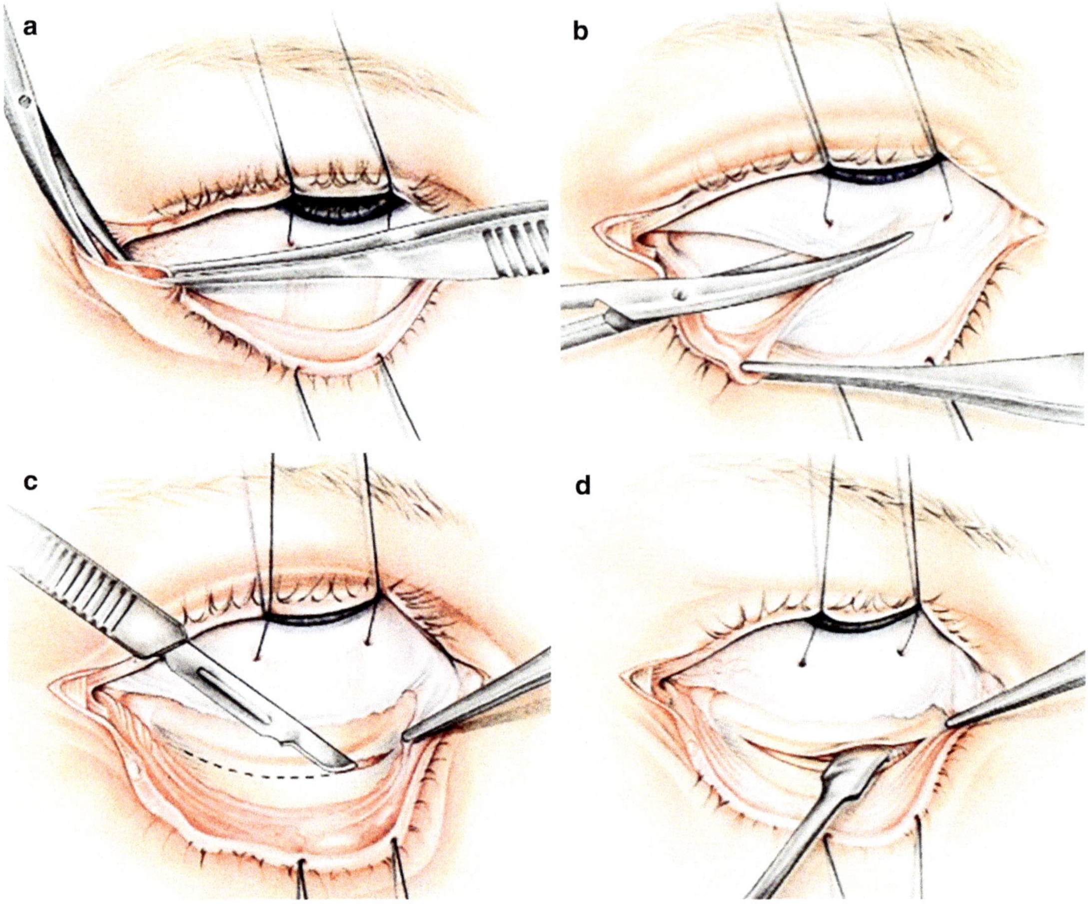

Fig. 12 Illustrations identifying steps involved in the conjunctival approach to the orbital floor and medial wall. (**a**) The lateral canthus is opened and a cantholysis performed to 'swing' the lower eyelid adequately. (**b**) The conjunctiva is opened at the lower border of the tarsus, with blunt dissection immediately posterior to the orbicularis muscle, keeping anterior to the septum, to expose the inferior orbital rim. (**c**) The periosteum is opened at the anterior inferior orbital rim. (**d**) A flat periosteal elevator is used to lift the periosteum off the orbital floor. This manoeuver is continued with a 16 mm malleable retractor to the posterior orbit. If required, the medial wall may be accessed via the same approach and the periosteum elevated superiorly to the level of the skull base

proptosis reduction and the risk of post-operative diplopia not only depends on anatomical factors and degree of intraorbital fibrosis, but also on the number of walls that are addressed, the location and extent of the bony windows, and the location and extent of periorbital opening. Experienced surgeons will consider these factors and will also evaluate the patient's appearance prior to the onset of TAO using old facial photographs, so that optimal results are obtained.

Intra-operative complications are generally due to haemorrhage from the undersurface of temporalis muscle or from vessels arising within the pterygo-palatine fossa. The cranial proximity way occasionally lead to dural exposure at the base of the trigonal bone removal, or at the frontal plate alongside upper bone removal; these rarely require treatment or cause any problem [36].

Surgery can be combined with intra-operative navigation to confirm anatomical positions and landmarks (see chapter "Navigation in Orbital Surgery").

Although masticatory oscillopsia has been described after the external-approach lateral decompression described above, few patients are

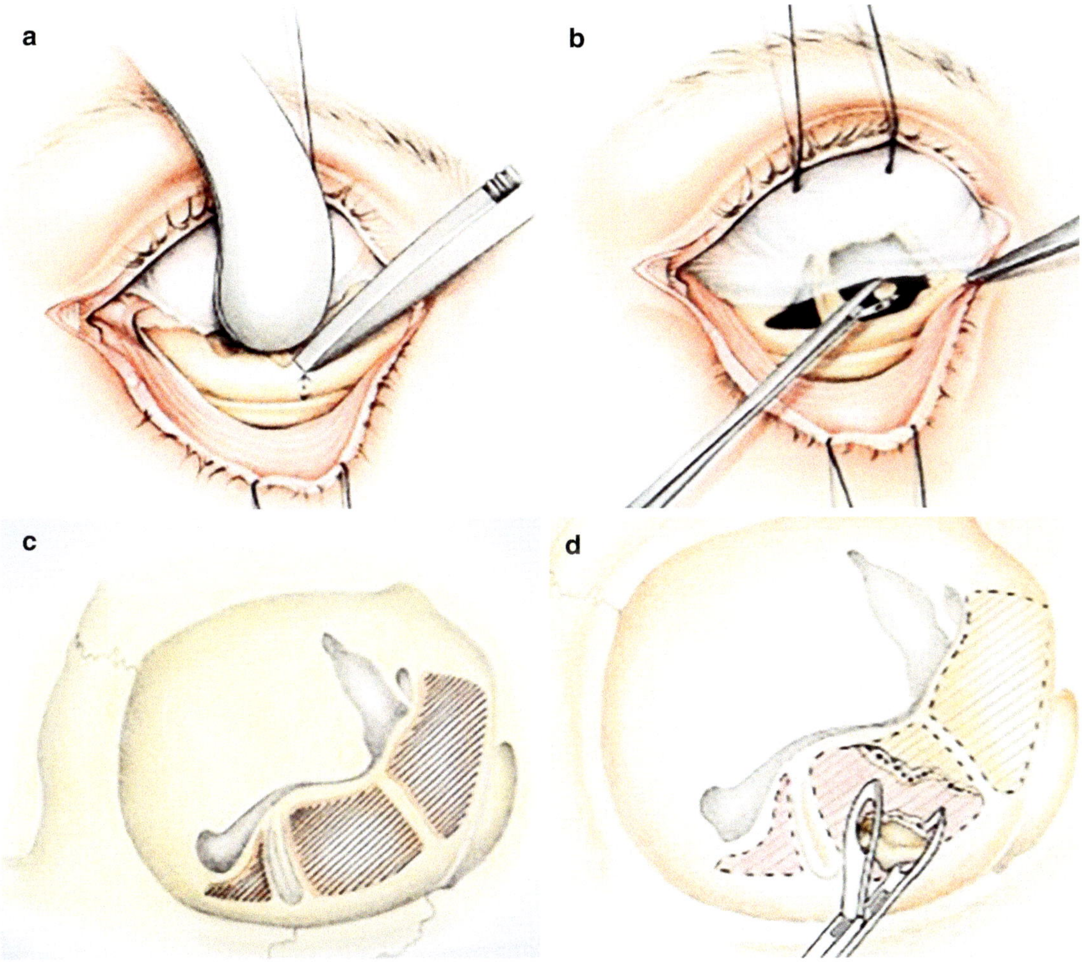

Fig. 13 Illustrations identifying access to the orbital floor and medial orbital wall. (**a**) The periosteum is elevated off the orbital floor using a malleable retractor and periosteal elevator. (**b**) The floor is readily in-fractured using an artery clip; the bony floor is then removed with an instrument such as a Watson Williams nasal polypus forceps, which has a wide 'bite' and readily enables bone to be removed to the posterior wall of the maxillary sinus. Note, in severe cases, the floor can also be decompressed *lateral* to the infraorbital nerve. The roof and floor of the bony infraorbital canal require complete removal to avoid 'pinching' of the infraorbital nerve over a posterior bony ledge. (**c**) The swinging lower eyelid approach affords access to the entire floor and medial orbital wall. (**d**) A Tilley-Henkle ethmoid punch can be used for bone removal, and is particularly suited to removal of the bony orbital wall, the soft tissues of the ethmoid sinuses, and the posterior half of the maxillo-ethmoid 'strut'—all essential components of an effective medial orbital wall decompression

troubled by it and almost all settle over a few months [41, 42]. Such post-operative masticatory oscillopsia is due to transmission of temporalis muscle contraction to the lateral orbital tissues.

For aesthetic rehabilitation, where only moderate degrees of decompression are required, the lateral wall approach is preferred by many—this approach addressing the problem of lacrimal gland prolapse, reducing upper and lower eyelid fullness, and having a very low incidence of new-onset diplopia (0–6%) [44].

For greater degrees of exophthalmos (~25–29 mm), a lateral and medial approach decompression is preferred by many surgeons. Although this carries an increased risk of new-onset diplopia, it also gives access to the orbital

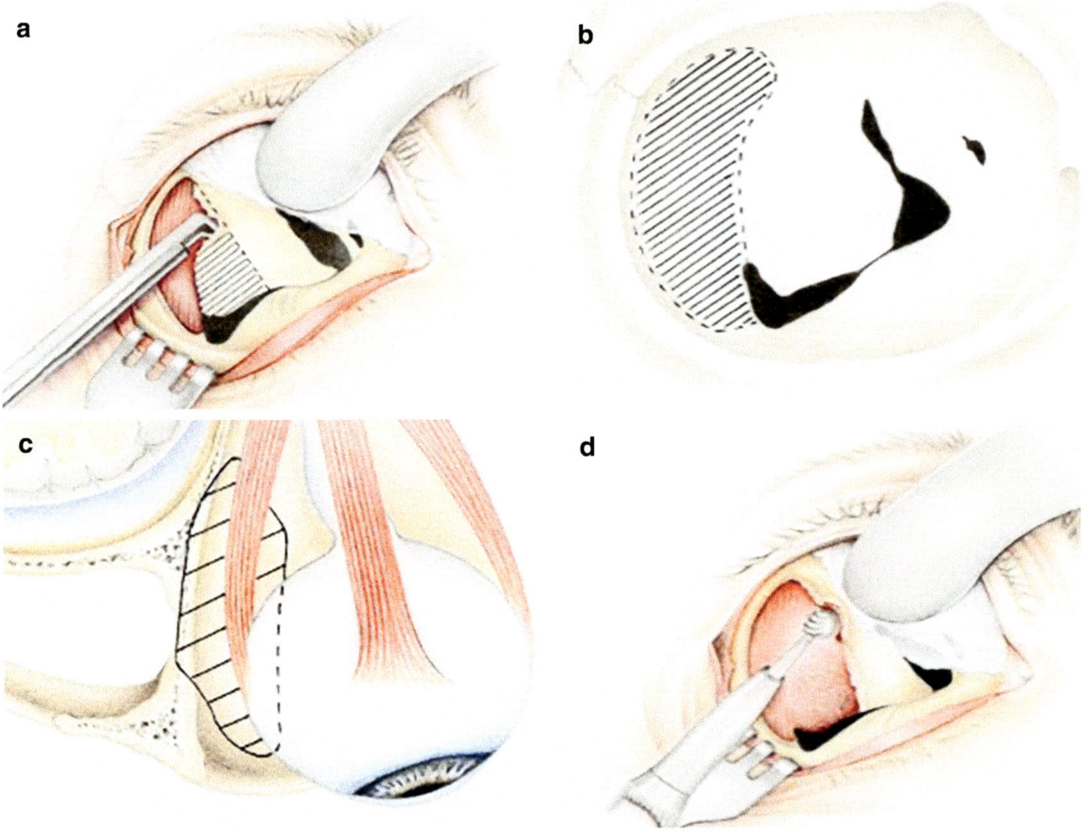

Fig. 14 Illustrations identifying the transconjunctival *ab interno* access to the lateral orbital wall. (**a–c**) Extent of bone removal of the lateral wall, posteriorly to the trigone of the sphenoid bone, and inferiorly to the inferior orbital fissure. (**d**) The most posterior bone removal is completed with a burr

floor should further decompression be desired. For more severe exophthalmos, a lower eyelid swing ("swinging eyelid") approach can be used for full access to the lateral wall and floor (Fig. 15); the medial wall can be accessed via the same incision, or via an additional retro-caruncular incision. Originally, orbital floor decompression involved removal of the entire floor, and in some cases, the nerve itself was removed [11]. Subsequent modifications largely prevented numbness and hypoglobus by removing the bony canal of the infraorbital nerve (but not the nerve), leaving the anterior 5–10 mm of the anterior floor intact to reduce the risk of hypoglobus (Fig. 16) [14], and preserving the infero-medial orbital 'strut' (Figs. 4, and 7) to prevent occlusion of drainage of the maxillary sinus (Fig. 9).

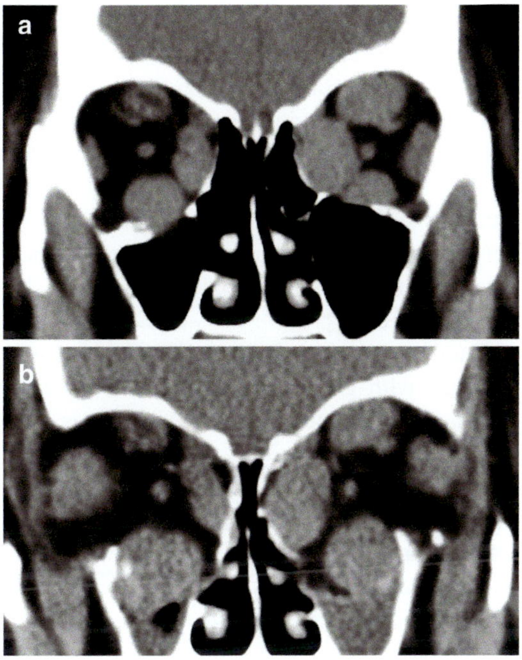

Fig. 15 Severe TAO with massive enlargement of the recti muscles and gross proptosis (radiology of patient shown in Fig. 8). (**a**) Pre-operative coronal CT image. (**b**) Post-operative CT views following three-wall decompression. Note prolapse of the massive recti muscles into the adjacent sinuses and lateral fenestrations (Courtesy of G. E. Rose and D. H. Verity)

4.3 Orbital Congestion: "Hydraulic Disease"

The concept of the 'hydraulic' variant of TAO is characterised by inactive disease, mild to moderate proptosis, and markedly increased orbital pressures. These pressures are associated with deep orbital vascular congestion, persistently raised intraocular pressures and, not infrequently, transient obscurations of vision associated with postural hypotension (especially in diabetics) [45]. Orbital decompression is very effective in this context, with immediate relief of obscurations, improvement in the intraocular pressure, and subjective and objective improvement in visual functions. It is important to emphasise that such patients are often subjected to prolonged (and ineffective) immunosuppression, being assumed to have active features of disease on account of the marked episcleral engorgement. However, this 'hydraulic' phase is well beyond the stage of active inflammation, and immunosuppression therefore has no value, while surgical decompression rapidly relieves orbital congestion [45].

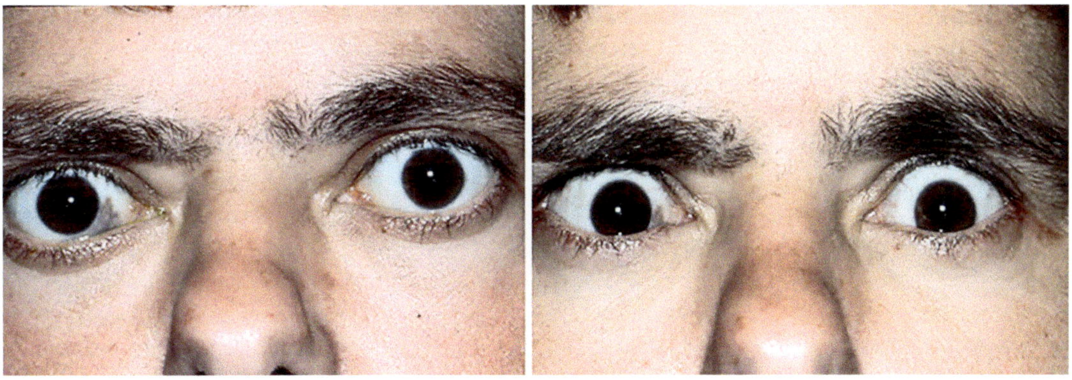

Fig. 16 Hypoglobus following excessive removal of the anterior orbital floor in orbital decompression (Pre-operative view *left*, post-operative view *right*)

5 Other Considerations

5.1 Choice of Decompression

The technique of decompression, and, for bony decompression, the sequence in which the walls are decompressed, varies according to indication and surgical preference. In 2009 a multi-centre Europe-wide study reported no fewer than 18 different techniques, with no clear consensus emerging on the optimal approach for a given indication [46]. A Cochrane review similarly noted a dearth of quality studies [47]. For patients *without* optic neuropathy, and mild-to-moderate exophthalmos, an *ab-externo* bone-removing, rim-sparing lateral orbital wall decompression is favoured by some. This approach avoids the risk of new-onset diplopia and hypoglobus, although about a third experience temporary post-operative oscillopsia (following the *ab-externo* approach). Where further reduction of proptosis is desired, medial wall and medial floor decompression remain surgical options. Others favour the *ab-interno* approach to the bony lateral wall [10, 43, 48] which also allows for deeper bone removal without exposing temporalis, this associated with a small (2.6%) risk of new-onset diplopia in primary gaze, and improvement in diplopia in 5% of those patients with pre-operative diplopia [10]. In addition, the internal approach to the lateral wall may cause less iatrogenic damage to the temporalis muscle and vasculature.

5.2 Orbital Fat Decompression

Orbital fat decompression was first described by Moore in 1920 [49], and later popularised by Olivari et al. and, as a treatment for stable exophthalmos without optic neuropathy, is both safe and fairly effective [50, 51] Richter et al. reported their experience over 20 years with a series of 3210 operations concluding that fat decompression is both effective and safe, with lower risks than bone decompression—particularly with respect to meningitis, CSF leak, vision loss, retrobulbar haemorrhage, paresis and periocular paresthesia [50]. Since the intraorbital soft tissue (excluding the globe) is approximately 14 cc in volume, 40% volumetric lessening of retro-bulbar tissue can be achieved by resecting 6 cc of fat [51]. A report in 2011 by Liao et al. confirmed a close correlation between the volume of excised fat and reduction of Hertel exophthalmometry with surgery [52], although such reduction is expected to be lower among patients whose proptosis is due to muscle enlargement. 4–6 mm proptosis reduction has been reported [53].

Fat decompression is more effective and safer in orbits with greater degrees of fat expansion. The safer inferolateral fat compartment is more easily accessible through a transconjunctival approach with or with canthotomy. Inferomedial fat can also be excised through a transconjunctival approach, and has also been described with endoscopic approaches. Deeper orbital fat removal is more effective than anterior fat, but has higher risks of complications. However, extraocular motility disturbance may occur after fat decompression, with new onset diplopia developing in 29% of 144 patients without *pre-*operative diplopia, this lasting more than 6 months in a fifth of these patients [50]. Finally, a risk with extensive orbital fat resection is volume depletion and hollowing in the upper and lower eyelids, especially with excessive anterior orbital fat removal.

5.3 Extraocular Muscles May (Seem to) Enlarge Following Orbital Decompression

Previous studies have indicated that the medial rectus muscle *expands* after medial decompression surgery, potentially limiting the decompressive effect [54]. Gupta et al have studied this effect following maximal deep lateral and medial balanced decompression in 48 patients (75 orbits) [55]. A significantly larger mean increase in the width of the lateral rectus muscle (2.7 mm) compared to the medial rectus muscle (0.7 mm) was noted. The precise mechanism remains elusive, but a number of theories have been proposed. These include possible disease reactivation [46], and post-operative (surgically-induced) myositis

[47]. Others have suggested that decompression results in reduced muscle compression, this favouring expansion of the (already hyperosmotic) muscles [50]. However, no similar expansion of the other extraocular muscles was observed, indicating either that no such mechanism exists, or that different pressure compartments occur in the orbit. Gupta et al. suggest that the discrepancy in the rectus expansion (lateral greater than medial) could be related to removal of deeper bone along the lateral wall [55]. Others consider that more bone is removed alongside the *medial* rectus (as far posteriorly as the annulus of Zinn) compared to the *lateral* rectus, and that a more likely explanation is that adequate decompression reverses the reduction of cross-sectional area of the muscles when they are elongated by exophthalmos [55].

6 Conclusions

The management of TAO and decompression is determined by the stage and severity of disease, as well as the indication for treatment.

Corticosteroids, increasingly given by the intravenous route, are indicated for active orbital disease with major congestion, diplopia or optic neuropathy. Patients with congestive optic neuropathy who show no major improvement in visual function after three weekly pulses of high-dose (500 mg–1 g) intravenous methylprednisolone, should be considered for medial wall and medial floor decompression with minimal further delay; we believe that such patients are frequently and unnecessarily exposed to the risks of chronic immunosuppression.

Thus, the indications for surgical treatment during the acute phase are optic neuropathy, major orbital congestion, and exposure keratopathy. During this early phase, urgent temporary tarsorrhaphy or eyelid lowering will address exposure keratopathy, while medial/floor decompression are effective for acute neuropathy and congestion.

For established disease, decompression will retroplace the globe, reduce exophthalmos, expand the orbital volume and address lacrimal gland prolapse. There is usually an improved eyelid position (especially lower eyelid) and improved prolapse of fat into the eyelid, making eyelid position and blepharoplasty surgery more effective when needed.

With respect to the lower eyelid, the term 'retraction' is often incorrectly used to describe displacement due to unaddressed exophthalmos. These can be addressed by other surgical procedures.

Strabismus surgery, when indicated, is followed by surgery to address eyelid fullness, contour and closure but despite all rehabilitative measures there is often a disparity between the surgical result and the final appearance desired by the patient. This so-called 'expectation gap' between desired, as compared to achievable, improvement is due both to the natural ageing process, and to the widespread change in distribution of facial adipose tissues.

Consideration should be given to orbital decompression for established exophthalmos before other rehabilitative measures, because it carries a risk of new-onset diplopia, and because the eyelid contour and fullness cannot be addressed if the tissues are displaced forwards by a proptotic eye. Indeed, all attempts to disguise significant degrees of proptosis with eyelid surgery alone (such as lateral tarsorrhaphy or eyelid lowering) will result in an unnatural appearance. Even if the eyelid retraction is corrected, the eyelids remain tightly 'pinched' around a prominent globe and the upper eyelid 'show' (the visible extent of skin in the primary position between the lash line and the skin crease) can be markedly increased due to the lack of an effective skin 'fold'. Furthermore, any attempts to reduce eyelid fullness with a blepharoplasty (in the presence of exophthalmos) tend to be futile due to unaddressed prolapse of the lacrimal gland from the lacrimal fossa onto the orbital rim; if decompression is subsequently performed, inappropriate debulking of the pre-aponeurotic fat pad can result in a hollow upper eyelid and sulcus.

In summary, the greatest two challenges to clinicians in treating TAO are dysthyroid optic neuropathy, and the subsequent aesthetic expectations of the patient once proptosis has been addressed. Considering optic neuropathy, where medical intervention with IVMP at the correct dose and frequency is ineffective, prompt orbital decompression, as described, will typically restore visual functions (and relieve congestion) without the need for prolonged immunosuppression. This advice may change in the future as newer targeted medical treatments become universally available. Nevertheless, in comparison with decompression surgery, such treatments remain relatively non-specific, and will be associated with side-effects in a significant minority of patients. Regarding the aesthetic expectations of the patient, the clinician should remember that all surgery tends to reduce the compliance of the eyelid tissues. Whilst such expectations are not unreasonable given the change of appearance due to TAO and the natural ageing process, the risk of ocular exposure due to a subtly impaired blink reflex should be carefully weighed against these expectations. Rather than improving appearance and function, surgery can be counterproductive, and a more conservative approach towards the end of treatment is often the best.

References

1. Douglas RS, Gupta S. The pathophysiology of thyroid eye disease: implications for immunotherapy. Curr Opin Ophthalmol. 2011;22:385–90.
2. Bahn RS, Heufelder AE. Pathogenesis of Graves' ophthalmopathy. N Engl J Med. 1993;329:1468–75.
3. Wiersinga WM, Bartalena L. Epidemiology and prevention of Graves' ophthalmopathy. Thyroid. 2002;12:855–60.
4. Krassas GE, Heufelder AE. Immunosuppressive therapy in patients with thyroid eye disease: an overview of current concepts. Eur J Endocrinol. 2001;144:311–8.
5. Verity DH, Rose GE. Acute thyroid eye disease (TED): principles of medical and surgical management. Eye (Lond). 2013;27:308–19.
6. Goldberg RA. Advances in surgical rehabilitation in thyroid eye disease. Thyroid. 2008;18:989–95.
7. Lyons CJ, Rootman J. Orbital decompression for disfiguring exophthalmos in thyroid orbitopathy. Ophthalmology. 1994;101:223–30.
8. Kikkawa DO, Pornpanich K, Cruz RC, et al. Graded orbital decompression based on severity of proptosis. Ophthalmology. 2002;109:1219–24.
9. Mehta P, Durrani OM. Outcome of deep lateral wall rim-sparing orbital decompression in thyroid-associated orbitopathy: a new technique and results of a case series. Orbit. 2011;30:265–8.
10. Paridaens DA, Verhoeff K, Bouwens D, van Den Bosch WA. Transconjunctival orbital decompression in Graves' ophthalmopathy: lateral wall approach ab interno. Br J Ophthalmol. 2000;84:775–81.
11. Dandy W. Results following the transcranial attack of orbital tumors. Arch Ophthalmol. 1942;25:191–6.
12. Alper MG. Pioneers in the history of orbital decompression for Graves' ophthalmopathy. Doc Ophthalmol. 1995;89:163–71.
13. Walsh TE, Ogura JH. Transantral orbital decompression for malignant exophthalmos. Trans Am Laryngol Rhino Otol Soc. 1957;59:56–81.
14. Kennedy DW, Goodstein ML, Miller NR, et al. Endoscopic transnasal orbital decompression. Arch Otolaryngol Head Neck Surg. 1990;116:275–82.
15. Baylis HI, Call NB, Shibata CS. The transantral orbital decompression (ogura technique) as performed by the ophthalmologists: a series of 24 patients. Ophthalmology. 1980;87:1005–12.
16. Anderson RL, Linberg JV. Transorbital approach to decompression in Graves' disease. Arch Ophthalmol. 1981;99:120–4.
17. McCord CD Jr. Current trends in orbital decompression. Ophthalmology. 1985;92:21–33.
18. Wulc AE, Popp JC, Bartlett SP. Lateral wall advancement in orbital decompression. Ophthalmology. 1990;97:1358–69.
19. Goldberg RA, Kim AJ, Kerivan KM. The Lacrimal keyhole, orbital door Jamb, and Basin of the inferior orbital Fissure. Three areas of deep bone in the lateral orbit. Arch Ophthalmol. 1998;116:1618–24.
20. Olivari N. Transpalpebral decompression of endocrine ophthalmopathy (Graves' disease) by removal of intraorbital fat: experience with 147 operations over 5 years. Plast Reconstr Surg. 1991;87:627–41; discussion 42-43
21. Trokel S, Kazim M, Moore S. Orbital fat removal. Decompression for Graves' orbitopathy. Opththalmology. 1993;100:674–82.
22. Rootman D. Orbital decompression for thyroid disease. Surv Ophthalmol. 2018;63:86–104.
23. Shorr N, Seiff SR. The four stages of surgical rehabilitations of the patient with dysthyroid ophthalmopathy. Ophthalmology. 1986;93:476–83.
24. Ben Simon GJ, Mansury AM, Schwarcz RM, et al. Simultaneous orbital decompression and correction of upper eyelid retraction versus staged procedures in thyroid-related orbitopathy. Ophthalmology. 2005;112:923–32.
25. Nair AA, Ediriwickrema LS, Dolman PJ, Law G, Harrison AR, Mokhtarzadeh A, Stewart K, Men C, Lucarelli MJ, van Landingham S, Wingelaar M, Verma R, Chen A, Selva D, Garrity J, Eckel L, Kazim M, Godfrey K, Baxter SL, Korn BS, Kikkawa DO. Predictive modeling of new-onset postoperative diplopia following orbital decompression for thyroid eye disease. Ophthalmic Plast Reconstr Surg. 2022;38:551–7.

26. Dolman PJ. Dysthyroid optic neuropathy: evaluation and management. J Endocrinol Invest. 2021;44:421–9.
27. Gupta A, Garcia MD, North V, Kazim M, Rose GE. Residual apical lamina papyracea as a cause for persistent dysthyroid optic neuropathy after orbital decompression. Ophthalmic Plast Reconstr Surg. 2023;39:e37–40.
28. Harvey JT. Orbital decompression for Grave's disease leaving the periosteum intact. Ophthal Plast Reconstr Surg. 1989;5:199–206.
29. Perry JD, Kadakia A, Foster JA. Transcaruncular orbital decompression for dysthyroid optic neuropathy. Ophthal Plast Reconstr Surg. 2003;19:353–8.
30. Liao SL, Chang TC, Lin LL. Transcaruncular orbital decompression: an alternate procedure for Graves ophthalmopathy with compressive optic neuropathy. Am J Ophthalmol. 2006;141:810–8.
31. McCann JD, Goldberg RA, Anderson RL, Burroughs JR, Ben Simon GJ. Medial wall decompression for optic neuropathy but lateral wall decompression with fat removal for non vision-threatening indications. Am J Ophthalmol. 2006;141:916–7.
32. McCord CD Jr, Putnam JR, Ugland DN. Pressure-volume orbital measurement comparing decompression approaches. Ophthal Plast Reconstr Surg. 1985;1:55–63.
33. Rootman J. Orbital surgery: a conceptual approach. 2nd ed. Philadelphia: Wolters Kluwer Health/Lippincott Williams & Wilkins; 2014.
34. Rose GE, Lund VJ. Clinical features and treatment of late enophthalmos after orbital decompression: a condition suggesting cause for idiopathic "imploding antrum" (silent sinus) syndrome. Ophthalmology. 2003;110:819–26.
35. McCormick CD, Bearden WH, Hunts JH, et al. Cerebral vasospasm and ischemia after orbital decompression for Graves ophthalmopathy. Ophthal Plast Reconstr Surg. 2004;20:347–51.
36. Isenberg SF, Scott JA. Management of massive haemorrhage during endoscopic sinus surgery. Otolaryngol Head Neck Surg. 1994;111:134–6.
37. Baldeschi L, Lupetti A, Vu P, Wakelkamp IM, Prummel MF, Wiersinga WM. Reactivation of Graves' orbitopathy after rehabilitative orbital decompression. Ophthalmology. 2007;114:1395–402.
38. McNab AA, Wright JE. Lateral orbitotomy—a review. Aust N Z J Ophthalmol. 1990;18:281–6.
39. Harris GJ, Logani SC. Eyelid crease incision for lateral orbitotomy. Ophthal Plast Reconstr Surg. 1999;15:9–16.
40. Graham SM, Brown CL, Carter KD, et al. Medial and lateral orbital wall surgery for balanced decompression in thyroid eye disease. Laryngoscope. 2003;113:1206–9.
41. Fayers T, Barker LE, Verity DH, Rose GE. Oscillopsia after lateral wall orbital decompression. Ophthalmology. 2013;120:1920–3.
42. Siah WF, Patel BC, Malhotra R. Surgical management of temple-related problems following lateral wall rim-sparing orbital decompression for thyroid-related orbitopathy. Br J Ophthalmol. 2016;100:1144–50.
43. Paridaens D, Lie A, Grootendorst RJ, van den Bosch WA. Efficacy and side effects of 'swinging eyelid' orbital decompression in Graves' orbitopathy: a proposal for standardised evaluation of diplopia. Eye (Lond). 2006;20:154–62.
44. Ben Simon GJ, Wang LL, McCann JD, et al. Primary gaze diplopia in patients with thyroid-related orbitopathy undergoing deep lateral orbital decompression with intraconal fat debulking: a retrospective analysis of treatment outcome. Thyroid. 2004;14:379–83.
45. Rose GE. Postural visual obscurations in patients with inactive thyroid eye disease; a variant of 'hydraulic' disease. Eye. 2006;20:1178–85.
46. European Group on Graves' Orbitopathy (EUGOGO), Mourits MP, Bijl H, Itea MA, et al. Outcome of orbital decompression for disfiguring proptosis in patients with Graves' orbitopathy using various surgical procedures. Br J Ophthalmol. 2009;93:1518–23.
47. Boboridis KG, Bunce C. Surgical orbital decompression for thyroid eye disease. Cochrane Database Syst Rev. 2011;12:CD007630.
48. Cruz AAV, Equiterio BSN, Cunha BSA, Caetano FB, Souza RL. Deep lateral orbital decompression for Graves orbitopathy: a systematic review. Int Ophthalmol. 2021;41:1929–47.
49. Moore RF. Exophthalmos and limitation of eye movements of Graves' disease. Lancet. 1920;ii:701.
50. Richter DF, Stoff A, Olivari N. Transpalpebral decompression of endocrine ophthalmopathy by intraorbital fat removal (Olivari technique): experience and progression after more than 3000 operations over 20 years. Plast Reconstr Surg. 2007;120:109–23.
51. Olivari N. Endocrine ophthalmopathy: surgical treatment. HNO. 2010;58:8–10.
52. Liao SL, Huang SW. Correlation of retrobulbar volume change with resected orbital fat volume and proptosis reduction after fatty decompression for Graves ophthalmopathy. Am J Ophthalmol. 2011;151:465–8.
53. Cheng AM, Wei Y-H, Tighe S, Sheha H, Liao S-L. Long-term outcomes of orbital fat decompression in Graves' orbitopathy. Br J Ophthalmol. 2018;102:69.
54. Wenz R, Levine MR, Putterman A, et al. Extraocular muscle enlargement after orbital decompression for Graves' ophthalmopathy. Ophthal Plast Reconstr Surg. 1994;10:34–41.
55. Gupta A, Nobori A, Wang Y, et al. Lateral rectus muscle expands more than medial rectus following maximal deep balanced orbital decompression. Ophthalmic Plast Reconstr Surg. 2018;34:140–2.

Strabismus in Thyroid-Associated Orbitopathy

Gustavo Savino, Andrea Papp, and Francesco M. Quaranta Leoni

Key Messages

- In patients with thyroid-associated orbitopathy (TAO), imaging identifies specific muscle involvement, the typical feature being enlargement of the belly of the muscle with sparing of tendinous insertion.
- Strabismus surgery should not be carried out until the angle of deviation is stable for at least 4 months. Observation may be advisable when diplopia is absent in primary or reading position or if strabismus is not stabilised. Fresnel prisms can provide relief, and can be definitive in patients with small angles of deviation.
- There is no nomogram for surgical dose-response in strabismus surgery for TAO. Patients should have realistic expectations about the treatment possibilities and the outcome, as more surgeries may be needed, binocular single vision might be achieved only in the primary and reading position, and proptosis may worsen after strabismus surgery.
- The main surgical procedure is recession of the restricted, fibrotic muscle(s). Undercorrection is the most common reported complication of horizontal strabismus surgery. Although strabismus surgery should be performed after decompression surgery, combined treatment may be proposed in selected patients.
- Botulinum toxin A (BTA) reduces muscle contraction and can be useful in the early, active phase of the disease, in the chronic phase in small angles of deviation and in the management of post-operative over- or undercorrection.
- Teprotumumab, a human monoclonal antibody that targets the insulin-like growth factor-1 receptor, has shown remarkable results in reduction of diplopia in multicenter, randomised placebo-controlled trials.

1 Background and Pathogenesis

Thyroid-associated orbitopathy (TAO), with either single or multiple extraocular muscle (EOM) enlargement, is the most frequent cause of restrictive strabismus [1]. Active TAO is characterised by infiltration of orbital tissues by immune cells (T lymphocytes, mast cells, B lymphocytes)

G. Savino (✉)
Department of Ophthalmology, Fondazione Policlinico Universitario A. Gemelli IRCCS, Rome, Italy
e-mail: gustavo.savino@unicatt.it

A. Papp
Department of Ophthalmology and Optometry, Medical University of Vienna, Vienna, Austria

F. M. Quaranta Leoni
Oftalmoplastica Roma, Rome, Italy

F. M. Quaranta Leoni et al. (eds.), *Oculoplastic, Lacrimal and Orbital Surgery*,
https://doi.org/10.1007/978-3-031-39638-0_37

and orbital remodelling, which gradually stabilises, leading to the inactive phase of the disease [2]. The extraocular muscles (EOM) are frequently involved, leading to impairment of ocular motility in the acute inflammatory phase followed by rapid fibrosis and reduced compliance [3].

The inferior rectus and medial rectus muscles are most commonly involved, followed by the superior rectus and lateral rectus. Typically, there is an enlargement of the muscle belly with sparing of the muscle tendon [2], this appearance being in contrast with myositis in which diffuse enlargement of the entire muscle from the origin to the tendon is observed [4] (Fig. 1).

The preponderance of inferior and medial rectus muscle involvement may reflect their higher density of resident macrophages [5]. However, the inferior rectus and inferior oblique muscles also have an extensive connective tissue system, this suggesting an alternative or further reason for increased involvement of the inferior rectus muscle [6].

According to a study by Wang et al. the most commonly involved solitary muscle group is that of the superior rectus and levator palpebrae muscles [7]. Patients presenting with enlargement of this group of muscles should therefore be investigated accordingly, this including thyroid stimulating immunoglobulin (TSI), TSH receptor autoantibodies (TRAb), and orbital imaging. Where these investigations are abnormal in the context of superior rectus/levator complex enlargement, TAO should be strongly considered [7].

Orbital fibroblasts are common to both EOM and orbital adipose tissue, and are thought to be a key target and effector cell in the pathogenesis of TAO. In patients with TAO, a heterogeneous population of orbital fibroblasts promotes the formation of mature extracellular matrix and hyaluronan, and interacts with mononuclear cells leading to local cytokine production and orbital inflammation, tissue remodelling, and fibrosis - all of which lead to orbital congestion, proptosis, and reduced eye motility [8, 9].

Although the pathophysiology of TAO remains incompletely understood, overexpression of insulin-like growth factor-1 (IGF-1R) and activation a of the IGF-1R/TSH-R complex are thought to play central roles, promoting the production of proinflammatory cytokines, including IL-6 and IL-8. TSH-Rs and IGF-IRs form physical and functional complexes leading to hyaluronan accumulation and cytokine expression. The ensuing inflammation, secondary oedema, and expansion of extraocular muscle and adipose tissues results in proptosis and restrictive strabismus [8, 10–12].

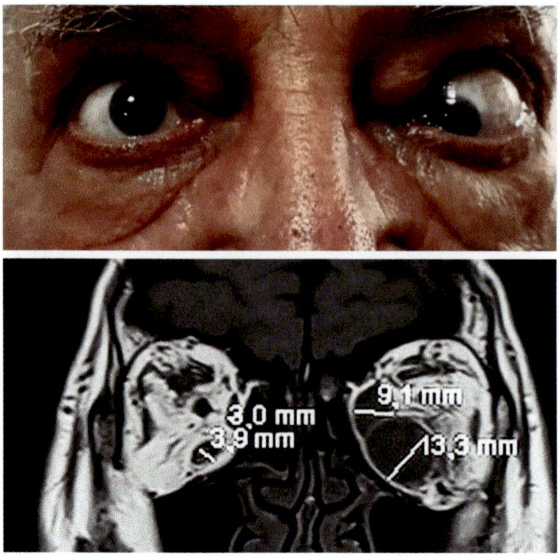

Fig. 1 Restrictive strabismus of the left eye, demonstrating marked esotropia and hypotropia. MRI (T1 coronal image) shows marked enlargement of the belly of both left inferior and medial recti

Histopathological studies implicate CD4+ and CD8+ T cells in the *initial* stages of active inflammatory disease, in addition to early activation of orbital fibroblasts [13]. Further observations include an increased macrophage expression in the early phases, and raised fibroblast HLA-DR expression at all stages of disease [13].

Studies of involved EOM in late disease—or after a period of immunosuppression—identify patchy lymphocytic infiltration and interstitial deposition of glycosaminoglycans (GAGs) by activated fibroblasts [10–12].

2 Clinical Assessment: Diagnosis, Imaging, Disease Staging

Involvement of the extraocular muscles in TAO varies greatly from one patient to another - being subclinical or overt, unilateral or bilateral, symmetrical or asymmetrical, and involving single or groups of muscles [4, 14, 15] Although proptosis and acquired restrictive strabismus commonly occur in TAO, they are also a feature of other conditions. Cranial nerve palsies, idiopathic myositis syndromes, mass lesions, and systemic diseases such as myasthenia gravis (MG) and chronic progressive external ophthalmoplegia (CPEO) should be considered. Variability and fatigue are suggestive of MG, whilst bilateral ptosis and progressive ophthalmoplegia suggest CPEO. Imaging and specific laboratory work-up can provide the clinician with clues to the most likely aetiology [4].

The *Corneal Light Reflex Test* is useful in assessing ocular alignment, and will identify both manifest and latent deviations (the latter by employing the cover-uncover test, *v.i.*). Note, it will not identify axial or non-axial displacement in the presence of fusion.

Examination of ductions (monocular eye movements) *and versions* (binocular eye movements in the same direction) is essential to establish which muscles are affected. Ductions are examined by covering one eye and asking the patient to fixate a small target from the primary position into all nine diagnostic positions of gaze. Note is made of restricted or delayed movements, and these can be quantified by an arc perimeter or Hess chart plot.

Versions are examined with both eyes open, and note is made of any ocular asymmetry in the different gaze positions.

Determination of vergences (binocular eye movements in the opposite direction) has an important prognostic value, as it provides information about the patient's ability to compensate a post-operative mild under- or overcorrection [16, 17]. Vergence movements are slow and tonic: the patient fixates a target, and a prism of increasing power is placed in front of one eye and slowly moved to elicit the fusional movement. If a manifest deviation is present, it should be neutralised before testing.

The *'cover'* and *'cover-uncover'* tests identify manifest and latent deviations respectively, and the direction of the deviation. For the test to be reliable, the acuity in each eye must be sufficient to fixate a small target for near and distance. The test should be done for near and distance in all diagnostic gaze positions, prioritising downgaze and primary position if vertical strabismus is present [17]. In the cover test, the eye is occluded while the patient looks at a small target; movement of the fellow eye to take up fixation indicates a manifest deviation. The alternate cover ('cover-uncover') test identifies the *total* angle of deviation. A cover is placed alternately in front of each eye while the patient maintains fixation; the amount of deviation is grossly estimated, and a prism with a power lower than that of the estimated deviation is placed in the appropriate position in front of one eye until no refixation is noted as each eye is covered in turn.

The *Forced Duction Test* (FDT) is performed intra-operatively under general or topical anaesthesia (4% lidocaine hydrochloride). The conjunctiva is grasped at the limbus with toothed forceps, and the eye is moved the opposite direction of the suspected mechanical restriction. Thus, to examine for restriction of the inferior rectus muscle, the limbus is grasped at the 3- and 9-o'clock positions and the eye moved in a superior direction, with resistance to such movement indicating inferior rectus restriction [18]. Note, where there is muscular paresis or paralysis, resistance is not encountered (Fig. 2).

Finally, torsional deficits can be assessed by means of a synoptophore after the correction of all vertical and horizontal deviations.

The *binocular single vision field (BSVF)* assessment identifies the binocular field of fusion, that is, the field without diplopia [19]. BSVF displays the areas of single and double vision and provides valuable longitudinal follow-up data.

Ultrasonography is a practical and inexpensive tool in evaluating anterior orbital changes in thyroid and non-thyroid myopathies. *Computed tomography* (CT) and *magnetic resonance imaging* (MRI) help to establish the degree of EOM enlargement and orbital fat expansion, exclude coexisting orbital pathology, and aid surgical planning [20]. EOM enlargement in TAO typically involves the belly of the muscle, sparing the tendinous insertions. Inflammatory changes within the orbital fat and EOMs are specifically evident in T2 and T1 post-contrast enhanced sequences of MRI studies [4] (Fig. 1).

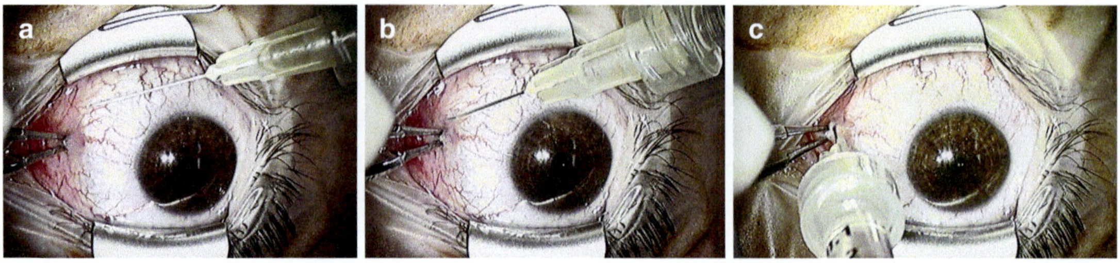

Fig. 2 Injection of Botulinum Toxin A reduces muscle contraction and may relieve restrictive diplopia in the active phase of TAO. (**a**) The patient is asked to look in the opposite direction of the muscle action and the needle is introduced parallel to the muscle. (**b**) The patient is asked to look towards the muscle to be injected. (**c**) The needle is brought to the vertical plane and the toxin injected slowly

Disease activity, and the response to anti-inflammatory treatment, can be evaluated with the clinical activity score (CAS), with MRI helping to differentiate between active and inactive TAO. Increased T2-weighted signal (occurring where there is increased water content of the muscles) is indicative of active inflammation [21], and short-tau inversion recovery (STIR) sequences suggest active inflammation [22].

In conclusion, the evaluation of ductions and versions helps to identify gross defects of ocular motility, and a quantitative study of the angle of deviation in all diagnostic positions of gaze is essential. Imaging will identify specific muscle involvement, and BSVF is helpful in pre-operative examination and post-operative follow-up.

3 The Role of Immunosuppressive Agents and Radiotherapy in Active Phase

Most patients with active moderate to severe TAO with ocular motility impairment benefit from immunosuppression. Glucocorticoids are the first-line treatment to reduce oedema and orbital inflammation, with improvement of extra-ocular motility and reduction of diplopia [23]. *Intravenous pulsed glucocorticoid administration* (methylprednisolone 500 mg/week for 6 weeks, followed by 250 mg/week for up to 6 weeks, depending on the clinical response) is preferred over oral administration (up to 100 mg of oral prednisone daily for 5 days, tapering to 20 mg within a month, and a slower taper thereafter), as it is more effective *and* has a safer profile [24–29]. However, high-dose systemic glucocorticoid therapy is associated with side effects such as hyperglycemia, hypertension, mood instability, and weight gain [29]. The maximum cumulative dose of IV methylprednisolone should not exceed 8 g to prevent acute liver damage [30].

Periocular and orbital glucocorticoid administration are alternative treatment options with fewer systemic side effects. A multicenter, randomised, controlled study found that patients who received four inferolateral orbital injections of 20 mg triamcinolone acetate experienced improvement in diplopia, with radiographic imaging showing a reduction in the size of extra-ocular muscles [31].

Orbital radiation therapy (OR) is a well-tolerated treatment option for active TAO [32]. OR has a nonspecific anti-inflammatory effect due to radiosensitive lymphocytes that infiltrate the orbit; OR also targets fibroblasts, leading to reduced glycosaminoglycan synthesis and secretion [32–34]. With a dose of 2 Gy daily for 2 weeks (20 Gy total), OR alone or in combination with steroids, was found to be effective in reducing diplopia and improving extraocular muscle motility [35–37].

Randomised trials evaluating the efficacy of OR are, however, limited, Furthermore, whilst a safe and effective treatment in cases of recent-onset diplopia, it is not effective in long-standing EOM dysfunction [33].

OR should be considered an option for TAO in patients showing active inflammatory myopathy, particularly before undergoing orbital decompression: patients treated with a combination of OR and IV steroids have less troublesome diplopia after decompression surgery than the patients treated with IV steroids alone, and this regime also reduces post-operative EOM enlargement [38].

Although some studies evaluating concomitant OR with glucocorticoids report different results [39–41], current evidence suggests that orbital radiation, used with or without corticosteroids, is indeed effective in improving motility restriction and decreasing clinical activity in TAO. Overall, the evidence indicates that OR modifies the active phase of TAO. Short-term risks of orbital radiation are minor, but long-term outcome data are lacking [42].

Recent advances in the understanding of the molecular basis of TAO have facilitated the development of novel, targeted molecular therapies. A study showed that *tocilizumab* (an IL-6 receptor monoclonal antibody) reduced inflammation in patients who were unable to tolerate glucocorticoids, with improved extraocular motility and resolution of diplopia in primary gaze in more than 50% of the patients [43]. However, in another randomised clinical trial, tocilizumab did not show significant improve of diplopia [44].

A retrospective study showed subjective improvement in diplopia, pain, and swelling in 40% of patients following 3 months of therapy with *adalimumab*, an anti-tumour necrosis factor-alpha agent, but with no significant improvement in extraocular movement restriction [45].

A case report showed that *infliximab* infusion improved ocular motility [46]. While these findings suggest that anti-tumour necrosis factor-alpha agents may be of benefit for selected patients with TAO, larger studies are still needed [47].

Teprotumumab, an insulin-like growth factor-1 receptor inhibiting novel human monoclonal antibody, reduces hyaluronan production and cytokine stimulation in orbital fibroblasts, leading to reduced intraorbital hyaluronan accumulation and reduced adipogenesis and muscle expansion [25, 26, 48–50]. In two multicenter, randomised placebo-controlled trials, patients receiving teprotumumab showed decreased proptosis, diplopia and inflammation following 24 weeks of treatment. In a recent study, orbital MRI imaging demonstrated decreased EOM volumes and orbital fat tissue volumes after treatment with teprotumumab [50, 51]. These findings may lead to a paradigm shift in the clinical management of TAO.

Unfortunately, despite prompt treatment with immunosuppressive agents and/or radiotherapy, strabismus still occurs in 15% of all patients in the active phase of TAO [52], resulting diplopia and interfering with the patient's quality of life [53].

4 Non-surgical Treatment

Non-surgical management options such as prism or botulinum toxin A (BTA) injection provide a temporary reduction, or even elimination, of intractable diplopia during the active phase.

Press-on (Fresnel) prisms are used temporarily both in horizontal and vertical diplopia to restore single binocular vision in primary and/or reading position [54], and may be definitive in patients with small angle strabismus.

BTA injection (10 - 25 units) - by reducing muscle contraction—results in relief of diplopia in selected cases and can reduce the amount of surgical recession needed at a later stage [55–58]. A large cohort analysis has shown that relatively *mild*, new onset TAO-associated strabismus has some chance for long-term benefits when treated with BTA, without the need for subsequent surgery.

On the other hand, for *severe* TAO-associated strabismus, there is only a slight, if any, chance of long term benefit. Although three quarters of the BTA injections led to a reduction in strabismus angle (by a mean 75% of the initial deviation), the average duration of this effect was only 2 months [59, 60]. In addition, relaxation of the inferior rectus muscle can result in decreased intraocular pressure [61].

4.1 Injection Technique of BTA

Forms

- onabotulinumtoxinA (Botox®; Allergan Inc., Dublin, Ireland)
- abobotulinumtoxinA (Dysport®; Ipsen, Paris, France)
- incobotulinumtoxinA (Xeomin®/Bocouture®; Merz Pharmaceuticals, Frankfurt, Germany).

Dose and Reconstitution

- 10–25U of Botox® in presence of fibrosis
- 2 mL of balanced salt solution (BSS) are injected into the bottle containing 50–100U of BTA in powder form to obtain 5U per 0.1 mL

Steps

1. Apply topical anaesthesia to the ocular surface (e.g. oxybuprocaine) 10 min before the procedure, followed by three more drops until the procedure starts.
2. Ensure aseptic conditions of the surgical field.
3. Place an eyelid speculum.
4. Ask the patient to look in the opposite direction of the muscle action to introduce the needle parallel to the muscle (Fig. 2a).
5. Ask the patient to look towards the muscle to be injected (Fig. 2b).
6. Verticalize the needle and inject the toxin slowly (Fig. 2c).
7. Slowly withdraw the needle.
8. Apply antibiotic ointment at the end of the procedure.

Patients should be reminded of the latency of the effects (2–7 days before becoming noticeable) as well as the potential adverse events (e.g. ptosis, hypercorrection of the deviation, subconjunctival haemorrhage).

Follow-up is recommended within the first 3 weeks to document the early effects of the toxin and later, after 4–8 months, to re-evaluate ocular alignment and need for re-injection.

5 Surgical Treatment: Indications and Timing

Approximately 0.6–20% of patients with TAO will require strabismus surgery [62, 63]. Although the aim of surgery is to restore binocular single vision (BSV), an optimal outcome may be challenging, especially in patients with combined horizontal and vertical deviations [14, 62–64]. The success rate of strabismus surgery in TAO patients varies, and reoperation rate is quoted as high as 45% of cases [64, 65].

Observation is advisable in cases with no double vision in primary or reading position, or if the strabismus is not stable. The indication for surgery depends on the angle of deviation in primary and reading position, BSVF assessment, anomalous head position, and aesthetic concerns [4, 14]. The main aim of surgery is to establish or to improve BSVF in primary gaze and reading position, and the evaluation of fusional vergences is useful to predict the likelihood of post-operative compensation of possible hypo- or hypercorrection.

It is advisable not to operate until the angle of deviation has been stable for at least 4 months. Furthermore, the thyroid function should be stable, and there should be no residual orbital inflammation [15, 66], as surgery in the active phase of TAO usually results in significant instability in surgical outcome [67]. Nevertheless, good short-term results in patients with stable measurements for *shorter* periods of time have also been reported, as well as a significant post-surgical change in the angle of deviation in 30% of patients who had been stable for at least 6 months [68].

Orbital decompression, if indicated, should be performed prior to strabismus surgery, as it can [69, 70] affect the initial deviation and/or results in new onset strabismus (less so with lateral wall decompression, but particularly so with medial decompression); horizontal strabismus surgery should therefore be performed 4–6 months after orbital decompression [69–73].

The literature concerning the incidence of strabismus after decompression is wide, varied, and technique-dependent. Following orbital decompression, new onset diplopia has been reported in various ranges, but improvement of pre-existing diplopia has been also described [69, 74–79]. One-wall decompression, medial and lateral wall decompression, and medial and inferior wall decompression, were associated with an esotropic shift [69]. To reduce this tendency, a balanced two-wall decompression (with preservation of the anterior maxillo–ethmoidal bony 'strut') has been suggested, as has the creation or maintenance of a periosteal 'sling' over the medial and inferior rectus muscles [69, 70, 78, 79]. However, these techniques rarely have been compared and the true value of small technical modifications is difficult to assess.

Eyelid surgery can be affected by both decompression and strabismus surgery, and should be performed after strabismus surgery [80–82] However, simultaneous decompression and strabismus surgery may be performed in selected cases to shorten patient rehabilitation [83, 84].

6 Surgical Techniques and the Role of Forced Duction Test

6.1 Surgical Management

Patients should be wisely counselled, and have realistic expectations. They are likely to need more than one operation, BSV may be achieved only in primary and reading positions, proptosis may increase, and lid-lag might worsen after strabismus surgery [85].

6.2 Forced Duction Test

As the extent of fibrosis of the involved muscles is highly variable, the conventional surgical dose-response tables are not reliable in TAO associated strabismus [86]. FDT, as mentioned, is a simple and method for evaluating the mechanical properties of extraocular muscles and is an important tool for planning and conducting strabismus surgery [87–89]. It should be performed before, during, and after strabismus surgery to assess the

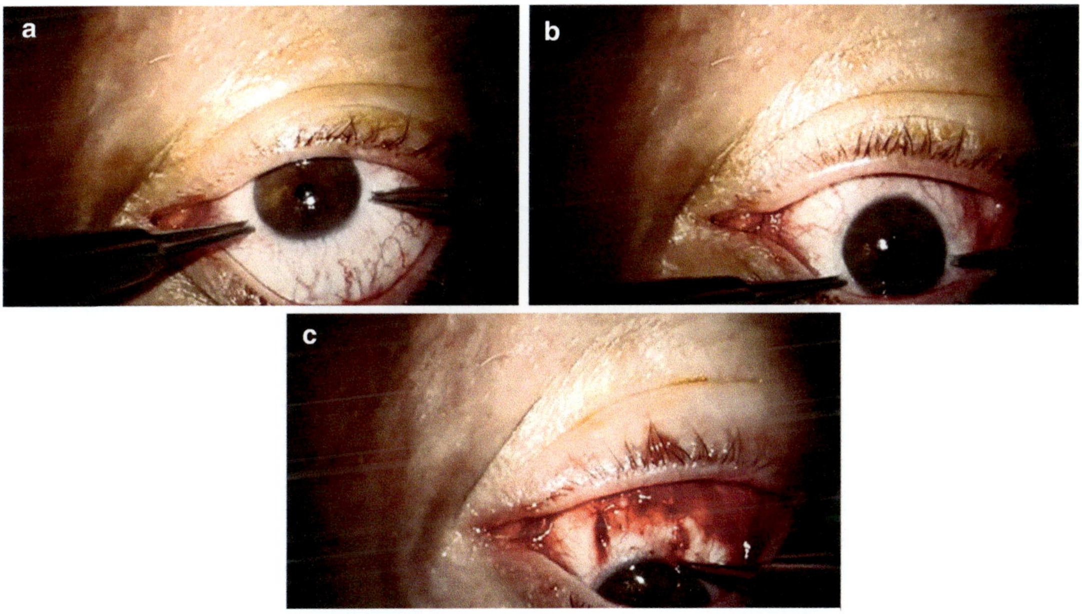

Fig. 3 Intra-operative forced duction test under general anaesthesia. (**a**, **b**) The forceps hold the limbus at the 3- and 9-o'clock positions and the eye is moved in sursumduction. The presence of resistance indicates IR restriction. (**c**) Intra-operative duction test after IR recession

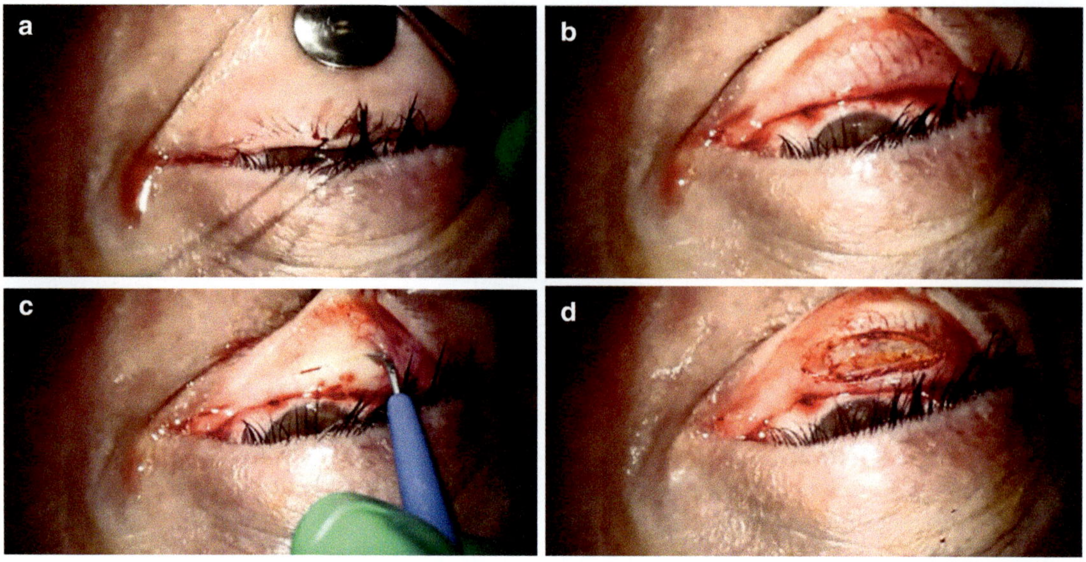

Fig. 4 Infratarsal lower eyelid retractor lysis. (**a**, **b**) A stay suture is placed through the lower tarsal plate close to the lid margin. The eyelid is everted over a Desmarres retractor. (**c**, **d**) An incision is made through the conjunctiva immediately below the lower border of the tarsal plate. The conjunctiva is dissected from the underlying lower eyelid retractors, and the retractors are divided from the lower border of the tarsus and recessed. A traction suture is placed in the lower lid and taped to the forehead for 24–48 h

amount of restriction (Fig. 3) [90]. Intra-operative FDT after disinsertion the inferior rectus muscle can be extremely useful in detecting masked restriction of the superior rectus muscle, as overlooking superior rectus fibrosis may determine post-operative overcorrection of the vertical deviation.

6.3 Basic Rules

- Thyroid function (TSH, fT4 and TrAb) should be assessed before strabismus surgery.
- Primary, secondary, and tertiary functions of each muscle should be considered at the time of planning the surgery of TAO-associated strabismus [91]. Ocular versions, ductions, FDT, assessment of ocular torsions and sensorimotor tests should be carried out pre-operatively. Orbital imaging is useful to show which muscles are involved [92].
- There is no standard nomogram for surgical dose-response for strabismus surgery in TAO [67].
- The main surgical procedure is recession of the restricted, fibrotic muscles. The inferior rectus is most commonly affected, followed by the medial rectus and superior rectus muscles [93].
- Restricted vertical muscles reduce the success of medial rectus recession surgery due to the secondary function (adduction) of the inferior rectus muscle [91].
- Bilateral inferior rectus recession of more than 6 mm may lead to post-operative A-pattern and exotropia in down-gaze. This is due to overaction of the superior oblique muscles in downgaze as a result of the decreased adduction caused by the weakening of the inferior rectus muscles [94–96]. To reduce this problem nasal transposition of both inferior recti have been suggested. This procedure collapses the A-pattern, but increases *in*cyclotorsion in downgaze.
- More than 4 mm of recession of the inferior rectus muscle may worsen lower lid retraction, Lockwood's ligament advancement and lower eyelid retractor lysis should be carried out at the time of strabismus surgery (Fig. 4) [97, 98].
- Muscle resection or plication is usually not the first choice in TAO, as it can result in overcor-

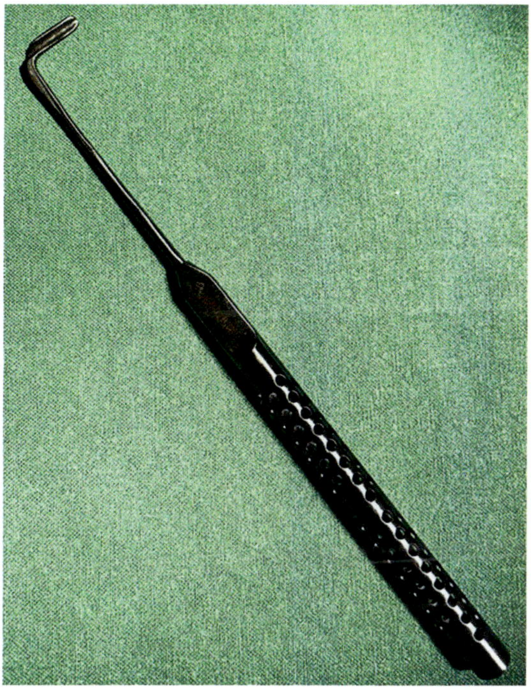

Fig. 5 Wright grooved hook. This instrument is useful to avoid rupture of a severely restricted extraocular muscle at surgery

rection and/or new onset deviation. However, successful, stable outcomes were reported with lateral rectus resection in cases of residual esotropia after maximal medial rectus muscle recession [99, 100].

- There is a risk of 'pulled-in-two syndrome' [95], a rupture of a tight extraocular muscle during surgery, that could be reduced with the use of a titanium muscle hook designed to reduce excessive traction (e.g. Wright grooved hook by Titan Surgical, Los Angeles, CA) (Fig. 5).
- The conjunctiva of these patients is usually thin and tears easily; it should be handled carefully during strabismus surgery.

Different surgical methods have been proposed for optimal surgical outcomes in TAO. As opposed to traditional planned (orthoptic-based surgery), intra-operative relaxed muscle positioning technique (in which muscles are recessed to the position where they rest freely on the globe without tension) has been reported to be successful in 78% of cases (Figs. 6 and 7) [101].

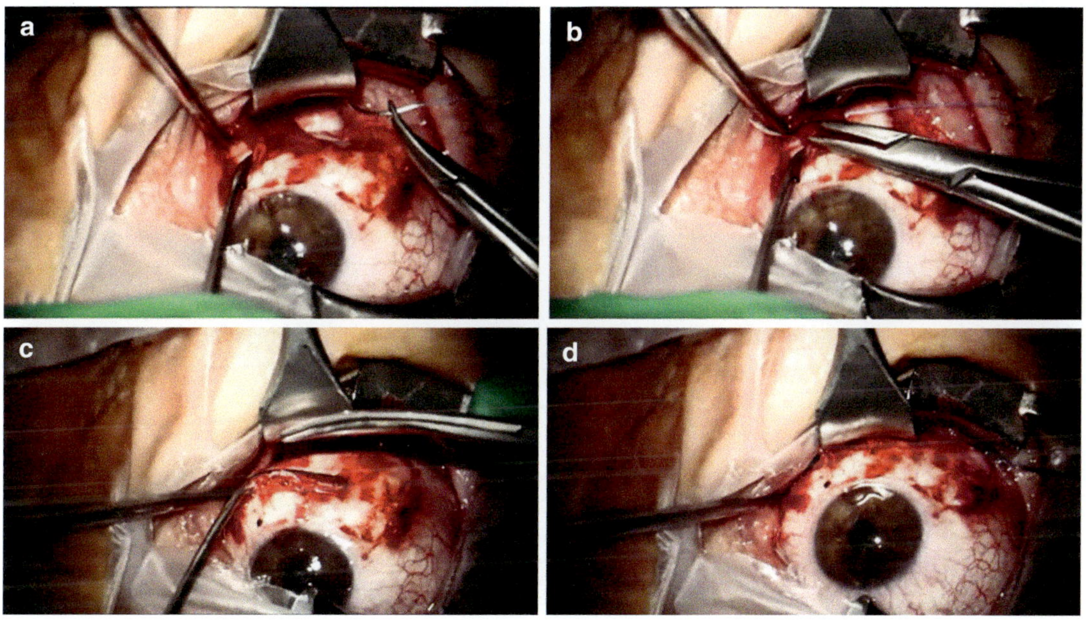

Fig. 6 Intra-operative relaxed muscle position technique: initial steps. (**a**, **b**) A polyglactin suture is placed within the muscle lying on the hook of the tight inferior rectus muscle. (**c**) The inferior rectus is disinserted from the sclera. (**d**) Position of the eye following the inferior rectus disinsertion

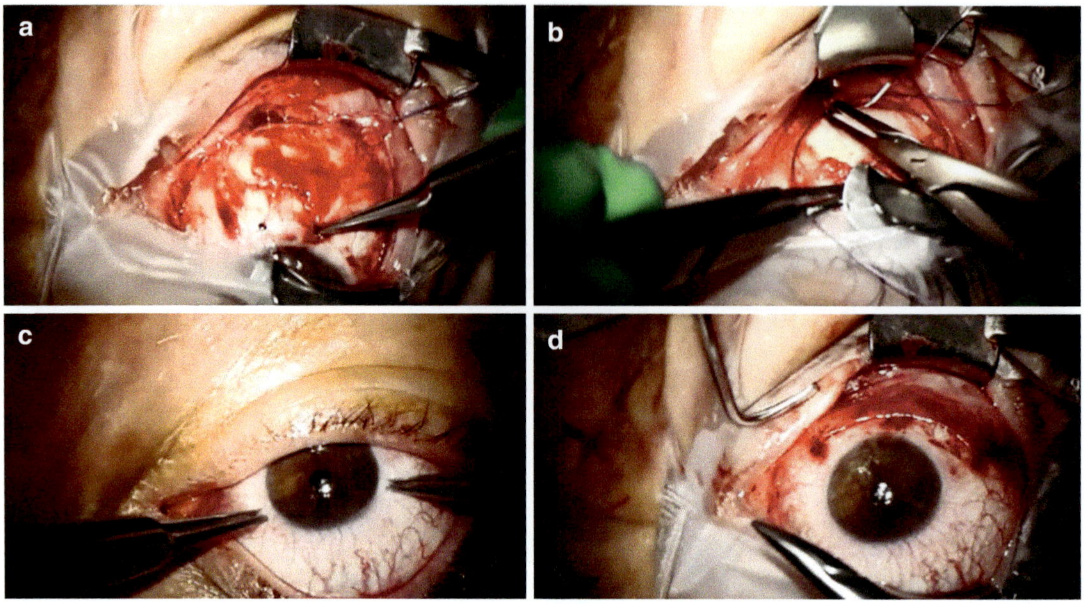

Fig. 7 Intra-operative relaxed muscle position technique: final steps. (**a**) Intra-operative forced duction test after the inferior rectus disinsertion from the sclera. (**b**) The inferior muscle is recessed to the position where it rests on the globe without tension. A long 6-0 absorbable suture is used. (**c**) Forced duction test before the muscle disinsertion (to be compared to **a**). (**d**) Eye position after inferior rectus and conjunctiva recession

Success rates of these two surgical techniques are similar but they are highly dependent on surgical experience. Additionally, the strabismus surgery in TAO should be individually tailored, and most surgeons therefore use a combination of both methods.

Variable suture techniques have been suggested to correct the TAO-associated strabismus and to prevent post-operative posterior shifting of the recessed thickened muscle tendons, these including adjustable sutures, semi-adjustable sutures, and fixed sutures [100, 102, 103]. One study reported overcorrection of the vertical deviation with adjustable sutures, whilst another found reported stable results [102, 103]. Kushner reported a 100% success rate in eliminating muscle slippage by using a semi-adjustable suture technique which comprises fixing two corners of the muscle to the sclera, and suspending the centre of the muscle on an adjustable suture [104]. According to another study, non-absorbable sutures can prevent a late overcorrection of the vertical deviation. However, non-absorbable sutures carry the risk of infection and a tendency for conjunctival exposure [105].

To maintain the arc of contact in large angle strabismus, tendon elongation with bovine pericardium in cases of severe esotropia after orbital decompression has been suggested as a safe procedure to correct esotropia up to 50 PD. [106]

Post-operative adhesion between muscles and surrounding tissues (fat, conjunctiva, Tenon's capsule) can limit surgical outcomes [107]. However, synthetic membranes to separate adhesions from the muscle and the sclera can increase scarring; local injections of corticosteroids are not effective, and 5-fluorouracil and mitomycin C [108, 109] can cause toxicity.

Amniotic membrane (AM) can act as a biological barrier between potentially adhesive surfaces, and its stromal matrix reduces inflammation, neovascularization, and scarring [108, 109]. AM transplantation has been carried out with success in several difficult restrictive strabismus cases series, and it can be considered as a useful adjuvant tool in the management in TAO associated strabismus [110, 111].

7 Combined Decompression and Strabismus Surgery

The most effective management for patients affected by moderate to severe TAO presenting with exophthalmos, strabismus, and eyelid retraction is a multi-sequenced approach, performed during the *inactive* stage of the disease as each surgery can affect subsequent stages [112].

A multi-staged approach requires as a longtime commitment, whereas addressing simultaneously the various aspects of the disease in one step may have benefits when access to surgical services is limited, or cost may be a concern [84].

Simultaneous lateral wall decompression, correction of eyelid retraction and strabismus surgery has been described in a limited number of patients with inactive TAO with a favourable outcome [113]. A retrospective study compared the outcome of simultaneous orbital decompression and vertical strabismus surgery with the outcome of staged decompression and vertical strabismus surgery in two different groups of patients with moderate to severe disease. In cases submitted to one-stage surgery, an endoscopic medial wall decompression was performed. This was followed by inferior rectus muscle recession, the extent of the recession being determined by marking the place of the released tendon, and varying from 4.5 to 6.5 mm, and the conjunctiva recessed following assessment of relieved restriction with a forced duction testing [114, 115]. The same approach was used in case of superior rectus recession. The lateral wall was decompressed through a lateral canthal incision in the same surgical session, if necessary. There were no reports of diplopia in both primary and reading position, and the reduction in post-operative exophthalmos was not significantly different between the two groups [84].

The opportunity for combined surgery was influenced by a transition towards an *endoscopic* surgical approach, and standardisation of restrictive strabismus surgery. Endoscopic decompression preserves the anterior inferomedial boney ‘strut’ between the maxillary antrum and the ethmoid air cells [116], and, if desired, preserves a thin sling of the periorbita of the medial orbital wall [117]. At the same time, with less tissue manipulation than traditional decompression approaches, vertical muscle surgery can be performed during the same surgical session [116]. The management of vertical strabismus aims to prioritise ocular alignment in downgaze and to avoid the risk of progressive overcorrection, and that this may be achieved with single-stage surgery [16, 113].

Medial rectus recession performed during the same session as endoscopic decompression might positively influence muscle restriction and reduce the rate of post-operative diplopia [118], but should preferably be corrected at a second stage, as extensive decompression and possible displacement of soft orbital tissues may determine or modify a pre-existing horizontal deviation [69, 84] (Fig. 8).

Moreover, the changes in horizontal strabismus after IR recession and IR nasal transposition are non-uniform in patients with TAO. Patients with a larger angle of pre-operative esotropia are expected to have a better improvement in esotropia after surgical correction of hypotropia, and a reduced amount of IR nasal transposition may be associated with an increased reduction in the angle of esotropia [119].

Orbital decompression combined with strabismus surgery may be performed in carefully selected cases during the active stage of TAO [84, 120]. Patients with superior rectus–levator complex enlargement and inferior visual field defects tend to have a lower threshold for early intervention and may need early decompression combined with muscle surgery [84, 121]. In patients with no light perception of up to 3 months of duration, decompression combined with vertical strabismus surgery may also be effective, as visual function might recover following extensive decompression combined with recession of extremely fibrotic muscles [84].

A single-stage approach can therefore be proposed as first-line therapy in selected patients with moderate to severe TAO who would refuse multiple procedures, with the only setback of a longer operating time [84].

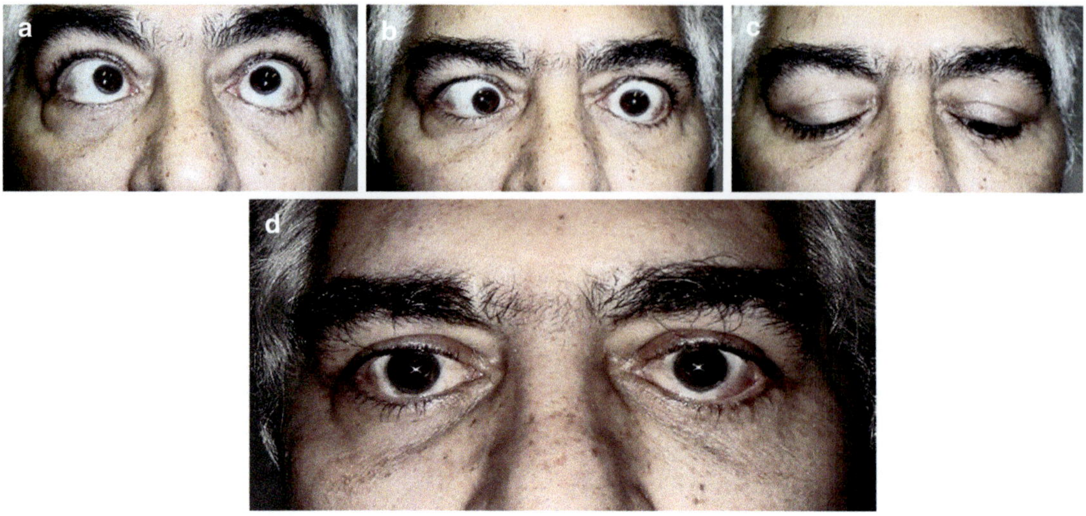

Fig. 8 Male patient with bilateral exophthalmos, right medial rectus restriction, bilateral inferior rectus restriction, left upper lid Müller's muscle fibrosis. (**a**) Pre-operatively, *upgaze*: attempted elevation with activation of both the superior recti and upper eyelid retractors, resulting in upper eyelid retraction. (**b**) Pre-operatively, *primary position*. (**c**) Pre-operatively, *downgaze*: left *lid lag* is due to Müller's muscle fibrosis. (**d**) Post-operatively: following bilateral endoscopic medial wall decompression and lateral wall decompression, bilateral inferior recti recession, left Müllerectomy (stage 1) and right medial rectus recession (stage 2, performed after 4 months)

8 Complications of Surgery and Management

The frequency of reoperation for strabismus in adults with TAO is reported to be as high as 26% [122, 123].

Under-correction is the most commonly reported complication of horizontal strabismus correction [91, 124], although simultaneous Tenon's recession improves the outcome [125].

Different options are available for under-corrected patients following large medial rectus muscles recession. Further recession may be extremely challenging due to muscle tightness and lack of space. Hang-back adjustable and non-adjustable sutures, and hang-back sutures with posterior fixation, have all been proposed in undercorrected patients [15, 126], as well as synthetic spacers (Silicon, Gore-Tex, Mersilene), and stored fascia lata, donor sclera, bovine pericardium and membrane [112, 127].

Some studies reported good outcomes of lateral rectus resection in patients with residual esotropia after medial rectus recession [99, 100]; lateral rectus resection may reduce proptosis, as opposed to medial rectus re-recession which usually *worsens* the exophthalmos [100].

Late over-correction may occur after inferior rectus recession and a post-operative mean drift toward overcorrection (from 1.9^D to 3^D) has been reported [117, 128]. Several factors have been associated with an increased risk of over-correction. Duration and severity of orbitopathy, impaired contralateral elevation and underestimation of increased ipsilateral superior rectus tone were reported as significant prognostic factors for overcorrection [129].

Furthermore, the progression of underlying thyroid myopathy after strabismus surgery, even in cases with a stable angle of deviation for 6 months, may result in late post-operative instability of deviation.

In addition, anatomical causes or an inadequate muscle scleral fixation can lead to muscle slippage or to a posterior shift of the IR scleral insertion. Predisposing factors for such post-operative complications are the gravitational forces, the short arc of contact in IR muscle, and the thickened tenon beneath the IR muscle in TAO patients [130].

Several surgical techniques have been proposed to prevent late overcorrection, including semi-adjustable hang-back approach for large recessions, non-absorbable sutures, long horizontal intrascleral simple hang-back for smaller recessions to prevent central sagging, meticulous Tenon's dissection, and reduction of the planned surgical dosage of the ipsilateral inferior rectus recession to reduce the risk of consecutive hypertropia [104].

Overcorrection after inferior rectus recession can be treated with recession of ipsilateral superior rectus, or contralateral restricted inferior rectus, or both. The angle deviation in all gaze positions, ocular ductions, forced intra-operative duction test, and orbital imaging help in surgical planning [14, 131].

Downgaze diplopia as a result of an early or late inferior rectus underaction after inferior rectus weakening is poorly tolerated [61]. The reversal of angle deviation is often related to an overlooked pre-operative incomitance between primary position and downgaze, often result of the mechanical imbalance between opposing muscle groups. When the overcorrection or the less common undercorrection in downgaze is limited, it can be treated conservatively with prisms on reading glasses, particularly in patients with a large vertical fusion range. Surgical treatment is reserved for large angles of deviation or for patients refusing conservative treatment. If a hypertropia with underaction of the inferior rectus (overcorrection) is present in down gaze after the inferior rectus recession, a posterior fixation suture (Faden operation) of the contralateral inferior rectus has been suggested [132].

As previously mentioned, inferior rectus muscle recession tends to result in a retraction of the inferior eyelid due to the anatomical association with Lockwood's ligament and the inferior eyelid retractors. Several surgical techniques have been recommended to correct lower lid retraction (see chapter "Management of Eyelid Retraction"). Lockwood ligament advancement and infratarsal lower eyelid retractor lysis (Fig. 3) at the same time of inferior rectus muscle recession tends to reduce the chance of this complication [97, 133].

References

1. Savino G, Petrone G, Volpe G, Midena G, Grimaldi G, Fiorentino V, Maceroni M. Vertical restrictive strabismus associated with proptosis: Similar clinical signs, different etiopathogenetic causes. A report of three patients. Eur J Ophthalmol. 2020:1120672120946929.
2. Garrity J, Bahn R. Pathogenesis of Graves ophthalmopathy: implications for prediction, prevention, and treatment. Am J Ophthalmol. 2006;142:147–53.
3. Bahn RS. Current insights into the pathogenesis of Graves' ophthalmopathy. Horm Metab Res. 2015;47:773–8.
4. Schotthoefer EO, Wallace DK. Strabismus associated with thyroid eye disease. Curr Opin Ophthalmol. 2007;18:361–5.
5. Van der Gaag R, Vernimmen R, Fiebelkorn N, et al. Graves'ophthalmopathy: what is the evidence for extraocular muscle specific autoantibodies. Int Ophthalmol. 1990;14:25–30.
6. Sergott RC, Glaser JS. Graves' ophhalmopathy. A clinical and immunologic review. Surv Ophthalmol. 1981;26:1–21.
7. Wang Y, Mettu P, Broadbent T, Radke P, Kevin Firl J, Banks Shepherd III, Couch SM, Nguyen A, Henderson AD, McCulley T, McClelland CM, Mokhtarzadeh A, Lee MS, Garrity JA, Harrison AR. Thyroid eye disease presenting with superior rectus/levator complex enlargement. Orbit. 2020;39:5–12.
8. Lee CE, Choi SH, Yoon JS. Chemokine expression during adipogenesis and inflammation in orbital fibroblasts from patients with Graves' orbitopathy. Korean J Ophthalmol. 2020;34:192–202.
9. Li H, Ma C, Liu W, He J, Li K. Gypenosides protect orbital fibroblasts in Graves ophthalmopathy via anti-inflammation and anti-fibrosis effects. Invest Ophthalmol Vis Sci. 2020;61:64.
10. Douglas RS, Gianoukakis AG, Kamat S, Smith TJ. Aberrant expression of the insulin-like growth factor-1 receptor by T cells from patients with Graves' disease may carry functional consequences for disease pathogenesis. J Immunol. 2007;178:3281–7.
11. Douglas RS. Teprotumumab, an insulin-like growth factor-1 receptor antagonist antibody, in the treatment of active thyroid eye disease: a focus on proptosis. Eye (Lond). 2019;33:183–90.
12. Douglas RS, Kahaly GJ, Patel A, Sile S, Thompson EHZ, Perdok R, Fleming JC, Fowler BT, Marcocci C, Marinò M, Antonelli A, Dailey R, Harris GJ, Eckstein A, Schiffman J, Tang R, Nelson C, Salvi M, Wester S, Sherman JW, Vescio T, Holt RJ, Smith TJ. Teprotumumab for the treatment of active thyroid eye disease. N Engl J Med. 2020;382:341–52.
13. Papp A, Lawson JM, Calder V, Fells P, Lightman S. T cells and fibroblasts in affected extraocular

muscles in early and late thyroid associated ophthalmopathy. Br J Ophthalmol. 2000;84:517–22.
14. Akbari MR, Mirmohammadsadeghi A, Mahmoudzadeh R, Veisi A. Management of thyroid eye disease-related strabismus. J Curr Ophthalmol. 2020;32:1–13.
15. Harrad R. Management of strabismus in thyroid eye disease. Eye (Lond). 2015;29:234–7.
16. Jefferis JM, Raoof N, Burke JP. Prioritising downgaze alignment in the management of vertical strabismus for thyroid eye disease: principles and outcomes. Eye (Lond). 2020;34:906–14.
17. Akbari M, Bayat R, Mirmohammadsadeghi A, Mahmoudzadeh R, Eshraghi B, Salabati M. Strabismus surgery in thyroid-associated ophthalmopathy; surgical outcomes and surgical dose responses. J Binocul Vis Ocul Motil. 2020;70:150–6.
18. Matlach J, Döllinger VKR, Eha J, Elflein HM, Weyer-Elberich V, Mildenberger P, Pitz S. Ocular ductions after rectus muscle recession and resection in thyroid eye disease. Strabismus. 2019;27:143–8.
19. Roper-Hall G. Evaluation of the field of binocular single vision in incomitant strabismus. Am J Ophthalmol. 1974;78:800–5.
20. Lo C, Ugradar S, Rootman D. Management of Graves myopathy: Orbital imaging in thyroid-related orbitopathy. J AAPOS. 2018;22:256.e1–9.
21. Politi LS, Godi C, Cammarata G, Ambrosi A, Iadanza A, Lanzi R, et al. Magnetic resonance imaging with diffusion-weighted imaging in the evaluation of thyroid-associated orbitopathy: getting below the tip of the iceberg. Eur Radiol. 2014;24:1118–26.
22. Kirsch EC, Kaim AH, De Oliveira MG, von Arx G. Correlation of signal intensity ratio on orbital MRI-TIRM and clinical activity score as a possible predictor of therapy response in Graves' orbitopathy—a pilot study at 1.5 T. Neuroradiology. 2010;52:91–7.
23. Bartalena L, Baldeschi L, Boboridis K, et al. The 2016 European Thyroid Association/European group on Graves' orbitopathy guidelines for the management of Graves' orbitopathy. Eur Thyroid J. 2016;5:9–26.
24. Bartalena L, Krassas GE, Wiersinga W, et al. Efficacy and safety of three different cumulative doses of intravenous methylprednisolone for moderate to severe and active Graves' orbitopathy. J Clin Endocrinol Metab. 2012;97:4454–63.
25. Marcocci C, Bartalena L, Tanda ML, Manetti L, Dell'Unto E, Rocchi R, Barbesino G, Mazzi B, Bartolomei MP, Lepri P, Cartei F, Nardi M, Pinchera A. Comparison of the effectiveness and tolerability of intravenous or oral glucocorticoids associated with orbital radiotherapy in the management of severe Graves' ophthalmopathy: results of a prospective, single-blind, randomized study. J Clin Endocrinol Metab. 2001;86:3562–7.
26. Zang S, Ponto KA, Kahaly GJ. Clinical review: Intravenous glucocorticoids for Graves' orbitopathy: efficacy and morbidity. J Clin Endocrinol Metab. 2011;96:320–32.
27. Minakaran N, Ezra DG. Rituximab for thyroid-associated ophthalmopathy. Cochrane Database Syst Rev. 2013;5:CD009226.
28. Hamed Azzam S, Kang S, Salvi M, Ezra DG. Tocilizumab for thyroid eye disease. Cochrane Database Syst Rev. 2018;11:CD012984.
29. Douglas RS, Gupta S. The pathophysiology of thyroid eye disease: implications for immunotherapy. Curr Opin Ophthalmol. 2011;22:385–90.
30. Le Moli R, Baldeschi L, Saeed P, Regensburg N, Mourits MP, Wiersinga WM. Determinants of liver damage associated with intravenous methylprednisolone pulse therapy in Graves' ophthalmopathy. Thyroid. 2007;17:357–62.
31. Ebner R, Devoto MH, Weil D, et al. Treatment of thyroid associated ophthalmopathy with periocular injections of triamcinolone. Br J Ophthalmol. 2004;88:1380–6.
32. Bartalena L, Pinchera A, Marcocci C. Management of Graves'ophthalmopathy: reality and perspectives. Endocr Rev. 2000;21:168–99.
33. Tanda ML, Bartalena L. Efficacy and safety of orbital radiotherapy for Graves' orbitopathy. J Clin Endocrinol Metab. 2012;97:3857–65.
34. Kahaly G, Beyer J. Immunosuppressant therapy of thyroid eye disease. Klin Wochenschr. 1988;66:1049–59.
35. Mourits MP, van Kempen-Harteveld ML, García MB, Koppeschaar HP, Tick L, Terwee CB. Radiotherapy for Graves' orbitopathy: randomised placebo-controlled study. Lancet. 2000;355:1505–9.
36. Prummel MF, Terwee CB, Gerding MN, et al. A randomized controlled trial of orbital radiotherapy versus sham irradiation in patients with mild Graves' ophthalmopathy. J Clin Endocrinol Metab. 2004;89:15–20.
37. Oeverhaus M, Witteler T, Lax H, et al. Combination therapy of intravenous steroids and orbital irradiation is more effective than intravenous steroids alone in patients with Graves' orbitopathy. Horm Metab Res. 2017;49:739–47.
38. Kim JW, Lee KH, Woo YJ, Kim J, Keum KC, Yoon JS. The effect of systemic steroids and orbital radiation for active Graves orbitopathy on postdecompression extraocular muscle volume. Am J Ophthalmol. 2016;171:11–7.
39. Bartalena L, Marcocci C, Chiovato L, et al. Orbital cobalt irradiation combined with systemic corticosteroids for Graves' ophthalmopathy: comparison with systemic corticosteroids alone. J Clin Endocrinol Metab. 1983;56:1139–44.
40. Ng CM, Yuen HK, Choi KL, et al. Combined orbital irradiation and systemic steroids compared with systemic steroids alone in the management of moderate-to-severe Graves' ophthalmopathy: a preliminary study. Hong Kong Med J. 2005;11:322–30.
41. Prummel MF, Mourits MP, Blank L, Berghout A, Koornneef L, Wiersinga WM. Randomized double-

blind trial of prednisone versus radiotherapy in Graves' ophthalmopathy. Lancet. 1993;342:949–54.
42. Sobel RK, Aakalu VK, Vagefi MR, Foster JA, Tao JP, Freitag SK, Wladis EJ, McCulley TJ, Yen MT. Orbital radiation for thyroid eye disease: A Report by the American Academy of Ophthalmology. Ophthalmology. 2022;129:450–5.
43. Pérez-Moreiras JV, Alvarez-López A, Gómez EC. Treatment of active corticosteroid-resistant Graves' orbitopathy. Ophthalmic Plast Reconstr Surg. 2014;30:162–7.
44. Perez-Moreiras JV, Gomez-Reino JJ, Maneiro JR, et al. Efficacy of tocilizumab in patients with moderate-to-severe corticosteroid-resistant Graves orbitopathy: a randomized clinical trial. Am J Ophthalmol. 2018;195:181–90.
45. Ayabe R, Rootman DB, Hwang CJ, Ben-Artzi A, Goldberg R. Adalimumab as steroid-sparing treatment of inflammatory-stage thyroid eye disease. Ophthalmic Plast Reconstr Surg. 2014;30:415–9.
46. Durrani OM, Reuser TQ, Murray PI. Infliximab: a novel treatment for sight-threatening thyroid associated ophthalmopathy. Orbit. 2005;24:117–9.
47. Wang Y, Patel A, Douglas RS. Thyroid eye disease: How a novel therapy may change the treatment paradigm. Ther Clin Risk Manage. 2019;15:1305–18.
48. Krieger CC, Neumann S, Place RF, Marcus-Samuels B, Gershengorn MC. Bidirectional TSH and IGF-1 receptor cross talk mediates stimulation of hyaluronan secretion by Graves' disease immunoglobins. J Clin Endocrinol Metab. 2015;100:1071–7.
49. Chen H, Mester T, Raychaudhuri N, et al. Teprotumumab, an IGF1R blocking monoclonal antibody inhibits TSH and IGF-1 action in fibrocytes. J Clin Endocrinol Metab. 2014;99:E1635–40.
50. Jain AP, Gellada N, Ugradar S, Kumar A, Kahaly G, Douglas R. Teprotumumab reduces extraocular muscle and orbital fat volume in thyroid eye disease. Br J Ophthalmol. 2022;106:165–71.
51. Douglas RS, Kahaly GJ, Patel A, et al. Teprotumumab for the treatment of active thyroid eye disease. N Engl J Med. 2020;382:341–52.
52. Skov C, Mazow M. Managing strabismus in endocrine eye disease. Can J Ophthalmol. 1984;19:269–74.
53. Yeatts RP. Quality of life in patients with Graves ophthalmopathy. Trans Am Ophthalmol Soc. 2005;103:368–411.
54. Gunton KB. Prism use in adult diplopia. Curr Opin Ophthalmol 2012; 23:400e404.
55. Dunn WJ, Arnold AC, O'Connor PS. Botolinum toxin for the treatment of dysthyroid ocular myopathy. Ophthalmology. 1986;93:470–5.
56. Scott AB. Botulinum toxin injection into extraocular muscles as an alternative to strabismus surgery. Ophthalmology. 1980;87:1044–9.
57. Lyons C, Vickers S, Lee J. Botulinum toxin therapy in dysthyroid strabismus. Eye. 1990;4:538–42.
58. Granet DB, Hodgson N, Godfrey KJ, et al. Chemodenervation of extraocular muscles with botulinum toxin in thyroid eye disease. Graefes Arch Clin Exp Ophthalmol. 2016;254:999e1.
59. Gair EJ, Lee JP, Khoo BK, Maurino V. What is the role of botulinum toxin in the treatment of dysthyroid strabismus? J AAPOS. 1999;3:272–4.
60. Lyons CJ, Vickers SF, Lee JP. Botulinum toxin therapy in dysthyroid strabismus. Eye (Lond). 1990;4:538–42.
61. Kikkawa DO, Cruz RC Jr, Christian WK, et al. Botulinum A toxin injection for restrictive myopathy of thyroid-related orbitopathy: effects on intraocular pressure. Am J Ophthalmol. 2003;135:427–31.
62. Bartley GB, Fatourechi V, Kadrmas EF, Jacobsen SJ, Ilstrup DM, Garrity JA, et al. The treatment of Graves' ophthalmopathy in an incidence cohort. Am J Ophthalmol. 1996;121:200–6.
63. Rajendram R, Bunce C, Adams GG, Dayan CM, Rose GE. Smoking and strabismus surgery in patients with thyroid eye disease. Ophthalmology. 2011;118:2493–7.
64. Jellema HM, Saeed P, Mombaerts I, Dolman PJ, Garrity J, Kazim M, et al. Objective and subjective outcomes of strabismus surgery in Graves' orbitopathy: A prospective multicentre study. Acta Ophthalmol. 2017;95:386–91.
65. Volpe NJ, Mirza-George N, Binenbaum G. Surgical management of vertical ocular misalignment in thyroid eye disease using an adjustable suture technique. J AAPOS. 2012;16:518–22.
66. Coats D, Paysse E, Plager D, Wallace D. Early strabismus surgery for thyroid ophthalmopathy. Ophthalmology. 1999;106:324–9.
67. Thomas SM, Cruz OA. Comparison of two different surgical techniques for the treatment of strabismus in dysthyroid ophthalmopathy. J AAPOS. 2007;11:258–61.
68. Lee YH, Oh SY, Hwang JM. Is 6 months of stable angle of strabismus enough to perform surgery in patients with strabismus related to thyroid ophthalmopathy? Br J Ophthalmol. 2010;94:955–6.
69. Rootman DB, Golan S, Pavlovich P, Rootman J. Postoperative changes in strabismus, ductions, exophthalmometry, and eyelid retraction after orbital decompression for thyroid orbitopathy. Ophthalmic Plast Reconstr Surg. 2017;33:289–93.
70. Zloto O, Ben Simon G, Didi Fabian I, Sagiv O, Huna-Baron R, Ben Zion I, et al. Association of orbital decompression and the characteristics of subsequent strabismus surgery in thyroid eye disease. Can J Ophthalmol. 2017;52:264–8.
71. Nardi M. Squint surgery in TED hints and fints, or why Graves' patients are difficult patients. Orbit. 2009;28:245–50.
72. Nunery WR, Nunery CW, Martin RT, Truong TV, Osborn DR. The risk of diplopia following orbital floor and medial wall decompression in subtypes of ophthalmic Graves' disease. Ophthalmic Plast Reconstr Surg. 1997;13:153–60.
73. Fabian ID, Rosen N, Ben Simon GJ. Strabismus after inferior-medial wall orbital decompres-

sion in thyroid-related orbitopathy. Curr Eye Res. 2013;38:204–9.
74. Chang M, Baek S, Lee TS. Long-term outcomes of unilateral orbital fat decompression for thyroid eye disease. Graefes Arch Clin Exp Ophthalmol. 2013;251:935–9.
75. Prat MC, Braunstein AL, Glass LRD, Kazim M. Orbital fat decompression for thyroid eye disease: Retrospective case review and criteria for optimal case selection. Ophthal Plast Reconstr Surg. 2015;31:215–8.
76. Richter DF, Stoff A, Olivari N. Transpalpebral decompression of endocrine ophthalmopathy by intraorbital fat removal (Olivari technique): Experience and progression after more than 3000 operations over 20 years. Plast Reconstr Surg. 2007;120:109–23.
77. European Group on Graves' Orbitopathy (EUGOGO), Mourits MP, Bijl H, Altea MA, et al. Outcome of orbital decompression for disfiguring proptosis in patients with Graves' orbitopathy using various surgical procedures. Br J Ophthalmol. 2009;93:1518–23.
78. Kacker A, Kazim M, Murphy M, et al. "Balanced" orbital decompression for severe Graves' orbitopathy: technique with treatment algorithm. Otolaryngol Head Neck Surg. 2003;182:228–35.
79. Sellari-Franceschini S, Berrettini S, Santoro A, et al. Orbital decompression in Graves' ophthalmopathy by medial and lateral wall decompression. Otolaryngol Head Neck Surg. 2005;133:185–9.
80. de Souza S, Lima LC, Velarde LG, Vianna RN, Herzog NG. The effect of horizontal strabismus surgery on the vertical palpebral fissure width. J AAPOS. 2011;15:473–5.
81. Fichter N, Krentz H, Guthoff RF. Functional and aesthetic outcome after bony lateral wall decompression with orbital rim removal and additional fat resection in Graves' orbitopathy with regard to the configuration of the lateral canthal region. Orbit. 2013;32:239–46.
82. Lagreze WA, Gerling J, Staubach F. Changes of the 1383 lid fissure after surgery on horizontal extraocular muscles. Am J Ophthalmol. 2005;140:1145–6.
83. Ben Simon GJ, Mansury AM, Schwarcz RM, Lee S, McCann JD, et al. Simultaneous orbital decompression and correction of upper eyelid retraction versus staged procedures in thyroid-related orbitopathy. Ophthalmology. 2005;112:923–32.
84. Quaranta-Leoni FM, Di Marino M, Leonardi A, Verrilli S, Romeo R. Single-stage orbital decompression, strabismus and eyelid surgery in moderate to severe thyroid associated orbitopathy. Orbit. 2022;41:184–92.
85. Gomi CF, Yang S-W, Granet DB, et al. Change in proptosis following extraocular muscle surgery: effects of muscle recession in thyroidassociated orbitopathy. J AAPOS. 2007;4:377–80.
86. Ponto KA, Hommel G, Pitz S, Elflein H, Pfeiffer N, Kahaly GJ. Quality of life in a German Graves orbitopathy population. Am J Ophthalmol. 2011;152:483–90.
87. Vishwanath M, Ansons A. Midoperative forced duction test as a guide to titrate the surgery for consecutive exotropia. Strabismus. 2009;17:41–4.
88. Kim S, Yang HK, Hwang JM. Surgical outcomes of unilateral recession and resection in intermittent exotropia according to forced duction test results. PLoS One. 2018;13:0200741.
89. Jung JH, Holmes JM. Quantitative intraoperative torsional forced duction test. Ophthalmology. 2015;122:1932–8.
90. Al Qahtani ES, Rootman J, Kersey J, Godoy F, Lyons CJ. Clinical pearls and management recommendations for strabismus due to thyroid orbitopathy. Middle East Afr J Ophthalmol. 2015;22: 307–11.
91. Lyu IJ, Lee JY, Kong M, Park KA, Oh SY. Surgical responses of medial rectus muscle recession in thyroid eye disease-related esotropia. PLoS One. 2016;11:0146779.
92. Nugent RA, Belkin RI, Neigel J, et al. Graves orbitopathy: correlation of CT and clinical findings. Radiology. 1990;177:675–82.
93. Dyer J. The oculorotary muscles in Graves' disease. Trans Am Ophthalmol Soc. 1976;74:425–56.
94. Kushner BJ. Torsion and pattern strabismus: potential conflicts in treatment. JAMA Ophthalmol. 2013;131:190–3.
95. Dagi LR, Elliott AT, Roper-Hall G, Cruz OA. Thyroid eye disease: honing your skills to improve outcomes. J AAPOS. 2010;14:425–31.
96. Del Monte MA. 2001 an ocular odyssey: lessons learned from 25 years of surgical treatment for Graves eye disease. Am Orthopt J. 2002;52:40e57.
97. Kushner BJ. A surgical procedure to minimize lower-eyelid retraction with inferior rectus recession. Arch Ophthalmol. 1992;110:1011–4.
98. Akbari MR, Raygan F, Ameri A, Jafari A, Eshraghi B, Fard MA. Lower eyelid retractor lysis versus Lockwood advancement to minimize lower eyelid retraction resulting from inferior rectus muscle recession. J AAPOS. 2013;4:445–7.
99. Weldy E, Kerr NC. Lateral rectus muscle resection following maximal recession of the medial rectus muscle in thyroid eye disease. J AAPOS. 2017;21:291–4.
100. Kim EY, Roper-Hall G, Cruz OA. Effectiveness of bilateral lateral rectus resection for residual esotropia in dysthyroid ophthalmopathy. Am J Ophthalmol. 2016;171:84–7.
101. Nicholson BP, De Alba M, Perry JD, Traboulsi EI. Efficacy of the intraoperative relaxed muscle positioning technique in thyroid eye disease and analysis of cases requiring reoperation. J AAPOS. 2011;15:321–5.

102. Cruz OA, Davitt BV. Bilateral inferior rectus muscle recession for correction of hypotropia in dysthyroid ophthalmopathy. J AAPOS. 1999;3:157–9.
103. Barker L, Mackenzie K, Adams GG, Hancox J. Long-term surgical outcomes for vertical deviations in thyroid eye disease. Strabismus. 2017;25:67–72.
104. Kushner BJ. An evaluation of the semiadjustable suture strabismus surgical procedure. J AAPOS. 2004;8:481–7.
105. Kerr NC. The role of thyroid eye disease and other factors in the overcorrection of hypotropia following unilateral adjustable suture recession of the inferior rectus (an American Ophthalmological Society thesis). Trans Am Ophthalmol Soc. 2011;109:168–200.
106. Oeverhaus M, Fischer M, Hirche H, Schluter A, Esser J, Eckstein AK. Tendon elongation with bovine pericardium in patients with severe esotropia after decompression in Graves' orbitopathy-efficacy and long-term stability. Strabismus. 2018;26:62–70.
107. Ozkan SB, Kir E, Culhaci N, Dayanir V. The effect of seprafilm on adhesions in strabismus surgery – an experimental study. J AAPOS. 2004;8:46–9.
108. Mora JS, Sprunger DT, Helveston EM, Evan AP. Intraoperative sponge 5-fluorouracil to reduce postoperative scarring in strabismus surgery. J AAPOS. 1997;1:92–7.
109. Minguini N, Monteiro de Carvalho KM, Akaishi PM, De Luca IM. Histologic effect of mitomycin C on strabismus surgery in the rabbit. Invest Ophthalmol Vis Sci. 2000;41:3399–401.
110. Kassem RR, El-Mofty RMA-M. Amniotic membrane transplantation in strabismus surgery. Curr Eye Res. 2019;44:451–64.
111. Strube YNJ, Conte F, Faria C, Yiu S, Wright KW. Amniotic membrane transplantation for restrictive strabismus. Ophthalmology. 2011;118:1175–9.
112. Shorr N, Seiff SR. The four stages of surgical rehabilitation of the patient with dysthyroid ophthalmopathy. Ophthalmology. 1986;93:476–83.
113. Choi SW, Lee JY, Lew H. Customized orbital decompression surgery combined with eyelid surgery or strabismus surgery in mild to moderate thyroid-associated ophthalmopathy. Korean J Ophthalmol. 2016;30:1–9.
114. Dal Canto AJ, Crowe S, Perry JD, Traboulsi EI. Intraoperative relaxed muscle positioning technique for strabismus repair in thyroid eye disease. Ophthalmology. 2006;113:2324–30.
115. Peragallo JH, Velez FG, Demer JL, Pineles SL. Postoperative drift in patients with thyroid ophthalmopathy undergoing unilateral inferior rectus muscle recession. Strabismus. 2013;21:23–8.
116. Finn AP, Bleier B, Cestari DM, Kazlas MA, Dagi LR, Lefebvre DR, et al. A retrospective review of orbital decompression for thyroid orbitopathy with endoscopic preservation of the inferomedial orbital bone strut. Ophthal Plast Reconstr Surg. 2017;33:334–9.
117. Jimenez-Chobillon MA, Lopez-Oliver RD. Transnasal endoscopic approach in the treatment of Graves ophthalmopathy: the value of a medial periorbital strip. Eur Ann Otorhinolaryngol Head Neck Dis. 2010;127:97–103.
118. Michel O, Oberlander N, Neugebauer P, Neugebauer A, Rüssmann W. Follow-up of transnasal orbital decompression in severe Graves' ophthalmopathy. Ophthalmology. 2001;108:400–4.
119. Vaidya A, Kakizaki H, Takahashi Y. Changes in horizontal strabismus after inferior rectus muscle recession with or without nasal transposition in thyroid eye disease: A retrospective, observational study. PLoS One. 2020;15:e0240019.
120. Tooley AA, Godfrey KJ, Kazim M. Evolution of thyroid eye disease decompression-dysthyroid optic neuropathy. Eye (Lond). 2019;33:206–11.
121. Oropesa S, Dunbar KE, Godfrey KJ, Callahan AB, Campbell AA, Kazim M. Predominant contribution of superior rectus–levator complex enlargement to optic neuropathy and inferior visual field defects in thyroid eye disease. Ophthal Plast Reconstr Surg. 2019;35:262–5.
122. Mocan MC, Ament C, Azar NF. The characteristics and surgical outcomes of medial rectus recessions in Graves' ophthalmopathy. J Pediatr Ophthalmol Strabismus. 2007;44:93–100.
123. Ha SG, Kim SH. Initial postoperative alignment in strabismus related to thyroid eye disease. J Pediatr Ophthalmol Strabismus. 2021;58:23–7.
124. Jellema HM, Saeed P, Braaksma-Besselink Y, Schuit A, Kloos R, Mourits MP. Unilateral and bilateral medial rectus recession in Graves' orbitopathy patients. Strabismus. 2014;22:182–7.
125. Scofield-Kaplan SM, Dunbar K, Stein G, Kazim M. improvement in both primary and eccentric ocular alignment after thyroid eye disease-strabismus surgery with tenon's recession. Ophthalmic Plast Reconstr Surg. 2018;34:S85–9.
126. Pineles SL, Chang MY, Holmes JM, Kekunnaya R, Özkan SB, Velez FG. Innovative techniques for the treatment of adult strabismus. J AAPOS. 2019;23:132–9.
127. Thorisdottir RL, Blohmé J, Malmsjö M. Clinical evidence supporting the use of donor sclera as spacer material in complicated cases of strabismus surgery - retrospective evaluation of surgical results in 117 patients with thyroid-associated ophthalmopathy or congenital strabismus. Acta Ophthalmol. 2019;97:74–9.
128. Honglertnapakul W, Cavuoto KM, McKeown CA, Capó H. Surgical treatment of strabismus in thyroid eye disease: characteristics, dose-response, and outcomes. J AAPOS. 2020;24:72.e1–7.
129. De Hoog J, Stravers S, Kalmann R. Recession of the inferior rectus muscle in Graves' orbitopathy. Eye (Lond). 2010;24:1011–7.

130. Chatzistefanou KI, Kushner BJ, Gentry LR. Magnetic resonance imaging of the arc of contact of extraocular muscles: Implications regarding the incidence of slipped muscles. J AAPOS. 2000;4:84–93.
131. Hudson HL, Feldon SE. Late overcorrection of hypotropia in Graves ophthalmopathy. Predictive factors. Ophthalmology. 1992;99:356–60.
132. Kushner BJ. Management of diplopia limited to down gaze. Arch Ophthalmol. 1995;113:1426–30.
133. Akbari MR, Raygan F, Ameri A, Jafari A, Eshraghi B, Fard MA. Lower eyelid retractor lysis versus Lockwood advancement to minimize lower eyelid retraction resulting from inferior rectus muscle recession. J AAPOS. 2013;17:445–7.

Management of Eyelid Retraction

Francesco M. Quaranta Leoni, David H. Verity, and Dion Paridaens

Key Messages

- Eyelid retraction has been suggested as one of the prime diagnostic criteria for thyroid-associated orbitopathy (TAO).
- Procedures to address upper eyelid retraction include both surgical interventions and conservative treatments, such as injections of triamcinolone acetonide, botulinum toxin type A and hyaluronic acid filler.
- The outcome of upper eyelid lengthening may be unpredictable, being unsatisfactory in about 20% of patients irrespective of surgical experience and of the type of surgical intervention, and the possibility of revisional surgery should be explained to patients.
- Lower eyelid 'retraction' is frequently a displacement due to globe position. Lower eyelid displacement in patients with TAO is often addressed by decompression, where indicated. Residual displacement can be corrected by retractor recession with or without a spacer material between the eyelid retractors and the lower tarsal border.
- No one spacer material is superior to another, each having relative advantages and disadvantages. Spacers are no longer routinely used for upper eyelid lengthening.
- Orbital decompression can influence the position of the lower eyelid, but does not address upper eyelid retraction.

1 Upper Eyelid Retraction

Upper eyelid retraction can be congenital or acquired. When acquired, it has been suggested as one of the prime diagnostic criteria for thyroid-associated orbitopathy (TAO), and in clinical practice TAO accounts for the vast majority of all cases.

Acquired causes of upper eyelid retraction include:

- Iatrogenic
  - Overcorrected ptosis
  - Excessive tissue excision in upper blepharoplasty
  - In association with lipodystrophy due to topical prostaglandin analogues [1]
- Neurogenic
  - VII nerve paresis or palsy
  - A feature of Brown's syndrome in certain directions of gaze

F. M. Quaranta Leoni (✉)
Oftalmoplastica Roma, Rome, Italy
e-mail: fquarantaleoni@gmail.com

D. H. Verity
Adnexal Service, Moorfields Eye Hospital, London, UK

St John of Jerusalem Eye Hospital Group, London, UK

D. Paridaens
Department of Oculoplastic, Orbital and Lacrimal Surgery, The Rotterdam Eye Hospital and Erasmus Medical Center, Rotterdam, The Netherlands

F. M. Quaranta Leoni et al. (eds.), *Oculoplastic, Lacrimal and Orbital Surgery*,
https://doi.org/10.1007/978-3-031-39638-0_38

  - Aberrant III nerve regeneration
  - Secondary compensatory elevation in the presence of contralateral ptosis
- Injury
  - Injuries to the upper eyelid lamellae, and/or to the retractor complex can be complicated by secondary tissue contracture
- Inflammation
  - TAO:

    Acute:

    Primary: Congestive changes within the levator complex

    Secondary: Overaction of the levator complex due to restricted upgaze resulting from congestion in the inferior rectus muscle

    Chronic:

    Primary retraction due to cicatricial changes within the levator complex

    Secondary: Overaction of the levator complex due to restricted upgaze with cicatricial changes in the inferior rectus muscle
  - Idiopathic inflammatory diseases with secondary contracture of the posterior lamella and entropion formation:

    Trachoma

    Mucous membrane pemphigoid

    Stevens Johnson syndrome

    Linear A disease
- Metastatic disease to the eyelid retractor complex (e.g. metastatic breast cancer)
- *Imploding antrum syndrome.* This characterised by enophthalmos and hypoglobus due to impaired aeration of the maxillary sinus and secondary collapse of the orbital floor. Patients present with pseudo-retraction of the upper eyelid due to a secondary hypoglobus [2].

The central upper eyelid margin normally rests 2 mm below the superior corneal limbus. Eyelid retraction is suspected when the margin is either level with, or above, the superior limbus (visible superior sclera being pathological in the great majority of cases, and termed *'superior scleral show'*, this in contradistinction to *'inferior scleral show'* which is typically a normal finding).

The upper eyelid position is documented with reference to the horizontal distance between the central corneal light reflex in the primary position of gaze, and the central upper lid margin (margin-reflex distance 1, MRD1) (Fig. 1). The measurement is inaccurate unless the examiner and patient are sat opposite each other, at the same level. Superior scleral show is measured by holding a ruler vertically at the lateral pupil border and recording the distance from the upper eyelid margin to the superior margin of the limbus with the eye in primary gaze.

In TAO, eyelid retraction may occur in isolation or in association with proptosis. It is a common finding that may involve the upper or lower eyelid and has been reported to be observed in about 90% of patients with TAO.

Typical features are:

- the Dalrymple sign (eyelid retraction in primary gaze)
- the Kocher sign (staring and frightened appearance of the eyes, particularly marked on attentive fixation)
- the von Graefe sign or *lid phase-lag* (delayed descent of the upper eyelid on downgaze) (Fig. 2).
- *lateral eyelid flare*, possibly due to eyelid inflammation and fibrosis of the lateral levator horn.

Upper eyelid retraction may present with ocular redness and irritation, symptoms of evaporative dry eye (particularly with periods of prolonged concentration such as reading), nocturnal lagophthalmos with ocular dryness on waking, and frank exposure keratitis. The 'staring' or 'startled' appearance also has marked psychosocial implications and can have a negative effect on the quality of life of affected patients [3].

The cause of upper eyelid retraction in TAO is multifactorial, and proposed mechanisms, which usually coexist, include adrenergic stimulation in uncontrolled hyperthyroidism, post-inflammatory fibrosis of the levator muscle–superior rectus complex and Muller's muscle, increased sympa-

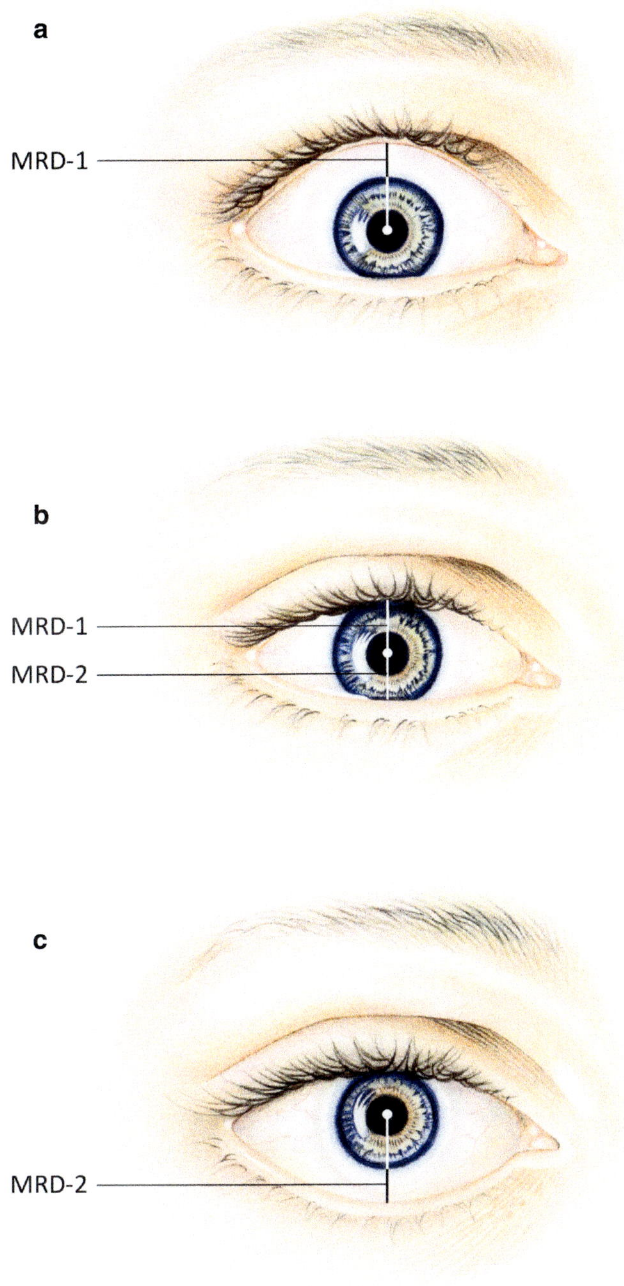

Fig. 1 Margin reflex distance-1 and margin reflex distance-2. (**a**) Upper eyelid retraction in primary position. MRD-1 describes the distance from the pupillary reflex to the upper eyelid margin. (**b**) Normal upper eyelid position. The eyelid covers about 1 mm of the upper and lower cornea in primary position. (**c**) Lower eyelid retraction in primary position: MRD-2 describes the distance from the pupillary reflex to the lower eyelid margin (Modified from: Pinas D, O B De Keizer R, Wubbels RJ, van den Bosch WA, Paridaens D. Results of surgical correction of upper eyelid retraction in Thyroid-Associated Orbitopathy. Acta Ophthalmol. 2021 Jun;99 (4):e608-e613)

thetic tone in Müller's muscle, scarring and/or inflammation of the orbital septum and anterior lamella, exophthalmos, contracture and restriction of the inferior rectus muscle with resultant increase in tone of the superior rectus and levator muscle (Fig. 3) [4].

In the absence of keratopathy, topical lubricants alone will control symptoms in the majority of patients. However, where there is evidence for

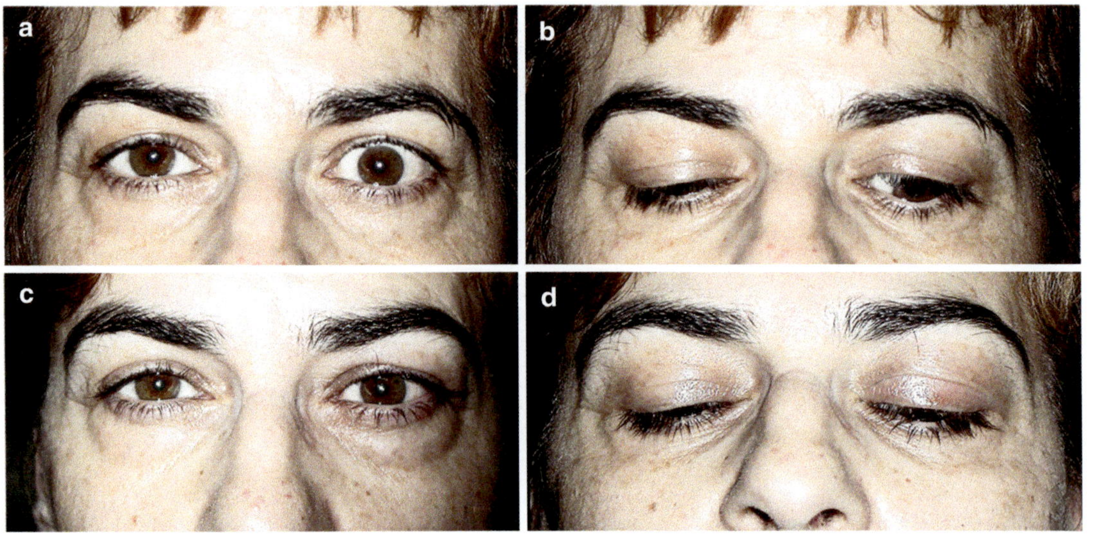

Fig. 2 (**a**) Left upper eyelid retraction in primary position. (**b**) Left *lid phase-lag* (delayed descent of the upper eyelid on downgaze). (**c**) Adequate correction of upper eyelid retraction following left posterior Müllerectomy. (**d**) *Lid lag* disappeared following Müllerectomy. The skin crease is slightly higher post-operatively

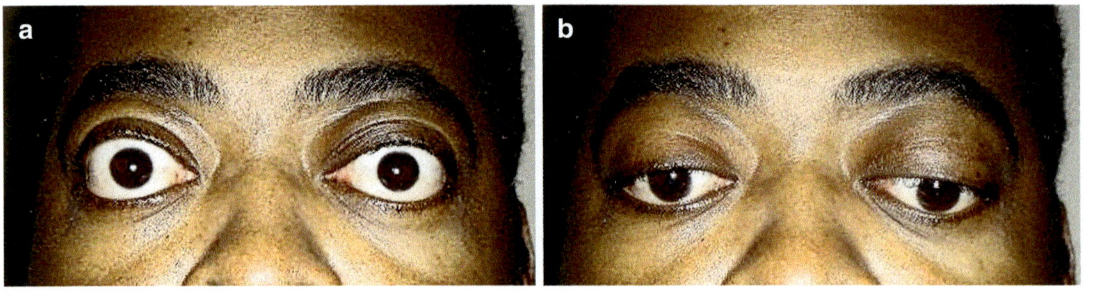

Fig. 3 (**a**) Bilateral secondary upper eyelid retraction. (**b**) Absence of lid retraction in downgaze. Upper eyelid retraction is determined by overaction of the levator complex due to restricted upgaze caused by fibrosis of the inferior recti muscles

punctate epithelial keratopathy, adjunctive measures are required to reduce the risk of infective keratopathy and chronic cicatricial changes. These include moisture chambers, swimming goggles, nocturnal antibiotic ointment, surgical and medical approaches to address the eyelid height, and—in extreme cases—temporary tarsorrhaphy where there is an acute and severe threat to a compromised ocular surface.

Procedures to address upper eyelid retraction include surgical intervention, injections of triamcinolone acetonide (TA), botulinum toxin type A (BTX-A), and hyaluronic acid filler. Some minimally invasive techniques are good temporary measures or reasonable choices for patients who refuse surgery or are poor surgical candidates. Although topical guanethidine eye drops have been employed, the results have been disappointing and are associated with miosis, undercorrection, and conjunctival hyperaemia [5].

In general, where the eyelid height and tissue compliance are sufficiently compromised, and ocular surface protection cannot be achieved with topical measures alone, surgical correction is preferred. Botulinum toxin to the levator muscle carries little advantage in the presence of major retraction, and is best avoided since it carries a risk to the integrity of the Bell's response and nocturnal corneal protection. In patients with major retraction and evidence for corneal compromise, urgent surgical correction is a more immediate and effective approach, both in the acute and chronic phases.

Several surgical procedures have been described to correct upper eyelid retraction. These comprise internal or external approach Müllerectomy, with or without graded levator muscle disinsertion, the use of hangback sutures, 'Z' myotomy (now largely superseded), spacer interposition and full-thickness eyelid blepharotomy [4]. However, both autogenous and non-autogenous spacers are associated with complications, these including post inflammatory scarring and resultant malposition, infection, extrusion, and asymmetry, and their use has largely fallen from favour.

In aesthetic rehabilitation for patients with TAO, eyelid surgery is formed as part of a staged sequence, with orbital decompression undertaken first, where indicated, followed by strabismus surgery. Simultaneous orbital decompression and eyelid retraction correction can be performed in selected cases to control moderate to marked ocular surface exposure, but further adjustment under local anaesthesia may be required at a later date. As anticipated, surgical correction carries a higher success rate in patients with stable, chronic disease than in patients with active disease, but early eyelid lowering is nevertheless indicated in patients presenting early in the course of disease with marked eyelid retraction [6].

Whether performed in the acute or chronic phase of TAO, surgical outcomes can be unpredictable, [7] with reoperation rates varying from 8.4 to 23% of eyelids, and with no technique considered consistently to yield superior results [8].

Less invasive options have their limitations as well, such as ptosis and vertical diplopia for BTX-A injections; potential lumps or oedema for filler injections, and relatively high cost of both.

According to a study, TAO-related upper eyelid retraction spontaneously improves in approximately 70% of patients by 12 months and 75% of patients by 24 months, without any surgery or other intervention to the eyelid. [9]

Therefore, the natural history of eyelid retraction is important in the management of these patients and it helps to decide on the best timing for surgery or the use of temporary measures. Milder cases may be managed conservatively since there is a downward trend in MRD1, with the most rapid improvement from presentation to 12 months, and continued but slower improvement from 12 to 48 months. There would be no significant difference in the natural course of upper eyelid retraction in patients with and without eyelid inflammation, and in patients with euthyroid or hypothyroid/hyperthyroid status at presentation, indicating that the improvement occurs regardless of disease activity and thyroid status, and the level of thyrotropin receptor autoantibodies (TRAb) apparently has no significant correlation.

This is contrary to what is originally believed that TAO patients would have an improvement in MRD1 after restoring a euthyroid state. Factors associated with a lower likelihood of normalisation are male sex, middle age, smoke, and a positive family history. [9]

2 Non-surgical Treatments

2.1 Transconjunctival Triamcinolone Injection

Transconjunctival triamcinolone acetonide (TA) injection can be an effective treatment option for TAO-related upper eyelid retraction, as a primary and adjunctive treatment, in active TAO patients [10]. It has been reported that the levator is enlarged in patients with TAO and upper eyelid retraction; thinning of the levator muscle after TA treatment was found during the MRI examinations. Steroids can reduce muscle and soft-tissue oedema, inhibit further inflammatory disease progression and prevent chronic fibrosis, thus decreasing the levator diameter with a consequent improvement of eyelid retraction.

Treatment can be undertaken in an outpatient setting under topical anaesthesia. A volume of 0.5 mL (40 mg/mL) triamcinolone acetonide (TA) solution is injected into the subconjunctival space 5 mm above the upper edge of the everted tarsus. The treatment can be repeated monthly and stopped if the retraction is completely resolved, noting that the degree and duration of active TAO may limit the effects of the treatment [11].

Patients must be monitored regularly for recurrences and side effects. Although effective in reducing eyelid retraction and inflammatory signs, TA injection carries the risk of induced ptosis, superior sulcus defect, raised intraocular pressure and vascular occlusion with resultant visual loss [10, 11].

2.2 Botulinum Toxin Type A Injection

Following topical anaesthesia, the upper eyelid is everted, the patient is asked to look down, and two injections are applied, one-third from the eyelid extremities. Botulinum toxin type A (BTX-A) is injected using a 30-gauge needle into the subconjunctival space at the superior margin of the tarsal plate. The concentration of BTX-A is 5 units per 0.1 mL. Doses between 2 and 15 units of BTX-A are injected depending on the severity of the retraction. Additional BTX-A injections can be performed on the tenth day in patients who had an undercorrection.

The effect of BTX-A remains for 4–5 months after a single session. Patients should be followed up every week for up to 6 months for signs of ocular surface disease and MRD1 measurements. [12]

Temporary complications, such as ptosis, ocular motility alterations with diplopia, and ecchymosis have been reported in some studies. There might be a decrease in flicking caused by BTX-A injection which could determine a dry eye and need of tear substitutes. [13, 14]

2.3 Hyaluronic Acid Injection

Topical eye drops are used to anaesthetise the conjunctiva. The conjunctiva just superior to the upper edge of the tarsus is exposed by everting the upper eyelid. A single bolus of 0.1–0.5 mL of hyaluronic acid (HA) is injected centrally in the subconjunctival plane using a 30-gauge needle, asking the patient to look down. The presence of a lateral flare may need additional filler injected temporally, transconjunctival or by external approach. Satisfactory results can usually be achieved with 1–2 injections in a single session.

Complications are typically temporary and minimal, including oedema, ecchymosis, and transient erythema at the injection site. Blue or dark colour changes, fluid build-up, contour irregularity and lumps may rarely occur. HA effectiveness by just a single injection has been reported for up to 15 months [15]. HA has usually better results, longer duration, and fewer side effects in comparison with Botox, and its effect can be reversible by injection of hyaluronidase [15, 16]. Foreign body sensation and skin pigment darkening have occasionally been described.

2.4 Teprotumumab

Teprotumumab is not specifically advocated in the treatment of eyelid retraction. However, soft tissue expansion of the face caused by TAO appears reduced following therapy, and volume decrease in the periorbital region can decrease MRD1, MRD2 and intercanthal distance [17].

3 Surgical Procedures

3.1 Posterior Approach Müllerectomy

This procedure is indicated for mild upper eyelid retraction up to 2.5 mm.

- Local anaesthesia is provided by local infiltration of the upper eyelid, placed subcutaneously with epinephrine supplementation, and subconjunctivally without epinephrine (Fig. 4a)
- The upper eyelid is everted on a Desmarres retractor (Fig. 4b) and the conjunctiva is incised along the superior tarsal margin.
- Dissection of the conjunctiva from Müller's muscle is performed superiorly for approximately 15 mm. Müller muscle is then cut from its superior tarsal insertion, dissected from the levator aponeurosis superiorly for 13–15 mm, transected near its origin from the inferior surface of the levator muscle. Alternatively, conjunctiva and Müller's muscle can be separated together from the aponeurosis (Fig. 4c), with Müller's muscle excised from the conjunctiva (Fig. 4d, e).

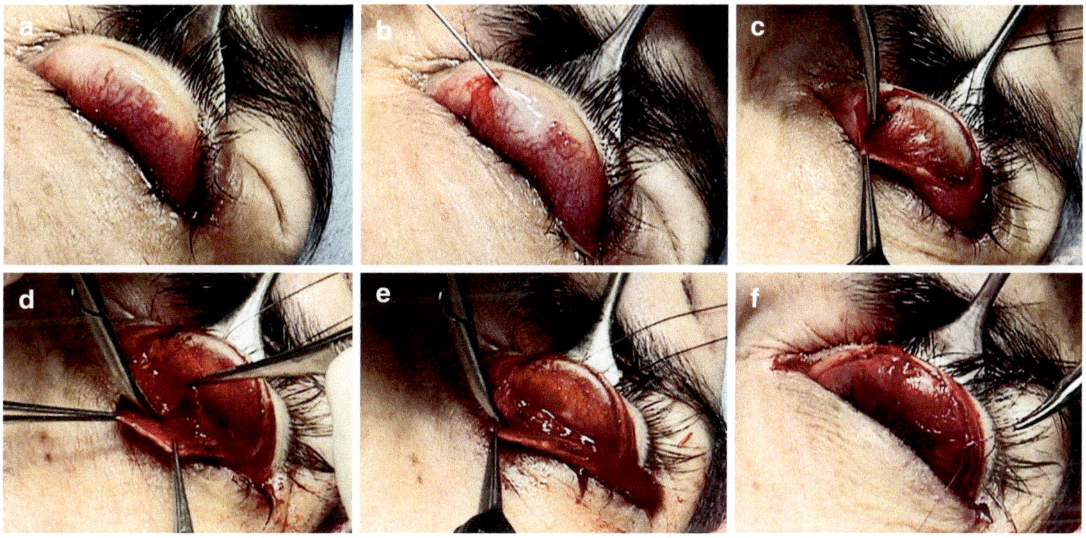

Fig. 4 Posterior Müllerectomy. (**a**) The eyelid is everted on a Desmarres retractor. (**b**) Local anaesthesia is provided subconjunctivally. (**c**) The conjunctiva is incised along the superior tarsal margin, and is separated together with Müller's muscle from the levator aponeurosis. (**d**) Müller's muscle is separated from the conjunctiva. (**e**) Müller's muscle is excised from the conjunctiva. (**f**) Following careful evaluation of eyelid height and contour, the conjunctiva is sutured with a continuous 7/0 absorbable suture

Care is taken to avoid damage to the lacrimal gland ducts by leaving the lateral extensions of Müller muscle intact.

- The conjunctiva is then repositioned and either sutured with a continuous 6-0 rapid polyglactin suture with knots buried (Fig. 4f) or allowed to heal primarily.

The patient's eyelid height and contour are evaluated during surgery to achieve the best possible symmetry with the contralateral side (Fig. 2).

4 Graded Anterior Levator Disinsertion/Reinsertion and Müllerectomy (ALDM)

This procedure is indicated for upper eyelid retraction greater than 2.5 mm, and when a lateral flare is present. The approach is graded and determined by the degree of eyelid retraction.

- The desired skin crease is marked, usually 10 mm above the eyelid margin, but it can be placed higher to match the skin crease of the contralateral eyelid or in case of proptosis. Where there is doubt, the surgeon errs on the lower side due to the tendency of the skin crease to rise with this procedure. If simultaneous excision of excess skin is planned, the marked line is extended laterally and the amount of skin to be excised is determined.
- After marking, 1–1.5 mL of local anaesthesia is administered subconjunctivally along the upper margin of the tarsal plate and subcutaneously in the plane between the orbicularis oculi muscle and the orbital septum at the level of the marked line.
- A skin incision is made along the marked line with a D-15 blade. Next, slight blunt upward dissection is performed in the plane between the orbicularis muscle and the orbital septum using Westcott scissors (Fig. 5a, b).
- The orbital septum is opened to expose the orbital fat overlying the levator aponeurosis, and the latter is dissected from the tarsal plate in upward direction. The central tarsal plate is exposed in the event that suture placement is required for subsequent height or contour control for later suture placement (Fig. 5c). The aponeurosis is then dissected from the underlying Müller's muscle (Fig. 5d).
- The lateral horn of the levator muscle is cut vertically (Fig. 5e); the nasal quarter of the levator

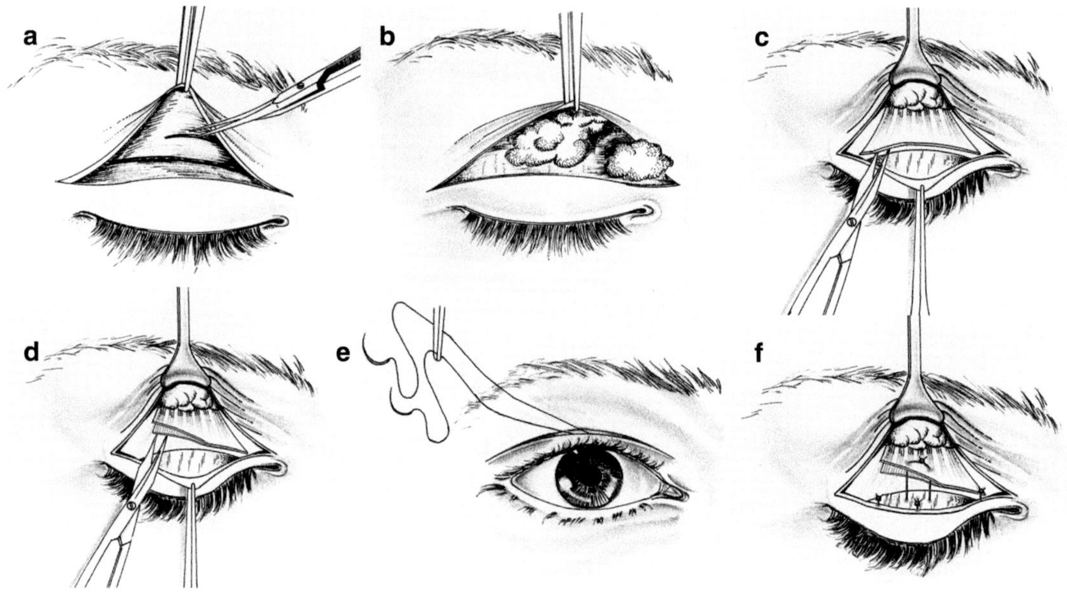

Fig. 5 Anterior levator disinsertion/reinsertion and Müllerectomy (ALDM). Surgical technique. (**a**) A skin and orbicularis incision has been made at the level of the skin crease. Slight blunt upward dissection behind the orbicularis muscle has been performed. Here, the orbital septum is opened. (**b**) After opening the orbital septum, orbital fat will generally prolapse. (**c**) Skin and fat are retracted upward with a Desmarres retractor and dissection of the levator aponeurosis is started laterally. The lateral horn of the levator muscle aponeurosis is cut vertically. Only the lateral and central part of the aponeurosis are dissected, the medial part is left intact. This prevents medial droop. (**d**) After dissection of the lateral part of the levator aponeurosis, the lateral and central part of Müller's muscle are cut just above the level of the horizontally running vessels and meticulously dissected off the underlying conjunctiva. Also, here, the medial part is untouched. (**e**) After placement of a temporary hangback suture, the upper eyelid position in primary direction of gaze is judged. The hangback suture is adjusted by gentle downwards pull until the upper eyelid position is adequate, that is at or slightly over the superior limbus, or, in unilateral cases, 0.5–1 mm higher than the contralateral upper eyelid. (**f**) Final situation prior to wound closure. A hangback suture has been placed above the pupil between the anterior surface of the tarsal plate and the disinserted levator aponeurosis. The dissected part of Müller's muscle remains disinserted. If the eyelid contour is inadequate, an additional temporal or medial hangback sutures can be applied. Eyelid crease reconstruction is performed through placement of at least three evenly spaced rapid polyglactin 6-0 sutures between the pretarsal orbicularis muscle and the superior part of the tarsal plate or, nasally, the levator aponeurosis. Then, the skin is closed with a running suture (polypropylene 6-0) (Modified from: Pinas D, O B De Keizer R, Wubbels RJ, van den Bosch WA, Paridaens D. Results of surgical correction of upper eyelid retraction in Graves' Orbitopathy. Acta Ophthalmol. 2021 Jun;99(4):e608-e613. (with permission of Wiley, publisher))

muscle is left intact. If indicated, additional local anaesthesia is injected into Müller's muscle.

- With Westcott scissors, from lateral to medial, two-thirds to three quarters of Müller's muscle is meticulously dissected from the underlying conjunctiva, leaving the medial insertion of this muscle to the underlying conjunctiva intact. If conjunctival buttonholes occur, no sutures are needed and they can be left to heal. The extent to which the temporal and central Müller's muscle is disinserted depends on the per-operative evaluation of eyelid contour and height.
- After adequate eyelid height and contour are obtained, a double-armed 5.0 Vicryl® suture is placed centrally in the tarsus, at about 2–3 mm from its upper edge (Fig. 5e). Both ends of the suture are passed through the posterior surface of the levator aponeurosis, and a loose knot is made in a 'hangback' fashion.
- The patient is asked to look directly at the surgeon to determine the upper eyelid position in primary gaze. If indicated, the knot is adjusted until the desired upper eyelid position is obtained (Fig. 5f). If the eyelid contour needs further adjustment, additional hangback sutures can be placed laterally or medially in similar fashion.
- Skin crease reformation may be performed with three evenly spaced single Vicryl® 6.0

rapidly reabsorbing sutures between the orbicularis muscle and the tarsal plate laterally and centrally, and the levator aponeurosis medially.

- The skin is closed with a running prolene 6.0 suture, that is removed after 5–7 days.

5 Anterior Approach Graded Blepharotomy

This procedure is indicated for significant upper eyelid retraction, although ALDM with hang-back sutures can be considered as well.

- Following 1–1.5 mL subcutaneous local anaesthesia, a skin crease incision is made with a D-15 blade at the desired level, to match the opposite side.
- The anterior tarsal surface exposed, and the orbital septum opened to allow the retractors to retract superiorly with minimal elevation of the final skin crease.
- The levator aponeurosis is then dissected off the tarsal surface, and Müller's muscle dissected meticulously off the conjunctiva, with frequent reassessment of the eyelid lowering achieved to that point.
- Where further lowering is required, the lateral horn is frequently divided in such cases, and in cases of marked retraction, the medial horn may also be divided to avoid a medially-oriented lid 'peak'.
- The conjunctiva is also opened medially with a full thickness incision, extending as far as the level of the upper punctum, but leaving a 3–4 mm centro-medial vertical 'bridge' of intact conjunctiva to avoid a 'flat' eyelid contour (Fig. 6).

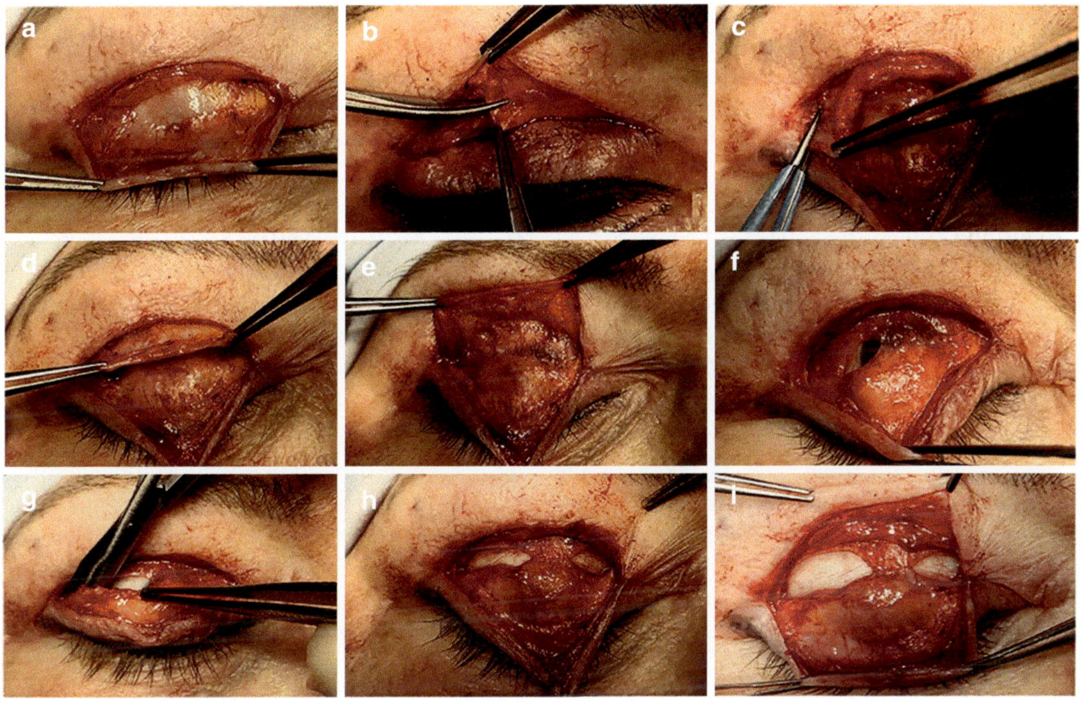

Fig. 6 Anterior approach graded blepharotomy. (**a**) A skin crease incision is made and the anterior tarsus is exposed. (**b**) The orbital septum is opened to allow the aponeurosis to rise without raising the skin crease. (**c**) The aponeurosis is dissected off the tarsus, and the lateral horn of the levator is divided if necessary. (**d**) The anterior aponeurosis is free of the septum. (**e**) The aponeurosis is dissected superiorly for up to 7 mm and the Müller's muscle is excised. (**f**) If insufficient eyelid lowering is achieved, the conjunctiva is opened, laterally first. (**g**) For marked retraction and lateral flare, the incision must be taken all the way to the orbital rim. (**h**) For residual central and medial retraction a small medial conjunctival opening is made as shown. (**i**) A centro-medial 4 mm *bridge* of intact conjunctiva is vital to avoid a flat upper eyelid contour

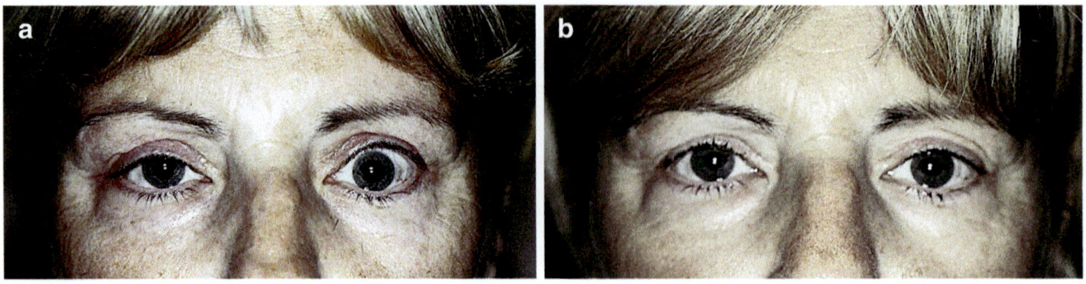

Fig. 7 (**a**) Left upper eyelid retraction; note right upper eyelid mild ptosis due to Hering's phenomenon (see chapter "Ptosis Repair in Cosmetic Surgery"). (**b**) Post-operative picture following left blepharotomy: adequate symmetry with no right upper eyelid ptosis

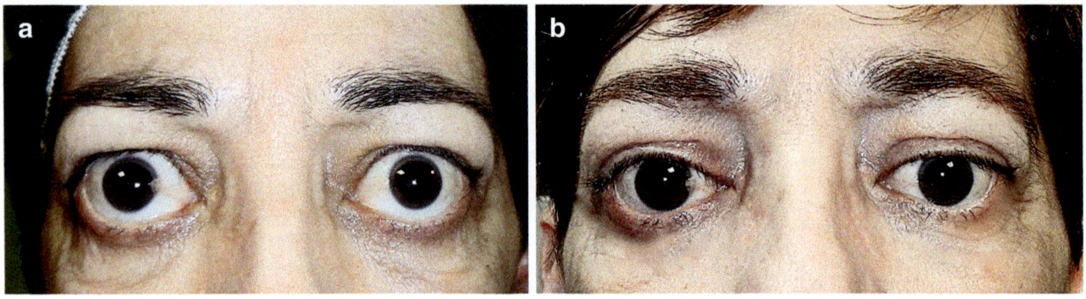

Fig. 8 Simultaneous orbital decompression and upper eyelid retraction correction. (**a**) Pre-operatively. (**b**) Post-operatively, following bilateral endoscopic medial wall decompression, lateral wall external decompression and bilateral anterior approach graded blepharotomy

- During surgery, the patient is checked in an upright position to evaluate the position of both upper eyelids, to achieve satisfactory symmetry. The upper eyelid is usually left covering the limbus by approximately 0.5–1 mm, based on the appearance of the contralateral eyelid, with no need for over-correction, and great care is taken in the final stages of retractor weakening and conjunctival opening to avoid a secondary ptosis (Fig. 7).
- Skin closure is achieved with a running interlocking 5-0 or 6.0 nylon or polypropylene suture, to be removed after about 10 days [18, 19].
- Where the conjunctiva has been opened, the overlying orbicularis should be closed first with an absorbable 6/0 suture to prevent fistula formation from the conjunctiva to the skin.

6 Simultaneous Orbital Decompression and Upper Eyelid Retraction Correction

A one-step approach is indicated in certain patients where there is both significant exophthalmos, and major eyelid retraction. Upper eyelid retraction correction (either Müllerectomy or graded blepharotomy) performed at the same time of the orbital decompression has been proposed by several authors, and the outcome appears unrelated to the amount of proptosis reduction [20–22].

Careful pre-operative evaluation usually allows reasonable results (Fig. 8), and possible over or undercorrections may be addressed at a second stage, performed under local anaesthesia, with the advantage of optimising eyelid contour.

Orbital decompression affects the lateral eyelid contour and diminishes the amount of lateral eyelid retraction surgery necessary to correct the flare sign, and in several cases the eyelid contour can be normalised with proptosis reduction only [23, 24].

In conclusion, the outcome of surgery for upper eyelid retraction can be unsatisfactory in about 20% of patients, irrespective of surgical experience and previous interventions, and the real likelihood of revisional surgery should be described at the outset. To improve the results, new tools are needed, such as local modulation of the healing process in the post-operative phase [4].

7 Lower Eyelid Retraction

Lower eyelid retraction can be congenital or acquired, although in the latter tends to represent eyelid *displacement* due to globe position, and not a retraction *per se*. Acquired causes of lower eyelid retraction include:

- Proptosis, due to orbital diseases, determining a vertical displacement
- Iatrogenic:
  - Excessive tissue excision in lower blepharoplasty
  - Inferior rectus recession—as the lower eyelid complex is intrinsically connected to the inferior oblique and rectus via the capsulopalpebral fascia [25]
- Neurogenic
  - VII nerve paresis or palsy
- Injury
  - Injuries to the lower eyelid can be complicated by secondary tissue contracture
- Inflammation
  - TAO:
    - Acute:
      - Inflammation or increased adrenergic stimulation of the lower eyelid complex, analogous to overaction of Müller's muscle
    - Chronic:
      - Lower eyelid retractors fibrosis
  - Idiopathic inflammatory diseases with secondary contracture of the posterior lamella

Lower eyelid position (margin reflex distance 2, MRD2) should be carefully recorded by measuring the distance from the central pupil light reflex to the central lower eyelid margin. Inferior scleral show can be measured recording the distance from the lower eyelid margin to the inferior margin of the limbus with the eye in primary gaze (Fig. 1).

The first procedures used to address lower eyelid retraction in patients with TAO included lateral and medial tarsorrhaphies, horizontal tightening, and lateral canthal elevation to counteract the retractors' contracture force [26].

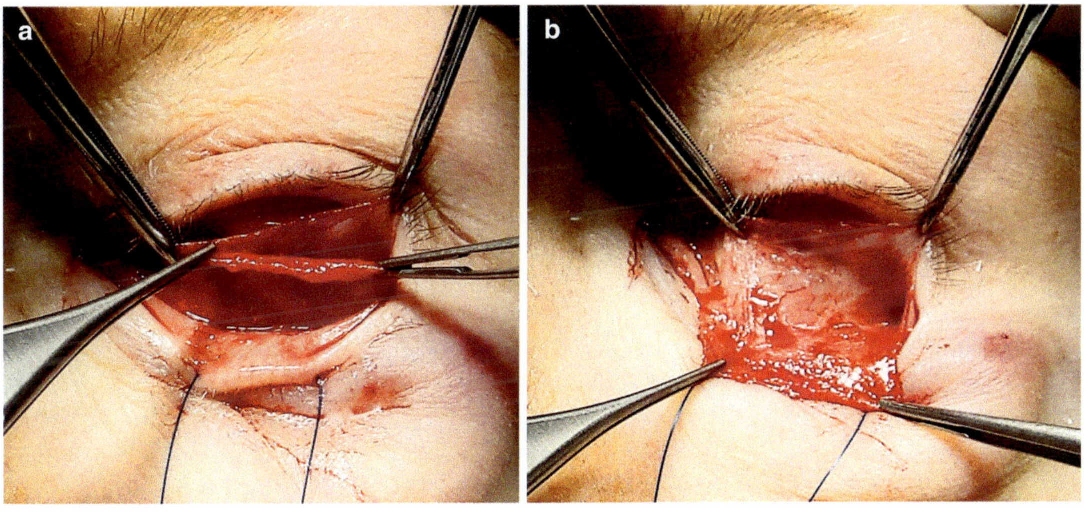

Fig. 9 Recession of lower eyelid retractors: transconjunctival approach. (**a**) The white sheet of the lower eyelid retractors is identified at the lower tarsal border and separated from the conjunctiva. (**b**) The retractors are carefully dissected from the conjunctiva of the lower eyelid and adequately recessed

Lower eyelid retraction can be successfully corrected in these patients by recessing the lower eyelid retractors (Fig. 9) and, in case of greater retraction, by positioning a graft or *spacer* between the retractors and the lower tarsal border. Horizontal eyelid laxity should be adequately corrected, orbicularis muscle should have residual function and there must be no shortage of lower eyelid skin [27]. Concomitant proptosis should be always considered and properly addressed: if present, orbital decompression should be advised.

As opposed to patients with cicatricial lower eyelid retraction, a subperiosteal midface suborbicularis oculi fat (SOOF) lifting is usually not necessary, as in most patients there is no need of additional lower eyelid anterior lamella. In patients with TAO skin should not be removed in case of simultaneous lower eyelid fat blepharoplasty.

8 Simultaneous Decompression and Lower Eyelid Retraction Correction

Orbital decompression can have effects on the position of lower eyelids [28–30]. The lower eyelid has been shown to elevate by approximately 0.5–1 mm after decompression with different techniques. This effect can be related to both surgical technique and to changes in orbital volume and axial globe position [30]. A greater reduction in proptosis is associated with greater improvement in MRD2, this being possibly attributed to reduction in the mechanical impedance from the curvature of the proptotic globe [31].

Improvement of lower eyelid position was demonstrated in patients undergoing simultaneous orbital decompression and correction of lower eyelid retraction, irrespective of the aetiology of lower eyelid retraction and proptosis or orbital decompression technique [32].

The disinsertion and release of the lower eyelid retractors may allow for greater elevation of the lower eyelid with respect to techniques in which the lower eyelid is not manipulated. It has been showed that there is not a significant difference in the quantity of change in MRD2 based on incisional approach, if additional release of lower eyelid retractors is not provided, when comparing transconjunctival and lateral decompression techniques [32].

Staged orbital decompression and lower eyelid retraction surgery may be unnecessary, and lower eyelid retraction correction performed at the time of orbital decompression may reduce the number of total procedures without compromising the results [22, 33].

9 Spacers: Materials, Surgical Technique and Complications

The use of a spacer allows for a greater elevation of the lower eyelid by supporting the eyelid itself and keeping lower eyelid retractors adequately recessed (Fig. 10) [27]

Spacers are classified in:

- **Autogenous**, such as hard palate mucosa (HPM), mucous membrane, dermis, ear or nasal cartilage, tarso-conjunctiva.
- **Non-autogenous**:

  Non-integrable, such as donor sclera, donor fascia, porcine dermal collagen (Permacol™ Medtronic), bioengineered acellular dermal matrix (BADM, AlloDerm™ LifeCell Corporation).

  Integrable (Medpor™).

Autogenous spacers do not retract and have a lower infection rate compared to allografts (donor sclera, donor fascia, BADM) but need harvesting.

Mucous membrane grafts are not thick enough to provide adequate eyelid support, and ear or nasal cartilage are too rigid. Tarso-conjunctiva from the homolateral or contralateral upper eyelid should preferably not be harvested in patients with TAO due to the consequent increase in upper eyelid retraction.

HPM grafts are widely used for lengthening the posterior lamella [34–37]. HPM grafts are composed of mucous membrane and firm stroma with a thickness and texture that matches tarsus.

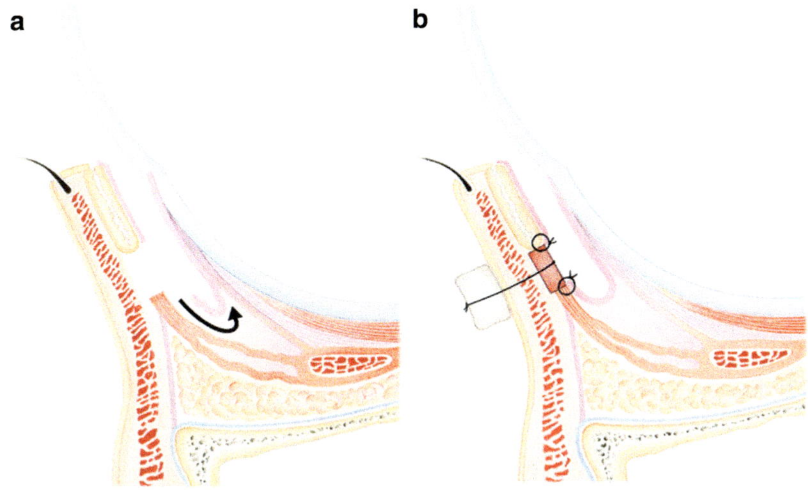

Fig. 10 (**a**) The lower eyelid retractors are disinserted from the lower edge of the tarsal plate and recessed. (**b**) Simultaneous positioning of an adequate spacer, that allows for a greater elevation of the lower eyelid by supporting the lower eyelid itself and keeping lower eyelid retractors adequately recessed. The spacer is sutured with buried interrupted 6-0 polyglactin sutures between the lower edge of the inferior tarsus and the upper edge of the spacer, and the lower edge of the spacer and the conjunctiva. If donor sclera is used, it should be covered by adequately mobilised conjunctiva. A bolster is usually applied and kept in place by means of double-armed 4-0 nonabsorbable sutures usually left in place for 7–10 days. No bolsters are needed for non-autogenous spacers such as donor sclera. In all cases the lower eyelid should be left on vertical traction for 2–4 days post-operatively

When harvesting HPM graft it is essential to avoid the greater palatine neurovascular bundle: it emerges from the greater palatine foramen which sits alongside the second and third molars in most people. The hard palate has a midline raphe and the area to be harvested must be medial to the greater palatine neurovascular bundle. Medially the graft should not reach the midline if a small graft is required or if the amount needed is for just one eyelid (Fig. 11). However, if large grafts are required it is safe to cross over the midline, although the midline mucosa is usually thinner and less useful for reconstruction. Local anaesthetic with adrenaline should be injected at the greater palatine foramen and at the incisive foramen to provide a greater palatine nerve block. Further anaesthetic should be injected below the graft area to improve haemostasis. The edges of the graft are cut with a 15 blade, and the graft is harvested by means of an ophthalmic crescent blade. The thickness required depends on the indication: usually mucosa and the underlying lamina propria are harvested, and the graft should not include the periosteum, as its removal may delay healing. Glandular tissue should be removed from the graft as it can continue to secrete, which is not desirable in the case where the graft is used for eyelid reconstruction. Diathermy is used to cauterise the donor site bed and an adrenaline soaked gauze pressure pack is left in situ while the graft is used at the donor site. A haemostatic mesh can be placed on the donor site and left in situ to dissolve. Alternatively, a palate protective device might be used.

Complications are rare: the most frequently observed complication is post-operative donor site bleeding that is minimised with careful surgical technique and the proper use of intra-operative cautery, and if needed post-operative pressure or diathermy. Sometimes the eyelid tends to become bulky with time, so extra care is needed in thinning the graft to make it homogeneously smooth.

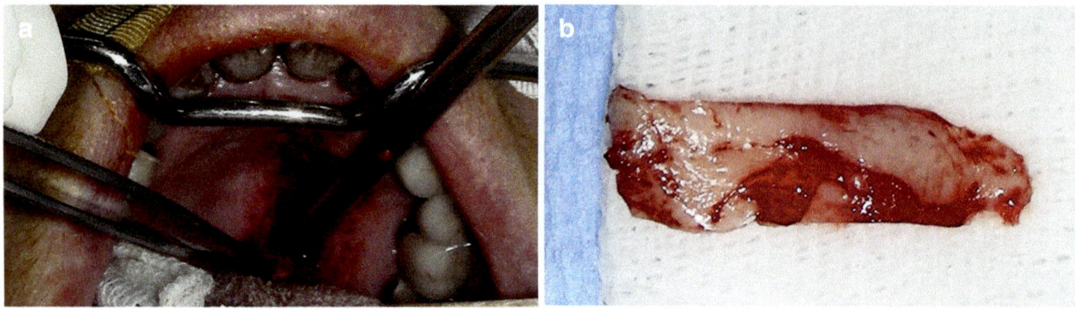

Fig. 11 Hard palate graft. (**a**) The hard palate is harvested medial to the greater palatine neurovascular bundle, and it should not reach the midline if the amount needed is for one eyelid. (**b**) Graft to be sutured at the conjunctival edges with buried 6-0 absorbable sutures

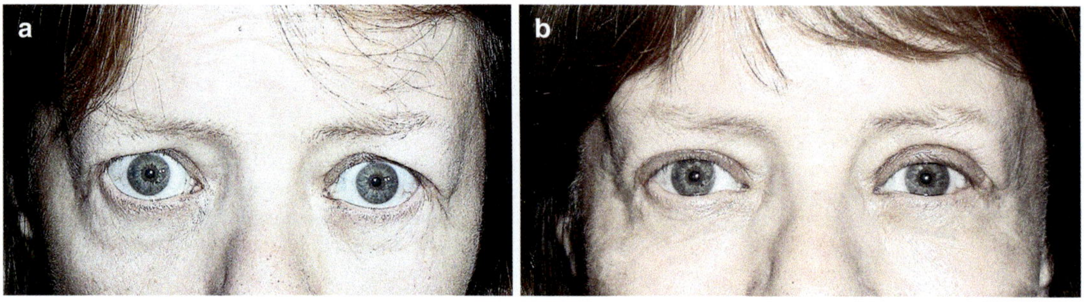

Fig. 12 (**a**) Bilateral upper and lower eyelid retraction persistent following bilateral orbital decompression. (**b**) Postoperatively, after bilateral Müllerectomy and bilateral lower eyelid retractors recession with positioning of a dermal graft

Posterior lamellar graft placement involves the placement of traction in the lower eyelid margin, recessing the conjunctiva and lower eyelid retractors, from just beneath the inferior edge of the tarsus, then suturing the graft in place to the tissue just at the conjunctival edges with buried 6-0 absorbable sutures. Adequate lateral support to the eyelid must be provided, by means of a lateral canthoplasty at the time of surgery, using deep 5-0 absorbable or non-absorbable sutures, being careful not to shorten the eyelid horizontally in an excessive fashion. Skin closure is usually made with interrupted 6-0 nonabsorbable sutures. Lower eyelid traction and padding for 24–48 h is useful in unilateral cases. Bilateral cases are helped by adequate positioning of self-adhesive tape (Steri-Strip™ 3M) and ice packs.

Dermis can be harvested from the abdominal, the inguinal or buttock region, and extra care should be taken to remove the fat to avoid bulkiness. Following the excision of the epidermis layer, dermis grafts can be conveniently left to conjunctivalize and may lead to good results (Fig. 12), but harvesting leaves an evident scar.

Porcine acellular dermal matrix has been used for permanent implantation in humans for the reconstruction, recontouring, and reformation of human soft connective tissue and as a supporting tissue in various surgical procedures. It is supplied as a 1-mm thick piece that can be cut to size and used in the lower eyelid as a substitute for HPM or other spacers [38]. It should be soaked in povidone-iodine for 5 min, then customised according to the nomogram 2:1 mm (graft height:inferior scleral show, ISS) [38]. The conjunctiva may be advanced over the graft, or sutured at the inferior edge of the graft with buried interrupted 6/0 polyglactin sutures, as with HPM, leaving it free to conjunctivalize. A protective contact lens may be left in place if need be.

In a recent study, both dermal grafts and porcine dermal collagen implant have shown to be effective to adequately correct lower eyelid retraction together with simultaneous orbital decompression and inferior rectus recession [22], although acellular dermis may contract significantly more than HPM when used as a lower eyelid spacer graft [39].

Medpor is integrable but relatively stiff, and it should be positioned through an anterior subciliary approach to reduce the chance of exposure, extrusion and granuloma formation [27]. However, due to the relatively high complication rate with this material for such surgery, its use has largely been superseded.

Although the current literature suggests that BADM grafts represent an implantation option for lower eyelid retraction repair and short-term results are favourable, long-term safety and efficacy remain unknown [40]. Longer follow-up is necessary to assess possible prion and other disease transmissions, as detection is elusive and may occur after decades of latency [41]. While AlloDerm has been used in Europe in the past, increasingly stringent regulations surrounding the sale of human tissue have made it recently unavailable in Europe [42].

Finally, it has been reported that lower eyelid retraction could be treated by the injection of HA under the orbicularis muscle. The filler can act as a lifter as it changes the balance of force of the lower eyelid, forcing it to shift upward to gain the new balance [43].

In conclusion, there is no single spacer material which is superior to all others [44], and there are advantages and disadvantages associated with the various available materials [40]. However, as technology continues to evolve, new devices may replace current available materials.

References

1. Sira M, Verity DH, Malhotra R. Topical Bimatoprost 0.03% and iatrogenic eyelid and orbital lipodystrophy. Aesthet Surg J. 2012;32:822–4.
2. Stryjewska-Makuch G, Goroszkiewicz K, Szymocha J, Lisowska G, Misiołek M. Etiology, early diagnosis and proper treatment of silent sinus syndrome based on review of the literature and own experience. J Oral Maxillofac Surg. 2022;80:113.e1–8.
3. Gaddipati RV, Meyer DR. Eyelid retraction, lid lag, lagophthalmos, and von Graefe's sign quantifying the eyelid features of Graves' ophthalmopathy. Ophthalmology. 2008;115:1083–8.
4. Pinas D, De Keizer ROB, Wubbels RJ, van den Bosch WA, Paridaens D. Results of surgical correction of upper eyelid retraction in Graves' orbitopathy. Acta Ophthalmol. 2021;99:e608–13.
5. Cruz AA, Ribeiro SF, Garcia DM, et al. Graves upper eyelid retraction. Surv Ophthalmol. 2013;58:63–76.
6. Soeters MR, van Zeijl CJJ, Boelen A, Kloos R, Saeed P, Vriesenkoop TM, Mourits MP. Optimal management of Graves' orbitopathy: a multidisciplinary approach. Neth J Med. 2011;69:302–8.
7. Kazim M, Gold KG. A review of surgical techniques to correct upper eyelid retraction associated with thyroid eye disease. Curr Opin Ophthalmol. 2011;22:391–3.
8. Golan S, Rootman DB, Goldberg RA. The success rate of TED upper eyelid retraction reoperations. Orbit. 2016;35:335–8.
9. Lee DC, Young SM, Kim YD, Woo KI. Course of upper eyelid retraction in thyroid eye disease. Br J Ophthalmol. 2020;104:254–9.
10. Young SM, Kim YD, Lang SS, Woo KI. Transconjunctival triamcinolone injection for upper lid retraction in thyroid eye disease—a new injection method. Ophthalmic Plast Reconstr Surg. 2018;34:587–93.
11. Xu DD, Chen Y, Xu HY, Li H, Zhang ZH, Liu YH. Long-term effect of triamcinolone acetonide in the treatment of upper lid retraction with thyroid associated ophthalmopathy. Int J Ophthalmol. 2018;11:1290–5.
12. Ozturk Karabulut G, Fazil K, Saracoglu Yilmaz B, Ozturker C, Günaydın ZK, Taskapili M, Kaynak P. An algorithm for Botulinum toxin A injection for upper eyelid retraction associated with thyroid eye disease: long-term results. Orbit. 2021;40:381–8.

13. Uddin JM, Davies PD. Treatment of upper eyelid retraction associated with thyroid eye disease with subconjunctival botulinum toxin injection. Ophthalmology. 2002;109:1183–7.
14. Träisk F, Tallstedt L. Thyroid associated ophthalmopathy: botulinum toxin A in the treatment of upper eyelid retraction—a pilot study. Acta Ophthalmol Scand. 2001;79:585–8.
15. Kohn JC, Rootman DB, Liu W, et al. Hyaluronic acid gel injection for upper eyelid retraction in thyroid eye disease: functional and dynamic high-resolution ultrasound evaluation. Ophthal Plast Reconstr Surg. 2014;30:400–4.
16. Hassan Hussien M, Abd El-Wahed Hassan E, El-Haddad NSEM. Comparison between hyaluronic acid filler and botulinum toxin type A in the treatment of thyroid upper eyelid retraction. Ther Adv Ophthalmol. 2020;12:2515841420979113.
17. Ugradar S, Braun J, Wang Y, Zimmerman E, Douglas RS. Facial and eyelid changes in thyroid eye disease are reversed by Teprotumumab. Plast Reconstr Surg Glob Open. 2021;9:e3809.
18. Elner VM, Hassan AS, Frueh BR. Graded full-thickness anterior blepharotomy for upper eyelid retraction. Trans Am Ophthalmol Soc. 2003;101:67–73.
19. Hintschich C, Haritoglou C. Full thickness eyelid transsection (blepharotomy) for upper eyelid lengthening in lid retraction associated with Graves' disease. Br J Ophthalmol. 2005;89:413–6.
20. Ben Simon GJ, Mansury AM, Schwarcz RM, Lee S, McCann JD, Goldberg RA. Simultaneous orbital decompression and correction of upper eyelid retraction versus staged procedures in thyroid-related orbitopathy. Ophthalmology. 2005;112:923–32.
21. Bernardini FP, Skippen B, Zambelli A, Riesco B, Devoto MH. Simultaneous aesthetic eyelid surgery and orbital decompression for rehabilitation of thyroid eye disease: the one-stage approach. Aesthet Surg J. 2018;38:1052–61.
22. Quaranta-Leoni FM, Di Marino M, Leonardi A, Verrilli S, Romeo R. Single-stage orbital decompression, strabismus and eyelid surgery in moderate to severe thyroid associated orbitopathy. Orbit. 2021;3:1–9.
23. Rootman DB, Golan S, Pavlovich P, Rootman J. Postoperative changes in strabismus, ductions, exophthalmometry, and eyelid retraction after orbital decompression for thyroid orbitopathy. Ophthal Plast Reconstr Surg. 2017;33:289–93.
24. Cruz AAV, Equitério B, Diniz SB, Garcia DM, Rootman DB, Goldberg RA, Galindo-Ferreiro A, Marqués-Fernández V, Sales-Sanz M. Upper eyelid contour changes after orbital decompression in Graves orbitopathy. Ophthalmic Plast Reconstr Surg. 2021;38:289–93.
25. Kakizaki H, Malhotra R, Madge SN, et al. Lower eyelid anatomy: an update. Ann Plast Surg. 2009;63:344–51.
26. Taban MR. Lower eyelid retraction surgery without internal spacer graft. Aesthet Surg J. 2017;37:133–6.
27. Collin JRO. Thyroid Eye Disease. In: Manual of Systematic Eyelid Surgery. 3rd Ed., Elsevier 2005;200–2.
28. Taban MR. Combined orbital decompression and lower eyelid retraction surgery. J Curr Ophthalmol. 2018;30:169–73.
29. Goncalves AC, Gupta S, Monteiro ML, Douglas RS. Customized minimally invasive orbital decompression surgery improves lower eyelid retraction and contour in thyroid eye disease. Ophthal Plast Reconstr Surg. 2017;33:446–51.
30. Rootman DB, Golan S, Pavlovich P, Rootman J. Postoperative changes in strabismus, ductions, exophthalmometry, and eyelid retraction after orbital decompression for thyroid orbitopathy. Ophthal Plast Reconstr Surg. 2016;33:289–93.
31. Rufer F, Schroder A, Erb C. White-to-white corneal diameter: normal values in healthy humans obtained with the Orbscan II topography system. Cornea. 2005;24:259–61.
32. Thorne AW, Rootman DB. Influence of surgical approach for decompression on lower eyelid position in thyroid eye disease. Orbit. 2020;39:84–6.
33. Norris JH, Ross JJ, O'Reilly P, Malhotra R. A review of combined orbital decompression and lower eyelid recession surgery for lower eyelid retraction in thyroid orbitopathy. Br J Ophthalmol. 2011;95:1664–9.
34. Siegel RJ. Palatal grafts for eyelid reconstruction. Plast Reconstr Surg. 1985;76:223–30.
35. Oestreicher JH, Pang NK, Liao W. Treatment of lower eyelid retraction by retractor release and posterior lamellar grafting: an analysis of 659 eyelids in 400 patients. Ophthalmic. Plast Reconstr Surg. 2008;24:207–12.
36. Puri K, Kumar A, Khatri M, Bansal M, Rehan M, Siddeshappa ST. 44-Year journey of palatal connective tissue graft harvest: A narrative review. J Indian Soc Periodontol. 2019;23:395–408.
37. McAlister CN, Oestreicher JH. Repeat posterior lamellar grafting for recalcitrant lower eyelid retraction is effective. Orbit. 2012;31:307–12.
38. McGrath LA, Hardy TG, McNab AA. Efficacy of porcine acellular dermal matrix in the management of lower eyelid retraction: case series and review of the literature. Graefes Arch Clin Exp Ophthalmol. 2020;258:1999–2006.
39. Sullivan SA, Dailey RA. Graft contraction: a comparison of acellular dermis versus hard palate mucosa in lower eyelid surgery. Ophthalmic Plast Reconstr Surg. 2003;19:14–24.
40. Tao JP, Aakalu VK, Wladis EJ, Sobel RK, Freitag SK, Foster JA, Yen MT. Bioengineered acellular dermal matrix spacer grafts for lower eyelid retraction repair: A Report by the American Academy of Ophthalmology. Ophthalmology. 2020;127:689–95.

41. Taban M, Douglas R, Li T, Goldberg RA, Shorr N. Efficacy of thick acellular human dermis (alloderm) for lower eyelid reconstruction. Arch Facial Plast Surg. 2005;7:38–44.
42. Zamanian K, Spicer J. Factors hampering adoption of biologic matrices in EU market for soft tissue reinforcement and regeneration. iData Research Inc.; 2015. (Guest Column, May 21, 2015, Retrieved 7 Feb 2021)
43. Xi W, Han S, Feng S, Li K, Brunetti B, Lazzeri D, Tong Y, Zhang Y. The injection for the lower eyelid retraction: a mechanical analysis of the lifting effect of the hyaluronic acid. Aesthetic Plast Surg. 2019;43:1310–7.
44. Park E, Lewis K, Alghoul MS. Comparison of efficacy and complications among various spacer grafts in the treatment of lower eyelid retraction: a systematic review. Aesthet Surg J. 2017;37:743–54.

Cosmetic Surgery for Thyroid-Associated Orbitopathy

Jonathan C. P. Roos, Rachna Murthy, and Dario Surace

Key Messages

- The aesthetic aspect of TAO should be a key aspect of patient assessment.
- Disfigurement from TAO confers an increased risk of death by suicide.
- An understanding of disease pathogenesis can permit aesthetic interventions without worsening the disease even in the active inflammatory phase.
- New therapies are addressing aesthetically significant aspects of TAO such as proptosis. This has led to a new emphasis on proptosis as an indicator of disease rather than inflammation. This will help towards aligning the perspective of patients and doctors more.
- The traditional staged surgical paradigm is often too conservative. A combined approach using surgical and non-surgical modalities will help reduce disfigurement and psychological harm.

J. C. P. Roos (✉) · R. Murthy
Face Restoration, Harley St, London, UK
e-mail: jr@facerestoration.com

D. Surace
LaVista Eye Center, Mestre, VE, Italy

1 Is TAO an Aesthetic Disease?

Ophthalmologists generally consider Thyroid Associated Orbitopathy (TAO) to be a self-limiting periocular autoimmune condition often resulting in diplopia and which can potentially threaten vision through corneal exposure or optic nerve compression. The inflammation follows Rundle's curve and will usually resolve by about 18 months, marking the end of the disease process for the patient.

This stands in some contrast with patients' views. For them, TAO is often primarily an aesthetic disease with disfigurement leading to loss of a sense of self and resulting in social isolation. Studies show that less than 5% of patients [1] consider themselves "cured" when the doctor feels the disease has run its course, and there is a significant increased risk of suicide associated with TAO [2] with a hazard ratio of 2.71. Though both views of this disease are accurate, it points to the importance of aesthetic interventions in the management of TAO—an area which has previously and perhaps understandably been neglected by eye doctors who are trained primarily to preserve vision. But all doctors are also taught to preserve life and quality of life and these areas have arguably been neglected in TAO. For the aesthetic consequences, as indicated above, lead directly to increased morbidity and mortality.

The effects of TAO on facial aesthetics are plentiful. TAO is associated with conjunctival

F. M. Quaranta Leoni et al. (eds.), *Oculoplastic, Lacrimal and Orbital Surgery*,
https://doi.org/10.1007/978-3-031-39638-0_39

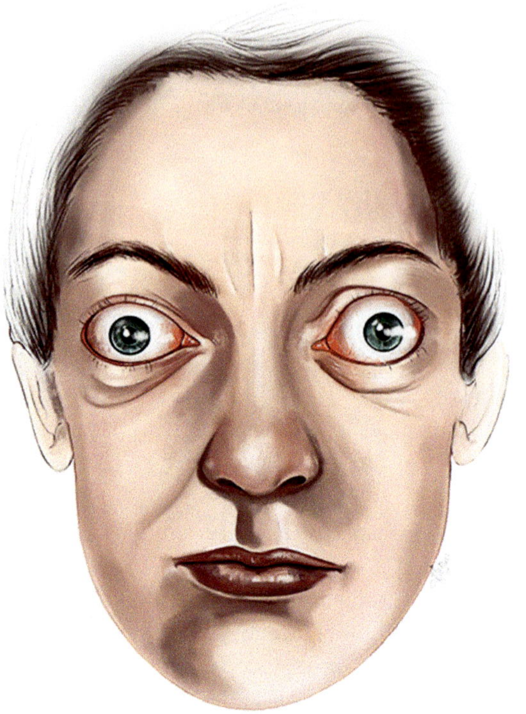

Fig. 1 Aesthetic sequelae of thyroid-associated orbitopathy: Upper and lower lid fullness, exophthalmos, upper lid retraction, lower lid displacement

chemosis and injection, corneal pannus, lid retraction, increased scleral show, upper lid swelling, periocular swelling, proptosis and strabismus. There is also a typical TAO glabellar frown and vertical furrowing of the central brow. These combine to create a staring and angry look as illustrated in Fig. 1. This in turn leads to difficult personal interactions as they are stared at by others [3], hence social withdrawal and depression [4] as well as lost job opportunities and reduced socioeconomic status.

This chapter is included here in the ESOPRS textbook as modern oculoplastic surgeons should be familiar with medical, surgical and non-surgical options available for the management of TAO, enabling them to provide early rehabilitation and mitigation.

2 Aesthetic Interventions for TAO

2.1 Optimal Thyroid Management and Control of Disease Drivers

Prevention is better than cure. This is the case even after the diagnosis of TAO has been established. Disease management of TAO can affect the severity and hence outcomes for patients with TAO—both visual [5] and aesthetic. Though we absolutely advocate for aesthetic intervention and rehabilitation one must not forget to control the disease. A complete approach to the modern management of TAO is covered elsewhere but should include a focus on:

- Strict thyroid endocrine control such as with a block and replace regimen. In addition to preventing deterioration euthyroid status can help resolve the corneal pannus seen in TAO.
- Cessation of smoking. Smoking is by far the most important modifiable risk factor for progression and severity of disease. Studies have shown that the circulating TSHR antibodies—which correlate with severity and indicate disease activity—persist far longer in those who smoke [6].
- Protection of the ocular surface.
- Consideration of antioxidant supplementation such as with selenium.
- Managing the microbiome and reducing any local inflammatory drivers such as nasal staphylococcal colonisation.
- Use of anti-inflammatory medication, both steroid and steroid sparing.
- Use of periocular surgery to reduce the orbital pressure—a known driver of disease severity.
- Early treatment with anti-proptotic drugs like teprotumumab.
- Judicious use of non-ocular surgery. For example, surgical thyroidectomy reduces circulating TRAb levels in TAO [6, 7] signifi-

cantly reduced proptosis in 12/15 patients in a prospective study [8] and reduces risk of TAO development when used for the treatment of Graves' disease [9].

2.2 Injectable Aesthetic Interventions

2.2.1 Dermal Fillers

Over the last decade there have been significant advances in the quality and structure of non-surgical injectables, with most companies now producing non-animal origin synthetic hyaluronic acid for aesthetic enhancement. More than seven million such injections are given per year world-wide and have replaced the older silicone, fat and collagen-based fillers.

Amongst the first to recognize the potential of these molecules to reduce morbidity in TAO lid retraction was Prof Goldberg and his team in California who treated both upper and lower lid retraction with minimal invasion [10]. As trauma to the periocular tissues can increase inflammation and exacerbate TAO treatments had been eschewed. But as a naturally occurring tissue substance with some reported anti-inflammatory biological properties, HA fillers are now used frequently in the US to reduce scleral show in TAO. This leads to an aesthetic improvement and serves to protect the eye from excess evaporation and dryness. Reports since indicate that this approach is associated with only minimal transient complications such as erythema oedema ecchymosis. The HA can be injected transcutaneously or transconjunctivally, usually a volume of around 0.5 mL being used. This has been reviewed recently [11].

2.2.2 Neurotoxin

Neuromodulation with botulinum toxin is also helpful in aesthetic management. As shown in Fig. 1, TAO is associated with vertical glabellar frown lines and an area of frontalis contraction giving a prominent and angry looking central forehead. Such an aggressive appearance likely contributes to the staring and social isolation experienced by TAO patients and can be mitigated with botulinum toxin injections. Reduction in frown lines will create a calmer appearance. Botox is given transcutaneously, requiring between 10 and 30 units centrally. It has few side effects and lasts around 3–4 months. Studies show that inducing a mild brow ptosis can help to reduce the MRD1 (and thus upper lid retraction induce scleral show) significantly, helping to soften the appearance further.

Though botulinum was first introduced into medicine for the treatment of strabismus—which are an aesthetic concern in TAO—neurotoxin cannot be used for aesthetic correction of strabismus in the TAO setting. This is because the squint is not caused by reduced or excessive muscle activity but scarring and muscle swelling, which the toxin will have little effect on.

2.2.3 Triamcinolone

Another injectable therapy with a proven track record is triamcinolone. This steroid can be given subconjunctivally or injected transcutaneously into the levator complex above the skin crease. A large retrospective study found that this effectively normalised upper lid MRD1 in well over 80% of patients [12] and did not affect intraocular pressure. This is helpful as triamcinolone is inexpensive compared to filler and widely available, including in resource poor countries or public payer healthcare systems.

2.3 Surgical Aesthetic Interventions

To put the surgical interventions in context it is important to understand the hierarchy of interventions. Patients requiring surgical interventions generally fall into two groups: (1) those with mild signs (no diplopia, mild proptosis, mild or absent eyelid retraction, some dermatochalasis, festoons) and (2) those with more severe degree of retraction and proptosis with evidence of diplopia. In the first group an aesthetic correction could be the only necessary treatment and a blepharoplasty alone may be the

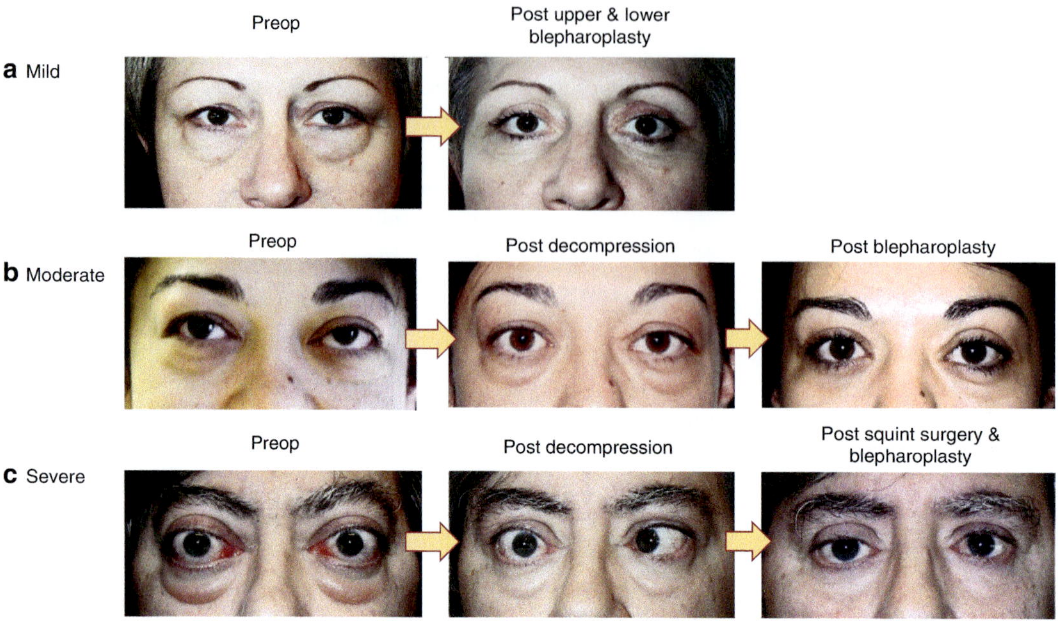

Fig. 2 Dysthyroid patients can have mild (**a**), severe (**b**), or more severe (**c**) disease. The former may require only a single procedure whilst the latter usually require a series of operations

only surgical intervention required. However for the second group, traditionally a series of four surgical steps are followed in sequence as part of the rehabilitative course [13]. The orbital decompression represents the first treatment to be performed in order to reduce proptosis. This is because decompression can worsen a pre-existent strabismus or generate a new-onset diplopia. If there is no diplopia, no squint surgery is needed. The third step is the correction of eyelid malpositions (mainly retraction but sometimes also blepharoptosis by tendon dehiscence). This comes after strabismus surgery as eyelid retraction (especially inferior) can be worsened or generated by a recession muscle surgery (more often the Inferior Rectus Muscle) even if eyelid retractor lysis is attempted at the time of the rectus muscle recession. The final step is the blepharoplasty to correct residual skin excess or festoons.

Therefore in the first group a blepharoplasty is often the only surgery to be performed (Fig. 2a), while in the second group the blepharoplasty represents the final step of a long rehabilitative course that in some cases requires four or more surgeries (Fig. 2b, c).

2.3.1 Eyelid Surgery

Eyelid Recession

Upper eyelid retraction is common in TAO and frequently requires a lid recession to reposition the lid in a more aesthetically appropriate position relative to the cornea. The aim is both to protect the ocular surface and to reduce the scleral show (which creates a staring appearance). There are a number of techniques [14] but the key is to ensure the lateral horn of levator is released as otherwise an unsightly lateral flare of the lid can occur. Also, as TAO is a scarring disease, recession must often exceed the target lid height as otherwise healing will reposition the lid with recurrence of scleral show. Often a lid recession can be performed by division of fibres from the conjunctival side but occasionally the retraction and scarring can be so severe that a dermis fat graft is required to act as a spacer to enable the lid to descend [15]. Interestingly, a recent study has demonstrated that unilateral retraction can be treated by contralateral Müller's muscle-conjunctiva resection; if a phenylephrine test on their normal eyes equalises the retracted lid a

Table 1 Particular blepharoplasty considerations in the context of TAO

Consideration	Advice
Ocular surface	Always perform an accurate evaluation of lacrimal function and surface integrity: TAO patients often suffer from dry eye on autoimmune basis and surgery can risk insufficient safe spontaneous lid occlusion
	At least 20 mm of residual skin should be left in place, and in any case lid occlusion should be naturally soft without needing force to close. A pinch test while drawing the lines of excision is recommendable
Masking of proptosis	Fat removal should be conservative and graded in relation with the entity of proptosis: the more is the proptosis, the less should be fat removal in order to mask the proptosis: an excess of depression in the bag area makes proptosis more visible. Excess fat removal can lead to skin tenting
Bleeding risk	Meticulous haemostasis with bipolar forceps during fat excision. TAO patients have a higher risk of bleeding due to the congestive orbitopathy related to the disease. Always cauterise before cutting. A history of anticoagulant use should be obtained and stopped prior to surgery if possible clinically

Müllerectomy can offer an effective alternative treatment with a predictable outcome [16].

Upper Blepharoplasty

Essentially a cosmetic upper blepharoplasty in a TAO patient differs little from a classical blepharoplasty, but some particular considerations are required in addition to those of a normal blepharoplasty. These are shown in Table 1.

See chapter "Upper Blepharoplasty" for the technique of upper blepharoplasty. Skin and orbicularis muscle can then be excised in a single layer [17] or as two separated flaps [18], making the muscular flap a little bit smaller in order to leave some muscle fibres concentric to the skin. This muscle can be cauterised without burning the skin in case of bleeding and can be utilised in order to anchor the wound to the periosteum as described below. A 5/0 Vicryl® suture can be placed laterally at the lateral canthus in order to anchor some fibres of the orbicularis muscle from the upper and lower edge of the wound to the periosteum of the orbital rim. The expected effect is to extend laterally the superior skin crease and to give support to the lateral eyebrow also avoiding the lateral skin to drop down. The retro orbicularis oculi fat (ROOF) differs from the orbital fat in that it is placed anteriorly to the orbital septum and posteriorly to the orbicularis muscle extending toward the eyebrow [19]. In TAO patients this compartment expands, giving a swollen appearance to the central and lateral part of the superior eyelid. Careful but not excessive sculpting or excision will help to achieve a good aesthetic result. A 6/0 nylon running suture can be used to close the skin.

Lower Blepharoplasty

A lower blepharoplasty can be helpful in addressing the expanded orbital fat compartment which will create lower lid malar oedema, festoons and fat prolapse. This surgery can be performed either through a transcutaneous or transconjunctival approach [20].

The transcutaneous approach is helpful when one wishes to excise skin [21]. Care should be taken to avoid excessive skin removal as this can lead to round eye, lagophthalmos or cicatricial ectropion. As shown in Fig. 3a–e, the skin is classically marked 1.5–2 mm below the lashes starting medially from the lower punctum level and continuing laterally into the "crow's feet" lateral skin creases. A small incision with a scalpel is performed and then the suborbicularis plane is identified and undermined with blunt scissors going medially. This skin muscle flap is cut with scissors, freeing it as far as the line of the inferior punctum. Just as with the upper blepharoplasty, skin and muscle can be undermined and excised separately in order to preserve more muscle in order to ensure good eyelid closure. The exposed septum is then incised and the surplus fat cauterised and removed. The skin muscle flap is finally laid and gently stretched up and laterally while opening the mouth, in order to determine the amount of excess skin to be taken away. A 6/0

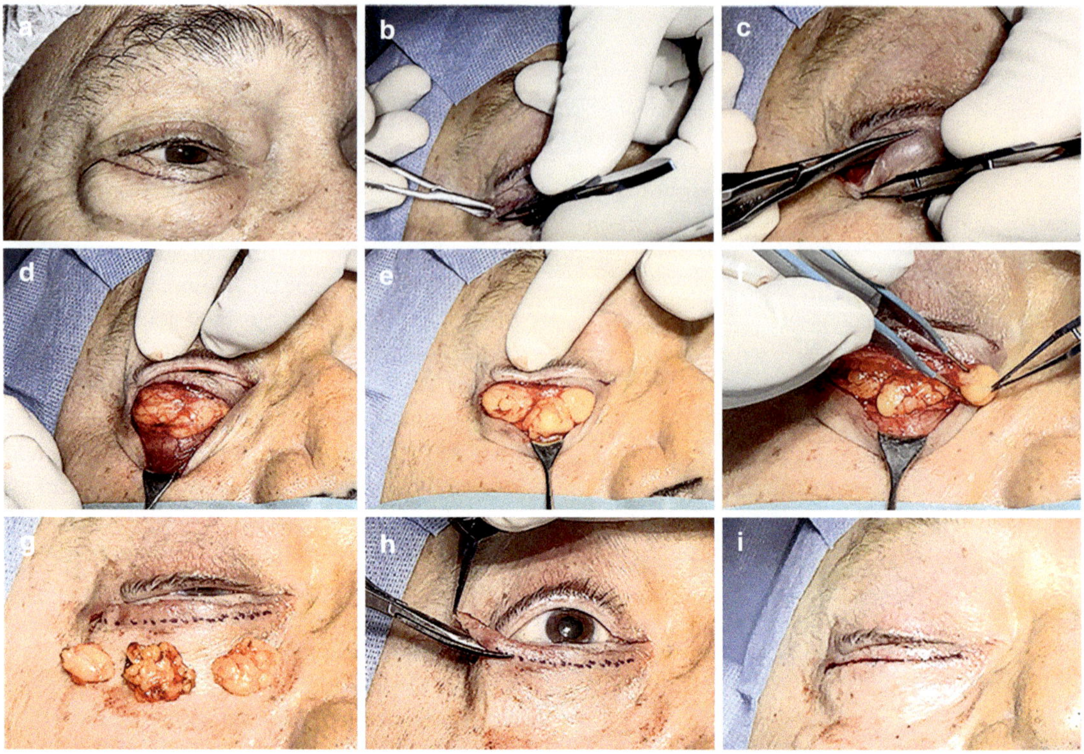

Fig. 3 Steps of transcutaneous lower blepharoplasty (see chapter "Brow Ptosis"). (**a**) Marking of the skin. (**b**) Detection of sub-orbicularis layer. (**c**) Undermining the sub-orbicularis layer and cutting the skin muscle flap. (**d**) Exposing the orbital septum. (**e**) Opening the orbital septum. (**f**) Excising orbital fat. (**g**) Amount of fat resection from the three pads. (**h**) Skin redraping and cutting. (**i**) Final appearance following skin excision

nylon suture is used to close the skin. A lower lid strengthening procedure such as a strip or pexy can be placed if there is eyelid laxity or risk of lid laxity detected during the pre-operative examination.

In contrast, the transconjunctival approach is thought to have a reduced risk of complications such as round eye or ectropion because the middle lamella is not disturbed [22]. It can also be less time-consuming, not requiring closure. However, the approach can be challenging with a tight eyelid, requiring surgery through a small opening [23]. This procedure is often appropriate for young patients with tight skin who do not require any skin excision. The procedure is performed by placing a Desmarres retractor in the lower eyelid, then the conjunctiva is incised half way between the tarsal border and the fornix. The capsulo-palpebral fascia is opened and the fat exposed. The conjunctival incision is extended to almost the total length of the eyelid, medial to lateral. Alternatively, two incisions can be performed leaving a small central bridge that covers the inferior rectus muscle and avoids a rare complication when retractors fail to reattach spontaneously. The herniated fat is resected: a gentle pushing on the globe simulates gravity and can help in calculating the amount of fat to be removed. Alternatively, instead of resecting, the fat can be redistributed and draped to fill the tear trough deformity.

Occasionally a transconjunctival blepharoplasty can be combined with a skin pinch technique to trim excess skin [24]. Though requiring two separate incisions, the advantage is that the middle lamella is untouched. The skin is pinched with forceps or hemostat in order to determine the amount that could be resected without risk of

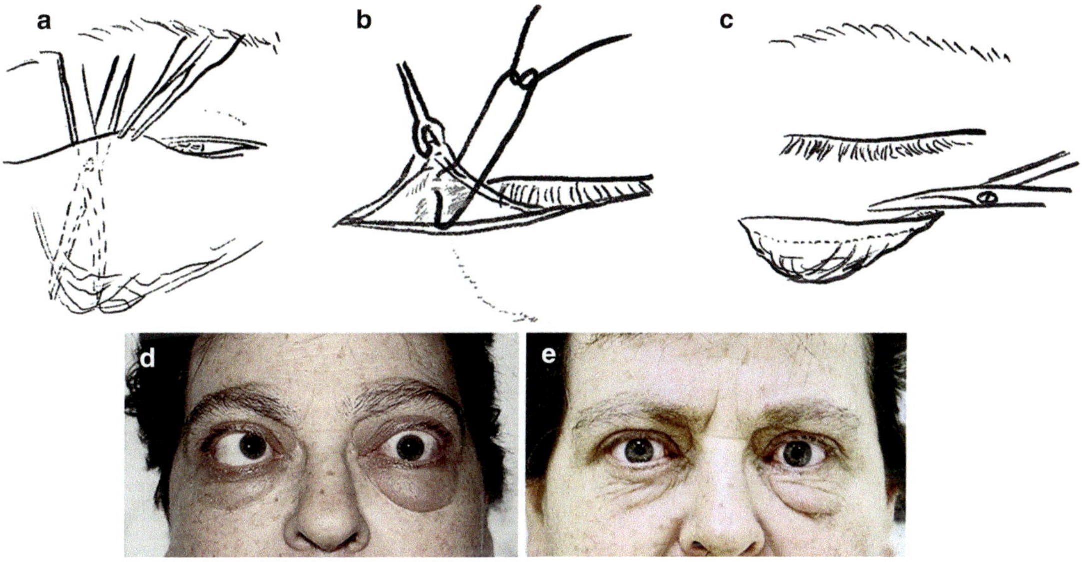

Fig. 4 Management of festoons. It is important to undermine skin generously (**a**) and then support the remaining tissue after skin excision with a periosteal anchor for the orbicularis (**b**) A direct skin excision of a festoon may be required (**c**) when there is inadequate lymphatic drainage, although this can leave a visible scar in the tear trough area. Following orbital decompression (**d**) there is usually a reduction of lower lid oedema but festoons may persist (**e**)

eyelid malposition [25]. Skin excision should be performed in a linear shape, not parallel to the inferior eyelid border at 5 mm from it [26]. Some surgeons prefer to follow the skin tension lines, where the skin fold forms. As the pinch does not incise the orbicularis muscle, the scar is usually not visible.

Alternatively chemical or laser skin resurfacing can be used together with a transconjunctival blepharoplasty in order to treat skin excess.

An alternative to the skin pinch is a mixed transcutaneous and transconjunctival approach. This is a transconjunctival blepharoplasty for the medial and central fat pad, associated with temporal skin-muscle flap and lateral fat pad excision. The creation of a skin-muscle flap in the lateral one third of the lid allows one to reach the lateral fat pad more easily and to stretch up and laterally the flap, removing part of it to correct skin excess.

Malar festoons form due inflammatory exudate or insufficient lymphatic drainage near the orbital rim and are usually due to excess skin and a weak low hanging orbicularis muscle. Extending the undermining of a skin-muscular flap beyond the inferior orbital rim (Fig. 4a) and re-draping the flap and anchoring the orbicularis muscle to the periosteum of the orbital rim (Fig. 4b), may minimise their appearance. If festoons originate from lymphedema, as in stabilised sequelae of TAO, direct resection may be required to correct this deformity (Fig. 4c). Though a scar is less disfiguring than a festoon, informed consent must be sought as some patients may otherwise be disappointed with the post-operative result. The dysthyroid patient shown in Fig. 4d showed a persistent left chronic malar festoon one year after orbital decompression and squint surgery (Fig. 4e), unlikely to resolve without an additional lower lid procedure.

2.3.2 Orbital Decompression

Orbital wall decompression has been reviewed at length (see chapter "Orbital Decompression Surgery") [27]. Decompression is performed in the acute setting for sight preservation [28] or in the quiescent phase as part of aesthetic rehabilitation where it can reduce proptosis and improve the appearance of the lids [29]. Though commonly performed, the risks of this surgery can be significant, including diplopia [5] and vision loss as well as pain or loss of sensation, particularly in the distribution of the infraorbital nerve. Adopting piezoelectric technology instead of mechanical drilling has been shown to be able to reduce this risk [30]. Decompression, performed as part of rehabilitative aesthetic care can also reactivate TAO [31]. Patients can also remain disappointed with the surgical results [32] and for this reason many clinicians may prefer to avoid decompression unless the proptosis is very noticeable. Though rare, orbital bones have been reported to regrow after decompression, resulting in recurrence of proptosis and need for repeat decompression [33].

2.3.3 Strabismus Surgery

Quality of life studies have shown that TAO patients greatly benefit from rehabilitative strabismus surgery [34]. However post TAO, extraocular muscles can remain scarred, stiff and enlarged. This makes the clinical result of surgery more difficult to predict. Rather than regular recessions, TAO strabismus surgery can require the use of spacer material such as donor sclera [35] or bovine pericardium [36]. A TAO clinic will therefore benefit from engaging with strabismus surgeon colleagues who have an interest in rehabilitative surgery following orbital inflammatory disease (see chapter "Strabismus in Thyroid-associated Orbitopathy").

2.4 Medical Interventions

2.4.1 IGF1 Receptor Blockade

Recently the FDA approved the first drug specifically aimed at treating TAO—the monoclonal antibody teprotumumab targeting the IGF1 receptor [37]. The clinical trials showed that this novel drug could achieve a marked reduction in proptosis: 82.9% of 41 teprotumumab-treated patients achieved a 2 mm or more reduction of proptosis compared with 9.5% of 42 placebo patients ($P < .001$) with few side-effects [38]. This was a remarkable medical orbital decompression. This medication therefore, in addition to being the first specific treatment aimed at TAO, also addresses the concerns important to patients with TAO. This has helped to shift the clinical goal posts in TAO to achieve an early cosmetic rehabilitation and one hopes increasingly without the need for decompression surgery. Proptosis very obviously affects the aesthetic appearance of patients. It is less evident that it can be used as a marker of diplopia or compromised vision—features which affect physical function. Though subsequent studies of teprotumumab have demonstrated some improvement in diplopia, the focus on a primarily aesthetic outcome rather than a functional one (ability to drive, squares of binocular single vision etc.) may complicate matters. As teprotumumab is also priced highly, it will undoubtedly lead to interesting debates in public payer health care systems where cost-benefit analyses are required prior to widespread adoption. Generic drugs targeting the same IGF1 receptor pathway further downstream may offer a cost-effective means by which to achieve the same aesthetic rehabilitation [39].

2.4.2 Immune Suppression

Standard medical immunosuppression can reduce the redness, swelling and proptosis seen in TAO and thereby offer some aesthetic improvement. Such drugs include steroids as well as steroid sparing agents such as cyclosporine, sirolimus, azathioprine etc. Treatment with steroids for aesthetic improvement must be weighed against the cushingoid facial features which patients may find distressing as well. It is important for oculoplastic surgeons caring for TAO patients to work as part of a team of clinicians so that all therapeutic avenues for improving facial aesthetic appearances are available—not just the surgical ones the oculoplastic surgeon is traditionally most well-placed to provide.

2.4.3 Prostaglandin Analogues

Prostaglandin analogues used in glaucoma, such as bimatoprost, were observed over a decade ago to cause periocular fat atrophy [40]. This has since also been confirmed in vitro: bimatoprost inhibits adipogenesis [41]. It was hoped therefore that treatment with bimatoprost might reduce the disfiguring fat expansion seen in TAO. Unfortunately, a recent randomised controlled trial failed to demonstrate efficacy [42]. This may have been because these drops fail to penetrate deep into the orbit where the adipocytes expand and that a small amount of anterior fat atrophy would have little observable effect on proptosis caused by deeper orbital fat compartment expansion. It is hoped that delivery to the affected fat compartment in a safe way may lead to a role for this medication for TAO.

2.4.4 Mental Health Interventions

Increasingly, clinicians have recognized the significant mental health burden caused by TAO. This has led to the development of quality of life scores which include psychometric assessments [43] and show good discriminant validity for severity in different cultures [44–46]. These batteries have confirmed that more than two thirds of TAO patients suffer some form of depression [4], and this may account for the increased mortality seen with TAO. The clinical team caring for patients with TAO should include input from psychologists [4] who can monitor the effects of aesthetic interventions on the well-being of TAO patients.

3 On the Timing of Aesthetic Interventions

The advent of fillers, neurotoxins and effective medical decompression in addition to improvements in surgical approaches provides the oculoplastic surgeon with an array of tools to provide aesthetic rehabilitation to TAO patients. But when should this be? Timing is very important in the management of this disease as traumatic interventions can rarely reactivate or exacerbate disease.

The non-surgical approaches outlined above, using neurotoxin and filler and triamcinolone, are thought to be far less likely to activate the disease and have been used to great effect even in the early active phase when traditionally interventions were precluded due to the risk of disease exacerbation.

Improved understanding of disease pathogenesis and clinical trials have also recently begun to upend the three-decade paradigm of sequential oculoplastic surgical rehabilitation for TAO, starting with decompression, followed by strabismus, lid positioning and then fat debulking. Recent studies demonstrated that orbital decompression combined with other surgical procedures, including aesthetic eyelid surgery in the same session, is safe and associated with high patient satisfaction [47, 48].

Earlier interventions targeting the aesthetic aspects of TAO with tools not shown to exacerbate disease can reduce the psychosocial burden of TAO [49]. Modern TAO care must be holistic and focus on prevention, mitigation and early aesthetic intervention to reduce the morbidity and mortality associated with this disfiguring autoimmune condition.

References

1. Sabini E, Leo M, Mazzi B, Rocchi R, Latrofa F, Nardi M, Vitti P, Marcocci C, Marinò M. Does Graves' orbitopathy ever disappear? Answers to an old question. Eur Thyroid J. 2017;6:263–70. (**This study shows how few patients with TED consider themselves cured)
2. Ferløv-Schwensen C, Brix TH, Hegedüs L. Death by suicide in Graves' disease and Graves' orbitopathy: A Nationwide Danish Register Study. Thyroid. 2017;27:1475–80. (** This study establishes TED as conferring a threat to life.)
3. Liao D, Ishii M, Darrach HM, Bater KL, Smith J, Joseph AW, Douglas RS, Joseph SS, Ishii LE. Objectively measuring observer attention in severe thyroid-associated orbitopathy: A 3D study. Laryngoscope. 2019;129:1250–4.

4. Charążka B, Suligowska A, Komorowski J, Siejka A. Quality of life in patients with orbitopathy—single center experience. Pol Merkur Lekarski. 2018;44:272–5.
5. Roos JCP, Murthy R. Comment on: A British Ophthalmic Surveillance Unit (BOSU) study into dysthyroid optic neuropathy in the United Kingdom. Eye (Lond). 2019;33:327–42.
6. Roos JCP, Paulpandian V, Murthy R. Serial TSH-receptor antibody levels to guide the management of thyroid eye disease: The impact of smoking, immunosuppression, radio-iodine, and thyroidectomy. Eye (Lond). 2019;33:212–7.
7. Erdoğan MF, Demir Ö, Ersoy RÜ, Gül K, Aydoğan Bİ, Üç ZA, Mete T, Ertek S, Ünlütürk U, Çakır B, Aral Y, Güler S, Güllü S, Çorapçıoğlu D, Dağdelen S, Erdoğan G. Comparison of early total thyroidectomy with antithyroid treatment in patients with moderate-severe Graves' orbitopathy: A randomized prospective trial. Eur Thyroid J. 2016;5:106–11.
8. Bhargav PRK, Sabaretnam M, Kumar SC, Zwalitha S, Devi NV. Regression of ophthalmopathic exophthalmos in Graves' disease after total thyroidectomy: A prospective study of a surgical series. Indian J Surg. 2017;79:521–6.
9. Stein JD, Childers D, Gupta S, et al. Risk factors for developing thyroid-associated ophthalmopathy among individuals with Graves disease. JAMA Ophthalmol. 2015;133:290–6.
10. Chang HS, Lee D, Taban M, Douglas RS, Goldberg RA. "En-glove" lysis of lower eyelid retractors with AlloDerm and dermis-fat grafts in lower eyelid retraction surgery. Ophthalmic Plast Reconstr Surg. 2011;27:137–41.
11. Grisolia ABD, Couso RC, Matayoshi S, et al. Non-surgical treatment for eyelid retraction in thyroid eye disease (TED). Br J Ophthalmol. 2018;102:158–63.
12. Young SM, Kim YD, Lang SS, Woo KI. Transconjunctival triamcinolone injection for upper lid retraction in thyroid eye disease-a new injection method. Ophthalmic Plast Reconstr Surg. 2018;34:587–93.
13. Bartalena L, Baldeschi L, Dickinson A, et al. Consensus statement of the European Group on Graves' orbitopathy (EUGOGO) on management of Graves' orbitopathy. Eur J Endocrinol. 2008;158:273–85.
14. Lee NG, Habib L, Hall J, Freitag SK. Simultaneous ipsilateral transconjunctival repair of upper and lower eyelid retraction in thyroid-associated ophthalmopathy. Orbit. 2019;38:124–9.
15. Kuzmanović Elabjer B, Miletić D, Bušić M, Biščan Tvrdi A, Bosnar D, Bjeloš M. Dermis-fat graft for correction of recurrent severe upper eyelid retraction in Graves' orbitopathy. Acta Clin Croat. 2018;57:173–6.
16. Saonanon P, Potita P. Contralateral Muller's muscle-conjunctiva resection: A therapeutic option in thyroid eye disease patients with unilateral eyelid retraction. Orbit. 2020;39:98–101.
17. Bosniak S. Upper lids: Anatomy and surgical techniques. In: Bosniak S, editor. Cosmetic blepharoplasty. Raven Press: New York; 1990. p. 37–58.
18. Carroll R, Manhanti R. En bloc resection in upper eyelid blepharoplasty. Ophthalmic Plast Reconstr Surg. 1992;8:47–9.
19. May J, Fears J, Zingarelli P. Retro-orbicularis oculus fat (ROOF) resection in aesthetic blepharoplasty: A 6-years study in 63 patients. Plast Reconstr Surg. 1990;86:682–9.
20. Bosniak S. Lower lids: Anatomy and surgical techniques. In: Bosniak S, editor. Cosmetic blepharoplasty. Raven Press: New York; 1990. p. 59–80.
21. Bourguet. Les hernies graisseuses de l'ôrbite: Notre traitement chirurgical. Bull Acad Natl Med. 1924;92:1270.
22. Baylis HI, Long JA, Groth MJ. Transconjunctival lower eyelid blepharoplasty. Technique and complications. Ophthalmology. 1989;96:1027–32.
23. Schwarz F, Randall P. Conjunctival incision for herniated orbital fat. Ophthalmic Surg. 1980;11:276.
24. Parkes ML, Bassiloios JI. Experience with the pinch technique in blepharoplasty. Laryngoscope. 1976;88:364–6.
25. Rosenfield LK. The pinch blepharoplasty revisited. Plast Reconstr Surg. 2005;115:1405–12.
26. Kim EM, et al. Power of the pinch: Pinch lower lid blepharoplasty. Ann Plast Surg. 2008;60:532–7.
27. Tooley AA, Godfrey KJ, Kazim M. Evolution of thyroid eye disease decompression-dysthyroid optic neuropathy. Eye (Lond). 2019;33:206–11. (*Excellent review of surgical decompression since its inception)
28. Liang QW, Yang H, Luo W, He JF, Du Y. Effect of orbital decompression on dysthyroid optic neuropathy: A retrospective case series. Medicine (Baltimore). 2019;98:e14162.
29. Park HH, Chun YS, Moon NJ, Kim JT, Park SJ, Lee JK. Change in eyelid parameters after orbital decompression in thyroid-associated orbitopathy. Eye (Lond). 2018;32:1036–41.
30. Naik MN, Nema A, Ali MH, Ali MJ. Piezoelectric surgery versus mechanical drilling for orbital floor decompression: Effect on infraorbital hypoaesthesia. Orbit. 2019;38:184–6.
31. Baldeschi L, Lupetti A, Vu P, Wakelkamp IM, Prummel MF, Wiersinga WM. Reactivation of Graves' orbitopathy after rehabilitative orbital decompression. Ophthalmology. 2007;114:1395–402.
32. Wickwar S, McBain H, Edmunds MR, Ezra DG, Rose GE, Newman SP. Patients' expectations for the functional and psychosocial outcomes of orbital decompression surgery for thyroid eye disease: A qualitative study. Psychol Health Med. 2018;23:475–84.
33. Ramesh S, Eichhorn K, Leibowitz S, Goldberg R. Bony regrowth after deep lateral orbital decompression. Ophthalmic Plast Reconstr Surg. 2018;34:533–5.
34. Schaut A, Cloché V, Mouna A, Angioi K, Berrod JP, Conart JB, Maalouf T. Évaluation par questionnaires

de l'amélioration de la qualité de vie des patients opérés de strabisme dans le cadre d'une maladie de Basedow. [Evaluation by quality of life questionnaires in patients undergoing strabismus surgery in Graves' disease]. J Fr Ophtalmol. 2018;41:814–22.

35. Thorisdottir RL, Blohmé J, Malmsjö M. Clinical evidence supporting the use of donor sclera as spacer material in complicated cases of strabismus surgery—retrospective evaluation of surgical results in 117 patients with thyroid-associated ophthalmopathy or congenital strabismus. Acta Ophthalmol. 2019;97:74–9.
36. Oeverhaus M, Fischer M, Hirche H, Schlüter A, Esser J, Eckstein AK. Tendon elongation with bovine pericardium in patients with severe esotropia after decompression in Graves' orbitopathy-efficacy and long-term stability. Strabismus. 2018;26:62–70.
37. Smith TJ, Kahaly GJ, Ezra DG, Fleming JC, Dailey RA, Tang RA, Harris GJ, Antonelli A, Salvi M, Goldberg RA, Gigantelli JW, Couch SM, Shriver EM, Hayek BR, Hink EM, Woodward RM, Gabriel K, Magni G, Douglas RS. Teprotumumab for thyroid-associated ophthalmopathy. N Engl J Med. 2017;376:1748–61. (**The most important therapeutic paper for TED in decades. Firmly establishes the role of the IGF1R as having a pathogenic role in TED)
38. Healio Ocular surgery News. Teprotumumab for treatment of thyroid eye disease meets endpoints in phase 3 study 1st March 2019. https://www.healio.com/ophthalmology/oculoplastics/news/online/%7B1a9105ba-7faf-449f-8969-478d876b07fe%7D/teprotumumab-for-treatment-of-thyroid-eye-disease-meets-endpoints-in-phase-3-study (Accessed 24 June 2019).
39. Roos JCP, Eglitis V, Murthy R. Inhibition of fibrotic contraction by sirolimus (rapamycin) in an ex vivo model of thyroid eye disease. Ophthalmic Plast Reconstr Surg. 2021;37:366–71.
40. Ipswich Star. Surgeon spots drug effect. 4 June 2009. https://www.ipswichstar.co.uk/news/surgeon-spots-drug-effect-1-172823. Accessed 23 June 2019.
41. Choi CJ, Tao W, Doddapaneni R, Acosta-Torres Z, Blessing NW, Lee BW, Pelaez D, Wester ST. The effect of prostaglandin analogue bimatoprost on thyroid-associated orbitopathy. Invest Ophthalmol Vis Sci. 2018;59:5912–23.
42. Draman MS, Morris DS, Evans S, Haridas A, Pell J, Greenwood R, Foy C, Taylor P, Pooprasert P, Muller I, Zhang L, Lane C, Okosieme O, Ludgate M, Dayan C. Prostaglandin F2-alpha eye drops (Bimatoprost) in Graves' orbitopathy: A randomized controlled double-masked crossover trial (BIMA Trial). Thyroid. 2019;29:563–72.
43. Wong MHY, Fenwick E, Aw AT, Lamoureux EL, Seah LL. Development and validation of the Singapore Thyroid Eye Disease Quality of Life Questionnaire. Transl Vis Sci Technol. 2018;7:14. (*An excellent example of the need to establish a patient's emotional well being).
44. Villagelin D, Romaldini J, Andrade J, Santos R, Milkos A, Teixeira PFDS, Ward LS. Evaluation of quality of life in the Brazilian Graves' disease population: Focus on mild and moderate Graves' orbitopathy patients. Front Endocrinol (Lausanne). 2019;10:192.
45. Zeng P, Fan SX, Li ZJ, Peng YY, Hu YX, Xu MT, Wang M. Evaluation of the Graves' Orbitopathy-Specific Quality of Life Questionnaire in the Mainland Chinese population. J Ophthalmol. 2019;2019:7602419.
46. Dietrich A, Taylor P, White P, Wilson V, Uddin J, Lee RWJ, Dayan C, Jackson S, CIRTED investigators. Establishing the usefulness of the GO-QOL in a UK hospital-treated population with thyroid eye disease in the CIRTED trial. Psychol Health Med. 2018;23:1341–55.
47. Bernardini FP, Skippen B, Zambelli A, Riesco B, Devoto MH. Simultaneous aesthetic eyelid surgery and orbital decompression for rehabilitation of thyroid eye disease: The One-Stage Approach. Aesthet Surg J. 2018;38:1052–61.
48. Quaranta-Leoni FM, Di Marino M, Leonardi A, Verrilli S, Romeo R. Single-stage orbital decompression, strabismus and eyelid surgery in moderate to severe thyroid associated orbitopathy. Orbit. 2022;41:184–92.
49. Douglas RS. Commentary on: Simultaneous aesthetic eyelid surgery and orbital decompression for rehabilitation of thyroid eye disease: The One-Stage Approach. Aesthet Surg J. 2018;38:1062–4.

Novel Immunomodulatory Treatment Modalities for Thyroid-Associated Orbitopathy

Diego Strianese, Dion Paridaens, Marco Sales-Sanz, and Santiago Ortiz-Pérez

Key Messages

- Intravenous glucocorticoids (IVGCs) are still considered the first-line treatment for active thyroid-associated orbitopathy (TAO).
- Combined with GCs, orbital radiotherapy is considered in patients with ocular motility disruption/diplopia or CON. ORT alone can be considered in patients who are steroid-resistant or intolerant.
- Cyclosporin, methotrexate, MMF, RTX, and Tocilizumab are considered second-line treatment options. Tocilizumab can be used as first choice treatment in patients who are steroid-resistant or intolerant.
- Teprotumumab is the only FDA approved drug for the treatment of TAO, but is currently not available in Europe

1 Introduction

Thyroid-associated orbitopathy (TAO), also known as thyroid eye disease and Graves' orbitopathy, is an autoimmune disease secondary to circulating auto-antibodies that activate receptors, namely Thyroid-Stimulating Hormone Receptors (TSHR) and Insulin-like Growth Factor-1 Receptors (IGF1-R), which are naturally expressed on orbital fibroblasts [1, 2]. The activation of these receptors is mostly systematically associated with Graves' hyperthyroidism with approximately 50% of these patients reporting symptoms of ophthalmopathy, but it can be rarely associated with autoimmune hypothyroidism or even euthyroidism [3]. TAO commonly affects women in their third to fifth decade, six times more than men [4]. Its hallmark is inflammation and enlargement of orbital muscles and orbital adipose tissue resulting in periorbital oedema, eyelid retraction, proptosis, chemosis, restrictive strabismus and diplopia. Three different phenotypes could be also identified based on the prevalence of the retroorbital tissue involved:

D. Strianese (✉)
Orbital Unit, University of Naples Federico II, Naples, Italy
e-mail: strianes@unina.it

D. Paridaens
Department of Oculoplastic, Orbital and Lacrimal Surgery, The Rotterdam Eye Hospital and Erasmus Medical Center, Rotterdam, the Netherlands

M. Sales-Sanz
Oculoplastic Surgery Unit, Ophthalmology Department, Hospital Universitario Ramón y Cajal, Madrid, Spain

Oculoplastic Surgery Unit, IMO Madrid, Grupo Miranza, Madrid, Spain

S. Ortiz-Pérez
Department of Ophthalmology, Hospital Universitario Virgen de las Nieves, Granada, Spain

Department of Surgery, University of Granada - Instituto de Investigación Biosanitaria ibs. GRANADA, Granada, Spain

F. M. Quaranta Leoni et al. (eds.), *Oculoplastic, Lacrimal and Orbital Surgery*,
https://doi.org/10.1007/978-3-031-39638-0_40

extraocular muscle predominance, fat predominance, mixture. Secondary vision-threatening complications include exposure keratopathy, corneal ulceration, and compressive optic neuropathy (CON). Clinically, TAO is typically divided into two phases "active/progressive" and "inactive/stable/fibrotic". The active phase of the disease lasts averagely between 6 months to 2 years [5]; however such dogmatic distinction has quite a number of exceptions. There are several ways to quantify TAO inflammation activity; the two most used assessment grading are Clinical Activity Score (CAS) and VISA parameters of I—inflammation [6]. The latter have also been validated. Both systems are based on clinical observation of certain clinical parameters which ultimately provide a quantitative numeric scoring useful for treatment decision making and evaluation of the outcome [7, 8]. TAO severity is classified into mild, moderate-to-severe, and vision-threatening based on the impairment of the visual function, appearance modification and impact of the disease on quality of life (Qol). Progression of the disease is also a crucial parameter to consider particularly in ITEDS assessment.

There is a general consensus that in patients with active moderate-to-severe TAO, systemic immunosuppressive therapy is indicated to suppress the immunological cascade, thereby preventing disease progression, preserving vision and improving Qol and [9]. Various Immunomodulatory agents have been used including glucocorticoids (GCs), antimetabolites, biologics (T-cell and B-cell inhibitors) and cytokine specific inhibitors [10]. To-date, there are no established guidelines on the use of the immunomodulatory agents in the treatment of TAO. New advances in TAO treatment are constantly emerging and the choice of immunomodulatory agents remains challenging, particularly for the frequency of disease recurrence, steroid resistance or dependence and fibrotic sequela [11] with the additional issue of the cost for some of those. In addition, concomitant morbidity such as diabetes or limited access to regular follow-up and cures as it was in the recent time because of the COVID-19 pandemic, may render management of TAO patients particularly harsh [12, 13].

In this chapter the most relevant up-to-date evidence on the medical and radiation treatment of moderate-to-severe TAO is presented with special concentration on clinically relevant issues. The effect of the currently available medications on the symptomatic improvement of TAO manifestations is explored in detail along with the side effects and complications. Apart from radiotherapy, categorization of the used local and systemic immunosuppressive agents will be based on the mechanism of action as following: anti-inflammatory agents (GCs), cytokine suppressors or inhibitors, cytostatic agents and monoclonal/polyclonal antibodies.

1.1 Systemic Glucocorticoids (GCs)

For more than 60 years, systemic GCs have been regarded as the mainstay of treatment of active moderate-to-severe TAO [14]. In 2016 and 2021, the published guidelines by the European Group on Graves' Orbitopathy (EUGOGO) recommended using high-dose intravenous glucocorticoids (IVGC) as the first line treatment for active moderate-to-severe TAO [15, 16]. The intravenous administration of glucocorticoids has been shown to be more effective than the oral route, and this might be attributed to higher blood concentrations that are attained faster. A recent systematic review, which included six clinical trials comparing the use of oral glucocorticoids (OGC) to IVGC in TAO, showed that the response rate was statistically more significant in the IVGC group (RR = 1.49, 95%CI: 1.25 ~ 1.77, $P < 0.00001$) [17]. In the current literature, IVGC achieved a higher response rate of 70–80% compared to only 50% in patients receiving OGC [15, 18–20]. The improvement in the CAS was also more pronounceable in the IVGC group [17]. Moreover, IVCG are better tolerated by patients with fewer adverse effects compared to OGC [15, 17, 21, 22]. Not all patients respond adequately to GCs as TAO flare-ups occurred in around 12–20% of patients after GCs cessation and 7.5%

progressed to the severe form manifesting CON [19, 23, 24].

Several doses and protocols regimen for IVGC administration have been reported; however, the most popular one for moderate-to-severe TAO includes a dose of 500 mg of intravenous methylprednisolone administered once weekly for six weeks and then tapered to 250 mg once weekly for another six weeks (cumulative dose of 4.5 g). Patients with more severe TAO may require a starting dose of 750 mg once weekly for 6 weeks and then 500 mg once weekly for another 6 weeks (cumulative dose of 7.8 g) [16]. A cumulative dose of 8 g should not be exceeded because such high doses may result in hepatic failure due to exacerbation of an underlying liver disease in addition to the possible cerebrovascular and cardiovascular morbidity [15]. Response to GCs treatment should be expected within 1–2 weeks [22].

When used early in the course of active disease, GCs may alter the natural history of TAO by switching off the immune cascade resulting in functional and aesthetic improvements which might reflect subsequently on patients' Qol [25].

GCs are well-known to alleviate the inflammatory signs of TAO such as eyelid and conjunctival swelling and redness as well as ocular motility dysfunction/diplopia. In terms of proptosis reduction, GCs showed conflicting results where several studies reported improvement ranging between 1–1.5 mm whereas a systematic review showed that neither OGCs nor IVGCs was a significant effect observed on proptosis [17, 25]. Lastly, GCs improved CON in more than two-thirds (77%) of TAO patients in clinical trials [25].

The adverse events of steroids are widely reported and documented in the medical literature. In one review of 1045 TAO patients treated with IVGCs, the cumulative morbidity was 6.5% while mortality reached 0.6%. Death occurred mainly in patients receiving high doses of IVGCs continuously for several days. Liver damage and even hepatic failure were reported previously with the use of high cumulative doses of GCs [25]. Hence, it is essential to screen patients for viral hepatitis and liver disease (liver ultrasound and liver function test) before commencing treatment. Fasting blood sugar and blood pressure should be evaluated before and during treatment routinely. Patients should be started on prophylactic proton pump inhibitors and calcium supplementation especially patients at risk of osteoporosis. GCs are generally contraindicated in patients with recent viral hepatitis or liver disease, uncontrolled hypertension and diabetes, severe cardiovascular disease, and psychiatric disorders [15].

1.2 Local Glucocorticoids

Periocular injection of Triamcinolone acetonide (TA) has been used for the treatment of TAO at the dose of 20 mg in 40 mg/mL concentration via subconjunctival or Kyretro-septal injection every 2–4 weeks. Studies showed marked improvement in CAS and reduction in eyelid retraction by at least 1 mm in TAO patients [26–30]. Rapid improvement in CAS after the first injection was reported proving a direct relationship between local steroid injection and symptoms' improvement in non-comparative prospective studies [26–28]. In one retrospective study, eyelid retraction was reduced by a mean difference of 2.31 mm (range of 0–7 mm) after local TA treatment; yet, the degree and duration of eyelid retraction were inversely related to the degree of improvement [31]. In another retrospective case series, only 12/97 patients (12.4%) showed no significant improvement in eyelid retraction with subconjunctival TA monthly injections while some of those who improved showed no benefit in upper eyelid position beyond 4 months from treatment [32]. Remarkably, Young et al. showed that both active and inactive diseases benefit from transconjunctival TA [30]. This observed improvement can be explained by the anti-inflammatory effect of steroids, degenerative atrophic changes in Muller's and levator muscles, steroid-induced ptosis, atrophy of Muller's muscle, and thinning or detachment of levator muscle [30, 32]. On the contrary, Lee et al. found that patients in the fibrotic phase showed no response to subconjunctival TA [33].

Improvement in EOM, specifically supraduction, was noted with periocular steroids; however, it did not prevent the need for future strabismus surgery [27, 28]. Muscle thickness reduction was assessed by ultrasound, computed tomography (CT) and magnetic resonance imaging (MRI) showing reduction in thickness of the recti muscles as well as the levator/superior rectus complex [26, 31, 32, 34].

One of the major advantages of local compared to systemic steroids is fewer side effects systemically. A prospective randomised trial comparing the efficacy of oral prednisolone to peribulbar TA showed a comparable reduction in proptosis and CAS. The study advocated the use of peribulbar steroid injection as it documented more adverse occurrences with oral prednisolone such as an increase in body weight, blood sugar, blood pressure, and gastritis without any significant superiority in TAO outcome [35].

Periorbital steroid injections were associated with serious vision-threatening complications including corneoscleral melting, globe perforation, and embolization resulting in vascular occlusion [36]. Elevation of intraocular pressure (IOP) was the commonest reported side effect, usually after the first injection in 4 and 10% of retro-septal and subconjunctival routes respectively [26–37]. All reported cases with IOP elevation were managed by topical medications apart from two cases that underwent selective laser trabeculoplasty [32]. Less common complications included cataract in elderly patients, periorbital hematoma, eyelid ptosis, menstrual cycle disturbances, hirsutism, and calf muscle cramps [27, 28, 32, 33].

1.3 Delivery of Steroids Through Nanotechnology

A recent Dutch pilot study was the first to employ nanotechnology for intravenous delivery of steroids (prednisolone wrapped in nanoparticles (liposomes)) to reduce systemic exposure. Such nanoparticles accumulate in areas of inflammation, such as the affected orbit(s) in patients with TAO, through a mechanism referred to as extravasation. The particles are smaller than blood cells and will migrate through the blood vessels in inflamed areas as these vessels have enlarged interstitial spaces. The authors showed a positive effect of long-circulating PEGylated liposomal prednisolone on the Clinical Activity Score in patients with moderate-to-severe TAO, resulting in fewer hospital visits and possibly fewer glucocorticoid-related side-effects. Further studies investigating the role of nano-medication (steroids or else) in TAO are needed [38].

1.4 Radiation Therapy

Orbital radiotherapy (ORT) has been in use for the treatment of TAO for many decades. It is usually administered on an outpatient basis where patients typically receive a total of 20 Gray (Gy) per orbit delivered in 10 fractions over 1–2 weeks to the retro-ocular tissues [15, 39, 40].

The effect of ORT is thought to result from the disruption of the DNA of orbital radio-sensitive proliferating cells provoked by ionising radiation. ORT may also limit the duration of TAO active phase which in turn curtails the duration of needed corticosteroid therapy and delays the need for rehabilitative surgery [41].

In the literature, numerous studies investigated the effect of ORT, alone or in combination with other agents, for the treatment of TAO. The current body of knowledge favours the use of ORT in patients with active moderate-to-severe TAO [40]. Two large studies comparing the effect of combined therapy (ORT with GCs) vs GCs alone demonstrated more reduction in the activity and severity of TAO with enhancement of ocular motility and reduction in EOM volume. The salient point to note from these studies is that patients receiving combined therapy in contrast to steroid monotherapy were considerably less likely to relapse or progress to CON [42, 43]. A meta-analysis reported the superiority of the concomitant regimen against ORT only in patients with moderate-to-severe TAO, especially during the first year of the disease [44]. In fact, a recent retrospective review of TAO patients presenting with clinical and radiological evidence of CON supported the use of combined therapy (2-week trial of steroids followed by adding ORT if there is response) as 94% (n = 98/104) of the cohort responded adequately and did not require urgent acute-phase orbital decompression, and ultimately, approximately one- third of these patients required rehabilitative surgeries during the fibrotic phase. A trend towards therapy failure was noticed in current or previous smokers and in patients with optic nerve stretching or absent apical crowdenning on imaging. The authors hypothesised that patients responding to steroids will likely respond to ORT, and the effect of ORT becomes evident as early as 4 weeks but the full effect may take up to 3 months [45]. Acute-phase orbital decompression is better reserved for patients with unresponsive CON or patients with stable disease for more predictable and enhanced cosmetic and functional results.

ORT is also an important treatment modality for patients who are steroid-resistant or patients with intractable diplopia [40]. A recent study looked at 40 patients with moderate-to-severe TAO resistant to steroids or patients suffering from severe diplopia. At 1 year after combined therapy, the CAS decreased in 70% of patients and EOM motility and diplopia improved in 42.5% and 32.5% respectively [46]. This further signifies the therapeutic role of combined therapy in patients with severe TAO or severe diplopia who are resistant to steroids or patients suffering from steroid-related morbidity. Generally, ORT is most efficient in improving ocular motility, soft tissue inflammation, and optic nerve compression with less effect on proptosis as inferred by the previous studies [42–46].

As far as safety is concerned, ORT carries a relatively very small risk of secondary malignancies in the irradiated field based on several studies with long-term follow-up [41]. Gillis et al. described a patient who presented with sphenoid wing meningioma 14 years after ORT, and the calculated risk of radiation-induced meningioma was 0.17% (n = 1/575). Three other patients in the same series developed hematologic malignancies which could be attributed to ORT and this increases the calculated risk up to 0.7% (n = 4/575) [47]. Ocular side effects including radiation retinopathy and accelerated cataract formation are theoretically possible as these ocular structures are radiosensitive with a high metabolic rate; nevertheless, these were rarely encountered [41]. One study demonstrated a possible association between radiation retinopathy and diabetes or uncontrolled hypertension [45, 48]. Another study suggested decreased risk of cataractogenesis when maintaining >0.5 cm space between the lens and anterior beam edge [49].

2 Cytokine Suppressors or Inhibitors

2.1 Cyclosporine

Cyclosporine is an immunomodulatory agent that inhibits the calcineurin pathway decreasing IL-2 cytokine secretion. It is usually administered at a starting dose of 5–7.5 mg/kg. The 2021 EUGOGO guideline advocated the use of cyclosporine plus oral OGCs in moderate-to-severe active orbitopathy that failed to respond to IVGCs alone [16]. The efficacy of this combination treatment proved to be superior to either medication alone with lower chances of disease recurrence [50, 51]. Cyclosporine combined with GCs resulted in improvement in inflammatory signs and symptoms, diplopia, and visual acuity. Proptosis improved by a mean of 3 mm with the aforementioned combination treatment [50, 52, 53]. Another advantage to the addition of cyclosporine is the reduction of muscle thickness that was objectively measured by CT scan [50–53]. It also resulted in complete resolution of TAO-associated CON in a series of eight patients [54]. Although the combination of cyclosporine and prednisolone proved superior to monotherapy, prednisolone was more effective than cyclosporine as a single therapy but with more adverse events in a single-blind randomised clinical trial (RCT) [51]. When cyclosporine was given alone, no marked improvement was noted in proptosis, visual acuity, EOM thickness, and patients' well-being [55, 56]. Relapse of TAO was also observed in some patients after medication discontinuation [50, 51]. Therefore, some experts argue that cyclosporine alone might not be a valid treatment option for TAO [56].

The commonest reported side effect of cyclosporine is a rise in creatinine levels in all patients. This is mostly reversible after discontinuation of treatment though irreversible nephropathy had been documented [50–52, 56]. Elevated liver enzymes and transient increase in androstenedione had also been reported [52, 56]. Hypertension is commonly reported with few patients requiring antihypertensive drugs; yet, blood pressure commonly normalises after medication cessation. Other less frequent side effects include hirsutism, behavioural change, weight gain and dose-dependent perioral, and distal paresthesia [51]. Seldom, predisposition to infection, i.e. Klebsiella pneumoniae was observed with cyclosporine administration [50].

2.2 Cytostatic Agents

2.2.1 Azathioprine

Azathioprine is a purine analog that disrupts the synthesis of nucleic acids (DNA and RNA) consequently reducing leukocytes' production. It is commonly administered at a dose of 100–200 mg daily for 45–48 weeks. When used in the treatment of TAO, there was no additional benefit of azathioprine in patients that had been treated with oral prednisolone. It showed no substantial improvement in CAS, exophthalmos, eyelid retraction, and visual acuity when compared to placebo [57, 58]. Only one retrospective study (n = 88) found that the addition of azathioprine aided in the reduction of steroid dose and facilitated its tapering. It documented improvement in CAS and diplopia; however, all these patients received radiotherapy so the efficacy of azathioprine in these parameters cannot be ascertained [59].

Azathioprine's adverse reactions include nausea, elevated liver enzymes, leukopenia, and mild infections [57, 58]. One case reported reactivation of Darier's disease, an inherited autosomal dominant dermatological condition resulting in multiple greasy papules, with the use of Azathioprine in TAO [60].

2.2.2 Methotrexate

Methotrexate inhibits the synthesis of DNA, RNA and protein by inhibiting dihydrofolate reductase enzyme resulting in immunosuppressive and anti-inflammatory properties [61]. It can be given orally or subcutaneously (SC) if not tolerated at a dose ranging between 7.5 and 25 mg/week along with folic acid supplements. It has been studied retrospectively as a second-line agent and as a steroid-sparing agent in the management of TAO. In severe active TAO refractory to GCs, improvement in VISA inflammatory scale to inactivity of TAO was established with methotrexate [62]. When the use of methotrexate plus methylprednisolone (n = 39) vs. methylprednisolone (n = 33) was compared in patients with CON, better visual improvement and VISA score were noted in the first 3 months with combined therapy; however, no difference was evident after 1 year when compared to methylprednisolone alone. Additionally, the dose of methylprednisolone was not successfully reduced when combined with methotrexate [63]. In a retrospective case series, which utilised methotrexate in 36 steroid intolerant patients, the CAS was markedly reduced in up to 94% of patients along with marked improvement in extraocular motility [64]. Methotrexate was also found to be an effective medication in all orbital inflammatory diseases including TAO. Patients had improvement in inflammatory signs and ocular motility and were able to taper or discontinue GCs intake; thus, reducing its associated side effects with improvement in overall Qol [65]. Methotrexate failed to improve TAO-associated proptosis and eyelid retraction [64].

Methotrexate was also used concomitantly with steroids for the treatment of TAO to reduce steroids' total dose. In 2018, a single-centre study from the UK assessed the feasibility of this first-line combination therapy where 23/24 patients with moderate-to-severe TAO received IVGCs plus methotrexate. It was noticed that most patients required a much lower GCs cumulative dose (mean of 2.72 g) to control their disease, and this suggests the efficacy of methotrexate. If this combination was not enough to suppress disease activity (observed in

42% of patients), other agents were further introduced including cyclosporine, azathioprine, and rituximab. A total of four patients eventually mandated orbital decompression surgery for CON which was not controlled medically. This study claimed benefit to its step-down approach; however, it should be interpreted cautiously because of its retrospective nature, limited sample size, absent control group and lack of elaboration on the improvement of clinical parameters [66]. Since methotrexate appears to have a favourable outcome in TAO treatment, it is worthwhile conducting clinical trials to validate its use as a steroid-sparing agent.

Elevated liver enzymes are frequently reported with the use of methotrexate; it is often transient, reversible and dose-dependent. Regular liver function tests and complete blood count are essential due to the potential hepatotoxicity and leukopenia. Fatigue and gastrointestinal disturbances are also common side effects. Gastrointestinal toxicity can be overcome by switching patients to the SC route. Arthralgia, cough, recurrent cystitis, headache, dry skin, and hair thinning were less frequently reported side effects [61–66].

2.2.3 Mycophenolate Mofetil (MMF)

MMF is another immunomodulatory agent that acts by depleting guanosine nucleotides from T and B cells resulting in inhibition of their proliferation. It is usually administered at a dose of 720 (mycophenolate sodium)—1000 (MMF) mg per day, divided into two doses, for 24 weeks. In a recent European multi-center trial (MINGO trial), IVGCs versus IVGCs plus MMF (360 mg twice daily) were assessed in the treatment of moderate-to-severe active TAO. The study showed no significant difference in the relapse rate between both groups at 12, 24 and 36 weeks and some patients from both groups progressed to CON with this occurring later in the combined therapy group. The combined therapy achieved an encouraging response rate at 24 and 36 weeks of follow-up, not to mention the noticeable improvement in inflammatory signs, CAS, and EOM (up-gaze and downgaze) but not proptosis [67].

In another RCT, patients with moderate-to-severe TAO that received MMF (1 g daily for 24 weeks) achieved better CAS reduction (reaching <3 in 93.8%), visual acuity, and proptosis improvement when compared to those that had received GCs. EOM motility was equally improved when given MMF or steroids [68]. In the aforementioned study, MMF was given at the dose of 360 mg twice daily, which might be a factor accounting for the discrepancy in results. A meta-analysis evaluating the efficacy of TAO treatments showed promising results with cyclosporine and MMF with good patient tolerance; however, such an outcome was not achieved with the combination of GCs and azathioprine. They concluded that IVGCs plus MMF provided better outcome than IVGCs plus cyclosporine but that was not superior to MMF monotherapy. In fact, IVGCs with MMF were ranked the second in efficacy after IVGCs plus ORT in the management of extraocular motility restriction.

Generally, the side effects of MMF are relatively mild, especially when compared with GCs and other immunomodulatory agents. These can range from the common gastrointestinal disturbances to mild hypokalemia, mild elevation in liver enzymes, and infections [68].

3 Mono- and Polyclonal Antibodies

3.1 Rituximab (RTX)

RTX is a chimeric mouse-human anti-CD20 monoclonal antibody that targets CD20 antigen on B lymphocytes resulting in inhibition of their proliferation and maturation producing 95% depletion of these cells [22, 69, 70] The use of RTX in the treatment of moderate-to-severe TAO was introduced around 15 years ago; thus, it is among the most studied biologic treatments for TAO [71–73].

Two double-masked RCTs studied the efficacy of RTX in TAO. The European trial compared RTX (n = 16) to IVGC (n = 16) in active moderate-to-severe TAO while the North American trial compared RTX (n = 13) to placebo (n = 12). The former trial showed a decline in disease activity with 100% response rate and no relapses at week 24 as well as less rehabilitative surgeries at 76 weeks of follow-up [74]. The later trial revealed no difference between both studied groups with respect to disease activity and clinical manifestations of the disease [75]. Both trials demonstrated no significant difference in proptosis at the end of the follow-up period. On the other hand, a recent RCT conducted by Li and associates in China aimed to evaluate the efficacy of combining RTX with radioiodine (^{131}I) therapy in patients with TAO and hyperthyroidism. The patients were assigned to receive either ^{131}I alone or ^{131}I in combination with IVGC or RTX. At 24 weeks post-therapy, patients in the RTX + ^{131}I group exhibited a statistically more significant reduction than the other groups in the following parameters: CAS, proptosis, palpebral fissure height, soft tissue inflammation, and fat/muscle volume appreciated on CT imaging. The Th1 and Th2 cytokines were almost normalised in these patients and this suggests that RTX might alter the natural course of the disease [76].

A recent systematic review, which included 11 studies (8 cohorts and 3 RCT, n = 167 patients) demonstrated that RTX was effective in reducing the CAS and this effect was maintained up to 12 months after the treatment. Moreover, a decrease in proptosis was shown at least one month after RTX and a decrease in thyroid receptor antibodies was evident at 6 and 12 months [69]. Another prospective randomised study compared the results of low-dose intraorbital RTX versus IVGC in patients with moderate-to-severe TAO. Interestingly, clinical improvement was evident in the RTX group at the first follow-up with depletion of peripheral lymphocytes. Only one patient (n = 1/10) in the RTX group advanced to severe TAO. The importance of this study lies in underscoring the therapeutic value of RTX in the treatment of active TAO [77]. Whether or not this route of administration carries less risk of adverse events and which patients are at risk of progression to CON are questions that remain unanswered until further studies become available.

The results of the above-cited studies are inconsistent, and this could be explained by the small sample size, variable patients' baseline characteristics, and different treatment regimens. However, these results emphasise the importance of appropriate patient selection and early treatment with RTX to achieve adequate immunosuppression.

Currently, the RTX dosage regimen for TAO is variable and centre dependent. In rheumatoid arthritis patients, 1000 mg of RTX is infused IV twice separated by 2 weeks. Some centres followed this protocol for TAO patients while others amended the second dose to 500 mg because complete peripheral B-cells depletion was achieved with much lower doses (100 mg) [74, 75]. Patients are usually pre-medicated prior to RTX with acetaminophen, antihistamine, and IV corticosteroids to prevent infusion reactions [74, 75].

Systemic adverse events associated with RTX are generally minor and reversible. The commonly reported adverse events were mild increase in temperature, nose and throat itching, headache, myalgia, and dyspepsia [69]. Regarding ocular side effects, orbital oedema, vision loss, and dysthyroid optic neuropathy (DON) were reported previously with RTX use [69, 70, 74, 75, 77]. It was proposed that patients developing ocular adverse events probably had subclinical DON which was further provoked by the immense release of cytokines (cytokine-release syndrome) after RTX infusion resulting in acute orbital oedema and consequent optic nerve compression [70]. However, firm conclusions are precluded since RTX was successful in treating six patients with DON while other reports demonstrated the failure of RTX in preventing or improving DON [77–79]. This confirms the role that other inflammatory pathways play in the pathogenesis of TAO unrelated to B-lymphocytes.

3.2 Tocilizumab

Tocilizumab, a recombinant humanised IgG1 monoclonal antibody, antagonises the Interleukin-6 (IL-6) receptor. It was initially approved by the Food and Drug Administration (FDA) for the treatment of rheumatoid arthritis, and since then it gained popularity and it is currently being used for the treatment of multiple systemic, ocular inflammatory, and autoimmune conditions such as juvenile idiopathic arthritis, giant cell arteritis, TAO and some uveitic entities [81, 82]. IL-6 appears to play a key role in the upregulation of the pathogenic process in TAO; therefore, blockage of its receptor will interrupt the inflammatory cascade [83]. Several small studies reported the promising results of IV or SC tocilizumab in the treatment of patients with steroid-intolerant or steroid-resistant TAO [83–85]. Nevertheless, there is only one double-masked RCT conducted at nine Spanish centres which demonstrated the efficacy of tocilizumab in the treatment of patients with moderate-to-severe TAO who did not respond adequately to the standard GCs therapy. The primary outcome, defined as an improvement in the CAS by at least 2 points at week 16 after receiving 4 infusions, was achieved by 93.3%, n = 14/15 patients in the tocilizumab group compared to 58.8%, n = 10/17 patients in the placebo group, $p = 0.04$. Significant improvement in proptosis in the treatment group was noted at week 16 (−1.5 mm vs 0 mm, $p = 0.01$), yet, this result was not sustained at week 40. The authors postulated that tocilizumab seems to be more effective in reducing soft tissue inflammation with less effect on proptosis, diplopia and eyelid aperture. In terms of tocilizumab safety, only two serious adverse events (moderate increase in transaminases at week 8 and acute pyelonephritis at week 32) were observed [24].

In another prospective interventional non-randomized study that included 18 patients who were resistant to corticosteroids, significant improvement in the CAS was seen in all 18 patients receiving tocilizumab with a follow-up period ranging from 9 to 27 months. Moreover, improvement in EOM motility and diplopia was noted in 83% and 54% of patients respectively whereas 72% demonstrated improvement in exophthalmos at a mean of -3.92 ± 1.54 mm, $p = 0.002$ [86]. A recent multicenter observational study including 48 steroid-resistant TAO patients treated with tocilizumab alone (n = 45) or in combination (n = 3) showed that 83.2% of eyes achieved a CAS ≤ 3 at a mean follow-up of 16 months [87].

When comparing the efficacy of tocilizumab to RTX in steroid-refractory TAO, a retrospective study showed that the primary outcome, ≥2 points reduction in baseline CAS, was achieved in 100% of patients receiving tocilizumab versus 64% of those on RTX (p = 0.17). An improvement in vision, proptosis and diplopia was noted in both groups. Relapse of disease was observed in 14% (1/7) of tocilizumab group vs 29% (4/14) of RTX group [88].

The optimum dose and route of administration of tocilizumab for the treatment of TAO are yet to be determined. The current dose and route of administration are actually based on the rheumatology literature and are as follows: IV infusion over 60 minutes of 8 mg/kg (not exceeding 800 mg) of tocilizumab every 4 weeks with a total of 4 infusions, or SC administration of a standardised single dose of 162 mg dose in 0.9 mL syringe biweekly for individuals <100 kg or weekly if >100 kg [85].

Adverse events associated with tocilizumab use include neutropenia, infections, costal osteitis, and gingival hyperplasia [87, 89]. In one study, 3 patients were diagnosed with breast ($n = 2$) and urothelial ($n = 1$) cancer one year after tocilizumab administration. Whether or not this is related to tocilizumab remains questionable given that TAO patients were observed to have a higher risk of certain malignancies. The authors proposed cancer surveillance in these patients, especially smokers, while on treatment [89].

Pre-treatment, it is essential to screen patients for latent tuberculosis in addition to laboratory evaluation including complete blood count, lipid panel, liver function test and hepatitis screening. Patients should be monitored routinely every 4–8 weeks during the treatment period for alterations in neutrophil count, platelets count, lipids, and hepatic transaminases as changes in these parameters were observed with tocilizumab [90]. The use of tocilizumab in pregnant ladies is better avoided as it may cross the placenta in the second and third trimester and the current evidence demonstrates its association with spontaneous miscarriage and preterm birth [91].

3.3 Anti-Tumor Necrosis Factor (Anti-TNF) Medications

Studies on TNF inhibitors in the treatment of TAO are scarce. Etanercept was the first ever used monoclonal antibody in 2005 by Paridaens et al. for the treatment of active TAO [92]. Etanercept, an anti-TNF agent given at a dose of 25 mg SC twice weekly for 12 weeks, was assessed in a small series of ten patients with active TAO where it showed a reduction of CAS, and two out of the six patients with diplopia improved on treatment [92]. In this study, no improvement in proptosis was noted. In contrast, a case report documented a minor 2 mm reduction in proptosis in a 37 years old lady with rheumatoid arthritis and TAO who received etanercept and methotrexate [93].

Infliximab is a chimeric anti-TNF-α medication that is partly mouse-derived and human-derived IgG1. It blocks the interaction of TNF-α with its receptor, eliminating cells expressing TNF-α [94]. Patients usually receive 3 mg/kg infusions every 8 weeks. Two TAO patients receiving infliximab showed rapid improvement in their inflammatory features (after one dose) and improvement in CAS [95, 96].

Adalimumab, a fully humanised anti-TNF-α antibody, is given at a single dose of 80 mg SC and then 40 mg biweekly. There was no reported improvement in proptosis and ocular motility in ten patients that received it. Although six patients had a reduction in their inflammatory score, there was no significant change after 3 months of Adalimumab treatment [97].

3.4 Teprotumumab

Teprotumumab is a new biologic drug that received the FDA approval in 2020 for the treatment of clinically active TAO. This drug is a fully human monoclonal antibody that blocks the IGF-1R, which plays an important role in the pathogenesis of TAO (Fig. 1). At the cellular

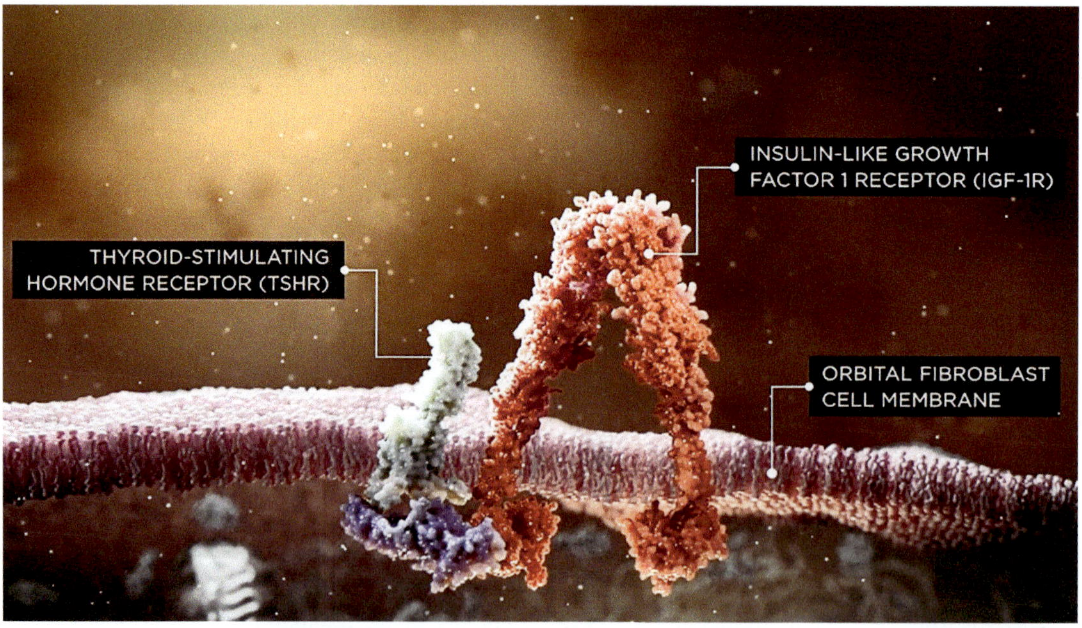

Fig. 1 Thyroid-stimulating hormone receptors (TSHR) and Insulin-like growth factor 1 receptors (IGF-1R) are co-localised on the cell membrane of orbital fibroblasts and form a signaling complex

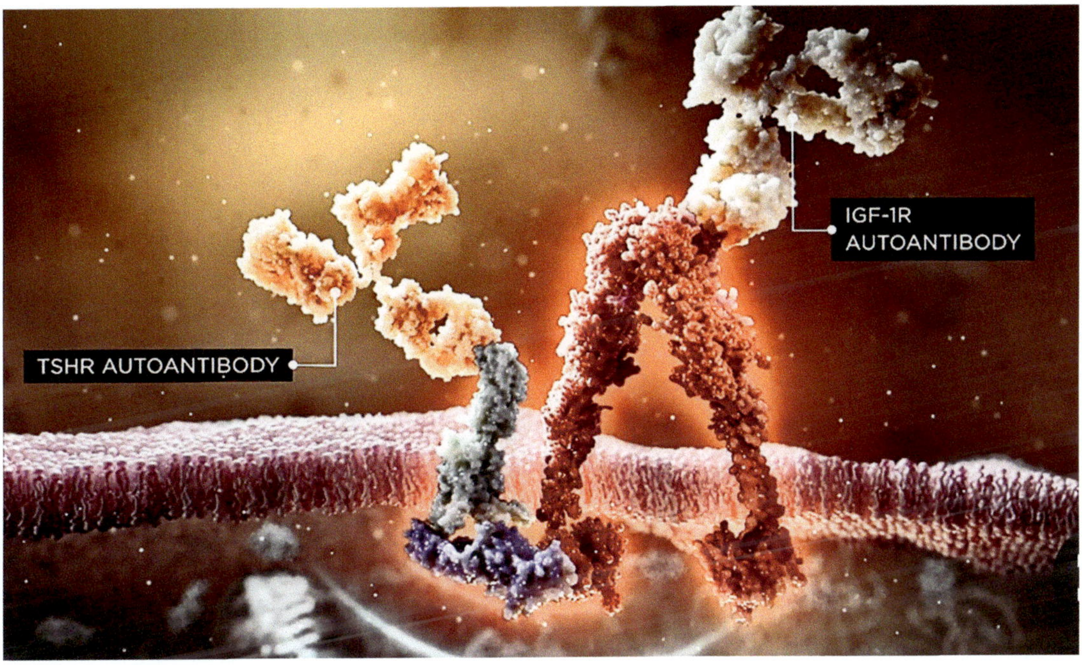

Fig. 2 Orbital fibroblasts overexpress IGF-1R. In thyroid-associated orbitopathy (TAO) this leads to severe inflammation and expansion of muscle and fat cells inside the orbit. Teprotumumab is an inhibitor of IGF-1R and turns off the signaling complex at the source of the disease

level, IGF-1R forms a complex with thyrotropin receptor to which the circulating TSHR antibodies bind resulting in the initiation of the inflammatory cascade (Fig. 2) [98, 99].

The FDA approval of this drug was based on phase 2 and 3 results of a randomised, double-masked, placebo-controlled clinical trial that was carried out in 13 different centres across Europe and the United States [100, 101]. These trials aimed to investigate the efficacy and safety of teprotumumab in patients with active moderate-to-severe TAO. The initial infusion dose of Teprotumumab was 10 mg/kg followed by 20 mg/kg for subsequent infusions once every 3 weeks for 21 weeks (a total of eight doses). The primary outcome at week 24 in the phase 3 trial was defined by the authors as a 2 mm or more reduction in proptosis without a corresponding increase of 2 mm or greater in the contralateral eye. Secondary end points included the overall response, CAS of 0 or 1, mean change in proptosis, diplopia response, and mean change in TAO-specific Qol. Patients in both groups had similar baseline characteristics. Remarkably, 83% (n = 34/41) of patients in the treatment group achieved a proptosis response occurring at a median of 6.4 weeks compared to only 10% (n = 4/42) in the placebo group. The mean reduction in proptosis was 3.32 mm at week 24. The proptosis response in the phase 2 trial was maintained for up to 48 weeks in the majority of patients receiving teprotumumab [101]. In addition, the key secondary endpoints were better in patients receiving teprotumumab versus placebo. Not only proptosis but also diplopia improved significantly at each follow-up visit and more than twice as many patients in the teprotumumab group had a diplopia response (68% vs 29%). Imaging in six patients demonstrated reduction in the volume of EOM and/or orbital fat volume (Fig. 3) [102]. The inferior rectus muscle, the most commonly affected muscle, demonstrated the greatest reduction in volume (n = 4/6 patients) [100]. Notably, none of the patients in the teprotumumab arm in both trials developed DON or visual field defects, and this further demonstrates the effectiveness of teprotumumab [100, 101].

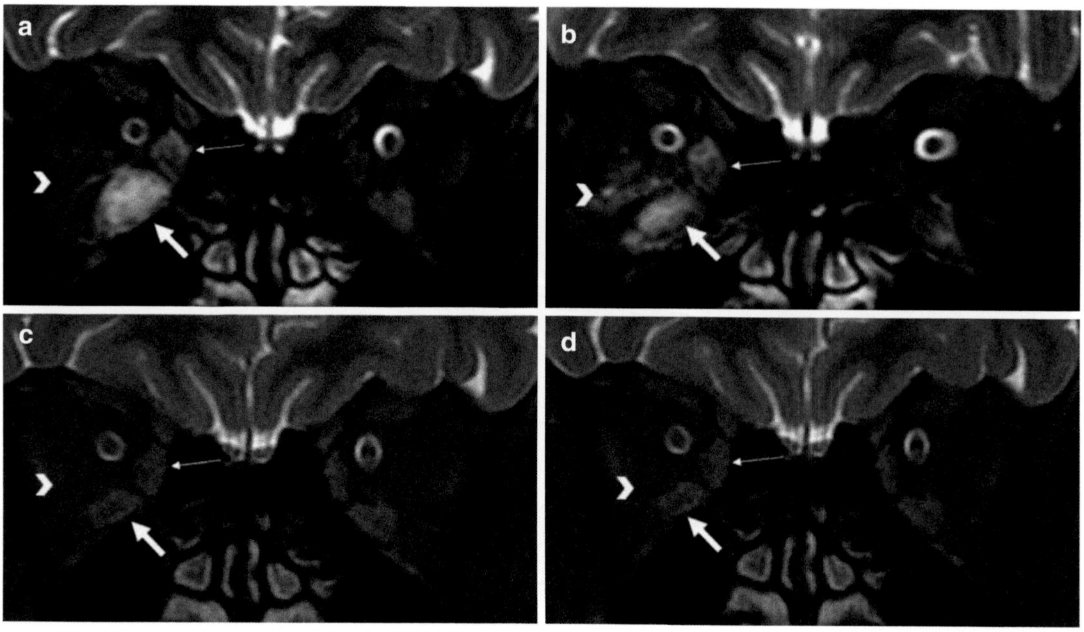

Fig. 3 MRI imaging of pre- and post-treatment EOM SIR. Sequential Coronal T2 fat saturation images. (**a**, **b**) Baseline images demonstrating enlargement and increased T2 signal (indicating inflammation) within the inferior rectus (*thick white arrow*), medial rectus (*thin white arrow*) and orbital fat (*arrowhead*). (**c**, **d**) After completion of teprotumumab therapy demonstrating reduction in the size and normalization of T2 signal (indicating resolution of inflammation) within the inferior rectus (*thick white arrow*), medial rectus (*thin white arrow*) and orbital fat (*arrowhead*). At baseline, this patient had Hertel exophthalmometry measurement of 23 mm, a Gorman diplopia score of 3 and clinical activity score (CAS) 5. At week 24 after teprotumumab therapy completion, the patient had proptosis measurement of 18 mm, Gorman diplopia score of 0 and a CAS of 0 (From: Jain AP, Gellada N, Ugradar S, Kumar A, Kahaly G, Douglas R. Teprotumumab reduces extraocular muscle and orbital fat volume in thyroid eye disease. Br J Ophthalmol. 2022 Feb;106(2):165-171. *Reproduced with permission from BMJ Journals*)

Pooled data analysis from these 2 trials showed that the number needed to treat (NNT) was 1.6 for proptosis response, 2.5 for diplopia response, 1.7 for overall response and 2.5 for disease inactivation ($p < 0.0001$). The authors divided the patients into subgroups to further assess diplopia and proptosis response (smokers, gender, duration of disease, age > 65 years, and others). Proptosis response was greater in teprotumumab vs placebo for all subgroups at 24 weeks follow up. Diplopia improvement was higher in those taking teprotumumab for all subgroups except smokers and those with baseline thyrotropin binding immunoglobulin levels <10 IU/L [103].

In 2021, Douglas et al. published the results of an Open-Label Clinical Extension Study (OPTIC-X) which is a continuation of the previously mentioned phase 3 trial. In this trial, teprotumumab (8 infusions over 24 weeks) was given to TAO patients who didn't respond to previously administered placebo treatment and to those who flared up at 48 weeks after taking teprotumumab. In the non-responders' group, proptosis improved in 89% (n = 33/37) of patients at a mean of −3.5 ± 1.7 mm. Diplopia also improved significantly where it resolved completely in 56.5% (n = 13/23) of patients. More than half of patients (n = 21/32) achieved a CAS of 0 or 1 at 24 weeks. These results paralleled OPTIC trial results and they were persistent in the majority of patients at 48 weeks of follow-up. Non-responders undergoing another course of teprotumumab treatment were few, but their proptosis response was less than the placebo group. In comparison, a second course of teprotumumab therapy for patients who flared up resulted in a proptosis response in 62.5% (n = 8/10) of patients at 24-weeks follow-up. These results proved that teprotumumab is also effective in patients with longer duration of TAO. In addition, re-treatment in those who did not respond initially or those who relapsed might add benefit without jeopardising safety [104].

Interestingly, Ugradar et al. in a recent publication showed that teprotumumab was also successful in reducing proptosis, diplopia, inflammation and orbital soft tissue volume in patients with chronic TAO (average of 7 years) receiving ≥3 infusions [105]. These results are encouraging and this effect is mostly related to the upregulation of IGF-1R even in the chronic stage of disease [106].

When studying the effect of teprotumumab in patients with asymmetric TAO, it was found to reduce proptosis, inflammation, and diplopia more in the orbit with worse manifestations resulting in reduced asymmetry [52].

The efficacy of teprotumumab was not limited to the orbit. In a prospective study on 23 TAO patients to evaluate teprotumumab effect on facial and eyelid changes, it was found that the mean reduction in full-face volume was 8.9 mL. The mean decrease in periorbital volume was 1.8 mL [107]. Reversal of these changes carries a positive influence on these patients' Qol.

All previously mentioned studies provided strong evidence on the efficacy of teprotumumab in reducing proptosis, improving diplopia, and enhancing the Qol of patients with TAO. This response was achieved regardless of the severity of proptosis or diplopia at baseline. A network metanalysis comparing the efficacies of 11 TAO treatments showed that teprotumumab was the most effective for proptosis reduction. It also achieved the second best response rate after IVGC+ORT [108].

Overall, teprotumumab seemed to be a safe drug as no deaths were reported in the treatment group in any of the previously cited studies. Most adverse events in both trials were graded mild to moderate. The most common reported side effects were as follows: muscle spasm, nausea, alopecia, diarrhoea, fatigue, hyperglycemia, hearing loss, dry skin, dysgeusia, and headaches. Hearing impairment occurred in a total of seven patients in both trials and it resolved spontaneously in almost all patients. In OPTIC-X study, hearing impairment (mild autophony and hypoacusis) was developed in two patients who previously experienced audiological symptoms in the first trial [104]. In both trials, hyperglycemia developed in a total of seven patients, mainly diabetics [100, 101]. In terms of serious adverse events, three patients developed drug-related infusion reactions [100, 104]. Two recent case reports documented the new onset of ulcerative colitis in patients receiving teprotumumab for TAO [109, 110]. However, teprotumumab might still be considered in patients with stable inflammatory bowel disease (IBD) along with close supervision by gastroenterologists [111].

Before commencing teprotumumab, patients should undergo a thorough medical evaluation paying special attention to the following: history of diabetes, symptoms/signs of a diagnosis of IBD, weight, and blood pressure. Routine investigations should include fasting blood sugar, HA1C, complete blood count, liver function test, and electrocardiogram. During the treatment course, fasting blood glucose should be monitored closely after the first two doses [111].

Although this medication opened the door to a new era in the treatment of TAO, further studies with longer follow-up durations are required to determine the long-term outcome and the future need for rehabilitative surgery in the treated patients.

4 Conclusions

- IVGCs are still considered the first-line treatment for active moderate-to-severe TAO, as they are well-known to improve inflammatory signs in this subset of patients. In addition, there is enough evidence that IVGCs demonstrated a good response rate in patients with TAO-related CON. A cumulative dose of 8 g should not be exceeded to prevent serious life and organ-threatening side effects. Patients should be monitored closely while on GCs, and treating physicians should withdraw treatment and consider other agents whenever serious life-threatening events occur. Patients receiving GCs may have disease recurrence in 20–30% of cases. To avoid threatening cumulative GCS doses, alternative or combined agents should be considered.

- Periorbital TA injections have shown certain effectiveness in the treatment of active TAO. The most notable improvement seems to be in eyelid retraction, particularly in patients with recent onset of eyelid retraction pre-treatment. Overall, local GCs do appear to play a role in the treatment of short-term eyelid retraction though this does not necessarily apply in long-standing retraction as the current opposing evidence precludes firm conclusions. Other parameters including CAS and proptosis also positively improved with periorbital TA injections. Extraocular motility improves to a lesser degree. Both retro-septal and subconjunctival injections showed similar outcomes; however, the incidence of IOP elevation is higher with subconjunctival injections. This latter, vision-threatening complication, taken together with other additional complications associated with the use of periorbital steroid injections such as corneoscleral melting, globe perforation, and retinal vascular occlusion constitutes the actual limitation in using TA injections.
- Nanotechnology for intravenous delivery of steroids (prednisolone wrapped in nanoparticles (liposomes)) to reduce the systemic exposure showed positive results in a pilot, but further study investigating the role of nanomedication (steroids or else) in TAO is needed
- ORT is an effective treatment option in patients with active TAO due to its disease-modifying effect even when administered solely. Some evidence advocates that in the active phase, the earlier ORT is commenced the more likely it will be effective, especially when combined with GCs which act synergistically, particularly in patients with ocular motility disruption/diplopia or CON. Eventually, ORT combined with GCs might be a feasible alternative in patients who are deemed steroid-resistant or intolerant. Treating physicians should weigh risks against benefits before instituting ORT because despite being minimal, potential risks exist and patients should be counselled accordingly. Patient's age may be considered a relevant factor in the decision making process.
- Cyclosporine is effective in treating TAO when used in combination with GCs. Results of its use as a single agent in TAO are not encouraging. Cyclosporine should be avoided in patients with nephropathy or uncontrolled hypertension.
- Methotrexate is effective in lowering inflammatory indices of TAO as it markedly improves CAS and even VISA scores. It is also useful in improving EOM motility and diplopia. It can be used in combination with GCs and may be used as a steroid-sparing agent although results of the latter are less definite. It is not very effective in reducing severe proptosis or eyelid retraction. Methotrexate is better avoided in patients with advanced liver disease.
- MMF in combination with GCs seems to be effective in the treatment of diplopia and EOM restriction and can be considered as an alternative treatment for patients that refuse radiotherapy. It also shows promising results as a monotherapy treatment in TAO, making it eligible as a second-line therapy, particularly considering that visual acuity, CAS, and proptosis have all shown improvement with MMF.
- RTX was found to improve CAS, proptosis, and orbital fat/muscle volume. However, until further large studies become available, the current preliminary evidence supports the use of RTX as a second-line agent in patients who are GCs resistant or intolerant. Nevertheless, its use in a late stage of the active stage seems to be uneventful. RTX should be avoided in patients at risk of CON.
- Preliminary results suggest that tocilizumab is effective in controlling the activity of TAO in patients who are resistant to corticosteroids. Currently, Tocilizumab should be considered as first choice in steroid-resistant patients when available and easily accessible for patients. Further evidence is required to elucidate its effect on proptosis, EOM, and eyelid aperture as a first-line treatment.

- To date, no large studies on the use of anti-TNF have been conducted to study the efficacy of anti-TNF medications in TAO.
- Teprotumumab is the only FDA approved drug for the treatment of TAO. It is effective in reducing CAS, proptosis, motility disturbance, and diplopia, orbital soft tissue and EOM volume and in improving patient's Qol. It appears to be the most effective treatment in reducing proptosis in patients with moderate-to-severe active TAO. It was also proven to be effective in patients with chronic TAO. It is generally a safe drug with mostly mild and reversible side effects. Current limitations in considering such medication as first-line treatment for TAO are the high cost and lacking data showing a significant lowering of recurrence rate in comparison to steroids.

References

1. Douglas RS, Gupta S. The pathophysiology of thyroid eye disease: Implications for immunotherapy. Curr Opin Ophthalmol. 2011;22:385–90.
2. Gianoukakis AG, Smith TJ. Recent insights into the pathogenesis and management thyroid-associated ophthalmopathy. Curr Opin Endocraniol Diabetes Obes. 2013;15:446–52.
3. Weetman A. Graves' disease. N Engl J Med. 2000;343:1236–48.
4. Bartley GB. The epidemiologic characteristics and clinical course of ophthalmopathy associated with autoimmune thyroid disease in Olmsted County, Minnesota. Trans Am Ophthalmol Soc. 1994;92:477–588.
5. Menconi F, Marcocci C, Marinò M. Diagnosis and classification of Graves' disease. Autoimmun Rev. 2014;13:398–402.
6. Mawn LA, Dolman PJ, Kazim M, et al. Soft tissue metrics in thyroid eye disease: An International Thyroid Eye Disease Society Reliability Study. Ophthalmic Plast Reconstr Surg. 2018;34:544–6.
7. Mourits MP, Prummel MF, Wiersinga WM, et al. Clinical activity score as a guide in the management of patients with Graves' ophthalmopathy. Clin Endocrinol (Oxf). 1997;47:9–14.
8. Barrio-Barrio J, Sabater AL, Bonet-Farriol E, et al. Graves' ophthalmopathy: VISA versus EUGOGO classification, assessment, and management. J OPHTHALMOL. 2015;2015:1–16.
9. Strianese D. Update on Graves disease: Advances in treatment of mild, moderate and severe thyroid eye disease. Curr Opin Ophthalmol. 2017;28:505–13.
10. Strianese D, Rossi F. Interruption of autoimmunity for thyroid eye disease: B-cell and T-cell strategy. Eye. 2019;33:191–9.
11. Strianese D, Piscopo R, Elefante A, et al. Unilateral proptosis in thyroid eye disease with subsequent contralateral involvement: Retrospective follow-up study. BMC Ophthalmol. 2013;13:21.
12. Lanni V, Iuliano A, Laezza MP, et al. Oculoplastic management of patients in the Covid-19 era: Experience from an Italian tertiary referral center. Orbit. 2020;39:391–3.
13. Al-Sharif E, Strianese D, AlMadhi NH, et al. Ocular tropism of coronavirus (CoVs): A comparison of the interaction between the animal-to-human transmitted coronaviruses (SARS-CoV-1, SARS-CoV-2, MERS-CoV, CoV-229E, NL63, OC43, HKU1) and the eye. Int Ophthalmol. 2021;41:349–62.
14. Hales IB, Thomas ID. Treatment of thyroid ophthalmopathy with corticoid analogues. Australas Ann Med. 1962;11:113–7.
15. Bartalena L, Baldeschi L, Boboridis K, et al. The 2016 European Thyroid Association/European Group on Graves' Orbitopathy Guidelines for the Management of Graves' Orbitopathy. Eur Thyroid J. 2016;5:9–26.
16. Bartalena L, Kahaly GJ, Baldeschi L, et al. The 2021 European Group on Graves' orbitopathy (EUGOGO) clinical practice guidelines for the medical management of Graves' orbitopathy. Eur J Endocrinol. 2021;185:G43–67.
17. Tu X, Dong Y, Zhang H, et al. Corticosteroids for Graves' ophthalmopathy: Systematic review and meta-analysis. Biomed Res Int. 2018;2018:1–9.
18. Aktaran Ş, Akarsu E, Erbağci İ, et al. Comparison of intravenous methylprednisolone therapy vs. oral methylprednisolone therapy in patients with Graves' ophthalmopathy: IVGC vs. OGC in Graves' ophthalmopathy. Int J Clin Pract. 2006;61:45–51.
19. Kahaly GJ, Pitz S, Hommel G, et al. Randomized, single blind trial of intravenous *versus* oral steroid monotherapy in Graves' orbitopathy. J Clin Endocrinol Metabol. 2005;90:5234–40.
20. van Geest RJ, Sasim IV, Koppeschaar HPF, et al. Methylprednisolone pulse therapy for patients with moderately severe Graves' orbitopathy: A prospective, randomized, placebo-controlled study. Eur J Endocrinol. 2008;158:229–37.
21. Zhao L-Q, Yu D-Y, Cheng J-W. Intravenous glucocorticoids therapy in the treatment of Graves' ophthalmopathy: A systematic review and meta-analysis. Int J Ophthalmol. 2019;12:1177–86.
22. Strianese D. Efficacy and safety of immunosuppressive agents for thyroid eye disease. Ophthal Plast Reconstr Surg. 2018;34:S56–9.
23. Bartalena L, Krassas GE, Wiersinga W, et al. Efficacy and safety of three different cumulative doses of intravenous methylprednisolone for moderate to severe and active Graves' orbitopathy. J Clin Endocrinol Metabol. 2012;97:4454–63.

24. Perez-Moreiras JV, Gomez-Reino JJ, Maneiro JR, et al. Efficacy of tocilizumab in patients with moderate-to-severe corticosteroid-resistant Graves orbitopathy: A randomized clinical trial. Am J Ophthalmol. 2018;195:181–90.
25. Zang S, Ponto KA, Kahaly GJ. Intravenous glucocorticoids for Graves' orbitopathy: Efficacy and morbidity. J Clin Endocrinol Metabol. 2011;96:320–32.
26. Hamed-Azzam S, Mukari A, Feldman I, et al. Fornix triamcinolone injection for thyroid orbitopathy. Graefes Arch Clin Exp Ophthalmol. 2015;253:811–6.
27. Bagheri A, Abbaszadeh M, Yazdani S. Intraorbital steroid injection for active thyroid ophthalmopathy. J Ophthalmic Vis Res. 2020;15:69–7.
28. Bordaberry M, Marques DL, Pereira-Lima JC, et al. Repeated peribulbar injections of triamcinolone acetonide: A successful and safe treatment for moderate to severe Graves' ophthalmopathy. Acta Ophthalmol. 2009;87:58–64.
29. Lee SJ, Rim THT, Jang SY, et al. Treatment of upper eyelid retraction related to thyroid-associated ophthalmopathy using subconjunctival triamcinolone injections. Graefes Arch Clin Exp Ophthalmol. 2013;251:261–70.
30. Young SM, Kim Y-D, Lang SS, et al. Transconjunctival triamcinolone injection for upper lid retraction in thyroid eye disease—a new injection method. Ophthal Plast Reconstr Surg. 2018;34:587–93.
31. Xu D, Liu Y, Xu H, et al. Repeated triamcinolone acetonide injection in the treatment of upper-lid retraction in patients with thyroid-associated ophthalmopathy. Can J Ophthalmol. 2012;47:34–41.
32. Xu D, Chen Y, Xu H, et al. Long-term effect of triamcinolone acetonide in the treatment of upper lid retraction with thyroid associated ophthalmopathy. Int J Ophthalmol. 2018;11:1290–5.
33. Lee JM, Lee H, Park M, et al. Subconjunctival injection of triamcinolone for the treatment of upper lid retraction associated with thyroid eye disease. J Craniofac Surg. 2012;23:1755–8.
34. Ebner R. Treatment of thyroid associated ophthalmopathy with periocular injections of triamcinolone. Br J Ophthalmol. 2004;88:1380–6.
35. Alkawas AA, Hussein AM, Shahien EA. Orbital steroid injection versus oral steroid therapy in management of thyroid-related ophthalmopathy: Orbital steroid injection versus oral steroid in TRO. Clin Experiment Ophthalmol. 2010;38:692–7.
36. Goldberg R. Orbital steroid injections. Br J Ophthalmol. 2004;88:1359–60.
37. Mo F, Xu D, Xu H, et al. Shallow periorbital injection of triamcinolone acetonide in treatment of lower eyelid entropion related to thyroid-associated ophthalmopathy: Three case reports. Medicine. 2020;99:e19026.
38. Detiger SE, Kremer TM, Dalm VASH, et al. A pilot study on the use of prednisolone-encapsulated liposomes for the treatment of moderate-to-severe Graves' orbitopathy with reduced systemic steroid exposure. Acta Ophthalmol. 2021;99:797–804.
39. Rajendram R, Bunce C, Lee RW, et al. Orbital radiotherapy for adult thyroid eye disease. Cochrane Database Syst Rev. 2012;7:CD007114.
40. Grassi P, Strianese D, Piscopo R, et al. Radiotherapy for the treatment of thyroid eye disease—a prospective comparison: Is orbital radiotherapy a suitable alternative to steroids? Ir J Med Sci. 2017;186:647–52.
41. Godfrey KJ, Kazim M. Radiotherapy for active thyroid eye disease. Ophthal Plast Reconstr Surg. 2018;4S Suppl 1:S98–S104.
42. Kim JW, Han SH, Son BJ, et al. Efficacy of combined orbital radiation and systemic steroids in the management of Graves' orbitopathy. Graefes Arch Clin Exp Ophthalmol. 2016;254:991–8.
43. Shams PN, Ma R, Pickles T, et al. Reduced risk of compressive optic neuropathy using orbital radiotherapy in patients with active thyroid eye disease. Am J Ophthalmol. 2014;157:1299–305.
44. Viani GA, Boin AC, De Fendi LI, et al. Radiation therapy for Graves' ophthalmopathy: A systematic review and meta-analysis of randomized controlled trials. Arq Bras Oftalmol. 2012;75:324–32.
45. Gold KG, Scofield S, Isaacson SR, et al. Orbital radiotherapy combined with corticosteroid treatment for thyroid eye disease-compressive optic neuropathy. Ophthal Plast Reconstr Surg. 2018;34:172–7.
46. Nicosia L, Reverberi C, Agolli L, et al. Orbital radiotherapy plus concomitant steroids in moderate-to-severe Graves' ophthalmopathy: Good results after long-term follow-up. Int J Endocrinol Metab. 2019;17:e84427.
47. Gillis CC, Chang EH, Al-Kharazi K, et al. Secondary malignancy following radiotherapy for thyroid eye disease. Rep Pract Oncol Radiother. 2016;21:156–61.
48. Wakelkamp I, Tan H, Saeed P, et al. Orbital irradiation for Graves' ophthalmopathy. Ophthalmology. 2004;111:1557–62.
49. Nanda T, Sanchez A, Purswani J, et al. Contour variability in thyroid eye disease with compressive optic neuropathy treated with radiation therapy Adv. Radiat Oncol. 2020;5:804–8.
50. Kahaly G, Schrezenmeir J, Krause U, et al. Ciclosporin and prednisone v. prednisone in treatment of Graves' ophthalmopathy: A controlled, randomized and prospective study. Eur J Clin Invest. 1986;16:415–22.
51. Prummel MF, Mourits MP, Berghout A, et al. Prednisone and cyclosporine in the treatment of severe Graves' ophthalmopathy. N Engl J Med. 1989;321:1353–9.
52. Weetman A, McGregor A, Ludgate M, et al. Cyclosporin improves Graves' ophthalmopathy. Lancet. 1983;2:486–9.
53. Dalmatova A, Grineva E. Evaluation of Methylprednisolone pulse therapy versus combined therapy with prednisolone and cyclosporine in the

treatment of infiltrative ophthalmopathy in Graves' disease. Probl Endokrinol (Mosk). 2007;53:27–30.
54. Weissel M, Zielinski C, Hauff W, et al. Combined therapy with cyclosporin a and cortisone in endocrine basedow endocrine orbitopathy: Successful use in compressive optic neuropathy. Acta Med Austriaca. 1993;20:9–13.
55. Witte A, Landgraf R, Markl A, et al. Treatment of Graves' ophthalmopathy with cyclosporin A. Klin Wochenschr. 1985;63:1000–4.
56. Kvetny J, Frandsen NE, Johnsen T, et al. Treatment of Graves' ophthalmopathy with Cyclosporin A. Acta Med Scand. 2009;220:189–91.
57. Rajendram R, Taylor PN, Wilson VJ, et al. Combined immunosuppression and radiotherapy in thyroid eye disease (CIRTED): A multicentre, 2 × 2 factorial, double-blind, randomised controlled trial. Lancet Diabetes Endocrinol. 2018;6:299–309.
58. Perros P, Weightman DR, Crombie AL, et al. Azathioprine in the treatment of thyroid-associated ophthalmopathy. Acta Endocrinol. 1990;122:8–12.
59. Chalvatzis NT, Tzamalis AK, Kalantzis GK, et al. Safety and efficacy of combined immunosuppression and orbital radiotherapy in thyroid-related restrictive myopathy: Two-center experience. Eur J Ophthalmol. 2014;24:953–9.
60. Levy SL, Salvi SM. Reactivation of Darier's disease following Azathioprine treatment for thyroid eye disease. Eye. 2013;27:568–9.
61. Bartalena L, Tanda ML, Medea A, et al. Novel approaches to the management of Graves' ophthalmopathy. Hormones (Athens). 2002;1:76–90.
62. Rubinov A, Zommer H, Aghazadeh H, et al. Role of methotrexate in thyroid-related orbitopathy. Can J Ophthalmol. 2018;53:34–8.
63. Yong K-L, Chng C-L, Ming Sie N, et al. Methotrexate as an adjuvant in severe thyroid eye disease: Does it really work as a steroid-sparing agent? Ophthal Plast Reconstr Surg. 2019;35:369–73.
64. Strianese D, Iuliano A, Ferrara M, et al. Methotrexate for the treatment of thyroid eye disease. J Ophthalmol. 2014;2014:1–5.
65. Grana ER, Phoebe L, Suhler EB, et al. Methotrexate as a corticosteroid-sparing agent for thyroid eye disease. J Clin Exp Ophthalmol. 2015;6:422.
66. Sipkova Z, Insull EA, David J, et al. Early use of steroid-sparing agents in the inactivation of moderate-to-severe active thyroid eye disease: A step-down approach. Clin Endocrinol (Oxf). 2018;89:834–9.
67. Kahaly GJ, Riedl M, König J, et al. Mycophenolate plus methylprednisolone versus methylprednisolone alone in active, moderate-to-severe Graves' orbitopathy (MINGO): A randomised, observer-masked, multicentre trial. Lancet Diabetes Endocrinol. 2018;6:287–98.
68. Ye X, Bo X, Hu X, et al. Efficacy and safety of mycophenolate mofetil in patients with active moderate-to-severe Graves' orbitopathy. Clin Endocrinol (Oxf). 2017;86:247–55.
69. Wang C, Ning Q, Jin K, et al. Does rituximab improve clinical outcomes of patients with thyroid-associated ophthalmopathy? A systematic review and meta-analysis. BMC Ophthalmol. 2018; 18:46.
70. Stan MN, Salvi M. MANAgement of endocrine disease: rituximab therapy for Graves' orbitopathy—lessons from randomized control trials. Eur J Endocrinol. 2017;176:R101–9.
71. Salvi M, Vannucchi G, Campi I, et al. Treatment of Graves' disease and associated ophthalmopathy with the anti-CD20 monoclonal antibody rituximab: An open study. Eur J Endocrinol. 2007;156:33–40.
72. Fassi DE, Nielsen CH, Hasselbalch HC, et al. Treatment-resistant severe, active Graves' ophthalmopathy successfully treated with B lymphocyte depletion. Thyroid. 2006;16:709–10.
73. Salvi M, Vannucchi G, Campi I, et al. Efficacy of rituximab treatment for thyroid-associated ophthalmopathy as a result of intraorbital B-cell depletion in one patient unresponsive to steroid immunosuppression. Eur J Endocrinol. 2006;154:511–7.
74. Salvi M, Vannucchi G, Currò N, et al. Efficacy of B-cell targeted therapy with rituximab in patients with active moderate to severe Graves' orbitopathy: A randomized controlled study. J Clin Endocrinol Metabol. 2015;100:422–31.
75. Stan MN, Garrity JA, Carranza Leon BG, et al. Randomized controlled trial of rituximab in patients with Graves' orbitopathy. J Clin Endocrinol Metabol. 2015;100:432–41.
76. Li J, Xiao Z, Hu X, et al. The efficacy of rituximab combined with ^{131}I for ophthalmic outcomes of Graves' ophthalmopathy patients. Pharmacology. 2017;99:144–52.
77. Savino G, Mandarà E, Gari M, et al. Intraorbital injection of rituximab versus high dose of systemic glucocorticoids in the treatment of thyroid-associated orbitopathy. Endocrine. 2015;48:241–7.
78. Krassas GE, Stafilidou A, Boboridis KG. Failure of rituximab treatment in a case of severe thyroid ophthalmopathy unresponsive to steroids: Letters to the Editor. Clin Endocrinol (Oxf). 2009;72:853–5.
79. Gess AJ, Silkiss RZ. Orbital B-Lymphocyte depletion in a treatment failure of rituximab for thyroid eye disease. Ophthal Plast Reconstr Surg. 2014;30:e11–3.
80. Salvi M, Vannucchi G, Beck-Peccoz P. Potential utility of rituximab for Graves' orbitopathy. J Clin Endocrinol Metabol. 2013;98:4291–9.
81. Kaneko A. Tocilizumab in rheumatoid arthritis: Efficacy, safety and its place in therapy. Ther Adv Chronic Dis. 2013;4:15–21.
82. Karkhur S, Hasanreisoglu M, Vigil E, et al. Interleukin-6 inhibition in the management of non-infectious uveitis and beyond. J Ophthalmic Inflamm Infect. 2019;9:17.
83. Jyonouchi SC, Valyasevi RW, Harteneck DA, et al. Interleukin-6 stimulates thyrotropin receptor expression in human orbital preadipocyte fibroblasts from

patients with Graves' ophthalmopathy. Thyroid. 2001;11:929–34.
84. Sy A, Eliasieh K, Silkiss RZ. Clinical response to tocilizumab in severe thyroid eye disease. Ophthal Plast Reconstr Surg. 2017;33:e55–7.
85. Copperman T, Kersten RC. Subcutaneous Tocilizumab for thyroid eye disease: Simplified dosing and delivery. Ophthal Plast Reconstr Surg. 2019;35:e64–6.
86. Pérez-Moreiras JV, Álvarez-López A, Gómez EC. Treatment of active corticosteroid-resistant Graves' orbitopathy. Ophthal Plast Reconstr Surg. 2014;30:162–7.
87. Sánchez-Bilbao L, Martínez-López D, Revenga M, et al. Anti-IL-6 receptor tocilizumab in refractory Graves' orbitopathy: National Multicenter Observational Study of 48 patients. J Clin Med. 2020;9:2816.
88. Bennedjaï A, Bouheraoua N, Gatfossé M, et al. Tocilizumab versus rituximab in patients with moderate to severe steroid-resistant Graves' orbitopathy. Ocul Immunol Inflamm 2022;30:500-505
89. Moi L, Hamedani M, Ribi C. Long-term outcomes in corticosteroid-refractory Graves' orbitopathy treated with tocilizumab. Clin Endocrinol (Oxf). 2022;97:363–70.
90. Actemra: Safety and lab monitoring guide with subcutaneous or intravenous administration. https://www.actemrahcp.com/content/dam/gene/actemrahcp/PDFs/ACT0002021800_Actemra_Lab_Monitoring_Guide_PDF_Reference.pdf. 2010.
91. Jones G, Panova E. New insights and long-term safety of tocilizumab in rheumatoid arthritis. Ther Adv Musculoskelet Dis. 2018;10:195–9.
92. Paridaens D, van den Bosch WA, van der Loos TL, et al. The effect of etanercept on Graves' ophthalmopathy: A pilot study. Eye. 2005;19:1286–9.
93. Boskovic O, Medenica S, Radojevic N, et al. Etanercept in the treatment of Graves' ophthalmopathy with primary hypothyroidism and rheumatoid arthritis. Cent Eur J Immunol. 2019;44:463–5.
94. Kapadia MK, Rubin PAD. The emerging use of TNF-A inhibitors in orbital inflammatory disease. Int Ophthalmol Clin. 2006;46:165–81.
95. Durrani O, Reuser T, Murray P. Infliximab: A novel treatment for sight-threatening thyroid associated ophthalmopathy. Orbit. 2005;24:117–9.
96. Komorowski J, Jankiewicz-Wika J, Siejka A, et al. Monoclonal anti-TNFalpha antibody (Infliximab) in the treatment of patient with thyroid associated ophthalmopathy. Klin Oczna. 2007;109:457–60.
97. Ayabe R, Rootman DB, Hwang CJ, et al. Adalimumab as steroid-sparing treatment of inflammatory-stage thyroid eye disease. Ophthal Plast Reconstr Surg. 2014;30:415–9.
98. Tsui S, Naik V, Hoa N, et al. Evidence for an association between thyroid-stimulating hormone and insulin-like growth factor 1 receptors: A tale of two antigens implicated in Graves' disease. J Immunol. 2008;181:4397–405.
99. Pritchard J, Han R, Horst N, et al. Immunoglobulin activation of T cell chemoattractant expression in fibroblasts from patients with Graves' disease is mediated through the insulin-like growth factor I receptor pathway. J Immunol. 2003;170:6348–54.
100. Douglas RS, Kahaly GJ, Patel A, et al. Teprotumumab for the treatment of active thyroid eye disease. N Engl J Med. 2020;382:341–52.
101. Smith TJ, Kahaly GJ, Ezra DG, et al. Teprotumumab for thyroid-associated ophthalmopathy. N Engl J Med. 2017;376:1748–61.
102. Jain AP, Gellada N, Ugradar S, et al. Teprotumumab reduces extraocular muscle and orbital fat volume in thyroid eye disease. Br J Ophthalmol. 2022;106:165–71.
103. Kahaly GJ, Douglas RS, Holt RJ, et al. Teprotumumab for patients with active thyroid eye disease: A pooled data analysis, subgroup analyses, and off-treatment follow-up results from two randomised, double-masked, placebo-controlled, multicentre trials. Lancet Diabetes Endocrinol. 2021;9:360–72.
104. Douglas RS, Kahaly GJ, Ugradar S, et al. Teprotumumab efficacy, safety, and durability in longer-duration thyroid eye disease and re-treatment. Ophthalmology. 2022;129:438–49.
105. Ugradar S, Kang J, Kossler AL, et al. Teprotumumab for the treatment of chronic thyroid eye disease. Eye (Lond). 2022;36:1553–9.
106. Ugradar S, Shi L, Wang Y, et al. Teprotumumab for non-inflammatory thyroid eye disease (TED): Evidence for increased IGF-1R expression. Eye. 2021;35:2607–12.
107. Ugradar S, Braun J, Wang Y, et al. Facial and eyelid changes in thyroid eye disease are reversed by teprotumumab. Plast Reconstr Surg Glob Open. 2021;9:e3809.
108. Xu N, Cui Y, Xie T, et al. Comparative efficacy of medical treatments for thyroid eye disease: A network meta-analysis. J Ophthalmol. 2018;2018:1–10.
109. Ashraf D, Jankovic I, El-Nachef N, et al. New-onset of inflammatory bowel disease in a patient treated with teprotumumab for thyroid associated ophthalmopathy. Ophthalmic Plast Reconstr Surg. 2021;37:e160–4.
110. Safo MB, Silkiss RZ. A case of ulcerative colitis associated with teprotumumab treatment for thyroid eye disease. Am J Ophthalmol Case Rep. 2021;22:101069.
111. Douglas RS, Wang Y, Dailey RA, et al. Teprotumumab in clinical practice: Recommendations and considerations from the OPTIC Trial Investigators. J Neuroophthalmol. 2021;41:461–8.

Quality of Life Studies in Thyroid-Associated Orbitopathy

Eyvind Rødahl, Sven Sahlin, and Maarten P. Mourits

Key Messages

- Health-related quality of life (HRQOL) is defined as "the physical, psychological and social domains of health, seen as distinct areas that are influenced by a person's experiences, beliefs, expectations and perceptions".
- To preserve or restore HRQOL may be seen as the ultimate goal of our efforts as physicians.
- HRQOL is usually assessed by questionnaires. Questionnaires were developed by researchers and patients in collaboration to find the most relevant themes and items. The themes most relevant for thyroid-associated orbitopathy (TAO) are consequences of visual functioning and psychosocial consequences of altered appearance.
- Questionnaires can be general, as the SF-36, or disease specific as the GO-QOL. General questionnaires have shown that the HRQOL in TAO is lower than in other severe chronic diseases. Reduced HRQOL has been linked to extraocular muscle involvement, soft tissue inflammation, proptosis and asymmetry, anxiety and depression. Specific questionnaires have demonstrated a significant improvement of HRQOL with therapies such as selenium treatment, corticosteroid treatment, immunomodulating therapy, decompressive surgery, lid surgery and squint surgery.
- The HRQOL assessment with instruments such as the GO-QOL could be used in daily clinical practice to improve follow-up and patient - physician interaction.
- The addition of HRQOL assessment to research studies will increase the value of obtained results. In order to make studies comparable, a standard instrument should be used. The GO-QOL has proven high validity, reliability and cultural applicability.

E. Rødahl (✉)
Department of Ophthalmology, Haukeland University Hospital, Bergen, Norway

Department of Clinical Medicine, University of Bergen, Bergen, Norway
e-mail: eyvind.rodahl@helse-bergen.no

S. Sahlin
Department of Clinical Neuroscience, Karolinska Institutet, Stockholm, Sweden

M. P. Mourits
Orbital Center, Department of Ophthalmology, Amsterdam University Medical Centers, Amsterdam, The Netherlands

1 Introduction

Quality of Life (QoL) is according to The World Health Organization (WHO) "an individual's perception of their position in life in the context of the culture and value systems in which they live and in relation to their goals, expectations, standards and concerns". Health-related QoL is

F. M. Quaranta Leoni et al. (eds.), *Oculoplastic, Lacrimal and Orbital Surgery*,
https://doi.org/10.1007/978-3-031-39638-0_41

defined as "the physical, psychological and social domains of health, seen as distinct areas that are influenced by a person's experiences, beliefs, expectations and perceptions" [1].

The discomfort, visual limitation and change of appearance in thyroid-associated orbitopathy (TAO) obviously impairs the individual's well-being. Studies of the impact of TAO on QoL first emerged a little more than two decades ago when Gerding, Terwee and their co-workers [2] assessed general quality of life using 24 questions from the Medical Outcomes Study (MOS-24) [3] and three subscales of the Sickness Impact Profile (SIP) [4]. To provide clinicians as well as researchers with a background for QoL assessment in patients with TAO, we have reviewed QoL studies reported for this group of patients. The theoretical basis for QoL studies has seen a major development over the past decades, but an in-depth discussion of this is beyond the scope of the present chapter.

2 Qualitative Studies

Qualitative studies are essential for the identification of items that are important for patients' perception of well-being. Such studies also allow a more detailed exploration of the psychosocial and emotional consequences of a disease.

Relatively few qualitative studies of TAO patients have been described. Estcourt and co-workers [5] used semi-structured interviews and thematic content analysis of 25 TAO patients, and identified three key themes that are major challenges for TAO patients: (a) development of an altered identity as a result of changes in appearance, abilities and roles due to physical consequences of TAO, (b) creation of coping strategies including denial, social avoidance, adjustment and stoicism, and (c) difficult interactions with healthcare practitioners due to uncertainty surrounding the diagnosis, prognosis and treatment choices, resulting in patients' disengagement, anger and frustration.

By in-depth interviews and participant observation of 13 individuals, Jensen and Harder [6] explored the consequences of bodily change on the patient's social behaviour in everyday situations. The main finding was the experience of "uncontrollable eyes". This resulted in (1) difficulties in using the eyes and face to communicate, (2) an experience of or being afraid that others would judge their personality from their appearance, (3) feeling clumsy, and (4) problems with reading, writing, and transporting themselves around that caused a feeling of being cut-off from the outside world. Patients developed coping strategies that included (1) telling others about their disease, (2) putting on a brave face, (3) minimising contact with people, (4) using camouflage like sunglasses or glasses, (5) adjusting to the bodily change, (6) changing shopping habits, and (7) opting out of activities. TAO was clearly life changing, and the authors recommend early identification of the impact of bodily change and planned support to help prevent serious QoL change.

In the development of a novel questionnaire for Asian patients, Wong and co-workers used focus groups and thematic saturation technique to identify items relevant for TAO patients [7]. Interestingly, many of the items conceived were quite similar to those included by Terwee and her colleagues in their Graves' Ophthalmopathy-Quality Of Life (GO-QOL) questionnaire (described below) [8], indicating that the problems facing TAO patients are similar across cultures and languages.

2.1 Physician Perceived QoL

Wang and co-workers asked 73 endocrinologists and 108 ophthalmologists to grade the QoL of American TAO patients with moderate to severe disease. Overall QoL was an average of 4.1 on a scale from 1 to 7, where 1 was not at all impaired and 7 was extremely impaired [9]. The overall QoL score progressively increased with the Clinical Activity Score (CAS) [10]. Ocular pain, strabismus and diplopia appeared to be the main drivers of physician perceived QoL impairment.

In the report by Watt and co-workers [11], physicians (n = 15) as well as patients with thyroid disease (n = 80, 17 suffering from TAO) contributed issues that they thought would be important in the assessment of thyroid-related QoL. Patients rated issues about psychosocial problems and impact on daily life as more relevant, whereas clinicians focused on thyroid-characteristic issues.

Although physicians tend to underestimate patient QoL impact, and place different emphasis than patients or their caregivers on which clinical signs and symptoms most impact QoL [12], physicians may still contribute complementary perspectives on patient QoL. It is also important to understand physician perceived QoL since that influences severity classification and guides treatment.

3 Quantitative Studies

Quantitative measures, usually in the form of questionnaires, are more easily adapted into routine clinical practice and clinical trials than qualitative studies. Questionnaires can be of a general nature or target specific consequences of a disease.

Development of a questionnaire is a stepwise process [13]. It is important to involve patients in the generation of relevant items. After the items have been identified, they are transcribed into carefully formulated questions. Finally, the performance of the questionnaire is scrutinised for different types of validity, reliability and responsiveness [14]. Two important requirements that must be considered for a questionnaire are uni-dimensionality and interval-level measurement. Uni-dimensionality means that only a single underlying item is measured. Many questionnaires are multidimensional, and uni-dimensionality is then achieved by separating the items into content areas or subscales. Interval-level measurement means that the distance between the steps on a rating scale should be equal. The response to many QoL questionnaires is an overall score derived by summative scoring of the items of the questionnaire. This is acceptable if all response categories have equal value. However, items may not have equal value. To ensure uni-dimensionality, and to resolve inequities in a scale arising from different difficulties of the items, psychometric methods like Rasch analysis can be of help.

3.1 General Health Related QoL Questionnaires

One of the most widely used questionnaires for assessing general health is the 36 item Short Form (SF-36) Health Status Survey. This questionnaire and a shorter 24-item form were developed as part of the Medical Outcome Study (MOS) [3].

SF-36 includes one multi-item scale that assesses eight health concepts: (1) limitations in physical activities because of health problems; (2) limitations in social activities because of physical or emotional problems; (3) limitations in usual role activities because of physical health problems; (4) bodily pain; (5) general mental health (psychological distress and well-being); (6) limitations in usual role activities because of emotional problems; (7) vitality (energy and fatigue); and (8) general health perceptions.

In the first study of TAO QoL in 1997. Gerding and co-workers [2] found low scores on the MOS-24, particularly on physical functioning and health perception, but also on role functioning, social functioning, mental health, and pain. The scores were lower than those reported for patients with other chronic diseases like diabetes, pulmonary emphysema, or heart failure. The scores did not correlate with the duration, severity, or activity of the disease.

In a German population, Kahaly and co-workers used SF-36 to assess QoL in patients with varying degrees of TAO [15]. Low scores were observed compared to a German reference group, especially for the items vitality, social functioning, mental health, health perceptions, and pain. As in the study by Gerding and co-workers, SF-36 scores did not correlate with the duration or severity of the eye disease.

In a study from Sweden, QoL in patients with Graves' disease treated with antithyroid drugs or radioiodine (without steroid prophylaxis) was assessed using SF-36 [16]. TAO developed in 23% among those receiving anti-thyroid drugs and 46% treated with radioiodine. Patients who developed or got worse from TAO at any time point during the study period had lower QoL.

3.2 Vision-related QoL Questionnaires

The Visual Function Questionnaire (VFQ) 25 is a 25 item questionnaire divided into 12 subscales that was developed by investigators at the US National Eye Institute to assess health related QoL in visually impaired individuals [17]. The VFQ-25 questionnaire has been translated to and validated for use in many languages. It was evaluated for use as a tool to assess health related QoL in patients with TAO by Bradley and co-workers [18]. Thirty individuals completed the questionnaire and were then interviewed to provide feedback on the questionnaire. Overall, a moderately impaired QoL was found in this study with the greatest impairments in the Mental Health and the Role Difficulties subscales. However, significant ceiling effects were seen in 7 of the 12 subscales, and more than two thirds of the participants perceived that the questionnaire lacked items relevant to their disease, in particular ocular discomfort and altered appearance.

Using a Chinese version of VFQ-25, Du and co-workers found that TAO patients with optic nerve involvement had lower scores than those without, in particular for Role Limitations and Mental Health subscales [19]. Ceiling effects were observed for three of the subscales.

Although VFQ-25 can be of some help in assessing vision-related QoL in TAO patients, it is recommended that a more disease-specific survey is used instead [20].

3.3 Thyroid Disease Related QoL Questionnaires

The most widely used instrument for assessing health related QoL in patients with thyroid disease is the thyroid-related patient reported outcome (ThyPRO), first developed by Watt and co-workers as an 85 item questionnaire [21], and later reduced to a shorter 39 item questionnaire [22].

One of 13 subscales is eye symptoms. In a systematic review of instruments used to assess health related QoL in patients with thyroid diseases, Wong and co-workers [23] found that the 85-item thyroid-specific patient-reported outcome measure (ThyPRO)showed the best methodological quality. GO-QOL was recommended for use in TAO patients.

3.4 Sinus Disease Questionnaires

The 22 item Sinonasal Outcomes Test (SNOT-22) has been developed to assess sinonasal-specific QoL. No questions on eye symptoms are included. In a study of 27 patients treated with endoscopic decompression, SNOT-22 was used to evaluate QoL before and one year after endoscopic decompression [24]. A significant improvement in total score and particularly for psychological and sleep dysfunction was observed.

3.5 Dry Eye Disease Questionnaires

In a study of meibomian gland dysfunction in TAO patients, Inoue evaluated QoL using a validated Japanese questionnaire for dry eye disease (DEQS) [25]. Dry eye disease QoL was worse in TAO patients than in healthy controls.

3.6 TAO Specific Questionnaires

3.6.1 GO-QOL

The Graves' orbitopathy-specific quality of life (GO-QOL) questionnaire was developed by Terwee and her colleagues in the Netherlands [8]. In their first report, they used a test consisting of 16 questions. Items considered relevant for TAO patients had been selected from existing vision-related quality-of-life instruments, including the Visual Function Index (VF-14) [26], Activities of Daily Vision Scale (ADVS) [27], and the Vision Related SIP [4]. Questions were added that explored the psychosocial consequences associated with changed appearance. The questions were subdivided into two subscales, each with eight questions. One was measuring the consequences of double vision and decreased visual acuity on visual functioning, while the other was measuring the psychosocial consequences of a changed appearance. The items were answered on a 3-point Likert scale and transformed to a 0 (worst) to 100 (best) scale. Construct validity and internal consistency was determined, based on principal component analysis, Cronbach alphas and correlations with MOS-24, three subscales of the SIP, demographic, and clinical measures. Mean scores (range 0–100) were 54.7 (SD 22.8) for visual functioning and 60.1 (SD 24.8) for appearance (higher score = better QoL). While overall quality of life was reduced on both subscales, severity of disease assessed by the NOSPECS [28] classification correlated only moderately with visual functioning and had low correlation with appearance.

In a follow-up study, test-retest reliability was assessed, and the original questionnaire was slightly modified to improve the validity of the subscale for visual appearance [29]. They also compared the effect of different treatments to define the minimal clinically important difference (MCID) in score on the GO-QOL [30]. Patients considered changes in GO-QOL scores of about 6–10 points as important improvements. The authors recommend that a mean change of at least 6 points should be required for less invasive procedures (strabismus and eyelid surgery) and at least 10 points for more invasive therapies (radiotherapy and orbital decompression).

The Persian translation of GO-QOL has been subjected to Rasch analysis and both visual functioning and appearance were found to have an acceptable internal consistency [31].

After its introduction, the GO-QOL has been translated to several languages including Chinese [32, 33], Danish, Dutch, English [34], French, Georgian, German [35], Greek, Hindi [36], Italian, Korean [37], Persian [31], Polish [38], Portuguese [39], Romanian, Russian, Serbian, Spanish [40], Swedish [41], Thai [42], and Turkish (see https://www.eugogo.eu/en/home/ for free downloads).

The questionnaire has been formally validated in English [43], Hindi [36], Persian [31] (Polish [38], Portuguese [39], and Thai [42].

Except for the item on bicycling [44, 45], the questions have been found to be relevant across cultures, and only minor modifications have been necessary for adopting the questionnaire in different populations.

3.6.2 TED-QOL

This is a 3-item questionnaire introduced by Fayers and Dolman. Overall quality of life, ability to carry out everyday activities, and satisfaction with your appearance are assessed on a scale from 1 (best) to 10 (worst). TED-QOL has similar validity and test-retest reliability as GO-QOL and GO-QLS (described below) [46]. Only a moderate correlation between items on the questionnaires and the severity of the eye disease as measured by VISA (Vision, Inflammation, Strabismus, Appearance) classification [47] was observed for the three tests. TED-QOL is a simple screening tool, but the authors acknowledge that more details on the patient's situation will be obtained when using the longer GO-QOL and GO-QLS.

3.6.3 GO-QLS

The GO-QLS is a 9-item questionnaire developed by Yeatts after analysis of the response from patients to a large questionnaire consisting of 105 items [45]. Included were items on (1) general and mental health from the Short Form, or SF-12, (2) self- perception and social functioning adapted from the Dermatology-Specific Quality of Life Questionnaire, or DSQL, (3) general visual function from the 51-item NEI-VFQ, and (4) visual function specific to TAO. One important issue that emerged from the development of the GO-QLS is that activities related to visual discrimination are strongly correlated with visual. These activities would include finding an object on a crowded shelf, recognizing facial features from across a room, or enjoying a movie or sporting event. In each of these visual activities, a patient is confronted with multiple visual stimuli or required to discriminate objects or features. Similar observations were made by Jensen and Harder [6]. The internal consistency of the scale was good (Cronbach's α of 0.89), and there was a reasonable correlation between GO-QLS and TAO severity scores.

3.6.4 TAO-QOL

The TAO-QOL is a questionnaire consisting of 90 items that was used in a German study on the effect of orbital decompression [48]. The questionnaire was constructed by clinicians without patient contributions. It has a relatively low internal consistency with a Cronbach's α of 0.63. The authors found a significant correlation between proptosis and the quality-of-life score, supporting that disfiguring proptosis is an important indication for decompression surgery.

3.6.5 OX-TED QOL

The Oxford-Thyroid Eye Disease QoL is a 7-item questionnaire used in one study to examine the effect of low-dose rituximab. Each question is scored from 1 to 10, with 1 indicating no concerns and 10 indicating major concerns. The higher the total score (maximum 70), the greater the impact of TAO on the patient's QoL [49]. How OX-TED was developed and validated, as well as its measurement properties was not described in detail. In 12 patients with active TAO who were treated early with low-dose rituximab, clinical activity and severity scores were significantly reduced. However, the average total OX-TED QOL score was 45 prior to treatment, decreasing non-significantly to 37 after treatment at an average follow-up of 6 months.

3.6.6 STED-QOL

In a recent report from Singapore, Wong and coworkers describe the construction of a questionnaire for Asian patients [7] using modern psychometric theory. In contrast to how the other TAO-specific questionnaires were developed, the authors first included patients in a qualitative study where relevant issues for item generation were identified using focus groups and a thematic saturation technique. For transcript generation, they adopted a constant comparative method, which involves coding each transcript for relevant themes, and iteratively comparing and contrasting these themes with subsequent transcripts, updating and refining the codes as each new transcript was analysed. A total of ten items across four QoL domains were generated: Activity Limitation (three items), Comfort (two items), Psychologic (four items), and Social (three items). The items were rated on a 5-point Likert-type scale. Rasch analysis [50] was used to explore the psychometric properties of the questionnaire. Interestingly, despite different sociocultural backgrounds, several of the items were similar to those included in the GO-QOL questionnaire. The scale showed good criterion validity, with scores decreasing as severity of TED worsened. The STED-QOL seems like a promising tool for QoL assessments, particularly in Asian patients.

4 Factors Important for Health Related QoL in TAO Patients

4.1 Clinical Features

The GO-QOL is the tool that has been used in most TAO quality-of-life studies. Correlations between disease activity measured by CAS and disease severity based on NOSPECS and European Group on Graves' Orbitopathy (EUGOGO) classifications have been reported for both subscales, but to a varying degree. This discrepancy can be explained in that the impact of the disease on each patient will be highly variable, and is dependent on many factors like expectations, coping ability, motivation, social support, and the physician-patient relationship [51].

Visual function subscale scores are reduced particularly in young individuals and in individuals with extraocular muscle involvement, soft tissue inflammation, and proptosis. Appearance subscale scores are reduced more frequently in females [52], and in individuals with soft tissue inflammation, asymmetry, and proptosis.

4.2 Interaction with Healthcare Practitioners

As reported by Estcourt and co-workers [5], difficult interactions with healthcare practitioners due to uncertainty surrounding the diagnosis, prognosis and treatment choices, may result in patients' disengagement, anger and frustration.

In an Australian study [34], Park and co-workers reported that a total of 74% of patients felt that education and counselling were inadequate and unhelpful in coping with and understanding TAO.

4.3 Thyroid Disease and Orbitopathy

In a study from Sweden, Ljunggren and co-workers [53] compared patients' views on therapy of their thyroid disease. A questionnaire was sent to 174 patients with hyperthyroidism. Twenty percent of the patients with TAO reported the eye problems to be much more troublesome and 14% somewhat more troublesome than the thyroid problems.

The effect on QoL of TAO in eu-/hypothyroid vs. hyperthyroid patients was examined by Ponto and co-workers. The authors found that compared with hyperthyroid TAO, QoL and working ability was less impaired in eu-/hypothyroid TAO [54].

Riguetto and co-workers examined QoL in Graves' disease patients using SF-36 and GO-QOL [55]. Eye involvement was a factor associated with a poor QoL.

4.4 Neuropsychiatric and Psychosocial Factors

Kahaly and co-workers examined German TAO patients combining the Hospital Anxiety and Depression Scale, a German adaptation of the Ways of Coping Checklist, and SF36 [56]. They found that psychosocial scales were considerably reduced in TAO patients compared to the reference group and to a group of diabetics, particularly in individuals with severe disease. Emotional distress, anxiety and depression was detected in 46, 41 and 24 individuals out of 102 examined, respectively, having a major impact on QoL.

Higher levels of anxiety (37%) and depression (26%) were observed among 123 TAO patients in the UK that had been scheduled for decompression [57] than in patients with other chronic disorders or disorders accompanied by facial disfigurement. Scores from the psychosocial questionnaires in the GO-QOL, the Hospital Anxiety and Depression Scale, and the Derriford Appearance Scale, were used in hierarchical multiple regression analyses to identify predictors of QoL. A total of 55% of the variance in GO-QOL visual function scores was explained by the regression model where age, asymmetrical TAO and depressed mood were significant unique contributors. For the GO-QOL appearance scores 75% of the variance was explained by the regression model. Here, gender, appearance-related cognitions and depressed mood were significant unique contributors.

In a study by Wang and co-workers where physicians were asked to grade QoL of American TAO patients with moderate to severe disease, [9] anxiety and/or depression was reported in 36% of the patients compared to the average 18.9% reported for the USA in 2017 by the US National Institute of Mental Health.

In a Korean study [58], SF-36 and Beck Depression Inventory (BDI) were used to assess QoL and depressive status in 49 patients. TAO patients scored lower than healthy controls on all subscales of the SF-36. When asked about the main cause for emotional distress with three possible answers: disfiguring change, functional impairment, or both, 20 patients responded with disfiguring change, 14 patients responded with functional impairment, and 15 patients reported both. Sixteen patients had BDI scores ≥16 indicative of clinical depression. These patients had significantly lower scores on the eight subscales and two summary scores of the SF-36, as well as higher clinical activity scores, as compared to the 33 patients with low BDI scores. No significant differences were observed between the high and low BDI score groups with respect to age, sex, duration of Graves' disease or TAO, or proptosis. There were no significant differences between patients with high and low BDI scores in terms of current severity stage by EUGOGO classification, main cause of distress, or history of optic neuropathy.

In a review of 15 studies to examine the psychosocial outcomes of treatment, Wickwar and co-workers [59] found that both major treatments such as surgery and other noninvasive treatments such as intravenous steroids could have a similar impact and show long-term benefits. Only three studies reviewed orbital decompressive surgery, which showed better psychosocial outcomes than other types of surgery. Clinicians should be aware when planning rehabilitative treatments such as surgery of the influence of psychosocial factors on QoL outcomes and the lack of a relationship with clinical factors such as disease severity.

Not only do patients with TAO frequently suffer from anxiety and depression, they also have a poorer self- image and significantly more disturbance in their sleep, social function, and work function than controls [45]. Individuals suffering from TAO are more likely to have psychotherapy [35], and are at higher risk for suicide [60] compared to the general population.

The pathogenic mechanisms behind the neuropsychiatric disorders in TAO are poorly understood. In a recent review, Bruscolini and co-workers summarised current evidence on neuropsychiatric abnormalities in Graves' disease [61]. The development of neuropsychiatric disorders in patients with TAO has been associated with both the detrimental effects of the altered circulating thyroid hormones on the nervous system, and with the psychological discomfort caused by poor quality of life, reduced social interactions and relapsing course of the disease. They remark the importance of a multidisciplinary approach and emphasise the potential benefit of neuropsychiatric approach on disease perception, patient compliance to medical and/or surgical treatment and clinical outcomes.

4.5 Occupational Aspects

Ponto and co-workers assessed occupational disability, income, and psychotherapy in a cohort of 250 German TAO patients [62] using a short questionnaire, in addition to the GO-QOL. Nearly half (45%) of the patients complained of restrictions in their daily activities, and 38% reported impaired self-perception. More than 1/3 (36%) were on sick leave because of TAO, 28% were disabled, 5% had retired early, and 3% had lost their job. Patients with severe TAO and motility disorders were on sick leave for longer times and were more likely to be disabled. 21% underwent psychotherapy. Patients who had been on sick leave for a long time and/or were disabled were more likely to undergo psychotherapy. The data indicate that patients with TAO suffer considerable emotional stress and occupational impairment and point to the need for preventive care and rapid rehabilitation.

4.6 Effect of Medical Treatment

The first incorporation of QoL in TAO clinical trials was reported by Terwee and co-workers. They evaluated the long-term effects of TAO and found that the QoL scores improved after immunosuppressive or surgical treatment, but the scores remained lower than those of healthy persons even many years after the final treatment [63]. Since then, the QoL measurements have been included in many clinical trials of different anti-inflammatory treatments and various surgical procedures.

4.6.1 Selenium

In a study comparing the effect of selenium, pentoxifylline and placebo, Marcocci and co-workers [64] found that after 6 months of treatment, GO-QOL scores among the 53 patients treated with selenium increased from baseline by 6 or more points for visual functioning in 33 patients (62%) and for appearance in 40 patients (75%). A significantly greater proportion of patients in the selenium group had an improved quality of life at 6 months, as compared with those given placebo. Moreover, the patients treated with selenium had a substantially lower rate of worsening of QoL (9 of 53 patients) as compared with those given placebo (20 of 46 patients).

4.6.2 Corticosteroids

Kahaly and co-workers examined the effect of oral vs. intravenous corticosteroids [65]. Intravenous therapy improved the physical and psychosocial components of the GO-QOL more than oral therapy.

Improvements in QoL after treatment with corticosteroids have been observed in several other studies [52]. Kashkouli and co-workers [66] observed that GO-QOL MCID was achieved in two-thirds of the patients. Hoppe and co-workers examined euthyroid, treatment-naïve patients with moderate to severe TAO who received i.v. methylprednisolone in a prospective trial [67]. Mean GO-QOL scores rose steadily, and sustained improvement from baseline was observed throughout the study period. There was a delay in the improvement of visual functioning which occurred after completion of treatment. On the contrary, appearance improved earlier at week 12, reached an apparent plateau after this, and was significantly better at weeks 24 and 36 than at baseline. The mean improvement in mean GO-QOL score and its subscales at week 36 vs. week 0 was around 6 points, considered a clinically important difference. Improvement was associated with response to treatment.

4.6.3 Teprotumumab

Assessments of QoL using the GO-QOL were included in studies of the response to teprotumumab [68, 69]. Compared to placebo, there were improvements with teprotumumab for GO-QOL total scores and on both subscales, more on visual functioning than appearance. The change from baseline was more than the MCID (6 points) for this type of intervention.

4.6.4 Radiotherapy

Some studies have found a positive effect of radiotherapy, while in a meta-analysis of four studies, no significant effect was found with no difference in QoL [70]. In a prospective trial of orbital irradiation and sham irradiation, QoL improved in both the irradiated and in the sham irradiated group [71].

4.7 Effect of Surgical Treatment

The TED-QOL was compared to GO-QOL in a study of the effect of rehabilitative surgery [72] in 56 patients that underwent 69 procedures for TAO (29 orbital decompressions, 15 strabismus operations, 25 eyelid procedures). The differences in scores between the three types of surgery (a measure of sensitivity) were statistically significant before and after surgery for all 3 TED-QOL scales and for both GO-QOL scales. The within-patient changes between the pre- and post-operative scores (a measure of responsiveness) were significant for the TED-QOL overall and appearance scales for each of the surgeries. The pre- and post-operative difference for the TED-QOL functioning scale was statistically significant for strabismus surgery but not for decompression or lid surgery. The change between the pre- and post-operative scores for the GO-QOL was significant for the functioning scale for strabismus and lid surgery and for the appearance scale for lid surgery but not for strabismus surgery or decompression.

4.7.1 Orbital Decompression

In a study of decompression surgeries in 139 patients across 11 European Centres administered by EUGOGO [73], the average pre-operative GO-QOL appearance score varied from 17.7 to 55.1. A few individuals had a lower score post-operatively, but most improved: the average change after surgery was +20.5. Variations in the average change of the appearance score were between 17.4 and 39.9 points, except for the translid and endoscopic approach, in which the change was no more than 1.8 points. A decrease of the visual functioning score was seen especially after the coronal approach, in which group de novo diplopia occurred most frequently.

In a study of orbital decompression surgery at Moorfields Eye Hospital by Wickar and co-workers [74], 123 patients completed the GO-QOL questionnaire before and at 6 weeks and 6 months after surgery. The GO-QOL visual function scores did not change significantly until 6 months after surgery. In contrast, GO-QOL appearance scores changed significantly by 6 weeks after surgery and continued to increase to 6 months, reaching a MCID for this scale. None of the changes in clinical or psychosocial outcomes significantly predicted change in GO-QOL visual function. However, a hierarchical regression model explained 79% of the variance in change in GO-QOL appearance, with change in subjective evaluation of appearance being the only unique predictor of change in appearance-related quality of life. It was suggested that psychosocial interventions targeting appearance-related cognitive processes, in particular personal evaluation of appearance, could enhance the QoL outcomes for patients with TAO undergoing orbital decompression surgery.

Iacobæus and Sahlin [41] examined 50 patients that underwent orbital decompression. They observed a significant, long-term, improvement in quality of life. The QoL-scores increased 28 ± 35 and 26 ± 31 points, respectively, on the two subscales, "visual functioning" and "appearance" (mean ± SD). The patient satisfaction questionnaire showed that 88% of the patients would recommend orbital decompression to a fellow patient. The GO-QOL questionnaire showed significant improvement in QoL-scores even many years after surgery.

Quality of life has also been shown to improve after fat decompression [75], and QoL assessments have been included in two studies on rim removal in lateral orbitotomies. One small study used GO-QOL before and after rim removal surgery, and found improvements both in the visual function and appearance subscale of the GO-QOL [76]. The other compared rim removal vs. rim sparing in 50 patients and found greater improvement in GO-QOL appearance score in the rim-sparing group supporting the use of the rim-sparing technique [77].

4.7.2 Strabismus Surgery

Jellema and co-workers examined 28 consecutive TAO patients who were scheduled for their first strabismus surgery [78]. The GO-QOL score for visual functioning was 46.3 ± 24.2 before surgery and 65.7 ± 30.5 after surgery. The GO-QOL score for appearance changed from 60.6 ± 25.9 to 69.5 ± 24.2. A weak correlation was found between the field of binocular single vision and the visual functioning score after surgery. A clinically relevant response was found in 20 (71%) patients. Those with a clinically relevant response showed a larger field of binocular single vision and better GO-QOL scores.

In a second study, the same group assessed 59 patients with two different tools (GO-QOL and TED-QOL) after one (n = 45) or two (n = 15) strabismus surgeries [79]. A moderate correlation was found between the field of binocular single vision and the GO-QOL visual functioning questionnaires. Both the GO-QOL and TED-QOL for visual functioning and appearance showed significantly higher scores after the treatment. The second surgery significantly expanded the field of binocular single vision and the QoL.

Campi and co-workers examined 66 patients treated with strabismus surgery at baseline and 12 weeks after surgery and found that GO-QOL score improved only in those without residual constant diplopia [80].

5 Recommendations

Several regulatory agencies like the US Food and Drug Administration require that QoL studies are included in clinical trials to assess both the effectiveness and side effects of novel treatments from the patients' perspective (https://www.fda.gov/regulatory-information/search-fda-guidance-documents/patient-reported-outcome-measures-use-medical-product-development-support-labeling-claims). Due to the observed substantial impairment in QoL in TAO patients, Wiersinga recommended in a review in 2012 [81] that GO-QOL should be incorporated as an independent primary outcome measure in randomized clinical trials, and also in the routine assessment of TAO in daily clinical practice. This was later followed by EUGOGO who recommended that the evaluation of QoL and psychological well-being by means of the GO-QOL questionnaire should be incorporated as an integral part of patient-focused management [82]. Use of the GO-QOL has also been included among the proposed standards of care for TAO patients in the UK [83]. A systematic review suggested that GO-QOL is the best disease-specific QoL assessment tool with its high validity, reliability, and cultural applicability [84]. Recently, Bartalena and Wiersinga [51] reviewed existing disease-specific quality-of-life (QoL) questionnaires for use in clinical trials of TAO patients, and also recommended the use of the GO-QOL.

References

1. Testa MA, Simonson DC. Assessment of quality-of-life outcomes. N Engl J Med. 1996;334:835–40.
2. Gerding MN, Terwee CB, Dekker FW, Koornneef L, Prummel MF, Wiersinga WM. Quality of life in patients with Graves' ophthalmopathy is markedly decreased: measurement by the medical outcomes study instrument. Thyroid. 1997;7:885–9.
3. Tarlov AR, Ware JE Jr, Greenfield S, Nelson EC, Perrin E, Zubkoff M. The Medical Outcomes Study. An application of methods for monitoring the results of medical care. JAMA. 1989;262:925–30.
4. Bergner M, Bobbitt RA, Carter WB, Gilson BS. The Sickness Impact Profile: development and final revision of a health status measure. Med Care. 1981;19:787–805.
5. Estcourt S, Vaidya B, Quinn A, Shepherd M. The impact of thyroid eye disease upon patients' well-being: a qualitative analysis. Clin Endocrinol (Oxf). 2008;68:635–9.
6. Jensen AL, Harder I. The impact of bodily change on social behaviour in patients with thyroid-associated ophthalmopathy. Scand J Caring Sci. 2011;25:341–9.
7. Wong MHY, Fenwick E, Aw AT, Lamoureux EL, Seah LL. Development and Validation of the Singapore Thyroid Eye Disease Quality of Life Questionnaire. Transl Vis Sci Technol. 2018;7:14.
8. Terwee CB, Gerding MN, Dekker FW, Prummel MF, Wiersinga WM. Development of a disease specific quality of life questionnaire for patients with Graves' ophthalmopathy: the GO-QOL. Br J Ophthalmol. 1998;82:773–9.
9. Wang Y, Sharma A, Padnick-Silver L, Francis-Sedlak M, Holt RJ, Foley C, et al. Physician-perceived impact of thyroid eye disease on patient quality of life in the United States. Ophthalmol Ther. 2021;10:75–87.
10. Mourits MP, Prummel MF, Wiersinga WM, Koornneef L. Clinical activity score as a guide in the management of patients with Graves' ophthalmopathy. Clin Endocrinol (Oxf). 1997;47:9–14.
11. Watt T, Hegedüs L, Rasmussen AK, Groenvold M, Bonnema SJ, Bjorner JB, et al. Which domains of thyroid-related quality of life are most relevant? Patients and clinicians provide complementary perspectives. Thyroid. 2007;17:647–54.
12. Wilson KA, Dowling AJ, Abdolell M, Tannock IF. Perception of quality of life by patients, partners and treating physicians. Qual Life Res. 2000;9:1041–52.
13. Guidance for industry. Patient-reported outcome measures: use in medical product development to support labeling claims: draft guidance. Health Qual Life Outcomes. 2006;4:79.
14. Pesudovs K, Burr JM, Harley C, Elliott DB. The development, assessment, and selection of questionnaires. Optom Vis Sci. 2007;84:663–74.
15. Kahaly GJ, Hardt J, Petrak F, Egle UT. Psychosocial factors in subjects with thyroid-associated ophthalmopathy. Thyroid. 2002;12:237–9.
16. Abraham-Nordling M, Wallin G, Träisk F, Berg G, Calissendorff J, Hallengren B, et al. Thyroid-associated ophthalmopathy; quality of life follow-up of patients randomized to treatment with antithyroid drugs or radioiodine. Eur J Endocrinol. 2010;163:651–7.

17. Mangione CM, Lee PP, Gutierrez PR, Spritzer K, Berry S, Hays RD. Development of the 25-item National Eye Institute Visual Function Questionnaire. Arch Ophthalmol. 2001;119:1050–8.
18. Bradley EA, Sloan JA, Novotny PJ, Garrity JA, Woog JJ, West SK. Evaluation of the National Eye Institute visual function questionnaire in Graves' ophthalmopathy. Ophthalmology. 2006;113:1450–4.
19. Du Y, Ye H, Li K, Xiao X, Chen R, He JF, et al. Vision-related quality of life tends to be more severely impaired in patients with dysthyroid optic neuropathy. Curr Eye Res. 2014;39:532–6.
20. Terwee CB, Wiersinga WM. Graves' quality of life. Ophthalmology. 2007;114:1416–7. Author reply 7-8
21. Watt T, Bjorner JB, Groenvold M, Rasmussen AK, Bonnema SJ, Hegedüs L, et al. Establishing construct validity for the thyroid-specific patient reported outcome measure (ThyPRO): an initial examination. Qual Life Res. 2009;18:483–96.
22. Watt T, Bjorner JB, Groenvold M, Cramon P, Winther KH, Hegedüs L, et al. Development of a short version of the thyroid-related patient-reported outcome ThyPRO. Thyroid. 2015;25:1069–79.
23. Wong CK, Lang BH, Lam CL. A systematic review of quality of thyroid-specific health-related quality-of-life instruments recommends ThyPRO for patients with benign thyroid diseases. J Clin Epidemiol. 2016;78:63–72.
24. Mueller SK, Miyake MM, Lefebvre DR, Freitag SK, Bleier BS. Long-term impact of endoscopic orbital decompression on sinonasal-specific quality of life. Laryngoscope. 2018;128:785–8.
25. Inoue S, Kawashima M, Arita R, Kozaki A, Tsubota K. Investigation of Meibomian gland function and dry eye disease in patients with Graves' ophthalmopathy. J Clin Med. 2020;9:2814.
26. Steinberg EP, Tielsch JM, Schein OD, Javitt JC, Sharkey P, Cassard SD, et al. The VF-14. An index of functional impairment in patients with cataract. Arch Ophthalmol. 1994;112:630–8.
27. Mangione CM, Phillips RS, Seddon JM, Lawrence MG, Cook EF, Dailey R, et al. Development of the 'Activities of Daily Vision Scale'. A measure of visual functional status. Med Care. 1992;30: 1111–26.
28. Werner SC. Modification of the classification of the eye changes of Graves' disease. Am J Ophthalmol. 1977;83:725–7.
29. Terwee CB, Gerding MN, Dekker FW, Prummel MF, van der Pol JP, Wiersinga WM. Test-retest reliability of the GO-QOL: a disease-specific quality of life questionnaire for patients with Graves' ophthalmopathy. J Clin Epidemiol. 1999;52:875–84.
30. Terwee CB, Dekker FW, Mourits MP, Gerding MN, Baldeschi L, Kalmann R, et al. Interpretation and validity of changes in scores on the Graves' ophthalmopathy quality of life questionnaire (GO-QOL) after different treatments. Clin Endocrinol (Oxf). 2001;54:391–8.
31. Kashkouli MB, Karimi N, Aghamirsalim M, Abtahi MB, Nojomi M, Shahrad-Bejestani H, et al. Measurement properties of the persian translated version of Graves Orbitopathy Quality of Life Questionnaire: A validation study. Ophthalmic Epidemiol. 2017;24:3–10.
32. Lin IC, Lee CC, Liao SL. Assessing quality of life in Taiwanese patients with Graves' ophthalmopathy. J Formos Med Assoc. 2015;114:1047–54.
33. Zeng P, Fan SX, Li ZJ, Peng YY, Hu YX, Xu MT, et al. Evaluation of the Graves' Orbitopathy-Specific Quality of Life Questionnaire in the Mainland Chinese Population. J Ophthalmol. 2019;2019:7602419.
34. Park JJ, Sullivan TJ, Mortimer RH, Wagenaar M, Perry-Keene DA. Assessing quality of life in Australian patients with Graves' ophthalmopathy. Br J Ophthalmol. 2004;88:75–8.
35. Ponto KA, Hommel G, Pitz S, Elflein H, Pfeiffer N, Kahaly GJ. Quality of life in a German Graves orbitopathy population. Am J Ophthalmol. 2011;152:483–90.e1.
36. Delampady K, Reddy SVB, Yadav SB. Assessing the quality of life in Indian Graves' orbitopathy patients and validation of Hindi version of GO-QOL questionnaire. Indian J Ophthalmol. 2020;68:1617–21.
37. Choi YJ, Lim HT, Lee SJ, Lee SY, Yoon JS. Assessing Graves' ophthalmopathy-specific quality of life in Korean patients. Eye (Lond). 2012;26:544–51.
38. Sawicka-Gutaj N, Bednarczuk T, Daroszewski J, Waligórska-Stachura J, Miśkiewicz P, Sowiński J, et al. GO-QOL—disease-specific quality of life questionnaire in Graves' orbitopathy. Endokrynol Pol. 2015;66:362–6.
39. Villagelin D, Romaldini J, Andrade J, Santos R, Milkos A, Teixeira P, et al. Evaluation of quality of life in the Brazilian Graves' Disease Population: Focus on mild and moderate Graves' orbitopathy patients. Front Endocrinol (Lausanne). 2019;10:192.
40. Delfino LC, Zunino A, Sapia V, Croome M, Ilera V, Gauna AT. Related quality of life questionnaire specific to dysthyroid ophthalmopathy evaluated in a population of patients with Graves' disease. Arch Endocrinol Metab. 2017;61:374–81.
41. Iacobæus L, Sahlin S. Evaluation of quality of life in patients with Graves' ophthalmopathy, before and after orbital decompression. Orbit. 2016;35:121–5.
42. Lumyongsatien M, Keeratidamkerngsakul B, Pornpanich K, Vangveeravong S, Saonanon P, Wiwatwongwana D, et al. Development and psychometric properties of the Thai Graves' ophthalmopathy quality of life (GO-QOL) questionnaire. J Patient Rep Outcomes. 2019;4:1.
43. Dietrich A, Taylor P, White P, Wilson V, Uddin J, Lee RWJ, et al. Establishing the usefulness of the GO-QOL in a UK hospital-treated population with thyroid eye disease in the CIRTED trial. Psychol Health Med. 2018;23:1341–55.
44. Stan MN, Holt R, Padnick-Silver L, Sile S. SAT-424 Assessing content validity of the Graves' Ophthalmopathy Quality of Life Questionnaire

(GO-QOL) in the United States. J Endocr Society. 2020;4:SAT-424.
45. Yeatts RP. Quality of life in patients with Graves ophthalmopathy. Trans Am Ophthalmol Soc. 2005;103:368–411.
46. Fayers T, Dolman PJ. Validity and reliability of the TED-QOL: a new three-item questionnaire to assess quality of life in thyroid eye disease. Br J Ophthalmol. 2011;95:1670–4.
47. Dolman PJ, Rootman J. VISA classification for Graves orbitopathy. Ophthalmic Plast Reconstr Surg. 2006;22:319–24.
48. Tehrani M, Krummenauer F, Mann WJ, Pitz S, Dick HB, Kahaly GJ. Disease-specific assessment of quality of life after decompression surgery for Graves' ophthalmopathy. Eur J Ophthalmol. 2004;14:193–9.
49. Insull EA, Sipkova Z, David J, Turner HE, Norris JH. Early low-dose rituximab for active thyroid eye disease: An effective and well-tolerated treatment. Clin Endocrinol (Oxf). 2019;91:179–86.
50. Cappelleri JC, Jason Lundy J, Hays RD. Overview of classical test theory and item response theory for the quantitative assessment of items in developing patient-reported outcomes measures. Clin Ther. 2014;36:648–62.
51. Bartalena L, Wiersinga WM. Proposal for standardization of primary and secondary outcomes in patients with active, moderate-to-severe Graves' orbitopathy. Eur Thyroid J. 2020;9:3–16.
52. Zloto O, Sagiv O, Priel A, Cukierman-Yaffe T, Tirosh A, Agmon-Levin N, et al. Gender differences in clinical presentation and prognosis of thyroid eye disease. Eur J Ophthalmol. 2021;31:2717–23.
53. Ljunggren JG, Törring O, Wallin G, Taube A, Tallstedt L, Hamberger B, et al. Quality of life aspects and costs in treatment of Graves' hyperthyroidism with antithyroid drugs, surgery, or radioiodine: results from a prospective, randomized study. Thyroid. 1998;8:653–9.
54. Ponto KA, Binder H, Diana T, Matheis N, Otto AF, Pitz S, et al. Prevalence, phenotype, and psychosocial well-being in euthyroid/hypothyroid thyroid-associated orbitopathy. Thyroid. 2015;25:942–8.
55. Riguetto CM, Neto AM, Tambascia MA, Zantut-Wittmann DE. The relationship between quality of life, cognition, and thyroid status in Graves' disease. Endocrine. 2019;63:87–93.
56. Kahaly GJ, Petrak F, Hardt J, Pitz S, Egle UT. Psychosocial morbidity of Graves' orbitopathy. Clin Endocrinol (Oxf). 2005;63:395–402.
57. Wickwar S, McBain HB, Ezra DG, Hirani SP, Rose GE, Newman SP. Which factors are associated with quality of life in patients with Graves' orbitopathy presenting for orbital decompression surgery? Eye (Lond). 2015;29:951–7.
58. Lee H, Roh HS, Yoon JS, Lee SY. Assessment of quality of life and depression in Korean patients with Graves' ophthalmopathy. Korean J Ophthalmol. 2010;24:65–72.
59. Wickwar S, McBain HB, Ezra DG, Hirani SP, Rose GE, Newman SP. What are the psychosocial outcomes of treatment for thyroid eye disease? A systematic review. Thyroid. 2014;24:1407–18.
60. Ferløv-Schwensen C, Brix TH, Hegedüs L. Death by suicide in Graves' disease and Graves' orbitopathy: A Nationwide Danish Register Study. Thyroid. 2017;27:1475–80.
61. Bruscolini A, Sacchetti M, La Cava M, Nebbioso M, Iannitelli A, Quartini A, et al. Quality of life and neuropsychiatric disorders in patients with Graves' Orbitopathy: Current concepts. Autoimmun Rev. 2018;17:639–43.
62. Ponto KA, Pitz S, Pfeiffer N, Hommel G, Weber MM, Kahaly GJ. Quality of life and occupational disability in endocrine orbitopathy. Dtsch Arztebl Int. 2009;106:283–9.
63. Terwee C, Wakelkamp I, Tan S, Dekker F, Prummel MF, Wiersinga W. Long-term effects of Graves' ophthalmopathy on health-related quality of life. Eur J Endocrinol. 2002;146:751–7.
64. Marcocci C, Kahaly GJ, Krassas GE, Bartalena L, Prummel M, Stahl M, et al. Selenium and the course of mild Graves' orbitopathy. N Engl J Med. 2011;364:1920–31.
65. Kahaly GJ, Pitz S, Hommel G, Dittmar M. Randomized, single blind trial of intravenous versus oral steroid monotherapy in Graves' orbitopathy. J Clin Endocrinol Metab. 2005;90:5234–40.
66. Kashkouli MB, Heidari I, Pakdel F, Jam S, Honarbakhsh Y, Mirarmandehi B. Change in quality of life after medical and surgical treatment of Graves' ophthalmopathy. Middle East Afr J Ophthalmol. 2011;18:42–7.
67. Hoppe E, Lee ACH, Hoppe D, Kahaly GJ. Predictive factors for changes in quality of life after steroid treatment for active moderate-to-severe Graves' orbitopathy: A Prospective Trial. Eur Thyroid J. 2021;9:313–20.
68. Smith TJ, Kahaly GJ, Ezra DG, Fleming JC, Dailey RA, Tang RA, et al. Teprotumumab for thyroid-associated ophthalmopathy. N Engl J Med. 2017;376:1748–61.
69. Douglas RS, Kahaly GJ, Patel A, Sile S, Thompson EHZ, Perdok R, et al. Teprotumumab for the treatment of active thyroid eye disease. N Engl J Med. 2020;382:341–52.
70. Rajendram R, Bunce C, Lee RW, Morley AM. Orbital radiotherapy for adult thyroid eye disease. Cochrane Database Syst Rev. 2012;7:Cd007114.
71. Prummel MF, Terwee CB, Gerding MN, Baldeschi L, Mourits MP, Blank L, et al. A randomized controlled trial of orbital radiotherapy versus sham irradiation in patients with mild Graves' ophthalmopathy. J Clin Endocrinol Metab. 2004;89:15–20.
72. Fayers T, Fayers PM, Dolman PJ. Sensitivity and responsiveness of the patient-reported TED-QOL to rehabilitative surgery in thyroid eye disease. Orbit. 2016;35:328–34.
73. Mourits MP, Bijl H, Altea MA, Baldeschi L, Boboridis K, Currò N, et al. Outcome of orbital decompression for disfiguring proptosis in patients with Graves'

orbitopathy using various surgical procedures. Br J Ophthalmol. 2009;93:1518–23.

74. Wickwar S, McBain H, Ezra DG, Hirani SP, Rose GE, Newman SP. The psychosocial and clinical outcomes of orbital decompression surgery for thyroid eye disease and predictors of change in quality of life. Ophthalmology. 2015;122: 2568–76.e1.
75. Cheng AM, Wei YH, Tighe S, Sheha H, Liao SL. Long-term outcomes of orbital fat decompression in Graves' orbitopathy. Br J Ophthalmol. 2018;102:69–73.
76. Fichter N, Krentz H, Guthoff RF. Functional and esthetic outcome after bony lateral wall decompression with orbital rim removal and additional fat resection in Graves' orbitopathy with regard to the configuration of the lateral canthal region. Orbit. 2013;32:239–46.
77. Zhang S, Li Y, Wang Y, Zhong S, Liu X, Huang Y, et al. Comparison of rim-sparing versus rim-removal techniques in deep lateral wall orbital decompression for Graves' orbitopathy. Int J Oral Maxillofac Surg. 2019;48:461–7.
78. Jellema HM, Merckel-Timmer E, Kloos R, Saeed P, Mourits MP. Quality of life improves after strabismus surgery in patients with Graves' orbitopathy. Eur J Endocrinol. 2014;170:785–9.
79. Jellema HM, Saeed P, Mombaerts I, Dolman PJ, Garrity J, Kazim M, et al. Objective and subjective outcomes of strabismus surgery in Graves' orbitopathy: a prospective multicentre study. Acta Ophthalmol. 2017;95:386–91.
80. Campi I, Currò N, Vannucchi G, Covelli D, Simonetta S, Fugazzola L, et al. Quantification of global ocular motility impairment in Graves' orbitopathy by measuring eye muscle ductions. Thyroid. 2021;31:280–7.
81. Wiersinga WM. Quality of life in Graves' ophthalmopathy. Best Pract Res Clin Endocrinol Metab. 2012;26:359–70.
82. Bartalena L, Baldeschi L, Boboridis K, Eckstein A, Kahaly GJ, Marcocci C, et al. The 2016 European Thyroid Association/European Group on Graves' Orbitopathy Guidelines for the Management of Graves' Orbitopathy. Eur Thyroid J. 2016;5:9–26.
83. Lee V, Avari P, Williams B, Perros P, Dayan C. A survey of current practices by the British Oculoplastic Surgery Society (BOPSS) and recommendations for delivering a sustainable multidisciplinary approach to thyroid eye disease in the United Kingdom. Eye (Lond). 2020;34:1662–71.
84. Lee THB, Sundar G. Quality of life in thyroid eye disease: a systematic review. Ophthalmic Plast Reconstr Surg. 2020;36:118–26.

Index

F. M. Quaranta Leoni et al. (eds.), *Oculoplastic, Lacrimal and Orbital Surgery*, https://doi.org/10.1007/978-3-031-39638-0

F

P

Q

R

T